Hydroxyzine	Meperidine	Metoclopramide	Midazolam	Morphine	Nalbuphine	Pentazocine	Pentobarbital	Perphenazine	Prochlorperazine	Promazine	Promethazine	Ranitidine	Scopolamine Hbr	Secobarbital	Thiethylperazine
C	C	C	C	C	C	C	C	C	C	C	C	C	C	I	
C	C	C	C	C		C	I	C	C		C		C	I	C
C	C	C	C	C		C	I	C	C	C	C	C	C	I	
							I							I	
I	I	I		I	I	I	I	I	I	I	I		I	I	I
I	C	C	I	C		C	I	C	I	I	I	C	C	I	
C	C	C	C	C		C	I	C	C	C	C	C	C	I	
C	C	C		C	C	C	I	C	C	C	C	C		C	I
C	C	C		C		C	I	C	C	C	C	C	C	C	I
C	C			C		I	I			C	C	C	C	C	I
	I			I		I					I				
■	C	C		C	C	C	I		C	C	C	I	C	I	
C	■	C		I		C	I	C	C	C	C	C	C	I	
C	C	■		C		C		C	C	C	C	C		I	
C		C	■	C	C			I	I	I	C	C		I	C
C	I	C		■		C	I	C	C	C	C	C	C	I	
C					■		I		C		*	C	C	I	C
C	C	C		C		■	I	C	C	C	C	-	C	C	I
I	I			I	I	I	■	I	I	I	I		C	I	
	C	C		C		C	I	■	C		C	C	C	I	I
C	C	C		C	C	C	I	C	■		C	C	C	C	
C	C	C		C		C	I		C	■	C		C	I	
C	C	C		C	C	C	I	C	C	C	■	C	C	I	
	C	C	I	C	C	C		C	C		C	■	C		C
C	C	C		C	C	C	C	C	C	C	C	■	I		
I	I	I		I	I	I	I	I	I	I	I		■	I	
				C				I				C		I	■

Parenteral compatibility occurs when two or more drugs are successfully mixed without liquefaction, deliquescence, or precipitation.

Drug Monographs New to This Edition
(See Appendix A, Selected New Drugs)

abacavir
alitretinoin
aminolevulinic acid
amprenavir
bexarotene
cilostazol
coagulation factor
  VIIa, recombinant
denileukin diftitox
dexmedetomidine
dofetilide
doxercalciferol
entacapone
epirubicin

exemestane
ganirelix
gatifloxacin
interferon alfa-n 1
  lymphoblastoid
levalbuterol
levetiracetam
levobupivacaine
lymphocyte immune
  globulin, (anti-
  thymocyte)
modafinil
moxifloxacin
nitric oxide

octreotide
orlistat
oseltamivir
perindopril
pioglitazone
poractant alfa
rabeprazole
rofecoxib
rosiglitazone
sirolimus
temozolomide
zaleplon
zanamivir

New Drugs in the 2002 Update

argatroban
arsenic trioxide
balsalazide
bivalirudin
cetrorelix
choriogonadotropin
colesevelam
gemtuzumab
insulin aspart/insulin glargine
iron sucrose
linezolid

meloxicam
mifepristone
pantoprazole
rivastigmine
tenecteplase
tinzaparin
triptorelin
verteporfin
ziprasidone
zonisamide

 GET CONNECTED!

Receive our FREE online drug updates!

Visit us at

  www.mosby.com/MERLIN/nursingdrugupdates/skidmore

and you'll be assured of receiving the most up-to-the-minute drug information, including*:

- Updates on recently approved drugs
- Names and brief descriptions of new drugs
- Drug alerts
- Updated drug information
- Hyperlinks to drug information websites

Visit our website today to get connected!

*Not every update will include each of these items. Information released by the FDA and other developments will determine the contents of each update.

Mosby's

Fourth Edition

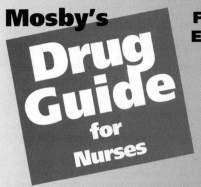

Drug Guide
for Nurses

Linda Skidmore-Roth, R.N., M.S.N., N.P.
Skidmore-Roth Publishing, Inc.
Englewood, Colorado
Formerly, Nursing Faculty,
New Mexico State University,
Las Cruces, New Mexico;
El Paso Community College,
El Paso, Texas

*Herbal Remedies CD-ROM to
accompany Mosby's Drug Guide
for Nurses by*
Steve Blake, N.D., D.Sc., M.H., M.T.

with 190 illustrations and 2 color inserts

 Mosby

A Harcourt Health Sciences Company

St. Louis   London   Philadelphia   Sydney   Toronto

Mosby

A Harcourt Health Sciences Company

Vice President, Nursing Editorial Director: Sally Schrefer
Executive Editor: N. Darlene Como
Developmental Editor: Tamara Myers
Project Manager: Deborah L. Vogel
Senior Production Editor: Sarah E. Fike
Designer: Bill Drone
Cover Illustrator: Ken Joudrey and Bill Drone

FOURTH EDITION
Copyright © 2001 by Mosby, Inc.

Previous editions copyrighted 1996, 1997, 1999

Notice
Pharmacology is an ever-changing field. Standard safety precautions must be followed, but as new research and clinical experience broaden our knowledge, changes in treatment and drug therapy may become necessary or appropriate. Readers are advised to check the most current product information provided by the manufacturer of each drug to be administered to verify the recommended dose, the method and duration of administration, and contraindications. It is the responsibility of the licensed prescriber, relying on experience and knowledge of the patient, to determine dosages and the best treatment for each individual patient. Neither the publisher nor the author assumes any liability for any injury and/or damages to persons or property arising from this publication.

No refund without mini CD-ROM

Mosby, Inc.
A Harcourt Health Sciences Company
11830 Westline Industrial Drive
St. Louis, Missouri 63146

Printed in the United States of America

Library of Congress Cataloging-in-Publication Data

Skidmore-Roth, Linda.
    Mosby's drug guide for nurses / Linda Skidmore-Roth. — 4th ed.
        p. ; cm.
    Includes bibliographical references and index.
    ISBN 0-323-01807-6
    1. Drugs—Handbooks, manuals, etc.   2. Nursing—Handbooks,
manuals, etc.   I. Title: Drug guide for nurses.   II. Title.
    [DNLM: 1. Pharmaceutical Preparations—administration & dosage—
Handbooks.   2. Pharmaceutical Preparations—administration & dosage—Nurses'
Instruction.   3. Drug Therapy—Handbooks.   4. Drug Therapy—Nurses'
Instruction. QV 39 S628mb 2001]
    RM301.12.S56   2001
    615′.1—dc21

01   02   03   04   GW/RDC   9   8   7   6   5   4   3

Consultants

Bob Aucker, Pharm.D
Clinical Pharmacist, St. Joseph Hospital,
Atlanta, Georgia

Jean Krajieck Bartek, Ph.D, A.R.N.P.
Associate Professor, University of Nebraska Medical Center
Colleges of Nursing and Medicine
Omaha, Nebraska

Barbara A. Brunow, R.N., M.S.N.
Instructor, Providence Hospital, School of Nursing,
Sandusky, Ohio

Marcia L. Buck, Pharm.D., F.C.C.P.
Clinical Pharmacy Specialist, Children's Medical Center
Clinical Associate Professor, Schools of Medicine and Nursing
University of Virginia
Charlottesville, Virginia

Connie L. Bush, R.N., M.S.
Associate Professor, Nursing, Niagara County Community College,
Sanborn, New York

Shari L. Clarke, R.N.C.
Nursing Unit Coordinator, Emory at Crawford Long Hospital,
Fayetteville, Georgia

Judy E. Davison, R.N., M.S., C.C.R.N.
Clinical Nurse Specialist, University of California San Diego Medical Center,
San Diego, California

Jane Doyle, R.N., B.S.N., M.S., M.B.A.
Nursing Faculty, Mount Wachusett Community College,
Gardner, Massachusetts

Laurel A. Eisenhauer, R.N., Ph.D.
Professor of Nursing, Boston College School of Nursing,
Chestnut Hill, Massachusetts

Tim Engelhardt, B.Sc., Pharm.D.
Manager, Pharmacy Services, Calgary District Hospital Group,
Calgary, Alberta, Canada

Linda A. Howe, R.N., M.S., M.A.E.
Director, Roper Hospital School of Nursing,
Charleston, South Carolina

Theresa M. Hulub, R.N., M.S.Ed., M.S.N.
Professor of Nursing Education, Niagara County Community College,
Sanborn, New York

Kimberly A. Hunter, Pharm.D.
Assistant Professor of Pharmacy Practice,
Washington State University College of Pharmacy;
Geriatric Clinical Pharmacist, Sacred Heart Medical Center,
Spokane, Washington

Natasha Leskovsek, R.N., M.B.A., J.D.
Fox, Bennett & Turner
Washington, DC

Jon E. Lewis, B.A., Ph.D.
Senior Research Scientist and Director,
Respiratory Diseases,
Marion Merrell Dow Research Institute,
Cincinnati, Ohio

Lori A. Martell, Ph.D.
Clinical Trials Coordinator,
Duke University Medical Center,
Durham, North Carolina

Edwina A. McConnell, R.N., Ph.D., FRCNA
Independent Nurse Consultant,
Gorham, Maine

Janet R. Paul, B.S.N., M.S.N., R.N.
Assistant Professor of Nursing,
Hahnemann University,
Philadelphia, Pennsylvania

Rosemary A. Pine, R.N., M.S.N.
Assistant Professor of Nursing,
Department Chair, ADN Program,
Houston Baptist University,
Houston, Texas

Norma Pinnell, R.N., B.S.N.
Instructor,
Kaplan Nursing,
St. Louis, Missouri

Carolyn Smith Powell, A.D.N., B.S.N., M.S.N.
Assistant Professor of Nursing,
Abraham Baldwin College,
Tifton, Georgia

Mary Quintas, R.N.
Miles Community College,
Department of Nursing,
Miles City, Montana

Robert T. Reilly, Pharm.D.
Associate Director of Pharmacy, Clinical Services,
Thomason Hospital,
El Paso, Texas

Roberta Roynayne, R.N., B.Sc.N., M.Sc.
Assistant Professor,
University of Ottawa,
School of Nursing,
Ottawa, Ontario

Carol Ruscin, R.N., B.S.
Level I Faculty,
Baptist Medical System,
School of Nursing,
Little Rock, Arkansas

Lori Schoonover, Pharm.D.
Assistant Professor, Pharmacy,
Washington State University,
Spokane, Washington

Roberta J. Secrest, Ph.D., Pharm.D., R.Ph.
Associate Scientist,
Marion Merrell Dow Research Institute,
Cincinnati, Ohio

Denice Sheehan, R.N., M.S.N., O.C.N.
Nursing Supervisor,
Hospice of the Western Reserve,
Mentor, Ohio

John R. White, Jr., Pharm.D.
Assistant Professor,
Washington State University,
College of Pharmacy,
Spokane, Washington

Preface

Mosby's Drug Guide for Nurses, fourth edition, presents more than 4000 generic and trade name drugs—those most commonly administered by students—as well as more than 2900 drug fact updates. To keep our readers up-to-date, the new edition also contains 38 detailed new monographs for drugs recently approved by the FDA, in addition to the 35 monographs comprising the 2000 update to the *Drug Guide,* which have been integrated into Section I of the book. The new drug monographs, which are found in Appendix A, "Selected New Drugs," include zaleplon (Sonata) used for short-term treatment of insomnia; rabeprazole (Aciphex) for erosive/ulcerative GERD; epirubicin (Ellence) used in breast cancer; and sirolimus (Rapamune) used to prevent organ rejection. In addition, Appendix B, "Recent FDA Drug Approvals," provides generic/trade names and uses for 8 of the most recently approved drugs, about which complete information was not yet available at the time this book went to press.

The fourth edition of *Mosby's Drug Guide for Nurses* also includes several other useful new features. Appendix G, "Herbal Products," lists 72 popular herbal supplements and their uses. A special new herbal product icon, ∅, appears throughout the text, highlighting more than 270 potential interactions between drugs and herbal products. Appendix E, "Rarely Used Drugs," provides abbreviated monographs for 39 infrequently used products. And Appendix D, "Combination Products," has been extensively revised to include 682 commonly used combination products. Presented in a new, easy-to-read format, this appendix has also been revised to include uses for all products. Also new to this edition is a "Do Not Confuse" icon, ∎, to identify look-alike/sound-alike drug names. This icon is incorporated into the monographs of nearly 200 pairs of drugs whose names may be easily confused. More than 100 "Nursing Alert" icons, ◆, highlight situations that potentially could put the patient at risk; and more than 60 "Do Not Crush" icons, ⊗, denote drugs that may not be administered in crushed form. A free mini-CD-ROM is included inside the back cover, providing detailed information on more than 30 of the most widely used herbal supplements. *Mosby's Drug Guide for Nurses* also includes free Internet updates on the Mosby website (www.mosby.com/MERLIN/nursingdrugupdates). The information found on this site will be updated periodically throughout the year to provide users with the very latest drug information.

Another new feature designed to help nurses identify common drugs and deliver high-quality patient care is a 16-page full-color insert containing 160 photographs of frequently prescribed tablets and capsules. The photos in this drug identification guide are arranged alphabetically by generic name, with common trade names and dosage strengths included. In addition, the 24-page, completely updated four-color photo atlas of drug administration will provide an invaluable resource for practitioners and students. Key drugs are highlighted with a special icon, **♥☞**, in the individual monograph and within the drug classifications section to call attention to important drugs. More than 60 drug classifications are provided.

Individual drug monographs also include **IV** content, featuring detailed coverage of both drug compatibilities and incompatibilities as well as site-specific information. The five-step nursing process format includes rationales. To aid application of the nursing process, therapeutic outcomes are prominently stated at the beginning of each monograph, and positive therapeutic outcomes are highlighted under the evaluation heading. Treatment of overdose is included after evaluation when appropriate.

Drug monographs are arranged in alphabetical order by generic name, and trade names are given for all medications commonly used in the United States and Canada. Drugs available only in Canada are identified by a maple leaf, **♣**. The following information is provided whenever possible for safe and effective administration of each drug:

Pronunciations: Pronunciations are provided to help the nursing student master the more complex generic names.

Functional and chemical classifications: All known broad functional and chemical classifications are given. These classifications allow the nurse to see similarities and dissimilarities among drugs that are in the same functional class and different chemical classes.

Pregnancy category: FDA pregnancy categories A, B, C, D, or X are noted at the beginning of the monograph and under *precautions* or *contraindications* depending on the FDA category. Appendix H provides a detailed explanation of each category.

Controlled substance schedule: Schedules are included for the United States (I, II, III, IV, V) and Canada (F, G, H). Appendix I provides a chart correlating the two systems with examples.

Action: Pharmacologic properties are described in detail. Action is discussed to the cellular level when known.

Therapeutic outcome: All possible results of medication use are detailed.

Uses: Provides drug application.

Investigational uses: Provides drug application for those uses a student may encounter in practice, although they are not FDA approved.

Dosage and routes: All available and approved dosages and routes are given for adult, pediatric, and geriatric patients.

Available forms: All available forms — including tablets, capsules, extended-release, injectables (**IV**, IM, SC, ID, IC), solutions, creams, ointments, lotions, gels, shampoos, elixirs, suspensions, suppositories, sprays, aerosols, and lozenges — are provided.

Adverse effects: Grouped by body system, common side effects are in *italic type,* and life-threatening reactions are in **boldface type,** allowing the student to quickly identify common and life-threatening reactions. All adverse effects are reported for an incidence of 1% or greater.

Contraindications: Contraindications are instances in which a medication absolutely should not be given. When the FDA has assigned pregnancy safety category D or X, it appears here.

Precautions: Special precautionary steps are given here, including FDA pregnancy safety categories A, B, and C. The new "Do Not Confuse" section with icon is appropriately placed just after "Precautions" in this new edition.

Pharmacokinetics: If known, onset, peak, and duration appear in an easily accessible chart format.

Pharmacodynamics: Absorption, distribution, elimination, and half-life are reported, when known, also in a handy chart format.

Interactions/incompatibilities: This section includes confirmed drug, food, and smoking interactions. The drugs are listed in alphabetical order, followed by the reaction(s) caused by that drug. Herbal interactions are included and identified by an icon to highlight potential interactions between herbal products and prescription or OTC drugs.

Lab test interferences: When known, lab test interferences are provided. Lab interference includes false negative and false positive results and increase or decrease interferences.

Nursing considerations: Highlighted nursing considerations are organized to foster use of the nursing process: Assessment; Nursing diagnoses; Implementation, including special instructions for administering drugs IM, **IV**, SC, PO, topically, and rectally; Patient/family education; and Evaluation, with positive therapeutic outcomes.

Treatment of overdose: Drugs and treatment for overdoses are provided for appropriate drugs.

Appendixes: The following appendixes are included to further enhance the usefulness of this reference: Selected New Drugs; Recent FDA Drug Approvals; Ophthalmic, Otic, Nasal, and Topical Products; Combination Products; Rarely Used Drugs; Less Frequently Used Antihistamines; Herbal Products; FDA Pregnancy Categories; Controlled Substance Chart; Commonly Used Abbreviations; IV Drug/Solution Compatibility Chart; and Nomogram for Calculation of Body Surface Area.

Disorders index: This book includes both a general index and a disorders index, both of which have been expanded in this edition. For easy application with integrated medical-surgical nursing courses, the disorders index lists major disorders and major drugs used in their management, followed by the page number for each drug listed.

Inside the covers: A syringe compatibility chart is printed inside the front cover for quick access, and installation instructions for the mini CD-ROM appear inside the back cover.

Design: This book features a functional, user-friendly, two-color design that includes alphabetical tabs; icons for key drugs ⚷, therapeutic outcome ➜, lifespan content 🅖 🅟, "Nursing Alert" ◆, and "Do Not Crush" ⊘; the new icons "Do Not Confuse" ◼ and "Herbal Interaction" ▨; colored monograph headings; and screened pages for the category drugs and index to facilitate information retrieval. The type and format of the book are spacious to enhance visual appeal and user-friendliness.

The following sources were consulted in the preparation of this edition:

American Society of Health-System Pharmacists: *American hospital formulary service drug information '99,* Bethesda, Md, 1999, The Society.

Clark J, Queener S, and Karb V: *Pharmacologic basis of nursing practice,* ed 5, St. Louis, 1998, Mosby.

Facts and Comparisons: *The review of natural products,* St. Louis, Mo. Updated monthly.

Facts and Comparisons, St. Louis, Mo. Updated monthly.

Gahart B: *Intravenous medications,* ed 13, St. Louis, 1999, Mosby.

Goodman A and others: *Goodman and Gilman's the pharmacological basis of therapeutics,* ed 10, New York, 1998, Pergamon Press.

McKenry LM and Salerno E: *Mosby's pharmacology in nursing,* ed 18, St. Louis, 1996, Mosby.

Trissel L: *Handbook on injectable drugs,* ed 10, Bethesda, Md, 1999, American Society of Hospital Pharmacists, Inc.

Acknowledgments

I am indebted to the nursing and pharmacology consultants who reviewed the manuscript, and I thank them for their thoughtful comments and encouragement. I would also like to thank Darlene Como and Dana Knighten, my editors, whose active encouragement and enthusiasm have made this book better than it might otherwise have been. In addition, I want to extend a special note of gratitude to Don Ladig, who has supported and encouraged my efforts since I began my relationship as an author with Mosby.

Linda Skidmore-Roth

Contents

abacavir
See Appendix A,
Selected New Drugs

---

acarbose (℞)
(a-kar′bose)
Prandese ✦, Precose
Func. class.: Oral antidiabetic
Chem. class.:
α-Glucosidase inhibitor
Pregnancy category **B**

Action: Delays the digestion of ingested carbohydrates, results in a smaller rise in blood glucose after meals; does not increase insulin production

▶**Therapeutic Outcome:**
Decreased blood glucose levels in diabetes mellitus

Uses: Stable adult-onset diabetes mellitus (type II) NIDDM, alone or in combination with a sulfonylurea

Dosage and routes
Initial dose
Adult: PO 25 mg tid with first bite of meal
Maintenance dose
Adult: PO may be increased to 50-100 mg tid; dosage adjustment at 4-9 wk intervals
Adult <60 kg: PO not to exceed 50 mg tid
Available forms: Tabs 50, 100 mg
Adverse effects
GI: Abdominal pain, diarrhea, flatulence, increased serum transaminase level

Contraindications: Hypersensitivity, diabetic ketoacidosis, cirrhosis, inflammatory bowel disease, colonic ulceration, partial intestinal obstruction, chronic intestinal disease, serum creatinine >2 mg/dl
Precautions: Pregnancy **B**,
P renal disease, lactation, children, hepatic disease

Pharmacokinetics	
Absorption	Unknown
Distribution	Unknown
Metabolism	GI tract
Excretion	Kidneys as intact drug
Half-life	Elimination 2 hrs

Pharmacodynamics
Unknown

Interactions
Individual drugs
Insulin: ↑ hypoglycemia
Isoniazid: ↑ hypoglycemia
Nicotinic acid: ↑ hypoglycemia
Phenytoin: ↑ hypoglycemia
Thyroid: ↑ hypoglycemia
Drug classifications
Calcium channel blockers: ↑ hypoglycemia
Corticosteroids: ↑ hypoglycemia
Digestive enzymes: ↓ effect of acarbose
Diuretics: ↑ hypoglycemia
Estrogens: ↑ hypoglycemia
Intestinal absorbents: ↓ effect of acarbose
Oral contraceptives: ↑ hypoglycemia
Phenothiazines: ↑ hypoglycemia
Sulfonylureas: ↑ hypoglycemia
Sympathomimetics: ↑ hypoglycemia
Herb/drug
Alfalfa: possible ↑ hypoglycemia
Lab test interferences
↑ AST, bilirubin
↓ calcium, Vit B$_6$

NURSING CONSIDERATIONS
Assessment
• Assess for hypoglycemia, hyperglycemia; even though this drug does not cause hypoglycemia, if on a sulfonylurea or insulin, hypoglycemia may be additive; if hypoglycemia occurs, treat with glucose or if severe, IV dextrose or IM glucagon
• Monitor 1 hr postprandial for establishing effectiveness, then glycosylated Hgb q3 mo.
• Monitor AST q3 mo × 1 yr, and periodically thereafter

Nursing diagnoses
☑ Nutrition altered, more than body requirements (uses)
☑ Nutrition altered, less than body requirements (adverse reactions)
☑ Knowledge deficit (teaching)
☑ Noncompliance (teaching)

Implementation
• Give tid with first bite of each meal
• Provide storage in tight container in cool environment

Patient/family education
• Teach patient the symptoms of hypoglycemia, hyperglycemia and what to do about each
• Instruct that medication must be taken as prescribed; explain consequences of discontinuing the medication abruptly
• Tell patient to avoid OTC medications unless approved by prescriber
• Teach patient that diabetes is a life-long illness; drug will not cure condition
• Instruct patient to carry/wear Medic Alert ID as diabetic
• Teach patient that diet and exercise regimen must be followed

Evaluation
Positive therapeutic outcome
• Decreased signs, symptoms of diabetes mellitus (polyuria, polydipsia, polyphagia, clear sensorium, absence of dizziness, stable gait)

---

acebutolol (℞)
(a-se-byoo' toe-lole)
Monitan ♣, Sectral
Func. class.: Antihypertensive
Chem. class.: Selective β_1-blocker; group II antidysrhythmic (II)
Pregnancy category **B**

Action: Competitively blocks stimulation of β-adrenergic receptors within vascular smooth muscle (decreases rate of SA node discharge, increases recovery time), slows conduction of AV node resulting in decreased heart rate (negative chronotropic effect), which decreases O_2 consumption in myocardium; also decreases renin-aldosterone-angiotensin system at high doses, inhibits β_2-receptors in bronchial system (high doses)

▷**Therapeutic Outcome:** Decreased B/P, heart rate, AV conduction, control of dysrhythmias

Uses: Mild to moderate hypertension, sinus tachycardia, persistent atrial extrasystoles, tachydysrhythmias

Investigational uses: Prophylaxis of MI, treatment of angina pectoris, tremor, mitral valve prolapse, thyrotoxicosis, idiopathic hypertrophic subaortic stenosis

---

☒ Herb/drug ◌ Do Not Crush ◆ Alert ☙ Key Drug **G** Geriatric **P** Pediatric

Dosage and routes
Hypertension
Adult: PO 400 mg qd or in 2 divided doses; may be increased to desired response; maintenance 200-1200 mg/qd in 2 divided doses

Ventricular dysrhythmia
Adult: PO 200 mg bid, may increase gradually; usual range 600-1200 mg daily; should be tapered over 2 wk before discontinuing

G ***Elderly:*** PO not to exceed 800 mg/qd

Renal dose
Creatinine clearance 50-25 ml/min, reduce dose by 50%; if <25 ml/min reduce dose by 75%

Available forms: Caps 200, 400 mg; tabs 200, 400 mg ✦

Adverse effects
CNS: Insomnia, fatigue, dizziness, mental changes, memory loss, hallucinations, depression, lethargy, drowsiness, strange dreams, catatonia
CV: **Profound hypotension, bradycardia, CHF,** cold extremities, postural hypotension, **2nd or 3rd degree heart block**
EENT: Sore throat, dry burning eyes
ENDO: Increased hypoglycemic response to insulin
GI: Nausea, diarrhea, vomiting, **mesenteric arterial thrombosis, ischemic colitis**
GU: Impotence, decreased libido, dysuria, nocturia
HEMA: **Agranulocytosis, thrombocytopenia, purpura**
INTEG: Rash, fever, alopecia, dry skin
MS: Joint pain, cramping
RESP: **Bronchospasm,** dyspnea, wheezing, cough

Contraindications: Hypersensitivity to β-blockers, cardiogenic shock, heart block (2nd or 3rd degree), sinus bradycardia, CHF, cardiac failure

Precautions: Major surgery, pregnancy **B,** lactation, diabetes mellitus, renal disease, thyroid disease, COPD, asthma, well-compensated heart failure, aortic or mitral valve, hepatic disease

Pharmacokinetics

Absorption	Well
Distribution	Crosses placenta, minimal CNS
Metabolism	Liver to diacetolol
Excretion	Kidneys, unchanged
Half-life	8-13 hr diacetolol, 3-4 hr acebutolol

Pharmacodynamics

	PO (ANTIHYPERTENSIVE)	PO (ANTIDYSRHYTHMIAS)
Onset	1-1½ hr	1 hr
Peak	2-4 hr	4-6 hr
Duration	12-24 hr	8-10 hr

Interactions
Individual drugs
Alcohol: ↑ hypotension (large amounts)
Diltiazem: ↑ hypotension, bradycardia
Hydralazine: ↑ hypotension, bradycardia
Insulin: ↑ hypoglycemia
Prazosin: ↑ hypotension, bradycardia
Thyroid: ↓ effectiveness
Verapamil: ↑ myocardial depression
Drug classifications
Antidiabetics, oral: ↑ hypoglycemic effect
Antihypertensives: ↑ hypertension
Cardiac glycosides: ↑ bradycardia

✦ Canada Only   Adverse effects: *italic* = common; **bold** = life-threatening

Diuretics: ↑ hypotension, bradycardia
Nitrates: ↑ hypotension
NSAIDs: ↓ antihypertensive effect
Theophyllines: ↓ bronchodilatation

☑ *Herb/drug*
Aloe: ↑ acebutolol effect
Buckthorn bark/berry: ↑ acebutolol effect
Cascara sagrada bark: ↑ acebutolol effect
Ephedra: ↑ dysrhythmia
Rhubarb root: ↑ acebutolol effect
Senna leaf/fruits: ↑ acebutolol effect
Lab test interferences
Positive: Antinuclear antibodies

NURSING CONSIDERATIONS
Assessment
• Monitor B/P during beginning treatment, periodically thereafter; pulse q4h; note rate, rhythm, quality; apical/radial pulse before administration; notify prescriber of any significant changes (pulse <60 bpm)
• Check for baselines in renal, liver function tests before therapy begins
• Assess for edema in feet, legs daily, monitor I & O, daily weight; check for jugular vein distention, rales bilaterally, dyspnea (CHF)
• Monitor skin turgor, dryness of mucous membranes for hydration status, especially **G** elderly

Nursing diagnoses
☑ Cardiac output, decreased (side effects)
☑ Injury, risk for physical (side effects)
☑ Knowledge deficit (teaching)
☑ Noncompliance (teaching)

Implementation
• Given ac, hs; tablet may be crushed or swallowed whole; give with food to prevent GI upset; reduced dosage in renal dysfunction; check pulse before giving, hold dose and notify prescriber if pulse is <60 bpm
• Store protected from light, moisture; place in cool environment

Patient/family education
◆• Teach patient not to discontinue drug abruptly, taper over 2 wk; may cause precipitate angina if stopped abruptly
• Teach patient not to use OTC products containing α-adrenergic stimulants (such as nasal decongestants, cold preparations); to avoid alcohol, smoking; to limit sodium intake as prescribed
• Teach patient how to take pulse and B/P at home, advise when to notify prescriber
• Instruct patient to comply with weight control, dietary adjustments, modified exercise program
• Tell patient to carry/wear Medic Alert ID to identify drug(s) that patient is taking, allergies; tell patient that drug controls symptoms but does not cure
• Caution patient to avoid hazardous activities if dizziness or drowsiness is present; that drug may cause sensitivity to cold
• Teach patient to report symptoms of CHF: difficult breathing, especially on exertion or when lying down, night cough, swelling of extremities or bradycardia, dizziness, confusion, depression, fever
• Teach patient to take drug as prescribed, not to double or

skip doses; take any missed doses as soon as remembered if several hours until next dose

Evaluation

Positive therapeutic outcome
• Decreased B/P in hypertension (after 1-2 wk)
• Absence of dysrhythmias

Treatment of overdose:

Lavage, **IV** atropine for bradycardia, **IV** theophylline for bronchospasm, digitalis, O₂, diuretic for cardiac failure, hemodialysis, **IV** glucose for hypoglycemia, **IV** diazepam (or phenytoin) for seizures

---

acetaminophen ⬦π
(OTC)
(a-seat-a-mee'noe-fen)
Abenol ✦, Acephen, Aceta, Actamin, Actimol, Aminofen, Apacet, APAP, Apo-Acetaminophen ✦, Aspirin-Free Pain Relief, Atasol ✦, Banesin, Children's Feverall, Dapa, Datril, Exdol ✦, FemEtts, Genapap, Genebs, Halenol, Liquiprin, Mapap, Maranox, Meda, Panadol, Redutemp, Robigesic ✦, Rounax ✦, Silapap, Snaplets-FR, St. Joseph Aspirin-Free, Tapanol, Tempra, Tylenol, Uni-Ace, Valorin

Func. class.: Nonnarcotic analgesic
Chem. class.: Nonsalicylate, paraaminophenol derivative

Pregnancy category **B**

Action: May block pain impulses peripherally that occur in response to inhibition of prostaglandin synthesis; does not possess antiinflammatory properties; antipyretic action results from inhibition of prostaglandins in the CNS (hypothalamic heat-regulating center)

➡**Therapeutic Outcome:**
Decreased pain, fever

Uses: Mild to moderate pain or fever

Dosage and routes
🄿 *Adult and child >12 yr:* PO/ Rect 325-650 mg q4h prn, not to exceed 4 g/day
🄿 *Child:* PO 10-15 mg/kg q4h
🄿 *Child 6-12 yr:* REC 325 mg q4-6h
🄿 *Child 3-6 yr:* REC 125 mg q4-6h
🄿 *Child 1-3 yr:* REC 80 mg q4h
🄿 *Child 3-11 mo:* REC 80 mg q6h

Available forms: Rec supp 120, 125, 325, 600, 650 mg; chewable tabs 80, 160 mg; caps 500 mg; elix 120, 160, 325 mg/5 ml; liq 120, 160 mg/5 ml, 500 mg/15 ml; sol 100 mg/1 ml, 120 mg/2.5 ml; tabs 160, 325, 500, 650 mg; granules 80 mg/pkg or cup

Adverse effects

CNS: Stimulation, drowsiness
GI: Nausea, vomiting, abdominal pain, **hepatotoxicity**
HEMA: Leukopenia, neutropenia, hemolytic anemia (long-term use), thrombocytopenia, pancytopenia
INTEG: Rash, urticaria, angioedema
SYST: **Anaphylaxis**
TOXICITY: Cyanosis, anemia, neutropenia, jaundice, pancytopenia, CNS stimulation, delirium followed

---

vascular collapse, convulsions, coma, death

Contraindications:
Hypersensitivity; intolerance to tartrazine (yellow dye no. 5), alcohol, table sugar, saccharin, depending on product

Precautions: Anemia, hepatic disease, renal disease, chronic alcoholism, pregnancy **B,** **G** elderly, lactation

Pharmacokinetics

Absorption	Well absorbed (PO), variable (rec)
Distribution	Widely distributed; crosses placenta in low concentrations
Metabolism	Liver 85%-95%; metabolites are toxic at high levels
Excretion	Kidneys—metabolites, breast milk
Half-life	3-4 hr

Pharmacodynamics

	PO	REC
Onset	½-1 hr	½-1 hr
Peak	1-3 hr	1-3 hr
Duration	3-4 hr	3-4 hr

Interactions
Individual drugs
Alcohol: ↑ hepatotoxicity, ↓ effect
Carbamazepine: ↓ effect, ↑ hepatotoxicity
Rifampin: ↓ effect, ↑ hepatotoxicity
Sulfinpyrazone; ↓ effect, ↑ hepatotoxicity
Warfarin: Hypoprothrombinemia; long-term use, high doses of acetaminophen
Zidovudine: ↑ bone marrow suppression
Drug classifications
Barbiturates: ↓ effect, ↑ hepatotoxicity
Hydantoins: ↓ effect, ↑ hepatotoxicity

Lab test interferences
Interference: Chemstrip G, Dextrostix, Visidex II, 5-HIAA

NURSING CONSIDERATIONS
Assessment
• Monitor liver function studies: AST, ALT, bilirubin, creatinine before therapy if long-term therapy is anticipated; may cause hepatic toxicity at doses >4 g/day with chronic use
• Monitor renal function studies: BUN, urine creatinine, occult blood; albumin indicates nephritis
• Monitor blood studies: CBC, pro-time if patient is on long-term therapy
• Check I&O ratio; decreasing output may indicate renal failure (long-term therapy)
• Assess for fever and pain: type of pain, location, intensity, duration, temperature, diaphoresis
• Assess for chronic poisoning: rapid, weak pulse, dyspnea, cold, clammy extremities; report immediately to prescriber
• Assess hepatotoxicity: dark urine, clay-colored stools, yellowing of skin and sclera; itching, abdominal pain, fever, diarrhea if patient is on long-term therapy
• Assess allergic reactions: rash, urticaria; if these occur, drug may have to be discontinued

Nursing diagnoses
☑ Pain (uses)
☑ Mobility, impaired physical mobility (uses)
☑ Injury, risk for (side effects)
☑ Knowledge deficit (teaching)

Implementation
• Administer to patient crushed or whole; chewable tabs may be chewed

• Give with food or milk to decrease gastric symptoms; give 30 min before or 2 hr after meals; absorption may be slowed

Patient/family education

⚠• Teach patient not to exceed recommended dosage; acute poisoning with liver damage may result; acute toxicity includes symptoms of nausea, vomiting, and abdominal pain; prescriber should be notified immediately

• Tell patient to read label on other OTC drugs; many contain acetaminophen and may cause toxicity if taken concurrently

• Teach patient to recognize signs of chronic overdose: bleeding, bruising, malaise, fever, sore throat

• Inform patient that urine may become dark brown as a result of phenacetin (metabolite of acetaminophen)

• Tell patient to notify prescriber for pain or fever lasting over 3 days

Evaluation

Positive therapeutic outcome
• Decreased pain
• Decreased fever

Treatment of overdose:
Drug level q4h, gastric lavage, activated charcoal; administer oral acetylcysteine to prevent hepatic damage (see acetylcysteine monograph, p. 11)

---

acetazolamide (℞)
(a-set-a-zole'-a-mide)
Apo-Acetazolamide ♣,
acetazolamide, Diamox,
Diamox Sequels, Hydrazol,
Func. class.: Diuretic carbonic anhydrase inhibitor; antiglaucoma agent, antiepileptic
Chem. class.: Sulfonamide derivative

Pregnancy category   C

Action: Decreases the aqueous humor in the eye, which lowers intraocular pressure by the inhibition of carbonic anhydrase; also inhibits carbonic anhydrase activity in proximal renal tubules to decrease reabsorption of water, sodium, potassium, bicarbonate; decreases carbonic anhydrase in CNS, increasing seizure threshold; prevents uric acid or cysteine buildup in the renal system by the decrease in pH causing alkaline urine

▶**Therapeutic Outcome:** Decreased intraocular pressure; control of seizures; prevention and treatment of acute mountain sickness; prevention of uric acid/cysteine renal stones; decreased edema in lung tissue and peripherally; decreased B/P

Uses: Open angle glaucoma, narrow angle glaucoma (preoperatively if surgery delayed), epilepsy (petit mal, grand mal, mixed), edema in CHF, drug-induced edema, acute mountain sickness

Investigational uses: Prevention of uric acid/cysteine renal stones, decrease CSF produc-

---

tion in infants with hydrocephalus

Dosage and routes
Closed angle glaucoma
Adult: PO/IM/**IV** 250 mg
q4h or 250 mg bid, to be used
for short-term therapy or 500
mg ES bid

Open angle glaucoma
Adult: PO/IM/**IV** 250 mg-
1g/day in divided doses for
amounts over 250 mg or
500 mg SR bid

Edema in CHF
Adult: IM/**IV** 250-375 mg/
day in AM

P *Child:* IM/**IV** 5 mg/kg/day
in AM

Seizures
Adult: PO/IM/**IV** 8-30 mg/
kg/day in 1-4 divided doses,
usual range 375-1000 mg/day
in divided doses tid or qid, or
300-900 mg/m²/day, not to
exceed 1.5 g/day

P *Child:* PO/IM/**IV** 8-30 mg/
kg/day in divided doses tid or
qid, or 300-900 mg/m²/day,
not to exceed 1 g/day

Mountain sickness
Adult: PO 250 mg q8-12h

Renal stones
Adult: PO 250 mg hs

P *Infants with hydrocephalus*
Infant: **IV** 5 mg/kg/day q6h,
may be increased up to 100
mg/kg/day if tolerated

Available forms: Tabs 125,
250 mg; caps ext rel 500 mg;
inj 500 mg

Adverse effects
CNS: Drowsiness, paresthesia,
anxiety, depression, headache,
dizziness, confusion, stimulation, fatigue, **convulsions,**
sedation, nervousness
EENT: Myopia, tinnitus

ENDO: Hyperglycemia, hypokalemia, hypocalcemia, hypomagnesemia, hyponatremia,
hyperchloremia
GI: Nausea, vomiting, anorexia, constipation, diarrhea,
melena, weight loss, **hepatic
insufficiency,** taste alterations
GU: Frequency, hypokalemia,
polyuria, **uremia,** glucosuria,
hematuria, dysuria, crystalluria,
renal calculi
HEMA: **Aplastic anemia,
hemolytic anemia, leukopenia, agranulocytosis, thrombocytopenia, purpura, pancytopenia**
INTEG: Rash, pruritus, urticaria, fever, **Stevens-Johnson
syndrome,** photosensitivity

Contraindications: Hypersensitivity to sulfonamides, severe
renal disease, severe hepatic
disease, electrolyte imbalances,
(hyponatremia, hypokalemia),
hyperchloremic acidosis, Addison's disease, long-term use in
narrow angle glaucoma

Precautions: Hypercalcemia,
pregnancy **C**

Do Not Confuse:
acetazolamide/acetohexamide,
Diamox/Trimox, Diamox/
Dobutrex

Pharmacokinetics	
Absorption	GI tract—65% if fasting, 75% with food); **IV**—complete
Distribution	Crosses placenta; widely distributed
Metabolism	None
Excretion	Kidneys, un-changed (80% within 24 hr); breast milk
Half-life	2½-5½ hr

Pharmacodynamics

	PO	PO–EXT REL	IV
Onset	1½ hr	2 hr	2 min
Peak	2-4 hr	3-6 hr	15 min
Duration	8-12 hr	18-24 hr	4-5 hr

Interactions
Individual drugs
Amphotericin B: ↑ hypokalemia
Aspirin: ↑ excretion of aspirin
Cyclosporine: ↑ toxicity
Diflunisol: ↑ side effects
Lithium: ↑ excretion of lithium
Methenamine: ↓ acetazolamide effect
Primidone: ↓ primidone level
Drug classifications
Amphetamines: ↑ action
Anticholinergics: ↑ anticholinergic action
Salicylates: ↑ toxicity
Lab test interferences
False positive: Urinary protein, 17-hydroxysteroids
Decrease: Thyroid iodine uptake

NURSING CONSIDERATIONS
Assessment
• Assess patient for tinnitus, hearing loss, ear pain; periodic testing of hearing is needed when high doses of this drug are given by **IV** route
• Monitor manifestations of hypokalemia: *RENAL:* acidic urine, reduced urine osmolality, nocturia, polyuria, polydipsia; *CARDIAC:* hypotension, broad T wave, U wave, ectopy, tachycardia, weak pulse; *NEURO:* muscle weakness, altered LOC, drowsiness, apathy, lethargy, confusion, depression; *GI:* anorexia, nausea, cramps, constipation, distention, paralytic ileus;

RESP: hypoventilation, respiratory muscle weakness
• Monitor for CNS, GI, cardiovascular, integumentary, neurologic manifestations of hypocalcemia: *CNS:* personality changes, anxiety, disturbances, depression, psychosis, nausea, vomiting; *GI:* constipation, abdominal pain from muscle spasm; *CV:* decreased contractility, decreased cardiac output, hypotension, lengthened ST segment, prolonged QT interval; *INTEG:* scaling eczema, alopecia, hyperpigmentation; *NEURO:* tetany, muscle twitching, cramping, grimacing, seizure, altered deep tendon reflexes, spasm
• Monitor for manifestations of hypomagnesemia: *CNS:* agitation; *NEURO:* muscle twitching, paresthesias, hyperactive reflexes, positive Babinski's reflex, dysphagia, nystagmus, seizures, tetany; *GI:* nausea, vomiting, diarrhea, anorexia, abdominal distention; *CARDIAC:* ectopy, tachycardia, broad, flat, or inverted T waves, depressed ST segment, prolonged QT, decreased cardiac output, hypotension
• Monitor for manifestations of hyponatremia: *CV:* increased B/P, cold, clammy skin, hypovolemia, or hypervolemia, vomiting, diarrhea, abdominal cramps; *NEURO:* lethargy, increased intracranial pressure, confusion, headache, seizures, coma, fatigue, tremors, hyperreflexia
• Monitor for manifestations of hyperchloremia: *NEURO:* weakness, lethargy, coma; *RESP:* deep, rapid breathing
• Assess fluid volume status: I&O ratio and record, count

or weigh diapers as appropriate, distended neck veins, crackles in lung, color, quality and sp gr of urine, skin turgor, adequacy of pulses, moist mucous membranes, bilateral lung sounds, peripheral pitting edema; dehydration symptoms of decreasing output, thirst, hypotension, dry mouth, and mucous membranes should be reported

• Monitor electrolytes: potassium, sodium, calcium, magnesium; also include BUN, blood pH, ABGs, uric acid, CBC, blood sugar

• Assess B/P before and during therapy with patient lying, standing, and sitting as appropriate; orthostatic hypotension can occur rapidly

• Monitor blood, urine glucose in diabetic patients; glucose levels may be increased

• Assess for eye pain, change in vision when using drug for intraocular pressure

• Assess neurologic status when using drug for seizures

• Assess for decreased symptoms of acute mountain sickness: headache, nausea, vomiting, dizziness, fatigue, drowsiness, shortness of breath, insomnia

• Assess for cross-sensitivity between other sulfonamides and this drug

Nursing diagnoses

☑ Sensory-perceptual alterations: visual (uses)

☑ Fluid volume deficit (side effects)

☑ Fluid volume excess (uses)

☑ Knowledge deficit (teaching)

Implementation

• Give in AM to avoid interference with sleep

• Administer fluids 2-3 L/day

to prevent renal calculi, unless contraindicated

• Potassium replacement if potassium level is <3.0

PO route

• Give with food, if nausea occurs, crush tabs and mix with sweet substance to counteract bitter taste; ES caps may be opened and sprinkled on food

🚫• Do not crush or chew caps

IV route

• Do not use solution that is yellow or has a precipitate or crystals

IV: Dilute 500 mg of drug/5 ml or more sterile water for inj; use within 24 hr

Direct IV: Give over 1 min or more

Intermittent infusion: May be added to NS, D_5W, $D_{10}W$, 0.45% NaCl; give over 4-8 hr

Additive compatibilities: Cimetidine, ranitidine

Additive incompatibilities: Multivitamins

Patient/family education

• Teach patient to take the medication early in the day to prevent nocturia

• Instruct patient to take with food or milk if GI symptoms of nausea and anorexia occur

• Teach patient to maintain a record of weight on a weekly basis and notify prescriber of weight loss of >5 lb

• Caution patient that this drug causes a loss of potassium, so food rich in potassium should be added to the diet; refer to a dietician for assistance in planning

• Advise patient to wear protective clothing and sunscreen in the sun to prevent photosensitivity

• Teach patient not to use alcohol or any OTC medica-

☑ Herb/drug   🚫 Do Not Crush   ◆ Alert   ⊶ Key Drug   **G** Geriatric   **P** Pediatric

tions without prescriber's approval; serious drug reactions may occur
• Emphasize the need to contact prescriber immediately if muscle cramps, weakness, nausea, dizziness, or numbness occurs
• Teach patient to take own B/P and pulse and record
• Teach patient to continue taking medication even if feeling better; this drug controls symptoms but does not cure the condition
• Teach patient to see ophthalmologist periodically; glaucoma is a slow process

Evaluation
Positive therapeutic outcome
• Decreased intraocular pressure
• Decreased edema
• Decreased seizures
• Prevention of mountain sickness
• Prevention of uric acid/ cysteine stones

Treatment of overdose:
Lavage if taken orally, monitor electrolytes, administer dextrose in saline, monitor hydration, CV, renal status

---

acetylcysteine ⚑ (℞)
(a-se-teel-sis'tay-een)
Mucomyst, Mucosal, Parvolex ♦
Func. class.: Mucolytic; antidote—acetaminophen
Chem. class.: Amino acid L-cysteine
Pregnancy category B

Action: Decreases viscosity of secretions in respiratory tract by breaking disulfide links of mucoproteins; increases hepatic glutathione, which is necessary to inactivate toxic metabolites in acetaminophen overdose

➔**Therapeutic Outcome:**
Decreased hepatotoxicity from acetaminophen overdose (PO); decreased viscosity of mucus in respiratory disorders (inh)

Uses: Acetaminophen toxicity; bronchitis; pneumonia; cystic fibrosis; emphysema; atelectasis; tuberculosis; complications of thoracic surgery and cardiovascular surgery; diagnosis in bronchial lab tests

Dosage and routes
Mucolytic
℗ *Adult and child:* INH 2-20 ml (10% sol) q1-4h prn, or 1-10 ml (20% sol)

Acetaminophen toxicity
℗ *Adult and child:* PO 140 mg/kg, then 70 mg/kg q4h × 17 doses to total 1330 mg/kg

Available forms: Sol 10%, 20%

Adverse effects
CNS: Dizziness, drowsiness, headache, fever, chills
CV: Hypotension
EENT: Rhinorrhea, tooth damage
GI: Nausea, stomatitis, constipation, vomiting, anorexia, **hepatotoxicity**
INTEG: Urticaria, rash, fever, clamminess
RESP: **Bronchospasm,** burning, **hemoptysis,** chest tightness

Contraindications: Hypersensitivity, increased intracranial pressure, status asthmaticus

Precautions: Hypothyroidism, Addison's disease, CNS depression, brain tumor, asthma, hepatic disease, renal disease, COPD, psychosis, alcoholism, convulsive disorders, lactation, pregnancy **B**

Pharmacokinetics

Absorption	Extensive (PO), locally (INH)
Distribution	Unknown
Metabolism	Liver
Excretion	Kidneys
Half-life	Unknown

Pharmacodynamics

	PO	INH
Onset	Unknown	1 min
Peak	Unknown	Unknown
Duration	up to 4 hr	5-10 min

Interactions
Individual drugs
Activated charcoal: ↓ absorption of acetylcysteine
Iron, copper, rubber: Do not use with acetylcysteine

NURSING CONSIDERATIONS
Assessment
Mucolytic use
• Assess cough: type, frequency, character, including sputum
• Assess characteristics, rate, rhythm of respirations, increased dyspnea, sputum; discontinue if bronchospasm occurs; ABGs for increased CO_2 retention in asthma patients
• Monitor VS, cardiac status including checking for dysrhythmias, increased rate, palpitations
Antidotal use
• Assess liver function tests, acetaminophen levels, protime, glucose, electrolytes; inform prescriber if dose is vomited or vomiting is persistent; provide adequate

hydration; decrease dosage in hepatic encephalopathy
• Assess for nausea, vomiting, rash; notify prescriber if these occur

Nursing diagnoses
☑ Injury, risk for physical (uses) (antidote)
☑ Impaired gas exchange (uses) (mucolytic)
☑ Airway clearance ineffective (uses) (mucolytic)
☑ Poisoning, risk for (uses) (antidote)
☑ Knowledge deficit (teaching)

Implementation
• Give decreased dosage to
G elderly patients; their metabolism may be slowed; give gum, hard candy, frequent rinsing of mouth for dryness of oral cavity
• Use only if suction machine is available
PO route: *Antidotal use*
• Lavage, then give within 24 hr; give with cola or soft drink to disguise taste; can be given with H_2O through tubes; use within 1 hr
INH route: *Mucolytic use*
• Use ac ½-1 hr for better absorption, to decrease nausea; only after patient clears airway by deep breathing, coughing
• Give by syringe 2-3 doses of 1-2 ml of 20% or 2-4 ml of 10% sol; 20% sol diluted with NS or water for injection; may give 10% sol undiluted
• Store in refrigerator: use within 96 hr of opening
• Provide assistance with inhaled dose: bronchodilator if bronchospasm occurs; wash face and rinse mouth after use to remove sticky feeling
• Use mechanical suction if cough insufficient to remove excess bronchial secretions

---

Patient/family education
Mucolytic use
• Tell patient to avoid driving or other hazardous activities until patient is stabilized on this medication; avoid alcohol, other CNS depressants; will enhance sedating properties of this drug
• Teach patient that unpleasant odor will decrease after repeated use; that discoloration of solution after bottle is opened does not impair its effectiveness; avoid smoking, smoke-filled rooms, perfume, dust, environmental pollutants, cleaners

Evaluation
Positive therapeutic outcome
• Absence of purulent secretions when coughing (mucolytic use)
• Clear lung sounds bilaterally (mucolytic use)
• Absence of hepatic damage (acetaminophen toxicity)
• Decreasing blood toxicology (acetaminophen toxicity)

activated charcoal (OTC)
Actidose, Actidose-Aqua, Charco-Aid 2000, CharcoCaps, Liqu-Char,
Func. class.:
Antiflatulent/antidote
Pregnancy category C

Action: Binds poisons, toxins, irritants; increases adsorption in GI tract; inactivates toxins and binds until excreted
➡ **Therapeutic Outcome:** Prevention of toxicity and death resulting from absorption of drugs
Uses: Poisoning

Dosage and routes
Poisoning
P Children should not get more than 1 dose of products with sorbitol
P *Adult and child:* PO 5-10 × weight of substance ingested; minimum dosage 30 g/250 ml of water; may give 20-40g q6h for 1-2 days in severe poisoning
Available forms: Powder 15, 25, 30, 40, 120, 125, 240 g/container; oral susp 12.5 g/60 ml, 15 g/72 ml, 15 g/120 ml, 25 g/120 ml, 30 g/120 ml, 50 g/240 ml; ♣ 15 g/120 ml, 25 g/125 ml, 50 g/225 ml, 50 g/250 ml

Adverse effects
GI: Nausea, black stools, vomiting, constipation, diarrhea

Contraindications: Hypersensitivity to this drug, unconsciousness, semiconsciousness, poisoning of cyanide, mineral acids, alkalies

Precautions: Pregnancy **C**

Pharmacokinetics

Absorption	None
Distribution	None
Metabolism	None
Excretion	Feces (unchanged)
Half-life	Unknown

Pharmacodynamics

Onset	1 min
Peak	Unknown
Duration	4-12 hr

Interactions
Individual drugs
Acetylcysteine: ↓ effectiveness of both drugs
Ipecac: ↓ effectiveness of both drugs

Food/drug
Dairy products: ↓ effect of activated charcoal

NURSING CONSIDERATIONS
Assessment
• Assess neurologic status including LOC, pupil reactivity, cough reflex, gag reflex, and swallowing ability before administration; do not give if neurologic status is impaired; aspiration may occur unless a protected airway is present
• Assess toxin, poison ingested, time of ingestion, and amount
• Monitor respiration, pulse, B/P to determine charcoal effectiveness if taken for barbiturate/narcotic poisoning

Nursing diagnoses
☑ Injury, risk for (uses)
☑ Poisoning, risk for (uses)
☑ Knowledge deficit (teaching)

Implementation
• Give after inducing vomiting unless vomiting contraindicated (i.e., cyanide or alkalies); mix with 8 oz water or fruit juice to form thick syrup; do not use dairy products to mix charcoal; repeat dose if vomiting occurs soon after dose
• Space at least 2 hr before or after other drugs, or absorption will be decreased; use a laxative to promote elimination; constipation occurs often
• Give alone; do not administer with ipecac; if patient unable to swallow, dilute to a less thick sol; keep container tightly closed to prevent absorption of gases
• Give through a nasogastric tube if patient unable to swallow

Patient/family education
• Tell patient stools will be black
• Teach patient about overdose/poison prevention and about keeping poison control chart available

Evaluation
Positive therapeutic outcome
• Alert, PERL (poisoning)
• Absence of distention
• Absence of odor in wounds

---

acyclovir ☜ (℞)
(ay-sye′kloe-ver)
Avirax ✦, Zovirax
Func. class.: Antiviral
Chem. class.: Acylic purine nucleoside analog
Pregnancy category   B

Action: Interferes with DNA synthesis by conversion to acyclovir triphosphate, causing decreased viral replication, time of lesional healing

▸**Therapeutic Outcome:** Decreased amount and time of healing of lesions

Uses: Mucocutaneous herpes simplex virus, herpes genitalis (HSV-1, HSV-2), herpes zoster; simple mucocutaneous herpes simplex in immunocompromised clients with initial herpes genitalis; herpes simplex encephalitis, cytomegalovirus, HSV after transplant

Dosage and routes
Renal disease
Lengthen dosing interval in renal disease if CrCl <50 ml/min

Herpes simplex
🄿**Adult and child >12 yr: IV** inf 5 mg/kg over 1 hr q8h × 5 days

---

☑ Herb/drug 🚫 Do Not Crush ✦ Alert ☜ Key Drug 🄖 Geriatric 🄿 Pediatric

P *Child <12 yr:* **IV** inf 250 mg/m² or 30 mg/kg day divided q8h over 1 hr × 5 days

Genital herpes
Adult: PO 200 mg q4h 5 times a day while awake × 5 days to 6 mo depending on whether initial, recurrent, or chronic

P *Adult and child:* TOP apply to all lesions q3h while awake, 6 times a day × 1 wk

Herpes simplex encephalitis
P *Child >6 mo:* **IV** 500 mg/m² q8h × 10-14 days

Herpes zoster
Adult: PO 800 mg q4h while awake × 7-10 days; **IV** 5 mg/kg q8h

Children with immunosuppression
P *Child >2 yr:* 20 mg/kg qid × 5 days

Varicella-zoster
Adult: PO 1000 mg q6h × 5 days or 600-800 mg q4h (5×/ day while awake); **IV** 500 mg/m² q8h or 10 mg/kg q8h × 7 days

P *Child:* PO 10-20 mg/kg (max 800 mg) qid × 5 days; **IV** 500 mg/m² q8h, or 10 mg/kg q8h × 7 days

Available forms: Caps 200 mg; tabs 400, 800 mg; inj **IV** 500 mg; top ointment 5% (50 mg/g); oral susp

Adverse effects
CNS: Tremors, confusion, lethargy, hallucinations, **convulsions,** *dizziness, headache,* encephalopathic changes
EENT: Gingival hyperplasia
GI: Nausea, vomiting, diarrhea, increased ALT, AST, abdominal pain, glossitis, colitis

GU: **Oliguria, proteinuria, hematuria,** vaginitis, moniliasis, **glomerulonephritis, acute renal failure,** changes in menses, polydipsia
INTEG: Rash, urticaria, pruritus, pain or phlebitis at **IV** site, unusual sweating, alopecia, stinging, burning, vulvitis
MS: Joint pain, leg pain, muscle cramps

Contraindications: Hypersensitivity

Precautions: Lactation, hepatic disease, renal disease, electrolyte imbalance, dehydration, pregnancy **B**

Pharmacokinetics

Absorption	Minimal (PO)
Distribution	Widely distributed, crosses placenta, CSF concentration 50% plasma
Metabolism	Liver, minimal
Excretion	Kidneys, 95% unchanged
Half-life	2.0-3.5 hr, increased in renal disease

Pharmacodynamics

	PO	IV	TOP
Onset	Unknown	Rapid	Unknown
Peak	1½-2½	Infusion's end	Unknown

Interactions
Individual drugs
Interferon: ↑ synergistic effect
Probenecid: ↑ neurotoxicity, nephrotoxicity
Zidovudine: ↑ drowsiness, side effects

NURSING CONSIDERATIONS
Assessment
• Monitor for signs of infection, type of lesions, area of body covered, purulent drainage

• Check I&O ratio; report hematuria, oliguria, fatigue, weakness; may indicate nephrotoxicity; check for protein in urine during treatment
• Monitor any patient with compromised renal system, since drug is excreted slowly in poor renal system function; toxicity may occur rapidly
• Monitor liver studies: AST, ALT
• Monitor blood studies: WBC, RBC, Hct, Hgb, bleeding time; blood dyscrasias may occur; drug should be discontinued
• Monitor renal studies: urinalysis, protein, BUN, creatinine, CrCl; increased BUN, creatinine indicates renal failure
• Obtain C&S before drug therapy; drug may be taken as soon as culture is taken; repeat C&S after treatment; determine the presence of other sexually transmitted diseases
• Monitor bowel pattern before, during treatment; if severe abdominal pain with bleeding occurs, drug should be discontinued
• Assess allergies before treatment, reaction of each medication; place allergies on chart in bright red letters; allergic reaction: burning, stinging, swelling, redness, rash, vulvitis, pruritus

Nursing diagnoses
☑ Infection, risk for (uses)
☑ Knowledge deficit (teaching)

Implementation
PO route
• Give with food to lessen GI symptoms
• Store at room temperature in dry place
Topical route
• Use finger cot or rubber glove to prevent further infection
• Enough medication to cover lesions completely
• After cleansing with soap and water before each application, dry well

Ⓜ IV route
• Provide increased fluids to 3 L/day to decrease crystalluria
• Give by int inf after reconstituting with 10 ml sterile water for injection/500 mg of drug (50 mg/ml); shake; dilute in 0.9% NaCl, LR, D_5W, D_5/0.25% NaCl, D_5/0.45% NaCl, D_5/0.9% NaCl (7 mg/ml); give over at least 1 hr (constant rate) by infusion pump to prevent nephrotoxicity; do not reconstitute with sol containing benzyl alcohol or parabens; check infusion site for redness, pain, induration; rotate sites
• Lower dosage in acute or chronic renal failure
• Store at room temperature for up to 12 hr after reconstitution; if refrigerated, sol may show a precipitate that clears at room temperature

Y-site compatibilities:
Allopurinol, amikacin, ampicillin, amphotericin B cholesteryl sulfate complex, cefamandole, cefazolin, cefonicid, cefoperazone, ceforanide, cefotaxime, cefoxitin, ceftazidime, ceftizoxime, ceftriaxone, cefuroxime, cephapirin, chloramphenicol, cimetidine, clindamycin, co-trimoxazole, dexamethasone sodium phosphate, dimenhydrinate, diphenhydramine, doxycycline, doxorubicin, erythromycin, famotidine, filgrastim, fluconazole, gallium, gentamicin, granisetron, heparin, hydrocortisone sodium succinate, hydromorphone,

imipenem/cilastatin, lorazepam, magnesium sulfate, melphalan, methylprednisolone sodium succinate, metoclopramide, metronidazole, multivitamin infusion, nafcillin, oxacillin, paclitaxel, penicillin G potassium, pentobarbital, perphenazine, piperacillin, potassium chloride, propofol, ranitidine, remifentanil, sodium bicarbonate, tacrolimus, teniposide, tetracycline, theophylline, thiotepa, ticarcillin, tobramycin, trimethoprim-sulfamethoxazole, vancomycin, zidovudine

Y-site incompatibilities:
Dobutamine, dopamine, ondansetron, verapamil

Additive compatibilities:
Fluconazole

Additive incompatibilities:
Blood products, protein-containing solutions, dobutamine, dopamine

Patient/family education
Topical route
• Tell patient not to use in eyes; for use when there is no evidence of infection; apply with glove to prevent further infection
• Instruct patient to avoid use of OTC creams, ointments, lotions unless directed by prescriber; may cause reinfection, delayed healing
• Teach patient to use asepsis (hand washing) before, after each application and avoid contact with eyes; to adhere strictly to prescribed regimen to maximize successful treatment outcome
PO route
• Teach patient that drug may be taken orally before infection

occurs; that drug should be taken when itching or pain occurs, usually before eruptions; that partners need to be told that patient has herpes; they can become infected, so condoms must be worn to prevent reinfections; that drug does not cure infection, just controls symptoms and does not prevent infection to others
◆• Tell patient to report sore throat, fever, fatigue; may indicate superinfection; that drug must be taken in equal intervals around the clock to maintain blood levels for duration of therapy
• Tell patient to notify prescriber of side effects: bruising, bleeding, fatigue, malaise; may indicate blood dyscrasias
• Tell patient to seek dental care during treatment to prevent gingival hyperplasia
• Teach female patients with genital herpes to have regular Pap smears to prevent undetected cervical cancer
⊘• Do not crush or chew caps

Evaluation
Positive therapeutic outcome
• Absence of itching, painful lesions
• Crusting and healed lesions

Treatment of overdose:
Discontinue drug, hemodialysis, resuscitate if needed

adenosine (℞)
(ah-den'oh-seen)
Adenocard
Func. class.: Antidysrhythmic misc.
Chem. class.: Endogenous nucleoside
Pregnancy category   C

Action: Slows conduction through AV node, can interrupt reentry pathways through AV node, and can restore normal sinus rhythm in patients with paroxysmal supraventricular tachycardia (PSVT)

➡**Therapeutic Outcome:**
Normal sinus rhythm in patients diagnosed with PSVT

Uses: PSVT

Dosage and routes
Adult: **IV** bol 6 mg; if conversion to normal sinus rhythm does not occur within 1-2 min, give 12 mg by rapid **IV** bol; may repeat 12 mg dose again in 1-2 min

🄿 *Infants and children:* 0.05 mg/kg; if not effective, increase dose by 0.05 mg/kg q2min to a max of 0.25 mg/kg or 12 mg

Available forms: Inj 3 mg/ml

Adverse effects
CNS: Lightheadedness, dizziness, arm tingling, numbness, apprehension, blurred vision, headache
CV: Chest pain, **atrial tachydysrhythmias,** sweating, palpitations, hypotension, *facial flushing*
GI: *Nausea,* metallic taste, throat tightness, groin pressure
RESP: *Dyspnea, chest pressure,* hyperventilation

Contraindications: Hypersensitivity, 2nd- or 3rd-degree heart block, AV block, sick sinus syndrome, atrial flutter, atrial fibrillation

Precautions: Pregnancy C,
🄿 lactation, children, asthma,
🄖 elderly

🄽 **Do Not Confuse:**
Adenocard/adenosine

Pharmacokinetics	
Absorption	Complete bioavailability
Distribution	Erythrocytes, cardiovascular endothelium
Metabolism	Liver, converted to inosine and adenosine monophosphate
Excretion	Kidneys
Half-life	10 sec

Pharmacodynamics	
Onset	Rapid
Peak	Unknown
Duration	1-2 min

Interactions
Individual drugs
Caffeine: ↓ effects of adenosine
Carbamazepine: ↑ heart block
Digoxin: ↑ ventricular fibrillation
Dipyridamole: ↑ effects of adenosine
Theophylline: ↓ effects of adenosine
Verapamil: ↑ ventricular fibrillation
Smoking
↑ tachycardia
🄳 *Herb/drug*
Aloe: may ↑ adenosine effect
Angelica: may ↑ adenosine effect
Buckthorn bark/berry: may ↑ adenosine effect
Cascara sagrada bark: may ↑ adenosine effect

🄳 Herb/drug   🄢 Do Not Crush   ◆ Alert   ☛ Key Drug   🄖 Geriatric   🄿 Pediatric

Rhubarb root: may ↑ adenosine effect

Senna leaf/fruits: may ↑ adenosine effect

NURSING CONSIDERATIONS
Assessment
• Monitor I&O ratio, electrolytes (potassium, sodium, chloride)

• Assess cardiac status: pulse, respiration, ECG intervals (PR, QRS, QT); check for transient dysrhythmias (PVCs, PACs, sinus tachycardia, AV block); B/P continuously for fluctuations

• Assess respiratory status: rate, rhythm, lung fields for rales, watch for respiratory depression; lung fields, bilateral rales may occur in CHF patient; if increased respiration, increased pulse occurs, drug should be discontinued

• Assess CNS effects: dizziness, confusion, paresthesias; drug should be discontinued

Nursing diagnoses
☑ Cardiac output, decreased (uses)
☑ Impaired gas exchange (adverse reactions)
☑ Knowledge deficit (teaching)

Implementation
• Give **IV** bol undiluted; give 6 mg or less by rapid inj; if using an **IV** line, use port near insertion site, flush with NS (50 ml); warm to room temperature before giving

Solution compatibilities:
D_5LR, D_5W, LR, 0.9% NaCl
• Store at room temperature; sol should be clear; discard unused drug

Patient/family education
• Tell patient to report facial flushing, dizziness, sweating, palpitations, chest pain

• Instruct patient to rise from sitting or standing slowly to prevent orthostatic hypotension

Evaluation
Positive therapeutic outcome
• Decreased B/P, dysrhythmias

---

alatrofloxacin (℞)
(ah-lat-troh-floks'ah-sin)
Trovan IV
trovafloxacin (℞)
(troh-vah-floks'ah-sin)
Trovan
Func. class.: Antiinfective
Chem. class.: Fluoroquinolone

Pregnancy category C

Action: Interferes with conversion of intermediate DNA fragments into high-molecular-weight DNA in bacteria; DNA gyrase inhibitor

▷**Therapeutic Outcome:** Bacterial action against the following: Nosocomial pneumonia: *Escherichia coli, Pseudomonas aeruginosa, Haemophilus influenzae, Staphylococcus aureus,* community-acquired pneumonia: *Staphylococcus pneumoniae, Haemophilus influenzae, Staphylococcus aureus, Klebsiella pneumoniae, Mycoplasma pneumoniae, Mycoplasma catarrhalis, Legionella pneumophilia, Chlamydia pneumoniae*

Uses: Nosocomial pneumonia, community-acquired pneumonia, chronic bronchitis, acute sinusitis, complicated intraabdominal infections, gyn/pelvic infection, skin/skin structure infections, UTIs, chronic bacterial prostatitis, urethral gonorrhea in males, PID, cervici-

---

tis caused by susceptible organisms

Dosage and routes
Adult: **IV**/PO 200-300 mg qd for 7-14 days, depending on infection

Available forms:
Sol for inj 5 mg/ml (alatrofloxacin); tabs 100, 200 mg (trovafloxacin)

Adverse effects
CNS: Headache, *dizziness,* insomnia, anxiety, psychosis, **seizures**
GI: Nausea, flatulence, vomiting, diarrhea, abdominal pain, **pseudomembranous colitis**
GU: Vaginitis, crystalluria ↑ BUN, creatinine
INTEG: Rash, pruritus, photosensitivity
HEMA: Anemia, **thrombocytopenia, leukopenia,** ↓ Hgb, Hct, ↑ platelets
MS: Arthralgia, myalgia

Contraindications: Hypersensitivity to quinolones, seizure disorders, cerebral atherosclerosis, photosensitivity

Precautions: Pregnancy **C,** lactation, children

Pharmacokinetics
Absorption	Unknown
Distribution	Unknown
Metabolism	Liver
Excretion	Kidneys, unchanged
Half-life	Unknown

Pharmacodynamics
Onset	Unknown
Peak	Unknown
Duration	Unknown

Interactions
Individual drugs
Citric acid/sodium citrate: ↓ absorption
Iron: ↓ absorption
Morphine IV: ↓ absorption
Sucralfate: ↓ absorption
Drug classifications
Antacids with aluminum/ magnesium: ↓ absorption

NURSING CONSIDERATIONS
Assessment
• Assess for previous sensitivity reaction to fluoroquinolones
• Monitor for signs and symptoms of infection: characteristics of sputum, WBC >10,000, fever; obtain baseline information before and during treatment
• Obtain C&S before beginning drug therapy to identify if correct treatment has been initiated
• Assess for allergic reactions: rash, urticaria, pruritus, chills, fever, joint pain; may occur a few days after therapy begins; epinephrine and resuscitation equipment should be available for anaphylactic reaction
• Assess bowel pattern qd; if severe diarrhea occurs, drug should be discontinued
• Assess for overgrowth of infection, perineal itching, fever, malaise, redness, pain, swelling, drainage, rash, diarrhea, change in cough, sputum
• Identify urine output; if decreasing, notify prescriber (may indicate nephrotoxicity); also check for increased BUN, creatinine
• Assess for CNS disorders; other fluoroquinolones cause seizures, stimulation
• Monitor blood studies: AST, ALT, CBC, Hct, bilirubin, LDH, alkaline phosphatase, Coombs' test monthly if patient is on long-term therapy
• Monitor electrolytes: potassium, sodium, chloride

☑ Herb/drug ◎ Do Not Crush ◆ Alert ✦☐ Key Drug ☐ Geriatric ☐ Pediatric monthly if patient is on long-term therapy

Nursing diagnoses
☑ Infection, risk for (uses)
☑ Diarrhea (side effects)
☑ Injury, risk for (side effects)
☑ Knowledge deficit (teaching)
☑ Noncompliance (teaching)

Implementation
IV route
• Check for irritation, extravasation, phlebitis daily

Incompatibilities:
Do not use with magnesium in the same IV line

Solution compatibilities
D_5, ½% NaCl, D_5/0.2% NaCl, LR

Patient/family education
• Teach patient to report sore throat, bruising, bleeding, joint pain; may indicate blood dyscrasias (rare)
• Advise patient to contact prescriber if vaginal itching, loose, foul-smelling stools, furry tongue occur, may indicate superinfection; report itching, rash, pruritus, urticaria
• Instruct patient to take all medication prescribed for the length of time ordered; drug must be taken around the clock to maintain blood levels; do not give medication to others
• Advise patient to notify prescriber of diarrhea with blood or pus, may indicate pseudomembranous colitis
• Advise patient to use sunscreen to prevent photosensitivity
• Teach patient that drug may be taken with or without food; separate sucralfate, antacids by ≥2 hr

Evaluation
Positive therapeutic outcome
• Absence of signs/symptoms of infection (WBC <10,000, temp WNL)
• Reported improvement in symptoms of infection

albumin, human (℞)
(al-byoo'min)
Albuminar 5%, Albutein 5%, Buminate 5%, Plasbumin 5%, Albuminar 25%, Albutein 25%, Buminate 25%, Plasbumin-25%
Func. class.: Blood derivative—volume expander
Chem. class.: Placental human plasma

Pregnancy category C

Action: Exerts colloidal oncotic pressure, which expands volume of circulating blood by pulling fluid from extravascular to intravascular spaces, and maintains cardiac output

➡ **Therapeutic Outcome:** Restoration of plasma volume by extravascular to intravascular fluid shift

Uses: Restores plasma volume in burns, hyperbilirubinemia, shock, hypoproteinemia, prevention of cerebral edema, cardiopulmonary bypass procedures, ARDS, hemorrhage; also replacement in nephrotic syndrome, hepatic failure

Dosage and routes
Burns
Adult: **IV** dose to maintain plasma albumin at 30-50 g/L, use 5% sol initially, then 25% sol after 24 hr

---

Shock
Adult: **IV** 500 ml of 5% sol
q30 min, as needed
P *Child:* 0.5-1 g/kg/dose

Hypoproteinemia
Adult: **IV** 1000-2000 ml of 5%
sol qd, not to exceed 5-10
ml/min or 25-100 g of 25%
sol qd, not to exceed 3 ml/
min, titrated to patient response

Hyperbilirubinemia/
erythroblastosis fetalis
P *Infant:* **IV** 1 g of 25% sol/kg
before transfusion

Available forms: Inj 50, 250
mg/ml (5%, 25%)

Adverse effects
CNS: Fever, chills, flushing,
headache
CV: **Fluid overload,** hypoten-
sion, erratic pulse, tachycardia
GI: Nausea, vomiting, in-
creased salivation
INTEG: Rash, urticaria
RESP: Altered respirations,
pulmonary edema

Contraindications: Hypersensitivity, CHF, severe anemia,
renal insufficiency

Precautions: Decreased salt
intake, decreased cardiac reserve, lack of albumin deficiency, hepatic disease, renal
disease, pregnancy **C**

Pharmacokinetics

Absorption	Complete bioavail-ability
Distribution	Intravascular spaces
Metabolism	Liver
Excretion	Unknown
Half-life	Unknown

Pharmacodynamics

Onset	15-30 min
Peak	Unknown
Duration	Unknown

Interactions: None
Lab test interferences
False: ↑ Alkaline phosphatase

NURSING CONSIDERATIONS
Assessment
• Monitor blood studies: Hct,
Hgb; if serum protein declines,
dyspnea, hypoxemia can result;
check for decreasing B/P,
erratic pulse, respiration
◆• Monitor CVP: pulmonary
wedge pressure will increase if
overload occurs; I&O ratio:
urinary output may decrease;
CVP reading: distended neck
veins indicate circulatory
overload; shortness of breath,
anxiety, insomnia, expiratory
rales, frothy blood-tinged
sputum, cough, cyanosis indicate pulmonary overload
• Assess for allergy: fever, rash,
itching, chills, flushing, urticaria, nausea, vomiting,
hypotension; requires discontinuation of infusion, use of
new lot if therapy reinstituted

Nursing diagnoses
☑ Fluid volume deficit (uses)
☑ Injury, risk for physical (uses)
☑ Fluid volume excess (adverse
   reactions)
☑ Knowledge deficit (teaching)

Implementation
• Check type of albumin; some
are stored at room temperature, some need to be
refrigerated; use only amber-
colored sol without precipitate;
solution should be clear
• Give **IV** slowly to prevent
fluid overload; 5% may be
given undiluted; 25% may be
given diluted (D_5W, 0.9%
NaCl) or undiluted; give over
4 hr, use infusion pump
• Provide adequate hydration
before, during administration;
whole blood may need to be

☑ Herb/drug 🚫 Do Not Crush ◆ Alert ⟐ Key Drug **G** Geriatric **P** Pediatric

given to prevent anemia; monitor hydration during treatment

Solution compatibilities:
LR, NaCl, Ringer's, D_5W, $D_{10}W$, $D_{2\frac{1}{2}}W$, dextrose/saline, dextran$_6$ D_5, dextran$_6$ NaCl 0.9%, dextrose/Ringer's, dextrose/LR

Y-*site compatibilities:* Diltiazem, lorazepam

Patient/family education
• Explain use, reason for albumin; provide information on what to report to prescriber (hypersensitivity, fluid overload)

Evaluation
Positive therapeutic outcome
• Increased B/P, decreased edema (shock, burns)
• Increased serum albumin levels
• Increased plasma protein (hypoproteinemia)

---

albuterol ⟳ (℞)
(al-byoo'ter-ole)
Airet, albuterol, Proventil, Proventil Repetabs, Ventolin, Ventolin Rotacaps, Volmax
Func. class.: Bronchodilator
Chem. class.: Adrenergic β_2-agonist, sympathomimetic, bronchodilator
Pregnancy category   C

Action: Causes bronchodilatation by action on β_2 (pulmonary) receptors by increasing levels of cyclic adenosine monophosphate (cAMP), which relaxes smooth muscle; produces bronchodilatation; CNS, cardiac stimulation, increased

diuresis, and increased gastric acid secretion; longer acting than isoproterenol

⊸Therapeutic Outcome: Increased ability to breathe because of bronchodilatation

Uses: Prevention of exercise-induced asthma, bronchospasm, bronchitis, emphysema, bronchiectasis, other pulmonary disease

Investigational uses: Hyperkalemia in dialysis patients

Dosage and routes
Prevention of exercise-induced bronchospasm
Adult: INH 2 puffs 15 min before exercising, NEB/IPPB 5 mg tid-qid; Volmax Ext Rel 8 mg q/2h; Repetabs 4-8 mg q/12h

P *Adult and child >4 yr:* 200 µg cap INH 15 min before exercises

G *Elderly:* 2 mg tid-qid, may increase gradually to 8 mg tid-qid

Other respiratory conditions
P *Adult and child ≥12 yr:* INH 1-2 puffs q4-6h; PO 2-4 mg tid-qid, not to exceed 8 mg

P *Child 2-6 yr:* INH 0.1 mg/kg tid (max 2 mg tid); may increase to 0.2 mg/kg tid (max 4 mg tid)

P *Adult and child >4 yr:* INH cap 200 µg cap inhaled q4-6h using Rotahaler

Available forms: Aerosol 90, 100 µg/actuation; tabs 2, 4 mg; oral sol 2 mg/5 ml, ♣ ext rel 4, 8 mg; inh sol 0.83, 1, ♣ 5 mg/ml; inh caps (Rotacaps) 200 µg

---

Adverse effects

CNS: *Tremors, anxiety,* insomnia, headache, dizziness, stimulation, *restlessness,* hallucinations, flushing, irritability
CV: *Palpitations, tachycardia, hypertension,* angina, hypotension, dysrhythmias
EENT: Dry nose, irritation of nose and throat
GI: *Heartburn, nausea, vomiting*
MISC: Flushing, sweating, anorexia, bad taste/smell changes
MS: Muscle cramps
RESP: Cough, wheezing, dyspnea, **bronchospasm,** dry throat

Contraindications: Hypersensitivity to sympathomimetics, tachydysrhythmias, severe cardiac disease, heart block

Precautions: Lactation, pregnancy **C,** cardiac disorders, hyperthyroidism, diabetes mellitus, hypertension, prostatic hypertrophy, narrow angle glaucoma, seizures, exercise-induced bronchospasm (aerosol) in children <12 years

Do Not Confuse:
Ventolin/Vantin, Proventil/Prinivil, albuterol/atenolol

Pharmacokinetics	
Absorption	Well absorbed (PO)
Distribution	Unknown
Metabolism	Liver extensively, tissues
Excretion	Unknown, breast milk
Half-life	3-4 hr

Pharmacodynamics			
	PO	PO–EXT REL	INH
Onset	½ hr	½ hr	5-15 min
Peak	2½ hr	2-3 hr	1-1½ hr
Duration	4-6 hr	12 hr	4-6 hr

Interactions

Drug classifications
β-Adrenergic blockers: Block therapeutic effect
Bronchodilators, aerosol: ↑ action of bronchodilator
Diuretics: ↑ ECG changes/ hypokalemia
MAOI: ↑ chance of hypertensive crisis
Oxytocics: Severe hypotension
Sympathomimetics: ↑ adrenergic side effects
Xanthines: ↑ toxicity

NURSING CONSIDERATIONS
Assessment
• Assess respiratory function: vital capacity, forced expiratory volume, ABGs, lung sounds, heart rate, rhythm (baseline and during therapy)
• Determine that patient has not received theophylline therapy before giving dose, to prevent additive effect; client's ability to self-medicate
• Monitor for evidence of allergic reactions; paradoxic bronchospasm; withhold dose; notify prescriber

Nursing diagnoses
☑ Airway clearance, ineffective (uses)
☑ Impaired gas exchange (uses)
☑ Knowledge deficit (teaching)

Implementation
PO route
• Give PO with meals to decrease gastric irritation; oral sol for children (no alcohol, sugar)
• In geriatric patients, a spacing device is advised
Aerosol route
• Give after shaking; have patient exhale and place mouthpiece in mouth, inhale slowly, hold breath, remove inhaler, exhale slowly; allow at least 1 min between inhalations

---

☑ Herb/drug   🚫 Do Not Crush   ◆ Alert   ☞ Key Drug   **G** Geriatric   **P** Pediatric

• Store in light-resistant container; do not expose to temperatures over 86° F (30° C)

Patient/family education

• Tell patient not to use OTC medications before consulting prescriber; excess stimulation may occur; instruct patient to use this medication before other medications and allow at least 5 min between each to prevent overstimulation; to limit caffeine products such as chocolate, coffee, tea, and cola

• Teach patient to use inhaler; review package insert with patient; to avoid getting aerosol in eyes or blurring may result; to wash inhaler in warm water and dry qd; to rinse mouth after using; to avoid smoking, smoke-filled rooms, persons with respiratory infections

♦• Teach patient that if paradoxic bronchospasm occurs to stop drug immediately and notify prescriber

• Instruct patient on administration of dose, not to use more than prescribed; serious side effects may occur; if taking PO regularly and dose is missed, take when remembered; space other doses on new time schedule; do not double doses

G• In geriatric patients, a spacing device is advised

Evaluation

Positive therapeutic outcome

• Absence of dyspnea and wheezing after 1 hr
• Improved airway exchange
• Improved ABGs

Treatment of overdose:
Administer a β₁-adrenergic blocker

---

aldesleukin (℞)
(al-dess-loo'kin)
interleukin-2, IL-2, Proleukin
Func. class.: Miscellaneous antineoplastics
Chem. class.: Interleukin-2, human recombinant, cytotine

Pregnancy category C

Action: Enhancement of lymphocyte mitogenesis and stimulation of IL-2–dependent cell lines; enhancement of lymphocyte cytotoxicity; induction of killer cell activity; induction of interferon-γ production; results in activation of cellular immunity and cytokines and inhibition of tumor growth

Therapeutic Outcome: Prevention of rapid growth of malignant cells

Uses: Metastatic renal cell carcinoma in adults, phase II for HIV in combination with zidovudine, melanoma

Investigational uses: Kaposi's sarcoma given with zidovudine, metastatic melanoma given with cyclophosphamide, non-Hodgkin's lymphoma given with lymphokine-activated killer cells, AIDS (phase I) given with zidovudine

Dosage and routes
Adult: **IV** inf 600,000 IU/kg (0.037 mg/kg) q8h over 15 min × 14 doses; off 9 days; repeat schedule for another 14 doses, for a maximum of 28 doses/course

Available forms: Powder for inj 2.2 million IU/vial

Adverse effects

CNS: Mental status changes, dizziness, sensory dysfunction, syncope, motor dysfunction, fever, chills, headache
CV: Hypotension, sinus tachycardia, dysrhythmias, bradycardia, PVCs, PACs, myocardial ischemia, **myocardial infarction, cardiac arrest,** capillary leak syndrome
GI: Nausea, vomiting, diarrhea, stomatitis, anorexia, GI bleeding, dyspepsia, constipation, **intestinal perforation/ileus,** jaundice, ascites
GU: Oliguria/anuria, proteinuria, hematuria, dysuria, renal failure
HEMA: Anemia, **thrombocytopenia, leukopenia, coagulation disorders, leukocytosis, eosinophilia**
INTEG: Pruritus, erythema, rash, dry skin, **exfoliative dermatitis,** purpura, petechiae, urticaria
MS: Arthralgia, myalgia
RESP: Pulmonary congestion, dyspnea, **pulmonary edema, respiratory failure,** tachypnea, pleural effusion, wheezing
SYST: Infection

Contraindications: Hypersensitivity, abnormal thallium stress test or pulmonary function tests, organ allografts

Precautions: CNS metastases, bacterial infections, renal/hepatic, cardiac/pulmonary disease, pregnancy **C,** lactation, [P] children, anemia, thrombocytopenia

[N] **Do Not Confuse:**
Proleukin/Prokine

Pharmacokinetics

Absorption	Complete bioavailability
Distribution	Rapid extracellular, intravascular
Metabolism	Kidneys (convoluted tubules)
Excretion	Kidneys
Half-life	85 min

Pharmacodynamics

Onset	4 wk
Duration	≤12 mo

Interactions
Individual drugs
Indomethacin: ↑ toxicity
Radiation: ↑ toxicity, bone marrow suppression
Drug classifications
Aminoglycosides: ↑ toxicity
Antihypertensives: ↑ hypotension
Antineoplastics: ↑ toxicity, bone marrow suppression
Corticosteroids: ↓ tumor effectiveness
Psychotropics: Unpredictable reactions
Lab test interferences
↑ Bilirubin, ↑ BUN, ↑ serum creatinine, ↑ transaminase, ↑ alkaline phosphatase, ↑ hypomagnesemia, ↑ acidosis hypocalcemia, ↑ hypophosphatemia, ↑ hypokalemia, ↑ hyperuricemia, ↑ hypoalbuminemia, ↑ hypoproteinemia, ↑ hyponatremia, ↑ hyperkalemia, ↑ alkalosis (toxic effect of drug)

NURSING CONSIDERATIONS
Assessment
• Monitor CBC, differential, platelet count weekly; withhold drug if WBC is <4000/mm³ or platelet count is <75,000/mm³; notify prescriber of these results; transfusion of RBCs, platelets may be required
⬦• Identify capillary leak syndrome (CLS), including a drop

in mean arterial pressure (2-12 hr after initiating therapy); hypotension and hypoperfusion will occur; monitor ECG, CVP in cardiac patients
• Monitor renal function studies: BUN, serum uric acid, urine CrCl, electrolytes before, during therapy; I&O ratio; report fall in urine output to <30 ml/hr
• Monitor temperature q4h; fever may indicate beginning infection
• Check liver function tests before, during therapy: bilirubin, AST, ALT, alkaline phosphatase as needed or monthly
• Monitor ECG; watch for ST-T wave changes, low QRS and T, possible dysrhythmias (sinus tachycardia, PVCs)
• Monitor baselines in pulmonary function; document FEV >2 L or ≥75% before therapy; check daily VS, pulse oximetry, dyspnea, rales, ABGs
• Obtain stress thallium study before therapy; document normal ejection fraction, unimpaired wall motion
• Assess for bleeding: hematuria, guaiac, bruising or petechiae, mucosa, or orifices q8h
• Assess for GI symptoms: frequency of stools, cramping
• Assess for acidosis, signs of dehydration: rapid respirations, poor skin turgor, decreased urine output, dry skin, restlessness, weakness
• Assess for cardiac status: B/P, pulse, character, rhythm, rate, ABGs, ECG
• Assess for infection: sore throat; antibiotics may be prescribed prophylactically

Nursing diagnoses
☑ Injury, risk for (adverse reactions)
☑ Body image disturbance (adverse reactions)
☑ Infection, risk for (adverse reactions)
☑ Knowledge deficit (teaching)

Implementation
• Give by intermittent **IV** inf after diluting 22 million IU (1.3 mg)/1.2 ml sterile (1.1 mg/ml) H_2O for inj at side of vial and swirl, do not shake; dilute dose with 50 ml D_5W and give over 15 min; use plastic bag; do not use an in-line filter; give through Y-tube or 3-way stopcock
• Give dopamine 1-5 kg/min before onset of hypotension; ↓ dose preserves kidney output
• Give hydrocortisone, dexamethasone, or sodium bicarbonate (1 mEq/1 ml) for extravasation, apply ice compresses
• Store in refrigerator any diluted drug; do not freeze; administer within 48 hr; bring to room temperature before infusing; discard unused portion

Y-site compatibilities:
Amikacin, **IV** fat emulsion, gentamicin, morphine, piperacillin, potassium chloride, ticarcillin, tobramycin, TPN #145, amphotericin B, calcium gluconate, diphenhydramine, dopamine, fluconazole, foscarnet, heparin, magnesium sulfate, metoclopramide, ondansetron, ranitidine, trimethoprim/sulfamethizole

Patient/family education
• Teach patient to avoid use of products containing aspirin or ibuprofen, razors, commercial mouthwash because bleeding may occur; to report symptoms of bleeding hematuria, tarry stools

---

- Tell patient to report signs of anemia: fatigue, headache, irritability, faintness, shortness of breath
- Tell patient to report any changes in breathing or coughing even several months after treatment
- Advise patient that contraception will be necessary during treatment; teratogenesis may occur
- Teach patient to report signs/symptoms of infection: fever, chills, sore throat; patient should avoid crowds or persons with known infections

Evaluation
Positive therapeutic outcome
- Decreased spread of malignancy

---

alendronate (℞)
(al-en′droe-nate)
Fosamax
Func. class.: Bone-resorption inhibitor
Chem. class.: Biphosphonate

Pregnancy category C

Action: Absorbs calcium phosphate crystal in bone and may directly block dissolution of hydroxyapatite crystals of bone; inhibits bone resorption, apparently without inhibiting bone formation and mineralization

➡ **Therapeutic Outcome:** Decreased symptoms of osteoporosis, Paget's disease

Uses: Osteoporosis in postmenopausal women, Paget's disease

Dosage and routes
Osteoporosis in postmenopausal women
🄶 *Adult and elderly:* PO 10 mg qd

Paget's disease
🄶 *Adult and elderly:* PO 40 mg qd × 6 mo

Available forms: Tabs 5, 10, 40 mg

Adverse effects
META: Anemia, hypokalemia, hypomagnesemia, hypophosphatemia
GI: Abdominal pain, anorexia, constipation, nausea, vomiting, esophageal ulceration
MS: Bone pain
CNS: Headache
CV: Hypertension
GU: UTI, fluid overload

Contraindications: Hypersensitivity to biphosphonates, hypocalcemia

🄿 **Precautions:** Children, lactation, pregnancy **C**, CrCl <35 ml/min, esophageal disease, ulcers, gastritis

Pharmacokinetics	
Absorption	Unknown
Distribution	Mainly to bones
Metabolism	Unknown
Excretion	Via kidneys
Half-life	Unknown

Pharmacodynamics
Unknown

Interactions
Individual drugs
Ranitidine: ↑ alendronate effect
Drug classifications
Antacids: ↓ absorption
Calcium supplements: ↓ absorption
NSAIDs: ↑ GI reactions

Salicylates: ↑ GI reactions
Food/drug
Food: ↓ absorption

NURSING CONSIDERATIONS
Assessment
• Monitor renal studies and Ca, P, Mg, K; confirm osteoporosis with bone density test before use
• Assess for hypercalcemia: paresthesia, twitching, laryngospasm, Chvostek's, Trousseau's signs
• Monitor alkaline phosphatase; level of 2× upper limit of normal is indicated for Paget's disease

Implementation
• Give PO for 6 mo to be effective in Paget's disease; take with 8 oz of water 30 min ac
• Store in cool environment out of direct sunlight

Patient/family education
• Teach patient to remain upright for 30 min after dose to prevent esophageal irritation
• Teach patient to take in AM before food, other meds, to take with 6-8 oz of water (no mineral water)
• To take calcium, vit D if dietary intake is lacking
• To use weight-bearing exercise to increase bone density

Evaluation
Positive therapeutic outcome
• Increased bone mass, absence of fractures

alfentanil (℞)
(al-fen'ta-nil)
Alfenta, Rapifen ✦
Func. class.: Narcotic analgesic
Chem. class.: Opiate, synthetic

Pregnancy category   C
Controlled substance schedule   II

Action: Inhibits ascending pain pathways in limbic system, thalamus, midbrain, hypothalamus by binding to opiate receptor sites; this alters pain perception and response

▶**Therapeutic Outcome:** Relief of pain (moderate, severe pain), anesthesia

Uses: In combination with other drugs in general anesthesia; as a primary anesthetic in general surgery usually used with barbiturates, oxygen, nitrous oxide, monitored anesthesia care (MAC)

Dosage and routes
Anesthesia <30 min
Combination
Adult: **IV** 8-50 µg/kg, may increase by 3-15 µg/kg

Anesthetic induction
Adult: **IV** 3-5 µg/kg, then 0.5-1.5 µg/kg/min; total dose is 8-40 µg/kg

Anesthesia 30-60 min
Induction
Adult: **IV** 20-50 µg/kg

Maintenance
Adult: **IV** 5-15 µg/kg; may give up to 75 µg/kg total dose

Continuous anesthesia >45 min
Induction
Adult: **IV** 50-75 µg/kg

Maintenance
Adult: **IV** 0.5-3.0 µg/kg/min; rate should be decreased by 30%-50% after 1 hr maintenance inf; may be increased to 4 µg/kg/min or bol doses of 7 µg/kg

Induction of anesthesia >45 min
Adult: **IV** 130-245 µg/kg, then 0.5-1.5 µg/kg/min or general anesthesia

MAC
Adult: **IV** duration ≤ ½ hr, 3-8 µg/kg; maintenance: 3-5 µg/kg at 5-20 min to 1 µg/kg/min; total dose 3-40 µg/kg

Available forms: Inj 500 µg/ml

Adverse effects
CNS: Drowsiness, dizziness, confusion, headache, sedation, euphoria, delirium, agitation, anxiety
CV: Palpitations, bradycardia, change in B/P, facial flushing, syncope, asystole
EENT: Tinnitus, blurred vision, miosis, diplopia
GI: Nausea, vomiting, anorexia, constipation, cramps, dry mouth
GU: Urinary retention, dysuria
INTEG: Rash, urticaria, bruising, flushing, diaphoresis, pruritus
MS: Rigidity
RESP: **Respiratory depression, apnea**

P **Contraindications:** Child <12 yr, hypersensitivity

Precautions: Pregnancy **C,** lactation, increased intracranial pressure, acute MI, severe heart disease, renal disease, hepatic disease, asthma, respiratory conditions, convulsive **G** disorders, elderly

Pharmacokinetics

Absorption	Complete
Distribution	Crosses placenta; 90% bound to plasma proteins
Metabolism	Liver, up to 100%
Excretion	Kidneys
Half-life	1-2 hr

Pharmacodynamics

Onset	Immediate
Peak	1-1½ min
Duration	30 min

Interactions
Individual drugs
Alcohol: ↑ respiratory depression, hypotension, ↑ sedation
Cimetidine: ↑ toxicity
Erythromycin: ↑ recovery time
Nalbuphine: ↓ analgesia
Pentazocine: ↓ analgesia
Drug classifications
Antihistamines: ↑ respiratory depression, hypotension
Benzodiazepines: ↑ hypotension
CNS depressants: ↑ respiratory depression, hypotension
MAOI: Do not use within 2 wk of alfentanil
Phenothiazines: ↑ respiratory depression, hypotension
Sedative/hypnotics: ↑ respiratory depression, hypotension
☑ *Herb/drug*
Kava: ↑ CNS depression
Lab test interferences
↑ Amylase, ↑ lipase

NURSING CONSIDERATIONS
Assessment
◆• Respiratory status: respiratory depression, character, rate, rhythm; notify prescriber if respirations are <12/min; CV status; bradycardia, syncope; monitor ECG continuously

---

☑ Herb/drug ◙ Do Not Crush ◆ Alert ⟳ Key Drug **G** Geriatric **P** Pediatric

Nursing diagnoses

☑ Pain (uses)
☑ Sensory perceptual alteration: visual, auditory (adverse reactions)
☑ Breathing pattern, ineffective (adverse reactions)
☑ Knowledge deficit (teaching) (preoperatively)

Implementation

General

• Administer pain medications for postoperative pain, since alfentanil effect is short; medication for severe pain may be required
• Benzodiazepines are given after surgery to reduce alfentanil dosage and reduce anesthesia recovery time

IV Direct IV

• Give direct **IV** over 1½-3 min; use tuberculin syringe for accurate dosing

IV Continuous IV

• Give cont **IV** by diluting 20 ml of drug in 230 ml of diluent (0.9% NaCl, D₅W, LR) (40 µg/ml); discontinue infusion 15 min before surgery is completed
• Store in light-resistant area at room temperature
Syringe compatibilities:
Atracurium
Y-site compatibilities:
Etomidate, propofol

Patient/family education

• Tell patients to avoid CNS depressants (alcohol, sedative/hypnotics) for at least 24 hr after use of this drug
• Discuss with patient that dizziness, drowsiness, and confusion are common; to avoid getting up without assistance
• Discuss in detail all aspects of the drug and the purpose of this drug and what to expect after anesthesia
• Tell patient to make position changes to lessen orthostatic hypotension

Evaluation

Positive therapeutic outcome

• Maintenance of anesthesia
• Absence of motor activity during surgery

Treatment of overdose: Narcan 0.2-0.8 **IV**, O₂, **IV** fluids, vasopressors; have resuscitation equipment available

---

alitretinoin

See Appendix A, Selected New Drugs

---

allopurinol (R)

(al-oh-pure′i-nole)
Generic allopurinol, Apo-Allopurinol ✦, Lopurin, Purinol ✦, Zyloprim
Func. class.: Antigout drug
Chem. class.: Xanthine enzyme inhibitor
Pregnancy category **C**

Action: Inhibits the enzyme xanthine oxidase, reducing uric acid synthesis

Therapeutic Outcome: Decreasing serum uric acid levels, decreasing joint pain

Uses: Chronic gout, hyperuricemia associated with malignancies, recurrent calcium oxalate calculi, Chaga's disease, cutaneous/visceral leishmaniasis

Dosage and routes
Gout/hyperuricemia
Adult: PO 200-600 mg qd depending on severity, not to exceed 800 mg/day

---

P *Child 6-10 yr:* 300 mg qd

P *Child <6 yr:* 150 mg qd

Impaired renal function
Adult, CrCl 30-40 ml/min:
PO 200 mg qd

Adult, CrCl <20 ml/min: PO
100 mg qd

Recurrent calculi
Adult: PO 200-300 mg qd

Uric acid nephropathy
prevention

P *Adult and child >10 yr:* PO
600-800 mg qd × 2-3 days

Available forms: Tabs,
scored, 100, 300 mg

Adverse effects

CNS: Headache, drowsiness,
neuritis, paresthesia

EENT: Retinopathy, cataracts,
epistaxis

GI: Nausea, vomiting, an-
orexia, malaise, metallic taste,
cramps, peptic ulcer, diarrhea,
stomatitis

HEMA: **Agranulocytosis,**
thrombocytopenia, aplastic
anemia, pancytopenia, leuko-
penia, bone marrow suppres-
sion, eosinophilia

INTEG: Fever, chills, dermatitis, pruritus, purpura, erythema, ecchymosis, alopecia

MISC: Myopathy, arthralgia,
hepatomegaly, **cholestatic**
jaundice, renal failure, exfoli-
ative dermatitis

Contraindications: Hypersensitivity

Precautions: Pregnancy C,
lactation, renal disease, hepatic

P disease, children

◩ Do Not Confuse:
allopurinol/apresoline,
Lopurin/Lupron

Pharmacokinetics

Absorption	80%
Distribution	Widely distributed
Metabolism	Liver to oxypurinol
Excretion	Kidneys
Half-life	2-3 hr, terminal 18-30 hr

Pharmacodynamics

Onset	Unknown
Peak	2-4 hr
Duration	Unknown

Interactions

Individual drugs

Ammonium chloride: ↑ kidney stone formation

Ampicillin: ↑ risk of rash

Azathioprine: ↑ action of
azathioprine

Bacampicillin: ↑ risk of rash

Chlorpropamide: ↑ action of
chlorpropamide

Cyclophosphamide: ↑ action
of allopurinol

Mercaptopurine: ↑ action of
mercaptopurine

Potassium/sodium
phosphate: ↑ kidney stone
formation

Theophylline: ↑ action of
allopurinol

Vitamin C: ↑ kidney stone
formation

Drug classifications

ACE inhibitors: ↑ action of
ACE inhibitors

Aluminum salts: ↓ effects of
allopurinol

Anticoagulants, oral: ↑ action
of oral anticoagulants

Antineoplastics: ↑ bone marrow suppression

Diuretics, thiazide: ↑ allopurinol toxicity

NURSING CONSIDERATIONS

Assessment

• Assess for pain including
location, characteristics, onset/
duration, frequency, quality,

---

intensity or severity of pain, precipitating factors
• Monitor uric acid levels q2wk; normal uric acid levels are 6 mg/dl or less; check I&O ratio; increase fluids to 2 L/day to prevent stone formation, toxicity
• Monitor CBC, AST, BUN, creatinine before starting treatment, monthly; check blood glucose in diabetic patients receiving oral antidiabetic agents
• Monitor nutritional status: discourage organ meat, sardines, salmon, legumes, gravies (high-purine foods), alcohol

Nursing diagnoses
✓ Nutrition, more than body requirements (uses)
✓ Knowledge deficit (teaching)

Implementation
• Give with meals to prevent GI symptoms; crush and mix with food or fluids for patients with swallowing difficulties
• Give a few days before antineoplastic therapy if using for hyperuricemia associated with malignancy

Patient/family education
• Tell patient to increase fluid intake to 2 L/day; to avoid taking large doses of vitamin C; kidney stone formation may occur; to maintain a diet enhancing urine alkalinity (e.g., milk, other dairy products); if taking for calcium oxalate stones, reduce dairy products, refined sugar, sodium, meat
• Tell patient to report skin rash, stomatitis, malaise, fever, aching; drug should be discontinued
• Advise patient to avoid hazardous activities if drowsiness or dizziness occurs; response may take several days to determine

• Tell patient to avoid alcohol, caffeine; these substances increase uric acid levels and decrease allopurinol levels
• Teach patient to report side effects and adverse reactions to prescriber, including rash, itching, nausea, vomiting

Evaluation
Positive therapeutic outcome
• Decreased pain in joints
• Decreased stone formation in kidney
• Decreased uric acid level to 6 mg/dl

alprazolam (℞)
(al-pray′zoe-lam)
Apo-Alpraz ✦, Novo-Alprazol ✦, Nu-Alpraz ✦, Xanax
Func. class.: Antianxiety/sedative/hypnotic
Chem. class.: Benzodiazepine
Pregnancy category **D**
Controlled substance schedule **IV**

Action: Depresses subcortical levels of CNS, including limbic system, reticular formation; potentiates GABA (γ-aminobutyric acid)

⇒**Therapeutic Outcome:** Decreased anxiety

Uses: Anxiety, panic disorders, anxiety with depressive symptoms

Investigational uses: Depression, social phobia, premenstrual syndrome

Dosage and routes
Anxiety disorder
Adult: PO 0.25-0.5 mg tid, not to exceed 4 mg/day in divided doses

G *Elderly:* PO 0.125-0.25 mg bid; increase by 0.125 mg as needed

Panic disorder
Adult: PO 0.5 mg may ↑ q 3-4 days by 1 mg/day or less

Premenstrual syndrome
Adult: PO 0.25 mg tid

Social phobia
Adult: PO 2-8 mg/day

Available forms: Tabs 0.25, 0.5, 1, 2 mg

Adverse effects
CNS: Dizziness, drowsiness, confusion, headache, anxiety, tremors, stimulation, fatigue, depression, insomnia, hallucinations
CV: Orthostatic hypotension, **ECG changes, tachycardia,** hypotension
EENT: Blurred vision, tinnitus, mydriasis
GI: Constipation, dry mouth, nausea, vomiting, anorexia, diarrhea
INTEG: Rash, dermatitis, itching

Contraindications: Hypersensitivity to benzodiazepines, narrow angle glaucoma, **P** psychosis, pregnancy **D**, child <18 yr

G Precautions: Elderly, debilitated, hepatic disease, renal disease

N Do Not Confuse:
alprazolam/lorazepam, Xanax/Lanoxin, Xanax/Tylox, Xanax/Zantac

Pharmacokinetics	
Absorption	Slow, complete
Distribution	Widely distributed; crosses placenta; crosses blood-brain barrier
Metabolism	Liver, to active metabolites
Excretion	Kidneys, breast milk
Half-life	12-15 hr

Pharmacodynamics	
Onset	1 hr
Peak	1-2 hr
Duration	4-6 hr, therapeutic response 2-3 days

Interactions
Individual drugs
Alcohol: ↑ CNS depression
Cimetidine: ↑ action of alprazolam
Disulfiram: ↑ action of alprazolam
Digoxin: ↑ digoxin levels
Levodopa: ↑ action of alprazolam
Drug classifications
Anticonvulsants: ↑ CNS depression
Antidepressants, tricyclics: ↑ CNS depression
Antihistamines: ↑ CNS depression
Oral contraceptives: ↑ action of alprazolam
Sedative/hypnotics: ↑ CNS depression
Ø *Herb/drug*
Kava: ↑ CNS depression
Lab test interferences
↑ AST/ALT, ↑ neutropenia

NURSING CONSIDERATIONS
Assessment
• Assess mental status: mood, sensorium, anxiety, affect, sleeping pattern, drowsiness, **G** dizziness, especially elderly; physical dependency, withdrawal symptoms: anxiety, panic attacks, agitation, con-

---

vulsions, headache, nausea, vomiting, muscle pain, weakness; suicidal tendencies; indications of increasing tolerance and abuse; withdrawl seizures may occur after rapid-decrease dose or abrupt discontinuation

• Monitor B/P (with patient lying, standing), pulse; if systolic B/P drops 20 mm Hg, hold drug, notify prescriber

• Monitor blood studies: CBC during long-term therapy; blood dycrasias have occurred rarely; decreased hematocrit, neutropenia may occur

• Monitor hepatic studies: AST, ALT, bilirubin, creatinine LDH, alkaline phosphatase, if on long-term treatment

• Monitor I&O; indicate renal dysfunction if on long-term treatment

Nursing diagnoses
✓ Anxiety (uses)
✓ Depression (uses)
✓ Injury, risk for (adverse reactions)
✓ Knowledge deficit (teaching)

Implementation

• Give with food or milk for GI symptoms; tab may be crushed, if patient is unable to swallow medication whole, and mixed with foods or fluids

• Give sugarless gum, hard candy, frequent sips of water for dry mouth

Patient/family education

• Tell patient that drug may be taken with food or fluids, and tabs may be crushed or swallowed whole

• Tell patient not to use for everyday stress or longer than 4 mo unless directed by prescriber; not to take more than prescribed amount; may

be habit forming; not to double doses or skip doses

• Tell patient to avoid OTC preparations unless approved by prescriber; alcohol and CNS depressants will increase CNS depression

• Tell patient to avoid driving, activities that require alertness, since drowsiness may occur; to avoid alcohol ingestion or other psychotropic medications; to rise slowly or fainting may occur, especially elderly; that drowsiness may worsen at beginning of treatment

• Tell patient not to discontinue medication abruptly after long-term use; withdrawal symptoms include vomiting, cramping, tremors, seizures

Evaluation
Positive therapeutic outcome

• Decreased anxiety, restlessness, sleeplessness (short-term treatment only)

Treatment of overdose:
Lavage, VS, supportive care

---

alprostadil (℞)
(al-pros'ta-dil)
Caverject, Edex, Muse, PGE₁ prostaglandin E₁, Prostin VR Pediatric, Prostin VR ♥
Func. class.: Hormone
Chem. class.: Prostaglandin E₁

Pregnancy category   C

Action: Relaxes smooth muscles of ductus arteriosus; results in increased O_2 content perfusion throughout body; causes erection by dilation of cavernosal arteries and relaxation of trabecular muscle, leads to the trapping of blood

➲ Therapeutic Outcome:
Maintenance of patent ductus arteriosus with increased O_2 in neonates with congenital heart defects

Uses: To maintain patent ductus arteriosus (temporary treatment), erectile dysfunction

Dosage and routes
Patent ductus arteriosus
🅿 **Infants:** IV/intraarterial inf 0.1 μg/kg/min, until desired response, then reduce to lowest effective amount; 0.4 μg/kg/min not likely to produce greater beneficial effects

Erectile dysfunction of vasculogenic or mixed etiology, psychogenic
Men: Intracavernosal 2.5 μg may increase by 2.5 μg, may then increase by 5-10 μg until adequate response occurs

Intraurethral
Men: Administer as needed to achieve erection

Available forms: Inj 500 μg/ml; lyopholized powder for inj 6.15, 11.9 μg/23.2 μg, 5, 10, 20, 40 μg/single dose vial; pellets 125, 250, 500, 1000 μg

Adverse effects
CNS: Fever, **convulsions,** lethargy, hypothermia, stiffness, hyperirritability, **cerebral bleeding**
CV: **Bradycardia, tachycardia, hypotension, CHF, ventricular fibrillation, shock,** flushing, **cardiac arrest,** edema
GI: Diarrhea, regurgitation, hyperbilirubinemia
GU: Oliguria, hematuria, **anuria**
HEMA: **DIC, thrombocytopenia,** anemia, **bleeding**
LOCAL (Caverject): Penile pain, prolonged erection, penile fibrosis, penile rash, edema, hematoma, ecchymosis
MISC: **Sepsis,** hypokalemia, **peritonitis,** hypoglycemia, hyperkalemia
MS: Deformities of long bones in neonates treated for prolonged period
RESP: **Apnea, bradypnea, wheezing, respiratory depression**
SYSTEMIC (Caverject): Headache, dizziness, flulike symptoms, sinusitis, nasal congestion, hypertension, back pain, prostatic disorder

Contraindications: Hypersensitivity, respiratory distress syndrome (RDS)

Precautions: Bleeding disorders, pregnancy **C**

Pharmacokinetics
Absorption	Complete bioavailability (**IV**)
Distribution	Unknown
Metabolism	80% lungs, rapidly
Excretion	Kidneys to metabolites
Half-life	Up to 10 min

Pharmacodynamics
Onset	1½-3 hr
Peak	Up to 11 hr
Duration	Infusion's end

Interactions: None

NURSING CONSIDERATIONS
Assessment
• Monitor ABGs, arterial pH, arterial pressure, continuous ECG; if arterial pressure decreases, reduce or stop drug; check for increased pH, B/P, urinary output, decreased ratio of PA to AP (restricted systemic blood flow)
• Assess neurologic status: level of consciousness, reflexes, muscle tone, response to

stimuli during administration; if convulsions, stiffness, or hyperirritability occurs, drug should be discontinued; have ☐ ventilator available; neonates <2 kg or infusion >48 hr means increased risk for CNS adverse reactions

• Assess respiratory and cardiac status: rate, rhythm, depth, and effort of respirations; check for bradypnea, tachypnea, apnea, wheezing, respiratory depression, be prepared to support ventilation; monitor arterial B/P by use of umbilical artery catheter, auscultation, Doppler transducer; check for bradycardia, hypotension

☐ • Assess neonate with bleeding tendencies for DIS

☐ • Check neonate for flushing, which indicates a need to reposition the intraarterial catheter

Nursing diagnoses
☑ Tissue perfusion, altered (cardiopulmonary, cerebral) (uses)
☑ Injury, risk for physical (uses, adverse reactions)
☑ Impaired gas exchange (uses)
☑ Knowledge deficit (teaching)

Implementation
• Give only with emergency equipment available by trained clinicians (patent ductus arteriosus)
• Administer by cont inf, after diluting with 0.9% NaCl or D_5W inj to a concentration of 500 µg/ml; dilute further with 0.9% NaCl, D_5W; 500 µg of drug/250 ml = 2 µg/ml; 0.1 µg/kg/min; run at 0.05 ml/kg/min, (2 µg/ml); at 0.02 ml/kg/min (5 µg/ml) use inf pump and arterial pressure measurement during inf; do not use sol with benzyl alcohol
◆ (fatal toxic syndrome may

occur); stable for 24 hr at room temperature
• Refrigerate drug; discard all mixed unused portion
• Do not mix with other drugs or sol

Patient/family education
• Teach family about diagnosis, prognosis, treatment; ☐ inform parents of neonate's condition
• Teach method for self-injection (erectile disorder), amount to be used, disposal of needle; there is little control over erection
• Teach patient to alternate sides of the penis with each inj; not to inject >3×/wk; to allow 24 hr between doses; to notify provider of new penile pain, nodules, or signs of infection

Evaluation
Positive therapeutic outcome
• Increased urine output (noncyanotic heart disease)
• Increased PO_2 (cyanotic heart disease)
• Absence of metabolic acidosis
• Erection (Caverject)

Treatment of overdose:
Discontinue drug, provide supportive measures

---

alteplase (℞)
(al-ti-plaze')
Activase, tissue plasminogin activator, t-PA, TPA
Func. class.: Thrombolytic enzyme
Chem. class.: Tissue plasminogen activator (TPA)
Pregnancy category   C

Action: Produces fibrin conversion of plasminogen to plasmin; able to bind to fibrin, convert plasminogen in thrombus to plasmin, which leads to local fibrinolysis, limited systemic proteolysis

⇒ **Therapeutic Outcome:** Lysis of thrombi in MI, pulmonary emboli (life threatening)

Uses: Lysis of obstructing thrombi associated with acute MI; conditions requiring thrombolysis, (e.g., PE, DVT, unclotting arteriovenous shunts), acute ischemic CVA

Investigational uses: Unstable angina

Dosage and routes
Adult >65 kg: **IV** a total of 100 mg; 6-10 mg given **IV** bol over 1-2 min, 60 mg given over 1st hr, 20 mg given over 2nd hr, 20 mg given over 3rd hr; or 1.25 mg/kg given over 3 hr for smaller patients

Accelerated inf
Adult: **IV** bol 15 mg; then 50 mg over ½ hr; 35 mg over 1 hr

Available forms: Powder for inj 20 mg (11.6 million IU/ vial), 50 mg (29 million IU/ vial), 100 mg (58 million IU/vial)

Adverse effects
CV: Sinus bradycardia, ventricular tachycardia, accelerated idioventricular rhythm
INTEG: Urticaria, rash
SYST: **GI, GU, intracranial, retroperitoneal bleeding, surface bleeding**

Contraindications: Hypersensitivity, active internal bleeding, recent CVA, severe uncontrolled hypertension, intracranial/intraspinal surgery/trauma, aneurysm

Precautions: Pregnancy **C**, lactation, children

⊠ Do Not Confuse:
alteplace/Altace

Pharmacokinetics	
Absorption	Complete
Distribution	Unknown
Metabolism	>80% liver
Excretion	Kidneys
Half-life	30 min

Pharmacodynamics	
Onset	Immediate
Peak	30-45 min
Duration	4 hr

Interactions
Individual drugs
Aspirin: ↑ bleeding
Dipyridamole: ↑ bleeding
Heparin: ↑ bleeding
Plicamycin: ↑ bleeding
Valproic acid: ↑ bleeding
Drug classifications
Anticoagulants, oral: ↑ bleeding
Cephalosporins: ↑ bleeding
NSAIDs: ↑ bleeding
Lab test interferences
↑ PT, ↑ APTT, ↑ TT

NURSING CONSIDERATIONS
Assessment
• Monitor VS q15 min, B/P, pulse, respirations (including peripheral), neurologic signs, temp at least q4h; temp >104° F (40° C) indicates internal bleeding; monitor rhythm closely; ventricular dysrhythmias may occur with hyperfusion; monitor heart, breath sounds, neurologic status, and peripheral pulses
◆• Assess for bleeding during first hr of treatment and 24 hr after procedure: hematuria, hematemesis, bleeding from mucous membranes, epistaxis, ecchymosis, puncture sites;

guaiac all body fluids and stools; obtain blood studies (Hct, platelets, PTT, PT, TT, APTT) before starting therapy; PT or APTT must be less than 2 times control before starting therapy; TT or PT q3-4h during treatment; draw CPK—MB drawn to identify drug effectiveness

• Assess allergy: fever, rash, itching, chills; mild reaction may be treated with antihistamines; report to prescriber

• Monitor ECG; on monitor, watch for segment changes, changes in rhythm: sinus bradycardia, ventricular tachycardia, accelerated idioventricular rhythm may occur due to reperfusion

Nursing diagnoses
✓ Pain (uses)
✓ Tissue perfusion, altered (uses)
✓ Injury, risk for (adverse reactions)

Implementation
• Give after reconstituting with provided diluent; add appropriate amount of sterile water for injection (no preservatives); 20-mg vial/20 ml or 50-mg vial/50 ml (1 mg/ml); mix by slow inversion or dilute with NaCl, D_5W to a concentration of 0.5 mg/ml further dilution; 1.5 to <0.5 mg/ml may result in precipitation of drug; use 18-gauge needle; flush line with NaCl after administration; use reconstituted **IV** sol within 8 hr or discard, within 6 hr of coronary occlusion for best results

❶• Do not use 150 mg or more total dose; intracranial bleeding may occur

• Give heparin therapy after thrombolytic therapy is discontinued and when TT, ACT, and APTT less than 2 times control (about 3-4 hr)

• Avoid invasive procedures, inj, rec temp; apply pressure for 30 sec to minor bleeding sites; 30 min to sites of atrial puncture, followed by pressure dressing; inform prescriber if this does not attain hemostasis; apply pressure dressing

• Store powder at room temperature or refrigerate; protect from excessive light

Y-site incompatibilities:
Dobutamine, dopamine, heparin, nitroglycerin

Y-site compatibilities:
Lidocaine, metoprolol, propranolol

Additive compatibilities:
Lidocaine, morphine, nitroglycerin

Patient/family education
• Teach patient reason for alteplase, signs and symptoms of bleeding, allergic reactions, when to notify prescriber

Evaluation
Positive therapeutic outcome
• Lysis of pulmonary thrombi
• Adequate hemodynamic state
• Absence of congestive heart failure

---

altretamine (℞)
(al-tret′a-meen)
Hexalen,
hexamethylmelamine,
Hexastat ✦
Func. class.: Misc. antineoplastic
Chem. class.: S-Triazine derivative (formerly known as hexamethylmelamine)
Pregnancy category **D**

Action: Products of metabolism form covalent bonds with tissue macromolecules including DNA, which may be responsible for cytotoxicity; activity is not cell cycle phase specific

⇒ Therapeutic Outcome: Prevention of rapid growth of malignant cells

Uses: Palliative treatment of recurrent, persistent ovarian cancer following first-line treatment with cisplatin or alkylating agent–based combination

Dosage and routes
Adult: PO 260 mg/m^2 day for 14 or 21 days in a 28-day cycle; give in 4 divided doses pc and hs

Available forms: Caps 50, 100 ✦ mg

Adverse effects
CNS: Peripheral sensory neuropathy, fatigue, **seizures,** mood disorders, disorders of consciousness, ataxia, dizziness, vertigo
GI: Nausea, anorexia, vomiting, increased alkaline phosphatase, **hepatic toxicity**
GU: Increased BUN, serum creatinine
HEMA: Leukopenia, thrombocytopenia, anemia
INTEG: Rash, pruritus, alopecia

Contraindications: Hypersensitivity, severe bone marrow depression, severe neurologic toxicity, pregnancy **D**

P Precautions: Lactation, children

Pharmacokinetics

Absorption	Well
Distribution	Concentrated in liver, kidneys, small intestine
Metabolism	Liver (99%)
Excretion	Kidneys
Half-life	4½-10½ hrs

Pharmacodynamics

Onset	Unknown
Peak	½-3 hr
Duration	Unknown

Interactions
Individual drugs
Cimetidine: ↑ toxicity
Radiation: ↑ toxicity
Drug classifications
Antineoplastics: ↑ bone marrow depression
MAOI: ↑ orthostatic hypotension

NURSING CONSIDERATIONS
Assessment
• Monitor CBC, differential, platelet count weekly; withhold drug if WBC is <4000 or platelet count is <75,000; granulocytes <1000 mm^3, notify prescriber of results; nadir (leukopenia/thrombocytopenia) occurs in 1 mo; resolves in 6 wk
• Monitor renal function studies: BUN, serum uric acid, urine CrCl before, during therapy; I&O ratio; report fall in urine output of 30 ml/hr;

---

monitor for decreased hyperuricemia
- Monitor for cold, fever, sore throat (may indicate beginning infection)
- Assess for bleeding: hematuria, guaiac, bruising or petechiae, mucosa or orifices q8h; no rec temp; identify inflammation of mucosa, breaks in skin; use viscous lidocaine (Xylocaine) for oral pain
- Identify food preferences; list likes, dislikes
- Identify edema in feet, joint or stomach pain, shaking
- Assess neurologic status: paresthesia, numbness, tingling; pyridoxine may minimize neurologic reaction

Nursing diagnoses
☑ Injury, risk for (adverse reactions)
☑ Infection, risk for (adverse reactions)
☑ Knowledge deficit (teaching)

Implementation
- Give 1 hr before or 2 hr after meals to lessen nausea and vomiting or antacid before oral agent; give drug after evening meal, before bedtime; antiemetic 30-60 min before giving drug to prevent vomiting
- Antibiotics for prophylaxis of infection may be prescribed, since infection potential is high
- Store in tight container

Patient/family education
- Tell patient that contraceptive measures are recommended during therapy; teratogenic effects occur
- Teach patient to avoid use of products containing alcohol, aspirin, or ibuprofen, razors, hard bristle toothbrush, and commercial mouthwash because bleeding may occur; to

report symptoms of bleeding (hematuria, tarry stools)
- Tell patient to report signs of anemia, (fatigue, headache, irritability, faintness, shortness of breath)
- Tell patient to report any changes in breathing or coughing even several months after treatment
- Tell patient that hair may be lost during treatment; a wig or hairpiece may make patient feel better; new hair may be different in color, texture
- Advise patient to avoid vaccinations during treatment; serious reactions may occur
- Teach patient to report signs/symptoms of infection: fever, chills, sore throat; patient should avoid crowds and persons with known infections

Evaluation
Positive therapeutic outcome
- Decreased size and spread of malignancy

aluminum hydroxide (OTC)
AlternaGEL, Alu-Cap, Alugel ✽, Aluminett, aluminum hydroxide, Alu-Tab, Amphojel, Basaljel, Dialume, Nephrox
Func. class.: Antacid, hypophosphatemic
Chem. class.: Aluminum product
Pregnancy category   C

Action: Neutralizes gastric acidity, binds phosphates in GI tract; these phosphates are excreted

Uses: Peptic, gastric, duodenal ulcers; hyperphosphatemia in

---

chronic renal failure; reflux esophagitis, hyperacidity

Investigational uses: stress ulcer, GI bleeding

➜**Therapeutic Outcome:** Decreased acidity, healing of ulcers; decreased phosphate levels in chronic renal failure

Dosage and routes
Adult: SUSP 5-10 ml 1 hr pc, hs; PO 600 mg 1 hr pc, hs, chewed with milk or water

GI bleeding
P *Infant:* PO 2-5 ml/dose q1-2h
P *Child:* PO 5-15 ml/dose q1-2h

Hyperphosphatemia in renal failure
Adult: Susp 500 mg-2 g bid-qid

Available forms
Caps 400, 500 mg; tabs 300, 500 mg; chewable tabs 600 mg; susp 450 mg/5 ml, 600 mg/5 ml; liq 320 mg/5 ml, 600 mg/5 ml, 675 mg/5 ml

Adverse effects
GI: Constipation, anorexia, **obstruction,** fecal impaction
META: Hypophosphatemia, hypercalciuria

Contraindications: Hypersensitivity to this drug or aluminum products, abdominal pain of unknown origin

G **Precautions:** Elderly, fluid restriction, decreased GI motility, GI obstruction, dehydration, renal disease, sodium-restricted diets, pregnancy **C**

Pharmacokinetics	
Absorption	Not usually absorbed
Distribution	Widely distributed if absorbed; crosses placenta
Metabolism	Unknown
Excretion	Feces, kidneys (small amounts), breast milk
Half-life	Unknown

Pharmacodynamics	
Onset	20-40 min
Peak	½ hr
Duration	½-1½ hr

Interactions
Individual drugs
Allopurinol: ↓ allopurinol effect
Amphetamine: ↑ levels
Chlorpromazine: ↓ absorption
Ciprofloxacin: ↓ effectiveness
Diflunisal: ↓ diflunisal effect
Isoniazid: ↓ absorption
Mexiletine: ↑ levels
Quinidine: ↑ levels
Salicylate: ↓ levels
Tetracycline: ↓ absorption
Ticlopidine: ↓ ticlopidine effect
Drug classifications
Corticosteroids: ↓ corticosteroid effect
H₂ antagonists: ↓ corticosteroid effect
Thyroid hormones: ↓ thyroid effect

NURSING CONSIDERATIONS
Assessment
• Assess pain symptoms: location, duration, intensity, alleviating precipitating factors
• Monitor phosphate levels, since drug is bound in GI system; urinary pH, calcium, electrolytes; hypophosphatemia: anorexia, weakness, fatigue, bone pain, hyperreflexia

---

- Monitor constipation; increase bulk in diet if needed

Nursing diagnoses

✓ Pain, chronic (uses)
✓ Constipation (adverse reactions)
✓ Knowledge deficit (teaching)

Implementation

- Give laxatives or stool softeners if constipation occurs, especially elderly
- Give after shaking liq; follow with water to facilitate passage
- Tab may be chewed if patient is unable to swallow; drink 8 oz of water after chewing; or by nasogastric tube if patient unable to swallow
- Give 1 hr before or after other medications to prevent poor absorption
- Give 15 ml 30 min pc and hs (esophagitis)
- May be given as prescribed q1-2 hr and given by gastric tube after diluting with water (peptic ulcer)

Patient/family education

- Instruct patient to increase fluids to 2000 ml/day unless contraindicated
- Instruct patient to avoid phosphate foods (most dairy products, eggs, fruits, carbonated beverages) during drug therapy; to add cheese, corn, pasta, plums, prunes, lentils after drug (hypophosphatemia)
- Instruct patient not to use for prolonged periods if serum phosphate is low or if on a low-sodium diet; CHF patients should check for sodium content and use sodium-reduced products
- Instruct patient that stools may appear white or speckled; constipation may result; to report black tarry stools, which indicate gastric bleeding

- Instruct patient to check with prescriber after 2 wk of self-prescribed antacid use; may be used for 4-6 wk after symptoms subside or as prescribed

Evaluation

Positive therapeutic outcome

- Absence of pain, decreased acidity
- Increased pH of gastric secretions
- Decreased phosphate levels

---

amantadine (℞)
(a-man′ta-deen)
amantadine HCl, Symadine, Symmetrel
Func. class.: Antiviral, antiparkinsonian agent
Chem. class.: Tricyclic amine

Pregnancy category   C

Action: Prevents uncoating of nucleic acid in viral cell, preventing penetration of virus to host; causes release of dopamine from neurons

⇒**Therapeutic Outcome:** Decreased Parkinson's symptoms, decreased symptoms of influenza type A or prevention

Uses: Prophylaxis or treatment of influenza type A, extrapyramidal reactions, parkinsonism, respiratory tract infections

Investigational uses: Neuroleptic malignant syndrome, cocaine dependency, enuresis

Dosage and routes
Influenza type A
℗*Adult and child >12 yr:* PO 200 mg/day in single dose or divided bid

℗*Child 9-12 yr:* PO 100 mg bid

P *Child 1-9 yr:* PO 4.4-8.8 mg/kg/day divided bid-tid, not to exceed 200 mg/day

Extrapyramidal reaction/ parkinsonism
Adult: PO 100 mg bid, up to 400 mg/day in EPS; give for 1 wk then 100 mg as needed up to 400 mg in parkinsonism

Renal dose
CrCl 40-50 ml/min 100 mg/day; CrCl 30 ml/min 200 mg 2×/wk; CrCl 20 ml/min 100 mg 3×/wk; CrCl <10 ml/min 100 mg alternating with 200 mg q7 days

Available forms: Caps 100 mg; syr 50 mg/5 ml

Adverse effects
CNS: Headache, dizziness, drowsiness, fatigue, *anxiety,* psychosis, *depression, hallucinations,* tremors, **convulsions,** confusion, *insomnia*
CV: Orthostatic hypotension, **CHF**
EENT: Blurred vision
GI: Nausea, vomiting, constipation, dry mouth
HEMA: **Leukopenia**
INTEG: Photosensitivity, dermatitis

Contraindications: Hypersen-
P sitivity, lactation, child <1 yr, eczematic rash

Precautions: Epilepsy, CHF, orthostatic hypotension, psychiatric disorders, hepatic disease, renal disease, peripheral
G edema, pregnancy **C**, elderly

N **Do Not Confuse:**
amantadine/ranitidine,
amantadine/rimantidine,
Symmetrel/Synthroid

Pharmacokinetics

Absorption	Well absorbed
Distribution	Crosses blood-brain barrier
Metabolism	Not metabolized
Excretion	Kidneys (90%) unchanged, breast milk
Half-life	24 hr

Pharmacodynamics

Onset	48 hr
Peak	2 wk
Duration	Unknown

Interactions
Individual drugs
Atropine: ↑ anticholinergic effects
Disopyramide: ↑ anticholinergic effects
Quinidine: ↑ anticholinergic effects
Drug classifications
Antidepressants, tricyclic: ↑ anticholinergic effects
Antihistamines: ↑ anticholinergic effects
Phenothiazines: ↑ anticholinergic effects
☑ *Herb/drug*
Belladonna leaf/root: ↑ anticholinergic effect
Henbane leaf: ↑ anticholinergic effect
Pheasant's eye herb: ↑ action/side effects
Quinine: ↑ action/side effects
Scopolia root: ↑ action/side effects

NURSING CONSIDERATIONS
Assessment
• Assess for drug toxicity: tremors, convulsions, lability, dysrhythmias; drug should be discontinued and physostigmine given
• Assess for symptoms of influenza A: increased temperature, malaise, aches and pains

---

- Check for mottling of skin, which disappears after several weeks of treatment
- Assess for skin eruptions, photosensitivity after administration of drug
- Monitor respiratory status: rate, character, wheezing, tightness in chest
- Assess for allergies before initiation of treatment, reaction of each medication

Nursing diagnoses
☑ Infection, risk for (uses)
☑ Knowledge deficit (teaching)

Implementation
- Give before exposure to influenza; continue for 10 days after contact
- Give at least 4 hr before hs to prevent insomnia
- Administer after meals for better absorption, to decrease GI symptoms; caps may be opened and mixed with food for easy swallowing
- Give in divided doses to prevent CNS disturbances: headache, dizziness, fatigue, drowsiness
- Store in tight, dry container

Patient/family education
- Teach patient to change body position slowly to prevent orthostatic hypotension
- Teach patient about aspects of drug therapy: the need to report dyspnea, weight gain, dizziness, poor concentration, dysuria, behavioral changes
- Teach patient to avoid hazardous activities if dizziness, blurred vision occur
- Teach patient to take drug exactly as prescribed; parkinsonian crisis may occur if drug is discontinued abruptly; drug should be tapered slowly
- Tell patient to avoid alcohol, OTC medications until discussed with prescriber, serious side effects can occur

Evaluation
Positive therapeutic outcome
- Absence of fever, malaise, cough, dyspnea in influenza A
- Decreased tremors, shuffling gait in Parkinson's disease, extrapyramidal symptoms

Treatment of overdose: Withdraw drug, maintain airway, administer epinephrine, aminophylline, O_2 **IV** corticosteroids, physostigmine

---

amifostine (℞)
(a-mi-foss'teen)
Ethyol
Func. class.: Cytoprotective agent for cisplatin
Pregnancy category **C**

Action: Binds and detoxifies damaging metabolites of cisplatin by converting this drug by aklaline phosphatase in tissue to an active free thiol compound

➡ **Therapeutic Outcome:** Decreased toxic reaction from cisplatin

Uses: Used to reduce renal toxicity when cisplatin is given in ovarian cancer

Dosage and routes
Adult: **IV** 910 mg/m² qd, within ½ hr before chemotherapy

Available forms: Powder for inj 500 mg/vial with 500 mg mannitol

Adverse effects
CNS: Dizziness, somnolence
CV: Hypotension
EENT: Sneezing
GI: Nausea, vomiting, hiccups
INTEG: Flushing

MISC: Hypocalcemia, rash, chills

Contraindications: Hypersensitivity to mannitol, aminothiol; hypotension, dehydration, lactation

G P Precautions: Elderly, CV disease, pregnancy **C,** children

Pharmacokinetics

Absorption	Complete
Distribution	Unknown
Metabolism	To free thiol compound
Excretion	Unknown
Half-life	5-8 min

Pharmacodynamics

Unknown

Interactions
Drug classifications
Antihypertensives: ↑ hypotension

NURSING CONSIDERATIONS
Assessment
• Assess fluid status before administration; administer antiemetic prior to administration to prevent severe nausea and vomiting; also, dexamethasone 20 mg **IV** and a serotonin antagonist such as ondanestron or granisetron
• Monitor calcium levels before and during treatment; calcium supplements may be given for low calcium levels
• Monitor blood pressure prior to and q5 min during infusion; if severe hypotension occurs, give **IV** 0.9% NaCl to expand fluid volume, place in Trendelenburg position

Nursing diagnoses
☑ Injury, risk for (uses)
☑ Knowledge deficit (teaching)

Implementation
• Give by **IV** intermittent INF after reconstituting with 9.5 ml of sterile 0.9% NaCl, further dilute with 0.9% NaCl to a concentration of 5-40 mg/ml, give at a rate over 15 min within ½ hr of chemotherapy

Y-site compatibilities: Amikacin, aminophylline, ampicillin, ampicillin/sulbactam, aztreonam, bleomycin, bumetanide, buprenorphine, butorphanol, calcium gluconate, carboplatin, carmustine, cefazolin, cefonicid, cefotaxime, cefotetan, cefoxitin, ceftazidime, ceftizoxime, ceftriaxone, cefuroxime, cimetidine, ciprofloxacin, clindamycin, cyclophosphamide, cytarabine, dacarbazine, dactinomycin, daunorubicin, dexamethasone, diphenhydramine, dobutamine, dopamine, doxorubicin, doxycycline, droperidol, enalaprilat, etoposide, famotidine, floxuridine, fluconazole, fludarabine, fluorouracil, furosemide, gallium, gentamicin, granisetron, haloperidol, heparin, hydrocortisone, hydromorphone, idarubicin, ifosfamide, imipenem-cilastatin, leucovorin, lorazepam, magnesium sulfate, mannitol, mechlorethamine, meperidine, mesna, methotrexate, methylprednisolone, metoclopramide, metronidazole, mezlocillin, mitomycin, mitoxantrone, morphine, nalbuphine, netilmicin, ondansetron, piperacillin, plicamycin, potassium chloride, promethazine, ranitidine, sodium bicarbonate, streptozocin, teniposide, thiotepa, ticarcillin, ticarcillin/clavulanate, tobramycin, trimethoprim-sulfamethoxazole, trimetrexate,

---

vancomycin, vinblastine, vincristine, zidovudine

Additive incompatibilities:
Do not mix with other drugs or solutions

Patient/family education
• Teach reason for medication and expected results
• Teach that side effects may cause severe nausea, vomiting, decreased B/P, chills, dizziness, somnolence, hiccups, sneezing

Evaluation
Positive therapeutic outcome
• Absence of renal damage

---

amikacin (R)
(am-i-kay'sin)
amikacin sulfate, Amikin
Func. class.: Antibiotic
Chem. class.: Aminoglycoside

Pregnancy category   D

Action: Interferes with protein synthesis in bacterial cell by binding to ribosomal subunit, which causes misreading of genetic code; inaccurate peptide sequence forms in protein chain, causing bacterial death

➤ **Therapeutic Outcome:**
Bactericidal effects for the following organisms: *Pseudomonas aeruginosa, Escherichia coli, Enterobacter, Acinetobacter, Providencia, Citrobacter, Staphylococcus, Serratia, Proteus*

Uses: Severe systemic infections of CNS, respiratory, GI, urinary tract, bone, skin, soft tissues

Investigational uses: *Mycobacterium avium* complex (intrathecal or intraventricular)

Dosage and routes
Severe systemic infections
🅟 *Adult and child:* **IV** inf 15 mg/kg/day in 2-3 divided doses q8-12h in 100-200 ml D_5W over 30-60 min, not to exceed 1.5 g; decreased dosages are needed in poor renal function as determined by blood levels, renal function studies; IM 15 mg/kg/day in divided doses q8-12h; qd or extended internal dosing as an alternative dosing regimen

🅟 *Neonates:* **IV** inf 10 mg/kg initially, then 7.5 mg/kg q12h in D_5W over 1-2 hr

Severe urinary tract infections
Adults: IM 250 mg bid

Adults with poor renal function: 5-7.5 mg/kg initially, then increased as determined by blood levels, renal function studies

Available forms: Inj IM, **IV** 50, 250 mg/ml

Adverse effects
CNS: Confusion, depression, numbness, tremors, **convulsions,** muscle twitching, **neurotoxicity,** dizziness, vertigo, tinnitus
CV: Hypotension or hypertension, palpitations
EENT: Ototoxicity, deafness, visual disturbances
GI: Nausea, vomiting, anorexia, increased ALT, AST, bilirubin, hepatomegaly, **hepatic necrosis,** splenomegaly
GU: **Oliguria, hematuria, renal damage, azotemia, renal failure, nephrotoxicity**
HEMA: **Agranulocytosis, thrombocytopenia, leukopenia, eosinophilia, anemia**
INTEG: Rash, burning, urticaria, dermatitis, alopecia

Contraindications: Mild to moderate infections, hypersensitivity to aminoglycosides, pregnancy **D**

P *Precautions:* Neonates, mild renal disease, myasthenia gravis, lactation, hearing deficits, **G** Parkinson's disease, elderly

N Do Not Confuse:
Amikin/Amicar

Pharmacokinetics

Absorption	Well absorbed (IM), complete absorbed (**IV**)
Distribution	Widely distributed in extracellular fluids, poor in CSF; crosses placenta
Metabolism	Minimal; liver
Excretion	Mostly unchanged (79%) in kidneys
Half-life **P**	2-3 hr, prolonged up to 7 hr in infants; increased in renal disease

Pharmacodynamics

	IM	IV
Onset	Rapid	Rapid
Peak	1-2 hr	1-2 hr

Interactions
Drug classifications
Anesthetics: ↑ neuromuscular blockade, respiratory depression
Aminoglycosides: ↑ ototoxicity, neurotoxicity, nephrotoxicity
Cephalosporins: Inactivation of amikacin
Diuretics, loop: ↑ ototoxicity
Nondepolarizing neuromuscular blockers: ↑ neuromuscular blockade, respiratory depression
Penicillins: Inactivation of amikacin

NURSING CONSIDERATIONS
Assessment
• Assess patient for previous sensitivity reaction
• Assess patient for signs and symptoms of infection, including characteristics of wounds, sputum, urine, stool, WBC >10,000, earache, temp; obtain baseline information and during treatment
• Obtain culture and sensitivity tests before beginning drug therapy to identify if correct treatment has been initiated
• Assess for allergic reactions: rash, urticaria, pruritus
• Identify urine output; if decreasing, notify prescriber (may indicate nephrotoxicity); also notify prescriber of increased BUN and creatinine, urine CrCl <80 ml/min; lower dosage should be given in renal impairment; urinalysis daily for protein, cells, casts
• Monitor blood studies: AST, ALT, CBC, Hct, bilirubin, LDH, alkaline phosphatase; Coombs' test monthly if patient is on long-term therapy
• Monitor electrolytes: potassium, sodium, chloride, magnesium monthly if patient is on long-term therapy
• Assess bowel pattern qd; if severe diarrhea occurs, drug should be discontinued
• Monitor for bleeding: ecchymosis, bleeding gums, hematuria, stool guaiac daily if on long-term therapy
• Assess for overgrowth of infection: perineal itching, fever, malaise, redness, pain, swelling, drainage, rash, diarrhea, change in cough, sputum
• Obtain weight before treatment; calculation of dosage is usually based on ideal body weight, but may be calculated on actual body weight
• Monitor VS during infusion, watch for hypotension, change in pulse

---

☑ Herb/drug ⓢ Do Not Crush ◆ Alert ⌖ Key Drug **G** Geriatric **P** Pediatric

• Assess **IV** site for thrombophlebitis including pain, redness, swelling q30 min; change site if needed; apply warm compresses to discontinued site
• Obtain serum peak, drawn 30-60 min after **IV** infusion or 60 min after IM injection; trough level drawn just before next dose; 20-30 μg/ml, trough 4-8 μg/ml, blood level should be 2-4 times bacteriostatic level
• Urine pH if drug is used for UTI; urine should be kept alkaline
◆• Deafness by audiometric testing, ringing, roaring in ears, vertigo; assess hearing before, during, after treatment
• Dehydration: high sp gr, decrease in skin turgor, dry mucous membranes, dark urine
• Vestibular dysfunction: nausea, vomiting, dizziness, headache; drug should be discontinued if severe

Nursing diagnoses
☑Infection, risk for (uses)
☑Diarrhea (side effects)
☑Knowledge deficit (teaching)
☑Injury, risk for (side effects)

Implementation
IM route
• Give deeply in large muscle mass
Ⓜ**IV route**
• Dilute 500 mg of drug in 100-200 ml of **IV** D₅W, D₅NaCl or 0.9% NaCl and give over ½-1 hr; flush after administration with D₅W or 0.9% NaCl

Syringe compatibilities:
Clindamycin, doxapram

Y-site compatibilities:
Acyclovir, amifostine, amiodarone, amsacrine, aztreonam, cisatracurium, cyclophospha-

mide, dexamethasone, diltiazem, enalamprilat, esmolol, filgrastim, fluconazole, fludarabine, foscarnet, furosemide, granisetron, idarubicin, IL-2, labetalol, lorazepam, magnesium sulfate, melphalan, midazolam, morphine, ondansetron, paclitaxel, perphenazine, remifentanil, sargramostim, teniposide, thiotepa, TPN #54, #61, #91, #203, #204, #212, vinorelbine, warfarin, zidovudine

Additive compatibilities:
Amobarbital, ascorbic acid inj, bleomycin, calcium chloride, calcium gluconate, cefepime, cefoxitin, chloramphenicol, chlorpheniramine, cimetidine, ciprofloxacin, clindamycin, cloxacillin, colistimethate, dimenhydrinate, diphenhydramine, epinephrine, ergonovine, fluconazole, furosemide, hydraluronidase, hydrocorticose, lincomycin, metaraminol, metronidazole, metronidazole/ sodium bicarbonate, norepinephrine, pentobarbital, phenobarbital, phytonadione, polymyxin B, prochlorperazine, promethazine, ranitidine, secobarbital, sodium bicarbonate, succinylcholine, vancomycin, verapamil

Patient/family education
• Teach patient to report sore throat, bruising, bleeding, joint pain; may indicate blood dyscrasias (rare)
• Advise patient to contact prescriber if vaginal itching, loose foul-smelling stools, furry tongue occur; may indicate superinfection

Evaluation
Positive therapeutic outcome
• Absence of signs/symptoms of infection: WBC <10,000,

temp WNL; absence of red draining wounds; absence of earache
• Reported improvement in symptoms of infection

Treatment of overdose: Withdraw drug; administer epinephrine, O_2, hemodialysis, exchange transfusion in the **P** newborn; monitor serum levels of drug; may give ticarcillin or carbenicillin

---

amiloride (℞)
(a-mill'oh-ride)
Amiloride HCl, Midamor
Func. class.: Potassium-sparing diuretic
Chem. class.: Pyrazine
Pregnancy category   B

Action: Acts primarily on proximal distal tubule by inhibiting reabsorption of sodium and water and increasing potassium retention and conserving hydrogen ions

▶Therapeutic Outcome: Diuretic and antihypertensive effect while retaining potassium

Uses: Diuretic-induced hypokalemia; used with other agents to treat edema, hypertension

Investigational uses: Cystic fibrosis (INH), lithium-induced polyuria

Dosage and routes
Adult: PO 5 mg qd; may be increased to 10-20 mg qd if needed

Available forms: Tabs 5 mg

Adverse effects
CNS: Headache, dizziness, fatigue, weakness, paresthesias, tremor, depression, anxiety

CV: Orthostatic hypotension, dysrhythmias, angina
EENT: Loss of hearing, tinnitus, blurred vision, nasal congestion, increased intraocular pressure
ELECT: **Hyperkalemia**
GI: Nausea, diarrhea, dry mouth, *vomiting, anorexia,* cramps, constipation, abdominal pain, jaundice, bleeding
GU: Polyuria, dysuria, frequency, impotence
HEMA: **Aplastic anemia, neutropenia (rare)**
INTEG: Rash, pruritus, alopecia, urticaria
RESP: Cough, dyspnea, shortness of breath

Contraindications: Anuria, hypersensitivity, hyperkalemia, impaired renal function

Precautions: Dehydration, pregnancy **B,** diabetes, acidosis, lactation, hepatic disease

Pharmacokinetics	
Absorption	Variable (10%-15%)
Distribution	Unknown
Metabolism	Unchanged in urine (50%) in feces (40%)
Excretion	Renal; breast milk
Half-life	6-9 hr

Pharmacodynamics	
Onset	2 hr
Peak	6-10 hr
Duration	24 hr

Interactions
Individual drugs
Lithium: ↑ Lithium toxicity
Drug classifications
ACE inhibitors: ↑ hyperkalemia
Antihypertensives: ↑ action
Diuretics, potassium-sparing: ↑ hyperkalemia

NSAIDs: ↓ effectiveness of amiloride
Potassium products: ↑ hyperkalemia
Salt substitutes: ↑ hyperkalemia
Food/drug
Potassium foods: ↑ hyperkalemia
Lab test interferences
Interference: GTT

NURSING CONSIDERATIONS
Assessment

• Monitor manifestations of hyperkalemia: *MS:* fatigue, muscle weakness; *CARDIAC:* dysrhythmias, hypotension; *NEURO:* paresthesias, confusion; *RESP:* dyspnea
• Monitor for manifestations of hyponatremia: *CV:* increased B/P, cold, clammy skin, hypovolemia or hypervolemia; *GI:* anorexia, nausea, vomiting, diarrhea, abdominal cramps; *NEURO:* lethargy, increased ICP, confusion, headache, seizures, coma, fatigue, tremors, hyperreflexia
• Monitor for manifestations of hyperchloremia: *NEURO:* weakness, lethargy, coma; *RESP:* deep rapid breathing
• Assess fluid volume status: I&O ratios and record, weight, distended red veins, crackles in lung, color, quality and sp gr of urine, skin turgor, adequacy of pulses, moist mucous membranes, bilateral lung sounds, peripheral pitting edema; dehydration symptoms of decreasing output, thirst, hypotension, dry mouth and mucous membranes should be reported
• Monitor electrolytes: potassium, sodium, calcium, magnesium; also include BUN, ABGs, uric acid, CBC, blood sugar

• Assess B/P before and during therapy with patient lying, standing, and sitting as appropriate; orthostatic hypotension can occur rapidly

Nursing diagnoses

☑ Fluid volume deficit (side effects)
☑ Fluid volume excess (uses)
☑ Knowledge deficit (teaching)

Implementation

• Give in AM to avoid interference with sleep
• With food; if nausea occurs, absorption may be increased

Patient/family education

• Teach patient to take medication early in the day to prevent nocturia
• Instruct patient to take with food or milk if GI symptoms of nausea and anorexia occur
• Teach patient to maintain a weekly record of weight and notify prescriber of weight loss >5 lb
• Caution patient that this drug causes an increase in potassium levels, so foods high in potassium should be avoided; refer to dietician for assistance, planning
• Caution patient not to exercise in hot weather or stand for prolonged periods since orthostatic hypotension will be enhanced
• Teach patient not to use alcohol or any OTC medications without prescriber's approval; serious drug reactions may occur
• Emphasize the need to contact prescriber immediately if muscle cramps, weakness, nausea, dizziness, or numbness occurs
• Teach patient to take own B/P and pulse and record

- Advise patient that dizziness and confusion may occur; avoid driving or other hazardous activities if alertness is decreased
- Teach patient to continue taking medication even if feeling better; this drug controls symptoms but does not cure the condition
- Advise patient with hypertension to continue other medical treatment (exercise, weight loss, relaxation techniques, cessation of smoking)

Evaluation
Positive therapeutic outcome
- Prevention of hypokalemia (diuretic use)
- Decreased edema
- Decreased B/P
- Increased diuresis

Treatment of overdose:
Lavage if taken orally; monitor electrolytes; administer **IV** fluids; monitor hydration, CV, renal status

---

amino acid (℞)
(a-mee′noe)
Injection: Aminess, Aminosyn, BranchAmin, NephrAmine, FreAmine HBC, HepatAmine Solution: Aminosyn, Aminosyn II, Aminosyn-PF, FreAmine III, Novamine, ProcalAmine, RenAmin, Travasol, Trophamine
Func. class.: Caloric agent
Chem. class.: Nitrogen product

Pregnancy category   C

Action: Needed for anabolism to maintain structure; decreases catabolism, promotes healing

▶**Therapeutic Outcome:**
Positive nitrogen balance, decreased catabolism

Uses: Hepatic encephalopathy, cirrhosis, hepatitis, nutritional support in cancer trauma, intestinal obstruction, short bowel syndrome, severe malabsorption

Dosage and routes
Amino acid inj
Adult: **IV** 80-120 g/day; 500 ml of amino acids/500 ml D_{50} given over 24 hr

Amino acid solution
Adult: **IV** 1-1.5 g/kg/day titrated to patient's needs

P *Child:* **IV** 2-3 g/kg/day titrated to patient's needs

Available forms: Inj **IV** 2.75%, 3.5%, 4.25%, 5%, 5.5%, 6%, 8.5%, 10%, 11.4%, 15% amino acids

Adverse effects
CNS: Dizziness, headache, confusion, **loss of consciousness**
CV: Hypertension, **CHF, pulmonary edema**
ENDO: Hyperglycemia, rebound hypoglycemia, electrolyte imbalances, hyperosmolar syndrome, hyperosmolar hyperglycemic nonketotic syndrome, alkalosis, acidosis, hypophosphatemia, hyperammonemia, dehydration, hypocalcemia
GI: Nausea, vomiting, liver fat deposits, abdominal pain
GU: Glycosuria, osmotic diuresis
INTEG: Chills, flushing, warm feeling, rash, urticaria, extravasation necrosis, phlebitis at injection site

Contraindications: Hypersensitivity, severe electrolyte im-

---

balances, anuria, severe liver damage, maple syrup urine disease, PKU

Precautions: Renal disease, pregnancy **C,** children, diabetes mellitus, CHF

Pharmacokinetics

Absorption	Complete bioavailability
Distribution	Widely distributed
Metabolism	Anabolism
Excretion	Kidney to urea nitrogen
Half-life	Unknown

Pharmacodynamics

Unknown

Interactions
Drug classifications
Diuretics: ↑ negative nitrogen balance
Glucocorticoids: ↑ negative nitrogen balance
Tetracyclines: ↑ negative nitrogen balance

NURSING CONSIDERATIONS
Assessment
• Monitor electrolytes (potassium, sodium, calcium, chloride, magnesium), blood glucose, ammonia, phosphate, ketones; renal, liver function studies: BUN, creatinine, ALT, AST, bilirubin; urine glucose q6h using Chemstrips, which are not affected by infusion substances; if BUN increases over 15%, therapy may need to be discontinued
• Check injection site for extravasation: redness along vein, edema at site, necrosis, pain; for a hard, tender area
• Monitor respiratory function q4h: auscultate lung fields bilaterally for crackles; monitor respirations for quality, rate, rhythm that indicates fluid overload
• Monitor temperature q4h for increased fever, indicating infection; if infection is suspected, infusion is discontinued and tubing bottle, catheter tip cultured; blood catheter may be obtained
⬥• Monitor for impending hepatic coma: asterixis, confusion, fetor, lethargy
• Hyperammonemia: nausea, vomiting, malaise, tremors, anorexia, convulsions; increased ammonia, ketone levels may occur

Nursing diagnoses
✓ Nutrition, less than body requirements (uses)
✓ Injury, risk for physical (uses, adverse reactions)
✓ Infection, risk for (adverse reactions)
✓ Knowledge deficit (teaching)

Implementation
• Give up to 40% protein and dextrose (up to 12.5%) via peripheral vein; stronger solutions require central **IV** administration; TPN only mixed with dextrose to promote protein synthesis
• Use immediately after mixing in pharmacy under strict aseptic technique using laminar flowhood; use infusion pump, in-line filter (0.22 μm) unless mixed with fat emulsion and dextrose (3 in 1)
⬥• Use careful monitoring technique; do not speed up infusion; pulmonary edema, glucose overload will result
• Storage depends on type of solution; consult manufacturer
• Change dressing and **IV** tubing to prevent infection q24-48h or q5-7 days if transparent dressing is used

Additive compatibilities:
Amikacin, aminophylline, aztreonam, calcium gluconate,

---

cefamandole, cefazolin, cefepime, cefotaxime, cefoxitin,
cefsulodin, ceftazidime, ceftriaxone, cefuroxime, cimetidine,
clindamycin, cyanocobalamin,
cyclophosphamide, cyclosporine, cytarabine, dopamine,
epoetin, erythromycin, famotidine, folic acid, fosphenytoin,
furosemide, heparin, insulin
(regular), isoproterenol, lidocaine, meperidine, metaraminol, methicillin, methotrexate,
methyldopa, methylprednisolone, metoclopramide, morphine, nafcillin, netilmicin,
nizatidine, norepinephrine,
ondansetron, oxacillin, penicillin G potassium, penicillin G
sodium, phytonadione, polymyxin B, sodium bicarbonate,
tacrolimus, tobramycin, vancomycin

Y-*site incompatibilities:*
Cephradine

Y-*site compatibilities:* Amikacin, aminophylline, amoxicillin, ampicillin, ascorbic acid inj,
atracurium, azlocillin, aztreonam, bumetanide, buprenorphine, calcium gluconate,
carboplatin, cefamandole,
cefazolin, cefonicid, cefoperazone, cefotaxime, cefotetan,
cefoxtin, ceftazidime, ceftizoxime, ceftriaxone, ce-
furoxime, cephalothin, cephapirin, chloramphenicol,
chlorpromazine, cimetidine,
clindamycin, clonazepam,
dexamethasone, diazepam,
digoxin, diphenhydramine,
dobutamine, dopamine, doxycycline, droperidol, enalaprilat,
epinephrine, erythromycin
lactobionate, famotidine, fentanyl, flucloxacillin, fluconazole,
folic acid, foscarnet, gentamicin, granisetron, haloperidol,
heparin, hydrocortisone, hydromorphone, hydroxyzine,
idarubicin, ifosfamide, IL-2,
imipenem/cilastatin, insulin
(regular), isoproterenol, kanamycin, leucovorin, levorphanol, lidocaine, lorazepam,
magnesium sulfate, mannitol,
meperidine, mesna, methicillin,
metronidazole, mezlocillin,
miconazole, morphine, moxalactam, multivitamins, nafcillin,
netilmicin, nitroglycerin, norepinephrine, octreotide, ofloxacin, ondansetron, oxacillin,
paclitaxel, penicillin G, penicillin G potassium, pentobarbital,
phenobarbital, piperacillin,
potassium chloride, prochlorperazine, ranitidine, salbuta-
mol, sargramostim, tacrolimus,
thiotepa, ticarcillin, ticarcillin/
clavulanate, tobramycin, tri-
methoprim/sulfamethoxazole,
urokinase, vancomycin, vecuronium, zidovudine

Patient/family education
• Teach reason for use of
amino acids as part of nutrition
(TPN)
• Instruct patient to report at
once to prescriber if chills,
sweating are experienced

Evaluation
Positive therapeutic outcome
• Weight gain
• Decreased jaundice in liver
disorders
• Increased LOC

aminoglutethimide (R)
(a-meen-oh-gloo-teth'i-mide)
Cytadren
Func. class.: Antineoplastic, adrenal steroid inhibitor
Chem. class.: Hormone
Pregnancy category D

Action: Acts by inhibiting DNA, RNA, protein synthesis; is derived from *Streptomyces verticillus;* replication is decreased by binding to DNA, which causes strand splitting; phase specific in G_2 and M phases; blocks biosynthesis of all steroid hormones (cortisol, androgens, progestins)

➡**Therapeutic Outcome:** Decreased spread of malignancy; decreased adrenal hormone in Cushing's syndrome

Uses: Suppression of adrenal function in Cushing's syndrome, adrenal cancer

Dosage and routes
Adult: PO 250 mg qid at 6-hr intervals; may increase by 250 mg/day q1-2 wk, not to exceed 2 g/day

Available forms: Tabs 250 mg

Adverse effects
CNS: Drowsiness, dizziness, headache, lethargy
CV: **Hypotension, tachycardia**
GI: Nausea, vomiting, anorexia, **hepatotoxicity**
INTEG: Rash, pruritus, hirsutism, *morbilliform skin rash*
HEMA: **Agranulocytosis, thrombocytopenia, transient leukopenia**

Contraindications: Hypersensitivity, hypothyroidism, pregnancy **D**
Precautions: Renal disease, hepatic disease, respiratory disease

Pharmacokinetics	
Absorption	Well absorbed
Distribution	Unknown
Metabolism	Liver (50%)
Excretion	Kidneys, unchanged (50%)
Half-life	13 hr initially

Pharmacodynamics
Unknown

Interactions
Individual drugs
Alcohol: ↑ effects of aminoglutethimide
Dexamethasone: ↑ metabolism, ↓ effect of dexamethasone
Digoxin: ↓ effects of digoxin
Medroxyprogesterone: ↓ effects of medroxyprogesterone
Theophylline: ↓ effects of theophylline
Warfarin: ↓ effects of warfarin
Lab test interferences
↓ plasma cortisol, ↓ thyroxine, ↓ urinary aldosterone, ↑ alkaline phosphatase, ↑AST, ↑TSH

NURSING CONSIDERATIONS
Assessment
• Monitor renal function studies: BUN, serum uric acid, urine CrCl, electrolytes before, during therapy; I&O ratio; report fall in urine output of 30 ml/hr
• Monitor temperature q4h; may indicate beginning infection
• Monitor liver function tests before, during therapy (bilirubin, AST, ALT, LDH) as

needed or monthly; RBC, Hct, Hgb, since these may be decreased
• Monitor inflammation of mucosa, breaks in skin, yellowing of skin and sclera, dark urine, clay-colored stools, itchy skin, abdominal pain, fever, diarrhea
• Assess symptoms indicating severe allergic reaction: rash, pruritus, urticaria, purpuric skin lesions, itching, flushing; if rash develops, drug may need to be discontinued
• Assess for Cushing's syndrome: buffalo hump, moon face, personality changes, hypertension, weakness, hirsutism

Nursing diagnoses
☑ Injury, risk for (adverse reactions)
☑ Body image disturbance (adverse reactions)
☑ Infection, risk for (adverse reactions)
☑ Knowledge deficit (teaching)

Implementation
• Give with food or fluids for GI upset
• Give in equal intervals q6h

Patient/family education
• Instruct patient to report side effects
• Advise patient to avoid use of alcohol, which potentiates this drug

Evaluation
Positive therapeutic outcome
• Prevention of rapid division of malignant cells, postmenopausal cancer, prostate cancer
• Suppression of adrenal function (Cushing's syndrome)

Treatment of overdose:
Induce vomiting, provide supportive care

aminolevulinic acid
See Appendix A, Selected New Drugs

aminophylline (℞)
(am-in-off'i-lin)
Aminophyllin, Phyllocontin, Truphylline
Func. class.: Bronchodilator
Chem. class.: Xanthine, ethylenediamine
Pregnancy category   C

Action: Relaxes smooth muscle of respiratory system by blocking phosphodiesterase, which increases cyclic AMP; increased cyclic AMP alters intracellular calcium ion movements; produces bronchodilatation, increased pulmonary blood flow, relaxation of respiratory tract

⇨**Therapeutic Outcome:** Increased ability to breathe

Uses: Bronchial asthma, bronchospasm, Cheyne-Stokes respirations

Investigational uses: Apnea
P in infancy for respiratory/ myocardial stimulation, Cheyne-Stokes respirations as a respiratory stimulant

Dosage and routes
Adult: PO 500 mg, then 250-500 mg q6-8h; cont **IV** 0.3-0.9 mg/kg/hr (maintenance); REC 500 mg q6-8h
P *Child:* PO 7.5 mg/kg, then 3-6 mg/kg q6-8h; **IV** 7.5 mg/kg, then 3-6 mg/kg q6-8h injected over 5 min; do

not exceed 25 mg/min; may give loading dose of 5.6 mg/kg over ½ hr; cont **IV** 1 mg/kg/hr (maintenance); for children/infants use drug without preservative of alcohol

Neonates: **IV**/PO 1 mg/kg initially for plasma increases of each 2 µg/ml, then 1 mg/kg q12h

Available forms: Inj 250 mg/10 ml, 500 mg/21 ml, 100 mg/100 ml in 0.45% NaCl; rect supp 250 mg, 500 mg; oral liq 105 mg/5 ml; tabs 100, 200 mg; con-rel tabs 225 mg

Pharmacokinetics

Absorption	Well absorbed (PO), slow (PO–ext rel), erratic (rec)
Distribution	Widely distributed; crosses placenta
Metabolism	Liver to caffeine
Excretion	Kidneys
Half-life	3-12 hr, increased in renal disease, CHF

Pharmacodynamics

	PO	PO–EXT REL	IV
Onset	15-60 min	Unknown	Immediate
Peak	1-2 hr	4-7 hr	Infusion's end
Duration	6-8 hr	8-12 hr	6-8 hr

Adverse effects

CNS: Anxiety, restlessness, insomnia, *dizziness,* **convulsions,** headache, lightheadedness, muscle twitching
CV: Palpitations, sinus tachycardia, hypotension, flushing, dysrhythmias, increased respiratory rate
GI: Nausea, vomiting, anorexia, diarrhea, bitter taste, dyspepsia, anal irritation (suppositories), epigastric pain
GU: Urinary frequency
INTEG: Flushing, urticaria, *rec supp (irritation)*
RESP: Tachypnea

Contraindications: Hypersensitivity to xanthines, tachydysrhythmias

Precautions: Elderly, CHF, cor pulmonale, hepatic disease, active peptic ulcer disease, diabetes mellitus, hyperthyroidism, hypertension, children, pregnancy **C,** glaucoma, prostatic hypertrophy

Interactions
Individual drugs
Adenosine: ↓ aminophylline effect
Allopurinol: ↓ metabolism, ↑ toxicity of aminophylline
Carbamazepine: ↑ or ↓ aminophylline levels
Cimetidine: ↓ metabolism, ↑ toxicity of aminophylline
Disulfiram: ↓ metabolism, ↑ toxicity of aminophylline
Halothane: ↑ risk of dysrhythmias
Interferon: ↓ metabolism, ↑ toxicity of aminophylline
Isoniazid: ↑ or ↓ aminophylline level
Lithium: ↓ effect of lithium
Methotrexate: ↑ effect of aminophylline
Mexiletine: ↓ metabolism, ↑ toxicity
Phenytoin: ↑ metabolism, ↓ effect of aminophylline
Rifampin: ↑ metabolism, ↓ effect of aminophylline
Thiabendazole: ↓ metabolism, ↑ toxicity
Drug classifications
Antibiotics, macrolide: ↑ aminophylline levels

Adverse effects: *italic* = common; **bold** = life-threatening

Barbiturates: ↓ effect of aminophylline

β-Adrenergic blockers: ↓ effect of aminophylline

Diuretics, loop: ↑ or ↓ aminophylline levels

Calcium channel blockers: ↑ aminophylline levels

Fluoroquinolones: ↓ metabolism, ↑ toxicity

Oral contraceptives: ↑ aminophylline levels

Sympathomimetics: ↑ CNS, CV adverse reactions

Smoking

↑ metabolism, ↓ effect

Food/drug

Caffeinated foods (cola, coffee, tea, chocolate): ↑ CNS, CV, adverse reactions

Charcoal-smoked foods: ↓ effect

Lab test interferences

↑ Plasma free fatty acids

NURSING CONSIDERATIONS
Assessment

• Monitor theophylline blood levels (therapeutic level is 10-20 µg/ml); toxicity may occur with small increase above

Ⓖ 20 µg/ml, especially elderly; determine whether theophylline was given recently (24 hr); check for toxicity: nausea, vomiting, anxiety, restlessness, insomnia, tachycardia, dysrhythmias, convulsions; notify prescriber immediately

• Monitor I&O; diuresis will occur; dehydration may result

Ⓖ in elderly or children in whom
Ⓟ diuresis is great

• Monitor respiratory rate, rhythm, depth; auscultate lung fields bilaterally; notify prescriber of abnormalities; check ECG for tachycardia, PVCs, PACs in patients with cardiac problems

• Monitor allergic reactions: rash, urticaria; if these occur, drug should be discontinued, prescriber notified

Nursing diagnoses

☑ Airway clearance, ineffective (uses)

☑ Activity intolerance (uses)

☑ Injury, risk for (uses, adverse reactions)

☑ Knowledge deficit (teaching)

Implementation
General

• Give around the clock to maintain blood (theophylline) levels

• If switching from **IV** to PO, give controlled-release dose at time of **IV** infusion discontinuation; if giving tab (immediate release), discontinue **IV** and wait >4 hr

PO route

• Give PO after meals or water to decrease GI symptoms; absorption may be affected with a full glass of water or food

Ⓢ• Do not crush or chew enteric-coated or controlled-release tabs

Ⓥ**IV route**

• Give **IV** after diluting in 5% dextrose to decrease burning sensation at inj site; only clear solutions; may be diluted for IV inf in 100-200 ml in D_5W, $D_{10}W$, $D_{20}W$, 0.9% NaCl, 0.45% NaCl, LR

• Avoid IM injection; pain and tissue damage may occur

• Only clear sol; flush **IV** line before dose; store diluted sol for 24 hrs if refrigerated

Syringe compatibilities:

Heparin, metoclopramide, pentobarbital, thiopental

Y-site compatibilities:

Allopurinol, amifostine, amphotericin B sulfate complex,

---

amrinone, aztreonam, ceftazidime, cimetidine, cladribine, doxorubicin liposome, enalaprilat, esmolol, famotidine, filgrastim, fluconazole, fludarabine, foscarnet, gallium, granisetron, heparin sodium with hydrocortisone sodium succinate, labetalol, melphalan, meropenem, morphine, netilmicin, paclitaxel, pancuronium, piperacillin/tazobactam, potassium chloride, propofol, ranitidine, remifentanil, sargramostim, tacrolimus, teniposide, thiotepa, tolazoline, vecuronium, Vit B with C

Y-site incompatibilities:
Dobutamine, hydralazine, ondansetron

Additive compatibilities:
Amobarbital, bretylium, calcium gluconate, chloramphenicol, cibenzoline, cimetidine, dexamethasone, diphenhydramine, dopamine, erythromycin lactobionate, esmolol, floxacillin, flumazenil, furosemide, heparin, hydrocortisone, lidocaine, mephentermine, meropenem, methyldopa, metronidazole/sodium bicarbonate, nitroglycerin, pentobarbital, phenobarbital, potassium chloride, ranitidine, secobarbital, sodium bicarbonate, terbutaline

Additive incompatibilities:
Ascorbic acid, bleomycin, cephalothin, cefotaxime, chlorpromazine, cimetidine, clindamycin, codeine, dimenhydrinate, dobutamine, doxorubicin, doxycycline, epinephrine, erythromycin glucceptate, hydralazine, hydroxyzine, insulin, isoproterenol, meperidine, methicillin, morphine, nafcillin, nitroprusside, norepinephrine, oxytetracycline, papaverine, penicillin G, pentazocine, phenobarbital, phenytoin, prochlorperazine, promazine, promethazine, sulfisoxazole, tetracycline, vancomycin

Rectal route
• Rec dose if patient is unable to take PO; retain rec dose for ½ hour

Patient/family education
• Teach patient to take doses as prescribed, not to skip dose; to check OTC medications, current prescription medications for ephedrine, which will increase CNS stimulation; advise patient not to drink alcohol or caffeine products (tea, coffee, chocolate, colas), which will increase action
• Teach patient to avoid hazardous activities; dizziness may occur
• Teach patient if GI upset occurs, to take drug with 8 oz water or food; absorption may be decreased
• Teach patient to remain in bed 15-20 min after rec supp is inserted to prevent removal
• Instruct patient that smoking increases metabolism; dosage may need to be increased
• Teach patient to obtain blood levels of drug every few months to prevent toxicity; not to change brands, since effect may not be the same
• Teach patient to increase fluids to 2 L/day to decrease viscosity of secretions

Evaluation
Positive therapeutic outcome
• Decreased dyspnea
• Respiratory stimulation in infants
• Clear lung fields bilaterally

amiodarone (℞)
(a-mee-o'da-rone)
Cordarone
Func. class.: Antidysrhythmic (Class III)
Chem. class.: Iodinated benzofuran derivative
Pregnancy category **D**

Action: Prolongs action potential duration and effective refractory period, slows sinus rate with increasing PR and QT intervals, noncompetitive α- and β-adrenergic inhibition; increases PR and QT intervals, decreases sinus rate

➡ **Therapeutic Outcome:** Decreased amount and severity of ventricular dysrhythmias

Uses: Severe ventricular tachycardia, supraventricular tachycardia, ventricular fibrillation or atrial fibrillation not controlled by 1st-line agents

Dosage and routes
Adult: PO loading dose 800-1600 mg/day × 1-3 wk; then 600-800 mg/day × 1 mo; maintenance 200-600 mg/day

Adult: **IV** loading dose (first rapid) 150 mg over the 1st 10 min (15 mg/min), add 3 ml (150 mg) to 100 ml D_5W, infuse 100 mg/ml, then slow 360 mg over the next 6 hr (1 mg/min), add 18 ml (900 mg) to 500 ml D_5W (1.8 mg/ml); maintenance at 540 mg given over the remaining 18 hr (0.5 mg/min), decrease rate of the slow inf to 0.5 mg/min

P *Child:* PO loading dose 10-15 mg/kg/day in 1-2 divided doses for 4-14 days, then 5 mg/kg/day

Available forms: Tabs 200 mg; inj 50 mg/ml

Adverse effects
CNS: Headache, dizziness, involuntary movement, tremors, peripheral neuropathy, malaise, fatigue, ataxia, paresthesias, insomnia
CV: Hypotension, **bradycardia, sinus arrest, CHF, dysrhythmias, SA node dysfunction**
EENT: Blurred vision, halos, photophobia, **corneal microdeposits,** dry eyes
ENDO: Hyperthyroidism or hypothyroidism
GI: Nausea, vomiting, diarrhea, abdominal pain, anorexia, constipation, **hepatotoxicity**
INTEG: Rash, photosensitivity, blue-gray skin discoloration, alopecia, spontaneous ecchymosis
MISC: Flushing, abnormal taste or smell, edema, abnormal salivation, coagulation abnormalities
MS: Weakness, pain in extremities
RESP: **Pulmonary fibrosis,** pulmonary inflammation

Contraindications: Sinus node dysfunction; 2nd-, 3rd-degree AV block; pregnancy **D**

Precautions: Goiter, Hashimoto's thyroiditis, SN dysfunction, 2nd- or 3rd-degree AV block, electrolyte imbalances, bradycardia, lactation

▨ **Do Not Confuse:** amiodarone/amrinone, Cordarone/Inocor

Pharmacokinetics	
Absorption	Slow, variable (PO) up to 65%
Distribution	Body tissues; crosses placenta
Metabolism	Liver
Excretion	Bile, kidney (minimal)
Half-life	15-100 days

Pharmacodynamics	
	PO
Onset	1-3 wk
Peak	Unknown
Duration	Up to months

Interactions
Individual drugs
Digitalis: ↑ bradycardia
Digoxin: ↑ blood levels, ↑ toxicity
Disopyramide: ↑ levels, ↑ toxicity
Flecainide: ↑ levels, ↑ toxicity
Lidocaine: Bradycardia, cardiac arrest
Mexiletine: ↑ levels, ↑ toxicity
Phenytoin: ↑ blood levels
Procainamide: ↑ levels, ↑ toxicity
Quinidine: ↑ levels, ↑ toxicity
Theophylline: ↑ levels
Warfarin: ↑ level, ↑ bleeding
Drug classifications
Antidysrhythmics: ↑ Torsades de pointes
Antihypertensives: ↑ hypotension
β-Adrenergic blockers: ↑ dysrhythmias, cardiac arrest
Calcium channel blockers: ↑ dysrhythmias, cardiac arrest
Herb/drug
Aloe: ↑ amiodarone effect
Buckthorn bark/berry: ↑ amiodarone effect
Cascara sagrada bark: ↑ amiodarone effect
Rhubarb root: ↑ amiodarone effect
Senna leaf/fruits: ↑ amiodarone effect

Lab test interference:
↑ T$_4$

NURSING CONSIDERATIONS
Assessment
• Monitor I&O ratio; monitor electrolytes: potassium, sodium, chloride
• Monitor chest x-ray, thyroid function tests
• Monitor liver function studies: AST, ALT, bilirubin, alkaline phosphatase
• Monitor ECG continuously to determine drug effectiveness; measure PR, QRS, QT intervals; check for PVCs, other dysrhythmias; monitor B/P continuously for hypotension, hypertension; check for rebound hypertension after 1-2 hr
• Monitor for dehydration or hypovolemia
• Assess for CNS symptoms: confusion, psychosis, numbness, depression, involuntary movements; if these occur, drug should be discontinued
• Assess for hypothyroidism: lethargy, dizziness, constipation, enlarged thyroid gland, edema of extremities, cool, pale skin
• Monitor hyperthyroidism: restlessness, tachycardia, eyelid puffiness, weight loss, frequent urination, menstrual irregularities, dyspnea, warm, moist skin
• Assess for pulmonary toxicity: dyspnea, fatigue, cough, fever, chest pain; drug should be discontinued if these occur
• Monitor cardiac rate, respiration: rate, rhythm, character, chest pain, ventricular tachycardia, supraventricular tachycardia or fibrillation
• Assess sight and vision before treatment and throughout

Adverse effects: *italic* = common; **bold** = life-threatening

therapy; microdeposits on the cornea may cause blurred vision, halos, and photophobia

Nursing diagnoses
☑ Cardiac output, decreased (uses)
☑ Gas exchange, impaired (adverse reactions)
☑ Knowledge deficit (teaching)

Implementation
PO route
• Give reduced dosage slowly with ECG monitoring only
• Give with meals for GI upset
Ⅳ **IV route**

Additive compatibilities: Dobutamine, lidocaine, potassium chloride, procainimide, verapamil

Y-site compatibilities: Amikacin, bretylium, clindamycin, dobutamine, dopamine, doxycycline, erythromycin, esmolol, gentamicin, insulin (regular), isoproterenol, labetalol, lidocaine, metaraminol, metronidazole, midazolam, morphine, nitroglycerin, norepinephrine, penicillin G potassium, phentolamine, phenylephrine, potassium chloride, procainamide, tobramycin, vancomycin

Solution compatibilities: D₅W, 0.9% NaCl

Patient/family education
• Instruct patient to report side effects immediately to prescriber
• Instruct patient that skin discoloration is usually reversible but skin may turn bluish on neck, face, arms when used for long periods
• Advise patient that dark glasses may be needed for photophobia

• Instruct patient to use sunscreen and protective clothing to prevent burning associated with photosensitivity
• Instruct patient to take medication as prescribed, not to double doses
• Instruct patient to complete follow-up appointment with health care provider including pulmonary function studies, chest x-ray, ophthalmic examinations

Treatment of overdose: Administer O₂, artificial ventilation, ECG, dopamine for circulatory depression, diazepam or thiopental for convulsions, isoproterenol

amitriptyline (℞)
(a-mee-trip'ti-leen)
amitriptyline HCl, Apo-Amitriptyline ♣, Elavil, Endep, Levate ♣, Novo-Triptyn ♣
Func. class.: Antidepressant—tricyclic
Chem. class.: Tertiary amine
Pregnancy category   C

Action: Blocks reuptake of norepinephrine, serotonin into nerve endings that increase action of norepinephrine, serotonin in nerve cells

Uses: Major depression

Investigational uses: Chronic pain management, prevention of cluster/migraine headaches

▶**Therapeutic Outcome:** Decreased symptoms of depression after 2-3 wk

---

☑ Herb/drug ⓢ Do Not Crush ◆ Alert ⊶ Key Drug ⓖ Geriatric ⓟ Pediatric

Dosage and routes
Depression
Adult: PO 30-100 mg hs; may increase to 200 mg qd, not to exceed 300 mg/day; IM 20-30 mg qid, or 80-120 mg hs

P *Adolescent:* PO 30 mg/day in divided doses; may be increased to 150 mg/day

G *Elderly:* Generally avoided because of anticholinergic side effects; if used, PO 10-25 mg at hs, increase by 10-25 mg/wk as tolerated

Cluster/migraine headaches
Adult: PO 50-150 mg/day

Chronic pain
Adult: PO 75-150 mg/day

Available forms: Tabs 10, 25, 50, 75, 100, 150 mg; inj IM 10 mg/ml; syrup 10 mg/ 5 ml ✦

Adverse effects
CNS: Dizziness, drowsiness, confusion, headache, anxiety, tremors, stimulation, weakness, insomnia, nightmares, EPS **G** (elderly), increased psychiatric symptoms, **hyperthermia**
CV: Orthostatic hypotension, **ECG changes, tachycardia, hypertension,** palpitations
EENT: Blurred vision, tinnitus, mydriasis, ophthalmoplegia
GI: Constipation, dry mouth, nausea, vomiting, **paralytic ileus,** increased appetite, cramps, epigastric distress, jaundice, **hepatitis,** stomatitis
GU: Retention
HEMA: **Agranulocytosis, thrombocytopenia, eosinophilia,** leukopenia
INTEG: Rash, urticaria, sweating, pruritus, photosensitivity

Contraindications: Hypersensitivity to tricyclic antidepressants, recovery phase of myocardial infarction, narrow-angle glaucoma

Precautions: Suicidal patients, convulsive disorders, prostatic hypertrophy, schizophrenia, psychosis, severe depression, increased intraocular pressure, narrow angle glaucoma, urinary retention, cardiac disease, hepatic/renal disease, hyperthyroidism, electroshock **P** therapy, elective surgery, child **G** <12 yr, pregnancy **C**, elderly

⚠ Do Not Confuse:
amitriptyline/nortriptyline, Elavil/Mellaril, Elavil/Oruvail

Pharmacokinetics

Absorption	Well absorbed
Distribution	Widely distributed; crosses placenta
Metabolism	Liver, extensively
Excretion	Kidneys, breast milk
Half-life	31-46 hr

Pharmacodynamics

	PO/IM
Onset	45 min
Peak	2-12 hr
Duration	Unknown

Interactions
Individual drugs
Alcohol: ↑ CNS depression
Cimetidine: ↑ levels, ↑ toxicity
Clonidine: ↑ hypertension; avoid use
Fluoxetine: ↑ levels, ↑ toxicity
Guanethidine: ↓ effects
Drug classifications
Antihypertensives: Blocked response to antihypertensive
Antithyroid agents: ↑ risk of agranulocytosis
Barbiturates: ↑ CNS effects
Benzodiazepines: ↑ CNS effects
CNS depressants: ↑ CNS effects

MAOI: Hypertensive crisis, convulsions
Oral contraceptives: ↑ effects, toxicity
Phenothiazines: ↑ amitriptylline levels, toxicity
Sympathomimetics, indirect acting: ↓ effects

☑ *Herb/drug*
Belladonna leaf/root: ↑ anticholinergic effect
Henbane leaf: ↑ anticholinergic effect
Kava: ↑ CNS depression
Scopolia root: ↑ amitriptyline action

Smoking
↑ metabolism, ↓ effects

Lab test interferences
↑ blood glucose, ↑ alkaline phosphatase

NURSING CONSIDERATIONS
Assessment
• Monitor B/P (with patient lying, standing), pulse q4h; if systolic B/P drops 20 mm Hg, hold drug, notify prescriber; take vital signs q4h in patients with cardiovascular disease
• Monitor blood studies: CBC, leukocytes, differential, cardiac enzymes if patient is receiving long-term therapy
• Monitor drug level: therapeutic 100-250 ng/ml; toxic >500 ng/ml
• Monitor hepatic studies: AST, ALT, bilirubin
• Check weight weekly; appetite may increase with drug
• Assess ECG for flattening of T wave, bundle branch block, AV block, prolongation of QTc interval, dysrhythmias in cardiac patients
• Assess for EPS primarily in
G elderly: rigidity, dystonia, akathisia
• Assess mental status: mood, sensorium, affect, suicidal

tendencies; increase in psychiatric symptoms: depression, panic
• Monitor urinary retention, constipation; constipation is
P more likely to occur in children
G or elderly
• Assess for withdrawal symptoms: headache, nausea, vomiting, muscle pain, weakness; do not usually occur unless drug was discontinued abruptly
• Identify alcohol consumption; if alcohol is consumed, hold dose until morning

Nursing diagnoses
☑ Coping, ineffective individual (uses)
☑ Injury, risk for physical (side effects)
☑ Knowledge deficit (teaching)
☑ Noncompliance (teaching)

Implementation
PO route
• Give with food or milk for GI symptoms
• Crush if patient is unable to swallow medication whole
• Give dosage hs if oversedation occurs during day; may
G take entire dose hs; elderly may not tolerate once/day dosing
• Store at room temp; do not freeze

Patient/family education
• Teach patient that therapeutic effects may take 2-3 wk
• Instruct patient to use caution in driving or other activities requiring alertness because of drowsiness, dizziness, blurred vision; to avoid rising quickly from sitting to
G standing, especially elderly
• Advise patient to avoid alcohol ingestion, other CNS depressants; overheating
• Teach patient not to discon-

tinue medication quickly after long-term use; may cause nausea, headache, malaise
• Advise patient to wear sunscreen or large hat, since photosensitivity occurs; hyperthermia can occur
• Teach patient to increase fluids, bulk in diet if constipation, urinary retention occur, G especially elderly
• Teach patient to take gum, hard sugarless candy, or frequent sips of water for dry mouth

Evaluation
Positive therapeutic outcome
• Decreased depression
• Absence of suicidal thoughts

Treatment of overdose: ECG monitoring, induce emesis, lavage, activated charcoal, administer anticonvulsant

---

amlodipine (R)
(am-loe'di-peen)
Norvasc
Func. class.: Antianginal, calcium channel blocker, antihypertensive
Chem. class.: Dihydropyridine

Pregnancy category C

Action: Inhibits calcium ion influx across cell membrane during cardiac depolarization; produces relaxation of coronary vascular smooth muscle, peripheral vascular smooth muscle; dilates coronary vascular arteries; increases myocardial oxygen delivery in patients with vasospastic angina

⇒**Therapeutic Outcome:** Decreased angina pectoris, dysrhythmias, B/P

Uses: Chronic stable angina pectoris, hypertension, vasospastic angina

Dosage and routes
Adult: PO 5-10 mg qd initially, may increase gradually to max 10 mg qd.
G *Elderly:* PO 2.5 mg qd
Available forms: Tabs 2.5, 5, 10 mg

Adverse effects
CNS: Headache, fatigue, dizziness, anxiety, depression, insomnia, paresthesia, somnolence, asthenia
CV: Dysrhythmia, edema, bradycardia, hypotension, palpitations, syncope, AV block
GI: Nausea, vomiting, diarrhea, gastric upset, constipation, abdominal cramps, flatulence, anorexia
GU: Nocturia, polyuria
INTEG: Rash, pruritus, urticaria, hair loss
MISC: Flushing, nasal congestion, sweating, shortness of breath, sexual difficulties, muscle cramps, cough, weight gain, tinnitus, epistaxis

Contraindications: Sick sinus syndrome, 2nd- or 3rd-degree heart block, hypotension less than 90 mm Hg systolic, hypersensitivity

Precautions: CHF, hypotension, hepatic injury, pregnancy
P **C,** lactation, children, renal
G disease, elderly

Do Not Confuse: Norvasc/Navane

Pharmacokinetics

Absorption	Well absorbed up to 90%
Distribution	Crosses placenta
Metabolism	Liver, extensively
Excretion	Kidneys to metabolites (90%)
Half-life	30-50 hr

Pharmacodynamics

Onset	Unknown
Peak	6-10 hr
Duration	24 hr

Interactions
Individual drugs
Alcohol: ↑ hypotension
Fentanyl: ↑ hypotension
Quinidine: ↑ hypotension
Drug classifications
Antihypertensives: ↑ hypotension
Nitrates: ↑ hypotension
NSAIDs: ↓ antihypertensive effect
Food/drug
Grapefruit: ↑ hypotension

NURSING CONSIDERATIONS
Assessment
• Assess fluid volume status: I&O ratio and record, weight, distended red veins, crackles in lung, color, quality and specific gravity of urine, skin turgor, adequacy of pulses, moist mucous membranes, bilateral lung sounds, peripheral pitting edema; dehydration symptoms of decreasing output, thirst, hypotension, dry mouth and mucous membranes should be reported
• Monitor B/P and pulse; if B/P drops, call prescriber
• Monitor ALT, AST, bilirubin daily; if these are elevated, hepatotoxicity is suspected
• Monitor if platelets are <150,000/mm^3; drug is usu-

ally discontinued and another drug started
• Monitor cardiac status: B/P, pulse, respiration, ECG

Nursing diagnoses
☑ Cardiac output, decreased (uses)
☑ Knowledge deficit (teaching)

Implementation
• Give once a day, with food for GI symptoms

Patient/family education
• Advise patient to avoid hazardous activities until stabilized on drug, dizziness is no longer a problem
• Instruct patient to avoid alcohol and OTC drugs unless directed by prescriber
• Advise patient to comply in all areas of medical regimen: diet, exercise, stress reduction, drug therapy; to notify prescriber of irregular heart beat, shortness of breath, swelling of feet and hands, pronounced dizziness, constipation, nausea, hypotension
• Teach patient to use as directed even if feeling better; may be taken with other cardiovascular drugs (nitrates, β-blockers)

Evaluation
Positive therapeutic outcome
• Decreased anginal pain
• Decreased B/P

Treatment of overdose:
Defibrillation, β-agonists, **IV** calcium inotropic agents, diuretics, atropine for AV block, vasopressor for hypotension

amoxapine (℞)
(a-mox′a-peen)
amoxapine, Asendin
Func. class.: Antidepressant—tetra
Chem. class.: Dibenzoxazepine derivative, secondary amine
Pregnancy category C

Action: Blocks reuptake of norepinephrine, serotonin into nerve endings, thereby increasing action of norepinephrine, serotonin in nerve cells

⇒**Therapeutic Outcome:** Decreased symptoms of depression after 2-3 wk

Uses: Depression

Dosage and routes
Adult: PO 50 mg tid; may increase to 100 mg tid on 3rd day of therapy; not to exceed 300 mg/day unless lower doses have been given for at least 2 wk; may be given daily dose hs; not to exceed 600 mg/day in hospitalized patients

G *Elderly:* PO 25 mg hs, may increase by 25 mg/wk, up to 150 mg/day in divided doses

Available forms: Tabs 25, 50, 100, 150 mg

Adverse effects
CNS: Dizziness, drowsiness, confusion, headache, anxiety, tremors, stimulation, weakness, insomnia, nightmares, EPS **G** (elderly), increased psychiatric symptoms, paresthesia, impairment of sexual functioning, **neuroleptic malignant syndrome**
CV: Orthostatic hypotension, ECG changes, tachycardia, hypertension, palpitations

EENT: Blurred vision, tinnitus, **A** mydriasis, ophthalmoplegia
GI: Dry mouth, constipation, nausea, vomiting, **paralytic ileus,** increased appetite, cramps, epigastric distress, jaundice, **hepatitis,** stomatitis
GU: Retention, **acute renal failure**
HEMA: **Agranulocytosis, thrombocytopenia, eosinophilia, leukopenia**
INTEG: Rash, urticaria, sweating, pruritus, photosensitivity

Contraindications: Hypersensitivity to tricyclic antidepressants, recovery phase of myocardial infarction, convulsive disorders, prostatic hypertrophy

Precautions: Suicidal patients, severe depression, increased intraocular pressure, narrow-angle glaucoma, urinary retention, cardiac disease, hepatic disease, hyperthyroidism, electroshock therapy, elective **G** surgery, elderly, pregnancy **C**

N **Do Not Confuse:**
amoxapine/amoxicillin,
amoxapine/Amoxil

Pharmacokinetics

Absorption	Well absorbed
Distribution	Widely distributed; crosses placenta
Metabolism	Liver, extensively
Excretion	Kidneys, breast milk
Half-life	8 hr

Pharmacodynamics

Onset	1-2 wk
Peak	2-6 wk
Duration	6-12 wk

Interactions
Individual drugs
Alcohol: ↑ CNS depression
Cimetidine: ↑ amoxapine levels, ↑ toxicity of amoxapine

Clonidine: Severe hypotension; avoid use
Fluoxetine: ↑ amoxapine levels, ↑ toxicity of amoxapine
Guanethidine: ↓ effects of amoxapine
Paroxetine: ↑ amoxapine level, ↑ toxicity
Sertraline: ↑ amoxapine level, ↑ toxicity

Drug classifications
MAOIs: Hypertensive crisis, convulsions
Barbiturates: ↑ effects of amoxapine
Benzodiazepines: ↑ effects of amoxapine
CNS depressants: ↑ effects of amoxapine
Sympathomimetics, indirect acting: ↓ effects of amoxapine
Oral contraceptives: ↑ effects, toxicity of amoxapine
Smoking
↑ metabolism, ↓ effects
☑ *Herb/drug*
Belladonna leaf/root: ↑ anticholinergic effect
Henbane leaf: ↑ anticholinergic effect
Kava: ↑ CNS depression
Scopolia root: ↑ amoxapine action
Lab test interferences
↑ blood glucose, ↑ alkaline phosphatase, ↑ prolactin

NURSING CONSIDERATIONS
Assessment
• Monitor B/P (with patient lying, standing), pulse q4h; if systolic B/P drops 20 mm Hg hold drug, notify prescriber; take vital signs q4h in patients with cardiovascular disease
• Monitor blood studies: CBC, leukocytes, differential, cardiac enzymes if patient is receiving long-term therapy
• Monitor blood level: therapeutic 20-100 ng/ml
• Monitor hepatic studies: AST, ALT, bilirubin
• Check weight weekly; appetite may increase with drug
• Assess ECG for flattening of T wave, bundle branch block, AV block, dysrhythmias in cardiac patients
• Assess for EPS primarily in **G** elderly: rigidity, dystonia, akathisia
• Assess mental status: mood, sensorium, affect, suicidal tendencies; increase in psychiatric symptoms: depression, **G** panic; confusion (elderly)
• Monitor urinary retention, constipation; constipation is **P** more likely to occur in **G** children and elderly
• Assess for withdrawal symptoms: headache, nausea, vomiting, muscle pain, weakness; do not usually occur unless drug was discontinued abruptly
• Identify alcohol consumption; if alcohol is consumed, hold dose until morning

Nursing diagnoses
✓ Coping, ineffective individual (uses)
✓ Injury, risk for physical (side effects)
✓ Knowledge deficit (teaching)
✓ Noncompliance (teaching)

Implementation
• Give with food or milk for GI symptoms
• Crush if patient is unable to swallow medication whole
• Store at room temp; do not freeze

Patient/family education
• Teach patient that therapeutic effects may take 2-3 wk
• Instruct patient to use caution in driving or other activities requiring alertness because

---

☑ Herb/drug Ⓢ Do Not Crush ◆ Alert ☗ Key Drug **G** Geriatric **P** Pediatric of drowsiness, dizziness, blurred vision; to avoid rising quickly from sitting to standing, especially elderly

G

• Teach patient to avoid alcohol ingestion, other CNS depressants

• Teach patient not to discontinue medication quickly after long-term use: may cause nausea, headache, malaise

• Teach patient to wear sunscreen or large hat, since photosensitivity occurs

• Teach patient to increase fluids, bulk in diet if constipation, urinary retention occur, especially elderly

G

• Advise patient to take gum, hard sugarless candy, or frequent sips of water for dry mouth

Evaluation
Positive therapeutic outcome
• Decreased depression
• Absence of suicidal thoughts

Treatment of overdose:
ECG monitoring, induce emesis, lavage, activated charcoal, administer anticonvulsant

---

amoxicillin (℞)
(a-mox-i-sill'in)
amoxicillin, Amoxil, Apo-Amoxi ✤, Novamoxin ✤, Nu-Amoxi ✤, Polymox, Trimox, Wymox
Func. class.: Broad-spectrum antiinfective
Chem. class.: Aminopenicillin

Pregnancy category   B

Action: Interferes with cell wall replication of susceptible organisms by binding to the bacterial cell wall; the cell wall, rendered osmotically unstable, swells and bursts from osmotic pressure

A

→Therapeutic Outcome:
Bactericidal effects for the following organisms: effective for gram-positive cocci *(Streptococcus pyogenes, S. faecalis, S. pneumoniae),* gram-negative cocci *(Neisseria gonorrhoeae, N. meningitidis, Escherichia coli),* gram-negative bacilli *(Haemophilus influenzae, Proteus mirabilis, Salmonella)*

Uses: Infections of respiratory tract, skin, skin structures, genitourinary tract, otitis media, meningitis, septicemia, sinusitis and endocarditis prophylaxis

Investigational uses: Lyme disease, *Chlamydia trachomatis* in pregnancy

Dosage and routes
Renal disease
CrCl 10-50 ml/min dose q12h; CrCl <10 ml/min dose q24h

Systemic infections
Adult: PO 750 mg-1.5 g qd in divided doses q8h

P *Child:* PO 20-50 mg/kg/day in divided doses q8h

Gonorrhea/urinary tract infections
Adult: PO 3 g given with 1 g probenecid as a single dose

Chlamydia trachomatis
Adult: PO 500 mg/d × 1 wk

Bacterial endocarditis prophylaxis
P *Child:* PO 50 mg/kg/hr before and 25 mg/kg 6 hr after procedure

Available forms: Caps 250, 500 mg; chewable tabs 125, 250 mg; powder for oral susp 50 mg/ml, 125, 250 mg/5 ml

---

✤ Canada Only   Adverse effects: *italic* = common; **bold** = life-threatening

Adverse effects
CNS: Headache, fever
GI: Nausea, vomiting, diarrhea, increased AST, ALT, abdominal pain, glossitis, colitis, **pseudomembranous colitis**
HEMA: Anemia, increased bleeding time, **bone marrow depression, granulocytopenia**
INTEG: Urticaria, rash
SYST: **Anaphylaxis, respiratory distress, serum sickness**

Contraindications: Hypersensitivity to penicillins; neonates

Precautions: Pregnancy **B,** hypersensitivity to cephalosporins, neonates, renal disease

Do Not Confuse:
amoxicillin/amoxapine, Amoxil/amoxapine, Amoxil/amoxicillin, Trimox/Diamox, Trimox/Tylox, Wymox/Tylox

Pharmacokinetics	
Absorption	Well absorbed (90%)
Distribution	Readily in body tissues, fluids, CSF; crosses placenta
Metabolism	Liver (30%)
Excretion	Breast milk, kidney, unchanged (70%)
Half-life	1-1.3 hr

Pharmacodynamics	
Onset	½ hr
Peak	2 hr

Interactions
Individual drugs
Probenecid: ↑ amoxicillin levels, ↓ renal excretion
Drug classifications
Oral anticoagulants: ↑ anticoagulant effects
Oral contraceptives: ↓ contraceptive effectiveness
Herb/drug
Khat: ↓ absorption

Lab test interferences
False positive: Urine glucose, urine protein

NURSING CONSIDERATIONS
Assessment
• Assess patient for previous sensitivity reaction to penicillins or other cephalosporins; cross-sensitivity between penicillins and cephalosporins is common
• Assess patient for signs and symptoms of infection, including characteristics of wounds, sputum, urine, stool, WBC >10,000, earache, fever; obtain baseline information and monitor symptoms during treatment
• Obtain C&S before beginning drug therapy to identify if correct treatment has been initiated
• Assess for allergic reactions during treatment: rash, urticaria, pruritus, chills, fever, joint pain; angioedema may occur a few days after therapy begins; epinephrine and resuscitation equipment should be available for anaphylactic reactions
• Identify urine output; if decreasing, notify prescriber (may indicate nephrotoxicity); also, increased BUN, creatinine, urinalysis, protein, blood
• Monitor blood studies: AST, ALT, CBC, Hct, bilirubin, LDH, alkaline phosphatase, Coombs' test monthly if patient is on long-term therapy
• Monitor electrolytes: potassium, sodium, chloride monthly if patient is on long-term therapy
• Assess bowel pattern qd; if severe diarrhea occurs, notify prescriber; drug should be

discontinued; may indicate pseudomembranous colitis
• Monitor for bleeding: ecchymosis, bleeding gums, hematuria, stool guaiac daily if on long-term therapy
• Assess for overgrowth of infection: perineal itching, fever, malaise, redness, pain, swelling, drainage, rash, diarrhea, change in cough, sputum

Nursing diagnoses
✓ Infection, risk for (uses)
✓ Diarrhea (side effects)
✓ Injury, risk for (side effects)
✓ Knowledge deficit (teaching)
✓ Noncompliance (teaching)

Implementation
• Give in even doses around the clock; if GI upset occurs, give with food; drug must be given for 10-14 days to ensure organism death and prevent superinfection; store in tight container
• The caps may be opened and contents taken with fluids
• Shake susp well before each dose; store in refrigerator for 7-10 days

Patient/family education
• Teach patient to report sore throat, bruising, bleeding, joint pain; may indicate blood dyscrasias (rare)
• Advise patient to contact prescriber if vaginal itching, loose, foul-smelling stools, diarrhea, sore throat, fever, fatigue, furry tongue occur; may indicate superinfection or agranulocytopenia
• Instruct patient to take all medication prescribed for the length of time ordered; not to double dose
• Advise patient to notify prescriber of diarrhea with blood or pus, which may indicate pseudomembranous colitis

Evaluation
Positive therapeutic outcome
• Absence of signs/symptoms of infection (WBC <10,000, temp WNL, absence of red draining wounds or earache)
• Reported improvement in symptoms of infection

Treatment of anaphylaxis:
Withdraw drug, maintain airway, administer epinephrine, aminophylline, O_2, **IV** corticosteroids

amoxicillin/ clavulanate (℞)
(a-mox-i-sill'in)
Augmentin, Clavulin ✦
Func. class.: Broad-spectrum antiinfective (extended spectrum)
Chem. class.: Amino-penicillin-β-lactamase inhibitor

Pregnancy category   B

Action: Interferes with cell wall replication of susceptible organisms; the cell wall, rendered osmotically unstable, swells and bursts from osmotic pressure; combination increases spectrum of activity, β-lactamase resistance

Therapeutic Outcome: Bactericidal effects for the following organisms: *Escherichia coli, Proteus mirabilis, Haemophilus influenzae, Streptococcus faecalis, S. pneumoniae;* and β-lactamase–producing organisms: *Neisseria gonorrhoeae, N. meningitis, Shigella, Salmonella, Enterococcus, Streptococcus*

Uses: Infections of respiratory tract, skin, skin structures, genitourinary tract; otitis media, meningitis, septicemia, sinusitis, and endocarditis prophylaxis

Dosage and routes
Renal disease
CrCl 10-30 ml/min dose q12h; CrCl <10 ml/min dose q24h

Adult: PO 250-500 mg q8h or 500-875 mg q12h depending on severity of infection

P *Child:* PO 20-40 mg/kg/day in divided doses q8h or 25-45 mg/kg/day in divided doses q12h

Available forms: Tabs 250, 500, 875 mg/125 mg clavulanate; chewable tabs 125, 200, 250, 400 mg; powder for oral susp 125, 200, 250, 400 mg/5 ml

Adverse effects
CNS: Headache, fever
GI: Nausea, diarrhea, vomiting, increased AST, ALT, abdominal pain, glossitis, colitis, black tongue, **pseudomembranous colitis**
GU: Oliguria, proteinuria, hematuria, *vaginitis, moniliasis,* **glomerulonephritis**
HEMA: Anemia, **bone marrow depression, granulocytopenia, leukopenia, eosinophilia, thrombocytopenic purpura**
INTEG: Rash, urticaria
META: Hyperkalemia, hypokalemia, alkalosis, hypernatremia
SYST: Anaphylaxis

Contraindications: Hypersensitivity to penicillins; neonates

P

Precautions: Pregnancy **B,** lactation, hypersensitivity to cephalosporins; neonates; renal disease

P

Pharmacokinetics	
Absorption	Well absorbed (90%)
Distribution	Readily in body tissues, fluids, CSF; crosses placenta
Metabolism	Liver (30%)
Excretion	Breast milk; kidney, unchanged (70%)
Half-life	1-1.3 hr

Pharmacodynamics	
Onset	½ hr
Peak	2 hr

Interactions
Individual drugs
Allopurinol: amoxicillin-induced skin rash
Probenecid: ↑ amoxicillin levels, decreased renal excretion
Drug classifications
Oral anticoagulants: ↑ anticoagulant effects
Oral contraceptives: ↓ contraceptive effectiveness
Herb/drug
Khat: ↓ absorption
Lab test interferences
False positive: Urine glucose, urine protein

NURSING CONSIDERATIONS
Assessment
• Assess patient for previous sensitivity reaction to penicillins or other cephalosporins; cross-sensitivity between penicillins and cephalosporins is common
• Assess patient for signs and symptoms of infection, including characteristics of wounds, sputum, urine, stool, WBC >10,000, earache, fever; obtain baseline information and during treatment
• Complete C&S before beginning drug therapy to identify if correct treatment has been initiated

---

☑ Herb/drug 🛇 Do Not Crush ◈ Alert ☞ Key Drug **G** Geriatric **P** Pediatric

- Assess for allergic reactions: rash, urticaria, pruritus, chills, fever, joint pain; angioedema may occur a few days after therapy begins; epinephrine and resuscitation equipment should be available for anaphylactic reaction
- Identify urine output; if decreasing, notify prescriber (may indicate nephrotoxicity)
- Monitor renal studies: urinalysis, protein, blood, BUN, creatinine
- Monitor blood studies: AST, ALT, CBC, Hct, bilirubin, LDH, alkaline phosphatase, Coombs' test monthly if patient is on long-term therapy
- Monitor electrolytes: potassium, sodium, chloride monthly if patient is on long-term therapy
- Assess bowel pattern qd; if severe diarrhea occurs, drug should be discontinued; may indicate pseudomembranous colitis
- Monitor for bleeding: ecchymosis, bleeding gums, hematuria, stool guaiac daily if on long-term therapy
- Assess for overgrowth of infection: perineal itching, fever, malaise, redness, pain, swelling, drainage, rash, diarrhea, change in cough, sputum

Nursing diagnoses
☑ Infection, risk for (uses)
☑ Injury, risk for (side effects)
☑ Diarrhea (side effects)
☑ Knowledge deficit (teaching)
☑ Noncompliance (teaching)

Implementation
- Give in even doses around the clock; if GI upset occurs, give with food; drug must be taken for 10-14 days to ensure organism death and prevent superinfection; store in tight container; cap can be opened and mixed with food or liq; chewable tabs should be chewed
- Administer only as directed; 2 250-mg tabs not equivalent to 1 500-mg tab due to strength of clavulanate
- Shake susp well before each dose, store in refrigerator for 2 wk or 1 wk at room temp

Patient/family education
- Teach patient to report sore throat, bruising, bleeding, joint pain; may indicate blood dyscrasias (rare)
- Advise patient to contact prescriber if vaginal itching, loose, foul-smelling stools occur; may indicate superinfection
- Instruct patient to take all medication prescribed for the length of time prescribed
- Advise patient to notify prescriber of diarrhea with blood or pus, which may indicate pseudomembranous colitis

Evaluation
Positive therapeutic outcome
- Absence of signs/symptoms of infection (WBC <10,000, temp WNL, absence of red draining wounds, earache)
- Reported improvement in symptoms of infection

Treatment of anaphylaxis:
Withdraw drug, maintain airway, administer epinephrine, aminophylline, O_2, **IV** corticosteroids

---

amphetamine (℞)
(am-fet′a-meen)
amphetamine sulfate
Func. class.: Cerebral stimulant
Chem. class.: Amphetamine

Pregnancy category C
Controlled substance schedule II

Action: Increases release of norepinephrine in nerve endings, dopamine in cerebral cortex to reticular activating system; increases CNS, respiratory stimulation, pupillary dilatation, vasoconstriction

➤ **Therapeutic Outcome:** Increased alertness, decreased fatigue, ability to stay awake (treatment of narcolepsy), increased attention span, decreased hyperactivity (ADHD)

Uses: Narcolepsy, ADHD

Dosage and routes
Narcolepsy
Adult: PO 5-60 mg qd in divided doses

P *Child >12 yr:* PO 10 mg qd increasing by 10 mg/day at weekly intervals

P *Child 6-12 yr:* PO 5 mg qd increasing by 5 mg/wk, max 60 mg/day

ADHD
P *Child >6 yr:* PO 5 mg qd-bid increasing by 5 mg/day at weekly intervals

P *Child 3-6 yr:* PO 2.5 mg qd increasing by 2.5 mg/day at weekly intervals

Available forms: Tabs 5, 10 mg

Adverse effects
CNS: Hyperactivity, insomnia, restlessness, talkativeness, dizziness, headache, chills, stimulation, dysphoria, irritability, aggressiveness, tremor, dependence, addiction
CV: Palpitations, **tachycardia,** hypertension, dysrhythmias, decreased heart rate
GI: Nausea, vomiting, anorexia, dry mouth, diarrhea, constipation, weight loss, metallic taste, cramps
GU: Impotence, change in libido
INTEG: Urticaria

Contraindications: Hypersensitivity to sympathomimetic amines, hyperthyroidism, hypertension, glaucoma, severe arteriosclerosis, drug abuse, cardiovascular disease, anxiety

Precautions: Gilles de la Tourette's syndrome, lactation, P child <6 yr, pregnancy **C**

Pharmacokinetics	
Absorption	Well absorbed within 3 hr
Distribution	Widely distributed; crosses placenta; high concentrations in brain
Metabolism	Liver
Excretion	Kidneys: pH dependent, increased pH leads to increased reabsorption; breast milk
Half-life	10-30 hr; increased when urine is alkaline, decreased when urine is acidic

Pharmacodynamics	
Onset	½ hr
Peak	1-3 hr
Duration	4-20 hr

A

Interactions
Individual drugs
Acetazolamide: ↓ excretion, ↑ effect
Ammonium chloride: ↓ effect
Ascorbic acid: ↓ effect
Haloperidol: Altered CNS effect
Meperidine: Hypertensive crisis
Sodium bicarbonate: ↓ excretion, ↑ effect
Thyroid: ↑ effects
Drug classifications
Antidepressants, tricyclics: ↑ dysrhythmias
β-Blockers: ↑ hypertension
Cardiac glycosides: ↑ dysrhythmias
MAOIs: Hypertensive crisis
Phenothiazines: Altered CNS effect
Sympathomimetics: ↑ effect
Food/drug
Cranberries/juice: ↑ amphetamine effect
Caffeine: ↑ amphetamine effect
Herb/drug
Kava: ↓ amphetamine effect
Lab test interferences
↑ plasma corticosteroids, **Interference:** urinary steroids

NURSING CONSIDERATIONS
Assessment
• Monitor VS, B/P, since this drug may reverse antihypertensives; check patients with cardiac disease more often for increased B/P
• Monitor CBC, urinalysis; in diabetes blood sugar, urine sugar; insulin changes may be required, since eating will decrease
• Monitor height and weight q3 mo, since growth rate in children may be decreased; appetite is suppressed, weight loss is common during the first few months of treatment
• Monitor mental status: mood, sensorium, affect, stimulation, insomnia; aggressiveness may occur; depression with crying spells may occur after drug has worn off
• Assess for physical dependency; should not be used for extended time except in ADHD; should be discontinued gradually to prevent withdrawal symptoms
• Assess for narcoleptic symptoms before medication and after; ability to stay awake should increase significantly
• In children or adults with ADHD, monitor for improved organizational skills, attention span, attending to tasks, impulse control, socialization, and ability to get along better with others
• Assess for withdrawal symptoms: headache, nausea, vomiting, muscle pain, weakness; drug tolerance develops after long-term use; dosage should not be increased if tolerance develops; this medication has a high abuse potential

Nursing diagnoses
☑ Thought processes, altered (uses, adverse reactions)
☑ Coping, impaired individual (uses)
☑ Knowledge deficit (teaching)
☑ Family coping, impaired individual (uses)

Implementation
• Give at least 6 hr hs to avoid sleeplessness; titrate to patient's response, lowest dosage should be used to control symptoms
• Use gum, hard candy, frequent sips of water for dry

mouth at beginning of treatment; these symptoms tend to lessen with time

Patient/family education

• Advise patient to decrease caffeine consumption (coffee, tea, cola, chocolate), which may increase irritability and stimulation; to avoid OTC preparations unless approved by prescriber; to avoid alcohol ingestion; these may cause serious drug interactions

• Instruct patient to taper off drug over several wks, or depression, increased sleeping, lethargy may occur

• Advise patient to avoid hazardous activities until stabilized on medication

• Instruct patient not to double doses if medication is missed; prescriber may suggest drug holidays (ADHD) during the school year to assess progress and determine continued drug necessity

• Instruct patient/family to notify health care provider if significant side effects occur: tremors, insomnia, palpitations, restlessness, drug changes may be needed

• Inform patient that if dry mouth occurs to use frequent sips of water, sugarless gum, hard candy during beginning therapy; dry mouth lessens with continued treatment

• Tell patient to get needed rest; patients feel more tired at end of day; to give last dose at least 6 hr hs to avoid insomnia

Evaluation

Positive therapeutic outcome

• Decreased activity in ADHD

• Absence of sleeping during day in narcolepsy

Treatment of overdose:

Administer fluids, hemodialysis, peritoneal dialysis, antihypertensives for increased B/P; ammonium chloride for increased excretion

---

amphotericin B deoxycholate (℞)

(am-foh-tehr'ih-sin de-ox-ee-kohl'ate)

Fungizone

amphotericin B cholesteryl (℞)

(koh-less'ter-il)

Amphotec

amphotericin B lipid complex (℞)

Abelcet

amphotericin B liposome (℞)

(lip'oh-sohm)

AmBisome

Func. class.: Antifungal

Chem. class.: Amphoteric polyene

Pregnancy category   B

Action: Increases cell membrane permeability in susceptible organisms by binding sterols in fungal cell membrane; decreases potassium, sodium, and nutrients in cell

▶**Therapeutic Outcome:** Fungistatic against histoplasmosis, blastomycosis, coccidioidomycosis, cryptococcosis, aspergillosis, phycomycosis, candidiasis, sporotrichosis

Uses: Treatment of severe, possibly fatal fungal infections (**IV**); treatment of topical fungal infections (top)

Investigational uses: Candiduria (bladder irrigation)

Dosage and routes
Deoxycholate
Adult: IV Give test dose of 1 mg; then 0.5 mg/kg, increase qd slowly to 0.5 mg/kg, may give 1 mg/kg/day or 1.5 mg/kg qid

P *Child:* IV 0.25 mg/kg infused initially, increase by 0.25 mg/kg qod to max of 1 mg/kg/day

P *Adult and child:* TOP apply 2-4 × daily

P *Adult and child:* 1 ml qid

Cholesteryl sulfate
P *Adult and child:* IV 3-4 mg/kg/day, max 6 mg/kg/day

Lipid complex
P *Adult and child:* IV 5 mg/kg/day

Liposome
P *Adult and child:* IV Fungal infections 3-5 mg/kg q24h

Visceral Leishmaniasis: 3 mg/kg q24h days 1-5, and 14 and 21; give 4 mg/kg on day 1-5, 10, 17, 24, 31 and 38 to immunocompromised patients

Available forms:
Amphotericin deoxycholate inj 50 mg vial, oral susp 100 mg/ml; *amphotericin B cholesteryl* powder for inj 50 mg/20 ml; 100 mg/50 ml; *amphotericin B lipid complex* susp for inj 100 mg/20 ml vial; *amphotericin B liposome* powder for inj 50 mg as liposome

Adverse effects
CNS: Headache, fever, chills, peripheral nerve pain, paresthesias, peripheral neuropathy, **convulsions,** dizziness
EENT: Tinnitus, deafness, diplopia, blurred vision
GI: Nausea, vomiting, anorexia, diarrhea, cramps, **hemorrhagic gastroenteritis, acute liver failure**
GU: Hypokalemia, axotemia, hyposthenuria, **renal tubular acidosis,** nephrocalcinosis, **permanent renal impairment, anuria, oliguria**
HEMA: Normochromic and normocytic anemia, **thrombocytopenia, agranulocytosis, leukopenia, eosinophilia,** hypokalemia, hyponatremia, hypomagnesemia
INTEG: Burning, irritation, pain, necrosis at inj site with extravasation, flushing, dermatitis, skin rash (top route)
MS: Arthralgia, myalgia, generalized pain, weakness, weight loss

Contraindications:
Hypersensitivity, severe bone marrow depression

Precautions:
Renal disease, pregnancy **B**

Pharmacokinetics
Absorption	Complete bioavailability (IV), rapidly absorbed (top)
Distribution	Body tissues
Metabolism	Liver
Excretion	Kidneys, detectable for several weeks
Half-life	Initial 24-48 hr, terminal 15 days

Pharmacodynamics
	IV	TOP
Onset	Immediate	Unknown
Peak	1-2 hr	Unknown

Interactions
Individual drugs
Flucytosine: ↑ synergistic effect
Mezlocillin: ↑ hypokalemia
Piperacillin: ↑ hypokalemia
Thiazides: ↑ hypokalemia
Ticarcillin: ↑ hypokalemia

Drug classifications
Diuretics: ↑ nephrotoxicity, hypokalemia
Glucocorticoids: ↑ hypokalemia
Nephrotoxic drugs: ↑ nephrotoxicity

☑ *Herb/drug*
Gossypol: ↑ risk of nephrotoxicity

NURSING CONSIDERATIONS
Assessment
• Monitor VS q15-30 min during first inf; note changes in pulse, B/P
• Monitor blood studies: Hgb, Hct, potassium, sodium, calcium, magnesium q2 wk; BUN, creatinine weekly; decreased Hgb, Hct, and magnesium are common with increased potassium
• Monitor weight weekly; if weight increases over 2 lb/wk, edema is present; renal damage should be considered
• Monitor for renal toxicity: increasing BUN, serum creatinine; if BUN is >40 mg/dl or if serum creatinine >3 mg/dl, drug may be discontinued or dosage reduced; I&O ratio: watch for decreasing urinary output, change in sp gr; discontinue drug to prevent permanent damage to renal tubules; provide hydration of 2-3 L/day
• Monitor for hepatotoxicity: increasing AST, ALT, alkaline phosphatase, bilirubin
• Monitor for allergic reaction: dermatitis, rash; drug should be discontinued, antihistamines (mild reaction) or epinephrine (severe reaction) administered; check inj site for thrombophlebitis
• Monitor for hypokalemia: anorexia, drowsiness, weakness, decreased reflexes, dizziness, increased urinary output, increased thirst, paresthesias; if these occur, drug should be decreased or discontinued and potassium administered

Top route
• Monitor for allergic reaction: burning, stinging, swelling, redness

Nursing diagnoses
☑ Infection, risk for (uses)
☑ Injury, risk for physical (adverse reaction)
☑ Knowledge deficit (teaching)

Implementation
Top route
• Provide enough medication to cover lesions completely; do not cover with occlusive dressing; apply liberally and rub thoroughly into affected area; administer after cleansing with soap, water before each application, dry well (as ordered), wear gloves during application
• Store at room temp in dry place

Ⅳ IV route
Deoxycholate
• Give after diluting 50 mg in 10 ml sterile water (no preservatives) (5 mg-1 ml); shake well, further dilute with 500 ml of D_5W to concentration of 0.1 mg/ml; do not use other diluents or sol; use large needle (20 G); change needle for each step; wear gloves
• Use test dosage of 1 mg/20 ml D_5W; give over 10-30 min; if no reaction, drug is administered as ordered
• Administer **IV** using in-line filter (mean pore diameter >1 μm) using distal veins; check for extravasation, necrosis q8h; use an inf pump; administer over 6 hr; rapid inf may result in circulation collapse; may also be given through central line

• Give acetaminophen and diphenhydramine 30 min before inf to reduce fever, chills, headache
• Give drug only after C&S confirm organism, drug needed to treat condition; make sure drug is used in life-threatening infections
• Store protected from moisture and light; diluted sol is stable for 24 hr at room temp, 1 wk refrigerated

Syrup compatibilities:
Heparin

Y-site compatibilities:
Aldesleukin, diltiazem, doxorubicin liposome, famotidine, remifentanil, tacrolimus, teniposide, thiotepa, zidovudine

Y-site incompatibilities:
Enalaprilat, fludarabine, foscarnet, ondansetron

Additive compatibilities:
Fluconazole, heparin, hydrocortisone, methylprednisolone, sodium bicarbonate

Solution compatibilities:
D_5W

Patient/family education
Top route
• Teach patient that skin and clothing may become discolored; to use asepsis (hand washing) before, after each application to prevent further infection
• Instruct patient to apply with glove to prevent further infection; not to cover with occlusive dressing; to continue even if condition improves
• Teach patient to avoid use of OTC creams, ointments, lotions, unless directed by prescriber
• Instruct patient to report increased itching, burning, rash, redness; ointment may

irritate most hairy areas; to report if condition worsens

IV IV route
• Advise patient that long-term therapy may be needed to clear infection (2 wk-3 mo depending on type of infection)
• Teach patient side effects and when to notify prescriber

Evaluation
Positive therapeutic outcome
• Decrease in size, number of lesions (top)
• Decreased fever, malaise, rash
• Negative C&S for infecting organism

---

ampicillin (Ŗ)
(am-pi-sill'in)
Amcil, Ampicin ✤, Apo-Ampi ✤, D-Amp ✤, Nu-Ampi ✤, NovoAmpicillin ✤, Penbriten ✤, Polycillin, Principen, Omnipen, Omnipen-N, Polycillin-N, Totacillin, Totacillin-N
Func. class.: Broadspectrum antiinfective
Chem. class.: Aminopenicillin

Pregnancy category   B

Action: Interferes with cell wall replication of susceptible organisms; the cell wall, rendered osmotically unstable, swells, bursts from osmotic pressure

➡**Therapeutic Outcome:**
Bactericidal effects for the following organisms: effective for gram-positive cocci *(Streptococcus pyogenes, Streptococcus faecalis, Streptococcus pneumoniae)*, gram-negative cocci *(Neisseria gonorrhoeae, N. meningitidis)*, gram-negative

bacilli *(Haemophilus influenzae, Proteus mirabilis, Salmonella, Shigella, Listeria monocytogenes)*, gram-positive bacilli

Uses: Infections of respiratory tract, skin, skin structures, genitourinary tract; otitis media, meningitis, septicemia, sinusitis, and endocarditis prophylaxis

Dosage and routes
Renal disease
CrCl 10-30 ml/min dose q6-12h; <10 ml/min dose q12h

Systemic infections
P *Adult and child ≥40 kg (88 lbs):* PO 250-500 mg q6h or 1-2 g qd in divided doses q6h; **IV**/IM 250-500 mg q6h, (up to 2 g q4h in severe infections) or 2-8 g qd in divided doses q4-6h

P *Child <40 kg:* PO 25-100 mg/kg/day in divided doses q6h; **IV**/IM 25-50 mg/kg/day in divided doses q8h for septicemia or bacterial meningitis

Meningitis
Adult: **IV** 8-14 g/day in divided doses q3-4h × 3 days
P *Child:* **IV** 100-200 mg/kg/day in divided doses q3-4h × 3 days

Gonorrhea
P *Adult and child ≥ 45 kg (99 lbs):* PO 3.5 g given with 1 g probenecid as a single dose or IM/**IV** 500 mg q 8-12 hr × 2 doses

Available forms: Powder for inj 125, 250, 500 mg, 1, 2 g; **IV** inf 500 mg, 1, 2 g; caps 250, 500 mg; powder for oral susp 100/ml, 125, 250, 500 mg/5 ml

Adverse effects
CNS: Lethargy, hallucinations, anxiety, depression, twitching, **coma, convulsions**
GI: Nausea, vomiting, diarrhea, **pseudomembranous colitis**
GU: Oliguria, proteinuria, hematuria, *vaginitis, moniliasis,* **glomerulonephritis**
HEMA: Anemia, increased bleeding time, **bone marrow depression, granulocytopenia**
INTEG: Rash, urticaria
SYST: **Anaphylaxis**

Contraindications: Hypersensitivity to penicillins

Precautions: Pregnancy **B**; hypersensitivity to cephalo-
P sporins; neonates; renal disease

N **Do Not Confuse:**
Omnipen/imipenem

Pharmacokinetics	
Absorption	Moderate, duodenum (35%-50%)
Distribution	Readily in body tissues, fluids, CSF; crosses placenta
Metabolism	Liver (30%)
Excretion	Breast milk; kidney unchanged (70%)
Half-life	50-110 min

Pharmacodynamics			
	PO	IM	IV
Onset	Rapid	Rapid	Rapid
Peak	2 hr	1 hr	Infusion's end

Interactions
Individual drugs
Allopurinol: ↑ ampicillin-induced skin rash
Disulfiram: ↑ ampicillin concentrations
Probenecid: ↑ ampicillin levels, ↓ renal excretion
Drug classifications
Oral contraceptives: ↓ contraceptive effectiveness

☑ Herb/drug ⬛ Do Not Crush ◆ Alert ⦵ Key Drug ⬛ Geriatric **P** Pediatric

⊘ *Herb/drug*
Khat: ↓ absorption
Lab test interferences
False positive: Urine glucose, urine protein

NURSING CONSIDERATIONS
Assessment

• Assess patient for previous sensitivity reaction to penicillins or other cephalosporins; cross-sensitivity between penicillins and cephalosporins is common

• Assess patient for signs and symptoms of infection, including characteristics of wounds, sputum, urine, stool, WBC >10,000, earache, fever; obtain baseline information and during treatment

• Obtain C&S before beginning drug therapy to identify if correct treatment has been initiated

• Assess for allergic reactions: rash, urticaria, pruritus, chills, fever, joint pain; angioedema may occur a few days after therapy begins; epinephrine and resuscitation equipment should be on unit for anaphylactic reaction; also, check for ampicillin rash: pruritic, red, raised

◆• Identify urine output; if decreasing, notify prescriber (may indicate nephrotoxicity)

• Monitor renal studies: urinalysis, protein, blood, BUN, creatinine

• Monitor blood studies: AST, ALT, CBC, Hct, bilirubin, LDH, alkaline phosphatase, Coombs' test monthly if patient is on long-term therapy

• Monitor electrolytes: potassium, sodium, chloride monthly if patient is on long-term therapy

• Assess bowel pattern qd; if severe diarrhea occurs, drug should be discontinued; may indicate pseudomembranous colitis

• Monitor for bleeding: ecchymosis, bleeding gums, hematuria, stool guaiac daily if on long-term therapy

• Assess for overgrowth of infection: perineal itching, fever, malaise, redness, pain, swelling, drainage, rash, diarrhea, change in cough, sputum

Nursing diagnoses
☑ Infection, risk for (uses)
☑ Injury, risk for (side effects)
☑ Diarrhea (side effects)
☑ Knowledge deficit (teaching)
☑ Noncompliance (teaching)

Implementation
PO route

• Give in even doses around the clock; drug must be taken for 10-14 days to ensure organism death and prevent superinfection; store caps in tight container

• Tabs may be crushed or caps opened and mixed with water

• Shake suspension well before each dose; store in refrigerator for 2 wk or 1 wk at room temp

IM route

• Reconstitute with 125 mg/ 0.9-1.2 ml; 250 mg/0.9-1.9 ml; 500 mg/1.2-1.8 ml; 1 g/2.4-7.4 ml; 2 g/6.8 ml

• Give deep in large muscle mass

IV route

• Reconstitute with 125 mg/ 0.9-1.2 ml; 250 mg/0.9-1.9 ml; 500 mg/1.2-1.8 ml; 1 g/2.4-7.4 ml; 2 g/6.8 ml

• Give by direct **IV** over 3-5 min in lower dosages (125-500 mg) or over 15 min in higher dosages (1-2 g)

• Give by intermittent inf after diluting with 0.9% NaCl, LR,

---

D_5W, D_5/0.45% NaCl; use 50 ml of sol and dilute to concentration of <30 mg/ml

Syringe incompatibilities:
Erythromycin, gentamicin, kanamycin, lincomycin, metoclopramide, oxytetracycline, streptomycin, tetracycline

Syringe compatibilities:
Chloramphenicol, colistimethate, heparin, procaine

Y-site incompatibilities:
Calcium gluconate, epinephrine, fluconazole, hetastarch, hydromorphone, hydralazine, ondansetron, sargramostim, verapamil, vinorelbine

Y-site compatibilities:
Acyclovir, amifostine, allopurinol, aztreonam, cyclophosphamide, doxorubicin liposome, enalaprilat, esmolol, famotidine, filgrastim, fludarabine, foscarnet, granisetron, heparin, regular insulin, labetalol, magnesium sulfate, melphalan, meperidine, morphine, multivitamins, oflaxacin, perphenazine, phytonadione, potassium chloride, propofol, remifentanil, thiotepa, tolazoline, vitamin B with C

Additive incompatibilities:
Amikacin, azetreonam, chlorpromazine, dopamine, gentamicin, hydralazine, hydrocortisone, prochlorperazine

Additive compatibilities:
Cefotiam, clindamycin, erythromycin, floxacillin, furosemide, tacrolimus, teniposide, theophylline, verapamil

Patient/family education
⬥• Teach patient to report sore throat, bruising, bleeding, joint pain; may indicate blood dyscrasias (rare)

• Advise patient to contact prescriber if vaginal itching, loose, foul-smelling stools, furry tongue occur; may indicate superinfection
• Instruct patient to take all medication prescribed for the length of time ordered
• Advise patient to notify prescriber of diarrhea with blood or pus, which may indicate pseudomembranous colitis
• Tab may be crushed; cap may be opened and mixed with water

Evaluation
Positive therapeutic outcome
• Absence of signs/symptoms of infection (WBC <10,000, temp WNL, absence of red draining wounds, earache)
• Reported improvement in symptoms of infection

Treatment of anaphylaxis:
Withdraw drug, maintain airway, administer epinephrine, aminophylline, O_2, **IV** corticosteroids

ampicillin/ sulbactam (℞)
(am-pi-sill'in/sul-bak'tam)
Unasyn
Func. class.: Broad-spectrum antiinfective
Chem. class.: Aminopenicillin

Pregnancy category   B
(ampicillin)

Action: Interferes with cell wall replication of susceptible organisms; the cell wall, rendered osmotically unstable, swells and bursts from osmotic pressure; this combination extends the spectrum of activ-

---

ity and inhibits β-lactamase that may inactivate ampicillin

Therapeutic Outcome:
Bactericidal against *Pneumococcus*, *Enterococcus*, *Streptococcus*, *Escherichia coli*, *Proteus mirabilis*, *Neisseria meningitidis*, *Neisseria gonorrhoeae*, *Shigella*, *Salmonella*, and *Haemophilus influenzae* organisms; use only with β-lactamase–producing strain of infection

Uses: Skin and structure infections, intraabdominal infections, gynecologic infections, soft tissue infections, otitis media, sinusitis, meningitis, septicemia

Dosage and routes
Renal disease
CrCl 15-29 ml/min dose q12h; CrCl 5-14 ml/min dose q24h

Adult and child >40 kg: **IV** 1 g ampicillin and 0.5 g sulbactam or 2 g ampicillin, and 1 g sulbactam q6h, not to exceed 4 g/day sulbactam

P *Child:* <40 kg **IV** 300 mg/ kg/day (ampicillin component) divided q6h

Available forms: Powder for inj 1.5 g (1 g ampicillin, 0.5 g sulbactam), 3 g (2 g ampicillin, 1 g sulbactam)

Adverse effects
CNS: Lethargy, hallucinations, anxiety, depression, twitching, **coma, convulsions**
GI: Nausea, vomiting, diarrhea, increased AST, ALT, abdominal pain, glossitis, colitis, **pseudomembranous colitis**
GU: Oliguria, proteinuria, hematuria, *vaginitis, moniliasis,* **glomerulonephritis**
HEMA: Anemia, increased

bleeding time, **bone marrow depression, granulocytopenia** *SYST:* **Anaphylaxis**

Contraindications: Hypersensitivity to penicillins

Precautions: Pregnancy **B,** hypersensitivity to cephalosporins, neonates, renal disease

Pharmacokinetics	
Absorption	Well absorbed (IM)
Distribution	Readily in body tissues, fluids, CSF; crosses placenta
Metabolism	Liver (10%-50%)
Excretion	Breast milk; kidney unchanged (75%)
Half-life	50-110 min (ampicillin)

Pharmacodynamics		
	IM	IV
Onset	Rapid	Immediate
Peak	1 hr	Infusion's end

Interactions
Individual drugs
Allopurinol: ampicillin-induced skin rash
Probenecid: ↑ ampicillin levels, ↓ renal excretion
Drug classifications
Oral contraceptives: ↓ contraceptive effectiveness
Herb/drug
Khat: ↓ absorption
Lab test interferences
False positive: Urine glucose, urine protein

NURSING CONSIDERATIONS
Assessment
• Assess patient for previous sensitivity reaction to penicillins or cephalosporins; cross-sensitivity between penicillins and cephalosporins is common
• Assess patient for signs and symptoms of infection; including characteristics of wounds,

sputum, urine, stool, WBC >10,000, earache, fever; obtain baseline information and during treatment

• Complete C&S before beginning drug therapy to identify if correct treatment has been initiated

• Assess for allergic reactions: rash, urticaria, pruritus, chills, fever, joint pain; angioedema may occur a few days after therapy begins; epinephrine and resuscitation equipment should be on unit for anaphylactic reaction

◆•• Identify urine output; if decreasing, notify prescriber (may indicate nephrotoxicity)

• Assess renal studies: urinalysis, protein, BUN, creatinine

• Monitor blood studies: AST, ALT, CBC, Hct, bilirubin, LDH, alkaline phosphatase, Coombs' test monthly if patient is on long-term therapy

• Monitor electrolytes: potassium, sodium, chloride monthly if patient is on long-term therapy

• Assess bowel pattern qd; if severe diarrhea occurs, drug should be discontinued; may indicate pseudomembranous colitis

• Monitor for bleeding: ecchymosis, bleeding gums, hematuria, stool guaiac daily if on long-term therapy

• Assess for superinfection: perineal itching, fever, malaise, redness, pain, swelling, drainage, rash, diarrhea, change in cough, sputum

Nursing diagnoses

☑ Infection, risk for (uses)
☑ Diarrhea (adverse reactions)
☑ Injury, risk for (adverse reactions)
☑ Knowledge deficit (teaching)
☑ Noncompliance (teaching)

Implementation

IM route

• Reconstitute by adding 3.2 ml/1.5 g or 6.4 ml/3 g; use sterile water, 0.5% or 2% lidocaine; give within 1 hr of preparation; give deep in large muscle mass

• Give after C&S completed; on empty stomach

IV IV route

• Give **IV** after diluting 1.5 g/4 ml or more sterile H_2O for inj (375 mg/ml); allow to stand until foaming stops; give directly over 15-30 min; dilute further in 50 ml of D_5W, D_5/10.45% NaCl, 10% invert sugar in water, LR, 6% sodium lactate, isotonic NaCl; administer within 1 hr after reconstitution; give as an intermittent inf over 15-30 min

Y-site incompatibilities:

Idarubicin, ondansetron, sargramostim

Y-site compatibilities:

Amifostine, aztreonam, cefepime, enalaprilat, famotidine, filgrastim, fluconazole, fludarabine, granisetron, heparin, regular insulin, meperidine, morphine, paclitaxel, remifentanil, tacrolimus, teniposide, theophylline, thiotepa

Additive incompatibilities:

Aminoglycosides

Additive compatibilities:

Aztreonam

Patient/family education

• Teach patient to report sore throat, bruising, bleeding, joint pain, persistent diarrhea; may indicate blood dyscrasias (rare) or superinfection

---

• Advise patient to contact prescriber if vaginal itching, loose, foul-smelling stools, furry tongue occur; may indicate superinfection

• Instruct patient to use another form of contraception other than oral contraceptives

Evaluation
Positive therapeutic outcome
• Absence of signs/symptoms of infection (WBC <10,000, temp WNL, absence of red draining wounds, earache)
• Reported improvement in symptoms of infection

Treatment of overdose: Withdraw drug, maintain airway, administer epinephrine, aminophylline, O_2, **IV** corticosteroids for anaphylaxis

---

amprenavir
See Appendix A,
Selected New Drugs

---

amrinone (℞)
(am'ri-none)
Inocor
Func. class.: Cardiac inotropic agent
Chem. class.: Bipyrimidine derivative

Pregnancy category   C

Action: Positive inotropic agent with vasodilator properties; reduces preload and afterload by direct relaxation of vascular smooth muscle; increases myocardial contractility

⊐ **Therapeutic Outcome:** Increased inotropic effect resulting in increased cardiac output

Uses: Short-term management of CHF that has not responded to other medication; can be used with digitalis products

Dosage and routes
🄟 *Adult and child:* **IV** bol 0.75 mg/kg given over 2-3 min; start inf of 5-10 μg/kg/min; may give another bol 30 min after start of therapy, not to exceed 10 mg/kg total daily dose

Available forms: Inj 5 mg/ml

Adverse effects
CV: Dysrhythmias, hypotension, headache, chest pain
ELECT: Hypokalemia
GI: Nausea, vomiting, anorexia, abdominal pain, **hepatotoxicity (rare), ascites,** jaundice, hiccups
HEMA: **Thrombocytopenia**
INTEG: Allergic reactions, burning at inj site
RESP: Pleuritis, **pulmonary densities, hypoxemia,** dyspnea

Contraindications: Hypersensitivity to this drug or bisulfites, severe aortic disease, severe pulmonic valvular disease, acute MI

Precautions: Lactation, preg-
🄟 nancy **C,** children, renal disease, hepatic disease, atrial
🄖 flutter/fibrillation, elderly

🄝 **Do Not Confuse:**
amrinone/amiodarone,
Inocor/Cordarone

Pharmacokinetics	
Absorption	Complete bioavailability
Distribution	Unknown
Metabolism	Liver, 50%
Excretion	Kidney, metabolites (60%-90%)
Half-life	4-6 hr, increased in CHF

Pharmacodynamics	
Onset	2-5 min
Peak	10 min
Duration	Variable

Interactions
Individual drugs
Disopyramide: ↑ hypotension
Drug classifications
Antihypertensives: ↑ hypotension
Cardiac glycosides: ↑ inotropic effect
⬚ Herb/drug
Aloe: ↑ amrinone action
Buckthorn bark/berry: ↑ amrinone action
Cascara sagrada: ↑ amrinone action
Ephedra: ↑ amrinone action
Senna pod/leaf: ↑ amrinone action
Lab test interferences
↓ Potassium, ↑ hepatic enzymes

NURSING CONSIDERATIONS
Assessment
• Monitor manifestations of hypokalemia: *renal:* acidic urine, reduced urine, osmolality, nocturia; *CV:* hypotension, broad T wave, U wave, ectopy, tachycardia, weak pulse; *neuro:* muscle weakness, altered LOC, drowsiness, apathy, lethargy, confusion, depression; *GI:* anorexia, nausea, cramps, constipation, distention, paralytic ileus; *resp:* hypoventilation, respiratory muscle weakness
• Assess fluid volume status:
G CVP in elderly, I&O ratio and record, weight, distended red veins, crackles in lung, color, quality and sp gr of urine, skin turgor, adequacy of pulses, moist mucous membranes, bilateral lung sounds, peripheral pitting edema; dehydration symptoms of decreasing output, thirst, hypotension, dry mouth, and mucous membranes should be reported
• Monitor electrolytes: potassium, sodium, calcium, magnesium; also include BUN, blood pH, ABGs
• Monitor B/P and pulse, PCWP, CVP, index, often during infusion; if B/P drops 30 mm Hg, stop infusion and call prescriber
• Monitor ALT, AST, bilirubin daily; if these are elevated, hepatoxicity is suspected
◆• If platelets are <150,000/mm³, drug is usually discontinued and another drug started
• Assess for extravasation: change site q48h

Nursing diagnoses
✓ Cardiac output, decreased (uses)
✓ Fluid volume excess (uses)
✓ Knowledge deficit (teaching)

Implementation
General
• Patients with low potassium levels (hypokalemia) should receive potassium supplements before amrinone administration
• Administer potassium supplements if ordered for potassium levels <3.0 mg/dl
Ⅳ IV route
• Do not mix directly with glucose sol; chemical reaction occurs over 24 hr; precipitate forms if amrinone and furosemide come in contact
Ⅳ Direct IV
• Administer into running dextrose inf through Y-connector or directly into tubing; may give undiluted over 2-3 min or dilute with NS to concentration of 1-3 mg/

ml; run at prescribed rate; another loading dose may be given in 30 min

IV Cont IV
• Give after diluting with 0.9%, or 0.45% NaCl (1-3 mg/ml); do not dilute with dextrose sol; decomposition of drug will occur; use inf pump; use sol within 24 hr of dilution; titrate to patient response

Syringe compatibilities: Propranolol, verapamil

Y-site compatibilities: Aminophylline, atropine, bretylium, calcium chloride, cimetidine, cisatracurium, digoxin, dobutamine, dopamine, epinephrine, famotidine, hydrocortisone, isoproterenol, lidocaine, metaraminol, methylprednisolone, nitroglycerin, nitroprusside, norepinephrine, phenylephrine, potassium chloride, procainamide, propranolol, remifentanil, verapamil

Y-site incompatibilities: Furosemide, sodium bicarbonate

Patient/family education
• Teach patient reason for medication and expected results
• Instruct patient to make position changes slowly; orthostatic hypotension may occur
• Teach patient signs and symptoms of hypersensitivity reactions and hypokalemia
• Advise patient that burning may occur at **IV** site

Evaluation
Positive therapeutic outcome
• Increased cardiac output
• Decreased PCWP, adequate CVP
• Decreased dyspnea, fatigue, edema, ECG

Treatment of overdose: Discontinue drug, support circulation

A

anagrelide (℞)
(a-na′gre-lide)
Agrylin
Func. class.: Antiplatelet
Chem. class.: Imidazoquinazolinone

Pregnancy category   C

Action: Reduces platelet count (mechanism not clear) and prevents early platelet shape changes in response to aggregating agents thus inhibiting platelet aggregation

Therapeutic Outcome: Inhibition of platelet aggregation

Uses: Essential thrombocythemia

Dosage and routes
Adult: PO 0.5 mg qid or 1 mg bid, may be adjusted after 1 wk, max 10 mg/day or 2.5 mg single dose

Available forms: Caps 0.5, 1.0 mg

Adverse effects
CNS: Headache, dizziness, seizures
CV: Postural hypotension, tachycardia, palpitations, **CHF, MI,** cardiomyopathy, cardiomegaly, **complete heart block, atrial fibrillation, arrhythmia**
HEMA: Anemia, **thrombocytopenia,** ecchymosis, lymphadenoma
INTEG: Rash

Contraindications: Hypersensitivity, hypotension

Precautions: Pregnancy **C**

Pharmacokinetics

Absorption	Unknown
Distribution	Unknown
Metabolism	Liver, extensively
Excretion	Feces/urine
Half-life	1.3 hr

Pharmacodynamics

Onset	Unknown
Peak	1 hr
Duration	>24 hr

Interactions
Individual drugs
Sucralfate: ↓ absorption
Food/drug
↓ absorption

NURSING CONSIDERATIONS
Assessment
• Monitor B/P, pulse baseline and during treatment until stable; take B/P with patient lying, standing; orthostatic hypotension is common
• Assess cardiac status: chest pain, what aggravates or ameliorates condition

Nursing diagnoses
☑ Cardiac output, decreased (uses)
☑ Knowledge deficit (teaching)

Implementation
• Give with 8 oz of water; to improve absorption give on an empty stomach
• Store at room temp

Patient/family education
• Teach patient that this medication is not a cure; that drug may have to be taken continuously in evenly spaced doses only as directed; if a dose is missed, take one when remembered up to 4 hr; do not double doses
• Inform patient that it is necessary to quit smoking to prevent excessive vasoconstriction
• Advise patient to rise slowly from sitting or lying down to prevent orthostatic hypotension
• Caution patient not to use alcohol or OTC medication unless approved by prescriber
• Caution patient to avoid hazardous activities until stabilized on medication; dizziness may occur
• Teach patient to report cardiac reactions, ↑ bruising/bleeding
• Advise patient to use contraception (female, child bearing)

Evaluation
Positive therapeutic outcome
• Absence of thrombo-cythemia

---

anastrozole (℞)
(an-ass-stroh′zole)
Arimidex
Func. class.: Antineoplastic
Chem. class.: Aromatase inhibitor
Pregnancy category   D

Action: Lowers serum estradiol concentrations; many breast cancers have strong estrogen receptors

➲**Therapeutic Outcome:** Prevention of rapidly growing malignant cells

Uses: Advanced breast carcinoma that has not responded to other therapy in estrogen-receptor-positive patients (usually postmenopausal)

Dosage and routes
Adult: PO 1 mg qd

Available forms: Tab 1 mg

Adverse effects
CNS: Hot flashes, headache, light-headedness, depression,

---

dizziness, confusion, insomnia, anxiety
CV: Chest pain, hypertension, thrombophlebitis
GI: Nausea, vomiting, altered taste, anorexia, diarrhea, constipation, abdominal pain, dry mouth
GU: Vaginal bleeding, pruritus vulvae
HEMA: Thrombocytopenia, leukopenia
INTEG: Rash, alopecia
MS: Bone pain, myalgia
RESP: Cough, sinusitis

Contraindications: Hypersensitivity, pregnancy **D**

Precautions: Leukopenia, thrombocytopenia, lactation, **P** cataracts, children, elderly, liver **G** disease, renal disease

Pharmacokinetics	
Absorption	Adequately absorbed
Distribution	Unknown
Metabolism	Liver
Excretion	Feces, urine
Half-life	50 hr

Pharmacodynamics	
Onset	Unknown
Peak	4-7 hr
Duration	Unknown

Interactions
Lab test interferences
↑ GGT, ↑ AST, ↑ ALT, ↑ alk phosphatase, ↑ cholesterol, ↑ LDL

NURSING CONSIDERATIONS
Assessment
• Monitor CBC, differential, platelet count weekly; withhold drug if WBC is <4000 or platelet count is <75,000; notify prescriber of results; monitor calcium levels (hypercalcemia is common)
• Assess for tumor flare: increase in bone, tumor pain

during beginning treatment; give analgesics as ordered to decrease pain
• Assess for bleeding: hematuria, guaiac, bruising or petechiae, mucosa or orifices, q8h; no rec temp

Nursing diagnoses
☑ Injury, risk for (adverse reactions)
☑ Knowledge deficit (teaching)

Implementation
• Give with food or fluids for GI upset; do not break, crush, or chew enteric products; repeat dose may be needed if vomiting occurs
• Store in light-resistant container at room temp

Patient/family education
• Instruct patient to report any complaints, side effects to health care prescriber; if dose is missed, do not double next dose
• Advise patient that vaginal bleeding, pruritus, hot flashes, can occur, and are reversible after discontinuing treatment
• Inform patient about who should be told about tamoxifen therapy
• Advise patient to report vaginal bleeding immediately; that tumor flare—increase in size or tumor, increased bone pain—may occur and will subside rapidly; may take analgesics for pain
• Caution patient to use sunscreen and protective clothing to prevent burns because photosensitivity is common
• Teach patient that hair loss may occur during treatment; a wig or hairpiece may make patient feel better; new hair may be different in color, texture
• Inform patient that rash or

lesions are temporary and may become large during beginning therapy

Evaluation
Positive therapeutic outcome
• Decreased spread of malignant cells in breast cancer

---

anistreplase (℞)
(an-is-tre-plaze′)
APSAC, Eminase
Func. class.: Thrombolytic enzyme
Chem. class.: Anisoylated plasminogen streptokinase activator complex
Pregnancy category   C

Action: Promotes thrombolysis by promoting conversion of plasminogen to plasmin; complex is a combination of plasminogen and streptokinase

⭢Therapeutic Outcome: Thrombolysis in coronary arteries

Uses: Management of acute MI; for lysis of coronary artery thrombi

Dosage and routes
Adult: **IV** inj 30 U over 4-5 min as soon as possible after onset of symptoms

Available forms: Powder, lyophilized 30 U/vial

Adverse effects
CNS: Headache, fever, sweating, agitation, dizziness, paresthesia, tremor, vertigo
CV: Hypotension, **dysrhythmias,** conduction disorders
GI: Nausea, vomiting
HEMA: Decreased Hct, **GI, GU, intracranial, retroperitoneal,** surface bleeding; **thrombocytopenia**

INTEG: Rash, urticaria, phlebitis at site, itching, flushing
MS: Low back pain, arthralgia
RESP: Altered respirations, dyspnea, **bronchospasm, lung edema**
SYST: **Anaphylaxis (rare)**

Contraindications: Hypersensitivity, active internal bleeding, intraspinal or intracranial surgery, neoplasms of CNS, severe hypertension, cerebral embolism, thrombosis, hemorrhage

Precautions: Arterial emboli from left side of heart, pregnancy **C,** ulcerative colitis/enteritis, renal disease, hepatic disease, hypocoagulation, COPD, subacute bacterial endocarditis, rheumatic valvular disease, intraarterial diagnostic procedure or surgery (10 days), recent major surgery, hypersensitivity to this drug or streptokinase

Pharmacokinetics	
Absorption	Complete bioavailability
Distribution	Unknown
Metabolism	Binds to plasmin
Excretion	Kidneys
Half-life	105 min

Pharmacodynamics	
Onset	Unknown
Peak	45 min
Duration	Unknown

Interactions
Individual drugs
Aspirin: ↑ bleeding potential
Dipyridamole: ↑ bleeding potential
Heparin: ↑ bleeding potential
Indomethacin: ↑ bleeding potential
Phenylbutazone: ↑ bleeding potential

Drug classifications
Anticoagulants: ↑ bleeding potential
NSAIDs: ↑ bleeding potential
🗲 *Herb/drug*
Bromelain: ↑ risk of bleeding
Lab test interferences
↑ PT, ↑ APTT, ↑ TT
↓ Fibrinogen, ↓ plasminogen

NURSING CONSIDERATIONS

Assessment

• Monitor VS, B/P, pulse, respirations, neurologic signs, temp at least q4h, temp >104° F (40° C) or indicators of internal bleeding, cardiac rhythm after intracoronary administration
• Assess for allergy: fever, rash, itching, chills; mild reaction may be treated with antihistamines; hypersensitivity reactions/dyspnea, wheezing, facial swelling should be treated with epinephrine
⬧• Monitor bleeding during 1st hr of treatment (hematuria, hematemesis, bleeding from mucous membranes, epistaxis, ecchymosis), continue to monitor for 24 hr after treatment; blood studies (Hct, platelets, PTT, PT, TT, APTT) before starting therapy; PT or APTT must be less than 2 × control before starting therapy; TT or PT q3-4h during treatment
• Monitor ECG, treat bradycardia, ventricular changes

Nursing diagnoses

✓ Tissue perfusion, decreased (uses)
✓ Injury, risk for (uses, adverse reactions)
✓ Knowledge deficit (teaching)

Implementation

• Give heparin therapy after thrombolytic therapy is discontinued, TT or APTT less than 2 × control (about 3-4 hr)
• Avoid invasive procedures: inj, rec temp; about 10% of patients have high streptococcal antibody titers, requiring increased loading doses
• Treat fever with acetaminophen
• Provide pressure for 30 sec to minor bleeding sites, 30 min to sites of arterial puncture followed by dressing; inform prescriber if hemostasis not attained; apply pressure dressing
• Give after reconstituting single-dose vial/5 ml sterile water for inj (not bacteriostatic water), and roll (not shake) to enhance reconstitution, try to minimize foaming; give over 2-5 min by direct **IV**, give within ½ hr of reconstitution or discard, do not add other meds to vial or syringe; give within 6 hr of thrombi identification for best results; cryoprecipitate or fresh frozen plasma if bleeding occurs; store powder in refrigerator; use within 30 min after reconstitution

Incompatibilities:
Do not mix with other drugs in sol or syringe

Patient/family education

• Teach patient action of drug and expected outcome; alert patient to possible hypersensitivity reactions and symptoms to report
• Advise patient bed rest is needed during entire course of treatment; handle patient as little as possible during therapy

Evaluation

Positive therapeutic outcome
• Absence of thrombolysis in MI
• Improved ventricular function

antihemophilic factor (AHF) (℞)
(an-tee-hee-moe-fill'ik)
Alphanate, antihemophilic factor, Helixate, Hemofilm, Humate-P, Koate-HP, Kogenate, Monoclate-P, Recombinate
Func. class.: Hemostatic, blood factor
Chem. class.: Factor VIII
Pregnancy category C

Action: Necessary for clotting. Activates factor X in conjunction with activated factor IX; transforms prothrombin to thrombin

➡ **Therapeutic Outcome:** Control of hemorrhage or excessive bleeding in factor VIII deficiency

Uses: Hemophilia A, patients with acquired circulating factor VIII inhibitors, factor VIII deficiency

Dosage and routes
Depends on severity of deficiency and level of antihemophilic factor

Massive hemorrhage
P *Adult and child:* **IV** 40-50 U/kg, then 20-25 U/kg q8-12h

Bleeding (overt)
P *Adult and child:* **IV** 15-25 U/kg, then 8-15 U/kg q8-12h × 4 days

Hemorrhage near vital organs
P *Adult and child:* **IV** 15 U/kg, then 8 U/kg q8h × 2 days, then 4 U/kg q8h × 2 days

Minor hemorrhage
P *Adult and child:* **IV** 8-10 U/kg/q24 hr × 2-3 days or 8 U/kg q12h × 2 days, then q24h × 2 days

Joint bleeding
P *Adult and child:* **IV** 5-10 U/kg q8-12h × 1-2 days

Available forms: Inj 250, 500, 1000, 1500 U/vial (number of units noted on label)

Adverse effects
CNS: Headache, *lethargy, chills, fever, flushing*
CV: Hypotension, tachycardia
GI: Nausea, vomiting, abdominal cramps, jaundice, **viral hepatitis**
HEMA: **Thrombosis, hemolysis, risk of hepatitis B, HIV**
INTEG: Rash, flushing, *urticaria,* stinging at inj site
RESP: **Bronchospasm**

Contraindications: Hypersensitivity, monoclonal antibody–derived factor VIII

P **Precautions:** Neonates/infants, hepatic disease, blood types A, B, AB, pregnancy **C**, factor VIII inhibitor

Pharmacokinetics	
Absorption	Complete availability
Distribution	Plasma
Metabolism	Not metabolized
Excretion	No excretion
Half-life	Biphasic 4 hr, 15 hr

Pharmacodynamics	
Onset	Immediate
Peak	Unknown
Duration	12 hr

Interactions: None

NURSING CONSIDERATIONS
Assessment
• Monitor blood studies (coagulation factors assay by % normal: 5% prevents spontaneous hemorrhage, 30%-50% for surgery, 80%-100% for severe hemorrhage; blood group of patient, donors (if applicable;

🅭 Herb/drug 🅢 Do Not Crush ◆ Alert ☞ Key Drug 🅖 Geriatric 🅟 Pediatric

most factor VIII not from specific blood group donors)
- Monitor I&O, urine color; notify prescriber if urine becomes orange, red; change in urine color signifying hemolytic reaction; patients other than blood type O are more at risk
- Monitor pulse: discontinue infusion if significant increase
- Obtain test for factor VIII inhibitors before starting treatment, may require concomitant antiinhibitor coagulant complex therapy; Hct, Coombs' test with blood types A, B, AB
- Assess for allergy: fever, rash, itching, jaundice, wheezing, tachycardia, nausea, vomiting; give diphenhydramine (Benadryl); continue therapy if reaction is mild, discontinue if severe; notify prescriber
✦• Monitor bleeding at ankles, knees, elbows, other joints; check for rebleeding after 15-30 min

Nursing diagnoses
☑ Tissue perfusion altered (uses)
☑ Injury, risk for (uses, adverse reactions)
☑ Knowledge deficit (teaching)

Implementation
- Administer **IV** slowly; use plastic syringe to reconstitute and administer; do not use glass, drug adheres to glass; use another needle as a vent when reconstituting; rotate gently to mix
- Administer after dilution with warm NS, D_5W, LR; give within 3 hr
- Administer by **IV** inf: give at ≤2 ml/min if concentration exceeds 34 U/ml; or over 3 min if concentration is less

than 34 U/ml; filter before using
- Store in refrigerator; do not freeze; after reconstitution, do not refrigerate; give within 3 hr

Additive compatibilities:
Do not mix with other drugs in sol or syringe

Patient/family education
- Advise patient to report any signs of bleeding: gums, under skin, urine, stools, emesis; review methods to prevent bleeding; to be checked q2-3 mo for HIV screen
- Instruct patient to avoid salicylates and ibuprofen; increases bleeding tendencies, decreases clotting
- Instruct patient to prepare, administer factor VIII concentrates at first sign of danger
- Instruct patient to advise health professionals of treatment for hemophilia
- Advise patient that immunization for hepatitis B may be given first
- Instruct patient to report hives, urticaria, chest tightness, hypotension; may be monoclonal antibody–derived factor VII; signs of viral hepatitis, AIDS
- Advise patient to carry identification describing disease process, drugs used

Evaluation
Positive therapeutic outcome
- Absence of bleeding
- Prevention of rebleeding

---

ardeparin (℞)
(are-de-pear'in)
Normiflo
Func. class.: Anticoagulant
Chem. class.: Low molecular weight heparin

Pregnancy category   C

Action: Prevents conversion of fibrinogen to fibrin and prothrombin to thrombin by enhancing inhibitory effects of antithrombin III

Therapeutic Outcome:
• Absence of deep vein thrombosis

Uses: Prevention of deep vein thrombosis after knee replacement surgery

Dosage and routes
Adult: SC 50 antifactor XaU/kg q12 h the evening of the day of knee replacement surgery or the following AM, continued until patient is fully ambulatory or 2 wk, whichever is first
• To be used SC only

Available forms: Inj 5000, 10,000 anti-XaU/0.5 ml

Adverse effects
CNS: **Intracranial bleeding,** fever
GI: Nausea, constipation, **hepatoxicity**
HEMA: **Thrombocytopenia,** anemia
INTEG: Pruritus, superficial wound infection, ecchymosis, rash
SYST: Hypersensitivity, **hemorrhage, anaphylaxis** possible

Contraindications: Hypersensitivity to this drug, pork products, heparin, or other anticoagulants; hemophilia, leukemia with bleeding, thrombocytopenic purpura, cerebrovascular hemorrhage, cerebral aneurysm, severe hypertension, other severe cardiac disease

G Precautions: Elderly, pregnancy **C,** hepatic disease, severe renal disease, blood dyscrasias, subacute bacterial endocarditis, acute nephritis, **P** lactation, child, recent childbirth, peptic ulcer disease, pericarditis, pericardial effusion, recent lumbar puncture, vasculitis, other diseases where bleeding is possible

Pharmacokinetics	
Absorption	Well
Distribution	Widely
Metabolism	Unknown
Half-life	Unknown

Pharmacodynamics
Unknown

Interactions
Drug classifications
Anticoagulants, oral: ↑ risk of bleeding
NSAIDs: ↑ risk of bleeding
Platelet inhibitors: ↑ risk of bleeding
Salicylates: ↑ risk of bleeding

NURSING CONSIDERATIONS
Assessment
• Assess for blood studies (Hct, occult blood in stools, CBC, platelets) during treatment since bleeding can occur
• Assess for bleeding gums, petechiae, ecchymosis, black tarry stools, hematuria, epistaxis, decrease in Hct, B/P; may indicate bleeding, possible hemorrhage; notify prescriber immediately, drug should be discontinued; protamine

should be equal to dose of drug given; 1 mg protamine = 100 anti-Xa U of drug
• Monitor for hypersensitivity: fever, skin rash, urticaria; notify prescriber immediately

Implementation
• Give by SC only; have patient sit or lie down; SC inj may be around the navel in a U-shape, upper outer side of thigh or upper outer quadrangle of the buttocks; rotate inj sites
• Changing needles is not recommended

Evaluation
• Therapeutic response: absence of deep vein thrombosis

Patient/family education
• Teach patient to avoid OTC preparations that may cause serious drug interactions unless directed by prescriber; may contain aspirin; other anticoagulants, NSAIDs
• Teach patient to use soft-bristle toothbrush to avoid bleeding gums, avoid contact sports, use electric razor, avoid IM injection
• Advise patient to report any signs of bleeding: gums, under skin, urine, stools; unusual bruising, hematoma at inj site

Treatment of overdose: Protamine sulfate 1% given **IV**

ascorbic acid (vitamin C) (OTC, ℞)
(as-kor'bic)
APO-C ♣, ascorbic acid, Ascorbicap, C-Span, Cebid, Cecon, Cenolate, Cetane, Cevalin, Cevi-Bid, Ce-Vi-Sol, C-Crystals, Dull-C, Flavorcee, Kamu-Jay ♣, Mega-C/A Plus, Ortho/CS, Redoxon ♣, Vita-C
Func. class.: Vitamin C, water-soluble vitamin
Pregnancy category C

Action: Needed for wound healing, collagen synthesis, antioxidant, carbohydrate metabolism, protein, lipid synthesis, prevention of infection

➤**Therapeutic Outcome:** Replacement and supplementation of vitamin C

Uses: Vitamin C deficiency, scurvy, delayed wound and bone healing, chronic disease, urine acidification, before gastrectomy; increased need: lactation, pregnancy, hyperthyroidism, emotional stress, trauma, burns

Investigational uses: Acidification of urine, common cold prevention

Dosage and routes
RDA
▪ *Neonates and up to 6 mo:* 30 mg
▪ *Infants 6 mo-1 yr:* 35 mg
▪ *Child 1-3 yr:* 40 mg
▪ *Child 4-10 yr:* 45 mg
▪ *Child 11-14 yr:* 50 mg
▪ *Adult and child ≥15 yr:* 60 mg
Pregnancy: 70 mg
Lactation: 90 mg

Scurvy
Adult: PO/SC/IM/**IV** 100 mg-500 mg qd, then 50 mg or more qd

P **Child:** PO/SC/IM/**IV** 100-300 mg qd, then 35 mg or more qd

Wound healing/chronic disease/fracture
Adult: SC/IM/**IV**/PO 200-500 mg qd

P **Child:** SC/IM/**IV**/PO 100-200 mg added doses

Urine acidification
Adult: 4-12 g qd in divided doses

P **Child:** 500 mg q6-8h

Available forms: Tabs 25, 50, 100, 250, 500, 1000, 1500 mg; effervescent tabs 1000 mg; chewable tabs 100, 250, 500 mg; timed release tabs 500, 750, 1000, 1500 mg; timed release caps 500 mg; crystals 4 g/tsp; powder 4 g/tsp; liq 35 mg/0.6 ml; sol 100 mg/ml; syr 20 mg/ml, 500 mg/5 ml; inj SC, IM, **IV** 100, 250, 500 mg/ml

Adverse effects
CNS: Headache, insomnia, dizziness, fatigue, flushing
GI: Nausea, vomiting, diarrhea, anorexia, heartburn, cramps
GU: Polyuria, urine acidification, oxalate or urate renal stones
HEMA: Hemolytic anemia in patients with G6PD

Contraindications: None significant

Precautions: Gout, pregnancy C, diabetes, renal calculi (large doses)

Pharmacokinetics	
Absorption	Actively absorbed (PO)
Distribution	Widely distributed; crosses placenta
Metabolism	Oxidation
Excretion	Kidneys, inactive; breast milk
Half-life	Unknown

Pharmacodynamics
Unknown

Interaction
Individual drugs
Deferoxamine: ↑ iron toxicity
Iron, oral: ↑ effect of oral iron
Mexiletine: ↑ excretion in acidic urine
Primadone: ↑ requirements for vitamin C
Drug classifications
Anticoagulants, oral: ↓ action of anticoagulants
Antidepressants, tricyclic: ↑ excretion in acidic urine
Estrogens: ↑ effect of estrogen
Salicylates: ↑ requirements of vitamin C
Smoking
Smoking decreases vitamin C levels
Lab test interferences
False positive: negatives in glucose tests (Clinitest, Tes-Tape)
False negative: occult blood (large dose)
↓ Bilirubin, ↓ urine oxalate, ↓ cysteine

NURSING CONSIDERATIONS
Assessment
• Assess nutritional status for inclusion of foods high in vitamin C: citrus fruits, cantaloupe, tomatoes
• Assess for vitamin C deficiency before, during, and after treatment; scurvy (gingivitis, bleeding gums, loose teeth); poor bone development

- Monitor I&O ratio, polyuria; in patients receiving large doses renal stones may occur
- Monitor ascorbic acid levels throughout treatment if continued deficiency is suspected
- Assess inj sites for inflammation, pain, redness

Nursing diagnoses

☑Nutrition, less than body requirements (uses)

☑Knowledge deficit (teaching)

Implementation

IV route

- Give undiluted by *direct* **IV** 100 mg over at least 1 min, rapid inf may cause fainting
- Give by intermittent inf after diluting with D$_5$W, D$_{10}$W, 0.9% NaCl, 0.45% NaCl, LR, Ringer's sol, dextrose/saline, dextrose/Ringer's combinations; temperature will increase pressure in ampules; wrap with gauze before breaking

Syringe incompatibilities: Cefazolin, doxapram

Syringe compatibilities: Metoclopramide

Additive incompatibilities: Bleomycin, cephapirin, nafcillin, sodium bicarbonate, warfarin

Additive compatibilities: Amikacin, calcium chloride, calcium gluceptate, calcium gluconate, cephalothin, chloramphenicol, chlorpromazine, colistimethate, cyanocobalamin, diphenhydramine, heparin, kanamycin, methicillin, methyldopa, penicillin G potassium, polymyxin B, prednisolone, procaine, prochlor-

perazine, promethazine, verapamil

Y-site compatibilities: Warfarin

PO route

- Mix **oral sol** with foods or fluids; **ext rel caps** should be swallowed whole

🚫• Do not crush, break, or chew

IM route

- Not to be diluted; give deep in large muscle mass

Patient/family education

- Teach patient necessary foods to be included in diet that are rich in vitamin C: citrus fruits, cantaloupe, tomatoes, chili peppers (red)
- Teach patient that, if oral contraceptives are taken, increased levels of vitamin C are needed; oral contraceptives deplete vitamin C
- Teach patient that smoking decreases vitamin C levels; not to exceed prescribed dose; increases will be excreted in urine, except time release
- Teach patient not to exceed RDA recommended dose, urinary stones may occur
- Teach patient using ascorbic acid for acidification of urine to test urine pH periodically

Evaluation

Positive therapeutic outcome

- Absence of anorexia, irritability, pallor, joint pain, hyperkeratosis, petechiae, poor wound healing
- Reversal of scurvy: bleeding gums, gingivitis, loose teeth

asparaginase (℞)
(a-spar'a-gin-ase)
Elspar, Kidrolase ✦
Func. class.: Antineoplastic
Chem. class.: *Escherichia coli* enzyme

Pregnancy category   C

Action: Indirectly inhibits protein synthesis in tumor cells; without amino acids, DNA, RNA synthesis is halted; asparagine, protein synthesis is halted; G_1 phase of cell cycle specific; a nonvesicant

▶**Therapeutic Outcome:** Prevention of rapidly growing malignant cells in leukemia

Uses: Acute lymphocytic leukemia in combination with other antineoplastics unresponsive to other agents

Investigational uses: Lymphosarcoma, other leukemias

Dosage and routes
In combination
Adult: **IV** 1000 IU/kg/day × 10 days given over 30 min; IM 6000 IU/m²/day

Sole induction
Adult: **IV** 200 IU/kg/day × 28 days

Available forms: Inj 10,000 IU

Adverse effects
CNS: Neuritis, dizziness, headache, **coma,** depression, fatigue, confusion, hallucinations
CV: Chest pain
ENDO: Hyperglycemia
GI: Nausea, vomiting, anorexia, cramps, stomatitis, **hepatotoxicity, pancreatitis**
GU: Urinary retention, **renal failure,** glycosuria, polyuria, azotemia, uric acid neuropathy
HEMA: **Thrombocytopenia,** leukopenia, myelosuppression, anemia, decreased clotting factors
INTEG: Rash, urticaria, chills, fever
RESP: **Fibrosis, pulmonary infiltrate**
SYST: **Anaphylaxis, hypersensitivity**

Contraindications: Hypersensitivity, infants, lactation, pancreatitis

Precautions: Renal disease, hepatic disease, pregnancy **C**

Pharmacokinetics	
Absorption	Complete bioavailability (**IV**)
Distribution	Intravascular spaces
Metabolism	Unknown
Excretion	Reticuloendothelial system
Half-life	8-30 hr (**IV**), 39-49 hr (IM)

Pharmacodynamics		
	IV	IM
Onset	Immediate	Immediate
Peak	14-24 hr	Unknown
Duration	3-5 wk	3-5 wk

Interactions
Individual drugs
Methotrexate: Blocked action of methotrexate
Vincristine: ↑ neurotoxicity
Drug classifications
Hepatotoxic agents: ↑ hepatotoxicity
Glucocorticosteroids: ↑ hyperglycemia
Lab test interferences
↓ Thyroid function tests

NURSING CONSIDERATIONS
Assessment
• Assess for signs and symptoms of pancreatitis (nausea, vomiting, severe abdominal pain), anaphylaxis (broncho-

spasm, dyspnea), cyanosis; monitor amylase, glucose
• Assess symptoms indicating severe allergic reaction: rash, pruritus, urticaria, purpuric skin lesions, itching, flushing; joint pain, bronchospasm, hypotension; epinephrine and crash carts should be nearby
• Monitor for frequency of stools, characteristics: cramping, acidosis; signs of dehydration: rapid respirations, poor skin turgor, decreased urine output, dry skin, restlessness, weakness
• Monitor CBC, differential, platelet count weekly; withhold drug if WBC count is <4000/mm^3 or platelet count is <100,000/mm^3, notify prescriber of results; also monitor PT, PTT, and TT, which may be increased
• Monitor pulmonary function tests, chest x-ray studies before, during therapy; chest x-ray film should be obtained q2 wk during treatment
• Monitor renal function studies: BUN, serum uric acid, ammonia urine CrCl, electrolytes before, during therapy
• Check I&O ratio; report fall in urine output of 30/ml/hr
• Monitor temperature q4h; may indicate beginning infection
• Obtain liver function tests before, during therapy (bilirubin, AST, ALT, LDH) as needed or monthly
• Monitor RBC, Hct, Hgb, since these may be decreased; serum, urine glucose levels
• Assess for bleeding: hematuria, guaiac, bruising or petechiae, mucosa, or orifices q8h
◆•• Assess for dyspnea, rales, nonproductive cough, chest

pain, tachypnea fatigue, increased pulse, pallor, lethargy, or swelling around eyes or lips; anaphylaxis may occur
• Assess for yellowing of skin and sclera, dark urine, clay-colored stools, itchy skin, abdominal pain, fever, diarrhea

Nursing diagnoses
☑ Injury, risk for (uses, adverse reactions)
☑ Body image disturbance (adverse reactions)

Implementation
• Give after intradermal skin testing and desensitization, give 0.1 ml (2 IU) intradermally after reconstituting with 5 ml sterile H_2O or 0.9% NaCl for injection; then add 0.1 ml of reconstituted drug to 9.9 ml diluent (20 IU/ml); observe for 1 hr, check for wheal
• Use allopurinol or sodium bicarbonate to reduce uric acid levels, alkalinization of urine

IM route
• Reconstitute with 2 ml NaCl/10,000 IU/vial, refrigerate, use within 8 hr

IV route
• Give by **IV** infusion using 21-, 23-, 25-gauge needle; administer by slow **IV** infusion via Y-tube or 3-way stopcock of flowing D_5W or NS infusion over 30 min after diluting 10,000 IU/5 ml of sterile H_2O or 0.9% NaCl (no preservatives) (2000 IU/ml); use of filter may be necessary if fibers are present

Y-site compatibilities:
Methotrexate, sodium bicarbonate

Patient/family education
• Teach patient to report any complaints or side effects to nurse or physician

---

- Teach patient to report any changes in breathing or coughing

Evaluation
Positive therapeutic response
- Decreased replication of leukemia cells

Treatment of anaphylaxis: Administer epinephrine, diphenhydramine, **IV** corticosteroids

---

aspirin ☦ (OTC)
(as´pir-in)
Acuprin, Artria S.R., A.S.A., Aspergum, Aspirin ✤, Aspir-Low, Aspirtab, Astrin ✤, Bayer, Easprin, Ecotrin, 8-Hour Bayer Timed Release, Empirin, Entrophen ✤, Halfprin, Norwich Extra-Strength, Novasen ✤, PMS-ASA ✤, Sloprin, St. Joseph Children's Supasa ✤, Therapy Bayer, ZORprin
Func. class.: Nonnarcotic analgesic
Chem. class.: Salicylate

Pregnancy category D
(3rd trimester)

Action: Blocks pain impulses in CNS, inhibition of prostaglandin synthesis; antipyretic action results from vasodilatation of peripheral vessels; decreases platelet aggregation

➡**Therapeutic Outcome:** Decreased pain, inflammation, fever; absence of MI, transient ischemic attacks, thrombosis

Uses: Mild to moderate pain or fever including rheumatoid arthritis, osteoarthritis, thromboembolic disorders, transient ischemic attacks in men, rheumatic fever, post-MI, prophylaxis of MI

Investigational uses: Prevention of cataracts (long-term use), prevention of pregnancy loss in women with clotting disorders

Dosage and routes
Arthritis
Adult: PO 2.6-5.2 g/day in divided doses q4-6h

P *Child:* PO 90-130 mg/kg/day in divided doses q4-6h

Kawasaki disease
P *Child:* PO 80-120 mg/kg/day in 4 divided doses, maintenance 3-8 mg/kg/day as a single dose × 8 wk

MI, stroke prophylaxis
Adult: PO 81-650 mg/day

Pain/fever
Adult: PO/REC 325-650 mg q4h prn, not to exceed 4 g/day

P *Child:* PO/REC 40-100 mg/kg/day in divided doses q4-6h prn

Thromboembolic disorders
Adult: PO 325-650 mg/day or bid

Transient ischemic attacks
Adult: PO 650 mg qid or 325 mg qid

Available forms: Tabs 325, 500, 650, 975 mg; chewable tabs 81 mg; cont rel tabs 800 mg; time-release tabs 650 mg; supp 120, 200, 300, 600 mg, 1.2 g; cream; gum 227.5 mg

Adverse effects
CNS: Stimulation, drowsiness, dizziness, confusion, **convulsion,** headache, flushing, hallucinations, **coma**
CV: Rapid pulse, pulmonary edema

EENT: Tinnitus, hearing loss
ENDO: Hypoglycemia, hyponatremia, hypokalemia
GI: Nausea, vomiting, **GI bleeding,** diarrhea, heartburn, anorexia, **hepatitis**
HEMA: **Thrombocytopenia, agranulocytosis, leukopenia, neutropenia, hemolytic anemia,** increased pro-time, PTT, bleeding time
INTEG: Rash, urticaria, bruising
RESP: Wheezing, hyperpnea
🄿 **SYST:** Reye's syndrome (children)

Contraindications: Hypersensitivity to salicylates, tartrazine (FDC yellow dye #5), GI bleeding, bleeding disorders, 🄿 children <12 yr, children with flulike symptoms, pregnancy **D** (3rd trimester), lactation, vitamin K deficiency, peptic ulcer

Precautions: Anemia, hepatic disease, renal disease, Hodgkin's disease, pre/postoperatively, gastritis, asthmatic patients with nasal polyps or aspirin sensitivity

Pharmacokinetics

Absorption	Well absorbed, small intestine (PO); erratic (enteric); slow (rec)
Distribution	Rapidly, widely distributed; crosses placenta
Metabolism	Liver, extensively
Excretion	Inactive metabolites, kidney; breast milk
Half-life	2-3 hr (low doses); 30 hr (high doses)

Pharmacodynamics

	PO	REC
Onset	15-30 min	Slow
Peak	1-2 hr	4-5 hr
Duration	4-6 hr	6-7 hr

Interactions
Individual drugs
Alcohol: ↑ bleeding
Ammonium chloride: ↑ salicylate level
Cefamandole: ↑ bleeding
Furosemide: ↑ toxic effects
Heparin: ↑ bleeding
Insulin: ↑ effects of insulin
Methotrexate: ↑ effects of methotrexate
Nizatidine: ↑ salicylate level
PABA: ↑ toxic effects
Phenytoin: ↑ effects of phenytoin
Plicamycin: ↑ bleeding
Probenecid: ↓ effects of probenecid
Spironolactone: ↓ effects
Sulfinpyrazone: ↓ effects
Drug classifications
Antacids: ↓ effects of aspirin
Anticoagulants: ↑ bleeding
Carbonic anhydrase inhibitors: ↑ toxic effects
Corticosteroids: ↓ effects of aspirin
NSAIDs: ↑ gastric ulcers
Penicillins: ↑ effects of penicillins
Salicylates: ↓ blood sugar levels
Steroids: ↓ effects of aspirin, ↑ gastric ulcers
Sulfonylamides: ↓ effects of sulfonylamides
Urinary acidifiers: ↑ salicylate levels
Urinary alkalizers: ↓ effects of aspirin
▨ *Herb/drug*
Horse chestnut: ↑ risk of bleeding
Kelpware: ↑ risk of bleeding
Lab test interferences
↑ Coagulation studies, ↑ liver function studies, ↑ serum uric acid, ↑ amylase, ↑CO_2, ↑ urinary protein
↓ Serum potassium, ↓ PBI, ↓ cholesterol

Interference: Urine catechol-amines, pregnancy test, urine glucose tests (Clinistix, Tes-Tape)

NURSING CONSIDERATIONS
Assessment
• Monitor liver function studies: AST, ALT, bilirubin, creatinine if patient is on long-term therapy
• Monitor renal function studies: BUN, urine creatinine if patient is on long-term therapy
• Monitor blood studies: CBC, Hct, Hgb, pro-time if patient is on long-term therapy
• Check I&O ratio; decreasing output may indicate renal failure (long-term therapy)
◆• Assess hepatotoxicity: dark urine, clay-colored stools, yellowing of the skin and sclera, itching, abdominal pain, fever, diarrhea if patient is on long-term therapy
• Assess for allergic reactions: rash, urticaria; if these occur, drug may have to be discontinued
• Assess for ototoxicity: tinnitus, ringing, roaring in ears; audiometric testing needed before, after long-term therapy
• Assess for visual changes: blurring, halos; corneal, retinal damage
• Check edema in feet, ankles, legs
• Identify prior drug history; there are many drug interactions
• Monitor pain: location, duration, type, intensity, before dose and 1 hr after
• Monitor musculoskeletal status: ROM before dose
• Identify fever: length of time and related symptoms

Nursing diagnoses
☑ Pain (uses)
☑ Mobility, impaired physical (uses)
☑ Injury, risk for (side effects)
☑ Knowledge deficit (teaching)

Implementation
PO route
• Administer to patient crushed or whole; chewable tab may be chewed
🚫• Do not crush enteric product
• Give with food or milk to decrease gastric symptoms; give 30 min before or 2 hr pc; absorption may be slowed
• Give antacids 1-2 hr after enteric products

Patient/family education
• Teach patient to report any symptoms of hepatotoxicity, renal toxicity, visual changes, ototoxicity, allergic reactions, bleeding (long-term therapy)
• Instruct patient to take with 8 oz of water and sit upright for 30 min after dose
• Instruct patient not to exceed recommended dosage; acute poisoning may result
• Advise patient to read label on other OTC drugs; many contain aspirin
• Inform patient that the therapeutic response takes 2 wk (arthritis)
• Teach patient to report tinnitus, confusion, diarrhea, sweating, hyperventilation
• Advise patient to avoid alcohol ingestion; GI bleeding may occur
• Advise patient with allergies that allergic reactions may develop
• Instruct patient to avoid buffered or effervescent products

---

- Teach patient not to give to children or teens with flu-like symptoms or chicken pox; Reye's syndrome may develop

Evaluation
Positive therapeutic outcome
- Decreased pain
- Decreased inflammation
- Decreased fever
- Absence of MI
- Absence of transient ischemic attacks, thrombosis

Treatment of overdose: Lavage, activated charcoal, monitor electrolytes, VS

---

atenolol (R)
(a-ten'oh-lole)
Apo-Atenolol ✦, atenolol, Nu-Atenol, Tenormin
Func. class.: Antihypertensive
Chem. class.: β-Blocker; $β_1$-; $β_2$-blocker (high doses)
Pregnancy category D

Action: Competitively blocks stimulation of β-adrenergic receptor within vascular smooth muscle; produces negative chronotropic activity, positive inotropic activity (decreases rate of SA node discharge, increases recovery time), slows conduction of AV node, decreases heart rate, decreases O_2 consumption in myocardium; also decreases renin-aldosterone-angiotensin system at high doses, inhibits $β_2$-receptors in bronchial system at higher doses

Therapeutic Outcome: Decreased B/P, heart rate, prevention of angina pectoris, MI

Uses: Mild to moderate hypertension, prophylaxis of angina pectoris, suspected or known MI

Investigational uses: Dysrhythmia, mitral valve prolapse, pheochromocytoma, hypertrophic cardiomyopathy, vascular headaches, thyrotoxicosis, tremors, alcohol withdrawal

Dosage and routes
Adult: IV 5 mg; repeat in 10 min if initial dose is well tolerated, then start PO dose 10 min after last IV dose

Adult: PO 50 mg qd, increasing q1-2 wk to 100 mg qd; may increase to 200 mg qd for angina

G *Elderly:* PO 25 mg/day initially
Renal disease
CrCl 15-35 ml/min, max 50 mg/day; CrCl <15 ml/min max dose 50 mg qod; hemodialysis 25-50 mg after dialysis

Available forms: Tabs 25, 50, 100 mg; IV 5 mg/10 ml

Adverse effects
CNS: Insomnia, fatigue, dizziness, mental changes, memory loss, hallucinations, depression, lethargy, drowsiness, strange dreams, catatonia
CV: **Profound hypotension, bradycardia, CHF, cold extremities, postural hypotension, 2nd- or 3rd-degree heart block**
EENT: Sore throat, dry burning eyes
ENDO: Increased hypoglycemic response to insulin
GI: Nausea, diarrhea, vomiting, **mesenteric arterial thrombosis, ischemic colitis**
GU: Impotence
HEMA: **Agranulocytosis, thrombocytopenia, purpura**

INTEG: Rash, fever, alopecia
RESP: **Bronchospasm,** dyspnea, wheezing

Contraindications: Hypersensitivity to β-blockers, cardiogenic shock, 2nd- or 3rd-degree heart block, sinus bradycardia, CHF, cardiac failure, pregnancy **D**

Precautions: Major surgery, lactation, diabetes mellitus, renal disease, thyroid disease, COPD, asthma, well-compensated heart failure

Do Not Confuse:
atenolol/albuterol, Tenormin/thiamine

Pharmacokinetics

Absorption	50%-60% (PO)
Distribution	Crosses placenta; protein binding (5%-15%)
Metabolism	Not metabolized
Excretion	Breast milk, kidneys (50%), feces (50%—unabsorbed drug)
Half-life	6-7 hr

Pharmacodynamics

	PO
Onset	1 hr
Peak	2-4 hr
Duration	24 hr

Interactions
Individual drugs
Alcohol: ↑ hypotension (large amounts)
Diltiazem: ↑ hypotension, bradycardia
Epinephrine: α-Adrenergic stimulation
Hydralazine: ↑ hypotension, bradycardia
Indomethacin: ↓ antihypertensive effect
Insulin: ↑ hypoglycemia
Methyldopa: ↑ hypotension, bradycardia

Prazosin: ↑ hypotension, bradycardia
Reserpine: ↑ hypotension, bradycardia
Thyroid: ↓ effectiveness of atenolol
Verapamil: ↑ myocardial depression
Drug classifications
Antidiabetics, oral: ↑ hypoglycemia
Antihypertensives: ↑ hypertension
β2-Agonist: ↓ bronchodilatation
Cardiac glycosides: ↑ bradycardia
Nitrates: ↑ hypotension
Theophyllines: ↓ bronchodilatation
Lab test interferences
Interference: Glucose insulin tolerance tests
↑ Uric acid, ↑ potassium, ↑ triglyceride, ↑ lipoproteins

NURSING CONSIDERATIONS
Assessment
• Monitor B/P during beginning treatment, periodically thereafter; pulse q4h; note rate, rhythm, quality: apical/radial pulse before administration; notify prescriber of any significant changes (pulse <50 bpm)
• Check for baselines in renal, liver function tests before therapy begins
• Assess for edema in feet, legs daily; monitor I&O, daily weight; check for jugular vein distention, rales bilaterally, dyspnea (CHF)
• Monitor skin turgor, dryness of mucous membranes for hydration status, especially
G elderly

Nursing diagnoses
✓ Cardiac output, decreased (uses)

☑ Injury, risk for physical (side effects)
☑ Knowledge deficit (teaching)
☑ Noncompliance (teaching)

Implementation
PO route
• Given ac, hs, tablet may be crushed or swallowed whole; give with food to prevent GI upset; reduced dosage in renal dysfunction
• Store protected from light, moisture; place in cool environment

Ⅳ IV route
• Give **IV** direct over 5 min or diluted in 10-50 ml D_5W, 0.9% NaCl, and give at prescribed rate

Y-*site compatibilities:*
Meperidine, meropenem, morphine

Patient/family education
• Teach patient not to discontinue drug abruptly; taper over 2 wk; may cause precipitate angina if stopped abruptly
• Teach patient not to use OTC products containing α-adrenergic stimulants (such as nasal decongestants, OTC cold preparations); to limit alcohol, smoking; to limit sodium intake as prescribed
• Teach patient how to take pulse and B/P at home; advise when to notify prescriber
• Instruct patient to comply with weight control, dietary adjustments, modified exercise program
• Advise patient to carry/wear Medic Alert ID for drugs and allergies; tell patient drug controls symptoms but does not cure
• Caution patient to avoid hazardous activities if dizziness, drowsiness is present

• Teach patient to report symptoms of CHF: difficult breathing, especially on exertion or when lying down, night cough, swelling of extremities or bradycardia, dizziness, confusion, depression, fever
• Teach patient to take drug as prescribed, not to double doses, skip doses; take any missed doses as remembered if at least 6 hr until next dose
• Advise patient that drug may mask symptoms of hypoglycemia in diabetic patients

Evaluation
Positive therapeutic outcome
• Decreased B/P in hypertension (after 1-2 wk)
• Absence of dysrhythmias
• Absence of MI
• Decreased angina

Treatment of overdose:
Lavage, **IV** atropine for bradycardia, **IV** theophylline for bronchospasm, digitalis, O_2, diuretic for cardiac failure, hemodialysis, **IV** glucose for hyperglycemia, **IV** diazepam (or phenytoin) for seizures

---

atorvastatin (℞)
(at-or′va-sta-tin)
Lipitor
Func. class.: Antilipidemic
Chem. class.: Synthetically derived fermentation product

Pregnancy category   X

Action: Inhibits HMG-CoA reductase enzyme, which reduces cholesterol synthesis

➡ **Therapeutic Outcome:** Decreased cholesterol levels and LDLs, increased HDLs

---

Uses: As an adjunct in primary hypercholesterolemia (types Ia, Ib), dysbetalipoproteinemia, elevated triglyceride levels

Dosage and routes
Adult: PO 10 mg qd, usual range 10-80, dosage adjustments may be made in 2-4 wk intervals

Available forms: Tabs 10, 20, 40 mg

Adverse effects
CNS: Headache
EENT: Lens opacities
GI: Dyspepsia, flatus, *liver dysfunction,* pancreatitis
INTEG: Rash, pruritus, alopecia
MS: Myalgia

Contraindications: Hypersensitivity, pregnancy **X,** lactation, active liver disease

Precautions: Past liver disease, alcoholism, severe acute infections, trauma, hypotension, uncontrolled seizure disorders, severe metabolic disorders, electrolyte imbalance

Pharmacokinetics

Absorption	Unknown
Distribution	Unknown
Metabolism	Liver
Excretion	Bile, feces, kidneys
Half-life	14 hr

Pharmacodynamics
Unknown

Interactions
Individual drugs
Cholestyramine: ↓ action of atorvastatin
Colestipol: ↓ action of atorvastatin
Cyclosporine: ↑ risk of rhabdomyolysis

Erythromycin: ↑ risk of rhabdomyolysis
Gemfibrozil: ↑ risk of rhabdomyolysis
Niacin: ↑ risk of rhabdomyolysis
Warfarin: ↑ action
Digoxin: ↑ action
Drug classifications
Azole antifungals: Possible rhabdomyolysis
Oral contraceptives: ↑ action

NURSING CONSIDERATIONS
Assessment
• Assess nutrition: fat, protein, carbohydrates; nutritional analysis should be completed by dietician before treatment
• Monitor bowel pattern daily; diarrhea may be a problem
• Monitor triglycerides, cholesterol at baseline and throughout treatment; LDL and VLDL should be watched closely; if increased, drug should be discontinued
• Monitor liver function studies q1-2 mo during the first 1½ yr of treatment; AST, ALT, liver function tests may be increased
• Monitor renal studies in patients with compromised renal system: BUN, I&O ratio, creatinine
• Assess eyes with slit lamp before, 1 mo after treatment begins, annually

Nursing diagnoses
☑ Diarrhea (adverse reactions)
☑ Knowledge deficit (teaching)
☑ Noncompliance (teaching)

Implementation
• Administer total daily dose at any time of day
• Store in cool environment in airtight, light-resistant container

---

Patient/family education
- Inform patient that compliance is needed for positive results to occur, not to double doses
- Teach patient that risk factors should be decreased: high-fat diet, smoking, alcohol consumption, absence of exercise
- Advise patient to notify prescriber if the GI symptoms of diarrhea, abdominal or epigastric pain, nausea, vomiting occur; or if chills, fever, sore throat occur
- Advise patient that treatment will take several years
- Advise patient that blood work and eye exam will be necessary during treatment
- Advise not to take if pregnant

Evaluation
Positive therapeutic outcome
- Decreased cholesterol levels, serum triglyceride
- Improved ratio of HDLs

---

atovaquone (℞)
(a-toe′va-kwon)
Mepron
Func. class.: Antiprotozoal
Chem. class.: Aromatic diamide derivative; analog of ubiquinone
Pregnancy category   C

Action: Interferes with DNA/RNA synthesis in protozoa, specifically ATP and nucleic acid synthesis

Therapeutic Outcome: Antiprotozoal for *Pneumocystis carinii* only

Uses: *Pneumocystis carinii* infections in patients intolerant of trimethoprim/sulfamethoxazole (co-trimoxazole)

Dosage and routes
Adult and adolescents 13-16 yrs: PO 750 mg bid with food tid for 21 days

Prevention of PCP
Adults and adolescents 13-16 yrs: PO 1500 mg qd with food

Available forms: 750 mg/5 ml

Adverse effects
CNS: Dizziness, headache, anxiety
CV: Hypotension
GI: Nausea, vomiting, diarrhea, anorexia, increased AST and ALT, acute pancreatitis, constipation, abdominal pain
HEMA: Anemia, **leukopenia**
INTEG: Pruritus, urticaria, *rash,* oral monilia
META: Hyperkalemia, hyperglycemia, hyponatremia

Contraindications: Hypersensitivity or history of developing life-threatening allergic reactions to any component of the formulation

Precautions: Blood dyscrasias, hepatic disease, diabetes mellitus, pregnancy **C,** lactation, children, elderly

Do Not Confuse:
Mepron (U.S.)/Mepron (meprobamate in Australia)

Pharmacokinetics	
Absorption	Poor; increased when taken with fatty foods
Distribution	Unknown
Metabolism	Hepatic recycling
Excretion	Feces, unchanged (94%)
Half-life	2-3 days

Pharmacodynamics	
Onset	Unknown
Peak	1-8 hr

Interactions
Individual drugs
Rifampin: ↓ effectiveness of atovaquone
Rifabutin: ↓ effectiveness of atovaquone
Drug classifications
Use cautiously with highly protein-bound drugs
Food/drug
↑ absorption of drug, especially fatty foods

NURSING CONSIDERATIONS
Assessment
• Assess for *Pneumocystis carinii:* monitor WBC, bilateral lung sounds, sputum for C&S; these should be checked before, periodically during, and after treatment; after collection of 1st sputum, therapy may begin
• Monitor for symptoms of hyponatremia: *CV:* increased B/P, cold, clammy skin, hypovolemia or hypervolemia; *GI:* anorexia, nausea, vomiting, diarrhea, abdominal cramps; *neuro:* lethargy, increased ICP, confusion, headache, seizures, coma, fatigue, tremors, hyperreflexia
• Monitor for symptoms of hypoglycemia/hyperglycemia in diabetic patients
• Monitor blood studies: blood glucose, CBC, platelets; I&O ratio; ECG for cardiac dysrhythmias, check B/P; liver studies: AST, ALT
• Monitor for signs of infection; anemia; monitor bowel pattern before, during treatment
• Monitor respiratory status: rate, character, wheezing, dyspnea
• Assess for dizziness, confusion, hallucination
• Assess for allergies before treatment, reaction of each medication; place allergies on chart; notify all people giving drugs

Nursing diagnoses
☑Infection, risk for (uses)
☑Diarrhea (adverse reactions)
☑Knowledge deficit (teaching)

Implementation
• Give with food (preferably fatty); increased absorption of the drug and higher plasma concentrations will occur; give tid × 3 wks

Patient/family education
• Instruct patient to take with food, preferably fatty foods, to increase plasma concentrations
• Advise patient to take drug exactly as prescribed

Evaluation
Positive therapeutic outcome
• Decreased temperature
• Ability to breathe
• Three negative sputum cultures

---

atracurium (℞)
(a-tra-cure′ee-um)
Tracrium
Func. class.: Neuromuscular blocker (nondepolarizing)
Chem. class.: Biquaternary ammonium ester

Pregnancy category   C

Action: Inhibits transmission of nerve impulses by binding with cholinergic receptor sites, antagonizing action of acetylcholine

---

☑ Herb/drug   🚫 Do Not Crush   ◆ Alert   ☛ Key Drug   🟦 Geriatric   🅿 Pediatric

A

→**Therapeutic Outcome:**
Skeletal muscle paralysis after anesthesia

Uses: Facilitation of endotracheal intubation; skeletal muscle relaxation during mechanical ventilation, surgery, or general anesthesia

Dosage and routes
P *Adult and child >2 yr:* **IV** bol 0.4-0.5 mg/kg, then 0.08-0.10 mg/kg 20-45 min after 1st dose if needed for prolonged procedures

P *Child 1 mo-2 yr:* **IV** bol 0.3-0.4 mg/kg

Available forms: Inj 10 mg/ml

Adverse effects
CV: Bradycardia, tachycardia, increased, decreased B/P
EENT: Increased secretions
INTEG: Rash, flushing, pruritus, urticaria
MS: Inadequate or prolonged block
RESP: Prolonged apnea, bronchospasm, cyanosis, respiratory depression

Contraindications: Hypersensitivity

Precautions: Pregnancy **C**, cardiac disease, lactation,
P children <2 yr, electrolyte imbalances, dehydration, neuromuscular disease, respiratory disease

Pharmacokinetics	
Absorption	Complete bioavailability
Distribution	Extracellular space, crosses placenta
Metabolism	Plasma
Excretion	Unknown
Half-life	Biphasic 2 min, 29 min

Pharmacodynamics	
Onset	2 min
Peak	5 min
Duration	20-60 min

Interactions
Individual drugs
Clindamycin: ↑ paralysis
Colistin: ↑ paralysis
Lidocaine: ↑ paralysis
Lithium: ↑ paralysis
Magnesium: ↑ paralysis
Polymyxin B: ↑ paralysis
Procainamide: ↑ paralysis
Quinidine: ↑ paralysis
Succinylcholine: ↑ paralysis
Drug classifications
Aminoglycosides: ↑ paralysis
β-Adrenergic blockers: ↑ paralysis
Diuretics, potassium-losing: ↑ paralysis
General anesthesia: ↑ paralysis
Magnesium salts: ↑ neuromuscular blockade
Opiates: ↑ neuromuscular blockade

NURSING CONSIDERATIONS
Assessment
• Assess for electrolyte imbalances (potassium, magnesium); may lead to increased action of this drug
• Monitor vital signs (B/P, pulse, respirations, airway) until fully recovered; rate, depth, pattern of respirations, strength of hand grip
• Monitor I&O ratio; check for urinary retention, frequency, hesitancy
• Assess recovery: decreased paralysis of face, diaphragm, leg, arm, rest of body
• Monitor allergic reactions: rash, fever, respiratory distress, pruritus; drug should be discontinued

Nursing diagnoses
☑ Breathing pattern, ineffective (uses)
☑ Communication, impaired verbal (adverse reactions)
☑ Fear (adverse reactions)

Implementation
- Anesthesiologist should use nerve stimulator to determine neuromuscular blockade
- Give anticholinesterase to reverse neuromuscular blockade
- Give undiluted direct **IV** over 5 min, or diluted in 10-50 ml of D$_5$W (½ NaCl or NS) and give as an inf at prescribed rate
- Give only by qualified person, usually an anesthesiologist; do not administer IM
- Give only slightly discolored solution
- Store in light-resistant area

Y-site compatibilities:
Cefazolin, cefuroxime, cimetidine, dobutamine, dopamine, epinephrine, esmolol, etomidate, fentanyl, gentamicin, heparin, hydrocortisone, isoproterenol, lorazepam, midazolam, morphine, nitroglycerine, ranitidine, sodium nitroprusside, trimethoprim/sulfamethoxazole, vancomycin

Y-site incompatibilities:
Diazepam

Additive compatibilities:
Bretylium, cimetidine, dobutamine, dopamine, esmolol, gentamicin, isoproterenol, lidocaine, morphine, potassium chloride, procainamide, vancomycin

Additive incompatibilities:
Barbiturates, sodium bicarbonate

Syringe compatibilities:
Alfantanil, fentanyl, midazolam, sufentanil

Patient/family education
- Provide reassurance if communication is difficult during recovery from neuromuscular blockade
- Provide explanation of all treatments and procedures before beginning

Evaluation
Positive therapeutic outcome
- Paralysis of jaw, eyelid, head, neck, rest of body

Treatment of overdose:
Edrophonium or neostigmine, atropine; monitor VS; may require mechanical ventilation

---

atropine ⚷ (Ṛ)
(a'troe-peen)
Atropine-1, Atropine Care Ophthalmic, Atropine Sulfate Ophthalmic, atropine sulfate S.O.P., Atropisol Ophthalmic, Isopto Atropine, Atropair, Atro-Pen, I-tropine, Minims Atropine ✿
Func. class.: Antidysrhythmic, anticholinergic parasympatholytic, mydriatic
Chem. class.: Belladonna alkaloid

Pregnancy category   C

Action: Blocks acetylcholine at parasympathetic neuroeffector sites; increases cardiac output, heart rate by blocking vagal stimulation in heart; dries secretions, decreases sweating, salivation in low doses; mydriasis, increased heart rate and cycloplegia occur at moderate

---

☑ Herb/drug Ⓢ Do Not Crush ◆ Alert ⚷ Key Drug Ⓖ Geriatric Ⓟ Pediatric doses; motility of GI, GU systems at high dose

➔Therapeutic Outcome: Drying of secretions, increased heart rate, cycloplegia, mydriasis

Uses: Bradycardia, bradydysrhythmia, anticholinesterase, insecticide poisoning, blocking cardiac vagal reflexes, decreasing secretions before surgery, antispasmodic with GU and biliary surgery, bronchodilator; opthalmically for cycloplegia, mydriasis

Dosage and routes
Bradycardia/ bradydysrhythmias
Adult: **IV** bol 0.5-1 mg given q3-5 min, not to exceed 2 mg

P *Child:* **IV** bol 0.01-0.03 mg/kg up to 0.4 mg or 0.3 mg/m²; may repeat q4-6h, min dose 0.1 mg to avoid paradoxical reaction

Insecticide poisoning
P *Adult and child:* IM/**IV** 2 mg qh until muscarinic symptoms disappear; may need 6 mg qh

Before surgery
Adult: SC/IM/**IV** 0.4-0.6 mg before anesthesia

P *Child:* SC 0.1-0.4 mg 30 min before surgery

Cycloplegic refraction
Adult: OPHTH ï-ïï gtt of 1% sol 1 hr before exam

P *Child:* OPHTH ï-ïï gtt of 0.5% sol bid-tid for up to 3 days before and 1 hr after exam

GI disorders
Adult: PO 0.3-1.2 mg q4-6h

Available forms: Inj 0.05, 0.1, 0.3, 0.4, 0.5, 0.8, 1 mg/ ml; tabs 0.4 mg; tabs 0.4, 0.6

mg; oint 1%; sol (ophth) 0.5%, 1%, 2%

Adverse effects
CNS: Headache, dizziness, involuntary movement, confusion, psychosis, anxiety, coma, flushing, drowsiness, insomnia, **G** weakness, delirium (elderly)
CV: Hypotension, paradoxic bradycardia, angina, PVCs, hypertension, tachycardia, ectopic ventricular beats
EENT: Blurred vision, photophobia, glaucoma, eye pain, pupil dilatation, nasal congestion
GI: Dry mouth, nausea, vomiting, abdominal pain, anorexia, constipation, paralytic ileus, abdominal distention, altered taste
GU: Retention, hesitancy, impotence, dysuria
INTEG: Rash, urticaria, contact dermatitis, dry skin, flushing
MISC: Suppression of lactation, decreased sweating

Contraindications: Hypersensitivity to belladonna alkaloids, angle closure glaucoma, GI obstructions, myasthenia gravis, thyrotoxicosis, ulcerative colitis, prostatic hypertrophy, tachycardia/ tachydysrhythmias, asthma, acute hemorrhage, hepatic disease, myocardial ischemia

Precautions: Pregnancy **C**, renal disease, lactation, CHF, tachydysrhythmias, hyperthyroidism, COPD, hepatic dis-
P ease, child <6 yr, hyperten-
G sion, elderly, intraabdominal infections, Down's syndrome, spastic paralysis, gastric ulcer

Pharmacokinetics

Absorption	Well absorbed (PO, SC, IM)
Distribution	Crosses blood-brain barrier, placenta
Metabolism	Liver
Excretion	Kidneys, unchanged (70%-90%); breast milk
Half-life	13-40 hr

Pharmacodynamics

	PO	IM/SC	IV	OPHTH
Onset	½ hr	15 min	2-4 min	½ hr
Peak	½-1 hr	30 min	2-4 min	30-60 min
Duration	4-6 hr	4-6 hr	4-6 hr	1-2 wk

Interactions
Individual drugs
Amantadine: ↑ anticholinergic effect
Disopyramide: ↑ anticholinergic effect
Ketoconazole: ↓ absorption
Levodopa: ↓ absorption
Methotrimeprazine: ↑ EPS
Potassium chloride, oral: ↑ GI lesions; wax-matrix tab
Quinidine: ↑ anticholinergic effect
Drug classifications
Antacids: ↓ absorption of atropine
Anticholinergics: ↑ anticholinergic effect
Antidepressants, tricyclic: ↑ anticholinergic effect
Antihistamines: ↑ anticholinergic effect
Antiparkinson agents: ↑ anticholinergic effects
MAOIs: ↑ anticholinergic effects
Phenothiazines: ↑ anticholinergic effects
☑ *Herb/drug*
Aloe: ↑ atropine action
Buckthorn bark/berry: ↑ atropine action
Cascara sagrada bark: ↑ atropine action

Rhubarb root: ↑ atropine action
Senna leaf/fruits: ↑ atropine action

NURSING CONSIDERATIONS
Assessment
• Monitor I&O ratio; check for urinary retention and daily output in elderly or postoperative patients 🄶
• Monitor ECG for ectopic ventricular beats, PVC, tachycardia in cardiac patients
• Monitor for bowel sounds; check for constipation; abdominal distention and constipation may occur
• Monitor respiratory status: rate, rhythm, cyanosis, wheezing, dyspnea, engorged neck veins
• Monitor for increased intraocular pressure: eye pain, nausea, vomiting, blurred vision, increased tearing; discontinue use if pain occurs (optic)
• Monitor cardiac rate: rhythm, character, B/P continuously
• Monitor allergic reaction: rash, urticaria
Nursing diagnoses
☑ Cardiac output, decreased (uses)
☑ Sensory-perceptual alteration: visual (adverse reactions)
☑ Constipation (adverse reactions)
☑ Knowledge deficit (teaching)
Implementation
🄸🄫 **IV route**
• Give **IV** undiluted or diluted with 10 ml sterile H_2O; give at a rate of 0.6 mg/min; give through Y-tube or 3-way stopcock; do not add to **IV** sol; may cause paradoxic bradycardia lasting 2 min

---

☑ Herb/drug   🅂 Do Not Crush   ✦ Alert   ☛ Key Drug   🄶 Geriatric   🄿 Pediatric

Syringe compatibilities:
Benzquinamide, butorphanol, chlorpromazine, cimetidine, dimenhydrinate, diphenhydramine, droperidol, fentanyl, glycopyrrolate, heparin, hydromorphone, hydroxyzine, meperidine, metoclopramide, midazolam, milrinone, morphine, nalbuphine, pentazocine, perphenazine, prochlorperazine, promazine, promethazine, propiomazine, ranitidine, scopolamine, sufentanil, Vit B with C

Y-site compatibilities:
Amrinone, etomidate, famotidine, heparin, hydrocortisone sodium succinate, meropenem, nafcillin, potassium chloride, sufentanil, vit B/C

Additive compatibilities:
Dobutamine, furosemide, meropenem, netilmicin, sodium bicarbonate, verapamil

PO route
• PO 30 min ac
• Give increased bulk, water in diet if constipation occurs (anticholinergic effect)

IM route
• Expect atropine flush 15-20 min after inj; it may occur in
P children and is not harmful

Patient/family education
• Advise patient not to perform strenuous activity in high temperatures; heat stroke may result
• Instruct patient to take as prescribed; not to skip doses
• Instruct patient to report change in vision; blurring or loss of sight; trouble breathing; sweating; flushing, chest pain, allergic reactions
• Caution patient not to operate machinery if drowsiness occurs
• Advise patient not to take

OTC products without approval of physician

Ophthalmic route
• Teach patient method of instillation: pressure on lacrimal sac for 1 min; do not touch dropper to eye
• Instruct patient that blurred vision will decrease with repeated use of drug; to omit next instillation if side effects are present
• Instruct patient not to perform hazardous tasks until able to see
• Advise patient to wait 5 min to use other drops; not to blink more than usual; use sunglasses to protect eyes

Evaluation

Positive therapeutic outcome
• Decreased dysrhythmias
• Increased heart rate
• Decreased secretions, GI, GU spasms
• Bronchodilatation
• Decrease in inflammation (iritis) or cycloplegic refraction (ophthalmic)

Treatment of overdose: O_2, artificial ventilation, ECG; administer dopamine for circulatory depression; administer diazepam or thiopental for convulsion; assess need for antidysrhythmics

attapulgite (OTC)
(at-a-pull'gite)
Diar Aid, Diasorb, Fowler's
Diarrhea Tablets ✦,
Hydrated Magnesium
Silicate, Kaopectate,
Kaopectate Advanced
Formula, Kaopectate
Maximum Strength,
Parepectolin, Rheaban,
St. Joseph Antidiarrheal
Func. class.: Antidiarrheal
Chem. class.: Hydrous
magnesium aluminum
silcate

Pregnancy class C

Action: Decreases gastric
motility, water content of
stool; adsorbent, demulcent

▷**Therapeutic Outcome:**
Decreased diarrhea

Uses: Diarrhea (cause undetermined), mild to moderate

Dosage and routes
Adult: PO 60-120 ml (45-90
ml conc) after each loose
bowel movement

P *Child >12 yr:* PO 60 ml after
each loose bowel movement

P *Child 6-12 yr:* PO 30-60 ml
(30 ml conc) after each loose
bowel movement

P *Child 3-6 yr:* PO 15-30 ml
(15 ml conc) after each loose
bowel movement

Available forms: Susp kaolin
0.87 g/5 ml, pectin 43 mg/5
ml; kaolin 0.98 g/5 ml, pectin
21.7 mg/5 ml

Adverse effects
GI: Constipation (chronic use)

Precautions: Pregnancy **C**

Pharmacokinetics

Absorption	Not absorbed
Distribution	Unknown
Metabolism	Unknown
Excretion	Unknown
Half-life	Unknown

Pharmacodynamics

Unknown

Interactions
All drugs: ↓ action of all other
drugs

Nursing diagnoses
☑ Diarrhea (uses)
☑ Constipation (adverse reac-
tions)
☑ Knowledge deficit (teaching)

NURSING CONSIDERATIONS
Assessment
• Assess bowel pattern before,
during, and after treatment;
check for rebound constipation
• Monitor for dehydration in
P children

Implementation
• For 48 hr only after each
diarrhea stool

Patient/family education
• Advise patient not to exceed
recommended dosage; notify
prescriber if symptoms continue
• Instruct patient to shake well
before administration

Evaluation
Positive therapeutic outcome
• Decreased diarrhea

---

auranofin (℞)
(au-ran'oh-fin)
Ridaura
Func. class.: Antiinflammatory (gold)
Chem. class.: Active gold compound (29%)
Pregnancy category **C**

Action: Antiinflammatory action unknown; may decrease phagocytosis, lysosomal activity or decrease prostaglandin synthesis; decreases concentration of rheumatoid factor, immunoglobulins

➔**Therapeutic Outcome:** Relief of pain, inflammation, slowing of rheumatoid arthritis resistant to other treatment

Uses: Rheumatoid arthritis unresponsive to other treatment

Investigational uses: SLE, psoriatic arthritis, pemphigus

Dosage and routes
Adult: PO 6 mg qd or 3 mg bid, may increase to 9 mg/day after 3 mo

Available forms: Caps 3 mg

Adverse effects
CNS: Dizziness, confusion, hallucinations, **seizures,** EEG abnormalities
GI: Diarrhea, abdominal cramping, stomatitis, nausea, vomiting, enterocolitis, anorexia, flatulence, metallic taste, dyspepsia, jaundice, increased AST, ALT, glossitis, gingivitis, melena, constipation
GU: **Proteinuria, hematuria,** increased BUN, creatinine, vaginitis
HEMA: **Thrombocytopenia, agranulocytosis, aplastic anemia, leukopenia, eosinophilia, neutropenia**
INTEG: Rash, pruritus, dermatitis, **exfoliative dermatitis,** urticaria, alopecia, photosensitivity
MISC: Iritis, corneal ulcers, gold deposits in ocular tissues
RESP: **Interstitial pneumonitis, fibrosis,** cough, dyspnea

Contraindications: Hypersensitivity to gold, necrotizing enterocolitis, bone marrow aplasia, child <6 yr, lactation, pulmonary fibrosis, exfoliative dermatitis, blood dyscrasias, recent radiation therapy, renal/hepatic disease, marked hypertension, uncontrolled CHF

Precautions: Elderly, CHF, diabetes mellitus, allergic conditions, ulcerative colitis, renal disease, liver disease, pregnancy **C**

Do Not Confuse:
Ridaura/Cardura

Pharmacokinetics	
Absorption	20%-30%
Distribution	Widely distributed; concentrated in joints
Metabolism	Unknown
Excretion	Kidneys slow (60%-90%); feces (10%-40%); breast milk
Half-life	1 mo (blood); up to 4 mo (tissue)

Pharmacodynamics	
Onset	Unknown
Peak	2 hr
Durations	8-16 wk (steady state)

Interactions
Individual drugs
Penicillamine: ↑ toxicity
Radiation: ↑ bone marrow toxicity

Drug classifications
Antineoplastics: ↑ bone marrow toxicity
Lab test interferences
False positive: TB skin test

NURSING CONSIDERATIONS
Assessment
• Assess symptoms of rheumatoid arthritis: pain in joints, stiffness, poor range of motion, inflammation
• Assess respiratory status: dyspnea, wheezing; if respiratory problems occur, drug should be discontinued; pneumonitis, fibrosis may occur
• Monitor urine; hematuria, proteinuria, increased BUN, creatinine may require decrease in dosage or discontinuation of treatment; I&O ratio
• Monitor blood studies: platelets, WBC, eosinophils, granulocytes monthly; drug should be discontinued if platelets <100,000/mm^3, WBC <4000 mm^3, eosinophils >5%, granulocytes <1500 mm^3
• Monitor hepatic test: ALT, AST, alkaline phosphatase monthly
• Monitor diarrhea stools; if severe, drug should be discontinued
• Assess allergy: rash, dermatitis, pruritus, angioneurotic edema, nitroid reactions; drug should be discontinued if any of these occur
◆• Assess gold toxicity: decreased Hgb, WBC <4000/mm^3, granulocytes <1500/mm^3, platelets <150,000/mm^3, severe diarrhea, stomatitis, hematuria, rash, itching, proteinuria; drug should be discontinued and dimercaprol (BAL) with glucocorticoids given

Nursing diagnoses
☑ Mobility, impaired (uses)
☑ Injury, risk for (adverse reactions)
☑ Diarrhea (adverse reactions)
☑ Knowledge deficit (teaching)

Implementation
• Give bid or may give as single dose qAM with food or drink to prevent GI symptoms
🚫• Do not chew, crush caps

Patient/family education
• Instruct patient that drug must be taken as prescribed to be useful; to obtain lab work monthly; that therapeutic effect may take 3-4 mo; patient should not double or skip doses
• Teach patient that diarrhea is common, but if blood appears in stools or urine, notify prescriber at once; that patient should check for bruising, hematemesis, hematuria, petechiae, bleeding gums, which indicate thrombocytopenia
• Advise patient to report abnormal skin conditions, stomatitis, fatigue, jaundice; may indicate blood dyscrasias; to notify prescriber of sore throat, fever, malaise; infection, gold toxicity: severe diarrhea, stomatitis, rash, itching; to avoid exposure to sunlight or ultraviolet light; to use sunscreen to prevent burns
• Teach patient to use dilute hydrogen peroxide for mild stomatitis, avoid hot spicy foods and food with high acidic content; use soft toothbrush, rinse more frequently, floss daily
• Teach patient that contraception should be used during treatment

---

Evaluation
Positive therapeutic outcome
- Ability to move joints with less pain
- Absence of stiffness, inflammation in joints

---

azathioprine 🔑 (℞)
(ay-za-thye'oh-preen)
Imuran
Func. class.: Immunosuppressant
Chem. class.: Purine analog
Pregnancy category D

Action: Produces immunosuppression by inhibiting purine synthesis, DNA, RNA in cells

⇒ Therapeutic Outcome: Absence of graft rejection, slowing of rheumatoid arthritis

Uses: Renal transplants to prevent graft rejection, often used with corticosteroids, cytotoxics; refractory rheumatoid arthritis, refractory ITP, glomerulonephritis, nephrotic syndrome, bone marrow transplant

Investigational uses: Myasthenia gravis, chronic ulcerative colitis, Crohn's disease, Behcet's syndrome

Dosage and routes
Renal dose
CrCl 10-50 ml/min 75% of dose; CrCl <10 ml/min 50% of dose

Prevention of rejection
P *Adult and child:* PO, **IV** 3-5 mg/kg/day, then maintenance (PO) of at least 1-2 mg/kg/day

Refractory rheumatoid arthritis
Adult: PO 1/mg/kg/day; may increase dosage after 2 mo by 0.5 mg/kg/day; not to exceed 2.5 mg/kg/day

Available forms: Tabs 50 mg; inj **IV** 100 mg

Adverse effects
GI: Nausea, vomiting, stomatitis, esophagitis, **pancreatitis, hepatotoxicity, jaundice**
HEMA: **Leukopenia, thrombocytopenia, anemia, pancytopenia**
INTEG: Rash
MS: Arthralgia, muscle wasting

Contraindications: Hypersensitivity, pregnancy **D**

Precautions: Severe renal disease, severe hepatic disease, **G** elderly

▧ Do Not Confuse:
Imuran/Imferon

Pharmacokinetics	
Absorption	Readily (PO)
Distribution	Crosses placenta
Metabolism	Liver to mercapto-purine
Excretion	Kidney, minimal
Half-life	3 hr

Pharmacodynamics		
	PO	IV
Onset	Unknown	Unknown
Peak	4 hr	Unknown
Duration	Unknown	Unknown

Interactions
Individual drugs
Allopurinol: ↑ toxicity
Cyclosporine: ↑ myelosuppression
Warfarin: ↓ action of warfarin
Drug classifications
Ace inhibitors: ↑ leukopenia

Antineoplastics: ↑ myelosuppression
Vaccines: ↓ immune response
Lab test interferences
↓ uric acid, ↑ LFTs
Interference: CBC, diff count

NURSING CONSIDERATIONS
Assessment
• Assess symptoms of rheumatoid arthritis: pain in joints, stiffness, poor range of motion, inflammation
• Monitor blood studies: Hgb, WBC, platelets during treatment monthly; if leukocytes are <3000/mm^3 or platelets <100,000/mm^3, drug should be discontinued or reduced; decreased Hgb level may indicate bone marrow suppression
• Monitor liver function studies: alkaline phosphatase, AST, ALT, amylase, bilirubin; and for hepatotoxicity: dark urine, jaundice, itching, light-colored stools; drug should be discontinued

Nursing diagnoses
☑ Mobility, impaired (uses)
☑ Infection, risk for (uses)
☑ Knowledge deficit (teaching)

Implementation
PO route
• Give all medications PO if possible, avoiding IM injections, since bleeding may occur
• Give with meals to reduce GI upset; nausea is common
• For several days before transplant surgery, patients should be placed in protective isolation

IV route
• Give after diluting 100 mg/10 ml of sterile water for inj; rotate to dissolve; may further dilute with 50 ml or more saline or glucose in saline given over >30 min (intermittent inf)

Solution compatibilities:
D$_5$W, NaCl 0.9%, NaCl 0.45%

Patient/family education
• Teach patient that therapeutic response may take 3-4 mo in rheumatoid arthritis; that drug is needed for life in renal transplant
• Instruct patient to report fever, rash, severe diarrhea, chills, sore throat, fatigue, since serious infections may occur; or clay-colored stools and cramping (hepatotoxicity)
• Advise patient to use contraceptive measures during treatment for 12 wk after ending therapy; drug is teratogenic
• Advise patient to avoid vaccinations
• Tell patient to avoid crowds and persons with known infections to reduce risk of infection
• Instruct patient not to use OTC medications without approval of prescriber
• To use soft-bristled toothbrush to prevent bleeding

Evaluation
Positive therapeutic outcome
• Absence of graft rejection
• Immunosuppression in autoimmune disorders
• Increased joint mobility without pain in rheumatoid arthritis

azelastine (℞)
(ay'ze-lass-teen)
Astelin
Func. class.: Leukotriene
synthesis inhibitor
Chem. class.: Phthalazi-
none derivative
Pregnancy category C

Action: Inhibits the synthesis
and release of leukotrienes;
antagonizes action of acetylcholine, histamine, serotonin

▶**Therapeutic Outcome:**
Decreased nasal stuffiness,
itching, swollen eyes

Uses: Seasonal allergic rhinitis

Dosage and routes
▣*Adult and child ≥12 yr:* Nasal
2 sprays/nostril bid

Available forms: Spray 137
µg/actuation

Adverse effects
CNS: Sedation (more common
with increased dosages),
drowsiness
MISC: Weight increase,
myalgia

Contraindications: Hypersensitivity

Precautions: Pregnancy C

Pharmacokinetics	
Absorption	Unknown
Distribution	Unknown
Metabolism	Liver, extensively
Excretion	Feces
Half-life	25-42 hr

Pharmacodynamics	
Onset	Unknown
Peak	4-5 hr
Duration	Unknown

Interactions
Individual drugs
Alcohol: ↑ CNS depression

Drug classifications
CNS depressants: ↑ CNS
depression
Narcotics: ↑ CNS depression
Sedative/hypnotics: ↑ CNS
depression

NURSING CONSIDERATIONS
Assessment
• Assess respiratory status:
rate, rhythm, increase in bronchial secretions, wheezing,
chest tightness; provide fluids
to 2 L/day to decrease secretion thickness

Nursing diagnoses
☑ Airway clearance, ineffective
(uses)
☑ Knowledge deficit (teaching)
☑ Noncompliance (teaching,
overuse)

Implementation
• Remove cap/safety clip from
spray pump
• Prime pump if using for first
time, push 4 times quickly,
away from face, blow your
nose, then place tip of pump
into one nostril, while holding
other nostril closed, tilt head
forward, and spray into nostril
• Put cover/safety clip back on

Patient/family education
• Teach patient all aspects of
drug uses; to notify prescriber
if confusion, sedation occur; to
avoid driving and other hazardous activity if drowsiness
occurs; to avoid alcohol and
other CNS depressants that
may potentiate effect
• Caution patient not to exceed recommended dosage;
dysrhythmias may occur

A

Evaluation
Positive therapeutic outcome
• Absence of running or congested nose

---

azithromycin (R)
(ay-zi-thro-my'sin)
Zithromax
Func. class.: Antiinfective
Chem. class.: Macrolide
(azalide)

Pregnancy category   B

Action: Binds to 50S ribosomal subunits of susceptible bacteria and suppresses protein synthesis; much greater spectrum of activity than erythromycin

Therapeutic Outcome: Bacteriostatic against the following susceptible organisms: *Moraxella catarrhalis, Streptococcus pneumoniae, Streptococcus pyogenes, Staphylococcus aureus, Haemophilus influenzae, Clostridium, Legionella pneumophila, Chlamydia trachomatis, Mycoplasma;* no effect on methicillin-resistant *S. aureus;* in children: acute otitis media *(H. influenzae, M. catarrhalis, S. pneumoniae) PO;* community-acquired pneumonia *(C. pneumoniae, H. influenzae, M. pneumoniae, S. pneumoniae) PO;* pharyngitis/tonsillitis *(S. pyogenes)*

Uses: Mild to moderate infections of the upper respiratory tract, lower respiratory tract; uncomplicated skin and skin structure infections, nongonococcal urethritis, or cervicitis; prophylaxis of disseminated *Mycobacterium avium* complex (MAC)

Dosage and routes
Adult: PO 500 mg on day 1, then 250 mg qd on days 2-5 for a total dose of 1.5 g; may give a one-time dose of 1 g for chlamydial infections; 1200 mg qwk for MAC prophylaxis; **IV** 500 mg qd $\geq$ 2 days, then 500 mg qd to complete 7-10 day therapy (community-acquired pneumonia); **IV** 500 mg qd × 2 days, then 250 mg qd to complete 7-day therapy (pelvic inflammatory disease (PID))

P *Child $\geq$2 yr:* 12 mg/kg qd for 5 days

P *Child <6 mo:* 10 mg/kg on day 1, then 5 mg/kg qd

Available forms: Caps 250 mg; tabs 250, 600 mg; powder for inj 500 mg; powder for oral susp 100 mg/5 ml, 200mg/5 ml, 1 gm/packet

Adverse effects
CNS: Dizziness, headache, vertigo, somnolence
CV: Palpitations, chest pain
GI: Nausea, vomiting, diarrhea, **hepatotoxicity,** abdominal pain, stomatitis, heartburn, dyspepsia, flatulence, melena, **cholestatic jaundice**
GU: Vaginitis, moniliasis, nephritis
INTEG: Rash, urticaria, pruritus, photosensitivity

Contraindications: Hypersensitivity to azithromycin or erythromycin

Precautions: Pregnancy **B,** lactation, hepatic/renal/
G cardiac disease, elderly, child
P <6 mo for otitis media, child <2 yr for pharyngitis, tonsillitis

Do Not Confuse: Zithromax/Zinacef

Herb/drug   Do Not Crush   Alert   Key Drug   G Geriatric   P Pediatric

Pharmacokinetics	
Absorption	Rapid, (PO) up to 50%
Distribution	Widely distributed
Metabolism	Unknown, minimal metabolism
Excretion	Unchanged (bile); kidneys, minimal
Half-life	11-70 hr

Pharmacodynamics	
Onset	Unknown
Peak	2-4 hr
Duration	24 hr

Interactions
Individual drugs
Astemizole: ↑ toxicity
Carbamazepine: ↑ toxicity
Ergotamine: ↑ toxicity
Pimozide: ↑ toxicity
Phenytoin: ↑ effects of oral anticoagulants
Theophylline: ↑ toxicity
Triazolam: ↓ clearance of triazolam
Drug classifications
Aluminum antacids: ↓ peak serum
Anticoagulants, orals: ↑ effect of oral anticoagulants
Magnesium antacids: ↓ levels of azithromycin
Food/drug
↓ absorption
Lab test interferences
↑ bilirubin, ↑ LDH, ↑ alk phosphatase, ↑ CPK, ↑ K, ↑ pro-time, ↑ BUN, ↑ creatinine, ↑ blood glucose, ↑ AST, ↑ ALT

NURSING CONSIDERATIONS
Assessment
• Assess for signs and symptoms of infection: drainage, fever, increased WBC >10,000 mm^3, urine culture positive, sore throat, sputum culture positive

• Monitor respiratory status: rate, character, wheezing, tightness in chest; discontinue drug if these occur
• Monitor allergies before treatment, reaction of each medication; place allergies on chart, notify all people giving drugs; skin eruptions, itching
• Monitor I&O ratio, renal studies; report hematuria, oliguria in renal disease; check urinalysis, protein, blood
• Monitor liver studies: AST, ALT, bilirubin, LDH, alkaline phosphatase; CBC with differential
• Monitor C&S before drug therapy; drug may be taken as soon as culture is taken; C&S may be repeated after treatment
• Monitor bowel pattern before, during treatment
• Assess for superinfection: sore throat, fever, fatigue

Nursing diagnoses
✓ Infection, risk for (uses)
✓ Diarrhea (adverse reactions)
✓ Knowledge deficit (teaching)

Implementation
• Provide adequate intake of fluids (2 L) during diarrhea episodes
• Give with a full glass of water; do not give with food; give caps/susp 1 hr before or 2 hr pc; tabs may be taken without regard to food; do not give with fruit juices
• Store at room temperature
• Reconstitute 1 gm packet for susp with 60 ml water, mix, rinse glass with more water and have patient drink to consume all medication
IV route
• Reconstitute 500 mg drug/ 4.8 ml sterile water for inj (100 mg/ml), shake, dilute with

≥250 ml 0.9% NaCl, 0.45% NaCl, or LR to 1-2 mg/ml
• Give 500 mg/1 hr or more, never give IM or as a bol

Patient/family education
• Instruct patient to report sore throat, black furry tongue, fever, loose foul-smelling stool, vaginal itching, discharge, fatigue; may indicate superinfection
• Caution patient not to take aluminum/magnesium-containing antacids or food simultaneously with this drug; blood levels of azithromycin will be decreased
• Instruct patient to notify prescriber of diarrhea stools, dark urine, pale stools, yellow discoloration of eyes or skin, severe abdominal pain; cholestatic jaundice is a severe adverse reaction
• Teach patient to take at evenly spaced intervals; complete dosage regimen; to notify prescriber if symptoms continue
• Teach patient that if pregnancy is suspected to notify prescriber
• Inform patient that sunburns may occur; wear protective clothing and sunscreen

Evaluation
Positive therapeutic outcome
• C&S negative for infection
• WBC within 5000-10,000 mm³

aztreonam (℞)
(az-tree'oh-nam)
azactam
Func. class.: Misc. antiinfective
Chem. class.: Monobactam

Pregnancy category B

Action: Inhibits organisms by inhibiting bacterial cell wall synthesis, which causes death of organism (bactericidal)

▷**Therapeutic Outcome:** Bactericidal action against susceptible organisms, specifically gram-negative aerobic organisms: *Escherichia coli, Serratia, Klebsiella, Enterobacter, Haemophilus influenzae, Shigella, Providencia, Salmonella, Neisseria gonorrhoeae, Pseudomonas aeruginosa,* including strains resistant to other drugs

Uses: Urinary tract infection; septicemia; skin, muscle, bone infection and other infections caused by gram-negative organisms

Investigational uses: May be used for acute uncomplicated gonorrhea in patients with penicillin-resistant gonococci, instead of spectinomycin

Dosage and routes
Urinary tract infections
Adult: **IV**/IM 500 mg-1 g q8-12h

Systemic infections
Adult: **IV**/IM 1-2 g q8-12h

🄿 *Child:* **IV**/IM 90-120 mg/ kg/day divided q6-8h

Severe systemic infections
Adult: **IV**/IM 2 g q6-8h; do not exceed 8 g/day
Continue treatment for 48 hr

---

after negative culture or until patient is asymptomatic

Available forms: Powder for inj 500 mg, 1, 2 g

Adverse effects

CNS: Lethargy, hallucinations, fever (pediatric), anxiety, depression, twitching, **coma, convulsions,** malaise

EENT: Tinnitus, diplopia, nasal congestion

GI: Nausea, vomiting, diarrhea, increased AST, ALT, abdominal pain, glossitis, colitis, pseudomembranous colitis

GU: Vaginal candidiasis, vaginitis, breast tenderness, increased BUN, creatinine

HEMA: Anemia, increased bleeding time, **bone marrow depression, granulocytopenia**

INTEG: Rash (pediatric)

Contraindications: Hypersensitivity

Precautions: Pregnancy **B,** lactation, children, impaired renal/hepatic function, elderly

Pharmacokinetics

Absorption	Well absorbed (IM)
Distribution	Widely distributed; crosses placenta
Metabolism	Liver, minimal
Excretion	Kidneys, unchanged (60%-70%); breast milk
Half-life	1.7 hr; increased in renal disease

Pharmacodynamics

	IM	IV
Onset	Rapid	Rapid
Peak	1 hr	Infusion's end

Interactions

Individual drugs

Cefoxitin: ↑ antagonist effect

Clindamycin: ↓ action of clindamycin

Furosemide: ↑ levels

Imipenem: ↑ antagonist effect

Probenecid: ↑ levels

Drug classifications

Aminoglycosides: ↑ nephrotoxicity

Antiinfectives: ↑ antagonist effect

Penicillins: ↑ or ↓ action of penicillins

Lab test interferences

Interference: Urine glucose using Clinitest/Benedict's reagent

Positive: Coombs' test

NURSING CONSIDERATIONS

Assessment

• Assess patient for previous sensitivity reaction to penicillins or cephalosporins; cross-sensitivity between penicillins, cephalosporins and this drug is common

• Assess patient for signs and symptoms of infection including characteristics of wounds, sputum, urine, stool, WBC >10,000, fever; obtain baseline information before and during treatment

• Complete C&S before beginning drug therapy to identify if correct treatment has been initiated

• Identify urine output; if decreasing, notify prescriber (may indicate nephrotoxicity); note color, character, pH of urine if drug is administered for urinary tract infection; output should be 800 ml less than intake; if urine is highly acidic, alkalinization may be needed

• Assess renal studies: urinalysis, protein, blood, serum creatinine, BUN

• Monitor blood studies: AST, ALT, CBC, Hct, bilirubin, LDH, alkaline phosphatase, Coombs' test monthly if pa-

tient is on long-term therapy
- Monitor electrolytes: potassium, sodium, chloride monthly if patient is on long-term therapy
- Assess bowel pattern daily; if severe diarrhea occurs, drug should be discontinued; may indicate pseudomembranous colitis
- Monitor for bleeding: ecchymosis, bleeding gums, hematuria, stool guaiac daily if on long-term therapy
- Assess for overgrowth of infection: perineal itching, fever, malaise, redness, pain, swelling, drainage, rash, diarrhea, change in cough, sputum

Nursing diagnoses
☑ Infection, risk for (uses)
☑ Diarrhea (side effects)
☑ Injury, risk for (side effects)
☑ Knowledge deficit (teaching)
☑ Noncompliance (teaching)

Implementation
IM route
- Reconstitute 1 g/3 ml or more of sterile water for inj 0.9% NaCl; may be diluted with 0.5% or 1% lidocaine to prevent pain; give deep in large muscle mass, massage; sol stable 1 wk refrigerated

IV route
- Check for irritation, extravasation, phlebitis daily; change **IV** site q72h
- For direct **IV**, dilute 1 g/10 ml or 2 g/20 ml sterile water for injection, shake, let stand until clear; give over 3-5 min into running **IV**
- For intermittent inf, further dilute with 50-100 ml of D_5W, $D_{10}W$, $D_5/0.25\%$ NaCl, $D_5/0.45\%$ NaCl, $D_5/0.9\%$ NaCl, 0.9% NaCl, D_5/LR, $D_5/0.02\%$, sodium bicarbonate, Ringer's or LR; give over

15-60 min into running **IV**

Syringe compatibilities:
Clindamycin

Y-site compatibilities:
Allopurinol, amifostine, amikacin, aminophylline, ampicillin, ampicillin/sulbactam, bleomycin, bumetanide, buprenorphine, butorphanol, calcium gluconate, carboplatin, carmustine, cefazolin, cefepime, cefonicid, cefoperazone, cefotaxime, cefotetan, cefoxitin, ceftazidime, ceftizoxime, ceftriaxone, cefuroxime, cimetidine, ciprofloxacin, cisatracurium, cisplatin, clindamycin, cyclophosphamide, cytarabine, dacarbazine, dactinomycin, dexamethasone, diltiazem, diphenhydramine, dobutamine, dopamine, doxorubicin, doxycycline, doxorubicin liposome, droperidol, enalaprilat, etoposide, famotidine, filgrastim, floxuridine, fluconazole, fludarabine, fluorouracil, foscarnet, furosemide, gallium, gentamicin, granisetron, haloperidol, heparin, hydrocortisone, hydromorphone, hydroxyzine, idarubicin, ifosfamide, imipenem-cilastatin, insulin (regular), leucovorin, magnesium sulfate, mannitol, mechlorethamine, melphalan, meperidine, mesna, methotrexate, methylprednisolone, metoclopramide, mezlocillin, minocycline, morphine, nalbuphine, netilmicin, ondansetron, piperacillin, piperacillin/tazobactam, plicamycin, potassium chloride, promethazine, propofol, ranitidine, remifentanil, sargramostim, sodium bicarbonate, teniposide, theophylline, thiotepa, ticarcillin, ticarcillin/clavulanate, to-

bramycin, trimethoprim-sulfamethoxazole, vinblastine, vincristine, vinorelbine, zidovudine

Y-site incompatibilities:
Vancomycin

Additive compatibilities:
Ampicillin/sulbactam, cefazolin, ciprofloxacin, clindamycin, gentamicin, tobramycin

Additive incompatibilities:
Nafcillin, cephradine, metronidazole

Patient/family education
• Teach patient to report sore throat, bruising, bleeding, joint pain; may indicate blood dyscrasias (rare)
• Advise patient to contact prescriber if vaginal itching, loose, foul-smelling stools, furry tongue occur; may indicate superinfection; report itching, rash, pruritus, urticaria
• Instruct patient to take all medication prescribed for the length of time ordered; drug must be taken around the clock to maintain blood levels; do not give medication to others
• Advise patient to notify prescriber of diarrhea with blood or pus

Evaluation
Positive therapeutic outcome
• Absence of signs/symptoms of infection (WBC <10,000, temp WNL, absence of red draining wounds), inflammation, temp
• Reported improvement in symptoms of infection

baclofen ⚕ (℞)
(bak'loe-fen)
baclofen, Lioresal, Lioresal Intrathecal
Func. class.: Skeletal muscle relaxant, central acting
Chem. class.: GABA chlorophenyl derivative

Pregnancy category C

Action: Inhibits synaptic responses in CNS by decreasing GABA, which decreases neurotransmitter function; decreases frequency, severity of muscle spasms

Therapeutic Outcome: Decreased spasticity of muscles

Uses: Spasticity in spinal cord injury, multiple sclerosis

Dosage and routes
Adult: PO 5 mg tid × 3 days, then 10 mg tid × 3 days, then 15 mg tid × 3 days, then 20 mg tid × 3 days, then titrated to response; not to exceed 80 mg/day

P *Child 2-8 yr:* 10-15 mg/kg/day divided q8h, titrate to max 40 mg/day

P *Child ≥ 8 yr:* As above, max 60 mg/day

Intrathecal
Use implantable intrathecal inf pump; use screening trial of 3 separate bol doses if needed (50 μg/ml, 75 μg/1.5 ml, 100 μg/2 ml); initially double screening dose that produced result and give over 24 hr; increase by 10%-30% q24h only; maintenance: 12-1500 μg/day

Available forms: Tabs 10, 20 mg, Intrathecal sol 10 mg/20 ml (500 μg/ml), 10 mg/5 ml (2000 μg/ml)

Adverse effects
CNS: Dizziness, weakness, fatigue, drowsiness, headache, *disorientation,* insomnia, paresthesias, tremors, **seizures**
CV: Hypotension, chest pain, palpitations, edema
EENT: Nasal congestion, blurred vision, mydriasis, tinnitus
GI: Nausea, constipation, *vomiting,* increased AST, alkaline phosphatase, abdominal pain, dry mouth, anorexia
GU: Urinary frequency
INTEG: Rash, pruritus

Contraindications: Hypersensitivity

Precautions: Peptic ulcer disease, renal disease, hepatic disease, stroke, seizure disorder, diabetes mellitus,
G pregnancy **C**, elderly

N **Do Not Confuse:**
Lioresal/Lotensin

Pharmacokinetics	
Absorption	Rapid
Distribution	Widely, crosses placenta
Metabolism	Liver, partially
Excretion	Kidney, unchanged
Half-life	2½-4 hr

Pharmacodynamics	
	PO
Onset	Unknown
Peak	2-3 hr
Duration	>8 hr

Interactions
Individual drugs
Alcohol: CNS depression
Drug classifications
Antidepressants, tricyclic: ↑ CNS depression
Barbiturates: ↑ CNS depression
Opiates: ↑ CNS depression

Sedative/hypnotics: ↑ CNS depression
Ⅾ *Herb/drug*
Kava: ↑ CNS depression
Lab test interferences
↑ AST, ↑ alkaline phosphatase, ↑ blood glucose

NURSING CONSIDERATIONS
Assessment
• Monitor B/P, weight, blood sugar, and hepatic function periodically
◆ • Check for increased seizure activity in epilepsy patient; this drug decreases seizure threshold, monitor EEG
• Check I&O ratio; check for urinary retention, frequency, hesitancy
• Allergic reactions: rash, fever, respiratory distress; severe weakness, numbness in extremities
• Assess CNS depression: dizziness, drowsiness, psychiatric symptoms
• Check dosage, as individual titration is required

Nursing diagnoses
☑ Mobility, impaired uses
☑ Injury, risk for (adverse reactions)
☑ Knowledge deficit (teaching)

Implementation
PO route
• Give with meals for GI symptoms; gum, frequent sips of water for dry mouth
• Store in airtight container at room temperature
Ⅳ **IV route**
• Titration is based on response
• Test dose: 50 mg/ml, give over 1 min or more

Additive compatibilities:
Morphine
IT route

• Do not use IT inj **IV**, IM, SC, epidural

Patient/family education
• Advise patient not to discontinue medication quickly; hallucinations, spasticity, tachycardia will occur; drug should be tapered off over 1-2 wk
• Advise patient not to take with alcohol, other CNS depressants
• Caution patient to avoid altering activities while taking this drug; to avoid hazardous activities if drowsiness or dizziness occurs
• Advise patient to avoid using OTC medication: cough preparations, antihistamines unless directed by prescriber
• Tell patient to increase fluid intake >2 L/day; to take with food

Evaluation
Positive therapeutic outcome
• Decreased pain, spasticity

Treatment of overdose: Induce emesis if conscious patient, lavage, dialysis

---

basiliximab (℞)
(bas-ih-liks'ih-mab)
Simulect
Func. class.: Immunosuppressive
Chem. class.: Murine/ human monoclonal antibody (Interleukin-2) receptor antagonist
Pregnancy category   B

Action: Binds to and blocks the IL-2 receptor, which is selectively expressed on the surface of activated T-lymphocytes; impairs the immune system to antigenic challenges

⊐**Therapeutic Outcome:** Prevention of graft rejection

Uses: Acute allograft rejection in renal transplant patients when used with cyclosporine and corticosteroids

Dosage and routes
Adult: **IV** 20 mg × 2 doses; 1st dose within 2 hr before transplant surgery; 2nd dose given 4 days after transplantation
P *Child 2-15 yr:* 12 mg/m^2 × 2 doses; 1st dose within 2 hr before transplant surgery; 2nd dose given 4 days after transplantation

Available forms: Powder for inj 20 mg

Adverse effects
CNS: Pyrexia, chills, tremors, headache, insomnia
CV: Chest pain, angina, **cardiac failure,** hypotension
GI: Vomiting, nausea, diarrhea, constipation, abdominal pain
MISC: Infection, moniliasis
MS: Arthralgia, myalgia
RESP: Dyspnea, wheezing, **pulmonary edema**

Contraindications: Hypersensitivity

Precautions: Pregnancy **B,**
G infections, elderly, lactation,
P children

Pharmacokinetics	
Absorption	Unknown
Distribution	Unknown
Metabolism	Unknown
Excretion	Unknown
Half-life	Unknown

Pharmacodynamics	
Onset	Unknown
Peak	Unknown
Duration	Unknown

Interactions
None known

NURSING CONSIDERATIONS
Assessment
• Monitor blood studies: Hgb, WBC, platelets during treatment qmo; if leukocytes are <3000/mm^3, drug should be discontinued
• Monitor liver function studies: alk phosphatase, AST, ALT, bilirubin
• Assess hepatotoxicity: dark urine, jaundice, itching, light-colored stools; drug should be discontinued

Nursing diagnoses
☑ Infection, risk for (adverse reactions)
☑ Knowledge deficit (teaching)

Implementation
• Administer all medications PO if possible; avoid IM injection, since infection may occur

IV **IV route**
• After adding 5 ml sterile water for inj, shake gently to dissolve, reconstitute to a vol of 50 ml with 0.9% NaCl or D$_5$, gently invert bag, do not shake

Patient/family education
• Instruct patient to report fever, chills, sore throat, fatigue, since serious infection may occur

Evaluation
Positive therapeutic outcome
• Absence of graft rejection

beclomethasone (℞)
(be-kloe-meth′a-sone)
Beclodisk ♣, Becloforte
Inhaler ♣, Beclovent,
Vanceril
Func. class.: Synthetic
glucocorticoid (long
acting)
Chem. class.: Beclomethasone diester

Pregnancy category   C

Action: Antiinflammatory; vasoconstrictive properties; also immunosuppressive

➔**Therapeutic Outcome:**
Decreased inflammation and normal immunity

Uses: Seasonal, perennial allergic rhinitis, nasal polyps, chronic steroid-dependent asthma

Dosage and routes
P *Adult and child >12 yr:*
INSTILL 1-2 sprays in each nostril bid-qid; INH 2-4 puffs tid-qid

P *Child 6-12 yrs:* INSTILL 1 spray in each nostril tid; INH 1-2 puffs tid-qid

Available forms: Aero 42 µg/spray (nasal); aero for inh 42 µg/activation; aerosol for nasal inh 0.042%

Adverse effects
CNS: Headache, paresthesia
EENT: Dryness, nasal irritation, burning, sneezing, secretions with blood, nasal ulcerations, **perforation of nasal septum,** candidal infection, earache, *hoarseness*
ENDO: **Adrenal suppression**
INTEG: Rash, urticaria, pruritus
RESP: **Acute status asthmaticus,** wheezing, cough

☑ Herb/drug 🚫 Do Not Crush ♦ Alert ⌖ Key Drug **G** Geriatric **P** Pediatric

MISC: **Angioedema adrenal insufficiency,** facial edema

Contraindications: Hypersensitivity, systemic corticosteroid therapy

Precautions: Pregnancy **C,** children <12, nasal ulcers, recurrent epistaxis

Pharmacokinetics

Absorption	Locally only
Distribution	Not distributed
Metabolism	Minimal
Excretion	Feces
Half-life	3-15 hr

Pharmacodynamics

	INH	NASAL
Onset	10 min	10 min
Peak	Unknown	Unknown
Duration	Unknown	Unknown

NURSING CONSIDERATIONS
Assessment
• Assess adrenal suppression: 17-KS, plasma cortisol for decreased levels, adrenal function periodically for HPA axis suppression during prolonged therapy; monitor growth and development
• Check nasal passages during long-term treatment for changes in mucus; check for burning, stinging; assess for glucocorticoid withdrawal: dizziness, hypotension, fatigue, muscle/joint pain; notify prescriber immediately
• Assess respiratory status: rest, rhythm, characteristics; auscultate lung bilaterally before and throughout treatment
• Assess for fungal infections in mucous membranes

Nursing diagnoses
☑Airway clearance, ineffective (uses)

☑Oral mucous membranes, altered (adverse reactions)
☑Knowledge deficit (teaching)
☑Noncompliance (teaching)

Implementation
• Give PO, using a spacer device for proper dose
• Use after cleaning aerosol top daily with warm water; dry thoroughly
• Store in cool environment; do not puncture or incinerate container

Patient/family education
• Teach patient to gargle/rinse mouth after each use to prevent oral fungal infections
• Teach patient that in times of stress, systemic corticosteroids may be needed to prevent adrenal insufficiency; do not discontinue oral drug abruptly, taper slowly
• Teach patient to continue using product even if mild nasal bleeding occurs; is usually transient
• Teach patient method of instillation after providing written instructions from manufacturer
• Teach patient to clear nasal passages before administration; use decongestant if needed; shake inhaler, invert, tilt head backward, insert nozzle into nostril, away from septum; hold other nostril closed and depress activator, inhale through nose, exhale through mouth

Evaluate
Positive therapeutic outcome
• Decrease in runny nose, improved symptoms of bronchial asthma

Adverse effects: *italic* = common; **bold** = life-threatening

benazepril (℞)
(ben-a′za-pril)
Lotensin
Func. class.: Antihypertensive
Chem. class.: ACE inhibitor

Pregnancy category
C (1st trimester)
D (2nd/3rd trimesters)

Action: Selectively suppresses renin-angiotensin-aldosterone system; inhibits ACE, preventing conversion of angiotensin I to angiotensin II; results in dilatation of arterial, venous vessels

➢Therapeutic Outcome: Decreased B/P in hypertension

Uses: Hypertension, alone or in combination with thiazide diuretics

Dosage and routes
Adult: PO 10 mg qd initially, then 20-40 mg/day divided bid or qd (without a diuretic); 5 mg PO qd (with a diuretic)

Renal dose: 5 mg qd with CrCl <30 ml/min/1.73 m^2; increase as needed to maximum of 40 mg/day

G *Elderly:* PO 5-10 mg/day initially

Available forms: Tabs 5, 10, 20, 40 mg

Adverse effects
CNS: Anxiety, hypertonia, insomnia, paresthesia, headache, dizziness, fatigue
CV: Hypotension, postural hypotension, syncope, palpitations, angina
GI: Nausea, constipation, vomiting, gastritis, melena
GU: Increased BUN, creatinine, decreased libido, impotence, urinary tract infection
HEMA: **Neutropenia, agranulocytosis**
INTEG: Rash, flushing, sweating
MISC: **Angioedema**
META: Hyperkalemia, hyponatremia
MS: Arthralgia, arthritis, myalgia
RESP: Cough, asthma, bronchitis, dyspnea, sinusitis

Contraindications: Hypersensitivity to ACE inhibitors, **D** (2nd/3rd trimesters), **P** lactation, children

Precautions: Impaired renal/liver function, dialysis patients, hypovolemia, blood dyscrasias, **G** CHF, COPD, asthma, elderly, bilateral renal artery stenosis; pregnancy **C** (1st trimester)

◤Do Not Confuse:
Lotensin/Lioresal, Lotensin/Loniten

Pharmacokinetics	
Absorption	<40%
Distribution	Unknown; crosses placenta
Metabolism	Liver metabolites; serum protein binding 97%
Excretion	Kidney, breast milk (minimal)
Half-life	10-11 hr (metabolite); increased in renal disease

Pharmacodynamics	
Onset	Unknown
Peak	½-1 hr
Duration	Unknown

Interactions
Individual drugs
Alcohol: ↑ hypotension (large amounts)
Lithium: ↑ serum levels

Drug classifications
Antihypertensives: ↑ hypotension
Diuretics: ↑ hypotension
Diuretics, potassium-sparing: ↑ hyperkalemia
Potassium supplements: ↑ toxicity
Sympathomimetics: ↑ toxicity
Lab test interferences
↑ BUN, ↑ creatinine, ↑ LFTs, ↑ bilirubin, ↑ uric acid, ↑ blood glucose

NURSING CONSIDERATIONS
Assessment
• Monitor blood studies: neutrophils, decreased platelets
• Monitor B/P at peak/trough level of drug, check for orthostatic hypotension, syncope; if changes occur, dosage change may be required
• Monitor renal studies: protein, BUN, creatinine; watch for increased levels that may indicate nephrotic syndrome and renal failure; monitor urine for protein; monitor renal symptoms: polyuria, oliguria, frequency, dysuria
• Establish baselines in renal, liver function tests before therapy begins
• Check potassium levels throughout treatment, although hyperkalemia rarely occurs
• Assess for allergic reactions: rash, fever, pruritus, urticaria; drug should be discontinued if antihistamines fail to help
Nursing diagnoses
✓ Cardiac output, decreased (uses)
✓ Injury, potential for (side effects)
✓ Knowledge deficit (teaching)
✓ Noncompliance (teaching)

Implementation
PO route
• Store in air-tight container at 86° F (30° C) or less
• Severe hypotension may occur after 1st dose of this medication; decreased hypotension may be prevented by reducing or discontinuing diuretic therapy 3 days before beginning benazepril therapy

Patient/family education
• Instruct patient not to discontinue drug abruptly; advise patient to tell all persons associated with care
• Teach patient not to use OTC products (cough, cold, allergy) unless directed by prescriber; serious side effects can occur; xanthines such as coffee, tea, chocolate, cola can prevent action of drug
• Emphasize the importance of complying with dosage schedule, even if feeling better; to continue with medical regimen to decrease B/P: exercise, cessation of smoking, decreasing stress, diet modifications
• Emphasize the need to rise slowly to sitting or standing position to minimize orthostatic hypotension; not to exercise in hot weather because increased hypotension can occur
• Teach patient to notify prescriber of mouth sores, sore throat, fever, swelling of hands or feet, irregular heartbeat, chest pain, coughing, shortness of breath
• Caution patient to report excessive perspiration, dehydration, vomiting, diarrhea; may lead to fall in B/P
• Caution patient that drug may cause dizziness, fainting, light-headedness; may occur

Adverse effects: *italic* = common; **bold** = life-threatening

during 1st few days of therapy; to avoid activities that may be hazardous

• Teach patient how to take B/P; teach normal readings for age group; ensure patient takes own B/P

• Advise patient to notify prescriber of pregnancy, drug will need to be discontinued

Evaluation
Positive therapeutic outcome
• Decreased B/P in hypertension

Treatment of overdose: 0.9% NaCl **IV** inf, hemodialysis

---

benztropine ⚷ (℞)
(benz'troe-peen)
Apo-Benztropin ✦,
Bensylate ✦, benztropine
mesylate, Cogentin, PMS-
Benztropine ✦
Func. class.: Cholinergic
blocker
Chem. class.: Tertiary
amine

Pregnancy category   C

Action: Blockade of central acetylcholine receptors in the CNS, neurotransmitters are balanced

▸**Therapeutic Outcome:** Decreased involuntary movements

Uses: Parkinsonian symptoms, extrapyramidal symptoms associated with neuroleptic drugs, acute dystonia

Dosage and routes
Drug-induced
extrapyramidal symptoms
Adult: IM/**IV** 1-4 mg qd/bid; give PO dose as soon as possible; PO 1-2 mg bid/tid; increase by 0.5 mg q5-6 days

P *Child:* IM/**IV** 0.02-0.05 mg/ kg/dose 1-2 × 1 day

G *Elderly:* PO 0.5 mg qd/bid, increase by 0.5 mg q5-6 days

Parkinsonian symptoms
Adult: PO 0.5-6 mg qd; increased 0.5 mg q5-6 days titrated to patient response

Acute dystonic reactions
Adult: IM/**IV** 1-2 mg, may increase to 1-2 mg bid (PO)

Available forms: Tabs 0.5, 1, 2 mg; inj IM, **IV** 1 mg/ml

Adverse effects
CNS: Confusion, anxiety, restlessness, irritability, delusions, hallucinations, headache, sedation, depression, incoherence, dizziness, memory loss; **G** delirium (elderly)
CV: Palpitations, tachycardia, hypotension, bradycardia
EENT: Blurred vision, photophobia, dilated pupils, difficulty swallowing, dry eyes, mydriasis, increased intraocular tension, angle closure glaucoma
GI: Dryness of mouth, constipation, nausea, vomiting, abdominal distress, **paralytic ileus,** epigastric distress
GU: Hesitancy, retention, dysuria
INTEG: Rash, urticaria, dermatoses
MISC: Increased temperature, flushing, decreased sweating, **hyperthermia, heat stroke,** numbness of fingers
MS: Muscular weakness, cramping

Contraindications: Hypersensitivity, narrow angle glaucoma, myasthenia gravis, **P** GI/GU obstruction, child <3 yr, peptic ulcer, megacolon, prostate hypertrophy

---

Precautions: Pregnancy **C,**
 elderly, lactation, tachycardia,
liver, kidney disease, drug
abuse history, dysrhythmias,
hypotension, hypertension,
 psychiatric patients, children

Pharmacokinetics

Absorption	Well (PO, IM), completely (**IV**) absorbed
Distribution	Unknown
Metabolism	Unknown
Excretion	Unknown
Half-life	Unknown

Pharmacodynamics

	IM/IV	PO
Onset	15 min	1 hr
Peak	Unknown	Unknown
Duration	6-10 hr	6-10 hr

Interactions
Individual drugs
Disopyramide: ↑ anticholinergic effects
Quinidine: ↑ anticholinergic effects
Drug classifications
Antacids: ↓ absorption of benzotropine
Antidepressants, tricyclic: ↑ anticholinergic effects
Antidiarrheals: ↓ absorption
Antihistamines: ↑ anticholinergic effects
Phenothiazines: ↑ anticholinergic effects

NURSING CONSIDERATIONS
Assessment
• Monitor I&O ratio; retention commonly causes decreased urinary output, distention, frequency, incontinence
• Assess for parkinsonism, extrapyramidal symptoms: shuffling gait, muscle rigidity, involuntary movements, pill rolling, muscle spasms, drooling before and during treatment

• Monitor for urinary hesitancy, retention; palpate bladder if retention occurs
• Monitor for constipation, cramping, pain in abdomen, abdominal distention; increase fluids, bulk, exercise if this occurs
• Assess for tolerance over long-term therapy; dosage may have to be increased or changed
• Assess for mental status: affect, mood, CNS depression, worsening of mental symptoms during early therapy
• Assess for benztropine "buzz" or "high," patients may imitate EPS

Nursing diagnoses
☑ Mobility, impaired (uses)
☑ Knowledge deficit (teaching)
☑ Noncompliance (teaching)

Implementation
PO route
• Give with or after meals to prevent GI upset; may give with fluids other than water; hard candy, frequent drinks, gum to relieve dry mouth
• Give hs to avoid daytime drowsiness in patient with parkinsonism
• May be crushed and mixed with food
• Store at room temperature
IM route
• Give in large muscle mass for dystonic symptoms
 IV route
• Give parenteral dose with patient recumbent to prevent postural hypotension; give undiluted 2 mg or less >1 min or more

Syringe compatibilities:
Chlorpromazine, fluphenazine, metoclopramide, perphenazine, thiothixene

---

Y-site compatibilities:
Fluconazole, tacrolimus

Patient/family education
• Teach patient to use caution in hot weather; drug may increase susceptibility to stroke since perspiration is decreased; patient should remain indoors
• Advise patient not to discontinue this drug abruptly; to taper off over 1 wk to prevent withdrawal symptoms (insomnia, involuntary movements, anxiety, tachycardias)
• Caution patient to avoid driving or other hazardous activities; drowsiness, dizziness may occur
• Teach patient to avoid OTC medication: cough, cold preparations with alcohol, antihistamines unless directed by prescriber; increased CNS depression may occur
• Advise patient to rise from sitting or recumbent position slowly to minimize orthostatic hypotension
• Teach patient to use gum, hard candy, frequent sips of water to decrease dry mouth; if dry mouth continues, saliva substitutes may be prescribed
• Instruct patient that doses should not be doubled, but missed dose may be taken up to 2 hr before next dose

Evaluation
Positive therapeutic outcome
• Absence of involuntary movements (pill rolling, tremors, muscle spasms)

bepridil (℞)
(be'pri-dil)
Bepadin, Vascor
Func. class.: Calcium channel blocker, antianginal, antihypertensive
Chem. class.: Angina

Pregnancy category C

Action: Inhibits calcium ion influx across cell membrane during cardiac depolarization; produces relaxation of coronary vascular smooth muscle, peripheral vascular smooth muscle; dilates coronary vascular arteries; increases myocardial oxygen delivery in patients with vasospastic angina

➤**Therapeutic Outcome:** Decreased angina pectoris

Uses: Chronic stable angina, used alone or in combination with propranolol

Dosage and routes
Adult: PO 200 mg qd, after 10 days may increase dose if needed; max dose 400mg/day

Available forms: Tabs, film-coated, 200, 300, 400 mg

Adverse effects
CNS: Headache, fatigue, drowsiness, dizziness, anxiety, depression, weakness, insomnia, confusion, lightheadedness, nervousness
CV: **Dysrhythmias,** edema, **CHF,** bradycardia, hypotension, palpitations, **AV block, torsades de pointes**
GI: Nausea, vomiting, diarrhea, gastric upset, constipation, increased levels in liver function studies
GU: Nocturia, polyuria
HEMA: **Agranulocytosis**

☑ Herb/drug ⬛ Do Not Crush ◆ Alert ⬤ᆵ Key Drug ⒼGeriatric ⓅPediatric

Contraindications: Sick sinus syndrome, 2nd- or 3rd-degree heart block, Wolff-Parkinson-White syndrome, hypotension less than 90 mm Hg systolic, cardiogenic shock, history of serious ventricular arrhythmias

Precautions: CHF, hypotension, hepatic injury, pregnancy **C**, lactation, children, renal disease, IHSS, concomitant β-blocker therapy

Do Not Confuse:
bepridil/Prepidil

Pharmacokinetics

Absorption	Well absorbed
Distribution	Plasma protein bound (99%), crosses placenta
Metabolism	Liver
Excretion	Urine, feces
Half-life	42 hr

Pharmacodynamics

Onset	1 hr
Peak	2-3 hr
Duration	24 hr

Interactions
Individual drugs
Fentanyl: ↑ hypotension
Drug classifications
Antidysrhythmics: ↑ prolongation of QT, depression of AV node
β-Adrenergic blockers: ↑ adverse reactions
Cardiac glycosides: ↑ prolongation of QT, depression of AV node
Food/drug
Grapefruit: ↑ hypotension
Lab test interferences
↑ Liver function tests, ↑ aminotransferase, ↑ CPK, ↑ LDH

NURSING CONSIDERATIONS
Assessment
• Assess fluid volume status: I&O ratio and record, weight, distended red veins, crackles in lung, color, quality, and sp gr of urine, skin turgor, adequacy of pulses, moist mucous membranes, bilateral lung sounds, peripheral pitting edema
• Assess cardiac status: B/P, pulse, respiration, ECG intervals (PR, QRS, QT), dysrhythmias
• Obtain digoxin levels if cardiac glycosides are given with bepridil

Nursing diagnoses
✓ Cardiac output, decreased (uses)
✓ Knowledge deficit (teaching)

Implementation
• Give once a day, with food for GI symptoms; adjust dose no more frequently than q10 days
• Do not break, chew, crush tabs

Patient/family education
• Instruct patient to avoid hazardous activities until stabilized on drug and dizziness is no longer a problem
• Instruct patient to limit caffeine consumption; to avoid alcohol and OTC drugs unless directed by prescriber
• Advise patient to comply in all areas of medical regimen: diet, exercise, stress reduction, drug therapy; to notify prescriber of irregular heart beat, shortness of breath, swelling of feet and hands, pronounced dizziness, constipation, nausea, hypotension
• Teach patient to use as directed even if feeling better; may be taken with other cardiovascular drugs (nitrates, β-blockers)

Evaluation
Positive therapeutic outcome
• Decreased anginal pain

Treatment of overdose:
Defibrillation, atropine for AV block, vasopressor for hypotension

---

betamethasone (℞)
(bay-tah-meth′ah-sone)
Betnelan ✦, Celestone
betamethasone acetate/ betamethasone sodium phosphate (℞)
Celestone Soluspan
betamethasone sodium phosphate (℞)
Celestone Phosphate, Selestoject
Func. class.: Corticosteroid, synthetic
Chem. class.: Glucocorticoid, long acting
Pregnancy category   C

Action: Decreases inflammation by suppression of migration of polymorphonuclear leukocytes, fibroblasts, reversal of increased capillary permeability and lysosomal stabilization

⇒**Therapeutic Outcome:**
Decreased inflammation and normal immunity

Uses: Immunosuppression, severe inflammation, prevention of neonatal respiratory distress syndrome (by administration to mother), chronic asthma, rhinitis (inh); psoriasis, eczema, contact dermatitis, pruritus (top)

Dosage and routes
Adult: PO 0.6-7.2 mg qd; IM/**IV** 0.6-7.2 mg qd in joint or soft tissue (sodium phosphate)

🅟 *Child:* PO 17.5 µg/kg/day in 3 divided doses; IM 17.5 µg/

kg/day in 3 divided doses every 3rd day or 5.8-8.75 µg/kg/day as a single dose (adrenal insufficiency)

🅟 *Child:* PO 62.5-250 µg/kg/day in 3 divided doses; IM 20.8-125 µg/kg/day of the base q12-24h (other uses)

🅟 *Adult and child:* TOP apply to affected area qid

Adult: INH 2-4 puffs tid-qid; not to exceed 20 inh/day

🅟 *Child: 6-12 yr:* INH 1-2 puffs tid-qid; not to exceed 10 inh/day

🅟 *Adult and child >12 yr:* INSTILL 1-2 sprays in each nostril bid-qid

Available forms:
betamethasone: tabs 500, 600 µg; tabs, effervescent 500 µg ✦; syrup 600 µg/5 ml; betamethasone acetate/ betamethasone sodium phosphate: inj susp acetate 3 mg/sodium phosphate (= to 3 mg base); betamethasone sodium phosphate: inj 4 mg (= to 3 mg base)/ml

Adverse effects
CNS: Depression, flushing, sweating, headache, ecchymosis, bruising, mood changes
CV: Hypertension, **circulatory collapse, thrombophlebitis, embolism,** tachycardia, **necrotizing angiitis, CHF**
EENT: Fungal infections, increased intraocular pressure, blurred vision
GI: Diarrhea, nausea, abdominal distention, **GI hemorrhage,** increased appetite, **pancreatitis**
HEMA: **Thrombocytopenia**
INTEG: Acne, poor wound healing, ecchymosis, bruising, petechiae

---

MS: Fractures, osteoporosis, weakness

Contraindications: Psychosis, hypersensitivity, idiopathic thrombocytopenia, acute glomerulonephritis, amebiasis, fungal infections, nonasthmatic bronchial disease, child <2 yr, AIDS, TB

Precautions: Pregnancy **C**, diabetes mellitus, glaucoma, osteoporosis, seizure disorders, ulcerative colitis, CHF, myasthenia gravis, renal disease, esophagitis, peptic ulcer

Pharmacokinetics

Absorption	Well absorbed (PO); systemic (top)
Distribution	Crosses placenta
Metabolism	Liver, extensively
Excretion	Kidney, breast milk
Half-life	3-5 hr, adrenal suppression 3-4 days

Pharmacodynamics

	PO	IM	IV	TOP
Onset	1-2 hr	Unknown	Rapid	Unknown
Peak	2 hr	4-8 hr	4-8 hr	Unknown
Duration	3 days	1-1½ days	1-1½ days	Unknown

Interactions
Individual drugs
Alcohol: ↑ GI bleeding
Amphotericin B: ↑ hypokalemia
Insulin: ↑ need for insulin
Mezlocillin: ↑ hypokalemia
Phenytoin: ↓ action, ↑ metabolism
Rifampin: ↓ action, ↑ metabolism
Ticarcillin: ↑ hypokalemia
Drug classifications
Barbiturates: ↓ action, ↑ metabolism
Diuretics: ↑ hypokalemia

Hypoglycemic agents: ↑ need for hypoglycemic agents
NSAIDs: ↑ GI bleeding
Salicylates: ↑ GI bleeding
Toxoids/vaccines: ↓ immune response
Herb/drug
Aloe: ↑ hypokalemia
Buckthorn bark/berry: ↑ hypokalemia
Cascara sagrada (bark): ↑ hypokalemia, chronic use/abuse
Lily of the Valley: ↑ side effects
Pheasant's eye: ↑ side effects
Rhubarb root: ↑ hypokalemia
Senna leaf/fruits: ↑ hypokalemia
Squill: ↑ side effects
Lab test interferences
↑ Cholesterol, ↑ sodium, ↑ blood glucose, ↑ uric acid, ↑ calcium, ↑ urine glucose
↓ calcium, ↓ potassium, ↓ T_4, ↓ T_3, ↓ thyroid ^{131}I uptake test, ↓ urine 17-OHCS, ↓ 17-KS, ↓ PBI
False negative: Skin allergy tests

NURSING CONSIDERATIONS
Assessment
Systemic route
• Monitor potassium, blood sugar, urine glucose while on long-term therapy; hypokalemia and hyperglycemia; check weight daily; notify prescriber of weekly gain >5 lb
• Monitor B/P q4h, pulse; notify prescriber if chest pain occurs
• Monitor I&O ratio; be alert for decreasing urinary output and increasing edema
• Check plasma cortisol levels during long-term therapy (normal level: 138-635 nmol/L [SI units] when drawn at 8 AM); adrenal function

periodically for HPA axis suppression

• Assess for symptoms of infection: increase temperature, WBC even after withdrawal of medication; drug masks infection symptoms

• Assess for symptoms of potassium depletion: paresthesias, fatigue, nausea, vomiting, depression, polyuria, dysrhythmias, weakness

• Monitor for edema, hypertension, cardiac symptoms

• Assess for mental status: affect, mood, behavioral changes, aggression

Top route

• Check temperature; if fever develops, drug should be discontinued

• Assess for systemic absorption: increased temperature, inflammation, irritation

Nursing diagnoses

☑ Infection, risk for (adverse reactions)

☑ Knowledge deficit (teaching)

☑ Noncompliance (teaching)

Implementation

Ⅳ **IV route**

• Give **IV** (only sodium phosphate product); give over >1 min; may be given by **IV** inf in compatible sol after shaking susp (parenteral)

• Give titrated dose; use lowest effective dose

Y-site compatibilities:

Heparin, hydrocortisone, potassium chloride, Vit B/C

IM route

• Give IM injection deep in large mass, rotate sites, avoid deltoid, use 21-G needle; in one dose in AM to prevent adrenal suppression; avoid SC administration; may damage tissue

PO route

• Give with food or milk to decrease GI symptoms

Inh route

• Give inh with water to decrease possibility of fungal infections; titrated dose; use lowest effective dose

• Use after cleaning aerosol top daily with warm water; dry thoroughly

• Store in cool environment; do not puncture or incinerate container

Top route

• Apply only to affected areas; do not get in eyes; apply medication, then cover with occlusive dressing (only if prescribed), seal to normal skin, change q12h; syst absorption may occur

• Apply only to dermatoses; do not use on weeping, denuded, or infected area

• Cleanse before applying drug; use treatment for a few days after area has cleared

• Store at room temperature

Patient/family education

Systemic route

• Advise patient that long-term therapy may be needed to clear infection (1-2 mo depending on type of infection); that ID as steroid user should be carried; dosage adjustment may be needed

🔶• Instruct patient to notify prescriber if therapeutic response decreases; caution patient not to discontinue abruptly; adrenal crisis can result

• Instruct patient to avoid OTC products: salicylates, alcohol in cough products, cold preparations unless directed by prescriber

---

☑ Herb/drug 🚫 Do Not Crush 🔶 Alert ☛ Key Drug 🅖 Geriatric 🅟 Pediatric

- Teach patient all aspects of drug usage including cushingoid symptoms
- Teach patient symptoms of adrenal insufficiency: nausea, anorexia, fatigue, dizziness, dyspnea, weakness, joint pain

Top route
- Caution patient to avoid sunlight on affected area; burns may occur

Evaluation

Positive therapeutic outcome
- Ease of respirations, decreased inflammation (systemic)
- Absence of severe itching, patches on skin, flaking (top)

---

bethanechol 🕮 (℞)
(be-than′e-kol)
bethanechol chloride,
Duvoid, Urebeth, Urecholine
Func. class.: Cholinergic stimulant
Chem. class.: Synthetic choline ester
Pregnancy category   C

Action: Stimulates muscarinic acetylcholine receptors directly; mimics effects of parasympathetic nervous system stimulation; stimulates gastric motility, micturition

➔Therapeutic Outcome: Absence of continued urinary retention

Uses: Urinary retention (postoperative, postpartum), neurogenic atony of bladder with retention

Dosage and routes
Adult: PO 10-50 mg bid-qid; SC 2.5-10 mg tid-qid prn
P *Child:* PO 0.6 mg/kg/day divided in 3-4 doses/day

Test dose
Adult: SC 2.5 mg repeated 15-30 min intervals × 4 doses to determine effective dose

Available forms: Tabs 5, 10, 25, 50 mg; inj SC 5 mg/ml

Adverse effects
CNS: Dizziness
CV: Hypotension, bradycardia, orthostatic hypotension, reflex tachycardia, **cardiac arrest, circulatory collapse**
EENT: Miosis, increased salivation, lacrimation, blurred vision
GI: Nausea, bloody diarrhea, belching, vomiting, cramps, fecal incontinence
GU: Urgency
INTEG: Rash, urticaria, flushing, increased sweating
RESP: **Acute asthma, dyspnea, bronchoconstriction**

Contraindications: Hypersensitivity, severe bradycardia, asthma, severe hypotension, hyperthyroidism, peptic ulcer, parkinsonism, seizure disorders, CAD, COPD, coronary occlusion, mechanical obstruction, peritonitis, recent urinary or GI surgery

Precautions: Hypertension,
P pregnancy **C**, lactation, child <8 yr, urinary retention

Pharmacokinetics	
Absorption	Poorly absorbed (PO); well absorbed (SC)
Distribution	Does not cross blood-brain barrier
Metabolism	Unknown
Excretion	Kidneys
Half-life	Unknown

Pharmacodynamics		
	PO	SC
Onset	30-90 min	5-15 min
Peak	1 hr	15-30 min
Duration	1-6 hr	2 hr

Interactions
Individual drugs
Donepezil: ↑ action of bethanechol

Procainamide: ↓ action of bethanechol

Quinidine: ↓ action of bethanechol

Drug classifications
Cholinergic agonists: ↑ action, ↑ toxicity

Ganglionic blockers: ↑ severe hypotension

Lab test interferences
↑ AST, ↑ lipase/amylase, ↑ bilirubin

NURSING CONSIDERATIONS
Assessment
• Monitor B/P, pulse, respirations; observe after parenteral dose for 1 hr
• Check I&O ratio; check for urinary retention or incontinence; if bladder emptying does not occur, notify prescriber; catheterization may be needed
• Assess for bradycardia, hypotension, bronchospasm, headache, dizziness, convulsions, sweating, cramping, respiratory depression; drug should be discontinued if toxicity occurs; atropine administration

Nursing diagnoses
☑ Urinary elimination, altered patterns (uses)
☑ Injury, risk for (adverse reactions)
☑ Knowledge deficit (teaching)

Implementation
SC route
◆• Give parenteral dose by SC route; use of IM, **IV** may result in cardiac arrest or cholinergic crisis (diarrhea with blood, cramping, hypotension, circulatory collapse)

◆• Administer only with atropine sulfate available for cholinergic crisis; give only after all other cholinergics have been discontinued
• Do not use sol with a precipitate, or if discolored

PO route
• Give increased doses if tolerance occurs as prescribed
• To avoid nausea and vomiting, take on an empty stomach; 1 hr ac or 2 hr pc
• Store at room temperature

Patient/family education
• Instruct patient to take drug exactly as prescribed; 1 hr ac or 2 hr pc; do not double doses; if dose is missed take within 1 hr of scheduled dose
• Caution patient to make position changes slowly; orthostatic hypotension may occur
• Instruct patient to report cramping, diarrhea with blood, flushing to prescriber

Evaluation
Positive therapeutic outcome
• Absence of urinary retention
• Absence of abdominal distention

Treatment of overdose:
Administer atropine 0.6-1.2 mg **IV** or IM (adult)

---

bexarotene
See Appendix A,
Selected New Drugs

---

bicalutamide (Ᵽ)
(bi-kal-yut′ah-mide)
Casodex
Func. class.: Antineoplastic hormone
Chem. class.: Non-steroidal antiandrogen
Pregnancy category X

Pharmacokinetics

Absorption	Well absorbed
Distribution	Unknown
Metabolism	Liver
Excretion	Urine, feces
Half-life	Unknown

Pharmacodynamics

Unknown

Action: Competitively inhibits the action to androgens by binding to cytosol androgen receptors in target tissue

Therapeutic Outcome: Prevention of growth of malignant cells

Uses: Prostate cancer in combination with luteinizing hormone-releasing hormone (LHRH) analog

Dosage and routes
Adult: PO 50 mg qd with LHRH

Available forms: Tab 50 mg

Adverse effects
GI: Diarrhea, constipation, nausea, vomiting, increased liver enzyme test
CV: Hot flashes, hypertension
CNS: Dizziness, paresthesia, insomnia
INTEG: Rash, sweating
GU: Nocturia, **hematuria,** UTI, impotence, gynecomastia, urinary incontinence
MISC: Infection, anemia, dyspnea, bone pain, headache, asthenia, back pain, flu syndrome

Contraindications: Hypersensitivity, pregnancy **X**

Precautions: Renal, hepatic disease, elderly, lactation

Interactions
Drug classifications
Anticoagulants: May be displaced from their binding sites
Lab test interferences
↑ AST, ↑ ALT, ↑ bilirubin, ↑ BUN, ↑ creatinine
↓ Hgb, ↓ WBC

NURSING CONSIDERATIONS
Assessment
• Assess for diarrhea, constipation, nausea, vomiting
• Assess for hot flashes, gynecomastia; assure patient that these are common side effects
• Monitor PSA (Prostate Specific Antigen), liver function studies

Nursing diagnoses
☑ Injury, risk for (uses, adverse reactions)
☑ Knowledge deficit (teaching)

Implementation
• Give at same time each day (for both drugs) either AM or PM with or without food
• Give only with LHRH treatment

Patient/family education
• Teach patient to recognize and report signs of anemia, hepatotoxicity, renal toxicity

Evaluation
Positive therapeutic outcome
• Decreased tumor size, spread of malignancy

---

biperiden (℞)
(bye-per′i-den)
Akineton
Func. class.: Cholinergic blocker, antiparkinsonian agent
Pregnancy category C

Action: Centrally acting competitive anticholinergic; blocks cholinergic responses in the CNS

➔**Therapeutic Outcome:** Decreased involuntary movements

Uses: Parkinsonian symptoms, extrapyramidal symptoms secondary to neuroleptic drug therapy

Dosage and routes
Extrapyramidal symptoms
Adult: PO 2 mg qd-tid; IM/**IV** 2 mg q30 min, if needed, not to exceed 8 mg/24 hr

Parkinsonian symptoms
Adult: PO 2 mg tid-qid; max 16 mg/24 hr

Available forms: Tabs 2 mg; inj IM/**IV** 5 mg/ml (lactate)

Adverse effects
CNS: Confusion, anxiety, restlessness, irritability, delusions, hallucinations, headache, sedation, depression, incoherence, dizziness, euphoria, tremors, memory loss
CV: Palpitations, tachycardia, postural hypotension, bradycardia
EENT: Blurred vision, photophobia, dilated pupils, difficulty swallowing, mydriasis, increased intraocular tension, angle closure glaucoma
GI: Dryness of mouth, constipation, nausea, vomiting, abdominal distress, **paralytic ileus**

GU: Hesitancy, retention, dysuria
INTEG: Rash, urticaria, dermatoses
MISC: Increased temperature, flushing, decreased sweating, **hyperthermia, heat stroke,** numbness of fingers
MS: Weakness, cramping

Contraindications: Hypersensitivity, narrow-angle glaucoma, myasthenia gravis, GI/GU obstruction, megacolon, stenosing peptic ulcers, prostatic hypertrophy

Precautions: Pregnancy **C**, ⒼG elderly, lactation, tachycardia, dysrhythmias, liver, kidney disease, drug abuse, hypotension, hypertension, psychiatric ⒫P patients, children

Pharmacokinetics	
Absorption	Well absorbed (PO, IM)
Distribution	Unknown
Metabolism	Unknown
Excretion	Unknown
Half-life	18-24 hr

Pharmacodynamics		
	IM/IV	PO
Onset	15 min	1 hr
Peak	Unknown	Unknown
Duration	6-10 hr	6-10 hr

Interactions
Individual drugs
Alcohol: ↑ sedation
Amantadine: ↑ anticholinergic effects
Digoxin: ↑ levels of digoxin
Levodopa: ↓ levels of levodopa
Haloperidol: ↑ schizophrenic symptoms
Drug classifications
Antacids: ↓ biperiden absorption

Antidepressants, tricyclic: ↑ anticholinergic effects
Antihistamines: ↑ anticholinergic effects
Phenothiazines: ↑ anticholinergic effects

NURSING CONSIDERATIONS
Assessment
• Monitor I&O ratio; retention commonly causes decreased urinary output, distention, frequency, incontinence
• Assess for parkinsonism, extrapyramidal symptoms: shuffling gait, muscle rigidity, involuntary movements, pill rolling, muscle spasms, drooling before and during treatment
• Assess patient response if anticholinergics are given
• Monitor for urinary hesitancy, retention; palpate bladder if retention occurs
• Monitor for constipation, cramping, pain in abdomen, abdominal distention; increase fluids, bulk, exercise if this occurs
• Assess for tolerance over long-term therapy; dosage may have to be increased or changed
• Assess for mental status: affect, mood, CNS depression, worsening of mental symptoms during early therapy

Nursing diagnoses
☑ Mobility, impaired (uses)
☑ Knowledge deficit (teaching)

Implementation
PO route
• Give with food or pc to prevent GI upset; may give with fluids other than water; hard candy, frequent drinks, gum to relieve dry mouth
• Give hs to avoid daytime drowsiness in patients with parkinsonism
• Store at room temp
IV IV route
• Give parenteral dose with patient recumbent to prevent postural hypotension; give undiluted 2 mg or less over 1 min or more

Patient/family education
• Teach patient to use caution in hot weather; drug may increase susceptibility to heat stroke since perspiration is decreased; patient should remain indoors
• Teach patient not to discontinue this drug abruptly; to taper off over 1 wk to prevent withdrawal symptoms (insomnia, involuntary movements, anxiety, tachycardias)
• Teach patient to avoid driving or other hazardous activities; drowsiness, dizziness may occur
• Teach patient to avoid OTC medication: cough, cold preparations with alcohol, antihistamines unless directed by prescriber; increased CNS depression may occur
• Caution patient to rise from sitting or recumbent position slowly to minimize orthostatic hypotension
• Teach patient to use gum, hard candy, frequent sips of water to decrease dry mouth; if dry mouth continues, saliva substitutes may be prescribed
• Instruct patient that doses should not be doubled, but missed dose may be taken up to 2 hr before next dose

Evaluation
Positive therapeutic outcome
• Absence of involuntary movements (pill rolling, tremors, muscle spasms)

✦ Canada Only   Adverse effects: *italic* = common; **bold** = life-threatening

bisacodyl (OTC)
(bis-a-koe'dill)
Bisc-Evac, Bisacolax ✦,
Bisco-Lax ✦, Carter's Little
Pills, Dacodyl, Deficol,
Dulcagen, Dulcolax, Fleet
Bisacodyl, Fleet Laxative,
Therelax
Func. class.: Laxative,
stimulant
Chem. class.: Diphenyl-
methane

Pregnancy category   C

Action: Acts directly on intestine by increasing motor
activity; thought to irritate
colonic intramural plexus;
increases water in the colon

➡ **Therapeutic Outcome:**
Decreased constipation

Uses: Short-term treatment of
constipation, bowel or rectal
preparation for surgery, examination

Dosage and routes
P *Adult ≥12 yr:* PO 5-15 mg in
PM or AM; may use up to 30 mg
for bowel or rec preparation;
REC 10 mg
P *Child >3 yr:* PO 5-10 mg as a
single dose
P *Child 2-11 yr:* RECT 10 mg
as a single dose
P *Child <2 yr:* RECT 5 mg as a
single dose

Available forms: Enteric
coated tabs 5 mg; rec supp 5,
10 mg; rect sol 10 mg/37 ml;
enema 0.33 mg/ml, 10 mg/5
ml; powder for rect sol 1.5 mg
bisacodyl/2.5 g tannic acid

Adverse effects
CNS: Muscle weakness
*GI: Nausea, vomiting, an-
orexia, cramps,* diarrhea, rectal
burning (supp)

META: Protein-losing enteropathy, alkalosis, hypokalemia,
tetany, electrolyte and fluid
imbalances

Contraindications: Hypersensitivity, rectal fissures, abdominal pain, nausea, vomiting,
appendicitis, acute surgical
abdomen, ulcerated hemor-
rhoids, acute hepatitis, fecal
impaction, intestinal/biliary
tract obstruction

Precautions: Pregnancy **C**

Pharmacokinetics	
Absorption	Poor
Distribution	Unknown
Metabolism	Liver, minimally
Excretion	Kidneys
Half-life	Unknown

Pharmacodynamics		
	PO	RECT
Onset	6-10 hr	15-60 min
Peak	Unknown	Unknown
Duration	Unknown	Unknown

Interactions
Drug classifications
Antacids: ↓ of enteric coating
of drugs
H$_2$-blockers: ↑ gastric irrita-
tion

☑ *Herb/drug*
Lily of the Valley: ↑ action/
side effects
Pheasant's eye: ↑ action/side
effects
Squill: ↑ action/side effects

NURSING CONSIDERATIONS
Assessment
• Monitor blood, urine electrolytes if used often by
patient; check I&O ratio to
identify fluid loss
• Assess cramping, rectal
bleeding, nausea, vomiting; if
these symptoms occur, drug
should be discontinued; iden-

tify cause of constipation; identify whether fluids, bulk, or exercise missing from lifestyle

Nursing diagnoses

☑ Constipation (uses)
☑ Diarrhea (side effects)
☑ Knowledge deficit (teaching)
☑ Noncompliance (teaching)

Implementation

PO route

• Give alone with water only for better absorption; do not take within 1 hr of antacids, milk

• Administer in AM or PM (oral dose)

🚫 • Do not chew; swallow tabs whole

Rectal route

• Lubricate before insertion, patient should retain for ½ hr

Patient/family education

• Discuss with the patient that adequate fluid and bulk consumption is necessary

• Advise patient that normal bowel movements do not always occur daily

• Teach patient not to use in presence of abdominal pain, nausea, vomiting; tell patient to notify prescriber if constipation unrelieved or if symptoms of electrolyte imbalance occur: muscle cramps, pain, weakness, dizziness, excessive thirst

Evaluation

Positive therapeutic outcome

• Decreased constipation within 3 days

---

bismuth subsalicylate (OTC)

(bis'meth sub-sa-li'si-late)

B

Bismatrol, Bismatrol Extra Strength, Bismed, Pepto-Bismol, Pepto-Bismol Maximum Strength, Pink Bismuth, PMS-Bismuth Subsalicylate

Func. class.: Antidiarrheal
Chem. class.: Salicylate

Pregnancy category   C

Action: Inhibits prostaglandin synthesis responsible for GI hypermotility; stimulates absorption of fluid and electrolytes; antimicrobial, antisecretory effects

⇥ **Therapeutic Outcome:** Absence of loose, watery stools

Uses: Diarrhea (cause undetermined); prevention of diarrhea when traveling; may be included to treat *H. pylori*

Dosage and routes
Adult: PO 30 ml or 2 tabs q30-60 min, not to exceed 8 doses per day for >2 days

🅟 *Child 10-14 yr:* PO 15 ml

Available forms: Chewable tabs 262 mg; susp 262 mg/15 ml, 524 mg/15 ml

Adverse effects
CNS: Confusion, twitching
EENT: Hearing loss, tinnitus, metallic taste, blue gums
GI: Increased fecal impaction (high doses), dark stools, constipation
HEMA: Increased bleeding time

🅟 **Contraindications:** Child <3 yr; impaction, children, teens with flulike symptoms, hyper-

---

sensitivity (aspirin), history of GI bleeding, renal disease

Precautions: Anticoagulant

G therapy, pregnancy **C**, elderly, lactation, gout, diabetes mellitus, immobility

Pharmacokinetics	
Absorption	Salicylate >90%
Distribution	None
Metabolism	None
Excretion	Feces (unchanged)
Half-life	Unknown

Pharmacodynamics	
Onset	1 hr
Peak	2 hr
Duration	4 hr

Interactions
Individual drugs
Aminosalicylic acid: ↑ side effects, ↑ toxicity
Tetracycline: ↓ absorption
Drug classifications
Anticoagulants, oral: ↑ effect of anticoagulants
Antidiabetics, oral: ↑ effect of antidiabetics
Salicylates: ↑ risk of salicylate toxicity
Lab test interferences
Interfere: Radiographic studies of GI system

NURSING CONSIDERATIONS
Assessment
• Monitor skin turgor; dehydration may occur in severe diarrhea; monitor electrolytes (potassium, sodium, chloride) if diarrhea is severe or continues long term
• Assess bowel pattern (frequency, consistency, shape, volume, color) before drug therapy, after treatment; check weight, bowel sounds; identify factors contributing to diarrhea (bacteria, diet, medications, tube feedings)

Nursing diagnoses
☑ Diarrhea (uses)
☑ Constipation (adverse reactions)
☑ Knowledge deficit (teaching)

Implementation
• Shake susp before use; chewable tabs should not be swallowed whole

Patient/family education
• Teach patient to stop use if symptoms do not improve within 2 days or become worse, or if diarrhea is accompanied by high fever
• Teach patient to increase fluids for rehydration
• Tell patient to chew or dissolve chewable tabs in mouth; do not swallow whole; shake susp before using
• Tell patient to avoid other salicylates unless directed by prescriber; not to give to

P children because of possibility of Reye's syndrome
• Tell patient that stools may turn gray; tongue may darken; impaction may occur in debilitated patients

Evaluation
Positive therapeutic outcome
• Decreased diarrhea

---

bisoprolol (Ṛ)
(bis-oh'pro-lole)
Zebeta
Func. class.: Antihypertensive
Chem. class.: β₁-Blocker (selective)

Pregnancy category   C

Action: Preferentially and competitively blocks stimulation of β₁-adrenergic receptor within cardiac muscle (decreases rate of SA node discharge, increases recovery time), slows conduction of AV node, decreases heart rate, which decreases O_2 consumption in myocardium; decreases renin-aldosterone-angiotensin system; inhibits β_2-receptors in bronchial and vascular smooth muscle at high doses

⇒**Therapeutic Outcome:**
Decreased B/P, heart rate

Uses: Mild to moderate hypertension

Investigational uses: Angina pectoris, supraventricular tachycardia

Dosage and routes
Renal/hepatic dose
2.5 mg PO, titrate upward

Hypertension
Adult: PO 2.5-5 mg qd; may increase if necessary to 20 mg once daily; may need to reduce dose in presence of renal or hepatic impairment

Available forms: Tabs 5, 10 mg

Adverse effects
CNS: Vertigo, headache, insomnia, fatigue, dizziness, mental changes, memory loss, hallucinations, depression, lethargy, drowsiness, strange dreams, catatonia, peripheral neuropathy
CV: **Ventricular dysrhythmias, profound hypotension, bradycardia, CHF,** cold extremities, postural hypotension, 2nd- or 3rd-degree heart block
EENT: Sore throat, dry burning eyes
ENDO: Increased hypoglycemic response to insulin
GI: Nausea, diarrhea, vomiting, **mesenteric arterial**

thrombosis, ischemic colitis, flatulence, gastritis, gastric pain
GU: Impotence, decreased libido
HEMA: **Agranulocytosis, thrombocytopenia,** purpura, **eosinophilia**
INTEG: Rash, fever, alopecia, pruritus, sweating
MISC: Facial swelling, weight gain, decreased exercise tolerance
MS: Joint pain, arthralgia
RESP: **Bronchospasm,** dyspnea, wheezing, cough, nasal stuffiness

Contraindications: Hypersensitivity to β-blockers, cardiogenic shock, heart block (2nd, 3rd degree), sinus bradycardia, CHF, cardiac failure

Precautions: Major surgery, pregnancy **C,** lactation, children, diabetes mellitus, renal or hepatic disease, thyroid disease, COPD, asthma, well-compensated heart failure, aortic or mitral valve disease, peripheral vascular disease, myasthenia gravis

⊠**Do Not Confuse:**
Zebeta/Diabeta

Pharmacokinetics	
Absorption	Well absorbed
Distribution	Unknown; protein binding (30%)
Metabolism	Liver, inactive metabolites
Excretion	Urine, unchanged (50%)
Half-life	9-12 hr

Pharmacodynamics	
Onset	Unknown
Peak	2-4 hr
Duration	24 hr

Interactions
Individual drugs
Alcohol: (large amounts) ↑ hypotension

Clonidine: Fatal reactions after discontinuing clonidine

Epinephrine: ↑ hypertension, then bradycardia

Flecainide: ↑ effects of both drugs

Guanethidine: ↑ hypotension

Haloperidol: ↑ effects of both drugs

Hydralazine: ↑ hypotension, bradycardia

Lidocaine: ↑ lidocaine toxicity

Quinidine: ↑ hypotension, bradycardia

Prazosin: ↑ hypotension, bradycardia

Reserpine: ↑ hypotension

Theophylline: ↓ bronchodilatation

Drug classifications
Barbiturates: ↓ antihypertensive effects

Calcium channel blockers: ↑ hypotension, myocardial depression

Contraceptives, oral: ↑ hypotension

Diuretics, loop: ↑ CV effects

MAOIs: ↑ bradycardia

NSAIDs: ↓ antihypertensive effect

Penicillins: ↓ antihypertensive effects

Salicylates: ↓ antihypertensive effects

Sulfonylureas: ↓ hypoglycemic effect

Lab test interferences
↑ AST, ↑ ALT

Interference: Glucose/insulin tolerance tests

NURSING CONSIDERATIONS
Assessment
• Monitor B/P during beginning treatment, periodically thereafter; pulse q4h: note rate, rhythm, quality; apical/radial pulse before administration; notify prescriber of any significant changes (pulse <50 bpm)

• Check for baselines in renal, liver function tests before therapy begins

• Assess for edema in feet, legs daily, monitor I&O, daily weight; check for jugular vein distention, rales bilaterally, dyspnea (CHF)

• Monitor skin turgor, dryness of mucous membranes for hydration status, especially
G elderly

Nursing diagnoses
☑ Cardiac output, decreased (uses)

☑ Injury, risk for (side effects)

☑ Knowledge deficit (teaching)

☑ Noncompliance (teaching)

Implementation
• Give qd; give with food to prevent GI upset; may be crushed

• Store protected from light, moisture; place in cool environment

Patient/family education
• Teach patient not to discontinue drug abruptly; may cause precipitate angina if stopped abruptly

• Teach patient not to use OTC products containing α-adrenergic stimulants (such as nasal decongestants, cold preparations); to avoid alcohol, smoking and to limit sodium intake as prescribed

• Teach patient how to take pulse and B/P at home; advise when to notify prescriber

• Instruct patient to comply with weight control, dietary adjustments, modified exercise program

• Tell patient to carry/wear

Medic Alert ID to identify drug being taken, allergies; tell patient drug controls symptoms but does not cure

• Caution patient to avoid hazardous activities if dizziness, drowsiness present

• Teach patient to take drug as prescribed, not to double doses, skip doses; take any missed doses as soon as remembered if at least 8 hr until next dose

Evaluation
Positive therapeutic outcome
• Decreased B/P in hypertension (after 1-2 wk)

Treatment of overdose: Lavage, **IV** atropine for bradycardia, **IV** theophylline for bronchospasm, digitalis, O_2, diuretic for cardiac failure, hemodialysis, **IV** glucose for hypoglycemia, **IV** diazepam (or phenytoin) for seizures

---

bitolterol (Ŗ)
(bye-tole′ter-ole)
Tornalate
Func. class.: Bronchodilator, β_2-adrenergic agonist; bronchodilator
Chem. class.: Acid ester of colterol

Pregnancy category C

Action: Causes bronchodilatation by action on β_2-receptors with increased synthesis of cyclic AMP; relaxes bronchial smooth muscle; inhibits mast cell degranulation; stimulates cilia to remove secretions with very little effect on heart rate

➤ **Therapeutic Outcome:** Ability to breathe without difficulty

Uses: Asthma, bronchospasm

Dosage and routes
P *Child >12 yr:* INH 2 puffs; wait 1-3 min before 3rd puff if needed; not to exceed 3 inh q6h or 2 inh q4h

Nebulization
P *Adult and child >12 yr:* INH 0.5 ml (1 mg) tid by intermittent flow or 1.25 mg tid by continuous flow

Available forms: Aerosol 0.37 mg/actuation; 0.2% neb sol

Adverse effects
CNS: Tremors, anxiety, insomnia, headache, dizziness, stimulation, restlessness, hallucinations
CV: Palpitations, tachycardia, hypertension, angina, hypotension
EENT: Dry nose, irritation of nose and throat
GI: Heartburn, nausea, vomiting, anorexia
MS: Muscle cramps
RESP: **Bronchospasm,** dyspnea

Contraindications: Hypersensitivity to sympathomimetics

Precautions: Lactation, pregnancy **C,** cardiac disorders, hyperthyroidism, diabetes mellitus

Pharmacokinetics	
Absorption	Unknown
Distribution	Unknown
Metabolism	Lungs to active metabolite
Excretion	Unknown
Half-life	Unknown

Pharmacodynamics	
Onset	3-4 min
Peak	½-1 hr
Duration	5-8 hr

Interactions
Drug classifications
β-**Adrenergic blockers:** Block therapeutic effect
Bronchodilators, aerosol: ↑ action of bronchodilator
MAOIs: ↑ chance of hypertensive crisis
Sympathomimetics: ↑ adrenergic side effects

NURSING CONSIDERATIONS
Assessment
• Monitor respiratory function: vital capacity, FEV, ABGs, lung sounds, heart rate, rhythm (baseline)
• Determine client's ability to self-medicate
• Monitor for evidence of allergic reactions; paradoxic bronchospasm; withhold dose; notify prescriber

Nursing diagnoses
☑ Impaired gas exchange (uses)
☑ Airway clearance, ineffective (uses)
☑ Knowledge deficit (teaching)

Implementation
• Give after shaking, exhale, place mouthpiece in mouth, inhale slowly, hold breath, remove, exhale slowly; allow at least 1 min between inh
• Store in light-resistant container; do not expose to temp over 86° F (30° C)

Patient/family education
• Tell patient not to use OTC medications; excess stimulation may occur; to use this medication before other medications and allow at least 5 min between each; to prevent overstimulation
• Teach patient use of inhaler; review package insert with patient; to avoid getting aerosol in eyes; blurring may result; to wash inhaler in warm water daily and dry well; to avoid smoking, smoke-filled rooms, persons with respiratory tract infections
• Teach patient that paradoxic bronchospasm may occur and to stop drug immediately and notify prescriber; to limit caffeine products such as chocolate, coffee, tea, and colas
• Instruct patient on administration of dose; not to use more than prescribed; serious side effects may occur; if taking regularly and dose is missed, take when remembered; space other doses on new time schedule

Evaluation
Positive therapeutic outcome
• Absence of dyspnea, wheezing after 1 hr
• Improved airway exchange
• Improved ABGs

Treatment of overdose:
Administer a β₂-adrenergic blocker

---

bleomycin ⚷ (Ŗ)
(blee-oh-mye′sin)
Blenoxane
Func. class.: Antineoplastic, antibiotic
Chem. class.: Glycopeptide
Pregnancy category   D

Action: Inhibits synthesis of DNA, RNA, protein; derived from *Streptomyces verticillus;* replication is decreased by binding to DNA, which causes strand splitting; phase specific in the G_2 and M phases; a nonvesicant

➡ **Therapeutic Outcome:** Prevention of rapidly growing malignant cells

---

Uses: Cancer of head, neck, penis, cervix, vulva of squamous cell origin, Hodgkin's disease, lymphosarcoma, reticulum cell sarcoma, testicular carcinoma, malignant pleural effusion

Dosage and routes
P *Adult and child:* SC/**IV**/IM 0.25-0.5 U/kg q1-2 wk or 10-20 U/m²; then 1 U/day or 5 U/wk; may also be given intraarterially; do not exceed total dose, 400 U in lifetime

Available forms: Powder for inj 15 U, 30 U

Adverse effects
CNS: Fever, chills
CV: Hypotension, peripheral vasoconstriction
GI: Nausea, vomiting, anorexia, stomatitis, weight loss
HEMA: Hypotension, peripheral vasoconstriction
INTEG: Rash, hyperkeratosis, nail changes, alopecia, fever and chills
RESP: **Fibrosis,** pneumonitis, wheezing, **pulmonary toxicity**
SYST: **Anaphylaxis**
IDIOSYNCRATIC REACTION: Hypotension, confusion, fever, chills, wheezing

Contraindications: Hypersensitivity, pregnancy **D**

Precautions: Renal, hepatic, respiratory disease

Pharmacokinetics	
Absorption	Well absorbed (IM, SC, intrapleural, intraperitoneal)
Distribution	Widely distributed
Metabolism	Liver, 30%
Excretion	Kidneys, unchanged (50%)
Half-life	2 hr; ↑ in renal disease

Pharmacodynamics	
Unknown	

Interactions
Individual drugs
Digoxin: ↓ digoxin level
Phenytoin: ↓ phenytoin levels
Radiation: ↑ toxicity, bone marrow suppression
Drug classifications
Antineoplastics: ↑ toxicity, bone marrow suppression

NURSING CONSIDERATIONS
Assessment
• Assess buccal cavity q8h for dryness, sores or ulceration, white patches, oral pain, bleeding, dysphagia; obtain prescription for viscous lidocaine (Xylocaine)
• Assess symptoms indicating severe allergic reaction: rash, pruritus, urticaria, purpuric skin lesions, itching, flushing
• Monitor CBC, differential, platelet count weekly; withhold drug if WBC count is <4000/mm³ or platelet count is <100,000/mm³; notify prescriber of results if WBC <20,000/mm³, platelets <150,000/mm³
• Monitor temp q4h (may indicate beginning of infection)
• Monitor liver function tests before and during therapy (bilirubin, AST, ALT, LDH) as needed or monthly
• Assess for bleeding: hematuria, stool guaiac, bruising or petechiae, mucosa or orifices q8h; inflammation of mucosa, breaks in skin
• Identify dyspnea, rales, unproductive cough, chest pain, tachypnea
• Identify effects of alopecia on body image; discuss feelings

about body changes; if edema in feet, joint pain, stomach pain, shaking present, prescriber should be notified; identify inflammation of mucosa, breaks in skin

Nursing diagnoses

☑ Injury, risk for (adverse reactions)

☑ Body image disturbance (adverse reactions)

☑ Infection, risk for (adverse reactions)

☑ Knowledge deficit (teaching)

Implementation

• Avoid contact with skin, very irritating; wash completely to remove

• Give fluids **IV** or PO before chemotherapy to hydrate patient

• Give antacid before oral agent; give antiemetic 30-60 min before giving drug to prevent vomiting and prn and antibiotics for prophylaxis of infection

• Provide liq diet: carbonated beverages, gelatin may be added if patient is not nauseated or vomiting

• Rinsing of mouth tid-qid with water, club soda; brushing of teeth bid-qid with soft brush or cotton-tipped applicators for stomatitis; use unwaxed dental floss

SC/IM route

• Reconstitute with 1-5 ml sterile water for inj; D_5W, 0.9% NaCl

IV **IV route**

• Drug should be prepared by experienced personnel using proper precautions

• Two test doses 2-5 U before initial dose; monitor for anaphylaxis

• Give by direct **IV** after reconstituting 15 U or less/5 ml or more of D_5W or 0.9% NaCl; give 15 U or less/10 min through Y-tube or 3-way stopcock initial dose; monitor for anaphylaxis

Intermittent inf

• Administer after diluting 50-100 ml 0.9% NaCl, D_5W and giving at prescribed rate

Syringe compatibilities:
Cisplatin, cyclophosphamide, doxorubicin, droperidol, fluorouracil, furosemide, heparin, leucovorin, methotrexate, metoclopramide, mitomycin, vinblastine, vincristine

Y-site compatibilities:
Allopurinol, amisostine, aztreonam, cisplatin, cyclophosphamide, doxorubicin, doxorubicin liposome, droperidol, filgrastim, fludarabine, fluorouracil, granisetron, heparin, leucovorin, melphalan, methotrexate, metoclopramide, mitomycin, ondansetron, paclitaxel, piperacillin/tazobactam, sargramostim, teniposide, thiotepa, vinblastine, vincristine, vinorelbine

Additive incompatibilities:
Aminophylline, ascorbic acid inj, carbenicillin, cefazolin, cephalothin, diazepam, hydrocortisone, methotrexate, mitomycin, nafcillin, penicillin G sodium, terbutaline

Additive compatibilities:
Amikacin, cephapirin, dexamethasone, diphenhydramine, fluorouracil, gentamicin, heparin, hydrocortisone, phenytoin, streptomycin, tobramycin, vinblastine, vincristine

Solution compatibilities:
0.9% NaCl

Patient/family education

• Teach patient to avoid use of products containing aspirin or

---

ibuprofen, razors, commercial mouthwash; bleeding may occur; to report symptoms of bleeding (hematuria, tarry stools)
• Instruct patient to report signs of anemia (fatigue, headache, irritability, faintness, shortness of breath)
• Instruct patient to report any changes in breathing or coughing even several months after treatment; to avoid crowds and persons with respiratory tract or other infections
• Inform patient that hair may be lost during treatment; a wig or hairpiece may make patient feel better; new hair may be different in color, texture
• Caution patient not to have any vaccinations without the advice of the prescriber; serious reactions can occur
• Advise patient contraception is needed during treatment and for several months after completion of therapy

Evaluation
Positive therapeutic outcome
• Prevention of rapid division of malignant cells

---

bretylium ⚕ (R)
(bre-til'ee-um)
Bretylate ✦, bretylium tosylate, Bretylol
Func. class.: Antidysrhythmic (Class III)
Chem. class.: Quaternary ammonium compound
Pregnancy category **C**

Action: After a transient release of norepinephrine, inhibits further release by postganglionic nerve endings; prolongs

action potential, duration, and effective refractory period

➡ **Therapeutic Outcome:** Absence of dysrhythmias

Uses: Serious ventricular tachycardia, cardioversion, ventricular fibrillation; for short-term use only

Dosage and routes
Renal disease
CrCl 10-50 ml/min 25%-50% dose; CrCl <10 ml/min avoid use

Severe ventricular fibrillation
Adult: **IV** bol 5 mg/kg; increase to 10 mg/kg repeated q15 min, up to 30 mg/kg; **IV** inf 1-2 mg/min or give 5-10 mg/kg over 10 min q6h (maintenance)

Ventricular tachycardia
Adult: **IV** inf 500 mg diluted in 50 ml D$_5$W or NS; infuse over 10-30 min; may repeat in 1 hr; maintain with 1-2 mg/min or 5-10 mg/kg over 10-30 min q6h; IM 5-10 mg/kg undiluted; repeat in 1-2 hr if needed; maintain with same dose q6-8h

Child: 2-5 mg/kg/dose

Available forms: Inj 50 mg/ml; 1, 2, 4 mg/ml prefilled syringes

Adverse effects
CNS: Syncope, dizziness, confusion, psychosis, anxiety
CV: Hypotension, postural hypotension, bradycardia, angina, PVCs, substernal pressure, transient hypertension, precipitation of angina
GI: Nausea, vomiting
RESP: Respiratory depression

Contraindications: Hypersensitivity, digitalis toxicity, aortic stenosis, pulmonary hyper- P tension, children

Precautions: Renal disease, pregnancy **C**, lactation, P children

Pharmacokinetics	
Absorption	Complete bioavailability (**IV**)
Distribution	Unknown
Metabolism	Not metabolized
Excretion	Kidneys, unchanged
Half-life	4-17 hr

Pharmacodynamics		
	IV	IM
Onset	5 min	½-2 hr
Peak	Infusion's end	Unknown
Duration	6-24 hr	6-24 hr

Interactions
Individual drugs
Caffeine: ↓ effects of adenosine
Carbamazepine: ↑ heart block
Dopamine: ↑ pressor effects
Norepinephrine: ↑ pressor effects
Drug classifications
Cardiac glycosides: ↑ toxicity
Sympathomimetics: ↑ sympathomimetic effect
☑ *Herb/drug*
Aloe: ↑ bretylium effect
Buckthorn bark/berry: ↑ bretylium effect
Cascara sagrada: ↑ bretylium effect
Rhubarb root: ↑ bretylium effect
Senna leaf/roots: ↑ bretylium effect

NURSING CONSIDERATIONS
Assessment
• Monitor ECG continuously to determine drug effectiveness; measure PR,

QRS, QT intervals; check for PVCs, other dysrhythmias; monitor B/P continuously for hypotension, hypertension; check for rebound hypertension after 1-2 hr

Nursing diagnoses
☑ Cardiac output, decreased (uses)
☑ Gas exchange, impaired (adverse reactions)
☑ Knowledge deficit (teaching)

Implementation
IM route
• Give in large muscle mass, rotate sites to prevent necrosis
IV **IV route**
Direct
• Give **IV** bol undiluted; give 6 mg or less over 1 min; if using an **IV** line, use port near insertion site, flush with normal saline (50 ml)
Intermittent inf
• Give by intermittent inf after diluting 500 mg/50 ml or more with 0.9% NaCl, D_5W, D_5/0.45% NaCl, D_5/0.9% NaCl, LR, ⅙ mol/L sodium lactate; run over >8 min
Cont inf
• Give by cont inf diluted in sol; give 1-2 mg/min; use inf site
• Store at room temp; sol should be clear

Additive compatibilities:
Aminophylline, atracurium, calcium chloride, calcium gluconate, digoxin, dopamine, esmolol, regular insulin, lidocaine, potassium chloride, quinadine verapamil

Additive incompatibilities:
Phenytoin

Y-site compatibilities:
Amiodarone, amrinone, cisatracurium, diltiazem, dobuta-

mine, famotidine, isoproterenol, ranitidine, remifentanil

Evaluation
Positive therapeutic outcome
• Decreased B/P, dysrhythmias, heart rate; normal sinus rhythm

---

bromocriptine (℞)
(broe-moe-krip′teen)
Parlodel
Func. class.: Antiparkinsonian agent; dopamine receptor agonist; ovulation stimulant
Chem. class.: Ergot alkaloid derivative

Pregnancy category **B**

Action: Inhibits prolactin release by activating postsynaptic dopamine receptors; activation of striatal dopamine receptors may be reason for improvement in Parkinson's disease

⇨Therapeutic Outcome: Decreased involuntary movements in Parkinson's disease; decreased lactation; decreased hormone levels in acromegaly; absence of amenorrhea in hyperprolactinemia

Uses: Female infertility, adjunct with levodopa in Parkinson's disease, prevention of postpartum lactation, amenorrhea caused by hyperprolactinemia, acromegaly

Dosage and routes
Hyperprolactinemic indications
Adult: PO 1.25-2.5 mg with meals; may increase by 2.5 mg q3-7 days; usual dosage 5-7.5 mg

Acromegaly
Adult: PO 1.25-2.5 mg/day × 3 days hs; may increase by 1.25-2.5 mg q3-7 days; usual range 20-30 mg/day; max 100 mg/day

Postpartum lactation
Adult: PO 2.5 mg qd-tid with meal × 14 or 21 days

Parkinson's disease
Adult: PO 1.25 mg bid with meals; may increase q2-4 wk by 2.5 mg/day; not to exceed 100 mg/day

Available forms: Caps 5 mg; tabs 2.5 mg

Adverse effects
CNS: Headache, depression, restlessness, anxiety, nervousness, confusion, **convulsions,** hallucinations, *dizziness,* fatigue, drowsiness, abnormal involuntary movements, psychosis
CV: Orthostatic hypotension, decreased B/P, palpitations, extrasystole, **shock,** dysrhythmias, bradycardia
EENT: Blurred vision, diplopia, burning eyes, nasal congestion
GI: Nausea, vomiting, anorexia, cramps, constipation, diarrhea, dry mouth, GI hemorrhage
GU: Frequency, retention, incontinence, diuresis
INTEG: Rash on face, arms, alopecia

Contraindications: Hypersensitivity to ergot, severe ischemic disease, severe peripheral vascular disease

Precautions: Lactation, hepatic disease, renal disease, children, pituitary tumors, pregnancy **B**

⊠ **Do Not Confuse:**
Parlodel/pindolol

Pharmacokinetics	
Absorption	Poorly absorbed
Distribution	Unknown
Metabolism	Liver, completely
Excretion	85%-98% feces
Half-life	4 hr (initial); 50 hr (terminal)

Pharmacodynamics	
Onset	½-1½ hr
Peak	1-3 hr
Duration	8-12 hr

Interactions
Individual drugs
Alcohol: ↑ disulfiram-like reaction
Haloperidol: ↓ levels of bromocriptine
Levodopa: ↑ neurologic effects
Loxapine: ↓ bromocriptine
Methyldopa: ↓ levels of bromocriptine
Metoclopramide: ↓ bromocriptine
Reserpine: ↓ effects of bromocriptine
Drug classifications
Analgesics, opioid: ↑ CNS depression
Antidepressants, tricyclics: ↓ levels of bromocriptine
Antihistamines: ↑ CNS depression
Antihypertensives: ↑ hypotension
Estrogens: ↓ bromocriptine effect
MAOIs: ↓ bromocriptine
Oral contraceptives: ↓ bromocriptine
Phenothiazines: ↓ levels of bromocriptine
Progestins: ↓ bromocriptine
Sedative/hypnotics: ↑ CNS depression

⊠ *Herb/drug*
Chaste tree fruit: ↓ bromocriptine effect
Lab test interferences
↑ Growth hormone, ↑ AST, ↑ ALT, ↑ BUN, ↑ uric acid, ↑ alkaline phosphatase

NURSING CONSIDERATIONS
Assessment
• Assess symptoms of Parkinson's disease (extrapyramidal symptoms): shuffling gait, muscle rigidity, involuntary movements, pill rolling, muscle spasms, drooling before and during treatment
• Assess for symptoms of suppression of lactation: decreasing breast tenderness and discomfort, decreasing milk production
• Monitor B/P; establish baseline, compare with other readings; this drug decreases B/P; patient should remain recumbent for 2-4 hr after first dose; supervise ambulation

Nursing diagnoses
☑ Mobility, impaired (uses)
☑ Knowledge deficit (teaching)

Implementation
• Give with meals or milk to prevent GI symptoms; crush tab if patient has swallowing difficulty
• Give hs so dizziness, orthostatic hypotension do not occur
• Store at room temp in airtight container

Patient/family education
• Advise patient to change position slowly to prevent orthostatic hypotension
• Tabs may be crushed and mixed with food
• Caution patient to use contraceptives during treatment with this drug; pregnancy may

---

occur; to use methods other than oral contraceptives

• Teach patient that therapeutic effect for Parkinson's disease may take 2 mo: galactorrhea, amenorrhea

• Caution patient to avoid hazardous activity if dizziness, drowsiness occurs during treatment start-up

• Advise patient to avoid alcohol and OTC medication unless approved by prescriber

• Teach patients with acromegaly to notify prescriber immediately if severe headache, nausea, vomiting, blurred vision occur; indicates change in enlargement of tumor

• Teach patients using drug for lactation suppression that treatment will last up to 3 wk and breast engorgement with milk production may occur after treatment is discontinued

Evaluation
Positive therapeutic outcome

• Parkinson's disease: decreased dyskinesia, decreased slow movements, decreased drooling

• Decreased breast engorgement with accompanied pain, tenderness

• Acromegly: decreased growth hormone levels

B

brompheniramine
(OTC, ℞)
(brome-fen-eer'a-meen)
Bromphen, brompheniramine, Chlorphed, Codimal-A, Conjec-B, Cophene-B, Dehist, Diamine T.D., Dimetane, Dimetane Extentabs, Dimetapp Allergy Liqui-Gels, Histaject Modified, Nasahist-B, ND-Stat Revised, Oraminic III, Veltane
Func. class.: Antihistamine
Chem. class.: Alkylamine, H_1-receptor antagonist
Pregnancy category B

Action: Acts on blood vessels, GI, respiratory system by competing with histamine for H_1-receptor site; decreases allergic response by blocking histamine

➡**Therapeutic Outcome:** Absence of allergy symptoms and rhinitis

Uses: Allergy symptoms, rhinitis, allergic dermatoses, nasal allergies, hypersensitivity reactions including blood transfusion reactions, anaphylaxis

Dosage and routes
Adult: PO 4-8 mg tid-qid, not to exceed 36 mg/day; TIME REL 8-12 mg bid-tid, not to exceed 36 mg/day; IM/**IV**/SC 5-20 mg q6-12h, not to exceed 40 mg/day

P *Child >6 yr:* PO 2 mg tid-qid, not to exceed 12 mg/day; IM/**IV**/SC 0.5 mg/kg/day divided tid or qid

---

P *Child <6 yr:* 1 mg q4-6h (not to exceed 6 mg/day)

Available forms: Tabs 4, 8, 12 mg; ext rel tabs 8, 12 mg; elix 2 mg/5 ml; inj 10 mg/ml

Adverse effects

CNS: Dizziness, drowsiness, poor coordination, fatigue, anxiety, euphoria, confusion, paresthesia, neuritis

CV: Hypotension, palpitations, tachycardia

EENT: Blurred vision, dilated pupils, tinnitus, nasal stuffiness, dry nose, throat, mouth

GI: Dry mouth, nausea, vomiting, anorexia, constipation, diarrhea

GU: Retention, dysuria, frequency, impotence

HEMA: **Thrombocytopenia, agranulocytosis, hemolytic anemia**

INTEG: Photosensitivity

RESP: Increased thick secretions, wheezing, chest tightness

Contraindications: Hypersensitivity to H_1-receptor antagonists, acute asthma attack, lower respiratory tract disease, **P** child <6 yr

Precautions: Increased intraocular pressure, renal disease, cardiac disease, hypertension, bronchial asthma, seizure disorder, stenosed peptic ulcers, hyperthyroidism, prostatic hypertrophy, bladder neck obstruction, pregnancy **B**

Pharmacokinetics	
Absorption	Well absorbed (PO, IM)
Distribution	Widely distributed; crosses blood-brain barrier
Metabolism	Liver, extensively
Excretion	Kidneys, metabolite; breast milk (minimal)
Half-life	12-34 hr

Pharmacodynamics			
	PO	SC/IM	IV
Onset	15-30 min	30 min	Immediate
Peak	2-5 hr	Unknown	Unknown
Duration	6-12 hr	8-12 hr	8-12 hr

Interactions

Individual drugs

Alcohol: ↑ CNS depression

Drug classifications

CNS depressants: ↑ CNS depression

MAOIs: ↑ anticholinergic effect

Opiates: ↑ CNS depression

Sedative/hypnotics: ↑ CNS depression

☑ *Herb/drug*

Henbane leaf: ↑ anticholinergic effect

Kava: ↑ CNS depression

Lab test interferences

False negative: Skin allergy tests (discontinue antihistamines before testing)

NURSING CONSIDERATIONS

Assessment

• Assess respiratory status: rate, rhythm, increase in bronchial secretions, wheezing, chest tightness; provide fluids to 2 L/day to decrease secretion thickness

• Monitor I&O ratio: be alert for urinary retention, frequency, dysuria, especially **G** elderly; drug should be discontinued if these occur

• Monitor CBC during long-term therapy; blood dyscrasias may occur but are rare

• **IV** administration may result in rapid drop in B/P, sweating, **G** dizziness, especially in elderly

Nursing diagnoses

✓ Airway clearance, ineffective (uses)

☑ Injury, risk for (side effects)
☑ Knowledge deficit (teaching)
☑ Noncompliance (teaching, overuse)

Implementation
PO route
• May give with food to prevent GI upset; absorption is not altered by food
• Store in tight, light-resistant container
IV IV route
• Give undiluted or dilute 10 mg/ml using 0.9% NaCl at a rate of 1 min or more
• May be further diluted in 0.9% NaCl, D_5W; give as intermittent inf at prescribed rate

Patient/family education
• Teach patient all aspects of drug use; to notify prescriber if confusion, sedation, hypotension occur; to avoid driving or other hazardous activity if drowsiness occurs; to avoid alcohol or other CNS depressants that may potentiate effect
• Instruct patient not to exceed recommended dosage; dysrhythmias may occur
• Teach patient hard candy, gum, frequent rinsing of mouth may be used for dryness

Evaluation
Positive therapeutic outcome
• Absence of running or congested nose, rashes

Treatment of overdose:
Administer ipecac syrup or lavage, diazepam, vasopressors, barbiturates (short acting)

bumetanide (Ⱥ)
(byoo-met′a-nide)
Bumex
Func. class: Loop diuretic
Chem. class.: Sulfonamide derivative

Pregnancy category   C

Action: Acts on the ascending loop of Henle in the kidney to inhibit the reabsorption of the electrolytes sodium and chloride, causing excretion of sodium, calcium, magnesium, chloride, water, and some potassium; also decreases reabsorption of sodium and chloride and increases the excretion of potassium in the distal tubule of the kidney; responsible for antihypertensive effect and peripheral vasodilatation

▶**Therapeutic Outcome:**
Decreased edema in lung tissue and peripherally; decreased B/P

Uses: Edema in congestive heart failure, nephrotic syndrome, ascites caused by hepatic disease, hepatic cirrhosis

Investigational uses: May be used alone or as adjunct with antihypertensives such as spironolactone, triamterene

Dosage and routes
Adult: PO 0.5-2 mg qd; may give 2nd or 3rd dose at 4-5 hr intervals; not to exceed 10 mg/day; may be given on alternate days or intermittently; **IV**/IM 0.5-1 mg/day; may give 2nd or 3rd dose at 2-3 hr intervals; not to exceed 10 mg/day

P *Child:* PO/IM/**IV** 0.02-0.1 mg/kg q12h, max 10 mg/day

Available forms: Tabs 0.5, 1, 2 mg; inj 0.25 mg/ml

Adverse effects

CNS: Headache, fatigue, weakness, vertigo, paresthesias

CV: Orthostatic hypotension, chest pain, ECG changes, circulatory collapse

EENT: Ear pain, tinnitus, blurred vision

ELECT: Hypokalemia, hypochlorsemic alkalosis, hypomagnesia, hyperuricemia, hypocalcemia, hyponatremia, metabolic alkalosis

ENDO: Hyperglycemia

GI: Nausea, diarrhea, dry mouth, vomiting, anorexia, cramps, oral and gastric irritations, pancreatitis

GU: Polyuria, **renal failure,** *glycosuria*

HEMA: **Thrombocytopenia, leukopenia, anemia**

INTEG: Rash, pruritus, purpura, urticaria

MS: Cramps, stiffness

Contraindications: Hypersensitivity to sulfonamides, anuria, electrolyte depletion

Precautions: Diabetes mellitus, dehydration, severe renal disease, pregnancy **C,** lactation

▧ Do Not Confuse:
Bumex/Buprenex

Pharmacokinetics

	PO/IM
Absorption	Rapidly, completely absorbed
	PO/IM/IV
Distribution	Crosses placenta
Metabolism	Liver (30%-40%)
Excretion	Breast milk, urine, feces
Half-life	1-1½ hr

Pharmacodynamics

	PO	IM	IV
Onset	½-1 hr	40 min	5 min
Peak	1-2 hr	Unknown	½ hr
Duration	4 hr	4 hr	2-3 hr

Interactions

Individual drugs

Alcohol: ↑ orthostatic hypotension

Ethacrynic acid: Combination may cause ↑ chance of arrhythmias (do not use together)

Indomethacin: ↓ diuretic and antihypertensive effects of bumetanide

Lithium: ↓ renal clearance causing ↑ toxicity

Metolazone: ↑ diuresis, electrolyte loss

Mezlocillin: ↑ hypokalemia

Probenecid: ↓ effect of bumetanide

Piperacillin: ↑ hypokalemia

Ticarcillin: ↑ hypokalemia

Drug classifications

Aminoglycosides: ↑ ototoxicity

Digitalis glycosides: ↑ potassium loss with relating arrhythmias

Glucocorticoids: ↑ hypokalemia

NSAIDs: ↓ diuretic effect

Potassium-wasting drugs: ↑ hypokalemia

NURSING CONSIDERATIONS

Assessment

• Assess patient for tinnitus, hearing loss, ear pain; periodic testing of hearing is needed when high doses of this drug are given by **IV** route

• Monitor for manifestations of hypokalemia: *Renal:* acidic urine, reduced urine osmolality, nocturia, polyuria, polydipsia; *CV:* hypotension, broad T wave, U wave, ectopy, tachycardia, weak pulse; *Neuro:* muscle weakness, altered LOC, drowsiness, apathy, lethargy, confusion, depression; *GI:* anorexia, nausea, cramps, constipation, distention, paralytic ileus; *Resp:* hypoventila-

tion, respiratory muscle weakness
• Monitor for manifestations of hypocalcemia: *CNS:* personality changes, anxiety, disturbances, depression, psychosis; *GI:* nausea, vomiting, constipation, abdominal pain from muscle spasm; *CV:* decreased contractility, decreased cardiac output, hypotension, lengthened ST segment, prolonged QT interval; *Integ:* scaling eczema, alopecia, hyperpigmentation; *Neuro:* tetany, muscle twitching, cramping, grimacing, seizure, altered deep tendon reflexes, spasm
• Monitor for manifestations of hypomagnesemia: *CNS:* agitation; *Neuro:* muscle twitching, paresthesias, hyperactive reflexes, positive Babinski's reflex, dysphagia, nystagmus, seizures, tetany; *GI:* nausea, vomiting, diarrhea, anorexia, abdominal distention; *CV:* ectopy, tachycardia, broad, flat, or inverted T waves, depressed ST segment, prolonged QT, decreased cardiac output, hypotension
• Monitor for manifestations of hyponatremia: *CV:* increased B/P, cold, clammy skin, hypovolemia or hypervolemia; *GI:* anorexia, nausea, vomiting, diarrhea, abdominal cramps; *Neuro:* lethargy, increased ICP, confusion, headache, seizures, coma, fatigue, tremors, hyperreflexia
• Monitor for manifestations of hyperchloremia: *Neuro:* weakness, lethargy, coma; *Resp:* deep rapid breathing
• Assess fluid volume status: I&O ratio and record, distended red veins, crackles in lung, color, quality and sp gr of urine, skin turgor, adequacy of pulses, moist mucous membranes, bilateral lung sounds, peripheral pitting edema; dehydration symptoms of decreasing output, thirst, hypotension, dry mouth and mucous membranes should be reported; if urinary output decreases or azotemia occurs, drug should be discontinued
• Monitor electrolytes: potassium, sodium, calcium, magnesium; also include BUN, blood pH, ABGs, uric acid, CBC, blood sugar
• Assess B/P before and during therapy with patient lying, standing, and sitting as appropriate; orthostatic hypotension can occur rapidly
• Monitor for digoxin toxicity in patients taking digoxin; lithium toxicity in those taking lithium

Nursing diagnoses
☑ Altered urinary elimination (side effects)
☑ Fluid volume deficit (side effects)
☑ Fluid volume excess (uses)
☑ Knowledge deficit (teaching)

Implementation
• Give in AM to avoid interference with sleep
• Potassium replacement if potassium level is <3.0 mg/dl whole, or use oral solutions; drug may be crushed if patient is unable to swallow

PO route
• With food, if nausea occurs; absorption may be reduced; the safest dosage schedule is on alternate days

IV route
• Do not use solution that is yellow or has a precipitate or crystals

---

IV **Direct IV**
• Give undiluted through Y-tube on 3-way stopcock; give 20 mg or less/min

Intermittent inf
• May be added to NS, D$_5$W, D$_{10}$W, D$_{20}$W, invert sugar 10% in electrolyte #1, LR, sodium lactate ⅙ mol/L; use within 24 hr to ensure compatibility; give through Y-tube or 3-way stopcock; give at 4 mg/min or less; use infusion pump

Y-site compatibilities:
Allopurinol, amifostine, aztreonam, cefepime, cisatracurium, cladribine, diltiazem, filgrastim, granisetron, lorazepam, morphine, piperacillin/tazobactam, propofol, remifantanil, teniposide, thiotepa, vinorelbine

Syringe compatibility:
Doxapram

Additive compatibilities:
Floxacillin, furosemide

Patient/family education
• Teach patient to take the medication early in the day to prevent nocturia
• Instruct the patient to take with food or milk if GI symptoms of nausea and anorexia occur
• Teach patient to maintain weekly record of weight and notify prescriber of weight loss of >5 lb
• Caution the patient that this drug causes a loss of potassium so food rich in potassium should be added to the diet; refer to a dietician for assistance in planning
• Caution the patient not to exercise in hot weather or stand for prolonged periods since orthostatic hypotension will be enhanced

• Teach patient not to use alcohol or any OTC medications without prescriber's approval; serious drug reactions may occur
• Emphasize the need to contact prescriber immediately if muscle cramps, weakness, nausea, dizziness, or numbness occurs
• Teach patient to take own B/P and pulse and record
• Caution the patient that orthostatic hypotension may occur; patient should rise slowly from sitting or reclining positions and lie down if dizziness occurs
• Teach patient to continue taking medication even if feeling better; this drug controls symptoms but does not cure the condition
• Advise the patient with hypertension to continue other medical treatment (exercise, weight loss, relaxation techniques, cessation of smoking)

Evaluation
Positive therapeutic outcome
• Decreased edema
• Decreased B/P
• Increased diuresis

---

buprenorphine (℞)
(byoo-pre-nor′feen)
Buprenex
Func. class.: Opioid analgesic
Chem. class.: Thebaine derivative
Pregnancy category **C**
Controlled substance schedule **V**

Action: Inhibits ascending pain pathways in limbic system, thalamus, midbrain, hypothala-

---

mus by binding to opiate receptor sites; this alters pain perception and response; generalized CNS depression

➲ **Therapeutic Outcome:** Relief of pain

Uses: Moderate to severe pain

Dosage and routes
Adult: IM/**IV** 0.3-0.6 mg q6h prn; may repeat dose after ½ hr; reduce dosage in elderly

🄶 *Elderly:* PO 0.15 mg q6h prn

Available forms: Inj 0.3 mg/ml (1 ml vials)

Adverse effects
CNS: Drowsiness, dizziness, confusion, headache, sedation, euphoria, **increased intracranial pressure**
CV: Palpitations, bradycardia, change in B/P, tachycardia
EENT: Tinnitus, blurred vision, *miosis,* diplopia
GI: Nausea, vomiting, anorexia, constipation, cramps
GU: Increased urinary output, dysuria
INTEG: Rash, urticaria, bruising, flushing, diaphoresis, pruritus
RESP: **Respiratory depression,** dyspnea, hypoventilation

Contraindications: Hypersensitivity, addiction (narcotic)

Precautions: Addictive personality, pregnancy **C,** lactation, increased intracranial pressure, MI (acute), severe heart disease, respiratory depression, hepatic disease, renal disease

🜲 **Do Not Confuse:**
Buprenex/Bumex

Pharmacokinetics

Absorption	Well absorbed (IM)
Distribution	Crosses placenta
Metabolism	Liver, extensively
Excretion	Kidneys, breast milk
Half-life	2½-3½ hr

Pharmacodynamics

	IM	IV
Onset	10-15 min	Immediate
Peak	1 hr	5 min
Duration	4 hr	2-5 hr

Interactions
Individual drugs
Alcohol: ↑ respiratory depression, hypotension, sedation
Drug classifications
Antihistamines: ↑ respiratory depression, hypotension
CNS depressants: ↑ respiratory depression, hypotension
MAOIs: Do not use within 2 wk
Opioids: ↑ CNS depression
Sedative/hypnotics: ↑ respiratory depression, hypotension
Herb/drug
Kava: ↑ **CNS depression**

NURSING CONSIDERATIONS
Assessment
• Assess pain characteristics: location, intensity, type before medication administration and following treatment
• Monitor VS after parenteral route; note muscle rigidity, drug history, liver, kidney function tests, respiratory dysfunction: respiratory depression, character, rate, rhythm; notify prescriber if respirations are <10/min
• Monitor CNS changes: dizziness, drowsiness, hallucinations, euphoria, LOC, pupil reaction; withdrawal in opioid dependent persons; if dependence occurs within 2 wk

of discontinuing drug, withdrawal symptoms will occur
• Monitor allergic reactions: rash, urticaria

Nursing diagnoses

☑ Pain (uses)

☑ Sensory-perceptual alteration: visual, auditory (adverse reactions)

☑ Breathing pattern, ineffective (adverse reactions)

☑ Knowledge deficit (teaching)

Implementation
• Give by inj (IM, **IV**), only with resuscitative equipment available; give slowly to prevent rigidity

IM route
• Give deep in large muscle mass; rotate sites of inj

IV **IV route**
• Give **IV** direct undiluted over 3-5 min; give slowly

Y-site compatibilities:
Allopurinol, amifostine, aztreonam, cefepime, cisatracurium, cladribine, filgrastim, granisetron, melphalan, piperacillin/tazobactam, propofol, remifentanil, teniposide, thiotepa, vinorelbine

Syringe compatibility:
Midazolam

Additive compatibilities:
Atropine, bupivacaine, diphenhydramine, droperidol, glycopyrrolate, haloperidol, hydroxyzine, promethazine, scopolamine

Additive incompatibilities:
Diazepam, floxacillin, furosemide, lorezepam

Patient/family education
• Instruct patient to report any symptoms of CNS changes, allergic reactions
• Caution patients to avoid CNS depressants: alcohol, sedative/hypnotics for at least 24 hr after taking this drug
• Discuss with patient that dizziness, drowsiness, and confusion are common; to avoid getting up without assistance
• Discuss in detail all aspects of the drug
• Instruct patient to change position slowly to prevent orthostatic hypotension
• Teach patient to turn, cough, deep breathe after surgery to prevent atelectasis

Evaluation
Positive therapeutic outcome
• Relief of pain

Treatment of overdose:
Narcan 0.2-0.8 **IV**, O_2, **IV** fluids, vasopressors

---

bupropion (℞)
(byoo-proe′pee-on)
Wellbutrin, Wellbutrin SR, Zyban
Func. class.: Misc. antidepressant, smoking deterrent
Chem. class.: Aminoketone
Pregnancy category   B

Action: Inhibits reuptake of dopamine, serotonin, norepinephrine

▸**Therapeutic Outcome:** Decreased symptoms of depression after 2-3 wk

Uses: Depression, smoking cessation

Dosage and routes
Depression
Adult: PO 100 mg bid initially, then increase after 3 days to 100 mg tid if needed; may increase after 1 mo to 150 mg tid

---

G *Elderly:* PO 50-100 mg/day, may increase by 50-100 mg q3-4 days

Smoking cessation
Adult: PO 150 mg bid, begin with 150 mg qd x 3 days then 300 mg/day continue for 7-12 wk

Available forms: Tabs 75, 100 mg; tabs, sus rel 100, 150 mg

Adverse effects
CNS: Headache, agitation, confusion, **seizures,** delusions, insomnia, sedation, tremors
CV: **Dysrhythmias,** hypertension, palpitations, tachycardia, hypotension
EENT: Blurred vision, auditory disturbance
GI: Nausea, vomiting, dry mouth, increased appetite, constipation
GU: Impotence, frequency, retention
INTEG: Rash, pruritus, sweating

Contraindications: Hypersensitivity, seizure disorder, eating disorders

Precautions: Renal and hepatic disease, recent MI, cranial trauma, pregnancy **B,** lactation, **P** children

Pharmacokinetics	
Absorption	Well absorbed; bioavailability poor
Distribution	Unknown
Metabolism	Liver extensively
Excretion	Kidneys
Half-life	8-24 hr, steady state 1½-5 wk

Pharmacodynamics	
Onset	Up to 4 wk
Peak	Unknown
Duration	Unknown

Interactions
Individual drugs
Alcohol: ↑ risk of seizures
Carbamazepine: ↓ bupropion effect
Cimetidine: ↑ levels, ↑ toxicity
Levodopa: ↑ risk of seizures
Phenytoin: ↑ toxicity
Theophylline: ↑ risk of seizures
Ritonavir: ↑ bupropion toxicity
Drug classifications
Antidepressants: ↑ risk of seizures
Antihistamines: ↑ CNS depression
Barbiturates: ↓ bupropion effects
Benzodiazepines: ↑ risk of seizures
CNS depressants: ↑ effects
MAOIs: Acute toxicity, risk of seizures
Phenothiazines: ↑ toxicity, risk of seizures
Steroids, systemic: ↑ risk of seizures
Herb/drug
Kava: ↑ CNS depression
Belladonna leaf/root: ↑ anticholinergic effect
Lab test interferences
↑ serum bilirubin, ↑ blood glucose, ↑ alkaline phosphatase ↓ VMA, ↓ 5-HIAA
False ↑ Urinary catecholamines

NURSING CONSIDERATIONS
Assessment
• Monitor B/P (with patient lying, standing), pulse q4h; if systolic B/P drops 20 mm Hg hold drug, notify prescriber; take vital signs q4h in patients with cardiovascular disease
• Assess smoking cessation progress after 7 wk, if progress has not been made, drug should be discontinued
• Assess for increased risk of seizures; if patient has used

CNS depressant or CNS stimulants, dosage of bupropion should not be exceeded
• Monitor blood studies: CBC, leukocytes, differential, cardiac enzymes if patient is receiving long-term therapy
• Monitor hepatic studies: AST, ALT, bilirubin if on long-term treatment
• Check weight weekly; appetite may increase with drug
• Assess ECG for flattening of T wave, bundle branch block, AV block, dysrhythmias in cardiac patients
• Assess for EPS primarily in **G** elderly: rigidity, dystonia, akathisia
• Assess mental status: mood, sensorium, affect, suicidal tendencies; increase in psychiatric symptoms: depression, panic
• Monitor urinary retention, constipation; constipation is **P** more likely to occur in children **G** or elderly
• Identify alcohol consumption; if alcohol was consumed, hold dose

Nursing diagnoses
☑ Coping, ineffective individual (uses)
☑ Injury, risk for (side effects)
☑ Knowledge deficit (teaching)
☑ Noncompliance (teaching)

Implementation
• Give with food or milk for GI symptoms
• Store at room temp; do not freeze

Patient/family education
• Teach patient that therapeutic effects may take 2-3 wk; not to increase dose without prescriber's approval; that treatment for smoking cessation lasts 7-12 wks
• Teach patient to use caution in driving or other activities requiring alertness because of drowsiness, dizziness, blurred vision; to avoid rising quickly from sitting to standing, **G** especially elderly
• Teach patient to avoid alcohol ingestion, obtain approval for other drugs
• Teach patient to increase fluids, bulk in diet if constipation, urinary retention occur, **G** especially elderly
• Teach patient to take gum, hard sugarless candy, or frequent sips of water for dry mouth
• Advise patient not to use with nicotine patches unless directed by prescriber, may increase B/P
• Teach patient that risk of seizures increases when dose is exceeded, or if patient has seizure disorder
• Teach patient to notify prescriber if pregnant

Evaluation
Positive therapeutic outcome
• Decrease in depression
• Absence of suicidal thoughts
• Smoking cessation

Treatment of overdose:
ECG monitoring, induce emesis, lavage, activated charcoal, administer anticonvulsant

buspirone (℞)
(byoo-spye′rone)
BuSpar
Func. class.: Antianxiety agent
Chem. class.: Azaspirodecanedione
Pregnancy category   B

Action: Acts by inhibiting the action of serotonin (5-HT) by binding to serotonin and dopamine receptors; also increases norepinephrine metabolism

⊃ **Therapeutic Outcome:** Decreased anxiety

Uses: Management and short-term relief of anxiety disorders

Dosage and routes
Adult: PO 5 mg tid; may increase by 5 mg/day q2-3 days; not to exceed 60 mg/day

Available forms: Tabs 5, 10, 15 mg

Adverse effects
CNS: Dizziness, headache, depression, stimulation, insomnia, nervousness, light-headedness, numbness, paresthesia, incoordination, tremors, excitement, involuntary movements, confusion, akathisia
CV: Tachycardia, palpitations, hypotension, hypertension, **CVA, CHF, MI**
EENT: Sore throat, tinnitus, blurred vision, nasal congestion, red, itching eyes, change in taste, smell
GI: Nausea, dry mouth, diarrhea, constipation, flatulence, increased appetite, rectal bleeding
GU: Frequency, hesitancy, menstrual irregularity, change in libido
INTEG: Rash, edema, pruritus, alopecia, dry skin
MISC: Sweating, fatigue, weight gain, fever
MS: Pain, weakness, muscle cramps, spasms
RESP: Hyperventilation, chest congestion, shortness of breath

Contraindications: Hypersensitivity, child <18 yr

Precautions: Pregnancy **B**, lactation, elderly, impaired hepatic/renal function

Pharmacokinetics

Absorption	Rapidly absorbed
Distribution	Unknown
Metabolism	Liver, extensively
Excretion	Feces
Half-life	2-3 hr

Pharmacodynamics

Unknown

Interactions
Individual drugs
Alcohol: ↑ CNS depression
Rifampin: ↓ buspirone effect
Drug classifications
MAOI: ↑ B/P, do not use together
Psychotropics: ↑ CNS depression
Food/drug
Grapefruit: ↑ buspirone effect
Herb/drug
Kava: ↑ CNS depression

NURSING CONSIDERATIONS
Assessment
• Assess anxiety reaction: inability to sleep, apprehension, dread, foreboding, or uneasiness related to unidentified source of danger
• Assess for previous drug dependence or tolerance; if patient is drug dependent or tolerant, amount of medication should be restricted
• Monitor B/P (lying, standing), pulse; if systolic B/P drops 20 mm Hg, hold drug, notify prescriber; check I&O; may indicate renal dysfunction
• Monitor mental status: mood, sensorium, affect, sleeping patterns, drowsiness, dizziness, suicidal tendencies
• Assess for CNS reaction, some reactions may be unpredictable

Nursing diagnoses
☑ Anxiety (uses)
☑ Knowledge deficit (teaching)
☑ Noncompliance (teaching)

Implementation
• Give with food or milk for GI symptoms; sugarless gum, hard candy, frequent sips of water for dry mouth
• May be crushed

Patient/family education
• Teach patient that drug may be taken with food; if dose is missed take as soon as remembered; do not double doses
• Caution patient to avoid OTC preparations unless approved by the prescriber; to avoid alcohol ingestion and other psychotropic medications unless prescribed; that 1-2 wk of therapy may be required before therapeutic effects occur
• Caution patient to avoid driving and activities requiring alertness, since drowsiness may occur; until medication response is known, tell patient that drowsiness may worsen at beginning of treatment
• Instruct patient not to discontinue medication abruptly after long-term use
• Advise patient to rise slowly or fainting may occur, espe-
🅖 cially in elderly

Evaluation
Positive therapeutic outcome
• Increased well-being
• Decreased anxiety, restlessness, sleeplessness, dread

Treatment of overdose:
Gastric lavage, VS, supportive care

---

busulfan (℞)
(byoo-sul'fan)
Myleran
Func. class.: Antineoplastic alkylating agent
Chem. class.: Nitrosourea

Pregnancy category D

Action: Changes essential cellular ions to covalent bonding with resultant alkylation; this interferes with normal biologic function of DNA; activity is not phase specific; action is due to myelosuppression

Therapeutic Outcome: Prevention of rapid growth of malignant cells in chronic myelocytic leukemia

Uses: Chronic myelocytic leukemia

Dosage and routes
Adult: PO 4-12 mg/day initially until WBC levels fall to 10,000/mm^3; then drug is stopped until WBC levels rise over 50,000/mm^3; then 1-3 mg/day

🅟 *Child:* PO 0.06-0.12 mg/kg or 1.8-4.6 mg/m^2/day; dosage is titrated to maintain WBC levels at 20,000/mm^3

Available forms: Tabs 2 mg

Adverse effects
GI: Nausea, vomiting, *diarrhea, weight loss*
GU: Impotence, sterility, amenorrhea, gynecomastia, *renal toxicity,* hyperuremia, adrenal insufficiency–like syndrome
HEMA: **Thrombocytopenia, leukopenia, pancytopenia, severe bone marrow depression**
INTEG: Dermatitis, hyperpigmentation, alopecia

RESP: **Irreversible pulmonary fibrosis,** pneumonitis
OTHER: **Chromosomal aberrations**

Contraindications: Radiation, chemotherapy, lactation, pregnancy **D** (3rd trimester), blastic phase of chronic myelocytic leukemia, hypersensitivity

Precautions: Childbearing age men and women, leukopenia, thrombocytopenia, anemia, hepatotoxicity, renal toxicity

Pharmacokinetics	
Absorption	Rapidly absorbed
Distribution	Unknown; crosses placenta
Metabolism	Liver, extensively
Excretion	Kidneys, breast milk
Half-life	Unknown

Pharmacodynamics
Unknown

Interactions
Individual drugs
Radiation: ↑ toxicity, bone marrow suppression
Drug classifications
Anticoagulants: ↑ risk of bleeding
Antineoplastics: ↑ toxicity, bone marrow suppression
Salicylates: ↑ risk of bleeding
Lab test interferences
False positive: Breast, bladder, cervix, lung cytology tests

NURSING CONSIDERATIONS
Assessment
• Monitor CBC, differential, platelet count weekly; withhold drug if WBC is <4000/mm³ or platelet count is <75,000/mm³; notify prescriber of results if WBC <20,000/mm³, platelets <150,000/mm³
• Monitor pulmonary function tests, chest x-ray films before, during therapy; chest film should be obtained q2 wk during treatment; check for dyspnea, rales, nonproductive cough, chest pain, tachypnea; pulmonary fibrosis may occur up to 10 yrs after treatment with busulfan
• Assess for increased uric acid levels, swelling, joint pain primarily in extremities; patient should be well hydrated to prevent urate deposits
• Monitor renal function studies: BUN, serum uric acid, urine CrCl before, during therapy; I&O ratio; report fall in urine output of 30 ml/hr; check for decreased hyperuricemia
• Monitor for cold, fever, sore throat (may indicate beginning infection); identify edema in feet, joint or stomach pain, shaking; prescriber should be notified
• Assess for bleeding: hematuria, guaiac, bruising or petechiae, mucosa or orifices q8h; no rectal temps

Nursing diagnoses
☑ Injury, risk for (adverse reactions)
☑ Body image disturbance (adverse reactions)
☑ Infection, risk for (adverse reactions)
☑ Knowledge deficit (teaching)

Implementation
• Give 1 hr before or 2 hr pc to lessen nausea and vomiting or give antacid before oral agent; give drug after evening meal, before bedtime; antiemetic 30-60 min before giving drug to prevent vomiting
• Give either allopurinol or sodium bicarbonate to maintain uric acid levels, alkalinization of urine; increase fluid intake to 2-3 L/day to prevent

urate deposits, calculus formation
- Administer antibiotics for prophylaxis of infection; may be prescribed since infection potential is high
- Store in tight container

Patient/family education
- Teach patient to avoid use of products containing aspirin or ibuprofen, razors, commercial mouthwash since bleeding may occur; to report symptoms of bleeding (hematuria, tarry stools)
- Instruct patient to report signs of anemia (fatigue, headache, irritability, faintness, shortness of breath)
- Instruct patient to report any changes in breathing or coughing even several months after treatment; to avoid crowds and persons with respiratory tract or other infections
- Teach patient that hair loss may occur; discuss the use of wigs or hair pieces
- Caution patient not to have any vaccinations without the advice of the prescriber; serious reactions can occur
- Advise patient that contraception is needed during treatment and for several months after the completion of therapy

Evaluation
Positive therapeutic outcome
- Decreased leukocytes to normal limits
- Absence of sweating at night
- Increased appetite, increased weight

---

butorphanol (℞)
(byoo-tor′fa-nole)
Stadol, Stadol NS
Func. class.: Narcotic analgesic
Chem. class.: Opiate
Pregnancy category **C**
Controlled substance schedule **IV**

Action: Inhibits ascending pain pathways in limbic system, thalamus, midbrain, hypothalamus by binding to opiate receptor sites; this alters pain perception and response

➡**Therapeutic Outcome:** Relief of pain

Uses: Moderate to severe pain, analgesia during labor, sedation preoperatively

Investigational uses: Migraine headache, pain

Dosage and routes
Adult: IM 1-4 mg q3-4h prn; **IV** 0.5-2 mg q3-4h prn; nasal spray in 1 nostril; may give another dose 1-1½ hr later; may repeat q3-4h

G *Elderly:* ½ adult dose at 2× the interval

Renal disease
CrCl 10-50 ml/min 75% dose; CrCl <10 ml/min 50% dose

Available forms: Inj 1, 2 mg/ml; intranasal 10 mg/ml

Adverse effects
CNS: Drowsiness, dizziness, confusion, headache, sedation, euphoria, weakness, hallucinations
CV: Palpitations, bradycardia, change in B/P
EENT: Tinnitus, blurred vision, miosis, diplopia
GI: Nausea, vomiting, anorexia, constipation, cramps

GU: Increased urinary output, dysuria, urinary retention
INTEG: Rash, urticaria, bruising, flushing, diaphoresis, pruritus
RESP: **Respiratory depression,** pulmonary hypertension

Contraindications: Hypersensitivity, addiction (narcotic), CHF, MI

Precautions: Addictive personality, pregnancy **C,** lactation, increased intracranial pressure, respiratory depression, hepatic disease, renal disease, child <18 yr

Do Not Confuse:
Stadol/Haldol

Pharmacokinetics

Absorption	Well absorbed (IM, Nasal); complete (**IV**)
Distribution	Crosses placenta
Metabolism	Liver, extensively
Excretion	Feces (10%-15%); kidneys, unchanged (small amounts)
Half-life	3-4 hr

Pharmacodynamics

	IM	IV	NASAL
Onset	10-30 min	1 min	15 min
Peak	½ hr	5 min	1-2 hr
Duration	3-4 hr	2-4 hr	4-5 hr

Interactions
Individual drugs
Alcohol: ↑ respiratory depression, hypotension, sedation
Drug classifications
Antihistamines: ↑ respiratory depression, hypotension
CNS depressants: ↑ respiratory depression, hypotension
MAOI: Do not use 2 wk before alfentanil
Sedative/hypnotics: ↑ respiratory depression, hypotension
Herb/drug
Kava: ↑ CNS depression

NURSING CONSIDERATIONS
Assessment
• Monitor VS after parenteral route; note muscle rigidity, drug history, liver, kidney function tests, respiratory dysfunction: respiratory depression, character, rate, rhythm; notify prescriber if respirations are <10/min
• Monitor CNS changes: dizziness, drowsiness, hallucinations, euphoria, LOC, pupil reaction
• Monitor allergic reactions: rash, urticaria

Nursing diagnoses
✓ Pain (uses)
✓ Sensory-perceptual alteration: visual, auditory (adverse reactions)
✓ Injury, risk for (adverse reactions)
✓ Knowledge deficit (teaching)

Implementation
• Store in light resistant container at room temp
IM route
• Give deeply in large muscle mass; rotate injection sites
Intranasal
• Give 1 spray in nostril
IV IV route
• Give **IV** undiluted at a rate of ≤2 mg/>3-5 min; titrate to patient response

Syringe compatibilities:
Atropine, chlorpromazine, cimetidine, diphenhydramine, droperidol, fentanyl, hydroxyzine, meperidine, methotrimeprazine, metoclopramide, midazolam, morphine, pentazocine, perphenazine, prochlorperazine, promethazine, scopolamine, thiethylperazine

Syringe incompatibilities:
Dimenhydrinate, pentobarbital

Y-site compatibilities:
Allopurinol, amifostine, azetreonam, cefepime, cisatracurium, cladribine, doxorubicin liposome, enalaprilat, esmolol, filgrastim, fludarabine, granisetron, labetalol, melphalan, paclitaxel, piperacillin/tazobactam, propofol, remifentanil, sargramostim, teniposide, thiotepa, vinorelbine

Patient/family education
• Instruct patient to report any symptoms of CNS changes, allergic reactions; to avoid CNS depressants: alcohol, sedative/hypnotics for at least 24 hr after taking this drug
• Discuss with patient that dizziness, drowsiness, and confusion are common; to avoid getting up without assistance
• Discuss in detail all aspects of the drug
Nasal route
• Teach patient to blow nose to clear both nostrils before using; remove clip and cover, prime before using until spray appears; pump must be re-primed q48h; close nostril with finger and spray once quickly; have patient sniff
• Patient should replace clip and cover after use; caution patient not to shake medication

Evaluation
Positive therapeutic outcome
• Pain relief

Treatment of overdose: Narcan 0.2-0.8 **IV**, O$_2$, **IV** fluids, vasopressors

calcitonin (human) (℞)
(kal-sih-toh′nin)
Cibacalcin
calcitonin (salmon) (℞)
Calcimir, Miacalcin, Miacalin Nasal Spray, Osteocalcin, Salmonine
Func. class.: Parathyroid agents (calcium regulator)
Chem. class.: Polypeptide hormone

Pregnancy category   C

Action: Decreases bone resorption, blood calcium levels by direct action on bone, GI system, and kidney; increases deposits of calcium in bones; renal excretion of calcium occurs

➡**Therapeutic Outcome:** Lowered calcium level, decreasing symptoms of Paget's disease

Uses: Paget's disease

Dosage and routes
Human
Paget's disease
Adult: SC 0.5 mg/day initially; may require 0.5 mg bid × 6 mo, then decrease until symptoms reappear

Salmon
Postmenopausal osteoporosis
Adult: SC/IM 100 IU/day; NASAL 200 IU qd alternating nostrils qd, activate pump before 1st dose

Paget's disease
Adult: SC/IM 100 IU qd, maintenance 50-100 IU qd or qod

Hypercalcemia
Adult: SC/IM 4 IU/kg q12h, increase to 8 IU/kg q12h if response is unsatisfactory

Available forms: Human: Inj (SC) 0.5 mg/vial; **Salmon:** Inj

---

☑ Herb/drug   🚫 Do Not Crush   ◆ Alert   ⟲ Key Drug   🄶 Geriatric   🄿 Pediatric

100 IU, 200 IU/ml, nasal spray 200 IU/actuation

Adverse effects
CNS: Headache, **tetany,** chills, weakness, dizziness
CV: Chest pressure
GI: Nausea, diarrhea, vomiting, anorexia, abdominal pain, salty taste, epigastric pain
GU: Diuresis
INTEG: Rash, flushing, pruritus of earlobes, edema of feet
MS: Swelling, tingling of hands
RESP: Dyspnea

Contraindications: Hypersensitivity

Precautions: Renal disease, children, lactation, osteogenic sarcoma, pregnancy **C**

Pharmacokinetics
Absorption	Completely absorbed
Distribution	Unknown
Metabolism	Rapid; kidneys, tissue, blood
Excretion	Kidneys, inactive metabolite
Half-life	1 hr

Pharmacodynamics
	SC
Onset	15 min
Peak	4 hr
Duration	8-24 hr

Interactions: None

NURSING CONSIDERATIONS
Assessment
• Assess for GI symptoms, polyuria, flushing, head swelling, tingling, headache; may indicate hypercalcemia; nervousness, irritability, twitching, seizures, spasm, paresthesia indicate hypocalcemia during beginning of treatment
• Identify nutritional status; check diet for sources of vitamin D (milk, some seafood), calcium (dairy products, dark green vegetables), phosphates
• Monitor BUN, creatinine, uric acid, chloride, electrolytes, urine pH, urinary calcium, magnesium, phosphate, urinalysis (calcium should be kept at 9-10 mg/dl; vitamin D 50-135 IU/dl), alkaline phosphatase baseline and q3-6 mo; check urine sediment for casts throughout treatment
• Assess for increased drug level, since toxic reactions occur rapidly; have calcium chloride or gluconate on hand if calcium level drops too low; check for tetany

Nursing diagnoses
☑ Injury, risk for (adverse reactions)
☑ Pain, chronic (uses)
☑ Knowledge deficit (teaching)

Implementation
• Store at <77° F (25° C); protect from light
SC route (human)
• Give by SC route only; rotate inj sites; use within 6 hr of reconstitution; give hs to minimize nausea, vomiting
IM route (salmon)
• After test dose of 10 IU/ml, 0.1 ml intradermally; watch 15 min; give only with epinephrine and emergency meds available
• IM injection in deep muscle mass slowly; rotate sites

Patient/family education
• Teach method of inj if patient will be responsible for self-medication
• Instruct patient to notify prescriber for hypercalcemic relapse: renal calculi, nausea, vomiting, thirst, lethargy, deep bone or flank pain
• Teach patient that warmth and flushing occur and last 1 hr

- Provide a low-calcium diet as prescribed (Paget's disease, hypercalcemia)
- Advise patients with osteoporosis to increase calcium and vitamin D in diet and to continue with moderate exercise to prevent continued bone loss
- Advise patients to report difficulty swallowing or change in side effects immediately to prescriber

Evaluation

Positive therapeutic outcome
- Calcium levels 9-10 mg/dl
- Decreasing symptoms of Paget's disease, including pain
- Decreased bone loss in osteoporosis

---

calcitriol (R)
(kal-si-tree′ole)
Calcijex, Rocaltrol, Vitamin D₃
Func. class.: Parathyroid agent (calcium regulator)
Chem. class.: Vitamin D hormone

Pregnancy category   C

Action: Increases intestinal absorption of calcium, provides calcium for bones, increases renal tubular resorption of phosphate

▶**Therapeutic Outcome:** Calcium at normal level

Uses: Hypocalcemia in chronic renal disease, hypoparathyroidism, pseudohypoparathyroidism

Dosage and routes
Hypocalcemia
Adult: PO 0.25 µg qd, may increase by 0.25 µg/day q4-8 wk; maintenance 0.25 µg qod-1 µg qd

Hypoparathyroidism/ pseudohypoparathyroidism
P*Adult and child >1 yr:* PO 0.25 µg qd; may be increased q2-4 wk; maintenance 0.25-2 µg qd

Available forms: Caps 0.25, 0.5 µg

Adverse effects
CNS: Drowsiness, headache, vertigo, fever, lethargy
GI: Nausea, diarrhea, vomiting, jaundice, anorexia, dry mouth, constipation, cramps, metallic taste
GU: Polyuria, hypercalciuria, hyperphosphatemia, hematuria
MS: Myalgia, arthralgia, decreased bone development

Contraindications: Hypersensitivity, hyperphosphatemia, hypercalcemia, vitamin D toxicity

Precautions: Pregnancy **C**, renal calculi, lactation, CV disease

▧ **Do Not Confuse:**
calcitriol/Calciferol

Pharmacokinetics	
Absorption	Well absorbed
Distribution	To liver, crosses placenta
Metabolism	Liver
Excretion	Bile
Half-life	3-6 hr

Pharmacodynamics	
Onset	2-6 hr
Peak	4 hr
Duration	Up to 5 days

Interactions
Individual Drugs
Cholestyramine: ↓ absorption of calcitriol
Phenytoin: ↑ Vit D metabolism
Verapamil: ↑ dysrhythmias

▨ Herb/drug ▧ Do Not Crush ✦ Alert ⚷ Key Drug ▣ Geriatric P Pediatric

Drug classifications
Antacids: ↑ hypermagnesemia
Diuretics, thiazide: ↑ hypercalcemia
Calcium supplements: ↑ hypercalcemia
Cardiac glycosides: ↑ dysrhythmias
Vitamin D products: ↑ toxicity
Vitamins, fat-soluble: ↓ calcitriol absorption
Lab test interferences
False: ↑ Cholesterol
Interference: Alk phos, electrolytes

NURSING CONSIDERATIONS
Assessment
• Assess GI symptoms, polyuria, flushing, head swelling, tingling, headache; may indicate hypercalcemia
• Identify nutritional status; check diet for sources of vitamin D (milk, some seafood), calcium (dairy products, dark green vegetables), phosphates
• Monitor BUN, creatinine, uric acid, chloride, electrolytes, urine pH, urinary calcium, magnesium, phosphate, urinalysis (calcium should be kept at 9-10 mg/dl; vitamin D 50-135 IU/dl), alkaline phosphatase baseline and q3-6 mo
◆• Assess for increased drug level, since toxic reactions occur rapidly; have calcium chloride on hand if calcium level drops too low; check for tetany

Nursing diagnoses
☑ Injury, risk for (adverse reactions)
☑ Pain, chronic (uses)
☑ Knowledge deficit (teaching)

Implementation
• Give with meals for GI symptoms
🚫• Do not crush or chew caps

Patient/family education
• Teach patient the symptoms of hypercalcemia and about foods rich in calcium
• Advise patient to avoid products with sodium: cured meats, dairy products, cold cuts, olives, beets, pickles, soups, meat tenderizers in chronic renal failure
• Advise patient to avoid products with potassium: oranges, bananas, dried fruit, peas, dark green leafy vegetables, milk, melons, beans in chronic renal failure
• Advise patient to avoid OTC products containing calcium, potassium, or sodium in chronic renal failure
• Instruct patient to avoid all preparations containing Vit D
• Instruct patient to monitor weight weekly

Evaluation
Positive therapeutic outcome
• Calcium levels 9-10 mg/dl

C

calcium carbonate
(PO-OTC, IV-℞)
Alka-Mints, Amitone, Apo-Cal ✦, BioCal, Calcarb, Calci-Chew, Calcilac, Calci-Mix, Calcite ✦, Calglycine ✦, Cal-Plus, Calsan ✦, Caltrate 600, Caltrate Jr., Chooz, Dicarbosil, Equilet, Gencalc, LIquid-Cal, Liquid-Cal-600, Maalox Antacid Caplets, Mallamint, Mylanta Lozenges ✦, Nephro-Calci, Nu-Cal ✦, Os-Cal 500, Oysco 500, Oystercal 500, Oyst-Cal 500, Rolaids Calcium Rich, Titralac, Tums, Tums E-X Extra Strength
Func. class.: Antacid, calcium supplement
Chem. class.: Calcium product

Pregnancy category   C

Action: Neutralizes gastric acidity

Therapeutic Outcome: Neutralized gastric acidity; calcium at normal levels

Uses: Antacid, calcium supplement; not suitable for chronic therapy

Dosage and routes
Adult: PO 350 mg-1.5 g or 2 pieces of gum 1 hr pc and hs

Available forms: Chewable tabs 350, 420, 500, 750, 850, 1000, 1250 mg; tabs 500, 600, 650, 1000, 1250 mg; gum 500 mg; susp 1250 mg/5 ml; lozenges 600 mg

Adverse effects
GI: Constipation, anorexia, nausea, vomiting, flatulence, diarrhea, rebound hyperacidity, eructation

Contraindications: Hypersensitivity, hypercalcemia, hyperparathyroidism, bone tumors

G Precautions: Elderly, fluid restriction, decreased GI motility, GI obstruction, dehydration, renal disease, pregnancy (C), lactation

Pharmacokinetics	
Absorption	Unknown
Distribution	Unknown
Metabolism	Unknown
Excretion	Feces
Half-life	Unknown

Pharmacodynamics	
Onset	20 min
Peak	Unknown
Duration	20-180 min

Interactions
Drug Classifications
Azole antiinfectives: ↓ levels of azole antiinfectives
Calcium channel blockers: ↓ levels of calcium channel blockers
Iron products: ↓ levels of iron products
Salicylates: ↓ levels of salicylates

NURSING CONSIDERATIONS
Assessment
• Monitor Ca⁺ (serum, urine), Ca⁺ should be 8.5-10.5 mg/dl, urine Ca⁺ should be 150 mg/day, monitor weekly
• Assess for milk-alkali syndrome: nausea, vomiting, disorientation, headache
• Assess for constipation; increase bulk in the diet if needed
• Assess for hypercalcemia: headache, nausea, vomiting, confusion

Implementation
PO route
- Administer as antacid 1 hr pc and hs
- Administer as supplement 1½ hr pc and hs
- Administer only with regular tablets or capsules; do not give with enteric-coated tablets
- Administer laxatives or stool softeners if constipation occurs

Evaluation
- Therapeutic response: absence of pain, decreased acidity

Patient/family education
- Advise patient to increase fluids to 2 L unless contraindicated, to add bulk to diet for constipation
- Advise patient not to switch antacids unless directed by prescriber
- Teach patient that therapeutic dose recommendations are figured as elemental calcium

calcium chloride/ calcium gluceptate/ calcium gluconate/ calcium lactate (PO, OTC; IV, ℞)
Func. class.: Electrolyte replacement—calcium product

Pregnancy category **C**

Action: Cation needed for maintenance of nervous, muscular, skeletal systems, enzyme reactions, normal cardiac contractility, coagulation of blood; affects secretory activity of endocrine, exocrine glands

▶**Therapeutic Outcome:** Calcium at normal level, absence of increased magnesium, potassium

Uses: Prevention and treatment of hypocalcemia, hypermagnesemia, hypoparathyroidism, neonatal tetany, cardiac toxicity caused by hyperkalemia, lead colic, hyperphosphatemia, vitamin D deficiency

Dosage and routes
Calcium chloride
Adult: **IV** 500 mg-1 g q1-3 days as indicated by serum calcium levels; give at <1 ml/ min; IAV 200-800 mg injected in ventricle of heart

Child: **IV** 25 mg/kg over several min

Calcium gluceptate
Adult: **IV** 5-20 ml; IM 2-5 ml

Newborn: 0.5 ml/100 ml of blood transfused

Calcium gluconate
Adult: PO 0.5-2 g bid-qid; **IV** 0.5-2 g at 0.5 ml/min (10% sol)

Child: PO/**IV** 500 mg/kg/ day in divided doses

Calcium lactate
Adult: PO 325 mg-1.3 g tid with meals

Child: PO 500 mg/kg/day in divided doses

Available forms: Many; check product listings

Adverse effects
CV: Shortened QT, heart block, hypotension, bradycardia, dysrhythmias, **cardiac arrest**
GI: Vomiting, nausea, constipation
HYPERCALCEMIA: Drowsiness, lethargy, muscle weakness, headache, constipation, **coma,** anorexia, nausea, vomiting, polyuria, thirst

INTEG: Pain, burning at **IV** site, severe venous thrombosis, necrosis, extravasation

Contraindications: Hypercalcemia, digitalis toxicity, ventricular fibrillation, renal calculi

Precautions: Pregnancy **C**, **P** lactation, children, renal disease, respiratory disease, cor pulmonale, digitalized patient, respiratory failure

Pharmacokinetics

Absorption	Complete bioavailability (**IV**)
Distribution	Readily extracellular; crosses placenta
Metabolism	Liver
Excretion	Feces (80%), kidney (20%), breast milk
Half-life	Unknown

Pharmacodynamics

	PO	IV
Onset	Unknown	Immediate
Peak	Unknown	Rapid
Duration	Unknown	½-1½ hr

Interactions

Individual drugs
Atenolol: ↓ effects of atenolol
Tetracycline: ↓ absorption of tetracycline (PO)
Verapamil: ↓ effects of verapamil

Drug classifications
Antacids: Milk-alkali syndrome (renal disease)
Cardiac glycosides: ↑ toxicity
Diuretics, thiazide: ↑ hypercalcemia
Fluoroquinolones: ↓ absorption of fluoroquinolones
Iron salts: ↓ absorption of iron

Food/drug
Calcium (dairy products): ↑ hypercalcemia

Lab test interferences
False ↓ Magnesium
↓ 17-OHCS

NURSING CONSIDERATIONS

Assessment

• Monitor ECG for decreased QT and T wave inversion: in hypercalcemia, drug should be reduced or discontinued
• Monitor calcium levels during treatment (9-10 mg/dl is normal level)
• Assess cardiac status: rate, rhythm, CVP, (PWP, PAWP if being monitored directly)

Nursing diagnoses

☑ Injury, risk for (uses, adverse reactions)
☑ Knowledge deficit (teaching)

Implementation

IV **IV route**

• Administer **IV** undiluted or diluted with equal amounts of 0.9% NaCl for inj to a 5% sol; give 0.5-1 ml/min
• Give through small-bore needle into large vein; if extravasation occurs, necrosis will result (**IV**); IM injection may cause severe burning, necrosis, and tissue sloughing; warm sol to body temp before administering
• Provide seizure precautions: padded side rails, decreased stimuli (noise, light); place airway suction equipment, padded mouth gag if calcium levels are low

Calcium chloride
Syringe compatibilities:
Milrinone

Y-site compatibilities:
Amrinone, dobutamine, epinephrine, esmolol, morphine, paclitaxel

Additive compatibilities:
Amikacin, ascorbic acid, bretylium, cephapirin, chloramphenicol, dopamine, hydrocortisone, isoproterenol, lidocaine, methicillin, norepinephrine,

penicillin, G potassium penicillin G sodium, pentobarbital, phenobarbital, sodium bicarbonate, verapamil, Vit B/C

*Calcium gluceptate
Additive compatibilities:*
Ascorbic acid inj, isoproterenol, lidocaine, norepinephrine, phytonadione, sodium bicarbonate

*Calcium gluconate
Additive compatibilities:*
Amikacin, aminophylline, ascorbic acid inj, bretylium, cephapirin, chloramphenicol, corticotropin, dimenhydrinate, erythromycin, furosemide, heparin, hydrocortisone, lidocaine, magnesium sulfate, methicillin, norepinephrine, penicillin G potassium, penicillin G sodium, phenobarbital, potassium chloride, tobramycin, vancomycin, verapamil, vit B/C

Syringe compatibilities:
Aldesleukin, allopurinol, amifostine, aztreonam, cefazolin, cefepime, ciprofloxacin, cladribine, dobutamine, enalaprilat, epinephrine, famotidine, filgrastim, granisetron, heparin/hydrocortisone, labetalol, melphalan, midazolam, netilmicin, piperacillin/tazobactam, potassium chloride, prochlorperazine, propofol, sargramostim, tacrolimus, teniposide, thiotepa, tolazoline, vinorelbine, vit B/C

PO route
• Give PO with or following meals to enhance absorption
• Store at room temp

Patient/family education
• Advise patient to remain recumbent 30 min after **IV** dose
• Caution patient to add food

high in vitamin D content; to add calcium-rich foods to diet: dairy products, shellfish, dark green leafy vegetables; decrease oxalate-rich and zinc-rich foods: nuts, legumes, chocolate, spinach, soy
• Advise patient to prevent injuries, avoid immobilization

Evaluation
Positive therapeutic outcome
• Decreased twitching, paresthesias, muscle spasms
• Absence of tremors, convulsions, dysrhythmias, dyspnea, laryngospasm, negative Chvostek's sign, negative Trousseau's sign

calcium polycarbophil (OTC)
(pol-i-kar'boe-fil)
Equalactin, Fiberall, FiberCon, Fiber-Lax, Mitrolan
Func. class.: Laxative, bulk-forming
Pregnancy category   C

Action: Attracts water, expands in intestine to increase peristalsis; also absorbs excess water in stool; decreases diarrhea

➡**Therapeutic Outcome:** Absence of constipation or diarrhea in irritable bowel syndrome

Uses: Constipation, irritable bowel syndrome (diarrhea), acute, nonspecific diarrhea

Dosage and routes
Adult: PO 1 g qd-qid prn, not to exceed 6 g/24 hr

🄿 *Child 6-12 yr:* PO 500 mg bid prn, not to exceed 3 g/ 24 hr

P *Child 3-6 yr:* PO 500 mg bid prn, not to exceed 1.5 g/24 hr

Available forms: Chewable tabs 500, 625, 1250 mg; tabs 500, 625 mg

Adverse effects
GI: **Obstruction,** abdominal distention, flatus, laxative dependence

Contraindications: Hypersensitivity, GI obstruction

Precautions: Pregnancy **C**

Pharmacokinetics	
Absorption	None
Distribution	None
Metabolism	Unknown
Excretion	Feces
Half-life	Not known

Pharmacodynamics	
Onset	12-24 hr
Peak	1-3 days
Duration	Unknown

Interactions
Individual drugs
Tetracycline: ↓ absorption of tetracycline

NURSING CONSIDERATIONS
Assessment
• Monitor blood, urine electrolytes if used often by patient; check I&O ratio to identify fluid loss
• Assess cramping, rectal bleeding, nausea, vomiting; if these symptoms occur, drug should be discontinued; identify cause of constipation; identify whether fluids, bulk, or exercise is missing from lifestyle

Nursing diagnoses
✓ Constipation (uses)
✓ Diarrhea (side effects)
✓ Knowledge deficit (teaching)
✓ Noncompliance (teaching)

Implementation
• Give alone for better absorption; give after mixing with water immediately before use; administer with 8 oz water or juice followed by another 8 oz of fluid
• Administer in AM or PM

Patient/family education
• Discuss with the patient that adequate fluid consumption is necessary; not to use laxatives long-term, laxative dependence will result
• Teach patient that normal bowel movements do not always occur daily
• Teach patient not to use in presence of abdominal pain, nausea, vomiting; tell patient to notify prescriber if constipation unrelieved or if symptoms of electrolyte imbalance occur: muscle cramps, pain, weakness, dizziness, excessive thirst

Evaluation
Positive therapeutic outcome
• Decreased constipation within 3 days
• Decreased diarrhea in colitis within 1 wk

---

calfactant (℞)
(cal-fak′tant)
Infasurf
Func. class.: Natural lung surfactant extract
Pregnancy category   N/A

Action: Replenishes surfactant and restores surface activity to
P the lungs in premature infants

➔ **Therapeutic Outcome:** Abil-
P ity of neonate to breathe without assistance

Uses: Prevention and treatment (rescue) of respiratory

---

distress syndrome in
P premature infants

Dosage and routes:
P **Newborn: INTRATRACHEAL
Instill**

3ml/kg of birth wt, given as 2
doses of 1.5 ml/kg, repeat
doses of 3 ml/kg of birth wt,
until up to 3 doses 12 hr apart
have been given

Available forms: Susp 35 mg
phospholipids/ml in 0.9%
NaCl with 0.65 mg proteins in
single-use vials containing 6 ml
susp

Adverse effects
RESP: **Pulmonary air leaks,
pulmonary interstitial emphysema, apnea, pulmonary
hemorrhage**
SYST: **Patent ductus arteriosus, intracranial hemorrhage,
severe intracranial hemorrhage, necrotizing enterocolitis, posttreatment sepsis,
posttreatment infection,**
bradycardia, oxygen desaturation, pallor, vasoconstriction,
hypotension, hypertension

Precautions: Bradycardia,
rales, infections

Pharmacokinetics

Absorption	Unknown
Distribution	Lung
Metabolism	Recycled
Excretion	Unknown
Half-life	Unknown

Pharmacodynamics

Onset	Few min
Peak	Unknown
Duration	Becomes lung associ-ated within hours of administration

Interactions
None

**NURSING CONSIDERATIONS
Assessment**
• Assess respiratory rate,
rhythm, character, chest expansion, color, transcutaneous
saturation, ABGs; moni-
tor ECG
• Check endotracheal tube
placement before dosing;
monitor for apnea after endotracheal administration
• Check for reflux of drug into
the endotracheal tube during
administration; stop drug
administration if this occurs,
and if needed increase peak
inspiratory pressure on the
ventilator by 4-5 cm H_2O until
tube is cleared
P • Assess infant for repeat dosing using radiographic confir-
mation of respiratory distress
syndrome; repeat doses should
be given as noted above; ventilator settings for repeat doses
F_{IO_2} are decreased by 0.2 or
amount to prevent cyanosis;
ventilator rate of 30/min;
inspiratory time <1 sec;
P if infant's pretreatment rate
was >30, leave unchanged
during dosing; resume usual
ventilator management after
dosing

Nursing diagnoses
✓ Gas exchange, impaired (uses)
✓ Knowledge deficit (teaching)

Implementation
• Administer after suctioning;
give by endotracheal administration only by persons trained
P in neonatal intubation and
ventilation
• Use a no. 5 Fr end-hole
catheter inserted into the
endotracheal tube with the tip
protruding just beyond the
end of the endotracheal tube;
shorten the catheter before
insertion; do not insert the

drug into the mainstream bronchus

- Divide each dose into quarters and administer with infant in different positions [P]
- Determine the dosing by weight of infant; slowly withdraw the contents into the plastic syringe through a 20-G needle; do not filter or shake; attach the premeasured no. 5 Fr catheter to syringe; fill with drug and discard excess through the catheter so only dose to be given remains in syringe [P]
- For prevention dosing, stabilize, weigh, and intubate the infant; give drug within 15 min of birth if possible; position infant and inj first quarter dose through catheter over 2-3 sec; remove catheter and manually ventilate with O_2 to prevent cyanosis (60 bpm) and sufficient positive pressure to promote adequate air exchange and chest wall excursion [P]
- For rescue dosing, give drug as soon as infant is placed on ventilator after birth; immediately before administering dose, change ventilator settings to 60/min, inspiratory time 0.5 sec, FIO_2; position infant and inj first quarter through catheter over 2-3 sec; remove catheter; return to mechanical ventilator [P]
- Ventilate infant for >30 sec or until stable after prevention or rescue strategy; reposition for next dose; same procedure for subsequent dosing; do not suction for at least 1 hr after dosing unless airway obstruction is evident; resume ventilator therapy after dosing [P]
- Reduce peak ventilator inspiratory pressures immediately if chest expansion improves substantially after dose
- Suction all infants before administration to prevent mucus plugging; if endotracheal tube obstruction is suspected, remove the obstruction and replace tube immediately [P]
- Store in refrigerator; protect from light; warm to room temp for >20 min or warm in hand 8 min before giving; do not use artificial warming methods; enter a vial only once; unopened, unused vials that have been warmed to room temp may be rerefrigerated within 8 hr of warming; do not warm and return to refrigerator more than once

Patient/family education

- Explain disease process and purpose of medication to parents; communicate neonate's progress [P]

Evaluation
Positive therapeutic outcome

- Significant improvement in respiratory status (oxygenation, arterial blood gases WNL)

---

candesartan (℞)
(can-deh-sar´tan)
Atacand
Func. class.: Antihypertensive
Chem. class.: Angiotensin II receptor (Type AT_1)

Pregnancy category C, 1st trimester; **D,** 2nd/3rd trimesters

---

Action: Blocks the vasoconstrictor and aldosterone-secreting effects of angiotensin II; selectively blocks the binding of angiotensin II to the AT_1 receptor found in tissues

→**Therapeutic Outcome:** Decreased B/P

Uses: Hypertension, alone or in combination

Dosage and routes
Adult: PO 16 mg qd initially in patients who are not volume depleted, range 8-32 mg/day; may be given with a diuretic

Available forms: Tabs 4, 8, 16, 32 mg

Adverse effects
CNS: Dizziness, fatigue, headache
CV: Chest pain, peripheral edema
EENT: Sinusitis, rhinitis, pharyngitis
GI: Diarrhea, nausea
MS: Arthralgia, pain
RESP: Cough, upper respiratory infection
SYST: Angioedema

Contraindications: Hypersensitivity; pregnancy **D** (2nd and 3rd trimesters)

Precautions: Hypersensitivity to ACE inhibitors; pregnancy **C** 1st trimester; lactation; children; elderly

Pharmacokinetics
Absorption	Well
Distribution	Bound to plasma proteins
Metabolism	Extensive
Excretion	Feces, urine, breast milk
Half-life	9 hr

Pharmacodynamics
Onset	Unknown
Peak	2 hr
Duration	24 hr

Interactions
None significant

NURSING CONSIDERATIONS
Assessment
• Assess B/P, pulse q4h; note rate, rhythm, quality
• Monitor electrolytes: potassium, sodium, chloride; total CO_2
• Obtain baselines in renal, liver function tests before therapy begins
• Assess blood studies: BUN, creatinine, LFTs before treatment
• Monitor for edema in feet, legs daily
• Assess for skin turgor, dryness of mucous membranes for hydration status
• Assess for pregnancy, this drug can cause fetal death when given in pregnancy
• Assess for adverse reactions, especially in renal disease
• Monitor for severe hypotension, place supine, give 0.9% NaCl **IV**

Nursing diagnoses
✓ Fluid volume deficit (side effects)
✓ Noncompliance (teaching)
✓ Knowledge deficit (teaching)

Implementation
PO route
• Administer without regard to meals

Patient/family education
• Teach patient not to take the drug if breastfeeding or pregnant, or have had an allergic reaction to this drug
• If a dose is missed, instruct patient to take as soon as possible, unless it is within an hour before next dose
• Advise patient to comply with dosage schedule, even if feeling better
• Teach patient to notify prescriber of fever, swelling of

hands or feet, irregular heart-beat, chest pain

• Advise patient excessive perspiration, dehydration, diarrhea may lead to fall in blood pressure—consult prescriber if these occur

• Inform patient that drug may cause dizziness, fainting; lightheadedness may occur

• Caution patient to rise slowly to sitting or standing position to minimize orthostatic hypotension

Evaluation
Positive therapeutic outcome
• Decreased B/P

---

capecitabine (℞)
(cap-eh-sit'ah-bean)
Xeloda
Func. class.: Antineoplastic, antimetabolite
Chem. class.: Fluoropyrimidine carbamate

Pregnancy category   **D**

Action: Competes with physiologic substrate of DNA synthesis, thus interfering with cell replication in the S phase of cell cycle (before mitosis); drug is converted to 5-FU

➥ **Therapeutic Outcome:**
Decreasing symptoms of breast cancer

Uses: Metastatic breast cancer

Dosage and routes:
Adult: PO 2500 mg/m^2/day in 2 divided doses q12h at end of meal ×2 wk, then 1 wk rest period; given in 3 wk cycles

Available forms: Tabs 150, 500 mg

Adverse effects
CNS: Dizziness, headache, *paresthesia, fatigue,* insomnia
GI: Nausea, vomiting, anorexia, diarrhea, stomatitis, abdominal pain, constipation, anorexia, dyspepsia, **intestinal obstruction**
HEMA: **Neutropenia, lymphopenia, thrombocytopenia, myelosuppression,** anemia
INTEG: Hand and foot syndrome, dermatitis, nail disorder
OTHER: Hyperbilirubinemia, eye irritation, pyrexia, edema, myalgia, limb pain, *pyrexia,* dehydration

Contraindications: Hypersensitivity to 5-fluorouracil, infants, pregnancy **D**

Precautions: Renal disease, hepatic disease, lactation, children, elderly

Pharmacokinetics	
Absorption	Readily, food ↓
Distribution	Unknown
Metabolism	Liver, extensively
Excretion	Kidneys
Half-life	45 min

Pharmacodynamics	
Onset	Unknown
Peak	1½ hr
Duration	Unknown

Interactions
Individual drugs
Leucovorin: ↑ toxicity
Drug classifications
Antacids: ↑ capecitabine

NURSING CONSIDERATIONS
Assessment
• Assess buccal cavity q8h for dryness, sores or ulceration, white patches, pain, bleeding, dysphagia; obtain prescription for viscous lidocaine (Xylocaine)

- Assess symptoms indicating severe allergic reation: rash, pruritus, urticaria, purpuric skin lesions, itching, flushing; drug should be discontinued
- Monitor CBC, differential, platelet count weekly; withhold drug if WBC count is <4000/mm^3 or platelet count is <100,000/mm^3; notify prescriber of results if WBC <20,000/mm^3, platelets <150,000/mm^3
- Monitor temp q4h (may indicate beginning of infection)
- Assess for hand/foot syndrome: paresthesia, tingling, painful/painless swelling, blistering, erythema with severe pain of hands/feet
- Assess for toxicity: severe diarrhea, nausea, vomiting, stomatitis
- Assess GI symptoms: frequency of stools, cramping; if severe diarrhea occurs, fluids/electrolytes may need to be given
- Monitor liver function tests before and during therapy (bilirubin, AST, ALT, LDH) as needed or monthly; note jaundice of skin or sclera, dark urine, clay-colored stools, itchy skin, abdominal pain, fever, diarrhea
- Assess for bleeding: hematuria, stool guaiac, bruising or petechiae, mucosa or orifices q8h; inflammation of mucosa, breaks in skin

Nursing diagnoses
✓ Injury, risk for (adverse reactions)
✓ Body image disturbance (adverse reactions)
✓ Infection, risk for (adverse reactions)
✓ Knowledge deficit (teaching)

Implementation
PO route
- Give antiemetic 30-60 min before giving drug to prevent vomiting and prn; give antibiotics for prophylaxis of infection
- Provide liq diet: carbonated beverages; gelatin may be added if patient is not nauseated or vomiting
- Help patient to rinse mouth tid-qid with water or club soda, brush teeth bid-qid with soft brush or cotton-tipped applicators for stomatitis, use unwaxed dental floss

Patient/family education
- Contraceptive measures are recommended during therapy; drug is teratogenic to fetus
- Advise patient to avoid use of products containing aspirin or ibuprofen, razors, commercial mouthwash, since bleeding may occur; to report symptoms of bleeding (hematuria, tarry stools)
- Instruct patient to report signs of anemia (fatigue, headache, irritability, faintness, shortness of breath)
- Advise patient not to become pregnant while taking this drug; to avoid using while lactating
- Advise patient not to double dose, if dose is missed
- Advise patient to report immediately severe diarrhea, vomiting, stomatitis, fever ≥100°, hand/foot syndrome, anorexia

Evaluation
Positive therapeutic outcome
- Prevention of rapid division of malignant cells

---

captopril ⚶ (℞)
(kap'toe-pril)
Capoten, Novo-Captopril ✦
Func. class.: Antihypertensive
Chem. class.: Angiotensin-converting enzyme (ACE) inhibitor
Pregnancy category C (1st trimester) D (2nd/3rd trimester)

Action: Selectively suppresses renin-angiotensin-aldosterone system; inhibits ACE; preventing conversion of angiotensin I to angiotensin II; results in dilatation of arterial, venous vessels

➡**Therapeutic Outcome:** Decreased B/P in hypertension; decreased preload, afterload in CHF

Uses: Hypertension, CHF, left ventricular dysfunction after MI, diabetic nephropathy

Dosage and routes
Malignant hypertension
Adult: PO 25 mg increasing q2h until desired response; not to exceed 450 mg/day

Hypertension
Adult:
Initial dose: PO 12.5 mg bid-tid; may increase to 50 mg bid-tid at 1-2 wk intervals; usual range 25-150 mg bid-tid; max 450 mg

P *Child:* PO 0.3-0.5 mg/kg/dose, titrate up to 6 mg/kg/day in 2-4 divided doses

CHF
Adult: PO 12.5 mg bid-tid given with a diuretic; may increase to 50 mg bid-tid; after 14 days may increase to 150 mg tid if needed

LVD after MI
Adult: PO 50 mg tid, may begin treatment 3 days after MI; give 6.25 mg as a single dose, then 12.5 mg tid, increase to 25 mg tid for several days, then 50 mg tid

Diabetic nephropathy
Adult: PO 25 mg tid

Available forms: Tabs 12.5, 25, 50, 100 mg

Adverse effects
CNS: Fever, chills
CV: Hypotension, postural hypotension, *tachycardia,* angina
GI: Loss of taste
GU: Impotence, dysuria, nocturia, **proteinuria, nephrotic syndrome, acute reversible renal failure,** polyuria, oliguria, frequency
HEMA: **Neutropenia, agranulocytosis, pancytopenia, thrombocytopenia,** anemia
INTEG: Rash, **angioedema**
MISC: **Angioedema,** hyperkalemia
RESP: **Bronchospasm,** *dyspnea, cough*

Contraindications: Hypersensitivity, lactation, heart block, **P** children, potassium-sparing diuretics, bilateral renal artery stenosis, **D** (2nd/3rd trimester)

Precautions: Dialysis patients, hypovolemia, leukemia, scleroderma, LE, blood dyscrasias, CHF, diabetes mellitus, pregnancy **C** (1st trimester), renal disease, thyroid disease, COPD, asthma

---

☑ Herb/drug   ◎ Do Not Crush   ◆ Alert   ⚶ Key Drug   **G** Geriatric   **P** Pediatric

Pharmacokinetics	
Absorption	Well absorbed
Distribution	Widely distributed; crosses placenta
Metabolism	Liver (50%)
Excretion	Kidneys, unchanged (50%)
Half-life	1½-2 hr

Pharmacodynamics	
Onset	¼-1 hr
Peak	1 hr
Duration	6-12 hr

Interactions
Individual drugs
Alcohol: ↑ hypotension (large amounts)
Allopurinol: ↑ hypersensitivity
Digoxin: ↑ serum levels
Indomethacin: ↓ antihypertensive effect
Insulin: ↑ hypoglycemia
Lithium: ↑ serum levels, toxicity
Tetracycline: ↓ absorption of tetracycline
Drug classifications
Antacids: ↓ absorption
Antidiabetics, oral: ↑ hypoglycemia
Antihypertensives: ↑ hypotension
Diuretics: ↑ hypotension
Diuretics, potassium-sparing: ↑ toxicity
NSAIDs: ↓ captopril effect
Potassium supplements: ↑ toxicity
Lab test interferences
False positive: Urine acetone

NURSING CONSIDERATIONS
Assessment
• May be crushed and mixed with food
• Monitor blood studies: neutrophils, decreased platelets
• Monitor B/P, check for orthostatic hypotension, syncope; if changes occur, dosage change may be required
• Monitor renal studies: protein, BUN, creatinine; watch for increased levels that may indicate nephrotic syndrome and renal failure; monitor renal symptoms: polyuria, oliguria, frequency, dysuria
• Establish baselines in renal, liver function tests before therapy begins; monitor for increased liver function studies
• Check potassium levels throughout treatment, although hyperkalemia rarely occurs
• Check for edema in feet, legs daily; monitor weight daily
• Assess for allergic reactions: rash, fever, pruritus, urticaria; drug should be discontinued if antihistamines fail to help

Nursing diagnoses
☑Cardiac output, decreased (uses)
☑Injury, risk for (side effects)
☑Knowledge deficit (teaching)
☑Noncompliance (teaching)

Implementation
• Store in air-tight container at 86° F (30° C) or less
• Severe hypotension may occur after 1st dose of this medication; decreasing hypotension may be prevented by reducing or discontinuing diuretic therapy 3 days before beginning captopril therapy
• Administer 1 hr ac or 1½ hr pc

Patient/family education
• Caution patient not to discontinue drug abruptly; advise patient to tell all persons associated with care
• Teach patient not to use OTC products (cough, cold, allergy) unless directed by

prescriber; serious side effects can occur; xanthines such as coffee, tea, chocolate, cola can prevent action of drug

• Teach patient importance of complying with dosage schedule, even if feeling better; to continue with medical regimen to decrease B/P: exercise, cessation of smoking, decreasing stress, diet modifications

• Emphasize the need to rise slowly to sitting or standing position to minimize orthostatic hypotension; not to exercise in hot weather or increased hypotension can occur

• Teach patient to notify prescriber of mouth sores, sore throat, fever, swelling of hands or feet, irregular heartbeat, chest pain, coughing, shortness of breath

• Caution patient to report excessive perspiration, dehydration, vomiting, diarrhea; may lead to fall in B/P

• Caution patient that drug may cause dizziness, fainting, lightheadedness; may occur during 1st few days of therapy; to avoid activities that may be hazardous

• Teach patient how to take B/P, and teach normal readings for age group; ensure patient takes regularly

• Advise patient to tell prescriber if pregnancy is suspected

Evaluation
Positive therapeutic outcome

• Decreased B/P in hypertension

Treatment of overdose: 0.9% NaCl **IV** infusion, hemodialysis

carbamazepine (℞)
(kar-ba-maz'e-peen)
Apo-Carbamazepine ✤, Atretol, Carbatrol, Epitol, Mazepine ✤, PMS-Carbamazepine ✤, Tegretol, Tegretol CR ✤, Tegretol-XR
Func. class.: Anticonvulsant
Chem. class.: Iminostilbene derivative

Pregnancy category   C

Action: Inhibits nerve impulses by limiting influx of sodium ions across cell membrane in motor cortex

Therapeutic Outcome: Absence of seizures; decreased trigeminal neuralgia pain

Uses: Tonic-clonic, complex-partial, mixed seizures; trigeminal neuralgia, diabetic neuropathy

Investigational uses: Diabetes insipidus, bipolar disorder, neurogenic pain, schizophrenia, psychotic behavior with dementia

Dosage and routes
Seizures
P *Adult and child >12 yr:* PO 200 mg bid; may be increased by 200 mg/day in divided doses q6-8h; maintenance 800-1200 mg/day; maximum 1200 mg/day; adjustment is needed to minimum dose to control seizures; ext rel give bid

P *Child <12 yr:* PO 10-20 mg/kg day in 3-4 divided doses

Trigeminal neuralgia
Adult: PO 100 mg/bid; may increase 100 mg q12h until pain subsides; not to exceed

---

☒ Herb/drug   Ⓢ Do Not Crush   ◆ Alert   ☛ Key Drug   Ⓖ Geriatric   Ⓟ Pediatric

1.2 g/day; maintenance is 200-400 mg bid

Available forms: Chewable tabs 100 mg; tabs 200 mg; oral susp 100 mg/5 ml; ext rel 100, 200 ♣, 400 ♣ mg; caps, ext rel 200, 300 mg

Adverse effects
CNS: Drowsiness, dizziness, confusion, fatigue, **paralysis,** headache, hallucinations, **worsening of seizures**
CV: **Hypertension, CHF,** hypotension, aggravation of CAD, dysrhythmias
EENT: Tinnitus, dry mouth, blurred vision, diplopia, nystagmus, conjunctivitis
🄖 *ENDO:* SIADH (elderly)
GI: Nausea, constipation, diarrhea, anorexia, vomiting, abdominal pain, stomatitis, glossitis, increased liver enzymes, **hepatitis**
GU: Frequency, retention, albuminuria, glycosuria, impotence
HEMA: **Thrombocytopenia, agranulocytosis, leukocytosis, neutropenia, aplastic anemia, eosinophilia,** increased pro-time
INTEG: Rash, **Stevens-Johnson syndrome,** urticaria
RESP: Pulmonary hypersensitivity (fever, dyspnea, pneumonitis)

Contraindications: Hypersensitivity to carbamazepine or tricyclic antidepressants, bone marrow depression, concomitant use of MAOIs

Precautions: Glaucoma, hepatic disease, renal disease, cardiac disease, psychosis, pregnancy **C,** lactation, 🄿 child <6 yr

🄝 **Do Not Confuse:**
Tegretol/Toradol

Pharmacokinetics

Absorption	Slow; completely absorbed
Distribution	Widely distributed
Metabolism	Extensively, liver
Excretion	Urine, feces, breast milk
Half-life	14-16 hr or more

Pharmacodynamics

Onset	2-4 day
Peak	4-8 hr
Duration	Unknown

Interactions
Individual drugs
Acetaminophen: ↑ metabolism, ↓ action
Benzodiazepines: ↓ effect of benzodiazepine
Clarithromycin: ↑ toxicity
Danazol: ↑ carbamazepine effect
Diltiazem: ↑ toxicity
Doxycycline: ↓ half-life
Felbamate: ↑ carbamazepine effect
Fluoxetine: ↑ carbamazepine effect
Fluvoxamine: ↑ carbamazepine effect
Haloperidol: ↓ serum levels, ↓ therapeutic efficacy
Lithium: ↑ CNS toxicity
Oral contraceptives: ↓ effect of oral contraceptives
Phenobarbital: ↑ effect
Phenytoin: ↑ and ↓ plasma levels, ↓ carbamazepine plasma levels
Quinine: ↑ carbamazepine levels
Theophylline: ↓ effect of theophylline, carbamazepine
Thyroid hormones: ↓ effect of thyroid hormones
Valproic acid: ↓ plasma levels, ↑ half-life of carbamazepine
Verapamil: ↑ toxicity
Warfarin: ↓ effect of warfarin

Drug classifications
Barbiturates: ↓ serum levels of carbamazepine
MAOIs: Fatal reaction; do not use together
Nondepolarizing muscle relaxants: Resistance to or reversal of effects of these agents
Posterior pituitary hormones: Potentiates antidiuretic effects
Succinimides: ↓ plasma levels
Food/drug
Grapefruit: ↓ carbamazepine level
Lab test interferences
↓ Thyroid function tests

NURSING CONSIDERATIONS
Assessment
• Monitor liver function tests (AST, ALT) and urine function tests, BUN, urine protein periodically during treatments
• Check blood levels during treatment or when changing dose; therapeutic level 4-12 µg/ml
• Assess for blood dyscrasias: fever, sore throat, bruising, rash, jaundice, epistaxis (long-term treatment only)
• Assess seizure activity including type, location, duration, and character; provide seizure precaution

Nursing diagnoses
☑ Injury, risk for (side effects)
☑ Knowledge deficit (teaching)

Implementation
• Give with food for GI symptoms
• Chew tab: tell patient to chew, not swallow whole
• Shake oral susp before use
• Mix an equal amount of water, D_5W, 0.9% NaCl when giving by NG tube, flush tube with 100 ml of above sol

Patient/family education
• Teach patient to carry Medic Alert ID stating patient's name, drugs taken, condition, prescriber's name, phone number
• Caution patient to avoid driving, other activities that require alertness until stabilized on medication
• Teach patient not to discontinue medication quickly after long-term use
• Teach patient to use a nonhormonal type of contraception to prevent harm to the fetus
• Advise patient to use sunscreen to prevent burns
• Teach patient to take exactly as prescribed, do not double or omit doses

Evaluation
Positive therapeutic outcome
• Decreased seizure activity

Treatment of overdose: Lavage, vital signs

---

carbidopa-levodopa (Ŗ)
(kar-bi-doe'pa lee-voe-doe'pa)
carbidopa/levodopa, Sinemet, Sinemet CR
Func. class.: Antiparkinsonism agent
Chem. class.: Catecholamine

Pregnancy category   C

Action: Decarboxylation of levodopa to periphery is inhibited by carbidopa; more levodopa is made available for transport to brain and conversion to dopamine in the brain

---

> **Therapeutic Outcome:** Absence of involuntary movements

Uses: Parkinsonism, restless leg syndrome, chronic manganese intoxication, cerebral arteriosclerosis

Dosage and routes
Adult: PO 3-6 tabs of 25 mg carbidopa/250 mg levodopa qd in divided doses, not to exceed 8 tabs/day; SUS REL 1 tab bid at intervals of not less than 6 hr; usual dosage 2-8 tabs/day at intervals of 4-8 hr

Available forms: Tabs 10/100, 25/100, 25 mg carbidopa/250 mg levodopa; sus rel tabs 50 mg/200 mg carbidopa/levodopa (Sinemet CR)

Adverse effects
CNS: Involuntary choreiform movements, hand tremors, fatigue, headache, anxiety, twitching, numbness, weakness, confusion, agitation, insomnia, nightmares, psychosis, hallucination, hypomania, severe depression, dizziness
CV: Orthostatic hypotension, tachycardia, hypertension, palpitation
EENT: Blurred vision, diplopia, dilated pupils
GI: Nausea, vomiting, anorexia, abdominal distress, dry mouth, flatulence, dysphagia, bitter taste, diarrhea, constipation
HEMA: **Hemolytic anemia, leukopenia, agranulocytosis**
INTEG: Rash, sweating, alopecia
MISC: Urinary retention, incontinence, weight change, dark urine

Contraindications: Hypersensitivity, narrow-angle glaucoma, undiagnosed skin lesions

Precautions: Renal disease, cardiac disease, hepatic disease, respiratory disease, MI with dysrhythmias, convulsions, peptic ulcer, pregnancy **C**

Pharmacokinetics	
Absorption	Well absorbed (PO); sus rel dose slow
Distribution	Widely distributed
Metabolism	Liver, extensively
Excretion	Kidneys, metabolites
Half-life	Levodopa (1 hr); carbidopa (1-2 hr)

Pharmacodynamics		
	PO	PO-SUS REL
Onset	Unknown	Unknown
Peak	1 hr	2½ hr
Duration	6-24 hr	Unknown

Interactions
Individual drugs
Metoclopramide: ↑ effects of levodopa
Papaverine: ↓ effects of levodopa
Pyridoxine: ↓ effects of levodopa
Drug classifications
Antacids: ↑ effects of levodopa
Anticholinergics: ↓ effects of levodopa
Antidepressants, tricyclics: ↑ hypotension
Benzodiazepines: ↓ effects of levodopa
Hydantoins: ↓ effects of levodopa
MAOIs: Hypertensive crisis
Lab test interferences
False positive: Urine ketones
False negative: Urine glucose
False ↑ Uric acid, ↑ urine protein, ↓ VMA, ↓ BUN, ↓ creatinine

---

Food/drug
Protein: ↓ absorption of levodopa
⊘ *Herb/drug*
Kava: ↑ parkinson symptoms

NURSING CONSIDERATIONS
Assessment
• Assess B/P, respiration, orthostatic B/P
• Monitor I&O ratio; retention commonly causes decreased urinary output, distention, frequency, incontinence; palpate bladder if retention occurs
• Assess for muscle twitching, blepharospasm that may indicate toxicity
• Monitor renal, liver, hematopoietic studies, also for diabetes, acromegaly during long-term therapy
• Assess for parkinsonism, shuffling gait, muscle rigidity, involuntary movements, pill rolling, muscle spasms, drooling before and during treatment
• Monitor for constipation, cramping, pain in abdomen, abdominal distention; increase fluids, bulk, exercise if this occurs
• Assess for tolerance over long-term therapy; dose may have to be increased or changed
• Assess for mental status: affect, mood, CNS depression, worsening of mental symptoms during early therapy

Nursing diagnoses
✓ Physical mobility, impaired (uses)
✓ Knowledge deficit (teaching)

Implementation
PO route
• Give drug until NPO before surgery; check with prescriber for continuing drug

• Adjust dosage depending on patient response
• Give with meals or pc to prevent GI symptoms; limit protein taken with drug
• Give only after MAOIs have been discontinued for 2 wk; if previously on levodopa, discontinue for at least 8 hr before change to levodopa-carbidopa
⊗ • Controlled-release tabs should be swallowed whole, not crushed or chewed

Patient/family education
• Teach patient to change positions slowly to prevent orthostatic hypotension
• Teach patient to report side effects: twitching, eye spasms, grimacing, protrusion of tongue, personality changes that indicate overdose
• Instruct patient to use drug exactly as prescribed; if drug is discontinued abruptly, parkinsonian crisis may occur; do not double doses; take missed dose as soon as remembered up to 2 hr before next dose
• Teach patient that urine, sweat may darken and is harmless
• Advise patient to use physical activities to maintain mobility and lessen spasms
• Instruct patient that OTC medications should not be used unless approved by prescriber
• Advise patient that drowsiness, dizziness are common; to avoid hazardous activities until response is known
• Explain that sips of water, hard candy, or gum may lessen dry mouth
• Teach patient to take with meals to prevent GI symptoms;

---

to limit protein intake, which impairs drug's absorption

Evaluation
Positive therapeutic outcome
• Decrease in akathisia
• Improved mood
• Decreased involuntary movements

---

carboplatin (Ŗ)
(kar'boe'pla-tin)
Paraplatin, Paraplatin-AQ ✦
Func. class.: Antineoplastic alkylating agent
Chem. class.: Platinum coordination compound
Pregnancy category **D**

Action: Produces interstrand DNA cross-links and to a lesser extent DNA-protein cross-links; activity is not cell cycle phase specific

➡ **Therapeutic Outcome:** Prevention of rapidly growing malignant cells

Uses: Palliative treatment of ovarian carcinoma recurrent after treatment with other antineoplastic agents, including cisplatin

Dosage and routes
(single agent)
Adult: **IV** inf 360 mg/m^2 given over 15 min on day 1 q4 wk; do not repeat single intermittent courses until neutrophil count is >2000/mm^3 and platelet count is >100,000/mm^3

Renal dose
CrCl 41-59 ml/min 250 mg/m^2, CrCl 16-40 ml/min 200 mg/m^2

Available forms: Inj 50, 150, 450 mg/vial

Adverse effects
CNS: **Convulsions, central neurotoxicity,** peripheral neuropathy
CV: Cardiac abnormalities
EENT: Tinnitus, hearing loss, *vestibular toxicity*
GI: Severe nausea, vomiting, diarrhea, weight loss
GU: **Renal tubular damage,** renal insufficiency, impotence, sterility, amenorrhea, gynecomastia
HEMA: **Thrombocytopenia, leukopenia, pancytopenia, neutropenia,** anemia, bleeding
INTEG: Alopecia, dermatitis, rash, erythema, pruritus, urticaria
META: Hypomagnesemia, hypocalcemia, hypokalemia, hyponatremia, hyperuremia
RESP: Mucositis

Contraindications: Hypersensitivity to this drug, platinum products, mannitol; severe bone marrow depression, significant bleeding, pregnancy **D**

Precautions: Radiation therapy within 1 mo, chemotherapy within 1 mo, lactation, liver disease

⬛ **Do Not Confuse:**
carboplatin/cisplatin

Pharmacokinetics	
Absorption	Complete
Distribution	Unknown
Metabolism	Liver
Excretion	Kidneys
Half-life	Initial 1-2 hr; postdistribution 2½-6 hr; increased in renal disease

Pharmacodynamics	
Onset	½ hr
Peak	Unknown
Duration	4-6 hr

Interactions
Individual drugs
Aspirin: ↑ risk of bleeding
Radiation: ↑ toxicity, bone marrow suppression
Drug classifications
Aminoglycosides: ↑ nephrotoxicity
Antineoplastics: ↑ toxicity, bone marrow suppression
Bone marrow–suppressing drugs: ↑ bone marrow suppression
Diuretics, loop: ↑ ototoxicity
Myelosuppressives: ↑ myelosuppression
Lab test interferences
↑ AST, ↑ BUN, ↑ alk phos, ↑ bilirubin, ↑ creatinine

NURSING CONSIDERATIONS
Assessment
• Monitor CBC, differential, platelet count weekly; withhold drug if WBC count is <4000/mm³ or platelet count is <100,000/mm³; notify prescriber of results if WBC <20,000/mm³, platelets <150,000/mm³
• Monitor renal function studies: BUN, creatinine, serum uric acid, urine CrCl before and during therapy; I&O ratio; report fall in urine output to <30 ml/hr
• Monitor temp q4h (may indicate beginning of infection)
• Monitor liver function tests before and during therapy (bilirubin, AST, ALT, LDH) as needed or monthly; note jaundice of skin or sclera, dark urine, clay-colored stools, itchy skin, abdominal pain, fever, diarrhea
• Assess for bleeding: hematuria, stool guaiac, bruising or petechiae, mucosa or orifices q8h; inflammation of mucosa, breaks in skin

• Identify dyspnea, rales, unproductive cough, chest pain, tachypnea
• Identify effects of alopecia on body image; discuss feelings about body changes

Nursing diagnoses
☑ Injury, risk for (adverse reactions)
☑ Body image disturbance (adverse reactions)
☑ Infection, risk for (adverse reactions)
☑ Knowledge deficit (teaching)

Implementation
• Antiemetic 30-60 min before giving drug to prevent vomiting, and prn
Ⅳ IV route
• Give **IV** after diluting 10 mg/ml of sterile water for inj, D₅W, NS (10 mg/ml); then further dilute with the same sol 1-4 mg/ml; give over 15 min or more (intermittent inf)
• Give **IV** inf over 5-6 hr; do not use needles or **IV** administration sets containing aluminum; may cause precipitate; diuretic (furosemide 40 mg **IV**) after infusion
• Store protected from light at room temp; reconstituted sol is stable for 8 hr at room temp

Y-site compatibilities:
Allopurinol, amifostine, aztreonam, cefepime, cladribine, doxorubicin liposome, filgrastim, fludarabine, granisetron, melphalan, ondansetron, paclitaxel, piperacillin/tazobactam, propofol, sargramostim, teniposide, thiotepa, vinorelbine

Additive compatibilities:
Cisplatin, etoposide, floxuridine, ifosfamide, ifosfamide/etoposide, paclitaxel

Additive incompatibilities:
Fluorouracil, mesna

Solution compatibilities:
D_5/0.2% NaCl, D_5/0.45% NaCl, D_5/0.9% NaCl, 0.9% NaCl, D_5W, sterile water for inj

Solution incompatibilities:
Sodium bicarbonate

Patient/family education
• Teach patient to avoid use of products containing aspirin or ibuprofen, razors, commercial mouthwash, since bleeding may occur; to report symptoms of bleeding (hematuria, tarry stools)
• Instruct patient to report signs of anemia (fatigue, headache, irritability, faintness, shortness of breath); sore throat, bleeding, bruising
• Instruct patient to report any changes in breathing or coughing even several months after treatment; to avoid crowds and persons with respiratory tract or other infections
• Advise patient that hair may be lost during treatment; a wig or hairpiece may make patient feel better; new hair may be different in color, texture
• Caution patient not to have any vaccinations without the advice of the prescriber; serious reactions can occur
• Teach patient that contraception is needed during treatment and for several months after the completion of therapy; not to breast feed during treatment

Evaluation
Positive therapeutic outcome
• Prevention of rapid division of malignant cells

---

carboprost (℞)
(kar′boe-prost)
Hemabate, Prostin/15M ✸
Func. class.: Oxytocic, abortifacient
Chem. class.: Prostaglandin
Pregnancy category   C

Action: Stimulates uterine contractions, causing complete abortion in approximately 16 hr

▶**Therapeutic Outcome:** Loss of fetus; decreased postpartum bleeding

Uses: Abortion between 13-20 wk gestation; postpartum hemorrhage caused by uterine atony not controlled by other methods

Dosage and routes
To induce abortion
Adult: IM 250 µg, then 250 µg q1½-3½ hr, may increase to 500 µg if no response, not to exceed 12 mg total dose

Postpartum hemorrhage
Adult: IM 250 µg, repeat at 15-90 min intervals, max total dosage 2 mg

Available forms: Inj 250 µg/ml

Adverse effects
CNS: Fever, chills, headache
GI: Nausea, vomiting, diarrhea

Contraindications: Hypersensitivity, severe hepatic disease, severe renal disease, PID, respiratory disease, cardiac disease

Precautions: Asthma, anemia, jaundice, diabetes mellitus, convulsive disorders, past uterine surgery, pregnancy **C**

Pharmacokinetics

Absorption	Well absorbed (nasal)
Distribution	Widely distributed (extracellular fluid)
Metabolism	Liver—rapidly
Excretion	Kidneys
Half-life	3-9 min

Pharmacodynamics

Onset	Unknown
Peak	16 hr
Duration	Unknown

Interactions
Drug classifications
Oxytocics: ↑ effects
⊘ *Herb/drug*
Ephedra: ↑ B/P, hypertension

NURSING CONSIDERATIONS
Assessment
• Monitor B/P, pulse; watch for change that may indicate hemorrhage
• Monitor respiratory rate, rhythm, depth; notify physician of abnormalities
• For length, duration of contraction; notify physician of contractions lasting over 1 min or absence of contractions
• Assess for incomplete abortion, pregnancy must be terminated by another method; drug is teratogenic

Nursing diagnoses
✓ Knowledge deficit (teaching)

Implementation
• Give IM in deep muscle mass; rotate injection sites if additional doses are given
• Have crash cart available on unit

Patient/family education
• Advise patient to report increased blood loss, abdominal cramps, increased temperature or foul-smelling lochia
• Teach methods of comfort control and pain control

Evaluation
Positive therapeutic outcome
• Loss of fetus
• Control of bleeding

---

carisoprodol (℞)
(kar-i-soe-proe′dole)
carisoprodol, Sodol, Soma, Vanadom
Func. class.: Skeletal muscle relaxant, central acting
Chem. class.: Meprobamate congener

Pregnancy category   C

Action: Depresses CNS by blocking interneuronal activity in descending reticular formation of spinal cord, producing sedation

⇒**Therapeutic Outcome:** Relaxation of skeletal muscles

Uses: Relieving pain, stiffness in musculoskeletal disorders

Dosage and routes
P *Adult and child >12 yr:* PO 350 mg tid-qid

Available forms: Tabs 350 mg

Adverse effects
CNS: Dizziness, weakness, drowsiness, headache, tremor, depression, insomnia, ataxia, irritability
CV: Postural hypotension, tachycardia
EENT: Diplopia, temporary loss of vision
GI: Nausea, vomiting, hiccups, epigastric discomfort
HEMA: Eosinophilia
INTEG: Rash, pruritus, fever, facial flushing, **erythema multiforme**
RESP: Asthmatic attack
SYST: Angioedema, **anaphylaxis**

Contraindications: P Hypersensitivity, child <12 yr, intermittent porphyria

Precautions: Renal disease, hepatic disease, addictive personality, pregnancy **C,** elderly G

Pharmacokinetics

Absorption	Well absorbed
Distribution	Crosses placenta
Metabolism	Liver, partially
Excretion	Kidney, unchanged; breast milk
Half-life	8 hr

Pharmacodynamics

Onset	½ hr
Peak	4 hr
Duration	4-6 hr

Interactions
Individual drugs
Alcohol: ↑ CNS depression
Drug classifications
Antidepressants, tricyclic: ↑ CNS depression
Barbiturates: ↑ CNS depression
Opioids: ↑ CNS depression
Sedative/hypnotic: ↑ CNS depression
Herb/drug
Kava: ↑ CNS depression
Lab test interferences
↑ AST, ↑ alkaline phosphatase, ↑ blood glucose

NURSING CONSIDERATIONS
Assessment
• Monitor ROM, atrophy, stiffness, and pain in muscles; assess throughout treatment
• Assess for idiosyncratic reaction within a few min or hr of administration (disorientation, restlessness, weakness, blurred vision); patient should be reassured that reaction is temporary
• Check for allergic reactions: rash, fever

Nursing diagnoses
☑ Mobility, impaired (uses)
☑ Injury, risk for (adverse reactions)
☑ Knowledge deficit (teaching)

Implementation
PO route
• Give with meals for GI symptoms
• Have patient use gum, frequent sips of water for dry mouth
• Store in tight container at room temp

Patient/family education
• Caution patient not to take with alcohol, other CNS depressants
• Advise patient to avoid altering activities while taking this drug
• Caution patient to avoid hazardous activities if drowsiness or dizziness occurs
• Caution patient to avoid using OTC medication such as cough preparations, antihistamines, unless directed by prescriber
• Advise patient not to discontinue rapidly after long-term use; insomnia, nausea, headache, spasticity, tachycardia may occur; taper over 1-2 wk

Evaluation
Positive therapeutic outcome
• Decreased pain, spasticity

Treatment of overdose:
Induce emesis of conscious patient, lavage, dialysis

C

---

carmustine (BCNU) (℞)
(kar-mus'teen)
BiCNU, BCNU, Gliadel
Func. class.: Antineoplastic alkylating agent
Chem. class.: Nitrosourea
Pregnancy category   D

Action: Alkylates DNA, RNA; inhibits enzymes that allow synthesis of amino acids in proteins; also responsible for cross-linking DNA strands; activity is not cell cycle phase specific

➡ Therapeutic Outcome: Prevention of rapidly growing malignant cells

Uses: Brain tumors such as glioblastoma, medulloblastoma, astrocytoma; multiple myeloma, Hodgkin's disease, other lymphomas; GI, breast, bronchogenic, and renal carcinomas

Dosage and routes
Adult: IV 75-100 mg/m^2 over 1-2 hr × 2 days or 200 mg/m^2 × 1 dose q6-8 wk; if WBC is 3000-3999/mm^3 give 50% of dose; if WBC is 2000-2999/mm^3 and platelets are 25,000-75,000/mm^3 give 25% of dose; withhold dose if WBC <2000/mm^3 and platelets <25,000/mm^3

Adult: Intracavitary 8 wafers inserted into resection cavity

Available forms: Powder for inj 100 mg; wafer 7.7 mg

Adverse effects
GI: Nausea, vomiting, anorexia, stomatitis, **hepatotoxicity**
GU: Azotemia, **renal failure**
HEMA: **Thrombocytopenia, leukopenia, myelosuppression, anemia**

INTEG: Burning, hyperpigmentation at inj site, alopecia
RESP: **Fibrosis, pulmonary infiltrate**

Contraindications: Hypersensitivity, leukopenia, thrombocytopenia, pregnancy **D**

Pharmacokinetics

Absorption	Completely absorbed
Distribution	Readily penetrates CSF
Metabolism	Liver, rapid
Excretion	Kidneys, breast milk
Half-life	Unknown

Pharmacodynamics
Unknown

Interactions
Individual drugs
Aspirin: ↑ risk of bleeding
Cimetidine: ↑ toxicity
Phenytoin: ↑ metabolism, ↓ effect
Radiation: ↑ toxicity, bone marrow suppression
Drug classifications
Anticoagulants: ↑ risk of bleeding
Antineoplastics: ↑ toxicity, bone marrow suppression
Bone marrow–suppressing drugs: ↑ bone marrow suppression
Live vaccines: ↑ adverse reactions, ↓ antibody reaction

NURSING CONSIDERATIONS
Assessment
• Assess buccal cavity q8h for dryness, sores or ulceration, white patches, pain, bleeding, dysphagia; obtain prescription for viscous lidocaine (Xylocaine)
• Assess symptoms indicating severe allergic reaction: rash, pruritus, urticaria, purpuric

---

skin lesions, itching, flushing; drug should be discontinued
• Monitor CBC, differential, platelet count weekly; withhold drug if WBC count is <2000/mm³ or platelet count is <25,000/mm³; notify prescriber of results if WBC <20,000/mm³, platelets <150,000/mm³
• Monitor renal function studies: BUN, creatinine, urine CrCl before and during therapy; I&O ratio; report fall in urine output to <30 ml/hr
• Monitor temp q4h (may indicate beginning of infection)
• Monitor liver function tests before and during therapy (bilirubin, AST, ALT, LDH) as needed or monthly; note yellowing of skin or sclera, dark urine, clay-colored stools, itchy skin, abdominal pain, fever, diarrhea; hepatotoxicity can be serious and fatal
• Assess for bleeding: hematuria, stool guaiac, bruising or petechiae, mucosa or orifices q8h; inflammation of mucosa, breaks in skin
• Identify effects of alopecia on body image; discuss feelings about body changes

Nursing diagnoses
☑ Injury, risk for (adverse reactions)
☑ Body image disturbance (adverse reactions)
☑ Infection, risk for (adverse reactions)
☑ Knowledge deficit (teaching)

Implementation
• Blood transfusion or RBC colony-stimulating factors to counter anemia may be required
• Give fluids **IV** or PO before chemotherapy to hydrate patient

• Provide antiemetic 30-60 min before giving drug to prevent vomiting, and prn; antibiotics for prophylaxis of infection
• Provide liq diet (carbonated beverages); gelatin may be added if patient is not nauseated or vomiting
• Give all medications PO, if possible, avoid IM inj if platelets <100,000/mm³

Wafer
• Foil pouches may be kept at room temp for 6 hr, if unopened
• If wafers are broken in several pieces, do not use

IV IV route
• Administer after diluting 100 mg/3 ml ethyl alcohol (provided); then further dilute 27 ml sterile water for inj; then dilute with 100-500 ml 0.9% NaCl or D₅W; give over 1 hr or more; use only glass containers; reduce rate if discomfort is felt
• Store reconstituted sol in refrigerator for 24h or room temp for 8h

Additive incompatibilities:
Sodium bicarbonate

Y-site compatibilities:
Amifostine, aztreonam, cefepime, filgrastim, fludarabine, granisetron, melphalan, ondansetron, piperacillin/tazobactam, sargramostim, teniposide, thiotepa, vinorelbine

Patient/family education
• Teach patient to avoid use of products containing aspirin or ibuprofen, razors, commercial mouthwash, since bleeding may occur; to report symptoms of bleeding (hematuria, tarry stools)

- Advise patient to avoid foods with citric acid, hot or rough texture if stomatitis is present
- Instruct patient to report signs of anemia (fatigue, headache, irritability, faintness, shortness of breath)
- Advise patient that hair may be lost during treatment; a wig or hair piece may make patient feel better; new hair may be different in color, texture
- Caution patient not to have any vaccinations without the advice of the prescriber; serious reactions can occur
- Advise patient that contraception is needed during treatment and for several months after completion of therapy; drug has teratogenic properties

Evaluation
Positive therapeutic outcome
- Prevention of rapid division of malignant cells

---

carteolol (℞)
(kar-tee′oe-lole)
Cartrol, Ocupress
Func.class.: Antihypertensive
Chem. class.: Nonselective β-blocker

Pregnancy category C

Action: Produces fall in B/P without reflex tachycardia or significant reduction in heart rate through mixture of alphablocking, beta-blocking effects and intrinsic sympathomimetic activity; elevated plasma renins are reduced; decreased intraocular pressure in glaucoma and intraocular hypertension

➡ **Therapeutic Outcome:** Decreased B/P, heart rate; decreased intraocular pressure

Uses: Mild to moderate hypertension; oph intraocular hypertension, open-angle glaucoma

Dosage and routes
Adult: PO 2.5 mg qd initially; may gradually increase to desired response, max 10 mg/day; oph ȋ gtt bid

Renal dose
CrCl >60 ml/min give dose q24h, CrCl 20-60 ml/min give dose q48h, CrCl <20 ml/min give dose q72h

Available forms: Tabs 2.5, 5 mg; oph sol 1%

Adverse effects
CNS: Dizziness, mental changes, drowsiness, fatigue, headache, catatonia, depression, anxiety, nightmares, paresthesia, lethargy, insomnia, decreased concentration
CV: Orthostatic hypotension, **bradycardia, CHF, chest pain, ventricular dysrhythmias, AV block, peripheral vascular insufficency,** palpitations
EENT: Tinnitus, visual changes, sore throat, double vision, dry, burning eyes
GI: Nausea, vomiting, diarrhea, dry mouth, flatulence, constipation, anorexia
GU: Impotence, dysuria, ejaculatory failure, urinary retention
HEMA: **Agranulocytosis, thrombocytopenic purpura (rare)**
INTEG: Rash, alopecia, urticaria, pruritus, fever
MS: Joint pain, arthralgia, muscle cramps, pain
OTHER: Facial swelling, decreased exercise tolerance, weight change, Raynaud's disease

---

RESP: **Bronchospasm,** dyspnea, wheezing, nasal stuffiness, pharyngitis

Contraindications: Hypersensitivity to β-blockers, cardiogenic shock, heart block (2nd or 3rd degree), sinus bradycardia, bronchial asthma

Precautions: Major surgery, pregnancy **C,** lactation, CHF, diabetes mellitus, renal disease, thyroid disease, COPD, well-compensated heart failure, nonallergic bronchospasm

Do Not Confuse:
Ocupress/Ocufen

Pharmacokinetics

Absorption	80%-90%
Distribution	Unknown; protein binding 23%-30%
Metabolism	Liver to active metabolite
Excretion	Kidneys, unchanged (50%-75%)
Half-life	Carteolol (6-8 hr); metabolite (8-12 hr); ↑ renal disease

Pharmacodynamics

	PO	OPH
Onset	Unknown	Unknown
Peak	1-3 hr	Unknown
Duration	Unknown	Unknown

Interactions
Individual drugs
Alcohol: ↑ hypotension (large amounts)
Clonidine: ↑ hypotension, bradycardia
Dopamine: ↓ CV effect
Dobutamine: ↓ CV effect
Epinephrine: α-Adrenergic stimulation
Insulin: ↑ hypoglycemia
Phenytoin (IV): ↑ myocardial depression

Reserpine: ↑ hypotension, bradycardia
Thyroid: ↓ effectiveness of carteolol
Verapamil: ↑ myocardial depression
Drug classifications
Amphetamines: ↑ hypertension, bradycardia
Anesthetics, general: ↑ hypotension
Antidiabetics, oral: ↑ hypoglycemia
Antihypertensives: ↑ hypertension
β$_2$-Agonists: ↓ bronchodilatation
Cardiac glycosides: ↑ bradycardia
MAOIs: ↑ hypertension
Nitrates: ↑ hypotension
NSAIDs: ↓ antihypertensive action
Theophyllines: ↓ bronchodilatation

NURSING CONSIDERATIONS
Assessment
• Monitor B/P during beginning treatment, periodically thereafter; pulse q4h; note rate, rhythm, quality: apical/radial pulse before administration; notify prescriber of any significant changes (pulse <50 bpm)
• Monitor blood glucose in those taking insulin, oral antidiabetics, dosage adjustment may be needed
• Check for baselines in renal, liver function tests before therapy begins
• Assess for edema in feet, legs daily; monitor I&O, daily weight; check for jugular vein distention and rales bilaterally, dyspnea (CHF)
• Monitor skin turgor, dryness of mucous membranes for

hydration status, especially
G elderly

Nursing diagnoses
☑ Cardiac output, decreased
(uses)
☑ Injury, risk for (side effects)
☑ Knowledge deficit (teaching)
☑ Noncompliance (teaching)

Implementation
PO route
• Give ac, hs; tab may be
crushed or swallowed whole;
give with food to prevent GI
upset
• Store protected from light,
moisture; placed in cool environment
Ophthalmic route
• Give bid, one drop in each
eye

Patient/family education
• Teach patient not to discontinue drug abruptly; taper over
2 wk; may cause precipitate
dysrhythmias, hypertension if
stopped abruptly
• Teach patient not to use
OTC products containing
α-adrenergic stimulants (such
as nasal decongestants, cold
preparations); to avoid alcohol,
smoking and to limit sodium
intake as prescribed
• Teach patient how to take
pulse and B/P at home; advise
when to notify prescriber
• Instruct patient to comply
with weight control, dietary
adjustments, modified exercise
program
• Advise patient to carry/wear
Medic Alert ID to identify
drug being taken, allergies; tell
patient drug controls symptoms but does not cure
• Caution patient to avoid
hazardous activities if dizziness,
drowsiness present
• Teach patient to report
symptoms of CHF; difficult

breathing, especially on exertion or when lying down, night
cough, swelling of extremities
or bradycardia, dizziness,
confusion, depression, fever
• Teach patient to take drug as
prescribed, not to double
doses, skip doses; take any
missed doses as soon as remembered if at least 4 hr until
next dose
• Teach patient method of
instillation for ophthalmic
route

Evaluation
Positive therapeutic outcome
• Decreased B/P in hyperten-
sion (after 1-2 wk)
• Lessened intraocular pressure
in glaucoma

Treatment of overdose:
Lavage, **IV** atropine for
bradycardia; **IV** theophylline
for bronchospasm, digitalis,
O_2, diuretic for cardiac failure;
IV glucose for hypoglycemia;
IV diazepam (or phenytoin) for
seizures

---

carvedilol (℞)
(kar-veh′dee-lol)
Coreg
Func. class.: α/β blocker
Pregnancy category **C**

Action: A mixture of nonselective β-blocking and α-blocking
activity; decreases cardiac output, exercise-induced tachycardia, reflex orthostatic
tachycardia; causes reduction
in peripheral vascular resistance
and vasodilation

▷**Therapeutic Outcome:** Decreased B/P in hypertension

Uses: Essential hypertension
alone or in combination with
other antihypertensives, CHF

Investigational uses: Angina pectoris, idiopathic cardiomyopathy

Dosage and routes
Essential hypertension
Adult: PO 6.25 mg bid × 7-14 days if tolerated well, then increase to 12.5 mg bid × 7-14 days if tolerated well, may be increased if needed to 25 mg bid, max 50 mg qd

Congestive heart failure
Adult: PO 3.125 mg bid × 2 wk; if well tolerated, give 6.25 mg bid × 2 wk, then double qwk to max dose

Angina pectoris
Adult: PO 25-50 mg bid

Idiopathic cardiomyopathy
Adult: PO 6.25-25 mg bid

Available forms: Tabs 3.125, 6.25, 12.5, 25 mg

Adverse effects
CNS: Dizziness, somnolence, insomnia, ataxia, hypesthesia, paresthesia, vertigo, depression
GI: Diarrhea, abdominal pain, ↑ alk phos, ↑ ALT/AST
CV: Bradycardia, postural hypotension, dependent edema, peripheral edema, **AV block, extrasystoles,** hypertension, hypotension, palpitations, peripheral ischemia
RESP: Rhinitis, pharyngitis, dyspnea
MISC: Fatigue, injury, back pain, UTI, viral infection, hypertriglyceridemia, **thrombocytopenia**

Contraindications: Hypersensitivity, bronchial asthma, class **IV** decompensated cardiac failure, 2nd or 3rd degree heart block, cardiogenic shock, severe bradycardia

Precautions: Cardiac failure, hepatic injury, peripheral vascular disease, anesthesia, major surgery, diabetes mellitus, G thyrotoxicosis, elderly, pregnancy **C**, P lactation, children, emphysema, chronic bronchitis, renal disease

C

Pharmacokinetics	
Absorption	Readily and extensively absorbed
Distribution	>98% bound to plasma proteins
Metabolism	Extensively liver
Excretion	Via bile into feces
G Half-life	Terminal half-life 5-9 hrs, increased in the elderly, hepatic disease

Pharmacodynamics
Unknown

Interactions
Individual drugs
Cimetidine: ↓ levels of carvedilol
Clonidine: ↓ heart rate, B/P
Digoxin: ↑ concentrations of digoxin
Reserpine: ↑ hypotension, bradycardia
Rifampin: ↓ levels of carvedilol
Drug classifications
Antidiabetic agents: ↑ hypoglycemia
Calcium channel blockers: ↑ conduction disturbance
MAOIs: ↑ bradycardia, hypotension

NURSING CONSIDERATIONS
Assessment
• Monitor renal studies including protein, BUN, creatinine; watch for increased levels that may indicate nephrotic syndrome; obtain baselines in renal and liver function studies before beginning treatment; if liver function studies are ele-

vated, drug should be discontinued
• Monitor I&O, weight daily
• Monitor B/P during beginning treatment and periodically thereafter, pulse q4h, note rate, rhythm, quality
• Monitor apical/radial pulse before administration; notify prescriber of significant changes
• Assess for edema in feet and legs daily

Nursing diagnoses
✓ Cardiac output, decreased (uses)
✓ Injury, risk for (adverse reactions)
✓ Knowledge deficit (teaching)
✓ Noncompliance (teaching)

Implementation
• Give PO ac, hs; tablets may be crushed or swallowed whole, give with food to ↓ orthostatic hypotension
• Administer reduced dosage in renal dysfunction

Patient/family education
• Tell patient to comply with dosage schedule even if feeling better, that improvement may take several weeks
• Teach patient to rise slowly to sitting or standing position to minimize orthostatic hypotension
• Encourage patient to report bradycardia, dizziness, confusion, depression, fever, weight gain, shortness of breath
• Teach patient to take pulse at home; advise when to notify prescriber
• Encourage patient not to discontinue drug abruptly, taper over 1-2 wk
• Advise patient to avoid hazardous activities until stabilized on medication, dizziness may occur

Evaluation
Positive therapeutic outcome
• Decreased B/P
• Decreased symptoms of CHF or angina

cascara sagrada/ cascara sagrada aromatic fluid extract/ cascara sagrada fluid extract (OTC)
(kas-kar′a)
Func. class.: Laxative
Chem. class.: Anthraquinone
Pregnancy category C

Action: Direct chemical irritation in colon; increases propulsion of stool; increases fluid in colon

➡**Therapeutic Outcome:** Decreased constipation; removal of bowel contents before surgery or diagnostic tests

Uses: Constipation; bowel or rectal preparation for surgery or examination

Dosage and routes
Adult: PO 325 mg hs; fluid 1 ml qd; aromatic fluid 5 ml qd
P *Child 2-12 yr:* PO/fluid/ aromatic fluid ½ adult dose
P *Child < 2 yr:* PO/fluid/ aromatic fluid ¼ adult dose

Available forms: tabs 325 mg; fluid extract 1 g/ml; aromatic fluid extract 1 g/ml

Adverse effects
GI: Nausea, vomiting, anorexia, cramps, diarrhea
META: Hypocalcemia, enteropathy, alkalosis, hypokalemia, **tetany**

Contraindications: Hypersensitivity, GI bleeding, obstruction, CHF, lactation, abdominal pain, nausea/vomiting, appendicitis, acute surgical abdomen, alcoholics (aromatic fluid extract)

Precautions: Pregnancy **C**

Pharmacokinetics

Absorption	Minimal
Distribution	Unknown
Metabolism	Liver, minimally
Excretion	Kidneys, feces
Half-life	Not known

Pharmacodynamics

Onset	6-12 hr
Peak	Unknown
Duration	Unknown

Interactions
Individual drugs
Digitalis: ↓ absorption
Nitrofurantoin: ↓ absorption
Drug classifications
Antibiotics: ↓ absorption
Oral anticoagulants: ↓ absorption
Salicylates: ↓ absorption
Tetracyclines: ↓ absorption
Herb/drug
Lily of the Valley: ↑ action, side effects
Pheasant's eye: ↑ action, side effects
Squill: ↑ action, side effects

NURSING CONSIDERATIONS
Assessment
• Monitor blood, urine electrolytes if drug used often by patient; check I&O ratio to identify fluid loss
• Assess cramping, rectal bleeding, nausea, vomiting; if these symptoms occur, drug should be discontinued; identify cause of constipation; identify whether fluids, bulk, or exercise is missing from lifestyle

Nursing diagnoses
☑ Bowel elimination, altered: constipation (uses)
☑ Bowel elimination, altered: diarrhea (side effects)
☑ Knowledge deficit (teaching)
☑ Noncompliance (teaching)

Implementation
• Give alone with water only for better absorption; do not administer with food; do not take within 1 hr of antacids, milk, or cimetidine
⊘ • Do not crush; swallow tabs whole
• Give in AM or PM (oral dose); evacuation will occur 6-12 hr later

Patient/family education
• Discuss with the patient that adequate fluid consumption is necessary
• Teach patient that normal bowel movements do not always occur daily
• Teach patient not to use in presence of abdominal pain, nausea, vomiting; tell patient to notify prescriber if constipation unrelieved or if symptoms of electrolyte imbalance occur: muscle cramps, pain, weakness, dizziness, excessive thirst

Evaluation
Positive therapeutic outcome
• Decreased constipation in 6-12 hr
• Removal of bowel contents

C

celecoxib (℞)
(cel-eh-cox'ib)
Celebrex
Func. class.: Nonsteroidal antiinflammatory
Pregnancy category   C

Action: Inhibits prostaglandin synthesis by decreasing enzyme needed for biosynthesis; analgesic, antiinflammatory, antipyretic properties

➡**Therapeutic Outcome:** Decreased pain, inflammation

Uses: Acute, chronic rheumatoid arthritis, osteoarthritis

Dosage and routes
Osteoarthritis
Adult: PO 200 mg/day as a single dose

Rheumatoid arthritis
Adult: PO 100-200 mg bid

Available forms: Caps 100, 200 mg

Adverse effects
CNS: Fatigue, anxiety, depression, nervousness, paresthesia
CV: **Tachycardia,** angina, **MI,** *palpitations, dysrhythmias, hypertension, fluid retention*
EENT: Tinnitus, hearing loss, blurred vision, glaucoma, cataract, conjunctivitis, eye pain
GI: Nausea, anorexia, vomiting, constipation, dry mouth, diverticulitis, gastritis, gastroenteritis, hemorrhoids, hiatal hernia, stomatitis, GI bleeding
GU: **Nephrotoxicity: dysuria, hematuria, oliguria, azotemia, cystitis,** UTI
HEMA: Blood dyscrasias, epistaxis, bruising, anemia
INTEG: Purpura *rash, pruritus, sweating, erythema, petechiae, photosensitivity, alopecia*
RESP: Pharyngitis, shortness of breath, pneumonia, coughing

Contraindications: Hypersensitivity to aspirin, iodides, other NSAIDs, asthma

Precautions: Pregnancy **C,**
🅿 lactation, children, bleeding disorders, GI disorders, cardiac disorders, hypersensitivity to other antiinflammatory agents

Pharmacokinetics	
Absorption	Well absorbed (PO)
Distribution	Crosses placenta, bound to plasma proteins
Metabolism	Liver
Excretion	Kidneys
Half-life	Unknown

Pharmacodynamics	
Onset	Unknown
Peak	3 hr
Duration	Unknown

Interactions
Individual drugs
Aspirin: ↓ effectiveness, ↑ adverse reactions
Coumadin: ↑ anticoagulant effects
Lithium: ↑ toxicity
Drug classifications
ACE inhibitors: may ↓ effects of ACE inhibitors
Anticoagulants: ↑ risk of bleeding
Antineoplastics: ↑ risk of hematologic toxicity
Glucocorticoids: ↑ adverse reactions
Diuretics: ↓ effectiveness of diuretics
NSAIDs: ↑ adverse reactions

NURSING CONSIDERATIONS
Assessment
• Assess for pain of rheumatoid arthritis, osteoarthritis; check

---

☑ Herb/drug 🅂 Do Not Crush ◆ Alert ↶ Key Drug 🅖 Geriatric 🅿 Pediatric

ROM, inflammation of joints, characteristics of pain

◆• Monitor blood counts during therapy; watch for decreasing platelets; if low, therapy may need to be discontinued, restarted after hematologic recovery; and for blood dyscrasias (thrombocytopenia): bruising, fatigue, bleeding, poor healing

Nursing diagnoses

☑ Pain (uses)
☑ Mobility, impaired physical (uses)
☑ Injury, risk for (side effects)
☑ Knowledge deficit (teaching)

Implementation
PO route

• Administer with food or milk to decrease gastric symptoms

⊘• Do not crush, dissolve, or chew caps

Patient/family education

• Teach patient that drug must be continued for prescribed time to be effective; to avoid other NSAIDs

• Caution patient to report bleeding, bruising, fatigue, malaise, since blood dyscrasias do occur

• Teach patient to take with a full glass of water to enhance absorption; do not crush, break, or chew

Evaluation
Positive therapeutic outcome

• Decreased pain in arthritic conditions

• Decreased inflammation in arthritic conditions

CEPHALOSPORINS

cefaclor
See cephalosporins—2nd generation
cefadroxil
cefazolin
See cephalosporins—1st generation
cefdinir
See cephalosporins—3rd generation
cefepime
cefixime
See cephalosporins—3rd generation
cefmandole
cefmetazole
cefonicid
See cephalosporins—2nd generation
cefoperazone
cefotaxime
See cephalosporins—3rd generation
cefotetan
cefoxitin
See cephalosporins—2nd generation
cefpodoxime
See cephalosporins—3rd generation
cefprozil
See cephalosporins—2nd generation
ceftazidime
ceftibuten
ceftizoxime
ceftriaxone
See cephalosporins—3rd generation
cefuroxime
See cephalosporins—2nd generation
cephalexin
cephalothin
cephapirin
cephradine
See cephalosporins—1st generation

CEPHALOSPORINS—1ST GENERATION

cefadroxil (℞)
(sef-a-drox'ill)
cefadroxil, Duricef, Ultracef
cefazolin (℞)
(sef-a'zoe-lin)
Ancef, cefazolin, Kefzol
cephalexin (℞)
(sef-a-lex'in)
Apo-Cephalex*, Cefanex, C-Lexin, cephalexin, Keflex, Keftab, Novo-Lexin*, Nu-Cephalex*
cephalothin (℞)
(sef-a-loe'thin)
cephalothin, Keflin
cephapirin (℞)
(sef-a-pye'rin)
Cefadyl, cephapirin
cephradine (℞)
(sef'ra-deen)
cephradine, Velosef
Func. class.: Antiinfective
Chem. class.: Cephalosporin (1st generation)

Action: Inhibits bacterial cell wall synthesis, rendering cell wall osmotically unstable, leading to cell death by binding to cell wall membrane

cefadroxil
⇒ Therapeutic Outcome:
Bactericidal effects for the following: gram-negative bacilli *Escherichia coli, Proteus mirabilis, Klebsiella* (UTI only); gram-positive organisms *Streptococcus pneumoniae, S. pyogenes, Staphylococcus aureus*

Uses: Upper, lower respiratory tract, urinary tract, skin infections; otitis media; tonsillitis, pharyngitis; particularly for UTI

cefazolin
⇒ Therapeutic Outcome
Bactericidal effects for the following: gram-negative organisms *Enterobacter* sp., *Haemophilus influenzae, Escherichia coli, Proteus mirabilis, Klebsiella*; gram-positive organisms *Streptococcus pneumoniae, S. pyogenes, Staphylococcus aureus*

Uses: Upper, lower respiratory tract, urinary tract, skin infections; bone, joint, biliary, genital infections; endocarditis, surgical prophylaxis, septicemia

cephalexin
⇒ Therapeutic Outcome:
Bactericidal effects for the following: gram-negative organisms *Haemophilus influenzae, Escherichia coli, Proteus mirabilis, Klebsiella*; gram-negative organisms *Haemophilus influenzae, Escherichia coli, Proteus mirabilis, Klebsiella*; gram-positive organisms *Streptococcus pneumoniae, S. pyogenes, Staphylococcus aureus*

Uses: Upper, lower respiratory tract, urinary tract, skin, bone infections; otitis media

cephalothin
⇒ Therapeutic Outcome:
Bactericidal effects for the following: gram-negative bacilli *Haemophilus influenzae, Escherichia coli, Proteus mirabilis, Klebsiella, Salmonella, Shigella*; gram-positive organisms *Streptococcus pneumoniae, S. pyogenes, Staphylococcus aureus*

Uses: Lower respiratory tract, urinary tract, skin and bone infections; septicemia, endocarditis; bacterial peritonitis

cephapirin
⇒ Therapeutic Outcome:
Bactericidal effects for the

following: gram-negative bacilli *Haemophilus influenzae, Escherichia coli, Proteus mirabilis, Klebsiella;* gram-positive organisms *Streptococcus pneumoniae, S. Viridans, Staphylococcus aureus*

Uses: Lower respiratory tract, urinary tract, skin infections; septicemia, endocarditis, bacterial peritonitis

cephradine
→**Therapeutic Outcome:** Bactericidal effects for the following: gram-negative bacilli *Haemophilus influenzae, Escherichia coli, Proteus mirabilis, Klebsiella;* gram-positive organisms *Streptococcus pneumoniae, S. pyogenes, Staphylococcus aureus*

Uses: Serious respiratory tract, urinary tract, skin infections; otitis media

Dosage and routes
cefadroxil
Adult: PO 1-2 g qd or q12h in divided doses, give a loading dose of 1 g initially

P *Child:* PO 30 mg/kg/day in divided doses

Renal dose: CrCl 25-50 ml/min 1g, then 500 mg q1/2h; CrCl 10-24 ml/min 500 mg q24h, CrCl <10 ml/min 500 mg q36h

Available forms: Caps 500 mg; tabs 1 g; oral susp 125, 250, 500 mg/5 ml

cefazolin
Life-threatening infections
Adult: IM/**IV** 1-2 g q6h

P *Child >1 mo:* IM/**IV** 100 mg/kg in 3-4 divided doses

Mild/moderate infections
Adult: IM/**IV** 250 mg-1 g q8h

P *Child >1 mo:* IM/**IV** 25-50 mg/kg in 3-4 equal doses

Renal dose: CrCl 35-54 ml/min: 250-1000 mg q12h; CrCl 10-34 ml/min: 125-500 mg q12h; CrCl <10 ml/min: 125-500 mg q24h

Available forms: Inj 500 mg, 1, 5, 10, 20 g

cephalexin
Renal dose: CrCl <40 ml/min give q8-12h; CrCl 5-10 ml/min give q12h; CrCl <5 ml/min give q24h

Moderate infections
Adult: PO 250-500 mg q6h

P *Child:* PO 25-50 mg/kg/day in 4 equal doses

Moderate skin infections
Adult: PO 500 mg q12h

Severe infections
Adult: PO 500 mg-1 g q6h

P *Child:* PO 50-100 mg/kg/day in 4 equal doses

Available forms: Caps 250, 500 mg; tabs 250, 500 mg, 1 g; oral susp 125, 250 mg/5 ml

cephalothin
Renal dose: CrCl 26-50 ml/min 1.5 g q6h; CrCl 10-25 ml/min 1 g q6h; CrCl <10 ml/min 500 mg q6h

Moderate infections
Adult: IM/**IV** 500 mg-1 g q4-6h

P *Child:* IM/**IV** 14-27 mg/kg q4h or 20-40 mg/kg q6h

Uncomplicated gonorrhea
Adult: IM 2 g as a single dose

Severe infections
Adult: IM/**IV** 1-2 g q4h

P *Child:* IM/**IV** 80-160 mg/kg/day in divided doses q4h

Available forms: Powder for inj 1, 2, 20 g

---

cephapirin
Adult: IM/**IV** 500 mg-1 g
q4-6h

P *Child:* IM/**IV** 40-80 mg/kg/
day in divided doses q6h or
10-20 mg/kg q6h

Renal dose: CrCl <10 ml/min
give q12h

Available forms: Powder for
inj 500 mg, 1, 2, 20 g; **IV** only
1, 2, 4 g

cephradine
Adult: PO 250 mg-1 g q6-12h

P *Child >1 yr:* PO 6-12 mg/kg
q6h

Renal dose: CrCl >20 ml/min
500 mg q6h; CrCl 5-20 ml/
min 250 mg q6h

Available forms: Caps 250,
500 mg; oral susp 125, 250
mg/5 ml

**Side effects/adverse
reaction**
CNS: Headache, dizziness,
weakness, paresthesia, fever,
chills
GI: Nausea, vomiting, *diarrhea, anorexia,* pain, glossitis,
bleeding; increased AST, ALT,
bilirubin, LDH, alk
phosphatase; abdominal pain,
pseudomembranous colitis
GU: Proteinuria, vaginitis,
pruritus, candidiasis, increased
BUN, **nephrotoxicity, renal
failure**
HEMA: **Leukopenia, thrombocytopenia, agranulocytosis,** anemia, **neutropenia,
lymphocytosis, eosinophilia,
pancytopenia, hemolytic
anemia**
INTEG: Rash, urticaria, dermatitis, **anaphylaxis**
RESP: Dyspnea

Contraindications: Hypersensitivity to cephalosporins,
P infants <1 mo

Precautions: Hypersensitivity
to penicillins, pregnancy **B,**
lactation, renal disease

N **Do Not Confuse:**
cephalexin/cefaclor,
cephapirin/cephradine,
Kefzol/Cefzil

cefadroxil

Pharmacokinetics

Absorption	Well absorbed
Distribution	Widely distributed; crosses placenta
Metabolism	Not metabolized
Excretion	Unchanged by kidneys; enters breast milk
Half-life	1½-2 hr

Pharmacodynamics

	PO
Onset	Rapid
Peak	1½-2 hr

cefazolin

Pharmacokinetics

Absorption	Well absorbed
Distribution	Widely distributed; crosses placenta
Metabolism	Not metabolized
Excretion	Unchanged by kidneys; enters breast milk
Half-life	1½-2½ hr

Pharmacodynamics

	IM	IV
Onset	Rapid	10 min
Peak	1-2 hr	Infusion's end

cephalexin

Pharmacokinetics

Absorption	Well absorbed
Distribution	Widely distributed; crosses placenta
Metabolism	Not metabolized
Excretion	Kidneys, unchanged; enters breast milk
Half-life	½-1 hr; increased in renal disease

Pharmacodynamics	
Onset	15-30 min
Peak	1 hr

cephalothin

Pharmacokinetics

Absorption	Well absorbed
Distribution	Widely distributed; crosses placenta
Metabolism	Not metabolized
Excretion	Kidneys, unchanged; enters breast milk
Half-life	½-1 hr

Pharmacodynamics

	IM	IV
Onset	Rapid	Immediate
Peak	½ hr	Infusion's end

cephapirin

Pharmacokinetics

Absorption	Well absorbed
Distribution	Widely distributed; crosses placenta
Metabolism	Not metabolized
Excretion	Kidneys, unchanged; enters breast milk
Half-life	½-1 hr

Pharmacodynamics

	IM	IV
Onset	Rapid	Immediate
Peak	½ hr	Infusion's end

cephradine

Pharmacokinetics

Absorption	Well absorbed
Distribution	Widely distributed; crosses placenta
Metabolism	Not metabolized
Excretion	Kidneys, unchanged; enters breast milk
Half-life	1-2 hr

Pharmacodynamics

	PO/IM	IV
Onset	Rapid	Immediate
Peak	1 hr	Infusion's end

Interactions
Individual drugs
Probenecid: ↓ excretion of drug and ↑ blood levels
Vancomycin: ↑ toxicity
Drug classifications
Aminoglycosides: ↑ toxicity
Lab test interferences
False: ↑ Creatinine (serum urine), ↑ urinary 17-KS
False positive: Urinary protein, direct Coombs' test, urine glucose
Interference: Cross-matching

NURSING CONSIDERATIONS
Assessment
• Assess patient for previous sensitivity reaction to penicillins or other cephalosporins; cross-sensitivity between penicillins and cephalosporins is common
• Assess patient for signs and symptoms of infection including characteristics of wounds, sputum, urine, stool, WBC >10,000, earache, fever; obtain baseline information and during treatment
• Obtain C&S before beginning drug therapy to identify if correct treatment has been initiated
• Assess for allergic reactions: rash, urticaria, pruritus, chills, fever, joint pain; angioedema may occur a few days after therapy begins; epinephrine and resuscitation equipment should be available for anaphylactic reaction
• Identify urine output; if decreasing, notify prescriber (may indicate nephrotoxicity); also check for increased BUN, creatinine
• Monitor blood studies: AST, ALT, CBC, Hct, bilirubin, LDH, alkaline phosphatase,

---

Coombs' test monthly if patient is on long-term therapy
• Monitor electrolytes: potassium, sodium, chloride monthly if patient is on long-term therapy
• Assess bowel pattern qd; if severe diarrhea occurs, drug should be discontinued; may indicate pseudomembranous colitis
• Monitor for bleeding: ecchymosis, bleeding gums, hematuria, stool guaiac daily if on long-term therapy
• Assess for superinfection: perineal itching, fever, malaise, redness, pain, swelling, drainage, rash, diarrhea, change in cough, sputum

Nursing diagnoses
✓ Infection, risk for (uses)
✓ Diarrhea (side effects)
✓ Fluid volume deficit, risk for (side effects)
✓ Injury, risk for (side effects)
✓ Knowledge deficit (teaching)
✓ Noncompliance (teaching)

cefadroxil
Implementation
• Give in even doses around the clock; if GI upset occurs, give with food; drug must be given for 10-14 days to ensure organism death and prevent superinfection
• Shake suspension, refrigerate, discard after 2 wks

cefazolin
Implementation
IM route
• Reconstitute 250-500 mg of drug with 2 ml sterile or bacteriostatic water for inj, or 0.9% NaCl; reconstitute 1 g of drug with 2.5 ml; give deep in large muscle mass, massage

IV IV route
• Check for irritation, extravasation, phlebitis daily, change site q72h
• For direct **IV** dilute in 10 ml of sterile water for injection; give over 5 min
• For intermittent inf dilute reconstituted sol (500 mg or 1 mg) in 50-100 ml D_5W, $D_{10}W$, D_5/0.25% NaCl, D_5/0.45% NaCl, D_5/0.9% NaCl, D_5/LR, or LR, 0.9% NaCl; give over 30-60 min; may be refrigerated up to 96 hr or stored 24 hr at room temp

Y-site incompatibilities:
Amiodarone, hetastarch, hydromorphone, idarubicin, vinorelbine tartrate

Y-site compatibilities:
Acyclovir, allopurinol, amifostine, atracurium, aztreonam, calcium gluconate, cyclophosphamide, diltiazem, enalaprilat, esmolol, famotidine, filgrastim, fluconazole, fludarabine, foscarnet, heparin, labetalol, lidocaine, magnesium sulfate, melphalan, meperidine, midazolam, morphine, multivitamins, ondansetron, perphenazine, pancuronium, regular insulin, sargramostim, tacrolimus, teniposide, theophylline, thiotepa, vecuronium, vit B/C

Syringe incompatibilities:
Ascorbic acid injection, cimetidine, lidocaine, vit B/C

Syringe compatibilities:
Heparin, vitamin B complex

Additive incompatibilities:
Amikacin, amobarbital, bleomycin, calcium gluceptate, calcium gluconate, colistimethate, erythromycin, kanamycin, oxytetracycline, pentobarbital, polymyxin B, tetracycline

---

☑ Herb/drug Ⓢ Do Not Crush ◆ Alert ☗ Key Drug Ⓖ Geriatric Ⓟ Pediatric

Additive compatibilities:
Aztreonam, clindamycin, famotidine, fluconazole, metronidazole, verapamil

cephalexin
Implementation
🚫 • Advise not to crush or chew caps
• Give in even doses around the clock; if GI upset occurs, give with food; drug must be taken for 10-14 days to ensure organism death and prevent superinfection
• Shake suspension, refrigerate, discard after 2 wks

cephalothin
Implementation
IM route
• Reconstitute 1 g/4 ml sterile water for inj; give deep in large muscle mass and massage
• IM route not preferred; causes intense pain and induration
IV IV route
• Check for irritation, extravasation, phlebitis daily; change site q72h
• For direct **IV** dilute in 1 g/10 ml or more sterile water for inj, D_5W, 0.9% NaCl; give over 3-5 min
• For intermittent inf, reconstitute 1-2 mg/50 ml sterile water for inj, D_5W, $D_{10}W$, D_5/LR, D_5/0.9% NaCl; 0.9% NaCl; may be further diluted in 50-100 ml D_5W, $D_{10}W$, 0.9% NaCl, or LR; give over 15-30 min
• For cont inf may be diluted in 500-1000 ml and run at prescribed rate; may use hydrocortisone 10-25 mg added to inf containing 4-6 g or more of cephalothin to decrease the incidence of thrombophlebitis
• Store refrigerated 96h, room temp 24h

Y-site incompatibilities:
Hetastarch
Y-site compatibilities:
Cyclophosphamide, famotidine, heparin, hydromorphone, magnesium sulfate, meperidine, morphine, multivitamins, perphenazine, potassium chloride, vit B/C

Syringe incompatibilities:
Metoclopramide
Syringe compatibilities:
Cimetidine

Additive incompatibilities:
Aminoglycosides, amikacin, aminophylline, amobarbital, bleomycin, calcium chloride, calcium gluceptate, calcium gluconate, colistimethate, diphenhydramine, doxorubicin, erythromycin, gentamicin, kanamycin, oxytetracycline, pentobarbital, penicillin G sodium, phenobarbital, polymyxin B, prochlorperazine, tetracycline

Additive compatibilities:
Ascorbic acid, chloramphenicol, clindamycin, fluorouracil, hydrocortisone, isoproterenol, magnesium sulfate, metaraminol, methicillin, methotrexate, potassium chloride, prednisolone, procaine, sodium bicarbonate, vit B/C

cephapirin
Implementation
IM route
• Reconstitute 1-2 g/1-2 ml of sterile water for inj; give deep in large muscle mass and massage
IV IV route
• Check for irritation, extravasation, phlebitis daily; change site q72h
• For intermittent inf, reconstitute 250 mg/2.4 ml, 500 mg/4.8 ml, 1 g/9.6 ml, 2

gm/19.2 ml sterile water for inj, D_5W, 0.9% NaCl; do not use sol with benzyl alcohol for

🅿 neonates; may be further diluted in 50-100 ml D_5W, $D_{10}W$, 0.9% NaCl, or LR; give over 30-60 min

• Store refrigerated 96h, room temp 24h

Y-site compatibilities:
Acyclovir, cyclophosphamide, famotidine, heparin, hydrocortisone, hydromorphone, magnesium sulfate, meperidine, morphine, multivitamins, perphenazine, potassium chloride, vit B/C

Additive incompatibilities:
Aminoglycosides, amikacin, ascorbic acid, epinephrine, gentamicin, kanamycin, mannitol, norepinephrine, oxytetracycline, phenytoin, tetracycline, thiopental

Additive compatibilities:
Bleomycin, calcium chloride, calcium gluconate, chloramphenicol, diphenhydramine, ergonovine maleate, heparin, hydrocortisone, metaraminol, oxacillin, penicillin G potassium, pentobarbital, phenobarbital, phytonadione, potassium chloride, sodium bicarbonate, succinylcholine, verapamil, warfarin, vitamin B complex

cephradine
Implementation
PO route
• May be given with food for GI symptoms
• When giving susp, shake well; refrigerate unused portion

IM route
• Reconstitute 250 mg/1.2 ml, 500 mg/ml, 1 g/4 ml sterile or bacterostatic water

for inj; give deep in large muscle mass, massage

Ⅳ IV route
• Check for irritation, extravasation, phlebitis daily; change site q72h
• Direct **IV** route 250-500 mg/5 ml sterile water, 0.9% NaCl, D_5W, or 1 g/10 ml, 2 g/20 ml; give over 3-5 min
• For intermittent inf, dilute 1 g/10 ml or more sterile water for inj, D_5W, $D_{10}W$, or D_5/0.9% NaCl; give over 30-60 min
• Store refrigerated 96h, room temp 24h

Additive incompatibilities:
Other antibiotics, calcium salts, D_5W, epinephrine, lidocaine, Ringer's or LR sol, NormosolR, NaCl, TPN #61, tetracycline

Patient/family education
• Teach patient to report sore throat, bruising, bleeding, joint pain; may indicate blood dyscrasias (rare)
• Advise patient to contact prescriber if vaginal itching, loose, foul-smelling stools, furry tongue occur; may indicate superinfection
• Instruct patient to take all medication prescribed for the length of time ordered
• Advise patient to notify prescriber of diarrhea with blood or pus, which may indicate pseudomembranous colitis

Evaluation
Positive therapeutic outcome
• Absence of signs/symptoms of infection (WBC <10,000, temp WNL, absence of red draining wounds, earache)
• Reported improvement in symptoms of infection
• Negative C&S

Treatment of anaphylaxis:
Epinephrine, antihistamines, resuscitate if needed

CEPHALOSPORINS— 2ND GENERATION

cefaclor (℞)
(sef′a-klor)
Ceclor
cefamandole (℞)
(sef-a-man′dole)
Mandol
cefmetazole (℞)
(sef-met′a-zole)
Zefazone
cefonicid (℞)
(se-fon′i-sid)
Monocid
cefotetan (℞)
(sef′oh-tee-tan)
Cefotan
cefoxitin (℞)
(se-fox′i-tin)
Mefoxin
cefprozil (℞)
(sef-proe′zill)
Cefzil
loracarbef (℞)
(lor-a-kar′beff)
Lorabid
Func. class.: Antiinfective
Chem. class.: Cephalosporin (2nd generation)

Action: Inhibits bacterial cell wall synthesis, rendering cell wall osmotically unstable, leading to cell death by binding to cell wall membrane

cefaclor
▷**Therapeutic Outcome:**
Bactericidal effects for the following: gram-negative bacilli *Haemophilus influenzae, Escherichia coli, Proteus mirabilis,* *Klebsiella;* gram-positive organisms *Streptococcus pneumoniae, Staphylococcus* beta-hemolytic; Streptococci, anaerobes, bacteroides sp.

Uses: Upper and lower respiratory tract, urinary tract, skin infections; otitis media; increased bone, joint, gynecologic infections; setpicemia

cefamandole
▷**Therapeutic Outcome:**
Bactericidal effects for the following: anaerobes *Bacteroides sp., Clostridium sp., Fusobacterium sp., Peptococcus sp., Peptostreptococcus sp.;* gram negative organisms *Haemophilus influenzae, Escherichia coli, Proteus mirabilis, Klebiella;* gram-positive organisms *Streptococcus pneumoniae, S. pyogenes, Staphylococcus aureus; Enterobacter sp., Morganella morganii, Proteus vulgaris, Providencia rettgeris*

Uses: Upper, lower respiratory tract, urinary tract, skin infections; peritonitis, septicemia, surgical prophylaxis

cefmetazole
▷**Therapeutic Outcome:**
Bactericidal effects for the following: anaerobes, including *Clostridium, Bacteroides sp., Fusobacterium sp.;* gram-negative organisms *Morganella morganii, Haemophilus influenzae, Escherichia coli, Proteus, Klebsiella, Bacteroides fragilis;* gram-positive organisms *Streptococcus pneumoniae, S. pyogenes, Staphylococcus aureus*

Uses: Infections of lower respiratory tract, urinary tract, skin, bone; intraabdominal infections

C

cefonicid
➡️ **Therapeutic Outcome:**
Bactericidal effects for the following: gram-negative organisms *Morganella morganii, Proteus vulgaris, Providencia vettger, Haemophilus influenzae, Escherichia coli, Proteus mirabilis, Klebsiella;* gram-positive organisms *Streptococcus pneumoniae, S. pyogenes, Staphylococcus aureus*

Uses: Lower respiratory tract, urinary tract, skin, bone, joint infections; otitis media, peritonitis, septicemia, preoperative prophylaxis

cefotetan
➡️ **Therapeutic Outcome:**
Bactericidal effects for the following: gram-negative organisms *Haemophilus influenzae, Escherichia coli, Enterobacter aerogenes, Proteus mirabilis, Klebsiella, Morganella morganii, Proteus vulgaris, Providencia, Enterobacter, Salmonella, Shigella, Acinetobacter, Bacteroides fragilis, Neisseria, Serratia;* gram-positive organisms *Streptococcus pneumoniae, S. pyogenes, Staphylococcus aureus;* anaerobes *Bacteroides, Clostridium, Fusobacterium, Peptococcus, Peptostreptococcus*

Uses: Serious upper or lower respiratory tract, urinary tract, gynecologic, skin, bone, joint, gonococcal, intraabdominal infections

cefoxitin
➡️ **Therapeutic Outcome:**
Bactericidal effects for the following: gram-negative bacilli *Haemophilus influenzae, Escherichia coli, Proteus, Klebsiella, Providencia, Neisseria gonorrhoeae;* gram-positive organisms *Streptococcus pneu-*

moniae, S. pyogenes, Staphylococcus aureus; anaerobes including *Clostridium, Bacteroides, Peptococcus, Peptostreptococcus*

Uses: Lower respiratory tract, urinary tract, skin, bone, gynecologic, gonococcal infections; septicemia, peritonitis

cefprozil
➡️ **Therapeutic Outcome:**
Bactericidal effects for the following: gram-negative bacilli *Haemophilus influenzae, Escherichia coli;* gram-positive organisms *Streptococcus pneumoniae, S. pyogenes, Staphylococcus aureus*

Uses: Upper and lower respiratory tract, urinary tract, skin infections; otitis media

loracarbef
➡️ **Therapeutic Outcome:**
Bactericidal effects for the following organisms: gram-negative *Haemophilus influenzae, Escherichia coli, Proteus mirabilis, Klebsiella;* gram-positive *Streptococcus pneumoniae, S. pyogenes, Staphyloccus aureus*

Uses: Upper and lower respiratory tract, urinary tract, skin infections; otitis media, pharyngitis, tonsillitis

Dosage and routes
cefaclor
Adult: PO 250-500 mg q8h, not to exceed 4 g/day or 375-500 mg (ext rel) q12h × 7-10 days

🄿 *Child <1 mo:* PO 20-40 mg/kg qd in divided doses q8h, or total daily dose may be divided and given q12h, not to exceed 1 g/day

---

Acute bacterial exacerbations of chronic bronchitis or acute bronchitis
Adult: 500 mg/12 hr × 1 wk (ext rel)

Pharyngitis/tonsillitis
Adult: 375 mg/12 hr × 10 days (ext rel)

Available forms: Caps 250, 500 mg; oral susp 125, 187, 250, 375 mg/5 ml; tabs, ext rel 375, 500 mg

cefamandole
Adult: IM/**IV** 500 mg-1 g q4-8h; may give up to 2 g q4h for severe infections

P *Child >1 mo:* IM/**IV** 8.3-16.7 mg/kg q4h, not to exceed adult dose

Renal dose: Dosage reduction indicated in renal impairment (CrCl <50 ml/min)

Available forms: Inj 1, 2, 10 g

cefmetazole
Adult: **IV** 2 g divided q6-12h × 5-14 days

Renal dose: CrCl <50 ml/min 1-2 g q12h; CrCl 10-29 ml/min 1-2 g q48h

Available forms: Powder for inj 1, 2 g/vial

cefonicid
Life-threatening infections
Adult: IM/**IV** BOL or INF 0.5-2 g/24 hr; divide in two doses if giving 2 g
• Dosage reduction indicated in renal impairment

Available forms: Inj 500 mg, 1, 10 g

cefotetan
Adult: **IV**/IM 1-2 g q12h × 5-10 days

Renal dose: CrCl 10-30 ml/min give q24h; CrCl <10 ml/min give q48h

Perioperative proplylaxis
Adult: **IV** 1-2 g ½-1 hr before surgery

Available forms: Inj 1, 2, 10 g

cefoxitin
Adult: IM/**IV** 1-2 g q6-8h

Renal dose: CrCl; <50 ml/min give q8-12h; CrCl 10-29 ml/min give q24h; CrCl <10 ml/min give q24-48h
• Dosage reduction indicated in renal impairment (CrCl <50 ml/min)
• Uncomplicated gonorrhea 2 g IM as single dose with 1 g PO probenecid at same time

Severe infections
Adult: IM/**IV** 2 g q4h

P *Child ≥3 mo:* IM/**IV** 80-160 mg/kg/day divided q4-6h; max 12 g/day

Available forms: Powder for inj 1, 2, 10 g

cefprozil
Renal dose: CrCl <30 ml/min 50% of dose

Upper respiratory infections
Adult: PO 500 mg q24h × 10 days

Otitis media
P *Child 6 mo-12 yr:* PO 15 mg/kg q12h × 10 days

Lower respiratory infections
Adult: PO 500 mg q12h × 10 days

Skin/skin structure infections
Adult: PO 250-500 mg q12h × 10 days

Available forms: Tabs 250, 500 mg; susp 125, 250 mg/5 ml

---

loracarbef

P *Adult and child >13:* PO 200-400 mg q12h

P *Child to 12 yr:* PO 15-30 mg/kg/day in 2 divided doses q12h

Renal dose: CrCl 10-49 ml/min 50% of dose; CrCl <10 ml/min q3-5 days

Available forms: Caps 200, 400 mg; 100, 200 mg/5 ml oral susp

Side effects/adverse reactions:

CNS: Dizziness, headache, fatigue, paresthesia, fever, chills, confusion

GI: Diarrhea, nausea, vomiting, anorexia, dysgeusia, glossitis, bleeding; increased AST, ALT, bilirubin, LDH, alk phosphatase; abdominal pain, loose stools, flatulence, heartburn, stomach cramps, colitis, jaundice

INTEG: Rash, urticaria, dermatitis, **Stevens-Johnson syndrome**

GU: Vaginitis, pruritus, candidiasis, increased BUN, **nephrotoxicity, renal failure,** pyuria, dysuria, reversible interstitial nephritis

HEMA: **Leukopenia, thrombocytopenia, agranulocytosis,** anemia, **neutropenia, lymphocytosis, eosinophilia, pancytopenia, hemolytic anemia, leukocytosis, granulocytopenia**

RESP: Dyspnea

SYST: **Anaphylaxis, serum sickness**

Contraindications Hypersensitivity to cephalosporins or related antibiotics, seizures

Precautions: Pregnancy **B,**
P lactation, children, renal disease

◼ Do Not Confuse:
cefaclor/cephalexin, Cefotan/Ceftin, cefprozil/Cafazolin, cefprozil/cefuroxime, Cefzil/Ceftin, Cefzil/Kefzol

cefaclor

Pharmacokinetics	
Absorption	Well absorbed
Distribution	Widely distributed; crosses placenta
Metabolism	Not metabolized
Excretion	Unchanged by kidneys (60%-80%); enters breast milk
Half-life	36-54 min; increased in renal disease

Pharmacodynamics	
Onset	15 min
Peak	½-1 hr

cefamandole

Pharmacokinetics	
Absorption	Well absorbed
Distribution	Widely distributed; crosses placenta
Metabolism	Not metabolized
Excretion	Unchanged by kidneys (60%-80%); enters breast milk
Half-life	½ to 1½ hr

Pharmacodynamics		
	IM	IV
Onset	Rapid	Immediate
Peak	½-2 hr	Infusion's end

cefmetazole

Pharmacokinetics

Absorption	Complete
Distribution	Widely distributed; crosses placenta
Metabolism	Not metabolized
Excretion	Kidneys, unchanged (85%); enters breast milk
Half-life	½-2 hr; increased in renal disease

Pharmacodynamics

Onset	Rapid
Peak	Infusion's end

cefonicid

Pharmacokinetics

Absorption	Well absorbed (IM)
Distribution	Widely distributed; crosses placenta
Metabolism	Not metabolized
Excretion	Kidneys, unchanged; enters breast milk
Half-life	4½ hr; increased in renal disease

Pharmacodynamics

	IM	IV
Onset	Rapid	5 min
Peak	1 hr	Infusion's end

cefotetan

Pharmacokinetics

Absorption	Well absorbed (IM)
Distribution	Widely distributed; crosses placenta
Metabolism	Not metabolized
Excretion	Kidneys, unchanged; enters breast milk
Half-life	5 hr; increased in renal disease

Pharmacodynamics

	IM	IV
Onset	Rapid	Immediate
Peak	1-3 hr	Infusion's end

cefoxitin

Pharmacokinetics

Absorption	Well absorbed (IM)
Distribution	Widely distributed; crosses placenta
Metabolism	Not metabolized
Excretion	Kidneys, unchanged; enters breast milk
Half-life	½-1 hr; increased in renal disease

Pharmacodynamics

	IM	IV
Onset	Rapid	Immediate
Peak	½ hr	Infusion's end

cefprozil

Pharmacokinetics

Absorption	Well absorbed (PO)
Distribution	Widely distributed; crosses placenta
Metabolism	Not metabolized
Excretion	Kidneys, unchanged; enters breast milk
Half-life	1-1½ hr; increased in renal disease

Pharmacodynamics

	PO
Onset	Unknown
Peak	Unknown

loracarbef

Pharmacokinetics

Absorption	Well absorbed
Distribution	Widely distributed; crosses placenta
Metabolism	Not metabolized
Excretion	Kidneys, unchanged; enters breast milk
Half-life	1 hr; increased in renal disease

Pharmacodynamics

Onset	Rapid
Peak	1 hr

C

Interactions
Individual drugs
Alcohol: Disulfiram reaction if ingested within 48-72 hr of cephalosporin
Plicamycin: ↑ bleeding
Probenecid: ↓ excretion of drug and ↑ blood levels
Sulfinpyrazone: ↑ toxicity
Valproic acid: ↑ bleeding
Vancomycin: ↑ toxicity
Drug classifications
Aminoglycosides: ↑ toxicity
Anticoagulants: ↑ bleeding
Thrombolytics: ↑ bleeding
Lab test interferences
False ↑ Creatinine (serum urine), false ↑ urinary 17-KS
False positive: Urinary protein, direct Coombs' test, urine glucose
Interference: Cross-matching

NURSING CONSIDERATIONS
Assessment
• Assess patient for previous sensitivity reaction to penicillins or other cephalosporins; cross-sensitivity between penicillins and cephalosporins is common
• Assess patient for signs and symptoms of infection including characteristics of wounds, sputum, urine, stool, WBC >10,000, earache, fever; obtain baseline information and during treatment
• Obtain C&S before beginning drug therapy to identify if correct treatment has been initiated
• Assess for allergic reactions: rash, urticaria, pruritus, chills, fever, joint pain; angioedema may occur a few days after therapy begins; epinephrine and resuscitation equipment should be available for anaphylactic reaction

• Identify urine output; if decreasing, notify prescriber (may indicate nephrotoxicity); also check for increased BUN, creatinine
• Monitor blood studies: AST, ALT, CBC, Hct, bilirubin, LDH, alkaline phosphatase, Coombs' test monthly if patient is on long-term therapy
• Monitor electrolytes: potassium, sodium, chloride monthly if patient is on long-term therapy
• Assess bowel pattern qd; if severe diarrhea occurs, drug should be discontinued; may indicate pseudomembranous colitis
• Monitor for bleeding: ecchymosis, bleeding gums, hematuria, stool guaiac daily if on long-term therapy
• Assess for overgrowth of infection: perineal itching, fever, malaise, redness, pain, swelling, drainage, rash, diarrhea, change in cough, sputum

Nursing diagnoses
☑ Infection, risk for (uses)
☑ Diarrhea (side effects)
☑ Fluid volume deficit, risk for (side effects)
☑ Injury, risk for (side effects)
☑ Knowledge deficit (teaching)
☑ Noncompliance (teaching)

Implementation
cefaclor
• Give in even doses around the clock; if GI upset occurs, give with food; drug must be given for 10-14 days to ensure organism death and prevent superinfection
• Shake suspension, refrigerate, discard after 2 wks
Ⓢ• Do not crush, cut, or chew ext rel tabs

☑ Herb/drug   Ⓢ Do Not Crush   ◆ Alert   ⊶ Key Drug   Ⓖ Geriatric   Ⓟ Pediatric

cefamandole
IM route
- Reconstitute with 3 ml sterile or bacteriostatic water for inj, 0.9% NaCl, or 0.5%-2.0% lidocaine HCl; give deep in large muscle mass, massage; check for redness, abscess at inj site

IV IV route
- Check for irritation, extravasation, phlebitis daily; change site q72h
- Direct **IV**: Dilute each g of drug with 10 ml of D_5W, 0.9% NaCl, or sterile water for inj; give over 5 min
- For intermittent inf further dilute with 100 ml of D_5W, $D_{10}W$, D_5/0.25% NaCl, D_5/0.45% NaCl, D^5/0.9% NaCl, D_5 LR, 0.9% NaCl; give over 15-30 min; may be refrigerated up to 96 hr or 24 hr at room temp
- For cont inf dilute with 500-1000 ml of above solutions; give over prescribed rate

Y-site incompatibilities:
Amiodarone, hetastarch

Y-site compatibilities:
Acyclovir, cyclophosphamide, hydromorphone, magnesium sulfate, meperidine, morphine, perphenazine

Syringe incompatibilities:
Cimetidine, gentamicin, tobramycin

Syringe compatibilities:
Heparin

Additive incompatibilities:
Aminoglycosides, calcium gluceptate, calcium gluconate, cimetidine, gentamicin

Additive compatibilities:
Clindamycin, floxacillin, furosemide, metronidazole, or verapamil

cefmetazole
- Check for irritation, extravasation, phlebitis daily; change site q72h
- For intermittent inf, reconstitute with sterile, bacteriostatic water for inj or 0.9% NaCl; may be further diluted with 0.9% NaCl, LR, D_5W (1-20 mg/ml); give over 30-60 min; may be refrigerated for 1 week or stored 24 hr at room temp

Additive compatibilities:
Famotidine, clindamycin, KCl

cefonicid
IM route
- Reconstitute 500 mg/2 ml of sterile water for inj (220 mg/ml) or 1000 mg/2.5 ml (325 mg/ml)
- Give deep in large muscle mass, massage

IV IV route
- Check for irritation, extravasation, phlebitis daily; change site q72h
- For direct **IV** give over 5 min
- For intermittent inf reconstituted sol should be further diluted in 50-100 ml D_5W, $D_{10}W$, D_5/LR, D_5/0.25% NaCl, D_5/0.45% NaCl, D_5/0.9% NaCl, 0.9% NaCl; or Ringer's, LR; give over 30 min; may be refrigerated up to 96 hr or stored 24 hr at room temp

Y-site incompatibilities:
Hetastarch, sargramostim

Y-site compatibilities:
Acyclovir, amifostine, aztreonam, teniposide, thiotepa

Additive incompatibilities:
Aminoglycosides

Additive compatibilities:
Clindamycin

---

cefotetan
IM route

• Reconstitute 1 g/2 ml or 2 g/3 ml of sterile or bacteriostatic water for inj; may be diluted with 0.5% of 1% lidocaine to prevent pain; give deep in large muscle mass, massage

IV **IV route**

• May be stored 96h refrigerated or 24h room temp
• Check for irritation, extravasation, phlebitis daily; change site q72h
• For direct **IV** dilute in 1 g/10 ml or more and give over 5 min
• For intermittent inf further dilute in 50-100 ml of 0.9% NaCl or D_5W; give over 3-5 min; discontinue primary line while running intermittent inf

Y-site compatibilities:
Allopurinol, amifostine, aztreonam, diltiazem, famotidine, filgrastim, fluconazole, fludarabine, heparin, regular insulin, melphalan, meperidine, morphine, paclitaxel, sargramostim, tacrolimus, teniposide, theophylline, thiotepa

Syringe incompatibilities:
Doxapram

Additive incompatibilities:
Aminoglycosides, tetracyclines, heparin

cefoxitin
IM route

• Reconstitute 1 g/2 ml of sterile water for inj; may be diluted with 0.5% or 1% lidocaine to prevent pain; give deep in large muscle mass, massage

IV **IV route**

• Check for irritation, extravasation, phlebitis daily; change site q72h

• For direct **IV**, dilute 1 g/10 ml or 2 g/20 ml sterile water for inj; shake, let stand until clear; give over 3-5 min
• For intermittent inf further dilute with 50-100 ml of D_5W, $D_{10}W$, D_5/0.25% NaCl, D_5/0.45% NaCl, D_5/0.9% NaCl, 0.9% NaCl D_5/LR, D_5/0.02%, sodium bicarbonate, Ringer's, or LR; give over 15-30 min; may store 96h refrigerated or 24h room temp
• For cont inf dilute in 500-1000 ml; give over prescribed rate

Y-site incompatibilities:
Hetastarch

Y-site compatibilities:
Acyclovir, amifostine, aztreonam, cyclophosphamide, diltiazem, famotidine, fluconazole, foscarnet, hydromorphone, magnesium sulfate, meperidine, morphine, ondansetron, perphenazine, temiposide, thiotepa

Additive compatibilities:
Amikacin, cimetidine, clindamycin, gentamicin, kanamycin, multivitamins, sodium bicarbonate, tobramycin, verapamil, vit B/C

Additive incompatibilities:
Aztreonam

Syringe compatibilities:
Heparin, insulin

cefprozil
IM route

• Reconstitute with 1 g/2 ml or 2 g/3 ml of sterile or bacteriostatic water for inj; may be diluted with 0.5% or 1% lidocaine to prevent pain; give deep in large muscle mass, massage

---

IV route
- Check for irritation, extravasation, phlebitis daily; change site q72h
- For direct **IV**, dilute 1 g/10 ml or more and give over 5 min
- For intermittent inf further dilute with 50-100 ml of 0.9% NaCl or D₅W; give over 3-5 min; discontinue primary line while running intermittent infusion

Y-site compatibilities: Famotidine, fluconazole, fludarabine, regular insulin, meperidine, morphine, sargramostim

Syringe incompatibilities: Doxapram

Additive incompatibilities: Aminoglycosides, tetracyclines, heparin

loracarbef
- Give on an empty stomach, 1 hr ac or 2 hr pc
- Do not crush, chew caps
- Oral susp should be shaken before administration; store for 2 wk at room temp, discard after 2 wk

Patient/family education
- Teach patient to report sore throat, bruising, bleeding, joint pain; may indicate blood dyscrasias (rare)
- Advise patient to contact prescriber if vaginal itching, loose, foul-smelling stools, furry tongue occur; may indicate superinfection
- Instruct patient to take all medication prescribed for the length of time ordered

- Advise patient to notify prescriber of diarrhea with blood or pus, which may indicate pseudomembranous colitis

Evaluation

Positive therapeutic outcome
- Absence of signs/symptoms of infection (WBC <10,000, temp WNL, absence of red draining wounds, earache)
- Reported improvement in symptoms of infection
- Negative C&S

Treatment of anaphylaxis: Epinephrine, antihistamines, resuscitate if needed

CEPHALOSPORINS— 3RD GENERATION

cefdinir (℞)
(sef'dih-ner)
Omnicef
cefepime (℞)
(sef'e-peem)
Maxipime
cefixime (℞)
(sef-icks'ime)
Suprax
cefoperazone (℞)
(sef-oh-per'a-zone)
Cefobid
cefotaxime (℞)
(sef-oh-taks'eem)
Claforan
cefpodoxime (℞)
(sef-poe-docks'eem)
Vantin
ceftazidime (℞)
(sef'tay-zi-deem)
Ceptaz, Fortaz, Magnacef ✦,
Pentacef, Tazicef, Tazidime
ceftibuten (℞)
(sef-ti-byoo'tin)
Cedax
ceftizoxime (℞)
(sef-ti-zox'eem)
Cefizox
ceftriaxone (℞)
(sef-try-ax'one)
Rocephin
moxalactam (℞)
(mox'a-lak-tam)
Moxam
Func. class.: Broad-spectrum antibiotic
Chem. class.: Cephalosporin (3rd generation)

Action: Inhibits bacterial cell wall synthesis, rendering cell wall osmotically unstable, leading to cell death

cefdinir
⇛**Therapeutic Outcome:** Bactericidal effects for the following: gram-negative organisms *Haemophilus influenzae,* gram-positive organisms *Streptococcus pneumoniae, S. pyogenes, Staphylococcus aureus*

Uses: Uncomplicated skin and skin structure infections, community-acquired pneumonia, acute exacerbations of chronic bronchitis, acute maxillary sinusitis, pharyngitis, tonsillitis

cefepime
⇛**Therapeutic Outcome:** Bactericidal effects for the following: gram-negative bacilli, *Escherichia coli, Proteus, Klebsiella;* gram-positive organisms *Streptococcus pneumoniae, S. pyogenes, Staphylococcus aureus*

Uses: Lower respiratory tract, urinary tract, skin, bone, gonococcal infections; septicemia, peritonitis

cefixime
⇛**Therapeutic Outcome:** Bactericidal effects for the following: *Escherichia coli, Proteus mirabilis, Streptococcus pyogenes, S. pneumoniae, Haemophilus influenzae, Moraxella catarrhalis*

Uses: Uncomplicated UTI, pharyngitis and tonsillitis, otitis media, acute bronchitis, and acute/exacerbations of chronic bronchitis

cefoperazone
➤ Therapeutic Outcome:
Bactericidal effects for the following: gram-negative organisms *Acinetobacter, Morganella morganii, Neisseria gonorrhea, Proteus vulgaris;* gram-positive organisms *Staphylococci, Streptococci, Streptococci* (beta-hemolytic), *Streptococcus pneumoniae, Haemophilus influenzae, Escherichia coli, Proteus mirabilis, Klebsiella, Enterobacter, Serratia, Citrobacter, Providencia, Pseudomonas aeruginosa;* anaerobes *Bacteroides, Clostridium, Eubacterium, Fusobacterium, Peptococcus, Peptostreptococcus*

Uses: Lower respiratory tract, urinary tract, skin, bone infections; bacterial septicemia, peritonitis, pelvic inflammatory disease (PID), endometritis

cefotaxime
➤ Therapeutic Outcome:
Bactericidal against some gram-negative and some gram-positive organisms: gram-negative organisms: *H. influenzae, E. coli, N. meningitidis, P. mirabilis, Klebsiella, Citrobacter, Serratia, Salmonella, Shigella;* gram-positive organisms: *Streptococcus pneumoniae, S. pyogenes, Staphylococcus aureus*

Uses: Lower serious respiratory tract, urinary tract, skin, bone, gonococcal infections; bacteremia, septicemia, meningitis

cefpodoxime
➤ Therapeutic Outcome:
Bactericidal effects for the following: gram-negative organisms *Neisseria gonorrhoeae, Haemophilus influenzae, Escherichia coli, Proteus mirabilis,* *Klebsiella;* gram-positive organisms *Streptococcus pneumoniae, S. pyogenes, Staphylococcus aureus*

Uses: Upper and lower respiratory tract, urinary tract, skin infections; otitis media, sexually transmitted diseases

ceftazidime
➤ Therapeutic Outcome:
Bactericidal effects for the following: gram-negative organisms *Haemophilus influenzae, Escherichia coli, Enterobacter aerogenes, Proteus mirabilis, Klebsiella, Citrobacter, Enterobacter, Pseudomonas aeruginosa, Shigella, Acinetobacter, Bacteroides fragilis, Neisseria;* gram-positive organisms *Streptococcus pneumoniae, S. pyogenes, Staphylococcus aureus*

Uses: Serious upper or lower respiratory tract, urinary tract, skin, gynecologic, bone, joint, intraabdominal infections; septicemia, meningitis

ceftibuten
➤ Therapeutic Outcome:
Bactericidal effects for the following: gram-negative bacilli *Haemophilus influenzae, Escherichia coli;* gram-positive organisms *Streptococcus pneumoniae, S. pyogenes, Staphylococcus aureus*

Uses: Upper and lower respiratory tract infections; otitis media

ceftizoxime
➤ Therapeutic Outcome:
Bactericidal effects for the following: gram-negative organisms *Haemophilus influenzae, Escherichia coli, Enterobacter aerogenes, Proteus mirabilis, Klebsiella, Acinetobacter, Neisseria gonorrhea, Providencia*

C

rettgeri, Pseudomonas aeruginosa, Serratia, Enterobacter; gram-positive organisms *Streptococcus pneumoniae, S. pyogenes, Staphylococcus aureus;* anaerobes *Bacteroides, Peptococcus, Peptostreptococcus*

Uses: Serious lower respiratory tract, urinary tract, skin, intraabdominal infections; septicemia, meningitis; bone, joint infections; pelvic inflammatory disease (PID) caused by *Neisseria gonorrhoeae*

ceftriaxone
⊃**Therapeutic Outcome:** Bactericidal effects on the following: gram-negative organisms *Haemophilus influenzae, Escherichia coli, Enterobacter aerogenes, Proteus mirabilis, Klebsiella, Citrobacter, Enterobacter, Pseudomonas aeruginosa, Neisseria, Serratia;* gram-positive organisms *Streptococcus pneumoniae, S. pyogenes, Staphylococcus aureus;* anaerobes *Bacteroides*

Uses: Serious lower respiratory tract, urinary tract, skin, gonococcal, intraabdominal infections; septicemia, meningitis; bone, joint infections

moxalactam
⊃**Therapeutic Outcome:** Bactericidal against some gram-negative and some gram-positive organisms

Uses: Gram-negative organisms: *H. influenzae, E. coli, P. mirabilis, Klebsiella, Citrobacter, Salmonella, Shigella, Serratia;* gram-positive organisms: *S. pneumoniae, S. pyogenes, S. aureus;* serious lower respiratory tract, urinary tract, skin, bone infections; septicemia, meningitis, intraabdominal infections

Dosage and routes
cefdinir
Uncomplicated skin and skin structure infections/community-acquired pneumonia
P **Adult and child ≥13 yr:** PO 300 mg q12h × 10 days
Acute exacerbations of chronic bronchitis/acute maxillary sinusitis
P **Adult and child ≥13 yr:** PO 300 mg q12h or 600 mg q24h × 10 days
Pharyngitis/tonsillitis
P **Adult and child ≥13 yr:** PO 300 mg q12h or 600 mg q24h × 10 days

Available forms: Caps 300 mg, oral susp 125 mg/ml
cefepime
Urinary tract infections (mild to moderate)
Adult: IV/IM 0.5-1 g q12h × 7-10 days
Urinary tract infections (severe)
Adult: IV 2 g q12h × 10 days
Pneumonia (moderate to severe)
Adult: IV 1-2 g q12h × 10 days
Dosage reduction indicated in renal impairment (CrCl <50 ml/min)
Uncomplicated gonorrhea
• IM 2 g as a single dose with 1 g PO probenecid at the same time

Available forms: Powder for inj 500 mg, 1, 2 g
cefixime
Adult: PO 400 mg qd as a single dose or 200 mg q12h
P **Child >50 kg or >12 yr:** PO use adult dosage

P *Child <50 kg or <12 yr:* PO 8 mg/kg/day as a single dose or 4 mg/kg q12h

Renal dose: CrCl 21-60 ml/min give 75% of dose; CrCl <20 ml/min give 50% of dose

Available forms: Tabs 200, 400 mg; powder for oral susp 100 mg/5 ml

cefoperazone
Adult: IM/**IV** 1-2 g q12h

Severe infections
Adult: IM/**IV** 6-12 g/day divided in 2-4 equal doses

Hepatic dose: give 50% of dose

Mild/moderate infections
Available forms: Inj 1, 2 g

cefotaxime
Adult: IM/**IV** 1-2 g q12h as a single dose

P *Child 1 mo-12 yr:* IM/**IV** 50-180 mg/kg/day divided q6h

Severe infections
Adult: IM/**IV** 2 g q4h, not to exceed 12 g/day

P *Child 1 mo-12 yr:* IM/**IV** 50 mg/kg q6h

Uncomplicated gonorrhea
Adult: IM 1 g
Dosage reduction indicated for severe renal impairment (CrCl <30 ml/min)

Available forms: Powder for inj 1, 2, 10 g; frozen inj 20, 40 mg/ml

cefpodoxime
P *Adult >13 yr: Pneumonia:* 200 mg q12h for 14 days; *uncomplicated gonorrhea:* 200 mg single dose; *skin and skin structure:* 400 mg q12h for 7-14 days; *pharyngitis and tonsillitis:* 100 mg q12h for 10 days; *uncomplicated UTI:* 100 mg q12h for 7 days; dosing

interval increased in presence of severe renal impairment

P *Child 5 mo-12 yr: acute otitis media:* 5 mg/kg q12h for 10 days; *pharyngitis/tonsillitis:* 5 mg/kg q12h (max 100 mg/dose or 200 mg/day) × 5-10 days

Renal dose: Reduce dose in renal disease

Available forms: Tabs 100, 200 mg/granules for susp 50, 100 mg/5 ml

ceftazidime
Adult: **IV**/IM 1-2 g q8-12h × 5-10 days

P *Child:* **IV** 30-50 mg/kg q8h not to exceed 6 g/day

P *Neonate:* **IV** 30-50 mg/kg q12h

Renal dose: CrCl <50 ml/min give q12h; CrCl 10-30 ml/min give q24h; CrCl <10 ml/min give q48h

Available forms: Inj 500 mg, 1, 2, 6 g

ceftibuten
Adult: PO 400 mg qd × 10 days

P *Child 6 mo-12 yr:* PO 9 mg/kg qd × 10 days

Renal dose: CrCl <50 ml/min give 200 mg q24h; CrCl 5-20 ml/min give 100 mg q24h

Available forms: Caps 400 mg; 90, 180 mg/5 ml

ceftizoxime
Adult: IM/**IV** 1-2 g q8-12h, may give up to 4 g q8h in life-threatening infections

P *Child <6 mo:* IM/**IV** 50 mg/kg q6-8h

Renal dose: CrCl <80 ml/min give 500-1500 mg q8h; CrCl 10-49 ml/min give 250-1000 mg q12h

---

Adverse effects: *italic* = common; **bold** = life-threatening

PID
Adult: IV 2 g q8h, may increase to 4 g q8h in severe infections

Available forms: Powder for inj 500 mg, 1, 2, 10 g; premixed 1 g, 2 g/50 ml

ceftriaxone
Reduce dosage in severe renal impairment (CrCl <10 ml/min)
Adult: IM/**IV** 1-2 g qd, max 2 g q12h
P **Child:** IM/**IV** 50-75 mg/kg/day in equal doses q12h

Uncomplicated gonorrhea
Adult: 250 mg IM as single dose

Meningitis
P **Adult and child:** IM/**IV** 100 mg/kg/day in equal doses q12h, max 4 g/day

Surgical prophylaxis
Adult: IV 1 g ½-2 hr preop
Available forms: Inj 500 mg, 1, 2, 10 g

moxalactam
Adult: IM/**IV** 2-4 g q8-12h

Mild infections
Adult: IM/**IV** 250-500 mg q8-12h

Severe infections
Dosage reduction indicated even for mild renal impairment (CrCl <80 ml/min)
Adult: IM/**IV** 2-6 g q8h
P **Child:** IM/**IV** 50 mg/kg q6-8h

Available forms: Powder for inj 1, 2, 10 g

Adverse effects
CNS: Headache, dizziness, weakness, paresthesia, fever, chills, seizures

GI: Nausea, vomiting, diarrhea, anorexia, pain, glossitis, **bleeding;** increased AST, ALT, bilirubin, LDH, alk phosphatase; abdominal pain, **pseudomembranous**
GU: **Proteinuria,** vaginitis, pruritus, candidiasis, increased BUN, **nephrotoxicity, renal failure**
HEMA: Leukopenia, **thrombocytopenia, agranulocytosis,** anemia, **neutropenia, lymphocytosis, eosinophilia, pancytopenia, hemolytic anemia**
INTEG: Rash, urticaria, dermatitis
RESP: Dyspnea
SYST: **Anaphylaxis** serum sickness

Contraindications: Hypersensitivity to cephalosporins, **P** infants <1 mo

Precautions: Hypersensitivity to penicillins, pregnancy **B,** lactation, renal disease, **P** children

Do Not Confuse:
Vantin/Ventolin, ceftazidime/ceftizoxime

cefdinir

Pharmacokinetics	
Absorption	Well absorbed
Distribution	Widely distributed; crosses placenta
Metabolism	Not metabolized
Excretion	Kidneys, unchanged; enters breast milk
Half-life	Unknown

Pharmacodynamics	
	PO
Onset	Unknown
Peak	Unknown

C

cefepime

Pharmacokinetics

Absorption	Well absorbed (IM)
Distribution	Widely distributed; crosses placenta
Metabolism	Not metabolized
Excretion	Kidneys, unchanged; enters breast milk
Half-life	2 hr; increased in renal disease

Pharmacodynamics

	IM	IV
Onset	Rapid	Immediate
Peak	79 mins	Infusion's end

cefixime

Pharmacokinetics

Absorption	40%-50% (PO: tab)
Distribution	Widely distributed
Metabolism	Not metabolized
Excretion	Kidneys, unchanged (50%); bile (10%); enters breast milk
Half-life	3-4 hr, increased in renal disease

Pharmacodynamics

Onset	15-30 min
Peak	1-2 hr

cefoperazone

Pharmacokinetics

Absorption	Well absorbed (IM)
Distribution	Widely distributed; crosses placenta
Metabolism	Not metabolized
Excretion	Bile; enters breast milk
Half-life	2 hr

Pharmacodynamics

	IM	IV
Onset	Rapid	5 min
Peak	1-2 hr	Infusion's end

cefotaxime

Pharmacokinetics

Absorption	Widely distributed
Distribution	Breast milk, small amounts
Metabolism	Liver, active metabolites
Excretion	40%-65% unchanged, kidney
Half-life	1 hr

Pharmacodynamics

	IV	IM
Onset	5 min	30 min
Peak	Unknown	Unknown
Duration	Unknown	Unknown

cefpodoxime

Pharmacokinetics

Absorption	Well absorbed (PO)
Distribution	Widely distributed; crosses placenta
Metabolism	Not metabolized
Excretion	Kidneys, unchanged; enters breast milk
Half-life	2-3 hr, increased in renal disease

Pharmacodynamics

	PO
Onset	Unknown
Peak	Unknown

ceftazidime

Pharmacokinetics

Absorption	Well absorbed (IM)
Distribution	Widely distributed; crosses placenta
Metabolism	Not metabolized
Excretion	Kidneys, unchanged; enters breast milk
Half-life	½-1 hr; increased in renal disease

Pharmacodynamics

	IM	IV
Onset	Rapid	Immediate
Peak	1 hr	Infusion's end

✦ Canada Only   Adverse effects: *italic* = common; **bold** = life-threatening

ceftibuten

Pharmacokinetics

Absorption	Well absorbed
Distribution	Widely distributed; crosses placenta
Metabolism	Not metabolized
Excretion	Kidneys, unchanged; enters breast milk
Half-life	1-1½ hr; increased in renal disease

Pharmacodynamics

Onset	Unknown
Peak	Unknown

ceftizoxime

Pharmacokinetics

Absorption	Well absorbed (IM)
Distribution	Widely distributed; crosses placenta
Metabolism	Not metabolized
Excretion	Kidneys, unchanged; enters breast milk
Half-life	1½-2 hr; increased in renal disease

Pharmacodynamics

	IM	IV
Onset	Rapid	Immediate
Peak	1 hr	Infusion's end

ceftriaxone

Pharmacokinetics

Absorption	Well absorbed
Distribution	Widely distributed; crosses placenta; enters CSF
Metabolism	Liver
Excretion	Kidneys, partly
Half-life	5-8 hr

Pharmacodynamics

	IM	IV
Onset	Rapid	Immediate
Peak	1 hr	Infusion's end

moxalactam

Pharmacokinetics

Absorption	Widely distributed
Distribution	Placenta, breast milk
Metabolism	Not metabolized
Excretion	60%-97% unchanged, urine
Half-life	1½-2½ hr

Pharmacodynamics

	IV	IM
Onset	5 min	½-2 hr
Peak	Unknown	Unknown
Duration	Unknown	Unknown

Interactions
Individual drugs
Probenecid: ↓ excretion of drug and ↑ blood levels
Vancomycin: ↑ toxicity
Drug classifications
Aminoglycosides: ↑ toxicity
Lab test interferences
False: ↑ Creatinine (serum urine), ↑ urinary 17-KS
False positive: Urinary protein, direct Coombs' test, urine glucose
Interference: Cross-matching

NURSING CONSIDERATIONS
Assessment
• Assess patient for previous sensitivity reaction to penicillins or other cephalosporins; cross-sensitivity between penicillins and cephalosporins is common
• Assess patient for signs and symptoms of infection including characteristics of wounds, sputum, urine, stool, WBC >10,000, fever; obtain baseline information and during treatment
• Obtain C&S before beginning drug therapy to identify if correct treatment has been initiated

---

• Assess for allergic reactions: rash, urticaria, pruritus, chills, fever, joint pain; angioedema may occur a few days after therapy begins; epinephrine and resuscitation equipment should be available for anaphylactic reaction

• Identify urine output; if decreasing, notify prescriber (may indicate nephrotoxicity); also check for increased BUN, creatinine

• Monitor blood studies: AST, ALT, CBC, Hct, bilirubin, LDH, alkaline phosphatase, Coombs' test monthly if patient is on long-term therapy

• Monitor electrolytes: potassium, sodium, chloride monthly if patient is on long-term therapy

• Assess bowel pattern qd; if severe diarrhea occurs, drug should be discontinued; may indicate pseudomembranous colitis

• Monitor for bleeding: ecchymosis, bleeding gums, hematuria, stool guaiac daily if on long-term therapy

• Assess for overgrowth of infection: perineal itching, fever, malaise, redness, pain, swelling, drainage, rash, diarrhea, change in cough, sputum

Nursing diagnoses
☑ Infection, risk for (uses)
☑ Injury, risk for (side effects)
☑ Diarrhea (side effects)
☑ Knowledge deficit (teaching)

Implementation
cefdinir
PO route
• Give oral suspension after adding 39 ml water to the 60 ml bottle; 65 ml water to the 12.0 ml bottle; discard unused portion after 10 days

cefepime
IM route
• Reconstitute 1 g/2 ml of sterile water for inj; may be diluted with 0.5% or 1% lidocaine to prevent pain; give deep in large muscle mass, massage
IV route
• Check for irritation, extravasation, phlebitis daily; change site q72h
• For intermittent inf dilute with 50-100 ml of D_5W, give over 30 min

Solution compatibilities: 0.9% NaCl, D_5, 0.5, 1.0% lidocaine, bacteriostatic water for inj with parabens/benzyl alcohol

cefixime
• Give in even doses around the clock; if GI upset occurs, give with food; drug must be given for 10-14 days to ensure organism death and prevent superinfection
• Shake suspension

cefoperazone
IM route
• Reconstitute 1 g/2.8 ml of sterile or bacteriostatic water for inj, or 2 g/5.4 ml; may be diluted further with 1 ml or 1.8 ml of 2% lidocaine to prevent pain; give deep in large muscle mass, massage
IV route
• Check for irritation, extravasation, phlebitis daily; change site q72h
• For intermittent inf, reconstituted sol should be further diluted 1 g/20-40 ml of 0.9% NaCl, D_5W, D_5/0.9% NaCl, D_5/LR, or LR; give over 15-30 min; may be refrigerated up to 96 hr or stored 24 hr at room temp

C

• For cont inf, final concentration is 2-25 mg/ml give at prescribed rate

Y-site incompatibilities: Gentamicin, hetastarch, labetalol, meperidine, ondansetron, perphenazine, sargramostim, tobramycin, vinorelbine tartrate

Y-site compatibilities: Acyclovir, allopurinol, aztreonam, cyclophosphamide, enalaprilat, esmolol, famotidine, foscarnet, fludarabine, hydromorphone, magnesium sulfate, melphalan, morphine, teniposide, thiotepa

Syringe incompatibilities: Doxapram

Syringe compatibilities: Heparin

Additive incompatibilities: Aminoglycosides

Additive compatibilities: Cimetidine, clindamycin, furosemide

cefotaxime
IV IV route

IV after diluting 1 g/10 ml D_5W, NS, sterile H_2O for inj and give over 3-5 min by Y-tube or 3-way stopcock; may be diluted further with 50-100 ml of normal saline or D_5W; run over ½-1 hr; discontinue primary inf during administration; or may be diluted in larger vol of sol and given as a cont inf over 6-24 hr
• For 10-14 days to ensure organism death, prevent superinfection

Additive compatibilities: Clindamycin, metronidazole, verapamil

Syringe compatibilities: Heparin, oflaxacin

Y-site compatibilities: Acyclovir, amifostine, aztreonam, cyclophosphamide, diltiazem, famotidine, fludarabine, hydromorphone, lorazepam, magnesium sulfate, melphalan, meperidine, midazolam, morphine, ondansetron, perphenazine, sargramostim, teniposide, thiotepa, tolazoline, vinorelbine

cefpodoxime
IM route
• Reconstitute 1 g/2 ml or 2 g/3 ml of sterile or bacteriostatic water for inj; may be diluted with 0.5% of 1% lidocaine to prevent pain; give deep in large muscle mass, massage

IV IV route
• Check for irritation, extravasation, phlebitis daily; change site q72h
• For direct **IV** dilute in 1 g/10 ml or more and give over 5 min
• For intermittent inf further dilute in 50-100 ml of 0.9% NaCl or D_5W; give over 3-5 min; discontinue primary line while running intermittent inf

Y-site compatibilities: Famotidine, fluconazole, fludarabine, regular insulin, meperidine, morphine, sargramostim

Syringe incompatibilities: Doxapram

Additive incompatibilities: Aminoglycosides, tetracyclines, heparin

ceftazidime
IM route
• Reconstitute 500 mg/1.5 ml or 1 g/3 ml of sterile or bacteriostatic water for inj; may be diluted with 0.5% or 1% lidocaine to prevent pain; give

---

deep in large muscle mass, massage

IV IV route

• Check for irritation, extravasation, phlebitis daily; change site q72h

• For direct **IV** dilute 500 mg/5 ml or 1 g/10 ml sterile water for inj; give over 3-5 min; do not use sol with benzyl alcohol for neonates

• For intermittent inf further dilute 1 g/10 ml or more 0.9% NaCl, D_5W, $D_{10}W$, D_5/0.25% NaCl, D_5/0.45% NaCl, D_5/0.9% NaCl, or LR; give over 30-60 min

• Store for 96h refrigerated, 24h room temp

Y-*site incompatibilities:*
Amsacrine, fluconazole, sargramostim, idarubicin

Y-*site compatibilities:*
Acyclovir, allopurinol, amifostine, aztreonam, ciprofloxacin, diltiazem, enalaprilat, esmolol, famotidine, filgrastim, fludarabine, foscarnet, granisetron, heparin, hydromorphone, labetalol, meperidine, melphalan, morphine, ondansetron, paclitaxel, rantidine, tacrolimus, teniposide, theophylline, thiotepa, vinorelbine tartrate, zidovudine

Additive *incompatibilities:*
Aminoglycosides, sodium bicarbonate

Additive *compatibilities:*
Ciprofloxacin, clindamycin, fluconazole, metronidazole, ofloxacin

ceftibuten
• Administer for 10 days to ensure organism death, prevent superimposed infection
• Administer after C&S

ceftizoxime
IM route

• Reconstitute 250 mg/0.9 ml, 500 mg/1.8 ml, 1 g/3.6 ml, 2 g/7.2 ml; may be diluted with 0.5% or 1% lidocaine to prevent pain; give deep in large muscle mass, massage

IV IV route

• Check for irritation, extravasation, phlebitis daily; change site q72h

• For intermittent inf reconstitute 250 mg/2.4 ml, 500 mg/4.8 ml, 1 g/9.6 mg/2 g/19.2 ml sterile water for inj, D_5W, or 0.9% NaCl; do not use sol with benzyl alcohol for neonates; may be further diluted in 50-100 ml D_5W, $D_{10}W$, 0.9% NaCl, or LR; give over 30-60 min

• May store 96h refrigerated, 24h room temp

Y-*site compatibilities:*
Acyclovir, allopurinol, amifostine, aztreonam, enalaprilat, esmolol, famotidine, fludarabine, foscarnet, hydromorphone, labetalol, melphalan, meperidine, morphine, ondansetron, sargramostim, teniposide, thiotepa, vinorelbine

Additive *incompatibilities:*
Aminoglycosides

Additive *compatibilities:*
Clindamycin, metronidazole

moxelactam
• For 10-14 days to ensure organism death, prevent superinfection

IV IV route

• **IV** after diluting 1 g/10 ml sterile H_2O, D_5, 0.9% NaCl; give through Y-tube over 3-5 min; may be further diluted 1 g/20 ml in D_5, 0.9% NaCl, give over ½ hr; may be

---

added to 500-1000 ml, give over 6-24 hr
• Vit K for bleeding (10 mg/wk)

Additive compatibilities: Metronidazole, ranitidine, verapamil

Syringe compatibilities: Heparin

Y-site compatibilities: Cyclophosphamide, hydromorphone, magnesium sulfate, meperidine, morphine, perphenazine

Patient/family education
• Teach patient to report sore throat, bruising, bleeding, joint pain; may indicate blood dyscrasias (rare)
• Advise patient to contact prescriber if vaginal itching, loose foul-smelling stools, furry tongue occur; may indicate superinfection
• Advise patient to notify prescriber of diarrhea with blood or pus, may indicate pseudomembranous colitis

Evaluation

Positive therapeutic outcome
• Absence of signs/symptoms of infection (WBC <10,000, temp WNL, absence of red draining wounds, earache)
• Reported improvement in symptoms of infection
• Negative C&S

Treatment of anaphylaxis: Epinephrine, antihistamines, resuscitate if needed

cerivastatin (℞)
(ser-iv'i-sta-tin)
Baycol
Withdrawn from market August 2001

Action: Inhibits biosynthesis of VLDL and LDL, which are responsible for cholesterol development

▶**Therapeutic Outcome:** Decreased cholesterol levels and LDLs, increased HDLs

Uses: As an adjunct in primary hypercholesterolemia (types IIa, IIb), mixed hyperlipidemia

Dosage and routes
(Patient should first be placed on a cholesterol-lowering diet)

Adult: 0.3 mg qd PM, may be given with a bile-acid–binding resin

Available forms: Tabs 0.2, 0.3, 0.4 mg

Adverse effects
CNS: Dizziness, headache
EENT: Blurred vision, dysgeusia, lens opacities
GI: Nausea, constipation, diarrhea, dyspepsia, flatus, abdominal pain, heartburn, **liver dysfunction**
INTEG: Rash, pruritis
MS: Muscle cramps, myalgia, **myositis, rhabdomyolysis**

Contraindications: Hypersensitivity, pregnancy **X,** lactation, active liver disease

Precautions: Past liver disease, alcoholism, severe acute infections, trauma, hypotension, uncontrolled seizure disorders, severe metabolic disorders,

---

electrolyte imbalances, visual
P condition, children

Pharmacokinetics

Absorption	Unknown
Distribution	Unknown
Metabolism	Unknown
Excretion	Unknown
Half-life	Unknown

Pharmacodynamics

Unknown

Interactions
Individual drugs
Cholestyramine: ↓ absorption
Colestipol: ↓ absorption
Cyclosporine: ↑ risk of myopathy
Erythromycin: ↑ risk of myopathy
Itraconazole: ↑ cerivistatin effect
Niacin: ↑ risk of myopathy
Propranolol: ↑ antihyperlipidemic activity
Lab test interferences
↑ CPK, ↑ liver function tests, bilirubin

NURSING CONSIDERATIONS
Assessment
• Assess nutrition: fat, protein, carbohydrates; nutritional analysis should be completed by dietician before treatment
• Monitor bowel pattern daily; diarrea may be a problem
• Monitor triglycerides, cholesterol at baseline and throughout treatment; LDL and VLDL should be watched closely; if increased, drug should be discontinued
Nursing diagnoses
☑ Diarrhea (adverse reactions)
☑ Knowledge deficit (teaching)
☑ Noncompliance (teaching)

Implementation
• Give with evening meal; if dosage is increased, take with breakfast and evening meal
• Store in cool environment in airtight, light-resistant container

Patient/family education
• Inform patient that compliance is needed for positive results to occur; not to double doses
• Teach patient that risk factors should be decreased: high-fat diet, smoking, alcohol consumption, absence of exercise
• Advise patient to notify prescriber if the GI symptoms of diarrhea, abdominal or epigastric pain, nausea, vomiting occur; or if chills, fever, sore throat occur
• Teach patient that effect may take up to 1 mo
• Advise patient not to use if pregnant or breast feeding

Evaluation
Positive therapeutic outcome
• Decreased cholesterol levels, serum triglyceride
• Improved ratio of HDLs

C

---

cetirizine (R)
(se-tear′i-zeen)
Zyrtec
Func. class: Antihistamine
Chem. class.: Piperazine, H_1 histamine antagonist
Pregnancy category   B

Action: Acts on blood vessels, GI, respiratory system by competing with histamine for H_1-receptor site; decreases allergic response by blocking pharmacologic effects of histamine; less sedation rate than with other antihistamines;

---

causes increased heart rate, vasodilatation, increased secretions

➡**Therapeutic Outcome:** Absence of allergy symptoms and rhinitis

Uses: Rhinitis, allergy symptoms

Dosage and routes
P *Child 6-12 yr:* PO 5-10 mg qd

P *Adult and child >12 yr:* PO 5-10 mg qd

G *Elderly:* PO 5 mg qd, may increase to 10 mg/day

Renal/hepatic dose
CrCl 11-31 ml/min 5 mg qd

Available forms: Tabs 5, 10 mg; syrup 5 mg/5 ml

Adverse effects
CNS: Headache, stimulation, *drowsiness,* sedation, *fatigue,* confusion, blurred vision, tinnitus, restlessness, tremors,
P paradoxical excitation in
G children or elderly
CV: Hypotension, palpitations, bradycardia, tachycardia, *dysrhythmias* (rare)
GI: Nausea, diarrhea, abdominal pain, *vomiting, constipation,* appetite increase, dry mouth
GU: Frequency, dysuria, urinary retention, impotence
HEMA: **Hemolytic anemia, thrombocytopenia, leukopenia, agranulocytosis, pancytopenia**
INTEG: Rash, eczema, photosensitivity, urticaria
RESP: Thickening of bronchial secretions; dry nose, throat

Contraindications: Hypersensitivity, newborn or premature
P infants, lactation, severe hepatic disease

Precautions: Pregnancy **B,**
G elderly, children, respiratory
P disease, narrow-angle glaucoma, prostatic hypertrophy, bladder neck obstruction, asthma

Pharmacokinetics	
Absorption	Well absorbed
Distribution	Protein binding 93%
Metabolism	Liver
Excretion	Kidneys
Half-life	8.3 hr

Pharmacodynamics	
Onset	Rapid
Peak	1-2 hr
Duration	Unknown

Interactions
Individual drugs
Alcohol: ↑ CNS depression
Theophylline: ↓ cetirizine clearance
Drug classifications
Anticoagulants, oral: ↓ action
CNS depressants: ↑ CNS depression
MAOI: ↑ anticholinergic effect
Opioids: ↑ CNS depression
Sedative/hyponotics: ↑ CNS depression
☑ *Herb/drug*
Kava: ↑ CNS depression
Food/drug
↓ absorption
Lab test interferences
False negative: Skin allergy tests (discontinue antihistamine 3 days before testing)

NURSING CONSIDERATIONS
Assessment
• Assess respiratory status: rate, rhythm; increase in bronchial secretions, wheezing, chest tightness; provide fluids to 2 L/day to decrease secretion thickness
• Monitor I&O ratio: be alert for urinary retention, fre-

☑ Herb/drug   ⊘ Do Not Crush   ◆ Alert   ⊶ Key Drug   G Geriatric   P Pediatric

quency, dysuria, especially
G elderly; drug should be discontinued if these occur
• Monitor CBC during long-term therapy; blood dyscrasias may occur but are rare

Nursing diagnoses
✓ Airway clearance, ineffective (uses)
✓ Injury, risk for (side effects)
✓ Knowledge deficit (teaching)
✓ Noncompliance (teaching overuse)

Implementation
• Give on an empty stomach 1 hr before or 2 hr pc to facilitate absorption
• Store in tight, light-resistant container

Patient/family education
• Teach all aspects of drug uses; to notify prescriber if confusion, sedation, hypotension occur; to avoid driving or other hazardous activity if drowsiness occurs; to avoid alcohol or other CNS depressants that may potentiate effect
• Instruct patient to take 1 hr before or 2 hr pc to facilitate absorption
• Instruct patient not to exceed recommended dose; dysrhythmias may occur
• Teach patient hard candy, gum, frequent rinsing of mouth may be used for dryness
• Advise patient to avoid using if breast feeding

Evaluation
Positive therapeutic outcome
• Absence of running or congested nose, rashes

Treatment of overdose:
Administer ipecac syrup or lavage diazepam, vasopressors, barbiturates (short acting)

---

chloral hydrate (℞)
(klor'al hye'drate)
Aquachloral, chloral hydrate, Noctec, Novochlorhydrate ✦, PMS-Chloral Hydrate
Func. class.: Sedative/hypnotic
Chem. class.: Chloral derivative

Pregnancy category **C**
Controlled substance schedule **IV** (USA), schedule **F** (Canada)

Action: Reduced to product trichloroethanol, which produces mild cerebral depression, causing sleep; generalized CNS depression

➡ Therapeutic Outcome: Ability to sleep, sedation

Uses: Sedation, insomnia, preoperative reduction of anxiety

Dosage and routes
Sedation
Adult: PO/rec 250 mg tid pc
P *Child:* PO 25-50 mg/kg tid, not to exceed 500 mg tid

Procedure sedation
P *Child:* PO/RECT 25-50 mg/kg, not to exceed 100 mg/kg or 2 g

Insomnia
Adult: PO/RECT 500 mg-1g 30 min before hs
P *Child:* PO/RECT 50-75 mg/kg (one dose)

Renal dose
CrCl <50 ml/min avoid use

Available forms: Caps 250, 500 mg; syr 250, 500 mg/5 ml; supp 325, 500, 650 mg

---

Adverse effects
CNS: Drowsiness, dizziness, stimulation, nightmares, ataxia, hangover (rare), lightheadedness, headache, paranoia
CV: Hypotension, **dysrhythmias**
GI: Nausea, vomiting, flatulence, diarrhea, unpleasant taste, **gastric necrosis**
HEMA: **Eosinophilia, leukopenia**
INTEG: Rash, urticaria, **angioedema,** fever, purpura, eczema
RESP: **Depression**

Contraindications: Hypersensitivity to this drug or triclofos, severe renal disease, severe hepatic disease, GI disorders (oral forms), gastritis

Precautions: Severe cardiac disease, depression, suicidal individuals, asthma, intermittent porphyria, pregnancy **C,** **G** lactation, elderly

Pharmacokinetics	
Absorption	Well absorbed (PO, rec)
Distribution	Widely distributed; crosses placenta
Metabolism	Liver to trichloroethanol
Excretion	Kidneys (inactive metabolite), feces, breast milk
Half-life	8-10 hr; active metabolite

Pharmacodynamics		
	PO	RECT
Onset	½-1 hr	Slow
Peak	Unknown	Unknown
Duration	4-8 hr	4-8 hr

Interactions
Individual drugs
Alcohol: ↑ CNS depression
Fluoxetine: ↑ action
Furosemide: ↑ diaphoresis, flushing

Phenytoin: ↓ levels of phenytoin
Propoxyphene: ↑ action
Drug classifications
Analgesics, opioid: ↑ CNS depression
Anticoagulants, oral: ↑ action of anticoagulants
Antidepressants: ↑ CNS depression
Antihistamines: ↑ CNS depression
Sedative/hypnotics: ↑ CNS depression
☑ *Herb/drug*
Kava: ↑ CNS depression
Lab test interferences
Interferences: Urine catecholamines, urinary 17-OHCS
False positive: Urine glucose (copper sulfate test), phentolamine test

NURSING CONSIDERATIONS
Assessment
• Assess patient's sleep pattern and note physical (sleep apnea, obstructed airway, pain/discomfort, urinary frequency) and psychologic (fear, anxiety) circumstances that interrupt sleep
• Assess patient's bedtime routine, presleep cues/props
• Assess potential for abuse; this drug may lead to physical and psychologic dependency; amount of drug should be limited
• Monitor blood studies: Hct, Hgb, RBCs, serum folate (if on long-term therapy), protime in patients receiving anticoagulants since action of anticoagulant may be increased
• Monitor mental status: mood, sensorium, affect, memory (long, short)
• Monitor physical dependency: more frequent

requests for medication, shakes, anxiety, pinpoint pupils
• Monitor respiratory dysfunction: respiratory depression, character, rate, rhythm; hold drug if respirations are <10/min or if pupils are dilated (rare)
• Assess for blood dyscrasias: fever, sore throat, bruising, rash, jaundice, epistaxis (rare)
• Assess previous history of substance abuse, cardiac disease, or gastritis

Nursing diagnoses
☑ Sleep pattern disturbance (uses)
☑ Anxiety (uses)
☑ Knowledge deficit (teaching)
☑ Noncompliance (teaching)

Implementation
General
• Regulate environmental stimuli (light, noise, temperature), remove foods and fluids that interfere with sleep
• Place side rails up after giving medication for hypnotic; remove cigarettes/matches from patient's environment to prevent fires
PO route
• Give ½-1 hr before hs for sleeplessness; give on empty stomach with full glass of water or juice for best absorption and to decrease corrosion (do not chew); after meals to decrease GI symptoms if used for sedation; dilute syr in 4 oz water or juice
🚫• Do not crush, chew caps
◆• Check dose of syrup carefully, fatal overdoses have occurred
Rectal route
• Store supp in dark container, in refrigerator; remove outer wrapper before insertion

Patient/family education
• Caution patient to avoid driving and other activities requiring alertness; to avoid alcohol ingestion or CNS depressants; serious CNS depression may result plus tachycardia, flushing, headache, hypotension
• Instruct patient not to discontinue medication quickly after long-term use; drug should be tapered over 1-2 wk; that effects may take 2 nights for benefits to be noticed; withdrawal symptoms include tremors, anxiety, hallucinations, delirium
• Teach patient alternate measures to improve sleep (reading, exercise several hours before hs, warm bath, warm milk, TV, self-hypnosis, deep breathing)
• Instruct the patient about factors that contribute to sleep pattern disturbances (lifestyle, shift work, long work hours, environmental factors, frequent napping)
• Teach patient to take drug as prescribed, not to double doses

Evaluation
Positive therapeutic outcome
• Ability to sleep at night
• Decreased amount of early morning awakening if taking drug for insomnia
• Sedation

Treatment of overdose: Lavage, activated charcoal; monitor electrolytes, vital signs

chlorambucil (R)
(klor-am′byoo-sil)
Leukeran
Func. class.: Antineoplastic
alkylating agent
Chem. class.: Nitrogen
mustard

Pregnancy category   D

Action: Alkylates DNA, RNA;
inhibits enzymes that allow
synthesis of amino acids in
proteins; activity is not cell
cycle phase specific

Therapeutic Outcome: Prevention of rapidly growing
malignant cells

Uses: Chronic lymphocytic
leukemia, Hodgkin's disease,
other lymphomas, macroglob-
ulinemia, nephrotic syndrome,
breast carcinoma, choreocarci-
noma, ovarian carcinoma

Dosage and routes
Adult: PO 0.1-0.2 mg/kg/
day × 3-6 wk initially, then 2-6
mg/day; maintenance 0.2
mg/kg × 2-4 wk; course may
be repeated at 2-4 wk intervals

P *Child:* PO 0.1-0.2 mg/kg/day
in divided doses or 4.5 mg/
m^2/day as 1 dose or in divided
doses

Available forms: Tabs 2 mg

Adverse effects
P *CNS:* **Convulsions**
*GI: Nausea, vomiting, diar-
rhea, weight loss,* **hepatotoxicity,**
jaundice
GU: Hyperuremia
HEMA: **Thrombocytopenia,
leukopenia, pancytopenia**
(prolonged use), **permanent
bone marrow suppression**

INTEG: Alopecia (rare), der-
matitis, rash, **Stevens-Johnson
Syndrome**
RESP: **Fibrosis, pneumonitis**

Contraindications: Radiation
therapy within 1 mo, chemotherapy within 1 mo, thrombocytopenia, smallpox vaccination, pregnancy **D**

Precautions: *Pneumococcus*
vaccination

Do Not Confuse:
Leukeran/leucovorin,
Leukeran/Leukine

Pharmacokinetics

Absorption	Rapidly, completely absorbed
Distribution	Crosses placenta
Metabolism	Liver, extensively
Excretion	Kidneys
Half-life	2 hr

Pharmacodynamics

Unknown

Interactions
Individual drugs
Radiation: ↑ toxicity, bone
marrow suppression
Drug classifications
Anticoagulants: ↑ risk of
bleeding
Antineoplastics: ↑ toxicity,
bone marrow suppression
**Bone marrow–suppressing
drugs:** ↑ bone marrow sup-
pression
Live vaccines: ↑ adverse reac-
tions, ↓ antibody reaction
Salicylates: ↑ risk of bleeding
Lab test interferences
↑ Uric acid

NURSING CONSIDERATIONS
Assessment
• Monitor CBC, differential,
platelet count weekly; withhold
drug if WBC is <2000 or gran-

ulocyte count <1,000/mm^3 notify prescriber of results if WBC <20,000/mm^3, platelets <50,000/mm^3
• Monitor pulmonary function tests, chest x-ray films before, during therapy; chest film should be obtained q2 wk during treatment; check for dyspnea, rales, unproductive cough, chest pain, tachypnea
• Assess for increased uric acid levels, swelling, joint pain primarily in extremities; patient should be well hydrated to prevent urate deposits
• Monitor renal function studies: BUN, serum uric acid, urine CrCl before, during therapy; I&O ratio; report fall in urine output of 30 ml/hr; monitor for decreased hyper-uricemia
• Assess for jaundice of skin, sclera, dark urine, clay-colored stools, itchy skin, abdominal pain, fever, diarrhea
• Monitor for cold, fever, sore throat (may indicate beginning infection); identify edema in feet, joint, stomach pain, shaking; prescriber should be notified
• Assess for bleeding: hematuria, guaiac, bruising or pete-chiae, mucosa or orifices q8h, no rect temp

Nursing diagnoses
☑ Injury, risk for (adverse reactions)
☑ Body image disturbance (adverse reactions)
☑ Infection, risk for (adverse reactions)
☑ Knowledge deficit (teaching)

Implementation
• Give 1 hr ac or 2 hr pc to lessen nausea and vomiting or antacid before oral agent, give

drug after evening meal, before hs; antiemetic 30-60 min before giving drug to prevent vomiting
• Give either allopurinol or sodium bicarbonate to maintain uric acid levels, alkalinization of urine; increase fluid intake to 2-3 L/day to prevent urate deposits, calculus formation
• Use of antibiotics for prophylaxis of infection may be prescribed, since infection potential is high
• Give all drugs PO if possible, avoid IM inj when platelets <100,000/mm^3
• Store in tight container

Patient/family education
• Teach patient to avoid use of products containing aspirin or ibuprofen, razors, commercial mouthwash, since bleeding may occur; to report symptoms of bleeding (hematuria, tarry stools)
• Instruct patient to report signs of anemia (fatigue, headache, irritability, faintness, shortness of breath)
• Instruct patient to report any changes in breathing or coughing even several mo after treatment; to avoid crowds and persons with respiratory tract or other infections
• Advise patient hair loss is common; discuss the use of wigs or hair pieces
• Caution patient not to have any vaccinations without the advice of the prescriber; serious reactions can occur
• Advise patient contraception is needed during treatment and for several months after the completion of therapy

Evaluation
Positive therapeutic outcome
- Decreased size of tumor
- Decreased spread of malignancy
- Improved blood values
- Absence of sweating at night
- Increased appetite, increased weight

---

chloramphenicol (R)
(klor-am-fen′i-kole)
Ak-Chlor, Chloracol, Chlorofair, chloramphenicol, Chloromycetin, Chloroptic, EconoChlor, Fenicol ✦, I-Chlor, Novochlorocap ✦, Pentamycetin ✦
Func. class.: Antiinfective, misc.
Chem. class.: Dichloroacetic acid derivative
Pregnancy category   C

Action: Binds to 50S ribosomal subunit, which interferes with or inhibits protein synthesis

⟹ **Therapeutic Outcome:** Bactericidal for *Haemophilus influenzae, Salmonella typhi, Rickettsia, Neisseria, Mycloplasma*

Uses: Meningitis, bacteremia, abdominal, skin, soft tissue infections; local infections of skin, ear, eye

Dosage and routes
Adult: PO/**IV** 12.5 mg/kg q6h, not to exceed 4 g/day

P *Children and infants >2 wk:* **IV**/PO 12 mg/kg q6h or 2.5 mg/kg q2hr

P *Infants <2 wk and premature:* **IV**/PO 6.25 mg/kg q6h

P *Adult and child:* Ophth 1-2 gtt of sol or ointment q 3-6 mo; otic 2-3 gtt bid or tid; top 1% cream tid or qid

P *Premature infants and neonates:* **IV**/PO 25 mg/kg/day in divided doses q6h

Available forms: Inj **IV** 100 mg/ml in 1 g vial; caps 250 mg; ophth ointment 10 mg/g; ophth sol 25 mg/15 ml, 5 mg/ml; top cream 1%; otic sol 0.5%

Adverse effects
CNS: Headache, **depression, confusion**
CV: **Gray syndrome in newborns: failure to feed, pallor, cyanosis, abdominal distention, irregular respiration, vasomotor collapse**
EENT: Optic neuritis, blindness
GI: Nausea, vomiting, diarrhea, abdominal pain, xerostomia, glossitis, colitis, pruritus ani
HEMA: **Anemia, bone marrow depression, thrombocytopenia, aplastic anemia, granulocytopenia, leukopenia** (rare)
INTEG: Itching, urticaria, contact dermatitis, rash

Contraindications: Hypersensitivity, severe renal disease, severe hepatic disease, minor infections

Precautions: Hepatic disease, P renal disease, infants, children, bone marrow depression (drug-induced), pregnancy **C**, lactation

---

chloramphenicol   243

Pharmacokinetics

Absorption	Well (PO) Completely (**IV**)
Distribution	Wide
Metabolism	Liver
Excretion	Kidneys, unchanged
Half-life	1½-4 hr

Pharmacodynamics

	PO	IV	TOP	OPH	OTIC
Onset	15 min	Rapid	Unkn	Unkn	Unkn
Peak	1-2 hr	Inf end	Unkn	Unkn	Unkn

Interactions
Individual drugs
Folic acid: ↓ action of folic acid
Iron: ↑ action of iron
Phenytoin: ↑ action of phenytoin
Rifampin: ↓ action of rifampin
Vitamin B$_{12}$: ↓ action of vitamin B$_{12}$
Drug classifications
Anticoagulants: ↑ prothrombin time
Barbiturates: ↑ levels of barbiturates
Penicillins: ↑ synergism

NURSING CONSIDERATIONS
Assessment
• Assess patient for previous sensitivity reaction to other antiinfectives; cross-sensitivity between penicillins and cephalosporins is common
• Assess patient for signs and symptoms of infection including characteristics of wounds, sputum, urine, stool, WBC >10,000, fever; obtain baseline information and during treatment
• Perform C&S testing before starting drug therapy to identify if correct treatment has been initiated
• Monitor drug level in impaired hepatic, renal systems; peak 15-20 mg/ml 3 hr after dose, trough 5-10 mg/ml prior to next dose
• Monitor blood studies: platelets q2 days, CBC
• Assess bowel pattern qd; if severe diarrhea occurs, drug should be discontinued
• Monitor for bleeding: ecchymosis, bleeding gums, hematuria, stool guaiac daily if on long-term therapy
• Assess for overgrowth of infection: perineal itching, fever, malaise, redness, pain, swelling, drainage, rash, diarrhea, change in cough, sputum

Nursing diagnoses
☑ Infection, risk for (uses)
☑ Diarrhea (adverse reaction)
☑ Injury, risk for (side effects)
☑ Knowledge deficit (teaching)
☑ Noncompliance (teaching)

Implementation
Top route
• Wash hands, clean area to be treated with soap and water before application
Ophthalmic route
• Apply a small amount of ointment in lower lid
• Have patient tilt head back before application
IV route
• Give after diluting 1 g/10 ml of sterile H$_2$O for inj or D$_5$W (10% sol); give >1 min
• May be further diluted in 50-100 ml of D$_5$W; give through Y-tube, 3-way stopcock, or additive inf set; run over ½-1 hr; store reconstituted solution at room temp for up to 30 days

Syringe compatibilities:
Ampicillin, cloxacillin, heparin, methicillin, penicillin G sodium

Y-site incompatibilities:
Fluconazole

❀ Canada Only   Adverse effects: *italic* = common; **bold** = life-threatening

Y-*site* compatibilities:
Acyclovir, cyclophosphamide, enalaprilat, esmolol, foscarnet, hydromorphone, labetalol, magnesium sulfate, meperidine, morphine, perphenazine, tacrolimus

Additive compatibilities:
Amikacin, aminophylline, ascorbic acid, calcium chloride/gluconate, cephalothin, cephapirin, colistimethate, corticotropin, cyanocobalamin, dimenhydrinate, dopamine, ephedrine, heparin, hydrocortisone, kanamycin, lidocaine, magnesium sulfate, metaraminol, methicillin, methyldopate, methylprednisolone, metronidazole, nafcillin, oxacillin, oxytocin, penicillin G potassium, penicillin G sodium, pentobarbital, phenylephrine, phytonadione, plasma protein fraction, potassium chloride, promazine, ranitidine, sodium bicarbonate, thiopental, verapamil, vit B

PO route
• Give oral form on empty stomach with full glass of water
🚫 • Do not crush or chew caps
• Store cap in airtight container at room temp

Patient/family education
• Teach patient all aspects of drug therapy; need to complete entire course of medication to ensure organism death (10-14 days); culture may be taken after complete course of medication
• Advise patient to report sore throat, fever, fatigue, unusual bleeding, or bruising; could indicate bone marrow depression (may occur weeks or months after termination of drug)
• Tell patient that drug must be taken at regular intervals around the clock to maintain blood levels

Evaluation
Positive therapeutic outcome
• Decreased symptoms of infection

---

chlordiazepoxide (℞)
(klor-dye-az-e-pox′ide)
Apo-Chlordiazepoxide ✤,
chlordiazepoxide HCl,
Libritabs, Librium,
Novopoxide ✤, Solium ✤
Func. class.: Antianxiety
Chem. class.: Benzodiazepine

Pregnancy category   D

Controlled substance schedule   IV

Action: Potentiates the actions of GABA, an inhibitory neurotransmitter, especially in the limbic system reticular formation, which depresses the CNS

➡ **Therapeutic Outcome:** Decreased anxiety, successful alcohol withdrawal, relaxation

Uses: Short-term management of anxiety, acute alcohol withdrawal, preoperative relaxation

Dosage and routes
Mild anxiety
Adult: PO 5-10 mg tid-qid

🅿 *Child >6 yr:* 5 mg bid-qid, not to exceed 10 mg bid-tid

Severe anxiety
Adult: PO 20-25 mg tid-qid

Preoperatively
Adult: PO 5-10 mg tid-qid on day before surgery; IM 50-100 mg 1 hr before surgery

Alcohol withdrawal
Adult: PO/IM/**IV** 50-100 mg, not to exceed 300 mg/day

Available forms: Caps 5, 10, 25 mg; tabs 5, 10, 25 mg; powder for IM inj 100 mg

Adverse effects
CNS: Dizziness, drowsiness, confusion, headache, anxiety, tremors, stimulation, fatigue, depression, insomnia, hallucinations
CV: Orthostatic hypotension, **ECG changes, tachycardia,** hypotension
EENT: Blurred vision, tinnitus, mydriasis
GI: Constipation, dry mouth, nausea, vomiting, anorexia, diarrhea
INTEG: Rash, dermatitis, itching

Contraindications: Hypersensitivity to benzodiazepines, narrow-angle glaucoma, psychosis, pregnancy **D,** child <18 yr

Precautions: Elderly, debilitated, hepatic disease, renal disease

Do Not Confuse:
Librium/Librax

Pharmacokinetics

Absorption	Well absorbed (PO); slow, erratic (IM)
Distribution	Widely distributed; crosses placenta, blood-brain barrier
Metabolism	Liver extensively
Excretion	Kidneys, breast milk
Half-life	5-30 hr (increased in elderly)

Pharmacodynamics

	PO	IM	IV
Onset	30 min	15-30 min	1-5 min
Peak	½ hr	Unknown	Unknown
Duration	4-6 hr	Unknown	Up to 1 hr

Interactions
Individual drugs
Alcohol: ↑ CNS depression
Cimetidine: ↑ action of cimetidine
Disulfiram: ↑ action of disulfiram
Fluoxetine: ↑ action of fluoxetine
Isoniazid: ↑ action of isoniazid
Ketoconazole: ↑ action of ketoconazole
Levodopa: ↓ action of levodopa
Metoprolol: ↑ action of metoprolol
Propoxyphene: ↑ action of propoxyphene
Propranolol: ↑ action of propranolol
Rifampin: ↓ action of chlordiazepoxide
Theophylline: ↓ sedative effects
Valproic acid: ↑ action of valproic acid
Drug classifications
Analgesics, opioid: ↑ CNS depression
Antidepressants: ↑ CNS depression
Antihistamines: ↑ CNS depression
Barbiturates: ↓ effect of chlordiazepoxide
Contraceptives, oral: ↑ effect of contraceptive
Herb/drug
Kava: ↑ CNS depression
Lab test interferences
↑↑ AST/ALT, serum bilirubin
False ↑ 17-OHCS
Decrease: RAIU
False positive: Pregnancy test (some methods)

NURSING CONSIDERATIONS
Assessment
• Assess anxiety reaction: inability to sleep, apprehension, dread, foreboding, or

---

uneasiness related to unidentified source of danger
• Assess for previous drug dependence or tolerance; if drug dependent or tolerant, amount of medication should be restricted
• Monitor B/P (with patient lying, standing), pulse; if systolic B/P drops 20 mm Hg, hold drug, notify prescriber
• Monitor blood studies: CBC during long-term therapy; blood dyscrasias have occurred rarely
• Monitor hepatic studies: AST, ALT, bilirubin, creatinine, LDH, alkaline phosphatase during long-term therapy
• Monitor mental status: mood, sensorium, affect, sleeping patterns, drowsiness, dizziness, suicidal tendencies

Nursing diagnoses
☑ Anxiety (uses)
☑ Knowledge deficit (teaching)
☑ Noncompliance (teaching)

Implementation
PO route
• Give with food or milk for GI symptoms, crushed if patient unable to swallow medication whole; do not open capsules; provide sugarless gum, hard candy, frequent sips of water for dry mouth
IM route
• Reconstitute with diluent provided (2 ml); agitate slowly, do not shake; give deep in large muscle mass to prevent severe pain; do not use IM diluent for **IV** route
Ⅳ IV route
• Reconstitute 100 mg/5 ml sterile water for inj or 0.9% NaCl; give over at least 1 min to prevent cardiac arrest, apnea, bradycardia

• Keep powder from light; refrigerate, mix when ready to use

Y-site compatibilities:
Heparin, hydrocortisone, potassium chloride, vitamin B with C

Solution compatibilities:
D_5W, 0.9% NaCl

Patient/family education
• Instruct patient that drug may be taken with food; if dose is missed take as soon as remembered; do not double doses
• Tell patient to avoid OTC preparations unless approved by prescriber; to avoid alcohol ingestion or other psychotropic medications unless directed by a prescriber
• Caution patient to avoid driving and activities requiring alertness, since drowsiness may occur; until medication response is known, tell patient that drowsiness may worsen at beginning of treatment
• Instruct patient not to discontinue medication abruptly after long-term use, drug should be tapered over 1 wk
• Caution patient to rise slowly or fainting may occur, especially in elderly
• Advise patient that drug should be avoided during pregnancy

Evaluation
Positive therapeutic outcome
• Increased well being
• Decreased anxiety, restlessness, sleeplessness, dread
• Successful alcohol withdrawal

Treatment of overdose:
Lavage, VS, supportive care

---

chloroquine 🔑π (℞)
(klor'oh-kwin)
Aralen HCl, Aralen
Phosphate, chloroquine
phosphate
Func. class.: Antimalarial
Chem. class.: Synthetic
4-aminoquinoline derivative

Pregnancy category C

Action: Inhibits parasite replications, transcription of DNA to RNA by forming complexes with DNA of parasite

▶**Therapeutic Outcome:** Decreased symptoms of malaria, amebiasis

Uses: Malaria caused by *Plasmodium vivax, P. malariae, P. ovale, P. falciparum* (some strains), amebiasis

Dosage and routes
Malaria suppression
🅿**Adult and child:** PO 5 mg base/kg/wk on same day of week, not to exceed 300 mg base; treatment should begin 1-2 wk before exposure and for 8 wk after; if treatment begins after exposure, 600 mg base for adult and 10 mg base/kg
🅿 for children in 2 divided doses 6 hr apart

Extraintestinal amebiasis
Adult: IM 160-200 mg base qd × 10-12 days or PO (HCl) 600 mg base qd × 2 days, then 300 mg base qd × 2-3 wk (phosphate)

🅿**Child:** IM/PO 10 mg/kg qd (HCl) × 2-3 wk, not to exceed 300 mg/day

Available forms: Tabs 250 mg (150 mg base), 500 mg (300 mg base) phosphate; inj 50 mg (40 mg base)/ml

HCl; inj 5 mg (200 mg base) phosphate

Adverse effects
CNS: Headache, stimulation, fatigue, **convulsion,** psychosis
CV: Hypotension, **heart block, asystole with syncope,** ECG changes
EENT: Blurred vision, corneal changes, retinal changes, difficulty focusing, tinnitus, vertigo, deafness, photophobia, corneal edema
GI: Nausea, vomiting, anorexia, diarrhea, cramps
HEMA: **Thrombocytopenia, agranulocytosis, hemolytic anemia, leukopenia**
INTEG: Pruritus, pigmentary changes, skin eruptions, lichen planus–like eruptions, eczema, **exfoliative dermatitis**

Contraindications: Hypersensitivity, retinal field changes, porphyria

Precautions: Pregnancy **C,**
🅿 children, blood dyscrasias, severe GI disease, neurologic disease, alcoholism, hepatic disease, G6PD deficiency, psoriasis, eczema, lactation, porphyria

Pharmacokinetics

Absorption	Well absorbed
Distribution	Widely
Metabolism	Liver
Excretion	Kidneys, feces
Half-life	3-5 days

Pharmacodynamics

	PO	IM
Onset	Rapid	Rapid
Peak	1-3 hr	30 min
Duration	6-8 hr	Unknown

Interactions
Individual drugs
Cimetidine: ↓ absorption
Kaolin: ↓ absorption

Drug classifications
Antacids, aluminum: ↓ absorption

NURSING CONSIDERATIONS
Assessment
• Monitor liver studies weekly: ALT, AST, bilirubin; renal status: before exposure, monthly thereafter: BUN, creatinine, output, sp gr, urinalysis
• Assess mental status often: affect, mood, behavioral changes; psychosis may occur
• Assess hepatic status: decreased appetite, jaundice, dark urine, fatigue
• Assess for toxicity: blurring vision, difficulty focusing, headache, dizziness, decreased knee, ankle reflexes, drug should be discontinued immediately

Nursing diagnoses
☑ Infection, risk for (uses)
☑ Diarrhea (side effects)
☑ Knowledge deficit (teaching)
☑ Noncompliance (teaching)
☑ Injury, risk for (side effects)

Implementation
PO route
• Give with meals to decrease GI symptoms; better to take on empty stomach 1 hr ac or 2 hr pc
• Give antiemetic if vomiting occurs
• Give after C&S is completed; monthly to detect resistance
IM route
• Give IM after aspirating to prevent inj into bloodstream

Additive compatibility:
Promethazine

Patient/family education
• Advise patient that compliance with dosage schedule, duration is necessary
• Instruct patient that scheduled appointments must be kept or relapse may occur
• Caution patient to avoid alcohol while taking drug
• Instruct diabetic to use blood glucose monitor to obtain correct result
• Teach patient to report weakness, fatigue, loss of appetite, nausea, vomiting, yellowing of skin or eyes, tingling/numbness of hands/feet
• Advise patient that urine may turn rust brown color
• Instruct patient to use sunglasses in bright sunlight to prevent photophobia

Evaluation
Positive therapeutic outcome
• Decreased symptoms of malaria

Treatment of overdose:
Induce vomiting, gastric lavage, administer barbiturate (ultrashort-acting), vasopressor; tracheostomy may be necessary

chlorothiazide (℞)
(klor-oh-thye′a-zide)
Diurigen, Diuril, Diuril Sodium, Diurigen
Func. class.: Diuretic, antihypertensive
Chem. class.: Thiazide; sulfonamide derivative
Pregnancy category B

Action: Acts on the distal tubule and thick ascending limb of the loop of Henle in the kidney, increasing excretion of sodium, water, chloride, magnesium, potassium, and bicarbonate

➡ **Therapeutic Outcome:** Decreased BP, decreased edema in tissues, peripherally, diuresis

Uses: Edema in congestive heart failure, nephrotic syndrome; may be used alone or as adjunct with antihypertensives; also for edema in corticosteroids, estrogen therapy

Dosage and routes
Edema, hypertension
Adult: PO/**IV** 500 mg-2 g qd in 2 divided doses

Diuresis
Ⓟ *Child >6 mo:* PO 20 mg/kg/day in 2 divided doses
Ⓟ *Child <6 mo:* PO up to 40 mg/kg/day in 2 divided doses

Available forms: Tabs 250, 500 mg; oral susp 250 mg/5 ml; inj 500 mg

Adverse effects
CNS: Drowsiness, paresthesia, anxiety, depression, headache, *dizziness, fatigue, weakness, fever, insomnia*
CV: Irregular pulse, orthostatic hypotension, palpitations, volume depletion
EENT: Blurred vision
ELECT: Hypokalemia, hypercalcemia, hyponatremia, hypochloremia, hypophosphatemia, hypomagnesemia, hyperlipidemia
GI: Nausea, vomiting, anorexia, constipation, diarrhea, cramps, pancreatitis, GI irritation, *hepatitis*
GU: Frequency, polyuria, *uremia,* glucosuria, hematuria
HEMA: Aplastic anemia, hemolytic anemia, leukopenia, agranulocytosis, thrombocytopenia, neutropenia
INTEG: Rash, urticaria, purpura, photosensitivity, alopecia
META: Hyperglycemia, *hyperuricemia,* hypomagnesemia, increased creatinine, BUN

Contraindications: Hypersensitivity to thiazides or sulfonamides, anuria, renal decompensation, lactation, hepatic coma

Precautions: Hypokalemia, renal disease, hepatic disease, gout, COPD, LE, diabetes Ⓖmellitus, pregnancy **B,** elderly, hyperlipidemia

Pharmacokinetics

	PO
Absorption	GI tract (10%-20%)
Distribution	Extracellular spaces; crosses placenta
Metabolism	Liver
Excretion	Urine, unchanged; breast milk
Half-life	1-2 hr

Pharmacodynamics

	PO	IV
Onset	2 hr	15 min
Peak	4 hr	½ hr
Duration	6-12 hr	2 hr

Interactions
Individual drugs
Allopurinol: ↑ toxicity
Cholestyramine: ↓ absorption of chlorothiazide
Colestipol: ↓ absorption of chlorothiazide
Diazoxide: ↑ hyperglycemia, hyperuricemia, hypotension
Digitalis: ↑ toxicity
Indomethacin: ↓ hypotensive response
Lithium: ↑ toxicity
Mezlocillin: ↑ hypokalemia
Piperacillin: ↑ hypokalemia
Ticarcillin: ↑ hypokalemia
Drug classifications
Anticoagulants: ↓ effects
Antidiabetics: ↓ effect of antidiabetic agent
Antihypertensives: ↑ antihypertensive effect
Glucocorticoids: ↑ hypokalemia

NSAIDs: ↓ hypotension
Nondepolarizing skeletal muscle relaxants: ↑ toxicity
Sulfonylureas: ↓ effect of sulfonylurea

Food/drug
↑ absorption

Lab test interferences
False negative: Phentolamine and tyramine tests
Interference: Urine steroid tests
↑ BSP retention, calcium, amylase, parathyroid test
↓ PBI, ↓ PSP

NURSING CONSIDERATIONS
Assessment
• Assess glucose in urine if patient is diabetic
• Monitor improvement in CVP q8h
• Check for rashes, temp elevation qd
 • Assess for confusion, especially in elderly; take safety precautions if needed
• Monitor manifestations of hypokalemia; *renal:* acidic urine, reduced urine, osmolality, nocturia; *CV:* hypotension, broad T wave, U wave, ectopy, tachycardia, weak pulse; *neuro:* muscle weakness, altered LOC, drowsiness, apathy, lethargy, confusion, depression; *GI:* anorexia, nausea, cramps, constipation, distention, paralytic ileus; *resp:* hypoventilation, respiratory muscle weakness
• Monitor for manifestations of hypomagnesemia; *CNS:* agitation, muscle twitching, paresthesias, hyperactive reflexes, positive Babinski reflex, dysphagia, nystagmus, seizures, tetany; *GI:* nausea, vomiting, diarrhea, anorexia, abdominal distention; *CV:* ectopy, tachycardia, broad, flat, or inverted T waves, depressed ST segment, prolonged QT, decreased cardiac output, hypotension
• Monitor for manifestations of hyponatremia: *CV:* increased B/P, cold, clammy skin, hypovolemia or hypervolemia; *GI:* anorexia, nausea, vomiting, diarrhea, abdominal cramps; *neuro:* lethargy, increased ICP, confusion, headache, seizures, coma, fatigue, tremors, hyperreflexia
• Monitor for manifestations of hyperchloremia: *neuro:* weakness, lethargy, coma; *resp:* coma, deep rapid breathing
• Assess fluid volume status: I&O ratios and record, count or weigh diapers as appropriate, weight, distended red veins, crackles in lung, color, quality and sp gr of urine, skin turgor, adequacy of pulses, moist mucous membranes, bilateral lung sounds, peripheral pitting edema; dehydration symptoms of decreasing output, thirst, hypotension, dry mouth and mucous membranes should be reported
• Monitor electrolytes: potassium, sodium, calcium, magnesium; also include BUN, blood pH, ABGs, uric acid, CBC, blood sugar
• Assess BP before and during therapy with patient lying, standing, and sitting as appropriate; orthostatic hypotension can occur rapidly

Nursing diagnoses
☑ Altered urinary elimination (adverse reactions)
☑ Fluid volume deficit
☑ Fluid volume excess (uses)
☑ Knowledge deficit (teaching)

Implementation
- Give in AM to avoid interference with sleep
- Potassium replacement if potassium level is 3.0
- Give whole, or use oral sol; drug may be crushed if patient is unable to swallow

PO route
- Give with food; if nausea occurs, absorption may be increased

IV route
- Do not use solution that is yellow, has a precipitate, or crystals
- Administer **IV** after diluting 0.5 g/18 ml or more of sterile water for inj; may be diluted further with dextrose or NaCl: give over 5 min; sol is stable at room temp for 24 hr

Additive incompatibilities:
Blood, blood products, amikacin, chlorpromazine, codeine, hydralazine, insulin, levorphanol, methadone, morphine, multivitamins, norepinephrine, polymyxin B, procaine, prochlorperazine, promazine, promethazine, streptomycin, tetracycline, triflupromazine, vancomycin

Additive compatibilities:
Cimetidine, lidocaine, nafcillin, sodium bicarbonate

Patient/family education
- Teach patient to take the medication early in the day to prevent nocturia
- Instruct patient to take with food or milk if GI symptoms of nausea and anorexia occur
- Teach patient to maintain a weekly record of weight and notify prescriber of weight loss >5 lb
- Caution patient that this drug causes a loss of potassium, so food rich in potassium should be added to the diet; refer to a dietician for assistance in planning
- Caution patient not to exercise in hot weather or stand for prolonged periods, since orthostatic hypotension will be enhanced; to use sunscreen to prevent burning
- Teach patient not to use alcohol or any OTC medications without prescriber's approval; serious drug reactions may occur
- Emphasize the need to contact prescriber immediately if muscle cramps, weakness, nausea, dizziness, or numbness occurs
- Teach patient to take own B/P and pulse and record
- Caution patient that orthostatic hypotension may occur; patient should rise slowly from sitting or reclining positions and lie down if dizziness occurs
- Teach patient to continue taking medication even if feeling better; this drug controls symptoms but does not cure the condition
- Advise the patient with hypertension to continue other medical treatment (exercise, weight loss, relaxation techniques, cessation of smoking)

Evaluation
Positive therapeutic outcome
- Decreased edema
- Decreased B/P
- Increased diuresis

Treatment of overdose:
Lavage if taken orally, monitor electrolytes; administer dextrose in saline; monitor hydration, CV, renal status

chlorpheniramine
(OTC, Ph)
(klor-fen-ir'a-meen)
Aller-Chlor, Allergy, Chlo-Amine, Chlor-100, Chlorate, Chlor-Niramine, chlorpheniramine maleate, Chlor-Pro, Chlortab, Chlor-Span, Chlor-Trimeton, Chlor-Tripolon ✦, Gon-Allerate, Novo-Pheniram ✦, PediaCare Allergy Formula, Pfeiffer's Allergy, Phenetron, Telachlor, Teldrin, Trymegen
Func. class.: Antihistamine
Chem. class.: Alkylamine, H_1-receptor antagonist

Pregnancy category **B**

Action: Acts on blood vessels, GI, respiratory system by competing with histamine for H_1-receptor site; decreases allergic response by blocking histamine

Therapeutic Outcome: Absence of allergy symptoms and rhinitis

Uses: Allergy symptoms, rhinitis, allergic dermatoses, nasal allergies, hypersensitive reactions including blood transfusion reactions, anaphylaxis

Dosage and routes
Adult: PO 2-4 mg tid-qid, not to exceed 36 mg/day; time rel 8-12 mg bid-tid, not to exceed 36 mg/day; IM/**IV**/SC 5-40 mg/day

P *Child 6-12 yr:* PO 2 mg q4-6h, not to exceed 12 mg/day; sus rel 8 mg hs or qd; sus rel not recommended for child <6 yr

P *Child 2-5 yr:* PO 1 mg q4-6h, not to exceed 4 mg/day

Available forms: Chewable tabs 2 mg; tabs 4 mg; time-rel tabs 8, 12 mg; time-rel caps 6, 8, 12 mg; syr 2 mg/5 ml; inj 10, 100 mg/ml

Adverse effects
CNS: Dizziness, drowsiness, poor coordination, fatigue, anxiety, euphoria, confusion, paresthesia, neuritis
EENT: Blurred vision, dilated pupils, tinnitus, nasal stuffiness, dry nose, throat, mouth
GI: Dry mouth, nausea, anorexia, diarrhea
GU: Retention, dysuria, frequency
HEMA: **Thrombocytopenia, agranulocytosis, hemolytic anemia**
INTEG: Photosensitivity
RESP: Increased thick secretions, wheezing, chest tightness

Contraindications: Hypersensitivity to H_1-receptor antagonists, acute asthma attack, lower respiratory tract disease

Precautions: Increased intraocular pressure, renal disease, cardiac disease, hypertension, bronchial asthma, seizure disorder, stenosed peptic ulcers, hyperthyroidism, prostatic hypertrophy, bladder neck obstruction, pregnancy **B**, **G** elderly

Do Not Confuse:
Teldrin/Tedral

Pharmacokinetics	
Absorption	Well absorbed (PO, SC, IM, **IV**)
Distribution	Widely distributed; crosses blood-brain barrier
Metabolism	Liver, mostly
Excretion	Kidneys, metabolite; breast milk (minimal)
Half-life	12-15 hr

 Herb/drug   Do Not Crush ✦ Alert ✦ Key Drug **G** Geriatric **P** Pediatric

Pharmacodynamics

	PO	SC	IM	IV
Onset	15-30 min	Unknown	Unknown	Immediate
Peak	1-2 hr	Unknown	Unknown	Unknown
Duration	6-12 hr	6-12 hr	6-12 hr	6-12 hr

Interactions
Individual drugs
Alcohol: ↑ CNS depression
Atropine: ↑ anticholinergic reactions
Disopyramide: ↑ anticholinergic reactions
Haloperidol: ↑ anticholinergic reactions
Quinidine: ↑ anticholinergic reactions
Drug classifications
Antidepressants: ↑ anticholinergic reactions
Antihistamines: ↑ anticholinergic reactions
CNS depressants: ↑ CNS depression
MAOIs: ↑ anticholinergic effect
Narcotics: ↑ CNS depression
Phenothiazines: ↑ anticholinergic reactions
Sedative/hypnotics: ↑ CNS depression
Herb/drug
Henbane leaf: ↑ anticholinergic effect
Kava: ↑ CNS depression
Lab test interferences
False negative: Skin allergy tests (discontinue antihistamines 3 days before testing)

NURSING CONSIDERATIONS
Assessment
• Assess respiratory status: rate, rhythm, increase in bronchial secretions, wheezing, chest tightness; provide fluids to 2 L/day to decrease secretion thickness

• Monitor I&O ratio: be alert for urinary retention, frequency, dysuria, especially elderly; drug should be discontinued if these occur
• **IV** administration may result in rapid drop in B/P, sweating, dizziness, especially in elderly

Nursing diagnoses
☑ Airway clearance, ineffective (uses)
☑ Injury, risk for (side effects)
☑ Knowledge deficit (teaching)
☑ Noncompliance (teaching, overuse)

Implementation
PO route
• May give with food to decrease GI upset; chewable tabs should be chewed and not swallowed whole; caps, time rel tabs should be swallowed whole
⊘ • Do not open or chew time rel tabs
• Store in tight, light-resistant container
SC/IM route
• Use only 20 mg/ml and 100 mg/ml strengths; does not need to be reconstituted or diluted
IV route
Give undiluted by direct **IV** (10 mg/ml strength only); administer 10 mg over 1 min or more

Additive incompatibilities:
Calcium chloride, kanamycin, norepinephrine, pentobarbital

Additive compatibilities:
Amikacin

Patient/family education
• Teach all aspects of drug use; to notify prescriber if confusion, sedation, hypotension, or difficulty voiding occur; to avoid driving and other hazardous activity if drowsiness

---

occurs; to avoid alcohol and other CNS depressants that may potentiate effect
• Teach patient not to exceed recommended dosage; dysrhythmias may occur
• Advise patient hard candy, gum, frequent rinsing of mouth may be used for dryness

Evaluation
Positive therapeutic outcome
• Absence of running or congested nose, rashes

Treatment of overdose: Administer ipecac syrup or lavage, diazepam, vasopressors, barbiturates (short acting)

chlorpromazine
Oⁿ (R)
(klor-proe'ma-zeen)
chlorpromazine HCl, Chlorpromanyl ✦, Oramazine, Thorazine, Thor-Prom
Func. class.: Antipsychotic/neuroleptic/antiemetic
Chem. class.: Phenothiazine, aliphatic
Pregnancy category   C

Action: Depresses cerebral cortex, hypothalamus, limbic system, which control activity aggression; blocks neurotransmission produced by dopamine at synapse; exhibits a strong α-adrenergic, anticholinergic blocking action; mechanism for antipsychotic effects is unclear

▶**Therapeutic Outcome:** Decreased signs and symptoms of psychosis; control of nausea, vomiting, intractable hiccups, decreased anxiety preoperatively

Uses: Psychotic disorders, mania, schizophrenia, anxiety, intractable hiccups, nausea, vomiting, preoperative relaxation, acute intermittent porphyria, behavioral problems in **P** children, nonpsychotic patients with dementia

Dosage and routes
Psychiatry
Adult: PO 10-50 mg q1-4h initially, then increase up to 2 g/day if necessary

Adult: IM 10-50 mg q1-4h

G *Elderly:* Use lowest effective dose

P *Child:* PO 0.5 mg/kg q4-6h

P *Child:* IM 0.5 mg/kg q6-8h

P *Child:* Rec 1 mg/kg q6-8h

Nausea and vomiting
Adult: PO 10-25 mg q4-6h prn; IM 25-50 mg q3h prn; rec 50-100 mg q6-8h prn, not to exceed 400 mg/day

P *Child ≥6 mo:* PO 0.55 mg/kg q4-6h; IM 0.55 mg/kg q6-8h; rect 1.1 mg/kg q6-8h, max IM ≤5 yr or ≤22.7 kg 40 mg; max IM 5-10 yr or 22.7-45.5 kg 75 mg

Adult: IV 25-50 mg qd-qid

P *Child:* IV 0.55 mg/kg q6-8h

Intractable hiccups
Adult: PO 25-50 mg tid-qid; IM 25-50 mg (used only if PO dose does not work); IV 25-50 mg in 500-1000 ml saline (only for severe hiccups)

Available forms: Tabs 10, 25, 50, 100, 200 mg; time rel caps 30, 75, 150, 200, 300 mg; syr 10 mg/5 ml; conc 30, 100 mg/ml; supp 25, 100 mg; inj 25 mg/ml

Adverse effects
CNS: **Neuroleptic malignant syndrome,** *extrapyramidal*

symptoms: pseudoparkinsonism, akathisia, dystonia, tardive dyskinesia, seizures, *headache*
CV: *Orthostatic hypotension,* hypertension, **cardiac arrest,** ECG changes, **tachycardia**
EENT: Blurred vision, glaucoma, dry eyes
GI: *Dry mouth, nausea, vomiting, anorexia, constipation,* diarrhea, jaundice, weight gain
GU: Urinary retention, enuresis, impotence, amenorrhea, gynecomastia, breast engorgement
HEMA: Anemia, **leukopenia, leukocytosis, agranulocytosis**
INTEG: *Rash,* photosensitivity, dermatitis
RESP: **Laryngospasm,** dyspnea, **respiratory depression**

Contraindications: Hypersensitivity, circulatory collapse, liver damage, cerebral arteriosclerosis, coronary disease, severe hypertension/hypotension, blood dyscrasias, coma, child <2 yr, brain damage, bone marrow depression, alcohol and barbiturate withdrawal

Precautions: Pregnancy **C,** lactation, seizure disorders, hypertension, hepatic disease, cardiac disease, elderly

Do Not Confuse:
chlorpromazine/chlorpropamide, chlorpromazine/prochlorperazine

Pharmacokinetics

Absorption	Variable (PO); well absorbed (IM)
Distribution	Widely distributed; crosses placenta
Metabolism	Liver, GI mucosa extensively
Excretion	Kidneys
Half-life	30 hr

Pharmacodynamics

	PO	REC	IM	IV
Onset	½1 hr	12 hr	Unkn	Rapid
Peak	Unkn	Unkn	Unkn	Unkn
Duration	4-6 hr*	3-4 hr	4-8 hr	Unkn

*Duration PO ext rel is 10-12 hr.

Interactions
Individual drugs
Alcohol: ↑ effects of both drugs, oversedation
Aluminum hydroxide: ↓ absorption
Bromocriptine: ↓ antiparkinsonian activity
Disopyramide: ↑ anticholinergic effects
Epinephrine: ↑ toxicity
Guanethidine: ↓ antihypertensive response
Levodopa: ↓ antiparkinsonian activity
Lithium: ↓ chlorpromazine levels, ↑ extrapyramidal symptoms, masking of lithium toxicity
Magnesium hydroxide: ↓ absorption
Norepinephrine: ↓ vasoresponse, ↑ toxicity
Phenobarbital: ↓ effectiveness, ↑ metabolism
Warfarin: ↓ anticoagulant effect
Drug classifications
Antacids: ↓ absorption
Anticholinergics: ↑ anticholinergic effects
Anticonvulsants: ↓ seizure threshold
Antidepressants: ↑ CNS depression
Antidiarrheals, adsorbent: ↓ absorption
Antihistamines: ↑ CNS depression
Antihypertensives: ↑ hypotension
Antithyroid agents: ↑ agranulocytosis

Barbiturate anesthetics:
↑ CNS depression
β-Adrenergic blockers: ↑
effects of both drugs
General anesthetics: ↑ CNS
depression
MAOI: ↑ CNS depression
Opioids: ↑ CNS depression
Sedative/hypnotics: ↑ CNS
depression
🗹 *Herb/drug*
Kava: ↑ CNS depression
Henbane leaf: ↑ anticholinergic effect
Lab test interferences
↑ Liver function tests, ↑ cardiac enzymes, ↑ cholesterol,
↑ blood glucose, ↑ prolactin,
↑ bilirubin, ↑ PBI, ↑ cholinesterase I, ↑ alkaline phosphatase, ↑ leukocytes, ↑ granulocytes, ↑ platelets
↓ Hormones (blood and
urine)
False positive: Pregnancy
tests, PKU, urine bilirubin
False negative: Urinary steroids, 17-OHCS

NURSING CONSIDERATIONS
Assessment
• Assess mental status: orientation, mood, behavior, presence
of hallucinations, and type
before initial administration
and monthly; this drug should
significantly reduce psychotic
behavior
• Assess any potentially reversible cause of behavior problems
🅖 in the elderly before and during therapy
• Check for swallowing of PO
medication; check for hoarding
or giving of medication to
other patients
• Monitor I&O ratio; palpate
bladder if low urinary output
🅖 occurs, especially in elderly;
urinalysis recommended before, during prolonged
therapy
• Monitor bilirubin, CBC,
liver function studies monthly
• Assess affect, orientation,
LOC, reflexes, gait, coordination, sleep pattern disturbances
• Monitor B/P with patient
sitting, standing, and lying;
take pulse and respirations q4h
during initial treatment; establish baseline before starting
treatment; report drops of 30
mm Hg; obtain baseline
ECG, Q wave, and T wave
changes
• Check for dizziness, faintness, palpitations, tachycardia
on rising; severe orthostatic
hypotension is common
◆• Identify for neuroleptic
malignant syndrome: hyperpyrexia, muscle rigidity, increased CPK, altered mental
status; drug should be discontinued
• Assess for extrapyramidal
symptoms including akathisia
(inability to sit still, no pattern
to movements), tardive dyskinesia (bizarre movements of
the jaw, mouth, tongue, extremities), pseudoparkinsonism
(rigidity, tremors, pill rolling,
shuffling gate); an antiparkinsonian drug should be prescribed
• Assess for constipation,
urinary retention daily; if these
occur, increase bulk, water in
diet
Nursing diagnoses
🗹 Thought processes, altered
(uses)
🗹 Coping, ineffective individual
(uses)
🗹 Knowledge deficit (teaching)
🗹 Noncompliance (teaching)

Implementation

PO route

- Give drug in liquid form mixed in glass of juice or cola if hoarding is suspected
- Periodically attempt dosage reduction in patients with behavioral problems
- Give with full glass of water, milk; or give with food to decrease GI upset
- 🚫 Do not crush, break, or chew time rel caps
- Store in tight, light-resistant container, oral sol in amber bottle

Rec route

- Give after placing in refrigerator for 30 min if too soft to insert; this route is used for nausea, vomiting, hiccups

IM route

- Inject in deep muscle mass; do not give SC; may be diluted with 0.9% NaCl, 2% procaine as prescribed; do not administer sol with a precipitate

IV IV route

- Give by direct **IV** by diluting with 0.9% NaCl to a concentration of 1 mg/1 ml; administer at a rate of 1 mg/2 min
- Give by cont inf after diluting 50 mg/500-1000 ml of D_5W, $D_{10}W$, 0.9% NaCl, 0.45% NaCl, LR, Ringer's or combinations (used for intractable hiccups)

Syringe incompatibilities:
Cimetidine, dimenhydrinate, heparin, pentobarbital, thiopental

Syringe compatibilities:
Atropine, benztropine, butorphanol, diphenhydramine, doxapram, droperidol, fentanyl, glycopyrrolate, hydromorphone, hydroxyzine, meperidine, metoclopramide, midazolam, morphine, pentazocine, perphenazine, prochlorperazine, promazine, promethazine, scopolamine

Y-site compatibilities:
Amsacrine, cisatracurium, cisplatin, cladribine, cyclophosphamide, cytarabine, doxorubicin, doxorubicin liposome, famotidine, filgrastim, fluconazole, granisetron, heparin, hydrocortisone, ondansetron, potassium chloride, propofol, teniposide, thiotepa, vinorelbine

Additive incompatibilities:
Aminophylline, amphotericin B, ampicillin, chloramphenicol, chlorothiazide, methicillin, methohexital, penicillin G, phenobarbital

Additive compatibilities:
Ascorbic acid, ethacrynate, netilmicin, theophylline, vit B/C

Patient/family education

- Teach patient to use good oral hygiene; frequent rinsing of mouth, sugarless gum for dry mouth
- Caution patient to avoid hazardous activities until drug response is determined; dizziness, blurred vision may occur
- Inform patient that orthostatic hypotension occurs often and to rise from sitting or lying position gradually, to remain lying down after IM injection for at least 30 min; tell patient to avoid hot tubs, hot showers, tub baths, since hypotension may occur; tell patient that in hot weather heat stroke may occur; take extra precautions to stay cool

- Advise patient to avoid abrupt withdrawal of this drug, or extrapyramidal symptoms may result; drug should be withdrawn slowly
- Teach patient to avoid OTC preparations (cough, hay fever, cold) unless approved by prescriber, since serious drug interactions may occur; avoid use with alcohol, CNS depressants, since increased drowsiness may occur
- Caution patient to use sunscreen and sunglasses to prevent burns
- Teach patient about extrapyramidal symptoms and necessity of meticulous oral hygiene, since oral candidiasis may occur
- Instruct patient to take antacids 2 hr before or after taking this drug
- Instruct patient to report sore throat, malaise, fever, bleeding, mouth sores; if these occur, CBC should be drawn and drug discontinued
- Teach that urine may turn pink or red
- Teach patient to use contraceptive measures

Evaluation

Positive therapeutic outcome
- Decrease in emotional excitement, hallucinations, delusions, paranoia
- Reorganization of patterns of thought, speech
- Increase in target behaviors

Treatment of overdose:
Lavage if orally ingested; provide airway, *do not induce vomiting or use epinephrine*

---

chlorthalidone (℞)
(klor-tha′li-doan)
Apo-Chlorthalidone ✿,
Novo-Thalidone ✿,
Uridon ✿, Hygroton,
Thalitone
Func. class.: Diuretic, antihypertensive
Chem. class.: Thiazide-like phthalimindine derivative
Pregnancy category   B

Action: Acts on the distal tubule and thick ascending limb of the loop of Henle in the kidney, increasing excretion of sodium, water, chloride, magnesium, potassium, and bicarbonate

➡ **Therapeutic Outcome:** Decreased B/P, decreased edema in lung tissues and peripherally, diuresis

Uses: Edema in congestive heart failure, nephrotic syndrome; may be used alone or as adjunct with antihypertensives; also for edema in corticosteroid, estrogen therapy

Dosage and routes
Adult: PO 25-200 mg/day or 200 mg every other day

 Elderly: PO 12.5 mg qd, initially

 Child: PO 2 mg/kg or 60 mg/m² 3 times a wk

Available forms: Tabs 15, 25, 50, 100 mg

Adverse effects
CNS: Paresthesia, headache, *dizziness, fatigue, weakness,* fever
ELECT: Hypokalemia, hypercalcemia, hyponatremia, hypochloremia, hypomagnesemia
EENT: Blurred vision

C

GI: *Nausea, vomiting, anorexia,* constipation, diarrhea, cramps, pancreatitis, GI irritation, **hepatitis**

GU: *Frequency,* polyuria, **uremia,** glucosuria

HEMA: **Aplastic anemia, leukopenia, agranulocytosis, thrombocytopenia, neutropenia**

INTEG: Rash, urticaria, purpura, photosensitivity

META: *Hyperglycemia, hyperuricemia,* increased creatinine, BUN

Contraindications: Hypersensitivity to thiazides or sulfonamides, anuria, renal decompensation, lactation

Precautions: Hypokalemia, renal disease, hepatic disease, gout, COPD, LE, diabetes mellitus, elderly, pregnancy **B,** hyperlipidemia

Do Not Confuse:
Uridon ♣/Vicodin, Hygroton/Regroton

Pharmacokinetics	
Absorption	Well absorbed
Distribution	Extracellular spaces; crosses placenta
Metabolism	Liver
Excretion	Urine, unchanged (30%-60%)
Half-life	40 hr

Pharmacodynamics	
Onset	2 hr
Peak	6 hr
Duration	24-72 hr

Interactions
Individual drugs
Alcohol: ↑ hypotensive effect
Allopurnol: ↑ toxicity
Amphotericin B: ↑ hypokalemia
Cholestyramine: ↓ absorption of chlorothalidone

Colestipol: ↓ absorption of chlorothalidone
Diazoxide: ↑ hyperglycemia, hyperuricemia, hypotension
Digitalis: ↑ toxicity
Lithium: ↑ toxicity
Mezlocillin: ↑ hypokalemia
Piperacillin: ↑ hypokalemia
Ticarcillin: ↑ hypokalemia
Drug classifications
Antidiabetics: ↓ effect of antidiabetic agent
Antihypertensives: ↑ antihypertensive effect
Nitrates: ↑ hypotension
Nondepolarizing skeletal muscle relaxants: ↑ toxicity
Glucocorticoids: ↑ hypokalemia
Sulfonylureas: ↓ effect of sulfonylurea
Food/drug
↑ absorption
Herb/drug
Aloe: Potassium deficiency
Buckthorn bark/berry: Potassium deficiency
Cascara sagrada bark: Potassium deficiency
Licorice root: Potassium deficiency
Senna pod/leaf: Potassium deficiency
Lab test interferences
↑ BSP retention, ↑ triglycerides, ↑ calcium, ↑ amylase
↓ PBI, ↓ PSP

NURSING CONSIDERATIONS
Assessment
• Monitor manifestations of hypokalemia; *CV:* hypotension, broad T wave, U wave, ectopy, tachycardia, weak pulse; *GI:* anorexia, nausea, cramps, constipation, distention, paralytic ileus; *Neuro:* muscle weakness, altered LOC, drowsiness, apathy, lethargy, confusion, depression; *Renal:* acidic urine, reduced urine, osmolality,

---

nocturia; *Resp:* hypoventilation, respiratory muscle weakness

• Monitor for manifestations of hypomagnesemia; *CNS:* agitation, muscle twitching, paresthesias, hyperactive reflexes, positive Babinski reflex, dysphagia, nystagmus seizures, tetany; *CV:* ectopy, tachycardia, broad, flat or inverted T waves, depressed ST segment, prolonged QT, decreased cardiac output, hypotension; *GI:* nausea, vomiting, diarrhea, anorexia, abdominal distention

• Monitor for manifestations of hyponatremia; *CV:* increased B/P, cold, clammy skin, hypovolemia or hypervolemia; *GI:* anorexia, nausea, vomiting, diarrhea, abdominal cramps; *Neuro:* lethargy, increased ICP, confusion, headache, seizures, coma, fatigue, tremors, hyperreflexia

• Monitor for manifestations of hyperchloremia; *Neuro:* weakness, lethargy, coma; *Resp:* coma, deep rapid breathing

• Assess fluid volumes status: I&O ratios and record, count or weigh diapers as appropriate, weight, distended red veins, crackles in lung, color, quality and sp gr of urine, skin turgor, adequacy of pulses, moist mucous membranes, bilateral lung sounds, peripheral pitting edema; dehydration symptoms of decreasing output, thirst, hypotension, dry mouth, and mucous membranes should be reported

• Monitor electrolytes: potassium, sodium, calcium, magnesium; also include BUN, blood pH, ABGs, uric acid, CBC, blood sugar

• Assess B/P before and during therapy with patient lying, standing, and sitting as appropriate; orthostatic hypotension can occur rapidly

Nursing diagnoses
☑ Altered urinary elimination (side effect)
☑ Fluid volume deficit (adverse reactions)
☑ Fluid volume excess (uses)
☑ Knowledge deficit (teaching)

Implementation
• Brand names Thalitone/ Hygroton should not be used interchangeably

• Give in AM to avoid interference with sleep

• Provide potassium replacement if potassium level is 3.0 mg/dl; give whole, or use oral solutions lightly; drug may be crushed if patient is unable to swallow

• Give with food; if nausea occurs, may crush tab and mix with fluids or applesauce for swallowing

Patient/family education
General
• Teach patient to take the medication early in the day to prevent nocturia

• Instruct patient to take with food or milk if GI symptoms of nausea and anorexia occur

• Teach patient to maintain weekly record of weight and notify prescriber of weight loss >5 lb

• Caution patient that this drug causes a loss of potassium, so food rich in potassium should be added to the diet; refer to a dietician for assistance in planning

• Caution the patient not to exercise in hot weather or stand for prolonged periods, since orthostatic hypotension will be enhanced; to use sunscreen to prevent burns

C

• Teach patient not to use alcohol, or any OTC medications without prescriber's approval; serious drug reactions may occur
• Emphasize the need to contact prescriber immediately if muscle cramps, weakness, nausea, dizziness, or numbness occurs
• Teach patient to take own B/P and pulse and record
• Caution patient that orthostatic hypotension may occur; patient should rise slowly from sitting or reclining positions and lie down if dizziness occurs
• Teach patient to continue taking medication even if feeling better; this drug controls symptoms but does not cure the condition
• Advise patient with hypertension to continue other medical treatment (exercise, weight loss, relaxation techniques, cessation of smoking)

Evaluation
Positive therapeutic outcome
• Decreased edema
• Decreased B/P
• Increased diuresis

Treatment of overdose:
Lavage if taken orally, monitor electrolytes; administer dextrose in saline; monitor hydration, CV, renal status

cholestyramine
⚿ (℞)
(koe-less-tear'a-meen)
Cholybar, LoCholest, Prevalite, Questran, Questran Light
Func. class.: Antilipemic
Chem. class.: Bile acid sequestrant
Pregnancy category   C

Action: Absorbs, combines with bile acids to form an insoluble complex that is excreted through feces; loss of bile acids lowers cholesterol levels

➡ Therapeutic Outcome: Decreasing cholesterol levels and low-density lipoproteins, decreased pruritus

Uses: Primary hypercholesterolemia, pruritus associated with biliary obstruction, diarrhea caused by excess bile acid, xanthomas

Dosage and routes
Adult: PO 4 g ac and hs, not to exceed 32 g/day
⊞ *Child:* PO 240 mg/kg/day in 3 divided doses; administer with food or drink

Available forms: Powder 4 g cholestyramine of 9 g or 5 g powder; tab 1 g

Adverse effects
CNS: Headache, dizziness, drowsiness, vertigo, tinnitus
GI: Constipation, abdominal pain, nausea, fecal impaction, hemorrhoids, flatulence, vomiting, steatorrhea, peptic ulcer
HEMA: Decreased vitamin A, D, K, red cell folate content, **hyperchloremic acidosis, bleeding,** decreased pro-time
INTEG: Rash, irritation of

perianal area, tongue, skin
MS: Muscle, joint pain
Contraindications: Hypersensitivity, biliary obstruction
Precautions: Pregnancy C, **P** lactation, children

Pharmacokinetics

Absorption	Not absorbed
Distribution	Not distributed
Metabolism	Not metabolized
Excretion	Binds with bile acids, feces
Half-life	Unknown

Pharmacodynamics

Onset	24-48 hr
Peak	1-3 wk
Duration	2-4 wk

Interactions
Individual drugs
Acetaminophen: ↓ absorption
Iron: ↓ absorption
Thyroid: ↓ absorption
Drug classifications
Anticoagulants, oral: ↓ absorption
β-Adrenergic blockers: ↓ absorption
Cardiac glycosides: ↓ absorption
Vitamins A,D,E,K: ↓ absorption
Lab test interferences
Interference: Cholecystography

NURSING CONSIDERATIONS
Assessment
• Assess nutrition: fat, protein, carbohydrates, nutritional analysis should be completed by dietician
• Assess skin integrity after patient has been receiving drug; itching, pruritus often occur from bile deposits on skin
• Monitor cardiac glycoside level if both drugs are being administered; cardiac glycoside levels will be decreased
• Monitor for signs of vitamin A, D, E, K deficiency; fasting LDL, HDL, total cholesterol, triglyceride levels, electrolytes if on extended therapy
• Monitor bowel pattern daily; increase bulk, water in diet if constipation develops

Nursing diagnoses
☑ Constipation (adverse reactions)
☑ Knowledge deficit (teaching)
☑ Noncompliance (teaching)

Implementation
• Give drug ac, hs; give all other medications 1 hr before cholestyramine or 4 hr after cholestyramine to avoid poor absorption; do not take dry; mix drug with applesauce or stir into beverage (2-6 oz); let stand for 2 min; avoid inhaling powder
• Provide supplemental doses of vitamin A, D, E, K, if levels are low

Patient/family education
◆• Teach patient symptoms of hypoprothrombinemia: bleeding mucous membranes, dark tarry stools, hematuria, petechiae; report immediately
• Teach patient importance of compliance, since toxicity may result if doses are missed; not to discontinue suddenly
• Teach patient that risk factors should be decreased: high-fat diet, smoking, alcohol consumption, absence of exercise
• Have patient mix drug with 6 oz of milk, water, fruit juice; do not mix with carbonated beverages; rinse glass to make sure all medication is taken or may mix drug in applesauce; allow to stand for 2 min before mixing

Evaluation
Positive therapeutic outcome
• Decreased cholesterol level (hyperlipidemia)
• Decreased diarrhea, pruritus (excess bile acids)

---

choline salicylate (℞)
(koe'leen sa-lis'ih-late)
Arthropan, Teejel ♣
Func. class.: Nonnarcotic analgesic
Chem. class.: Salicylate
Pregnancy category   C

Action: Blocks pain impulses in CNS that occur in response to inhibition of prostaglandin synthesis; antipyretic action results from inhibition of hypothalamic heat-regulating center to produce vasodilatation to allow heat dissipation

⇒Therapeutic Outcome: Decreased pain, inflammation, fever

Uses: Mild to moderate pain or fever including arthritis, juvenile rheumatoid arthritis

Dosage and routes
Arthritis
Adult and child >12 yrs: PO 870-1740 mg qid; max 6 times a day

Pain/fever
Adult: PO 870 mg q3-4h prn

Available forms: Liq 870 mg/5 ml

Adverse effects
CNS: Stimulation, drowsiness, dizziness, confusion, **convulsion,** headache, flushing, hallucinations, **coma**
CV: Rapid pulse, pulmonary edema
EENT: Tinnitus, hearing loss

ENDO: Hypoglycemia, hyponatremia, hypokalemia
GI: Nausea, vomiting, GI bleeding, diarrhea, heartburn, anorexia, **hepatitis**
HEMA: **Thrombocytopenia, agranulocytosis, leukopenia, neutropenia, hemolytic anemia,** increased pro-time
INTEG: Rash, urticaria, bruising
RESP: Wheezing, hyperpnea

Contraindications: Hypersensitivity to salicylates, GI bleeding, bleeding disorders, children <3 yr, vitamin K deficiency, children with flulike symptoms

Precautions: Anemia, hepatic disease, renal disease, Hodgkin's disease, pregnancy **C,** lactation

Pharmacokinetics
Absorption	Well absorbed
Distribution	Widely distributed; crosses placenta
Metabolism	Liver, extensively
Excretion	Kidney, active metabolites; breast milk
Half-life	2-3 hr (low doses); 15-30 hr (high doses)

Pharmacodynamics
Onset	15-30 min
Peak	1-3 hr
Duration	3-6 hr

Interactions
Individual drugs
Alcohol: ↑ bleeding
Cefamandole: ↑ bleeding
Furosemide: ↑ toxic effects
Heparin: ↑ bleeding
Insulin: ↑ effects
Methotrexate: ↑ effects
PABA: ↑ toxic effects
Penicillins: ↑ effects
Phenytoin: ↑ effects
Plicamycin: ↑ bleeding
Probenecid: ↓ effects

Spironolactone: ↓ effects
Sulfinpyrazone: ↓ effects
Valproic acid: ↑ effects,
↑ bleeding
Vancomycin: ↑ ototoxicity
Drug classifications
Antacids: ↓ effects of choline
salicylate
Anticoagulants: ↑ effects
**Carbonic anhydrase
inhibitors:** ↑ toxic effects
NSAIDs: ↑ gastric ulcers
Penicillins: ↑ effects
Salicylates: ↓ blood sugar
levels
Steroids: ↓ effects of choline
salicylate, ↑ gastric ulcers
Sulfonylamides: ↓ effects
Urinary acidifiers: ↑ salicylate
levels
Urinary alkalizers: ↓ effects of
choline salicylate
Food/drug
Foods that acidify the urine ↑
salicylate level
Lab test interferences
↑ Coagulation studies, ↑ liver
function studies, ↑ serum uric
acid, ↑ amylase, ↑ CO_2, ↑
urinary protein
↓ Serum potassium, ↓ PBI,
↓ cholesterol
Interference: Urine catecholamines, pregnancy test, urine
glucose tests (Clinistix, Tes-Tape)

NURSING CONSIDERATIONS
Assessment
• Monitor pain: location,
duration, type, intensity, prior
to dose and 1 hr after
• Monitor musculoskeletal
status: ROM before dose
• Identify fever, length of time
and related symptoms
• Monitor liver function
studies: AST, ALT, bilirubin,
creatinine if patient is on long-term therapy

• Monitor renal function
studies: BUN, urine creatinine
if patient is on long-term therapy
• Monitor blood studies:
CBC, Hct, Hgb, pro-time if
patient is on long-term therapy
• Check I&O ratio; decreasing
output may indicate renal
failure (long-term therapy)
◆• Assess hepatotoxicity: dark
urine, clay-colored stools,
yellowing of the skin and
sclera, itching, abdominal pain,
fever, diarrhea if patient is on
long-term therapy
• Assess for allergic reactions:
rash, urticaria; if these occur,
drug may have to be discontinued
• Assess for ototoxicity: tinnitus, ringing, roaring in ears;
audiometric testing needed
before, after long-term therapy
• Assess for visual changes:
blurring, halos; corneal, retinal
damage
• Check edema in feet, ankles,
legs
• Identify prior drug history;
there are many drug interactions

Nursing diagnoses
☑ Pain (uses)
☑ Mobility, impaired physical
(uses)
☑ Knowledge deficit (teaching)
☑ Injury, risk for (side effects)

Implementation
• Administer to patient
crushed or whole
• Give with food or milk to
decrease gastric symptoms;
give 30 min ac or 2 hr pc;
absorption may be slowed
• Give antacids 1-2 hr after
enteric products

Patient/family education
- Teach patient to report any symptoms of hepatotoxicity, renal toxicity, visual changes, ototoxicity, allergic reactions, bleeding (long-term therapy)
- Advise patient to take with 8 oz of water and sit upright for 30 min after dose
- Caution patient not to exceed recommended dosage; acute poisoning may result
- Caution patient to read label on other OTC drugs; many contain aspirin products
- Inform patient that the therapeutic response takes 2 wk (arthritis)
- Teach patient to report tinnitus, confusion, diarrhea, sweating, hyperventilation
- Caution patient to avoid alcohol ingestion; GI bleeding may occur
- Teach patient that patients who have allergies may develop allergic reactions
- Caution patient to avoid buffered or effervescent products
- Teach patient not to give to children; Reye's syndrome may develop

Evaluation
Positive therapeutic outcome
- Decreased pain
- Decreased inflammation
- Decreased fever
- Increased mobility

Treatment of overdose:
Lavage, activated charcoal, monitor electrolytes, VS

---

cidofovir (℞)
(si-doh-foh'veer)
Vistide
Func. class.: Antiviral
Chem. class.: Nucleotide analog
Pregnancy category   C

Action: Suppresses cytomegalovirus (CMV) replication by selective inhibition of viral DNA synthesis

Therapeutic Outcome: Decreased symptoms of CMV

Uses: CMV retinitis in patients with AIDS

Dosage and routes
Dilute in 100 ml 0.9% saline sol before administration; probenecid must be given PO 2 g 3 hr prior to the cidofovir infusion and 1 g at 2 and 8 hr after ending the cidofovir infusion; give 1 L of 0.9% saline sol **IV** with each INF of cidovovir, give saline INF over 1-2 hr period immediately prior to cidofovir; patient should be given a second L if the patient can tolerate the fluid load; second L given at time of cidofovir or immediately afterward and should be given over a 1-3 hr period
Renal dose
CrCl <50 ml/min reduce dose
Induction
Adult: IV Inf 5 mg/kg given over 1 hr at a constant rate qwk × 2 consecutive wk
Maintenance
Adult: IV Inf 5 mg/kg given over 1 hr q2 wk

Available forms: Inj

Adverse effects
CNS: Fever, chills, **coma,** confusion, abnormal thought, *dizziness,* bizarre dreams, *head-*

ache, psychosis, tremors, somnolence, paresthesia, *amnesia, anxiety, insomnia,* **seizures**
CV: **Dysrhythmias,** hypertension/hypotension
EENT: Retinal detachment in CMV retinitis
GI: Abnormal LFTs, nausea, vomiting, anorexia, diarrhea, abdominal pain, **hemorrhage**
GU: **Hematuria,** increased creatinine, BUN, **nephrotoxicity**
HEMA: **Granulocytopenia, thrombocytopenia, irreversible neutropenia, anemia, eosinophilia**
INTEG: Rash, alopecia, pruritus, acne, urticaria, pain at inj site, phlebitis
RESP: Dyspnea

Contraindications: Hypersensitivity to this drug or probenecid, sulfa drugs

Precautions: Preexisting cytopenias, renal function impairment, pregnancy **C,** lactation, children <6 mo, elderly, platelet count <25,000/mm³

Pharmacokinetics
Unknown

Pharmacodynamics
Unknown

Interactions
Individual drugs
Amphotericin B: ↑ nephrotoxicity
Foscarnet: ↑ nephrotoxicity
Pentamidine IV: ↑ nephrotoxicity
Drug classifications
Aminoglycosides: ↑ nephrotoxicity

NURSING CONSIDERATIONS
Assessment
• Obtain culture before treatment is initiated; cultures of blood, urine, and throat may all be taken; CMV is not confirmed by this method; the diagnosis is made by an ophth exam
• Monitor kidney, liver function, increased hemopoietic studies and BUN; serum creatinine, AST, ALT, creatinine, AST, ALT, creatinine clearance, A-G ratio, baseline and drip treatment, blood counts should be done q2wk; watch for decreasing granulocytes, Hgb; if low, therapy may have to be discontinued and restarted after hematologic recovery; blood transfusions may be required
• Assess for GI symptoms: severe nausea, vomiting, diarrhea; severe symptoms may necessitate discontinuing drug
• Assess electrolytes and minerals: calcium, phosphorous, magnesium, sodium, potassium; watch closely for tetany during first administration
• Assess for symptoms of blood dyscrasias (anemia, granulocytopenia); bruising, fatigue, bleeding, poor healing
• Assess allergic reactions: flushing, rash, urticaria, pruritus
• Assess for leukopenia, neutropenia, thrombocytopenia: WBCs, platelets q2d during 2 ×/day dosing and qwk thereafter; check for leukopenias, with qd WBC count in patients with prior leukopenia, with other nucleoside analogs, or for whom leukopenia counts are <1000 cells/mm³ at start of treatment

---

• Monitor serum creatinine or creatinine clearance at least q2wk; give only to those with creatinine levels ≤1.5 mg/dl, CrCl >55 ml/min, urine protein <100 mg/dl

Nursing diagnoses
☑ Infection, risk for (uses)

Implementation
• Mix under strict aseptic conditions using gloves, gown and mask, and using precautions for antineoplastics
• Administer after diluting in 100 ml 0.9% NaCl
• Give slowly; do not give by bolus **IV**, **IV**, SC inj
• Use diluted sol within 12 hr, do not refrigerate or freeze; do not use sol with particulate matter or discoloration

Patient/family education
• Advise to notify prescriber if sore throat, swollen lymph nodes, malaise, fever occur, may indicate other infections
• Advise to report perioral tingling, numbness in extremities, and paresthesias
• Teach that serious drug interactions may occur if OTC products are ingested; check first with prescriber
• Teach that drug is not a cure, but will control symptoms
• Advise that regular ophth exams must be continued
• Advise that major toxicities may necessitate discontinuing drug
• Advise to use contraception during treatment and that infertility may occur; men should use barrier contraception for 90 days after treatment

Evaluation
Positive therapeutic outcome
• Decreased symptoms of CMV

Treatment of overdose:
Discontinue drug; use hemodialysis, and increase hydration

cilostazol
See Appendix A, Selected New Drugs

C

cimetidine ⚓ (R, OTC)
(sye-met′i-deen)
Apo-Cimetidine ✦,
Tagamet, Tagamet HBL,
Tagamet HCl, Tagamet TiHab
Func. class.: H_2-receptor antagonist
Chem. class.: Imidazole derivative
Pregnancy category **B**

Action: Inhibits histamine at H_2-receptor site in the gastric parietal cells, which inhibits gastric acid secretion

⮞**Therapeutic Outcome:** Healing of duodenal or gastric ulcers; prevention of duodenal ulcers; decreases symptoms of gastroesophageal reflux disease (GERD) and Zollinger-Ellison syndrome

Uses: Short-term treatment of duodenal and gastric ulcers and maintenance; management of GERD and Zollinger-Ellison syndrome

Investigational uses: Prevention of aspiration pneumonitis, stress ulcers, upper GI bleeding, herpes infection, hirsutism, urticaria

Dosage and routes
Treatment of active ulcers
P *Adult and child:* PO 300 mg qid with meals, hs × 8 wk or 400 mg bid, 800 mg hs; after 8 wk give hs dose only; **IV** bol

---

✦ Canada Only   Adverse effects: *italic* = common; **bold** = life-threatening

300 mg/20 ml 0.9% NaCl over 1-2 min q6h; **IV** inf 300 mg/50 ml D$_5$W over 15-20 min; IM 300 mg q6h, not to exceed 2400 mg

P *Child:* 20-40 mg/kg/day

Prophylaxis of duodenal ulcer
P *Adult and child >16 yr:* 400 mg hs

GERD
Adult: PO 800-1600 mg/day in divided doses

Hypersecretory conditions (Zollinger-Ellison syndrome)
Adult: PO/IM/**IV** 300-600 mg q6h; may increase to 12 g/day if needed

Upper GI bleeding prophylaxis
Adult: **IV** 50 mg/hr; lowered in renal disease

Aspiration pneumonitis prophylaxis
Adult: **IV** 300 mg 1 hr before anesthesia, then 300 mg **IV** q4h until patient is alert

Renal dose
CrCl 20-40 ml/min 300 mg q8h; CrCl <20 ml/min 300 mg q12h

Available forms: Tabs 100, 200, 300, 400, 800 mg; liq 300 mg/5 ml; inj 300 mg/2 ml, 300 mg/50 ml 0.9% NaCl

Adverse effects
CNS: Confusion, headache, depression, dizziness, anxiety, weakness, psychosis, tremors, **convulsions**
CV: Bradycardia, tachycardia
GI: Diarrhea, abdominal cramps, **paralytic ileus,** *jaundice*
GU: Gynecomastia, galactorrhea, impotence, increase in BUN, creatinine

HEMA: **Agranulocytosis, thrombocytopenia, neutropenia, aplastic anemia, increase in pro-time**
INTEG: Urticaria, rash, alopecia, sweating, flushing, **exfoliative dermatitis**

Contraindications: Hypersensitivity

Precautions: Pregnancy **B,**
P lactation, child <16 yr, organic brain syndrome, hepatic dis-
G ease, renal disease, elderly

Pharmacokinetics	
Absorption	Well absorbed (PO, IM); completely absorbed (**IV**)
Distribution	Widely distributed; crosses placenta
Metabolism	Liver (30%)
Excretion	Kidneys, unchanged (70%); breast milk
Half-life	1½-2 hr; increased in renal disease

Pharmacodynamics		
	PO	IV/IM
Onset	½ hr	10 min
Peak	45-90 min	½ hr
Duration	4-5 hr	4-5 hr

Interactions
Individual drugs
Ketoconazole: ↓ absorption of cimetidine
Lidocaine: ↑ toxicity
Procainamide: ↑ toxicity
Quinidine: ↑ toxicity
Warfarin: ↑ toxicity
Drug classifications
Antacids: ↓ absorption of cimetidine
Anticoagulants, oral: ↑ toxicity
Antidepressants, tricyclic: ↑ toxicity
Benzodiazepines: ↑ toxicity
β-Adrenergic blockers: ↑ toxicity

Iron salts: ↓ absorption of iron salts
Phenytoins: ↑ toxicity
Theophyllines: ↑ toxicity
Lab test interferences
↑ Alkaline phosphatase, ↑ AST, ↑ creatinine, prolactin
False positive: Gastroccult
False negative: Skin allergy tests

NURSING CONSIDERATIONS
Assessment
• Assess patient with ulcers or suspected ulcers: epigastric or abdominal pain, hematemesis, occult blood in stools, blood in gastric aspirate before and/or throughout treatment; monitor gastric pH (5 or > should be maintained)
• Monitor I&O ratio, BUN, creatinine, CBC with differential monthly

Nursing diagnoses
☑ Pain (uses)
☑ Knowledge deficit (teaching)

Implementation
PO route
• Give with meals for lengthened drug effect; antacids 1 hr before or 1 hr after cimetidine
IV route
• Give by direct **IV** after diluting 300 mg/20 ml of normal saline for inj; give over 2 min or more
• Give intermittent **IV** by diluting 300 mg/50 ml of D_5W; run over 15-20 min
• Give by cont inf after using total daily dose (900 mg) diluted in 100-1000 ml D_5W given over 24 hr
• Store diluted sol at room temp up to 48 hr

Syringe compatibilities:
Atropine, butorphanol, cephalothin, diazepam, diphenhydramine, doxapram, droperidol, fentanyl, glycopyrrolate, heparin, hydromorphone, hydroxyzine, lorazepam, meperidine, midazolam, morphine, nafcillin, nalbuphine, penicillin G sodium, pentazocine, perphenazine, prochlorperazine, promazine, promethazine, scopolamine

Syringe incompatibilities:
Cefamandole, cefazolin, chlorpromazine, pentobarbital, secobarbital

Y-site compatibilities:
Acyclovir, amifostine, aminophylline, amrinone, atracurium, aztreonam, cisatracurium, cisplatin, cladribine, cyclosphosphamide, cytarabine, diltiazem, doxorubicin, doxorubicin liposome, enalaprilat, esmolol, filgrastim, fluconazole, fludarabine, foscarnet, gallium, granisetron, haloperidol, heparin, hetastarch, idarubicin, labetalol, melphalan, meropenem, methotrexate, midazolam, ondansetron, paclitaxel, pancuronium, piperacillin/tazobactam, propofol, sargramostim, tacrolimus, teniposide, theophylline, thiotepa, tolazoline, vecuronium, vinorelbine, zidovudine

Y-site incompatibilities:
Amsacrine

Additive compatibilities:
Acetazolamide, amikacin, aminophylline, atracurium, cefoperazone, cefoxitin, chlorothiazide, clindamycin, colistimethate, dexamethasone, digoxin, epinephrine, erythromycin, ethacrynate, floxacillin, flumazenil, furosemide, gentamicin, insulin, isoproterenol, lidocaine, lincomycin, meropenem, metaraminol, methylprednisolone, norepinephrine,

penicillin G potassium, phytonadione, polymyxin B, potassium chloride, protamine, quinidine, tacrolimus, tetracycline, vancomycin, verapamil, vitamin B complex, vit B/C

Additive incompatibilities:
Amphotericin B

Patient/family education

• Advise patient that any gynecomastia or impotence that develops is reversible after treatment is discontinued

• Caution patient to avoid driving, other hazardous activities until stabilized on this medication; drowsiness or dizziness may occur

• Advise patient to avoid black pepper, caffeine, alcohol, harsh spices, extremes in temp of food; tell patient to avoid OTC preparations: aspirin, cough, cold preparations; condition may worsen

• Advise patient that smoking decreases the effectiveness of the drug; smoking cessation should be considered

• Teach patient that drug must be continued for prescribed time to be effective and taken exactly as prescribed; doses are not to be doubled; to take missed dose when remembered up to 1 hr before next dose

• Instruct patient to report bruising, fatigue, malaise; blood dyscrasias may occur

• Have patient report to prescriber immediately any diarrhea, black tarry stools, sore throat, dizziness, confusion, or delirium

Evaluation
Positive therapeutic outcome
• Decreased pain in abdomen
• Healing of ulcers

• Absence of gastroesophageal reflux
• Gastric pH of 5 or >

---

ciprofloxacin ⊙ᴨ (℞)
(sip-ro-floks′a-sin)
Cipro, Cipro IV
Func. class.: Urinary anti-infectives
Chem. class.: Fluoroquinolone antibacterial
Pregnancy category **C**

Action: Interferes with conversion of intermediate DNA fragments into high-molecular-weight DNA in bacteria; DNA gyrase inhibitor

▶**Therapeutic Outcome:** Bactericidal action against the following: gram-positive organisms *Staphylococcus epidermidis,* methicillin-resistant strains of *Staphylococcus aureus, Streptococcus pyogenes, S. pneumoniae;* gram-negative organisms *Escherichia coli, Klebsiella* species, *Enterobacter, Salmonella, Shigella, Proteus vulgaris, Providencia stuartii, P. retgeri, Morganella morganii, Pseudomonas aeruginosa, Serratia, Haemophilus, Acinetobacter, Neisseria gonorrhoeae, meningitidis, Branhamella catarrhalis, Yersinia, Vibrio, Brucella, Campylobacter, Aeromonas*

Uses: Adult urinary tract infections (including complicated); chronic bacterial prostatitis; acute sinusitis; lower respiratory, skin, bone, joint infections; infectious diarrhea; conjunctivitis, corneal ulcers (ophthalmic)

Dosage and routes
Uncomplicated urinary tract infections
Adult: PO 250 mg q12h; **IV** 200 mg q12h

Complicated/severe urinary tract infections
Adult: PO 500 mg q12h; **IV** 400 mg q12h

Respiratory, bone, skin, joint infections
Adult: PO 500 mg q12h

Corneal ulcers, conjunctivitis
Adult: Ophth 1-2 gtts q15-30 min until infection is controlled, then 1-2 gtts 4-6 times daily

Renal dose
CrCl <50 ml/min PO 250-500 mg q12h; CrCl 5-29 ml/min PO 250-500 mg q18h; **IV** 200-400 mg q18-24h

Available forms: Tabs 250, 500, 750, mg; 200 mg/100 ml D$_5$, 400 mg/200 ml D$_5$; 200, 400 mg vial; oph sol

Adverse effects
CNS: Headache, dizziness, fatigue, insomnia, depression, *restlessness*
GI: Nausea, constipation, increased ALT, AST, flatulence, insomnia, heartburn, *vomiting, diarrhea,* oral candidiasis, dysphagia
INTEG: Rash, pruritus, urticaria, photosensitivity, flushing, fever, chills
MS: Tremor, arthralgia, tendon rupture

Contraindications: Hypersensitivity to quinolones

Precautions: Pregnancy **C**, **P** lactation, children, renal disease

Pharmacokinetics

Absorption	Well absorbed (75%) (PO)
Distribution	Widely distributed
Metabolism	Liver (15%)
Excretion	Kidneys (40%-50%)
Half-life	3-4 hr; increased in renal disease

Pharmacodynamics

	PO	IV
Onset	Rapid	Immediate
Peak	1 hr	Infusion's end

Interactions
Individual drugs
Caffeine: ↓ levels
Cyclosporine: ↑ nephrotoxicity ↑ effect
Didanosine: ↓ absorption
Enteral feeding: ↓ absorption
Nitrofurantoin: ↓ effectiveness
Probenecid: ↑ blood levels
Sucralfate: ↓ absorption of ciprofloxacin
Theophylline: ↑ levels
Warfarin: ↑ warfarin effect
Zinc sulfate: ↓ absorption of ciprofloxacin
Drug classifications
Antacids: ↓ absorption of ciprofloxacin
Anticoagulants, oral: ↑ effect of anticoagulants
Antineoplastics: ↓ ciprofloxacin levels
Iron salts: ↓ absorption of ciprofloxacin
Herb/drug
Yerba mate: ↑ toxicity
Food/drug
Dairy products: ↓ absorption
Food: ↓ absorption
Lab test interferences
↑ AST, ↑ ALT, ↑ BUN, ↑ creatinine, ↑ alkaline phosphatase

NURSING CONSIDERATIONS
Assessment
• Assess patient for previous sensitivity reaction
• Assess patient for signs and symptoms of infection including characteristics of wounds, sputum, urine, stool, WBC >10,000, fever; obtain baseline information before and during treatment
• Obtain C&S before beginning drug therapy to identify if correct treatment has been initiated
• Assess for allergic reactions: rash, urticaria, pruritus, chills, fever, joint pain; may occur a few days after therapy begins; epinephrine and resuscitation equipment should be available for anaphylactic reaction
• Identify urine output; if decreasing, notify prescriber (may indicate nephrotoxicity); also check for increased BUN, creatinine
• Monitor blood studies: AST, ALT, CBC, Hct, bilirubin, LDH, alkaline phosphatase, Coombs' test monthly if patient is on long-term therapy
• Monitor electrolytes: potassium, sodium, chloride monthly if patient is on long-term therapy
• Assess bowel pattern qd; if severe diarrhea occurs, drug should be discontinued
• Monitor for bleeding: ecchymosis, bleeding gums, hematuria, stool guaiac daily if on long-term therapy
• Assess for overgrowth of infection: perineal itching, fever, malaise, redness, pain, swelling, drainage, rash, diarrhea, change in cough, sputum

Nursing diagnoses
☑ Infection, risk for (uses)
☑ Diarrhea (side effects)
☑ Injury, risk for (side effects)
☑ Knowledge deficit (teaching)
☑ Noncompliance (teaching)

Implementation
PO route
• Give around the clock to maintain proper blood levels
• Administer 2 hr before or 2 hr after antacids, zinc, iron, calcium

Ⅳ IV route
• Check for irritation, extravasation, phlebitis daily
• For intermittent inf, dilute to 1-2 mg/ml of D_5W, 0.9% NaCl; give over 60 min; it will remain stable under refrigeration for 2 wks

Y-site incompatibilities:
Heparin, mezlocillin

Y-site compatibilities:
Amifostine, amino acids, aztreonam, calcium gluconate, ceftazidime, cisatracurium, digoxin, diltiazem, diphenhydramine, dobutamine, dopamine, doxorubicin liposome, gallium, gentamicin, granisetron, hydroxyzine, lidocaine, lorazepam, metoclopramide, midazolam, midodrine, piperacillin, potassium acetate, potassium chloride, potassium phosphates, prednisolone, promethazine, propofol, ranitidine, remifentanil, Ringer's, sodium chloride, tacrolimus, teniposide, thiotepa, tobramycin, verapamil

Additive compatibilities:
Amikacin, aztreonam, ceftazidime, cyclosporine, gentamicin, metronidazole, netilmicin, piperacillin, potassium acetate, potassium chloride, potassium phosphates, prednisolone,

---

promethazine, propofol, raniti-dine, Ringer's, sodium chloride, tobramycin, vit B/C

Additive incompatibilities: Aminophylline, amoxicillin, clindamycin, floxacillin, mezlocillin

Patient/family education
• Teach patient to report sore throat, bruising, bleeding, joint pain; may indicate blood dyscrasias (rare)
• Teach patient to contact prescriber if adverse reaction occurs or if inflammation or pain in tendon occurs
• Advise patient to contact prescriber if vaginal itching, loose, foul-smelling stools, furry tongue occur; may indicate superinfection; report itching, rash, pruritus, urticaria
• Instruct patient to take all medication prescribed for the length of time ordered; drug must be taken around the clock to maintain blood levels; do not give medication to others
• Advise patient to notify prescriber of diarrhea with blood or pus

Evaluation
Positive therapeutic outcome
• Absence of signs/symptoms of infection (WBC <10,000, temp WNL, absence of red draining wounds)
• Reported improvement in symptoms of infection

---

cisatracurium (℞)
(sis-a-tra-cyoor'ee-um)
Nimbex
Func. class.: Neuromuscular blocker (nondepolarizing)

Pregnancy category B

Action: Inhibits transmission of nerve impulses by binding with cholinergic receptor sites, antagonizing action of acetylcholine

Therapeutic Outcome: Paralysis of body for administration of anesthesia

Uses: Facilitation of endotracheal intubation, skeletal muscle relaxation during mechanical ventilation surgery, or general anesthesia

Dosage and routes
Adult: **IV** 0.15 and 0.2 mg/kg depending on desired time to intubate and length of surgery: use peripheral nerve stimulation to evaluate dosage

P *Child 2-12 yr:* **IV** 0.1 mg/kg over 5-10 sec with halothane or opioid anesthesia

Available forms: Inj 2, 10 mg/ml

Adverse effects
CV: Bradycardia, tachycardia; increased, decreased B/P
EENT: Increased secretions
RESP: **Prolonged apnea, bronchospasm, cyanosis, respiratory depression**
INTEG: Rash, flushing, pruritus, urticaria

Contraindications: Hypersensitivity

Precautions: Pregnancy **B**, **P** cardiac disease, lactation, children <2 yr electrolyte imbalances, dehydration, neuromus-

---

cular disease, respiratory disease

Pharmacokinetics	
Unknown	

Pharmacodynamics	
Onset	1-3 min
Peak	2-5 min
Duration	30-40 min

Interactions
Individual drugs
Carbamazepine: ↓ duration of neuromuscular blockade
Lithium: ↑ neuromuscular blockade
Isoflurane: ↑ neuromuscular blockade
Phenytoin: ↓ duration of neuromuscular blockade
Succinylcholine: ↓ neuromuscular blockade
Drug classifications
Aminoglycosides: ↑ neuromuscular blockade
Antibiotics, polymix: ↑ neuromuscular blockade
β-Adrenergic blockers: ↑ neuromuscular blockade
Opioids: ↑ neuromuscular blockade

NURSING CONSIDERATIONS
Assessment
• Assess for electrolyte imbalances (K, Mg), may lead to increased action of this drug
• Assess vital signs (B/P, pulse, respirations, airway) until fully recovered; rate, depth, pattern of respirations; strength of handgrip
• Assess I&O ratio: check for urinary retention, frequency, hesitancy
• Assess recovery: decreased paralysis of face, diaphragm, legs, arms, rest of body
• Assess allergic reactions: rash, fever, respiratory distress, pruritus; drug should be discontinued

Nursing diagnoses
☑ Breathing pattern, ineffective (uses)
☑ Communication, impaired (adverse reactions)
☑ Knowledge deficit (teaching)

Implementation
IV route
• Use nerve stimulator by anesthesiologist to determine neuromuscular blockade
• Give anticholinesterase to reverse neuromuscular blockade
• Give by slow **IV** only by qualified person, do not administer IM
• Store in light-resistant area
• Reassure if communication is difficult during recovery from neuromuscular blockage

Evaluation
Positive therapeutic outcome
• Paralysis of jaw, eyelid, head, neck, rest of body

Treatment of overdose:
Endrophonium or neostigmine, atropine, monitor VS; mechanical ventilation

cisplatin (R)
(sis′pla-tin)
Platinol, Platinol-AQ
Func. class.: Antineoplastic alkylating agent
Chem. class.: Inorganic heavy metal
Pregnancy category **D**

Action: Alkylates DNA, RNA; inhibits enzymes that allow synthesis of amino acids in proteins; activity is not cell cycle phase specific

▶ **Therapeutic Outcome:** Prevention of rapidly growing malignant cells

Uses: Advanced bladder cancer; adjunctive in metastatic testicular cancer and metastatic ovarian cancer; head, neck, esophageal, prostatic, lung, and cervical cancer; lymphoma

Dosage and routes
Testicular cancer
Adult: IV 20 mg/m^2 qd × 5 days, repeat q3 wk for 3 cycles or more, depending on response

Bladder cancer
Adult: IV 50-70 mg/m^2 q3-4 wk

Ovarian cancer
Adult: IV 100 mg/m^2 q4 wk or 50 mg/m^2 q3 wk with cyclophosphamide therapy; mix with 2 L of NaCl and 37.5 g mannitol over 6 hr

Available forms: Inj 0.5 ♣, /mg/ml

Adverse effects
CNS: **Convulsions,** peripheral neuropathy
CV: Cardiac abnormalities
EENT: Tinnitus, hearing loss, vestibular toxicity
GI: Severe nausea, vomiting, diarrhea, weight loss
GU: **Renal tubular damage,** renal insufficiency, impotence, sterility, amenorrhea, gynecomastia, hyperuremia
HEMA: **Thrombocytopenia, leukopenia, pancytopenia**
INTEG: Alopecia, dermatitis
META: Hypomagnesemia, hypocalcemia, hypokalemia, hypophosphatemia
RESP: **Fibrosis**
SYST: **Hypersensitivity reaction**

Contraindications: Radiation therapy within 1 mo, chemotherapy within 1 mo, thrombocytopenia, smallpox vaccination, pregnancy **D**

Precautions: Pneumococcal vaccination

⚠ **Do Not Confuse:**
cisplatin/carboplatin

Pharmacokinetics
Absorption	Complete bioavailability
Distribution	Widely distributed
Metabolism	Liver
Excretion	Kidneys
Half-life	30 hr

Pharmacodynamics
Unknown

Interactions
Individual drugs
Aspirin: ↑ risk of bleeding
Radiation: ↑ toxicity, bone marrow suppression
Drug classifications
Aminoglycosides: ↑ nephrotoxicity
Antineoplastics: ↑ toxicity, bone marrow suppression
Bone marrow–suppressing drugs: ↑ bone marrow suppression
Diuretics, loop: ↑ ototoxicity
Lab test interferences
↑ uric acid, ↑ BUN, ↑ creatinine, ↓ creatinine clearance, ↓ calcium, ↓ phosphate, ↓ potassium, ↓ magnesium

NURSING CONSIDERATIONS
Assessment
• Monitor CBC, differential, platelet count weekly; withhold drug if WBC count is <4000/mm^3 or platelet count is <100,000/mm^3; notify prescriber of results if WBC <20,000/mm^3, platelets <150,000/mm^3
• Monitor renal function studies: BUN, creatinine, serum uric acid, urine CrCl before and during therapy; I&O ratio; report fall in urine output to <30 ml/hr; dose

should not be given if BUN <25 mg/dl; creatinine <1.5 mg/dl
• Monitor temp q4h (may indicate beginning of infection)
• Monitor liver function tests before and during therapy (bilirubin, AST, ALT, LDH) as needed or monthly; note yellowing of skin or sclera, dark urine, clay-colored stools, itchy skin, abdominal pain, fever, diarrhea
• Assess for increased uric acid levels, swelling, joint pain primarily in extremities; patient should be well hydrated to prevent urate deposits
• Assess for bleeding: hematuria, stool guaiac, bruising or petechiae, mucosa or orifices q8h; note inflammation of mucosa, breaks in skin
• Identify dyspnea, rales, nonproductive cough, chest pain, tachypnea
• Identify effects of alopecia on body image; discuss feelings about body changes
• Identify edema in feet, joint pain, stomach pain, shaking; prescriber should be notified

Nursing diagnoses
☑Injury, risk for (adverse reactions)
☑Body image disturbance (adverse reactions)
☑Infection, risk for (adverse reactions)
☑Knowledge deficit (teaching)

Implementation
• Hydrate patient with 0.9% NaCl over 8-12 hr before treatment
• Give all medications PO, if possible, avoid IM inj when platelets <100,000/mm³
• Give epinephrine, antihistamines, corticosteroids for hypersensitivity reaction; anti-emetic 30-60 min before giving drug to prevent vomiting, and prn; allopurinol or sodium bicarbonate to maintain uric acid level, alkalinization of urine; antibiotics for prophylaxis of infection; diuretic (furosemide 40 mg **IV**) or mannitol after infusion
• After diluting 10 mg/10 ml or 50 mg/50 ml sterile water for inj; withdraw prescribed dose, dilute ½ dose with 1000 ml D₅ 0.2 NaCl or D₅ 0.45 NaCl with 37.5 g mannitol; **IV** inf is given over 3-4 hr; use a 0.45 μm filter; total dose 2000 ml over 6-8 hr; check site for irritation, phlebitis; do not use equipment containing aluminum

Y-site compatibilities:
Allopurinol, aztrenonam, bleomycin, chlorpromazine, cimetidine, cladribine, cyclophosphamide, dexamethasone, diphenhydramine, doxapram, doxorubicin, doxorubicin liposome, droperidol, famotidine, filgrastim, fludarabine, fluorouracil, furosemide, ganciclovir, granisetron, heparin, hydromorphone, leucovorin, lorazepam, melphalan, methotrexate, methylprednisolone, metoclopramide, mitomycin, morphine, ondansetron, paclitaxel, prochlorperazine, promethazine, propofol, ranitidine, sargramostim, teniposide, vinblastine, vincristine, vinorelbine

Syringe compatibilities:
Bleomycin, cyclophosphamide, doxapram, doxorubicin, droperidol, fluorouracil, furosemide, heparin, leucovorin, methotrexate, metoclopramide, mitomycin, vinblastine, vincristine

---

☑ Herb/drug   ⓢ Do Not Crush   ◈ Alert   ☞ Key Drug   ⒼGeriatric   ⓅPediatric

Additive incompatibilities:
Fluorouracil, mesna, thiotepa

Additive compatibilities:
Carboplatin, cyclophosphamide with etoposide, etoposide, etoposide with floxuridine, floxuridine, floxuridine with leucovorin, hydroxyzine, ifosfamide, ifosfamide with etoposide, leucovorin, magnesium sulfate, mannitol, ondansetron

Solution incompatibilities:
Sodium bicarbonate 5%, 0.1% NaCl, water

Solution compatibilities:
D_5/0.225% NaCl, D_5/0.45% NaCl, D_5/0.9% NaCl, D_5/0.45% NaCl with mannitol 1.875%, D_5/0.33% NaCl with mannitol 1.875%, D_5/0.33% NaCl with KCl 20 mEq and mannitol 1.875%, 0.9% NaCl, 0.45% NaCl, 0.3% NaCl, 0.225% NaCl, water

Patient/family education
• Teach patient to avoid use of products containing aspirin or ibuprofen, razors, commercial mouthwash, since bleeding may occur; to report symptoms of bleeding (hematuria, tarry stools)
• Instruct patient to report signs of anemia (fatigue, headache, irritability, faintness, shortness of breath)
• Instruct patient to report any changes in breathing or coughing even several months after treatment; to avoid crowds and persons with respiratory tract or other infections
• Advise patient that hair may be lost during treatment; a wig or hair piece may make patient feel better; new hair may be different in color, texture
• Tell patient not to have any

vaccinations without the advice of the prescriber; serious reactions can occur
• Caution patient contraception is needed during treatment and for several months after the completion of therapy

Evaluation
Positive therapeutic outcome
• Prevention of rapid division of malignant cells

citalopram (℞)
(sigh-tal'oh-pram)
Celexa
Func. class.: Antidepressant
Chem class.: Selective serotonin reuptake inhibitor (SSRI)
Pregnancy category   B

Action: Inhibits CNS neuron uptake of serotonin but not of norepinephrine

Therapeutic Outcome:
Decreased symptoms of depression after 2-3 wk

Uses: Major depressive disorder

Dosage and routes
Adult: PO 20 mg qd AM or PM, may increase if needed to 40 mg/day after 1 wk; maintenance: after 6-8 wk of initial treatment, continue for 24 wk (32 wk total), reevaluate long-term usefulness

Available forms: Tabs 20, 40 mg

Adverse effects
CNS: Headache, nervousness, insomnia, drowsiness, anxiety, tremor, dizziness, fatigue, sedation, poor concentration, abnor-

mal dreams, agitation, **convulsions**
CV: Hot flashes, palpitations,
angina pectoris, **hemorrhage,**
hypertension, first-degree
tachycardia
EENT: Visual changes, ear/
eye pain, photophobia, tinnitus
*GI: Nausea, diarrhea, dry
mouth, anorexia, dyspepsia,
constipation, cramps, vomiting,
taste changes, flatulence, decreased appetite*
*GU: Dysmenorrhea, decreased
libido, urinary frequency, urinary tract infection,* amenorrhea, cystitis, impotence
INTEG: Sweating, rash, pruritus, acne, alopecia, urticaria
MS: Pain, arthritis, twitching
*RESP: Infection, pharyngitis,
nasal congestion, sinus headache, sinusitis, cough, dyspnea,
bronchitis,* asthma, hyperventilation, pneumonia
*SYST: Asthenia, viral infection,
fever, allergy, chills*

Contraindications: Hypersensitivity

P **Precautions:** Pregnancy **B,**
G lactation, children, elderly

Pharmacokinetics

Absorption	Well absorbed
Distribution	Unknown
Metabolism	Liver
Excretion	Kidneys, steady state 28-35 days
Half-life	Unknown

Pharmacodynamics

Onset	Unknown
Peak	Unknown
Duration	Unknown

Interactions
Individual drugs
Alcohol: ↑ CNS depression
Carbamazepine: ↑ toxicity
Lithium: ↑ toxicity

Drug classifications
Antifungals, azole: ↑ citalopram levels
Barbiturates: ↑ CNS depression
Benzodiazepines: ↑ CNS depression
β-Adrenergic blockers: ↑ plasma levels of β-blockers
CNS depressants: ↑ CNS depression
Macrolides: ↑ citalopram levels
MAOIs: Hypertensive crisis, convulsions
Sedative/hypnotics: ↑ CNS depression
• Do not use with MAOIs

Lab test interferences:
↑ Serum bilirubin, ↑ blood glucose, ↑ alk phosphatase, ↓ VMA, ↓ 5-HIAA, ↓ blood glucose
False: ↑ Urinary catecholamines

NURSING CONSIDERATIONS
Assessment
• Monitor B/P (lying, standing), pulse q4h; if systolic B/P drops 20mm hg, hold drug and notify prescriber; take vital signs q4h in patients with cardiovascular disease
• Monitor blood studies: CBC, leukocytes, differential, cardiac enzymes if patient is receiving long-term therapy; check platelets, bleeding can occur
• Monitor hepatic studies: AST, ALT, bilirubin
• Check weight qwk; appetite may increase with drug
• Assess ECG for flattening of T wave, bundle branch block, AV block, dysrhythmias in cardiac patients
• Assess EPS primarily in
G elderly: rigidity, dystonia, akathisia

☑ Herb/drug   ⊗ Do Not Crush   ◆ Alert   ⛐ Key Drug   G Geriatric   P Pediatric

- Assess mental status: mood, sensorium, affect, suicidal tendencies; increase in psychiatric symptoms: depression, panic
- Monitor urinary retention, constipation; constipation is **P** more likely to occur in children **G** or elderly
◆• Assess for withdawal symptoms: headache, nausea, vomiting, muscle pain, weakness; do not usually occur unless drug is discontinued abruptly
- Identify patient's alcohol consumption; if alcohol is consumed, hold dose until AM

Nursing diagnoses
☑ Coping, ineffective individual (uses)
☑ Injury, risk for (side effects)
☑ Knowledge deficit (teaching)
☑ Noncompliance (teaching)

Implementation
- Give with food or milk for GI symptoms
- Give dosage hs if oversedation occurs during day
- Store at room temp; do not freeze

Patient/family education
- Teach patient that therapeutic effects make take 2-3 wk
- Instruct patient to use caution in driving or other activities requiring alertness because of drowsiness, dizziness, blurred vision; to avoid rising quickly from sitting to stand-**G** ing, especially elderly
- Caution patient to avoid alcohol ingestion, other CNS depressants
- Advise patient not to discontinue medication quickly after long-term use: may cause nausea, headache, malaise
- Instruct patient to increase fluids, bulk in diet if constipa-

tion, urinary retention occur, **G** especially elderly
- Advise patient to take gum, hard sugarless candy, or frequent sips of water for dry mouth

Evaluation
Positive therapeutic outcome
- Decrease in depression
- Absence of suicidal thoughts

---

clarithromycin (℞)
(clare-i-thro-mye′sin)
Biaxin
Func. class.: Antiinfective
Chem. class.: Macrolide

Pregnancy category   C

Action: Binds to 50S ribosomal subunits of susceptible bacteria and suppresses protein synthesis

➡**Therapeutic Outcome:** Bactericidal action against the following: *Streptococcus pneumoniae, S. pyogenes, Mycoplasma pneumoniae, Corynebacterium diphtheriae, Bordetella pertussis, Listeria monocytogenes, Haemophilus influnzae, Staphylococcus aureus, Mycobacterium avium (MAC), M. intracellulare,* complex infections in AIDS patients, *Helicobacter pylori* in combination with omeprazole

Uses: Mild to moderate infections of the upper respiratory tract, lower respiratory tract; uncomplicated skin and skin structure infections

Dosage and routes
Adult: PO 250-500 mg bid × 7-14 days; 500 mg bid continues for *M. avium* (MAC)

P *Child:* PO 15 mg/kg/day (max 1000 mg) divided q12h × 10 days

H. pylori infection
Adult: PO 500 mg qd plus omeprazole 2 × 20 mg q AM (day 1-14) then omeprazole 20 mg q AM (days 15-28)

Available forms: Tabs 250, 500 mg; granules for oral susp 125 mg/5 ml, 250 mg/5 ml

Adverse effects
CV: Ventricular dysrhythmias
GI: Nausea, vomiting, diarrhea, **hepatotoxicity,** abdominal pain, stomatitis, heartburn, anorexia, abnormal taste, **pseudomembranous colitis**
GU: Vaginitis, moniliasis
HEMA: Leukopenia, thrombocytopenia, increased INR
INTEG: Rash, urticaria, pruritus, **Stevens-Johnson Syndrome**
MISC: Headache

Contraindications: Hypersensitivity

Precautions: Pregnancy **C,** lactation, hepatic/renal disease

Pharmacokinetics	
Absorption	50%
Distribution	Widely distributed
Metabolism	Liver
Excretion	Kidneys, unchanged (20%-30%)
Half-life	4-6 hr

Pharmacodynamics	
Onset	Unknown
Peak	2 hr

Interactions
Individual drugs
Carbamazepine: ↑ toxicity, from ↑ levels of carbamazepine
Clindamycin: ↓ action of clindamycin

Delavirdine: ↑ clarithromycin levels
Digoxin: ↑ blood levels of digoxin, ↑ digoxin effects
Fluconazole: ↑ clarithromycin levels
Pimozide: ↑ effect, ↑ dysrhythmias
Rifampin: ↓ action of rifampin
Tacrolimus: ↑ effects of tacrolimus
Theophylline: ↑ toxicity from ↑ levels of theophylline
Triazolam: ↑ effects of triazolam
Zidovudine: ↑ or ↓ action
Drug classifications
Oral anticoagulants: ↑ effects of oral anticoagulants
Lab test interferences
False ↑ 17-OHCS/17-KS, false ↑ AST, false ↑ ALT, BUN, creatinine, LDH, total bilirubin ↓ Folate assay

NURSING CONSIDERATIONS
Assessment
• Assess patient for signs and symptoms of infection including characteristics of wounds, sputum, urine, stool, WBC >10,000, earache, fever; obtain baseline information before and during treatment
• Obtain C&S before beginning drug therapy to identify if correct treatment has been initiated
• Monitor blood studies: AST, ALT, CBC, Hct, bilirubin, LDH, alkaline phosphatase, Coombs' test monthly if patient is on long-term therapy
• Assess bowel pattern qd; if severe diarrhea occurs, drug should be discontinued
• Assess for overgrowth of infection: perineal itching, fever, malaise, redness, pain,

swelling, drainage, rash, diarrhea, change in cough, sputum

Nursing diagnoses
- ✓ Infection, risk for (uses)
- ✓ Diarrhea (side effects)
- ✓ Knowledge deficit (teaching)
- ✓ Noncompliance (teaching)

Implementation
- Ensure adequate fluid intake (2 L) during diarrhea episodes
- Give q12h to maintain serum level

Patient/family education
- Advise patient to contact physician if vaginal itching, loose, foul-smelling stools, furry tongue occur; may indicate superinfection
- Instruct patient to take all medication prescribed for the length of time ordered

Evaluation
Positive therapeutic outcome
- Absence of signs/symptoms of infection (WBC <10,000, temp WNL, absence of red draining wounds)
- Reported improvement in symptoms of infection

---

clemastine (℞)
(klem'as-teen)
Antihist-1, Contac Allergy 12 Hour, Tavist
Func. class.: Antihistamine
Chem. class.: Ethanolamine derivative, H_1-receptor antagonist

Pregnancy category B

Action: Acts on blood vessels, GI, respiratory system by competing with histamine for H_1-receptor site; decreases allergic response by blocking histamine

Therapeutic Outcome: Absence of allergy symptoms and rhinitis

Uses: Allergy symptoms, rhinitis, allergic dermatoses, nasal allergies, hypersensitive reactions including blood transfusion reactions, anaphylaxis

Dosage and routes
Adult and child >12 yr: PO 1.34-2.68 mg bid-tid, not to exceed 8.04 mg/day

Available forms: Tabs 1.34, 2.68 mg; syr 0.67 mg/ml

Adverse effects
CNS: Dizziness, drowsiness, poor coordination, fatigue, anxiety, euphoria, confusion, paresthesia, neuritis, paradoxic excitement (child)
CV: Hypotension, palpitations, tachycardia
EENT: Blurred vision, dilated pupils, tinnitus, nasal stuffiness, dry nose, throat, *mouth*
GI: Constipation, dry mouth, nausea, vomiting, anorexia, diarrhea
GU: Retention, dysuria, frequency
*HEMA: **Thrombocytopenia, agranulocytosis, hemolytic anemia***
INTEG: Rash, urticaria, photosensitivity, sweating
RESP: Increased thick secretions, wheezing, chest tightness

Contraindications: Hypersensitivity to H_1-receptor antagonists, acute asthma attack, lower respiratory tract disease

Precautions: Increased intraocular pressure, renal disease, cardiac disease, hypertension, bronchial asthma, seizure disorder, stenosed peptic ulcers, hyperthyroidism, prostatic hypertrophy, bladder neck

---

obstruction, pregnancy **B**,
G elderly

Pharmacokinetics
Absorption	Well absorbed
Distribution	Widely distributed
Metabolism	Liver, extensively
Excretion	Kidneys, breast milk (high)
Half-life	Unknown

Pharmacodynamics
Onset	15-60 min
Peak	1-2 hr
Duration	12 hr

Interactions
Individual drugs
Alcohol: ↑ CNS depression
Drug classifications
CNS depressants: ↑ CNS depression
MAOI: ↑ anticholinergic effect
Opioids: ↑ CNS depression
Sedative/hypnotics: ↑ CNS depression
Herb/drug
Henbane leaf: ↑ anticholinergic effect
Kava: ↑ CNS depression
Lab test interferences
False negative: Skin allergy tests (discontinue antihistamines 3 days before testing)

NURSING CONSIDERATIONS
Assessment
• Assess respiratory status: rate, rhythm, increase in bronchial secretions, wheezing, chest tightness; provide fluids to 2 L/day to decrease secretion thickness
• Monitor I&O ratio: be alert for urinary retention, frequency, dysuria, especially
G elderly; drug should be discontinued if these occur

Nursing diagnoses
☑ Airway clearance, ineffective (uses)
☑ Injury, risk for (side effects)
☑ Knowledge deficit (teaching)
☑ Noncompliance (teaching, overuse)

Implementation
• May give with food to decrease GI upset
🚫 • Do not crush or chew caps
• Store in tight, light-resistant container

Patient/family education
• Teach all aspects of drug uses; to notify prescriber if confusion, sedation, hypotension occur; to avoid driving and other hazardous activity if drowsiness occurs; to avoid alcohol and other CNS depressants that may potentiate effect
• Instruct patient to take 1 hr ac or 2 hr pc to facilitate absorption
• Caution patient not to exceed recommended dosage; dysrhythmias may occur
• Teach patient hard candy, gum, frequent rinsing of mouth may be used for dryness
• Tell patient if EENT or CNS symptoms occur (blurred vision, severe dry mouth, dry throat, confusion, dizziness, poor coordination, euphoria), prescriber should be notified

Evaluation
Positive therapeutic outcome
• Absence of running or congested nose, rashes

Treatment of overdose:
Administer ipecac syrup or lavage, diazepam, vasopressors, barbiturates (short acting)

clindamycin HCl (Ŗ)
(klin-dah-my′sin)
Cleocin HCl
clindamycin palmitate (Ŗ)
Cleocin Pediatric, Dalacin C Palmitate
clindamycin phosphate (Ŗ)
Cleocin Phosphate, Dalacin C, Dalacin C Phosphate
Func. class.: Antiinfective, misc.
Chem. class.: Lincomycin derivative

Pregnancy category   B

Action: Binds to 50S subunit of bacterial ribosomes; suppresses protein synthesis

Therapeutic Outcome: Absence of infection

Uses: Infections caused by staphylococci, streptococci, *Rickettsia, Fusobacterium, Actinomyces, Peptococcus, Clostridium*

Dosage and routes
Adults: PO 150-450 mg q6hr; IM/**IV** 1.2-1.8 g/day in 2-4 divided doses mg q6-12hr, not to exceed 4800 mg/day

Vaginal route
Adult: 5 g applicatorful at bedtime × 1 wk

Topical route
Adult: Sol 1% apply bid

PID: Adult **IV** 600 mg q6h plus gentamicin

P *Child <1 mo:* 15-20 mg/kg/day divided q6-8h

P *Child >1 mo:* PO 8-20 mg/kg/day in divided doses q6-8hr; IM/**IV** 20-40 mg/kg/day in divided doses q6-8hr in 3-4 equal doses

Available forms: Phosphate: Inj 150, 300, 600 mg base/4 ml; 900 mg base/ml; 900 mg base/60 ml; inj Inf in D$_5$ 300, 600, 900 mg; HCL: caps 75, 150, 300 mg; palmitate: oral sol 75 mg/ml

Adverse effects
EENT: Rash, urticaria, pruritus, erythema, pain, abscess at injection site
GI: Nausea, vomiting, abdominal pain, diarrhea, **pseudomembranous colitis,** *anorexia, weight loss*
GU: Increased AST, ALT, bilirubin, alk phosphatase, jaundice, *vaginitis,* urinary frequency
HEMA: **Leukopenia, eosinophilia, agranulocytosis, thrombocytopenia, polyarthritis**

Contraindications: Hypersensitivity to this drug or lincomycin, ulcerative colitis/enteritis

Precautions: Renal disease, liver disease, GI disease, elderly, pregnancy **B**, lactation, tartrazine sensitivity

Pharmacokinetics

Absorption	Well absorbed (PO, IM), minimal (top)
Distribution	Widely distributed; crosses placenta
Metabolism	Liver, extensively
Excretion	Kidneys, breast milk
Half-life	2½ hr

Pharmacodynamics

	PO	IM	IV	TOP	VAG
Onset	Rapid	Rapid	Rapid	Rapid	Rapid
Peak	½-1 hr	1½ hr	Infusion's end	Unknown	Unknown

Interactions
Individual drugs
Chloramphenicol: ↓ action of chloramphenicol
Erythromycin: ↓ action of clindamycin
Kaolin: ↓ absorption

Drug classifications
Neuromuscular blockers: ↑ neuromuscular blockade

Lab test interferences
↑ Alk phosphatase, ↑ bilirubin, ↑ CPK, ↑ AST, ↑ ALT

NURSING CONSIDERATIONS
Assessment
• Assess any patient with compromised renal system; drug is excreted slowly in poor renal system function; toxicity may occur rapidly
• Assess patient for signs and symptoms of infection including characteristics of wounds, sputum, urine, stool, WBC >10,000, fever; obtain baseline information before and during treatment
• Complete culture and sensitivity testing before beginning drug therapy; this will identify if correct treatment has been initiated
• Assess for allergic reactions: rash, urticaria, pruritus, chills, fever, joint pain; may occur a few days after therapy begins; epinephrine and resuscitation equipment should be available in case of an anaphylactic reaction
• Identify urine output; if decreasing, notify prescriber (may indicate nephrotoxicity); also look for increased BUN and creatinine levels
• Monitor blood studies: AST, ALT, CBC, Hct, bilirubin, LDH, alk phosphatase, Coombs' test monthly if patient is on long-term therapy
• Monitor electrolytes: potassium, sodium, chloride monthly if patient is on long-term therapy
• Assess bowel pattern qd; if severe diarrhea occurs, drug should be discontinued; may indicate pseudomembranous colitis
• Monitor for bleeding: ecchymosis, bleeding gums, hematuria, stool guaiac daily if on long-term therapy
• Assess for overgrowth of infection: perineal itching, fever, malaise, redness, pain, swelling, drainage, rash, diarrhea, change in cough, sputum

Nursing diagnoses
☑ Infection, risk for (uses)
☑ Diarrhea (adverse reactions)
☑ Injury, risk for (adverse reaction)
☑ Knowledge deficit (teaching)
☑ Noncompliance (teaching)

Implementation
PO route
• Give with 8 oz of water; give with meals for GI symptoms
• Shake liquids well
• Do not refrigerate oral preparations; stable at room temperature for 2 wks
🚫• Do not crush, chew caps
IM route
• If more than 600 mg must be given, divide into two injections
• Give deeply in large muscle mass; rotate sites
Ⅳ IV route
• Give by infusion only; do not administer bolus dose; dilute 300 mg or more/50 ml or more of D$_5$W, NS
• May be further diluted in greater amounts of D$_5$W, 0.9% NaCl and given as a cont inf in acute pelvic inflammatory disease (PID); give first dose

---

☑ Herb/drug   🚫 Do Not Crush   ◆ Alert   ⟔ Key Drug   🄶 Geriatric   🄿 Pediatric

10 mg/min over ½ hr, then 0.75 mg/min; increased rates may be used to keep serum blood levels higher; run over >10 min; no more than 120 mg in a 1 hr inf

Syringe compatibilities:
Amikacin, aztreonam, gentamicin, heparin

Syringe incompatibilities:
Tobramycin

Y-site incompatibilities:
Idarubicin

Y-site compatibilities:
Amifostine, amiodarone, amphotericin B cholesteryl, amsacrine, aztreonam, cisatracurium, cyclophosphamide, diltiazem, doxorubicin liposome, enalaprilat, esmolol, fludarabine, foscarnet, granisetron, heparin, hydromorphone, labetolol, magnesium sulfate, melphalan, meperidine, midazolam, morphine, multivitamins, odansetron, perphenazine, piperacillin/tazobactam, propofol, remifentanil, sargramostim, tacrolimus, teniposide, theophylline, thiotepa, vinorelbine, vit B/C, zidovudine

Additive compatibilities
Amikacin, ampicillin, aztreonam, cefamandole, cefazolin, cefepine, cefonicid, cefoperazone, cefotaxime, cefoxitin, ceftazidime, ceftizoxime, cefuroxime, cephalothin, cimetidine, fluconazole, heparin, hydrocortisone, kanamycin, methylplednisolone, metoclopramide, metronidazole, netilmicin, ofloxacin, penicillin G, pipercillin, potassium chloride, sodium bicarbonate, tobramycin, verapamil, vit B/C

Additive incompatibilities:
Ciprofloxacin

Top route
• Avoid contact with eyes, mucous membranes, and open cuts during topical application; if accidental contact occurs, rinse with cool water
• Wash affected areas with warm water and soap, rinse, pat dry before application

Patient/family education
• Tell patient to take oral drug with full glass of water; may take with food if GI symptoms occur; antiperistaltic drugs may worsen diarrhea
• Teach patient aspects of drug therapy: need to complete entire course of medication to ensure organism death (10-14 days); culture may be taken after medication course has been completed
• Advise patient to report sore throat, fever, fatigue; may indicate superimposed infection
• Advise patient that drug must be taken at equal intervals around clock to maintain blood levels

Evaluation
Positive therapeutic outcome
• Decreased temperature, negative C&S

Treatment of hypersensitivity: Withdraw drug; maintain airway; administer epinephrine, aminophylline, O₂, **IV** corticosteroids

---

clofazimine (℞)
(kloe-faz′i-meen)
Lamprene
Func. class.: Leprostatic
Pregnancy category   C

Action: Inhibits mycobacterial growth, binds to mycobacterial DNA; exerts antiinflammatory

---

properties in controlling leprosy reactions

→**Therapeutic Outcome:** Decreased infection of leprosy

Uses: Lepromatous leprosy, dapsone-resistant leprosy, lepromatous leprosy complicated by erythema nodosum leprosum

Dosage and routes
Erythema nodosum leprosum
Adult: PO 100-200 mg qd × 3 mo, then taper dosage to 100 mg when disease is controlled; do not exceed 200 mg/day

Dapsone-resistant leprosy
Adult: PO 100 mg/day in combination with at least one other antileprosy drug × 3 yr, then 100 mg qd clofazimine only

Available forms: Caps 50 mg

Adverse effects
CNS: Dizziness, headache, fatigue, drowsiness
EENT: Pigmentation of cornea and conjunctiva, drying, burning, itching, irritation
GI: Diarrhea, nausea, vomiting, abdominal pain, intolerance, **GI bleeding, obstruction,** anorexia, constipation, **hepatitis,** jaundice
INTEG: Pink or brown discoloration, dryness, pruritus, rash, photosensitivity, acne, monilial cheilosis
MISC: Discolored urine, feces, sputum, sweat

Contraindications:
Hypersensitivity to this drug

Precautions: Pregnancy C, **P** lactation, children, abdominal pain, diarrhea, depression

Pharmacokinetics
Absorption	Partially
Distribution	Crosses placenta
Metabolism	Liver
Excretion	Feces, bile
Half-life	70 days

Pharmacodynamics
Unknown

Interactions
Individual drugs
Alcohol: ↑ toxicity
Carbamazepine: ↑ toxicity
Cycloserine: ↑ toxicity
Ethionamide: ↑ toxicity
Rifampin: ↑ toxicity
Drug classifications
Antacids, aluminum: ↓ absorption
Lab test interferences
↑ albumin, ↑ bilirubin, ↑ AST, ↑ eosinophilia, ↑ hypokalemia, ↑ glucose, ↑ ESR

NURSING CONSIDERATIONS
Assessment
• Perform liver studies weekly: ALT, AST, bilirubin
• Monitor renal status: before initiation of therapy, then monthly: BUN, creatinine, output, sp gr, urinalysis
• Assess mental status often: affect, mood, behavioral changes; psychosis may occur
• Monitor hepatic status: decreased appetite, jaundice, dark urine, fatigue

Nursing diagnoses
☑ Infection, risk for (uses)
☑ Diarrhea (side effects)
☑ Injury, risk for (side effects)
☑ Knowledge deficit (teaching)

Implementation
• Give with meals to decrease GI symptoms

☑ Herb/drug　🚫 Do Not Crush　🔶 Alert　⚕ Key Drug　🄶 Geriatric　🄿 Pediatric

- Provide antiemetic if vomiting occurs

🚫 • Do not crush, chew caps

Patient/family education
- Teach patient that compliance with dosage schedule, duration is necessary
- Teach patient that scheduled appointments must be kept or relapse may occur
- Caution patient to avoid alcohol while taking drug
- Teach diabetic patients to use blood glucose monitor to obtain correct result
- Advise patient to report weakness, fatigue, loss of appetite, nausea, vomiting, yellowing of skin or eyes, tingling/numbness of hands/feet

Evaluation
Positive therapeutic outcome
- Decreased symptoms of leprosy

---

clomiphene (℞)
(kloe'mi-feen)
Clomid, clomiphene citrate, Milophene, Serophene
Func. class.: Ovulation stimulant
Chem. class.: Nonsteroidal antiestrogenic
Pregnancy category X

Action: Increases LH, FSH release from the pituitary, which increase maturation of ovarian follicle, ovulation, development of corpus luteum

➡️**Therapeutic Outcome:** Pregnancy

Uses: Female infertility (ovulatory failure)

Dosage and routes
Adult: PO 50-100 mg qd × 5 days or 50-100 mg qd beginning on day 5 of cycle; may be repeated until conception occurs or 3 cycles of therapy have been completed

Available forms: Tabs 50 mg

Adverse effects
CNS: Headache, depression, restlessness, anxiety, nervousness, fatigue, insomnia, dizziness, flushing
CV: Vasomotor flushing, phlebitis, **deep vein thrombosis**
EENT: Blurred vision, diplopia, photophobia
GI: Nausea, vomiting, constipation, abdominal pain, bloating
GU: Polyuria, frequency of urination, **birth defects, spontaneous abortions,** multiple ovulation, breast pain, oliguria, abnormal uterine bleeding
INTEG: Rash, dermatitis, urticaria, alopecia

Contraindications: Hypersensitivity, pregnancy **X,** hepatic disease, undiagnosed uterine bleeding, uncontrolled thyroid or adrenal dysfunction, intracranial lesion, ovarian cysts

Precautions: Hypertension, depression, convulsions, diabetes mellitus

🚫 **Do Not Confuse:**
clomiphene/clomipramine

Pharmacokinetics	
Absorption	Well distributed
Distribution	Unknown
Metabolism	Liver, extensively
Excretion	Feces
Half-life	5 days

Pharmacodynamics
Unknown

Interactions: None
Lab test interferences
↑ FSH/LH, ↑ BSP, ↑ thyroxine, ↑ TBG

NURSING CONSIDERATIONS
Assessment
• Determine liver function tests before therapy: AST, ALT, alkaline phosphatase
• Monitor serum progesterone, urinary excretion of pregnanediol to identify occurrence of ovulation
• Pelvic examination should be done to determine ovarian size, cervical condition
• Endometrial biopsy may be done in women over 35 to rule out endometrial carcinoma

Nursing diagnoses
☑Sexual dysfunction (uses)
☑Knowledge deficit (teaching)

Implementation
• Give after discontinuing estrogen therapy
• Give at same time qd to maintain drug level; begin on 5th day of menstrual cycle

Patient/family education
• Advise patient that multiple births are common after drug is taken
• Instruct patient to notify prescriber immediately if low abdominal pain occurs; may indicate ovarian cyst, cyst rupture
• Advise patient to notify prescriber of photophobia, blurred vision, diplopia
• Teach patient if dose is missed, double at next time; if more than one dose is missed, call prescriber
• Instruct patient that response usually occurs 4-10 days after last day of treatment
• Teach patient method for taking, recording basal body temp to determine whether ovulation has occurred; if ovulation can be determined (there is a slight decrease in temp, then a sharp increase for ovulation), to attempt coitus 3 days before and qod until after ovulation
• Teach patient if pregnancy is suspected, to notify prescriber immediately

Evaluation
Positive therapeutic outcome
• Fertility

---

clomipramine (℞)
(klom-ip′ra-meen)
Anafranil
Func. class.: Tricyclic antidepressant
Chem. class.: Tertiary amine
Pregnancy category   C

Action: Potent inhibitor of serotonin uptake; also increases dopamine metabolism

▸**Therapeutic Outcome:** Decreased signs and symptoms of obsessive-compulsive disorder, decreased depression

Uses: Depression, dysphoria, anxiety, agoraphobia and other phobias, obsessive-compulsive disorder

Dosage and routes
Obsessive-compulsive disorder
Adult: PO 25 mg hs; increase gradually over 4 wk to a dosage of 75-300 mg/day in divided doses

▣ *Child 10-18 yr:* PO 25-50 mg/day gradually increased or 3 mg/kg/day whichever is smaller; not to exceed 200 mg/day

Depression
Adult: PO 50-150 mg/day in a single or divided dose

Anxiety/agoraphobia
Adult: PO 25-75 mg/day
Available forms: Caps 25, 50, 75 mg

Adverse effects
CNS: Dizziness, tremors, ma-nia, **seizures**, aggressiveness
CV: Hypotension, tachycardia, **cardiac arrest**
ENDO: Galactorrhea, hyper-prolactinemia
GI: Constipation, dry mouth, nausea, dyspepsia
GU: Delayed ejaculation, anor-gasmy, retention
HEMA: **Agranulocytosis, neutropenia, pancytopenia**
INTEG: Diaphoresis
META: Hyponatremia

Contraindications: Hypersen-sitivity

Precautions: Seizures, suicidal patients, elderly, pregnancy C

Do Not Confuse:
clomipramine/clomiphene, clomipramine/desipramine

Pharmacokinetics	
Absorption	Well absorbed
Distribution	Widely distributed
Metabolism	Liver, extensively
Excretion	Kidneys, breast milk
Half-life	19-37 hr; steady state 1-2 wk

Pharmacodynamics	
Onset	≥2 wk
Peak	2-6 hr

Interactions
Individual drugs
Alcohol: ↑ CNS depression
Cimetidine: ↑ clomipramine level
Clonidine: Severe hypertension; avoid use
Epinephrine: Severe hyperten-sion, avoid use

Fluoxetine: ↑ clomipramine level
Fluvoxamine: ↑ clomipramine level
Guanethidine: ↓ effects
Norepinephrine: Severe hy-pertension, avoid use
Sertraline: ↑ clomipramine level

Drug classifications
Barbiturates: ↓ clomipramine levels
Benzodiazepines: ↑ effects
CNS depressants: ↑ effects
MAOIs: Hypertensive crisis, convulsions
Sympathomimetics, indirect-acting: ↓ effects
Oral contraceptives: ↑ effects, toxicity

Herb/drug
Belladonna leaf/root: ↑ anticholinergic effect
Henbane leaf: ↑ anticholiner-gic effect
Kava: ↑ CNS depression
Scopolia root: ↑ clomipramine effect

Lab test interferences
↑ Serum bilirubin, ↑ blood glucose, ↑ alkaline phosphatase ↓ VMA, ↓ 5-HIAA
False ↑ Urinary catechola-mines

NURSING CONSIDERATIONS
Assessment
• Monitor B/P (with patient lying, standing), pulse q4h; if systolic B/P drops 20 mm Hg hold drug, notify prescriber; take vital signs q4h in patients with cardiovascular disease
• Monitor blood studies: CBC, leukocytes, differential, cardiac enzymes if patient is receiving long-term therapy
• Monitor hepatic studies: AST, ALT, bilirubin
• Check weight weekly; appe-tite may increase with drug

• Assess ECG for flattening of T wave, QTc prolongation bundle branch block, AV block, dysrhythmias in cardiac patients

G • Assess for EPS primarily in elderly: rigidity, dystonia, akathisia

• Assess mental status: mood, sensorium, affect, suicidal tendencies; increase in psychiatric symptoms: depression, panic

P **G** • Monitor urinary retention, constipation; constipation is more likely to occur in children or elderly

• Assess for withdrawal symptoms: headache, nausea, vomiting, muscle pain, weakness; do not usually occur unless drug was discontinued abruptly

• Identify alcohol consumption; if alcohol is consumed, hold dose until morning

Nursing diagnoses

✓ Coping, ineffective individual (uses)

✓ Injury, risk for physical (side effects)

✓ Knowledge deficit (teaching)

✓ Noncompliance (teaching)

Implementation

• Give with food or milk for GI symptoms

🚫 • Do not crush, chew caps

• Store at room temp; do not freeze

Patient/family education

• Teach patient that therapeutic effects may take 2-3 wk

• Teach patient to use caution in driving or other activities requiring alertness because of drowsiness, dizziness, blurred vision; to avoid rising quickly from sitting to standing, especially elderly **G**

• Teach patient to avoid alcohol ingestion, other CNS depressants

• Teach patient not to discontinue medication quickly after long-term use: may cause nausea, headache, malaise

• Teach patient to wear sunscreen or large hat, since photosensitivity occurs

• Teach patient to increase fluids, bulk in diet if constipation, urinary retention occur, especially elderly **G**

• Teach patient to take gum, hard sugarless candy, or frequent sips of water for dry mouth

Evaluation

Positive therapeutic outcome

• Decrease in depression

• Absence of suicidal thoughts

Treatment of overdose:

ECG monitoring, induce emesis, lavage, activated charcoal, administer anticonvulsant

---

clonazepam (℞)

(kloe-na′zi-pam)

Klonopin, Rivotril, Syn-Clonazepam ✦

Func. class.: Anticonvulsant

Chem. class.: Benzodiazepine derivative

Pregnancy category **D**

Controlled substance schedule **IV**

Action: Inhibits spike, wave formation in absence seizures (petit mal), decreases amplitude, frequency, duration, spread of discharge in minor motor seizures

---

➔**Therapeutic Outcome:** Decreased frequency, severity of seizures

Uses: Absence, atypical absence, akinetic, myoclonic seizures, Lennox-Gastaut syndrome

Investigational uses: Parkinsonian dysarthrias, acute mania, adjunct in schizophrenia, neuralgias, multifocal tic disorders, restless leg syndrome

Dosage and routes

Adult: PO not to exceed 1.5 mg/day in 3 divided doses; may be increased 0.5-1 mg q3 days until desired response; not to exceed 20 mg/day

🅿 *Child <10 yr or 30 kg:* PO 0.01-0.03 mg/kg/day in divided doses q8h, not to exceed 0.05 mg/kg/day; may be increased 0.25-0.5 mg q3 days until desired response; not to exceed 0.1-0.2 mg/kg/day

Available forms: Tabs 0.5, 1, 2 mg

Adverse effects

CNS: Drowsiness, dizziness, confusion, behavioral changes, tremors, insomnia, headache, suicidal tendencies, slurred speech

CV: Palpitations, bradycardia

EENT: Increased salivation, nystagmus, diplopia, abnormal eye movements

GI: Nausea, constipation, polyphagia, anorexia, xerostomia, diarrhea, gastritis, sore gums

GU: Dysuria, enuresis, nocturia, retention

HEMA: **Thrombocytopenia, leukocytosis, eosinophilia**

INTEG: Rash, alopecia, hirsutism

RESP: **Respiratory depression,** dyspnea, congestion

Contraindications: Hypersensitivity to benzodiazepines, acute narrow-angle glaucoma, pregnancy **D**

Precautions: Open-angle glaucoma, chronic respiratory disease, renal/hepatic disease, 🅖elderly

🚫**Do Not Confuse:**

Klonopin/clonidine

Pharmacokinetics

Absorption	Well absorbed
Distribution	Crosses blood-brain barrier, placenta
Metabolism	Liver
Excretion	Kidneys
Half life	18-50 hr

Pharmacodynamics

Onset	½-1 hr
Peak	1-2 hr
Duration	6-12 hr

Interactions
Individual drugs

Alcohol: ↑ CNS depression

Carbamazepine: ↓ effectiveness

Cimetidine: ↓ metabolism, ↑ action

Disulfiram: ↓ metabolism, ↑ action

Fluoxetine: ↓ metabolism, ↑ action

Isoniazid: ↓ metabolism, ↑ action

Ketoconazole: ↓ metabolism, ↑ action

Metoprolol: ↓ metabolism, ↑ action

Phenytoin: ↓ clonazepam levels

Propoxyphene: ↓ metabolism, ↑ action

Propranolol: ↓ metabolism, ↑ action

Valproic acid: ↑ seizures
Drug classifications

Antidepressants: ↑ CNS depression

Anticonvulsants: ↑ CNS depression

Antihistamines: ↑ CNS depression

Barbiturates: ↑ CNS depression, ↓ effect of clonazepam

General anesthetics: ↑ CNS depression

Hypnotics: ↑ CNS depression

Opiates: ↑ CNS depression

Oral contraceptives: ↓ metabolism, ↑ action

Sedatives: ↑ CNS depression

⚗ *Herb/drug*

Kava: ↑ CNS depression

Lab test interferences

↑ AST, ↑ alkaline phosphatase

NURSING CONSIDERATIONS
Assessment

• Assess mental status: mood, sensorium, affect, memory

G (long, short), especially elderly

• Assess for blood dyscrasias: fever, sore throat, bruising, rash, jaundice, epistaxis (long-term treatment only)

• Monitor blood level: therapeutic level 20-80 ng/ml

• Assess seizure activity including type, location, duration, and character; provide seizure precaution

• Assess renal studies: urinalysis, BUN, urine creatinine

• Monitor blood studies: RBC, Hct, Hgb, reticulocyte counts weekly for 4 wk then monthly

• Monitor hepatic studies: ALT, AST, bilirubin, creatinine

• Monitor drug levels during initial treatment

• Assess for signs of physical withdrawal if medication suddenly discontinued

• Assess eye problems: need for ophthalmic examinations before, during, after treatment (slit lamp, fundoscopy, tonometry)

• Assess allergic reaction: red raised rash; if this occurs, drug should be discontinued

• Monitor for toxicity: bone marrow depression, nausea, vomiting, ataxia, diplopia, cardiovascular collapse

Nursing diagnoses

☑ Injury, risk for (side effects)

☑ Knowledge deficit (teaching)

Implementation

• Give on empty stomach for best absorption

Patient/family education

• Teach patient to carry ID card or Medic Alert bracelet stating patient's name, drugs taken, condition, physician's name, phone number

• Caution patient to avoid driving, other activities that require alertness

• Caution patient to avoid alcohol ingestion or CNS depressants; increased sedation may occur

• Teach patient not to discontinue medication quickly after long-term use; taper off over several weeks

Evaluation

Positive therapeutic outcome

• Decreased seizure activity

Treatment of overdose:

Lavage, activated charcoal, VS, monitor electrolytes

---

clonidine ⟋ (R̶)
(klon'i-deen)
Catapres, Catapres-TTS,
clonidine HCl, Dixarit ✦,
Duraclon
Func. class.: Antihypertensive, analgesic
Chem. class.: Central
α-adrenergic agonist
Pregnancy category   C

Action: Inhibits sympathetic vasomotor center in CNS, which reduces impulses in sympathetic nervous system; B/P, pulse rate, cardiac output decreased

▶**Therapeutic Outcome:** Decreased B/P in hypertension

Uses: Mild to moderate hypertension; used alone or in combination

Investigational uses: Narcotic withdrawal, prevention of vascular headaches, treatment of menopausal symptoms, dysmenorrhea, attention deficit disorder

Dosage and routes
Hypertension
Adult: PO/trans 0.1 mg bid, then increase by 0.1 mg/day or 0.2 mg/day until desired response; range 0.2-0.8 mg/day in divided doses

🄶*Elderly:* PO 0.1 mg hs, may increase gradually

🄿*Child:* 5-10 μg/kg/day in divided doses q8-12h, max 0.9 mg/day

Opioid withdrawal
Adult: PO 0.3-1.2 mg/day; decreased dosage given over several days

Severe pain
Adult: Cont epidural Inf 30 μg/hr

ADHD
🄿*Child:* 0.05 mg/day; titrate up to max 0.4 mg/day

Available forms: Tabs 0.025 ✦, 0.1, 0.2, 0.3 mg; trans sys 2.5, 5, 7.5 mg delivering 0.1, 0.2, 0.3 mg/24 hr, respectively

Adverse effects
CNS: Drowsiness, sedation, headache, fatigue, nightmares, insomnia, mental changes, anxiety, depression, hallucinations, delirium
CV: Orthostatic hypotension, palpitations, **CHF,** ECG abnormalities
EENT: Taste change, parotid pain
ENDO: Hyperglycemia
GI: Nausea, vomiting, malaise, constipation, dry mouth
GU: Impotence, dysuria, *nocturia,* gynecomastia
INTEG: Rash, alopecia, facial pallor, pruritus, hives, edema, burning papules, excoriation (trans patches)
MS: Muscle, joint pain, leg cramps

Contraindications: Hypersensitivity

Precautions: MI (recent), diabetes mellitus, chronic renal failure, Raynaud's disease, thyroid disease, depres-
🄿sion, COPD, child <12 (patches), asthma, pregnancy
🄶C, lactation, elderly, noncompliant patients

◨ **Do Not Confuse:**
clonidine/Klonopin,
Catapres/Cataflam

C

Pharmacokinetics

Absorption	Well absorbed (PO, trans)
Distribution	Widely distributed; crosses blood-brain barrier
Metabolism	Liver, extensively
Excretion	Kidneys, unchanged (30%)
Half-life	12-16 hr

Pharmacodynamics

	PO	TRANS
Onset	½-1 hr	3 days
Peak	2-4 hr	Unknown
Duration	8 hr	8 hr (after removal)

Interactions
Individual drugs
Alcohol: ↑ CNS depression
Levodopa: ↓ levodopa effect
Verapamil: AV block
Drug classifications
Amphetamines: ↓ hypotensive effects
Anesthetics: ↑ CNS depression
Antidepressants, tricyclic: ↓ hypotensive effects
β-Adrenergic blockers: ↑ bradycardia
Cardiac glycosides: ↑ bradycardia
Diuretics: ↑ hypotensive effects
Hypnotics: ↑ CNS depression
Nitrates: ↑ hypotensive effects
Opiates: ↑ CNS depression
Sedatives: ↑ CNS depression
Lab test interferences
↑ Blood glucose
↓ VMA, ↓ catecholamines, ↓ aldosterone

NURSING CONSIDERATIONS
Assessment
• Perform blood studies: neutrophils, decreased platelets
• Perform renal studies: protein, BUN, creatinine; watch for increased levels that may indicate nephrotic syndrome: polyuria, oliguria, frequency

• Monitor baselines in renal, liver function tests before therapy begins; check potassium levels, although hyperkalemia rarely occurs
• Monitor B/P, pulse if the drug is being used for hypertension; notify prescriber of changes
• Assess for opiate withdrawal in patients receiving the drug for opioid withdrawal, including fever, diarrhea, nausea, vomiting, cramps, insomnia, shivering, dilated pupils, weakness
• Check for edema in feet, legs daily; monitor I&O; check for decreasing output
• Note allergic reaction: rash, fever, pruritus, urticaria; drug should be discontinued if antihistamines fail to help
• Note allergic reaction from patches: rash, urticaria, angioedema; should not continue to use
• Assess for symptoms of CHF: edema, dyspnea, wet rales, B/P, weight gain
Nursing diagnoses
☑ Injury, potential for physical (side effects)
☑ Knowledge deficit (teaching)
☑ Noncompliance (teaching)
Implementation
PO route
• PO: give last dose at hs
Trans route
• Apply patch weekly; remove old patch and wash off residue; apply to site without hair; best absorption over chest or upper arm; rotate sites with each application; clean site before application; apply firmly, especially around edges
• Store patches in cool environment, tabs in tight container

☒ Herb/drug 🚫 Do Not Crush ◆ Alert ⚭ Key Drug 🅖 Geriatric 🅟 Pediatric

Patient/family education
• Instruct patient not to discontinue drug abruptly, or withdrawal symptoms may occur: anxiety, increased B/P, headache, insomnia, increased pulse, tremors, nausea, sweating
• Caution patient not to use OTC (cough, cold, or allergy) products unless directed by prescriber
• Caution patient to avoid sunlight or wear sunscreen, protective clothing if in sunlight; photosensitivity may occur
• Teach patient to comply with dosage schedule even if feeling better; drug controls symptoms, does not cure
• Caution patient to change position slowly, to rise slowly to sitting or standing position to minimize orthostatic hypotension, especially elderly
• Instruct patient to notify physician of mouth sores, sore throat, fever, swelling of hands or feet, irregular heartbeat, chest pain, signs of angioedema, increased weight
• Teach patient about excessive perspiration, dehydration, vomiting; diarrhea may lead to fall in B/P; consult prescriber if these occur
• Tell patient that drug may cause dizziness, fainting; lightheadedness may occur during 1st few days of therapy; use hard candy, saliva product, or frequent rinsing of mouth for dry mouth
• Advise patient that compliance is necessary; not to skip or stop drug unless directed by prescriber
• Teach patient that drug may cause skin rash or impaired perspiration

• Teach patient that response may take 2-3 days if drug is given trans; instruct on administration of patch; return demonstration
• Teach patient to avoid hazardous activities, since drug may cause drowsiness, dizziness
• Teach patient to administer 1 hr ac

Evaluation
Positive therapeutic outcome
• Decrease in B/P in hypertension
• Decrease in withdrawal symptoms
• Decrease in pain
• Decrease in vascular headaches
• Decrease in dysmenorrhea
• Decrease in menopausal symptoms

Treatment of overdose:
Supportive treatment; administer tolazoline, atropine, dopamine prn

clopidogrel (Ŗ)
(klo-pid′oh-grel)
Plavix
Func. class.: Platelet aggregation inhibitor
Chem. class.: Thienopyridine derivative
Pregnancy category **B**

Action: Inhibits first and second phases of ADP-induced effects in platelet aggregation

Therapeutic Outcome:
Decreased stroke by decreasing platelet aggregation

Uses: Reducing the risk of stroke in high-risk patients

Dosage and routes
Adult: PO 75 mg qd with or without food

Available forms: Tabs 75 mg

Adverse effects
CV: Edema, hypertension
CNS: Headache, dizziness
GI: Nausea, vomiting, diarrhea, GI discomfort
HEMA: Epistaxis, purpura
INTEG: Rash, pruritus
MISC: UTI, depression, hypercholesterolemia, chest pain, fatigue, **intracranial hemorrhage**
MS: Arthralgia, back pain
RESP: Upper respiratory tract infection, dyspnea, rhinitis, bronchitis, cough

Contraindications: Hypersensitivity, active bleeding

Precautions: Past liver disease, pregnancy **B**, lactation, P children, increased bleeding risk, neutropenia, agranulocytosis

Pharmacokinetics	
Absorption	Well absorbed
Distribution	Unknown
Metabolism	Liver, extensively
Excretion	Kidneys, unchanged drug
Half-life	Platelets 11 days

Pharmacodynamics	
Onset	Unknown
Peak	1-3 hr
Duration	Unknown

Interactions
Individual drugs
Aspirin: ↑ bleeding tendencies

Drug classifications
Anticoagulants: ↑ bleeding tendencies
NSAIDs: ↑ bleeding tendencies

NURSING CONSIDERATIONS
Assessment
• Monitor liver function studies: AST, ALT, bilirubin, creatinine if patient is on long-term therapy (4 mo or more)
• Monitor blood studies: CBC, Hct, Hgb, pro-time if patient is on long-term therapy; thrombocytopenia, neutropenia may occur

Nursing diagnoses
☑ Injury, risk for (uses)
☑ Knowledge deficit (teaching)

Implementation
• Give with food to decrease gastric symptoms

Patient/family education
• Advise patient that blood work will be necessary during treatment
• Advise patient to report any unusual bleeding to prescriber
• Instruct patient to take with food or just after eating to minimize GI discomfort
• Caution patient to report side effects such as diarrhea, skin rashes, subcutaneous bleeding

Evaluation
Positive therapeutic outcome
• Absence of stroke

clorazepate (R)
(klor-az'e-pate)

Apo-clorazepate ✦,
clorazepate dipotassium,
Gen-XENE, Tranxene,
Tranxene-SD, Tranxene
T-TAB

Func. class.: Antianxiety,
anticonvulsant

Chem. class.: Benzodiazepine

Pregnancy category D

**Controlled substance
schedule IV**

Action: Potentiates the actions
of GABA; especially in limbic
system, reticular formation has
anticonvulsant effects

⇒Therapeutic Outcome: Decreased anxiety, restlessness,
insomnia

Uses: Anxiety, acute alcohol
withdrawal, adjunct in seizure
disorders

Dosage and routes
Anxiety
Adult: PO 15-60 mg/day

G *Elderly:* PO 7.5 mg qd bid

Alcohol withdrawal
Adult: PO 30 mg then day 1,
30-60 mg in divided doses; day
2, 45-90 mg in divided doses;
day 3, 22.5-45 mg in divided
doses; day 4, 15-30 mg in
divided doses; then reduce
daily dose to 7.5-15 mg

Seizure disorders
P *Adult and child >12 yr:* PO
7.5 mg tid; may increase by 7.5
mg/wk or less, not to exceed
90 mg/day

P *Child 9-12 yr:* PO 7.5 mg bid;
may increase by 7.5 mg/wk or
less, not to exceed 60 mg/day

Available forms: Caps 3.75,
7.5, 15 mg; tabs 3.75, 7.5, 15
mg; single-dose tab 11.25,
22.5 mg

Adverse effects

CNS: Dizziness, drowsiness,
confusion, headache, anxiety,
tremors, stimulation, fatigue,
depression, insomnia, hallucinations, lethargy

CV: Orthostatic hypotension,
ECG changes, tachycardia,
hypotension

EENT: Blurred vision, tinnitus,
mydriasis

GI: Constipation, dry mouth,
nausea, vomiting, anorexia,
diarrhea

INTEG: Rash, dermatitis,
itching

Contraindications: Hypersensitivity to benzodiazepines,
narrow-angle glaucoma, psychosis, pregnancy **D,** child
<18 yr

G Precautions: Elderly, debilitated, hepatic disease, renal
disease

Pharmacokinetics	
Absorption	Well absorbed
Distribution	Widely distributed; crosses placenta
Metabolism	Liver
Excretion	Kidneys, breast milk
Half-life	30-100 hr

Pharmacodynamics	
Onset	15 min
Peak	1-2 hr
Duration	4-6 hr

Interactions
Individual drugs
Alcohol: ↑ CNS depression
Cimetidine: ↑ effects of clo-
razepate
Disulfiram: ↑ effects of clo-
razepate
Fluoxetine: ↑ clorazepate
effects

Ketoconazole: ↑ clorazepate effects

Valproic acid: ↑ effects of clorazepate

Drug classifications

CNS depressants: ↑ CNS depression

MAOI: ↑ effects of clorazepate

Oral contraceptives: ↑ effects of clorazepate

Herb/drug

Kava: ↑ CNS depression

Lab test interferences

↑ AST/ALT

NURSING CONSIDERATIONS
Assessment

• Monitor B/P (with patient lying, standing), pulse; if systolic B/P drops 20 mm Hg, hold drug, notify prescriber

• Monitor blood studies: CBC during long-term therapy; blood dyscrasias have occurred rarely

• Monitor hepatic studies: AST, ALT, bilirubin, creatinine, LDH, alkaline phosphatase

• Monitor I&O; may indicate renal dysfunction

• Monitor mental status: mood, sensorium, affect, sleeping pattern, drowsiness, dizziness, physical dependency; withdrawal symptoms: headache, nausea, vomiting, muscle pain, weakness after long-term use; suicidal tendencies

Nursing diagnoses

✓ Coping, ineffective individual (uses)

✓ Knowledge deficit (teaching)

✓ Noncompliance (teaching)

Implementation

• Give with food or milk for GI symptoms

🚫 • Do not chew, crush caps

• Use sugarless gum, hard candy, frequent sips of water for dry mouth

• Check to see PO medication has been swallowed

Patient/family education

• Teach patient that drug may be taken with food

• Teach patient not to use for everyday stress or longer than 4 mo, unless directed by a prescriber; not to take more than prescribed amount; may be habit forming

• Caution patient to avoid OTC preparations unless approved by a prescriber

G • Caution patient to avoid driving, activities that require alertness; drowsiness may occur, especially in elderly

• Advise patient to avoid alcohol ingestion or other psychotropic medications, unless prescribed

• Advise patient not to discontinue medication abruptly after long-term use

• Advise patient to rise slowly or fainting may occur

• Teach patient that drowsiness may worsen at beginning of treatment

Evaluation

Positive therapeutic outcome

• Decreased anxiety, restlessness

• Decreased seizure activity

Treatment of overdose:

Lavage, VS, supportive care, flumazenil

---

cloxacillin (℞)

(klox-a-sill'in)
Apo-Cloxi ✤, Bactopen ✤,
cloxacillin sodium, Cloxapen,
Novo-cloxin ✤, Orbenin ✤
Func. class.: Broad-
spectrum antiinfective
Chem. class.: Penicillinase-
resistant penicillin
Pregnancy category B

Action: Interferes with cell wall
replication of susceptible organisms; the cell wall, rendered
osmotically unstable, swells,
bursts from osmotic pressure

▣ **Therapeutic Outcome:**
Bactericidal effects for the
following: gram-positive cocci
*Staphylococcus aureus, S. epider-
mis,* penicillinase-producing
staphylococci

Uses: Penicillinase-producing
staphylococci, streptococci;
respiratory tract, skin, skin
structure infections; sinusitis
Dosage and routes
Adult: PO 1-4 g/day in divided doses q6h or 250 mg-1 g
q6h
▣ *Child:* PO 50-100 mg/kg in
divided doses q6h, max 4
g/day
Available forms: Caps 250,
500 mg; powder for oral susp
125 mg/5 ml
Adverse effects

CNS: Lethargy, hallucinations,
anxiety, depression, muscle
twitching, **coma, convulsions**
*GI: Nausea, vomiting, diar-
rhea,* increased AST, ALT,
abdominal pain, glossitis,
pseudomembranous colitis
GU: **Oliguria, proteinuria,**
hematuria, *vaginitis, moniliasis,*
glomerulonephritis

HEMA: Anemia, **increased
bleeding time, bone marrow
depression, granulocytopenia**
SYST: Anaphylaxis
Contraindications: Hypersensitivity to penicillins; neonates,
severe renal, hepatic disease
Precautions: Pregnancy **B,**
hypersensitivity to cephalosporins

Pharmacokinetics	
Absorption	Moderate (35%-60%)
Distribution	Widely distributed; crosses placenta
Metabolism	Liver (up to 22%)
Excretion	Breast milk; kidneys, unchanged (30%-45%)
Half-life	0.5-1.1 hr, increased in hepatic/renal disease

Pharmacodynamics	
Onset	½ hr
Peak	½-2 hr

Interactions
Individual drugs

Aspirin: ↑ cloxacillin concentrations
Disulfiram: ↑ cloxacillin concentrations
Probenecid: ↑ cloxacillin
concentrations, ↓ renal excretion
Drug classifications

Oral anticoagulants: ↑ anticoagulant effects
Oral contraceptives: ↓ action
of oral contraceptives
Food/drug

**Food, carbonated drinks,
citrus fruit juices:** ↓ absorption
▣ *Herb/drug*

Khat: ↓ absorption, separate
by ≥2 hr
Lab test interferences

False positive: Urine glucose,
urine protein

NURSING CONSIDERATIONS
Assessment

• Assess patient for previous sensitivity reaction to penicillins or other cephalosporins; cross-sensitivity between penicillins and cephalosporins is common
• Assess patient for signs and symptoms of infection including characteristics of wounds, sputum, urine, stool, WBC >10,000, fever; obtain baseline information and during treatment
• Obtain C&S before beginning drug therapy to identify if correct treatment has been initiated
• Assess for allergic reactions: rash, urticaria, pruritus, chills, fever, joint pain may occur a few days after therapy begins; epinephrine and resuscitation equipment should be available for anaphylactic reaction
◆• Identify urine output; if decreasing, notify prescriber (may indicate nephrotoxicity); also check for increased BUN, creatinine
• Monitor blood studies: AST, ALT, CBC, Hct, bilirubin, LDH, alkaline phosphatase, Coombs' test monthly if patient is on long-term therapy
• Monitor electrolytes: potassium, sodium, chloride monthly if patient is on long-term therapy
• Assess bowel pattern qd; if severe diarrhea occurs, drug should be discontinued; may indicate pseudomembranous colitis
• Monitor for bleeding: ecchymosis, bleeding gums, hematuria, stool guaiac daily if on long-term therapy
• Assess for overgrowth of infection: perineal itching, fever, malaise, redness, pain, swelling, drainage, rash, diarrhea, change in cough, sputum

Nursing diagnoses

☑ Infection, risk for (uses)
☑ Diarrhea (side effects)
☑ Injury, risk for (side effects)
☑ Knowledge deficit (teaching)
☑ Noncompliance (teaching)

Implementation

• Give in even doses around the clock; if GI upset occurs, give with food; drug must be given for 10-14 days to ensure organism death and prevent superinfection; store in airtight container
🚫• Do not crush, chew caps
• Shake susp well before each dose; store in refrigerator for 2 wk, 1 wk at room temp

Patient/family education

• Teach patient to report sore throat, bruising, bleeding, joint pain; may indicate blood dyscrasias (rare)
• Advise patient to contact prescriber if vaginal itching, loose, foul-smelling stools, furry tongue occur; may indicate superinfection
• Instruct patient to take all medications prescribed for the length of time ordered
• Advise patient to notify prescriber of diarrhea with blood or pus, which may indicate pseudomembranous colitis

Evaluation

Positive therapeutic outcome
• Absence of signs/symptoms of infection (WBC <10,000, temp WNL, absence of red, draining wounds)
• Reported improvement in symptoms of infection

Treatment of anaphylaxis:

Withdraw drug, maintain airway, administer epinephrine,

☑ Herb/drug   🚫 Do Not Crush   ◆ Alert   ☗ Key Drug   🅖 Geriatric   🅟 Pediatric aminophylline, O_2, **IV** corticosteroids

clozapine (℞)
(kloz'a-peen)
clozapine, Clozaril
Func. class.: Antipsychotic
Chem. class.: Tricyclic dibenzodiazepine derivative
Pregnancy category **B**

Action: Interferes with dopamine receptor binding with lack of extrapyramidal symptoms and tardive dyskinesia; also acts as an adrenergic, cholinergic, histaminergic, serotonergic antagonist

➡ **Therapeutic Outcome:** Decreased psychotic behavior

Uses: Management of psychotic symptoms in schizophrenic patients for whom other antipsychotics have failed

Dosage and routes
Adult: PO 25 mg qd or bid; may increase by 25-50 mg/day; normal range 300-450 mg/day after 2 wk; do not increase dosage more than 2 times/wk; do not exceed 900 mg/day; use lowest dosage to control symptoms

Available forms: Tabs 25, 100 mg

Adverse effects
CNS: Sedation, salivation, dizziness, headache, tremors, sleep problems, akinesia, fever, **seizures,** *sweating, akathisia, confusion, fatigue, insomnia, depression, slurred speech, anxiety,* **neuroleptic malignant syndrome**
CV: Tachycardia, hypotension, hypertension, chest pain, ECG changes

GI: Drooling or excessive salivation, constipation, nausea, abdominal discomfort, vomiting, diarrhea, anorexia
GU: Urinary abnormalities, incontinence, ejaculation dysfunction, frequency, urgency, retention
HEMA: Leukopenia, neutropenia, agranulocytosis, eosinophilia
MS: Weakness; pain in back, neck, legs; spasm
RESP: Dyspnea, nasal congestion, throat discomfort

Contraindications: Hypersensitivity, myeloproliferative disorders, severe granulocytopenia, CNS depression, coma, narrow-angle glaucoma

Precautions: Pregnancy **B**, lactation, children <16, hepatic, renal, cardiac disease, seizures, prostatic enlargement, elderly

🚫 **Do Not Confuse:**
Clozaril/Clinoril

Pharmacokinetics	
Absorption	Well absorbed
Distribution	Widely distributed; crosses blood-brain barrier, placenta; 95% bound to plasma proteins
Metabolism	Liver
Excretion	Kidneys, feces (metabolites)
Half-life	8-12 hr

Pharmacodynamics	
Onset	Unknown
Peak	Steady state 2½ hr
Duration	4-12 hr

Interactions
Individual drugs
Alcohol: ↑ effects of both drugs, oversedation
Digoxin: ↑ plasma concentration of digoxin

Warfarin: ↑ plasma concentrations
Drug classifications
Antacids: ↓ absorption
Anticholinergics: ↑ anticholinergic effects
Antidepressants: ↑ CNS depression
Antihistamines: ↑ CNS depression
Antihypertensives: ↑ hypotension
Antineoplastics: ↑ bone marrow suppression
Food/drug
Caffeine: ↓ clozapine levels
☑ *Herb/drug*
Kava: ↑ CNS depression
Lab test interferences
↑ Liver function tests, ↑ cardiac enzymes, ↑ cholesterol, ↑ blood glucose, ↑ prolactin, ↑ bilirubin, ↑ PBI, ↑ cholinesterase,^{131}I
False positive: Pregnancy tests, PKU
False negative: Urinary steroids, 17-OHCS

NURSING CONSIDERATIONS
Assessment
• Assess mental status: orientation, mood, behavior, presence of hallucinations, and type before initial administration and monthly; this drug should significantly reduce psychotic behavior
• Check for swallowing of PO medication; check for hoarding or giving of medication to other patients
• Monitor I&O ratio, palpate bladder if low urinary output
🜨 occurs, especially in elderly; urinalysis recommended before, during prolonged therapy
• Monitor bilirubin, CBC, liver function studies monthly; discontinue treatment if WBC <3000/mm^3 or if granulocyte <1500/mm^3; test q wk
• Assess affect, orientation, LOC, reflexes, gait, coordination, sleep pattern disturbances
• Monitor B/P with patient sitting, standing, and lying; take pulse and respirations q4h during initial treatment; establish baseline before starting treatment; report drops of 30 mm Hg
• Check for dizziness, faintness, palpitations, tachycardia on rising
• Identify for neuroleptic malignant syndrome: hyperpyrexia, muscle rigidity, increased CPK, altered mental status; drug should be discontinued
• Assess for extrapyramidal symptoms including akathisia (inability to sit still, no pattern to movements), tardive dyskinesia (bizarre movements of the jaw, mouth, tongue, extremities), pseudoparkinsonism (rigidity, tremors, pill rolling, shuffling gate)
• Assess for constipation, urinary retention daily; if these occur, increase bulk, water in diet
Nursing diagnoses
☑ Thought processes, altered (uses)
☑ Coping, ineffective individual (uses)
☑ Knowledge deficit (teaching)
☑ Noncompliance (teaching)
Implementation
🜨 • Decrease dosage in elderly since metabolism is slowed
• Give with full glass of water, milk; or give with food to decrease GI upset
• Store in tight, light-resistant container; oral sol in amber bottle

---

Patient/family education
• Teach patient to use good oral hygiene; frequent rinsing of mouth, sugarless gum for dry mouth
• Caution patient to avoid hazardous activities until drug response is determined
• Inform patient that orthostatic hypotension occurs often and to rise from sitting or lying position gradually
• Caution patient to avoid hot tubs, hot showers, tub baths, since hypotension may occur
• Teach patient to avoid OTC preparations (cough, hay fever, cold) unless approved by prescriber, since serious drug interactions may occur; avoid use with alcohol, CNS depressants; increased drowsiness may occur
• Teach patient about extrapyramidal symptoms and necessity of meticulous oral hygiene, since oral candidiasis may occur
• Teach patient to report sore throat, malaise, fever, bleeding, mouth sores; if these occur, CBC should be drawn and drug discontinued
• Advise patient that in hot weather, heat stroke may occur; take extra precautions to stay cool
• Teach patient symptoms of agranulocytosis and need for blood test q wk; report flu-like symptoms

Evaluation
Positive therapeutic outcome
• Decrease in emotional excitement, hallucinations, delusions, paranoia
• Reorganization of patterns of thought, speech

Treatment of anaphylaxis: Withdraw drug, maintain airway

---

coagulation factor VIIa, recombinant
See Appendix A, Selected New Drugs

---

codeine ⚷ (℞)
(koe'deen)
Paveral ✦, Codeine
Narcotic analgesics
Func. class.: Opiate, phenanthrene derivative

Pregnancy category **C**
Controlled substance schedule **II, III, IV, V**
(depends on route)

Action: Depresses pain impulse transmission at the spinal cord level by interacting with opioid receptors; decreases cough reflex, GI motility

Therapeutic Outcome: Pain relief, decreased cough, decreased diarrhea depending on route

Uses: Moderate to severe pain, nonproductive cough

Investigational uses: Diarrhea

Dosage and routes
Pain
Adult: PO 15-60 mg q4h prn; IM/SC 15-60 mg q4h prn
P *Child:* PO 3 mg/kg/day in divided doses q4h prn

Cough
Adult: PO 10-20 mg q4-6h, not to exceed 120 mg/day
P *Child:* PO 1-1.5 mg/kg/day in 4 divided doses, not to exceed 60 mg/day

Diarrhea
Adult: PO 30 mg; may repeat qid prn

✦ Canada Only   Adverse effects: *italic* = common; **bold** = life-threatening

Renal dose
CrCl 10-50 ml/min 75% of dose; CrCl <10 ml/min 50% of dose

Available forms: Inj 15, 30, 60 mg/ml; tabs 15, 30, 60 mg; oral sol 10mg/5 ml ♣, 15 mg/5 ml

Adverse effects
CNS: Drowsiness, sedation, dizziness, agitation, dependency, lethargy, restlessness
CV: Bradycardia, palpitations, orthostatic hypotension, tachycardia
GI: Nausea, vomiting, anorexia, constipation
GU: Urinary retention
INTEG: Flushing, rash, urticaria
RESP: **Respiratory depression, respiratory paralysis**

Contraindications: Hypersensitivity to opiates, respiratory depression, increased intracranial pressure, seizure disorders, severe respiratory disorders

G Precautions: Elderly, cardiac dysrhythmias, pregnancy **C**

N Do Not Confuse:
codeine/Lodine

Pharmacokinetics

Absorption	Complete (IM)
Distribution	Widely distributed; crosses placenta
Metabolism	Liver, extensively
Excretion	Kidneys (up to 15%), breast milk
Half-life	3-4 hr

Pharmacodynamics

	PO	IM	SC
Onset	30-45 min	15-30 min	15-30 min
Peak	1-2 hr	30-60 min	Unknown
Duration	4 hr	4 hr	4 hr

Interactions
Individual drugs
Alcohol: ↑ respiratory depression, hypotension, ↑ sedation
Drug classifications
Antihistamines: ↑ respiratory depression, hypotension
CNS depressants: ↑ respiratory depression, hypotension
MAOI: Use with caution
Phenothiazines: ↑ respiratory depression, hypotension
Sedative/hypnotics: ↑ respiratory depression, hypotension
✓ Herb/drug
Kava: ↑ CNS depression
Lab test interferences
↑ Amylase, ↑ lipase

NURSING CONSIDERATIONS
Assessment
• Assess pain: intensity, type, alleviating factors
• Monitor VS after parenteral route; note muscle rigidity, drug history, liver, kidney function tests, respiratory dysfunction: respiratory depression, character, rate, rhythm; notify prescriber if respirations are <10/min
• Monitor CNS changes: dizziness, drowsiness, hallucinations, euphoria, LOC, pupil reaction
• Monitor allergic reactions: rash, urticaria
Nursing diagnoses
✓ Pain (uses)
✓ Sensory perceptual alteration: visual, auditory (adverse reactions)
✓ Breathing pattern, ineffective (adverse reactions)
✓ Knowledge deficit (teaching)
Implementation
• Give with antiemetic if nausea, vomiting occur
• Administer when pain is beginning to return, determine

---

dosage interval by patient response; continuous dosing of medication is more effective given prn; explain analgesic effect

• Medication should be slowly withdrawn after long-term use to prevent withdrawal symptoms

• Store in light-resistant container at room temp

PO route
• May be given with food or milk to lessen GI upset

IM/SC route
• Do not give if cloudy, or a precipitate has formed

IV route
• Give slowly by direct inj

Syringe compatibilities: Glycopyrrolate, hydroxyzine

Y-site compatibilities: Cefmetazole

Additive incompatibilities: Aminophylline, amobarbital, chlorothiazide, heparin, methicillin, pentobarbital, phenobarbital, phenytoin, secobarbital, thiopental

Patient/family education
• Teach patient to report any symptoms of CNS changes, allergic reactions; to avoid CNS depressants: alcohol, sedative/hypnotics for at least 24 hr after taking this drug

• Discuss with patient that dizziness, drowsiness, and confusion are common

• Advise patient to avoid getting up without assistance

• Discuss in detail all aspects of the drug

Evaluation
Positive therapeutic outcome
• Decreased pain
• Decreased cough

Treatment of overdose: Narcan 0.2-0.8 **IV**, O$_2$, **IV** fluids, vasopressors

colchicine ⚘ (℞)
(kol′chi-seen)
Func. class.: Antigout agent
Chem. class.: Colchicum autumnale alkaloid
Pregnancy category
C(PO), **D**(IV)

Action: Inhibits microtubule formation of lactic acid in leukocytes, which decreases phagocytosis and inflammation in joints

Therapeutic Outcome: Decreased pain, inflammation of joints

Uses: Gout, gouty arthritis (prevention, treatment); to arrest progression of neurologic disability in multiple sclerosis

Investigational uses: Hepatic cirrhosis, familial Mediterranean fever

Dosage and routes
Prevention
Adult: PO 0.5-1.8 mg qd depending on severity; **IV** 0.5-1 mg qd-bid

Treatment
Adult: PO 0.5-1.2 mg, then 0.5-1.2 mg q1h, until pain decreases or side effects occur; **IV** 2 mg, then 0.5 mg q6h, not to exceed 4 mg/24 hr

Available forms: Tabs 0.5, 0.6 mg; inj **IV** 1 mg/2 ml

Adverse effects
GI: Nausea, vomiting, anorexia, malaise, metallic taste, cramps, peptic ulcer, diarrhea

GU: Hematuria, **oliguria, renal damage**
HEMA: **Agranulocytosis, thrombocytopenia, aplastic anemia, pancytopenia**
INTEG: Chills, dermatitis, pruritus, purpura, erythema
MISC: Myopathy, alopecia, reversible azoospermia, peripheral neuritis

Contraindications:
Hypersensitivity; serious GI, renal, hepatic, cardiac disorders; blood dyscrasias, pregnancy **D (IV)**

Precautions: Severe renal disease, blood dyscrasias, pregnancy **C** (PO), hepatic disease, elderly, lactation, children

Pharmacokinetics

Absorption	Well absorbed
Distribution	WBCs
Metabolism	Deacetylates in liver
Excretion	Feces (metabolites/active drug)
Half-life	20 min

Pharmacodynamics

	PO
Onset	Unknown
Peak	½-2 hr
Duration	Unknown

Interactions
Individual drugs
Cyclosporine: ↑ bone marrow depression
Erythromycin: ↑ colchicine effect
Phenylbutazone: ↑ blood dyscrasias
Radiation: ↑ bone marrow depression
Vitamin B$_{12}$: ↓ action of vitamin B$_{12}$, may cause reversible malabsorption

Drug classifications
Acidifiers: ↓ action of colchicine

Alkalinizers: ↑ action of colchicine
Bone marrow depressants: ↑ bone marrow depression
CNS depressants: ↑ action of CNS depressants
Diuretics, loop: ↓ colchicine effect
NSAIDs: ↑ GI effects
Sympathomimetics: ↑ action of sympathomimetics

Lab test interferences
↑ Alkaline phosphatase, ↑ AST/ALT
False positive: RBC, Hgb

NURSING CONSIDERATIONS
Assessment
• Assess pain and mobility of joints
• Monitor I&O ratio; observe for decrease in urinary output; CBC, platelets, reticulocytes before, during therapy (q 3 mo): Coombs' test to determine Coombs' negative hemolytic anemia
• Assess for toxicity: weakness, abdominal pain, nausea, vomiting, diarrhea

Nursing diagnoses
☑ Pain, chronic (uses)
☑ Immobility, impaired (uses)
☑ Knowledge deficit (teaching)

Implementation
PO route
• Give on empty stomach (1 hr ac or 2 hr pc) for better absorption
IV IV route
• Give **IV** undiluted or diluted 1 mg/10-20 ml normal saline or sterile water for inj; give over 2-5 min
• Do not give IM or SC
• Wait ≥wk after giving a full course of **IV** colchicine, before giving more doses

---

Patient/family education
• Teach patient to increase fluids to 3-4 L/day
• Caution patient to avoid alcohol, OTC preparations that contain alcohol; skin rashes have occurred
• Instruct patient to report any pain, redness, or hard area, usually in legs
• Teach patient importance of complying with medical regimen; bone marrow depression may occur

Evaluation
Positive therapeutic outcome
• Decreased stone formation on x-ray
• Decreased pain in kidney region
• Absence of hematuria
• Decreased pain in joints

Treatment of overdose:
D/C medication, may need opioids to treat diarrhea

---

colestipol (℞)
(koe-les´ti-pole)
Colestid
Func. class.: Antilipemic
Chem. class.: Bile sequestrant, resin exchange agent

Pregnancy category B

Action: Absorbs, combines with bile acids to form an insoluble complex that is excreted through feces; loss of bile acids lowers cholesterol levels

➡Therapeutic Outcome: Decreasing cholesterol levels and low-density lipoproteins, decreased pruritus

Uses: Primary hypercholesterolemia, xanthomas, digitalis

toxicity, pruritus due to biliary obstruction, diarrhea due to bile acids

Dosage and routes
Adult: PO 15-30 g/day in 2-4 divided doses; 2-8 tabs/day

Available forms: Granules 300 g, 500 g bottles, 5 g packets, tabs 1 g

Adverse effects
GI: Constipation, abdominal pain, nausea, fecal impaction, hemorrhoids, flatulence, vomiting, steatorrhea, peptic ulcer
HEMA: Decreased vitamin A, D, E, K, red folate content; **hyperchloremic acidosis, bleeding, decreased pro-time**
INTEG: Rash, irritation of perianal area, tongue, skin

Contraindications: Hypersensitivity, biliary obstruction

Precautions: Pregnancy **B,** lactation, children, bleeding disorders

Pharmacokinetics
Absorption	Not absorbed
Distribution	Not distributed
Metabolism	Not metabolized
Excretion	Binds with bile acids, feces
Half-life	Unknown

Pharmacodynamics
Unknown

Interactions
Individual drugs
Acetaminophen: ↓ absorption of acetaminophen
Amiodarone: ↓ absorption of amiodarone
Methotrexate: ↓ absorption of methotrexate
Naproxen: ↓ absorption of naproxen
Phenylbutazone: ↓ absorption of phenylbutazone

Piroxicam: ↓ absorption of piroxicam

Propranolol: ↓ absorption of propanolol

Thyroid: ↓ absorption of thyroid

Ursodiol: ↓ absorption of ursodiol

Drug classifications
Anticoagulants, oral: ↓ absorption

Antidiabetics, oral: antagonize colestipol

Cardiac glycosides: ↓ absorption

Diuretics, thiazide: ↓ absorption

NSAIDs: ↓ absorption

Vitamins A,D,E,K: ↓ absorption

Lab test interferences
↑ Liver function studies, ↑ Cl, ↑ PO_4

NURSING CONSIDERATIONS
Assessment
• Assess nutrition: fat, protein, carbohydrates; nutritional analysis should be completed by dietician
• Assess skin integrity after patient has been receiving drug; itching, pruritus often occur from bile deposits on skin
• Monitor cardiac glycoside level, if both drugs are being administered; cardiac glycoside levels will be decreased
• Monitor for signs of vitamin A, D, E, K deficiency; check serum cholesterol, triglyceride levels, electrolytes if on extended therapy
• Monitor bowel pattern daily; increase bulk, water in diet if constipation develops

Nursing diagnoses
☑ Constipation (adverse reactions)
☑ Knowledge deficit (teaching)
☑ Noncompliance (teaching)

Implementation
• Give drug ac, hs; give all other medications 1 hr before or 4 hr after colestipol to avoid poor absorption; give drug mixed with applesauce or stirred into beverage (2-6 oz), let stand for 2 min; do not take dry
• Provide supplemental doses of vitamins A, D, E, K, if levels are low
🚫• Tabs should be swallowed whole; do not crush, chew

Patient/family education
• Teach patient symptoms of hypoprothrombinemia: bleeding mucous membranes, dark, tarry stools, hematuria, petechiae; report immediately
• Teach patient importance of compliance, since toxicity may result if doses are missed; not to discontinue suddenly
• Teach patient that risk factors should be decreased: high-fat diet, smoking, alcohol consumption, absence of exercise
• Tell patient to mix drug with 6 oz of milk, water, fruit juice; may be mixed with carbonated beverages; rinse glass to make sure all medication is taken or may mix drug in applesauce; allow to stand for 2 min before mixing

Evaluation
Positive therapeutic outcome
• Decreased cholesterol level (hyperlipidemia)
• Decreased diarrhea, pruritus (excess bile acids)

corticotropin (℞)
(kor-ti-koe-troe′pin)
ACTH, Acthar, corticotropin,
Duracton ✤, H.P. Acthar Gel
Func. class.: Pituitary
hormone
Chem. class.: Adrenocorti-
cotropic hormone
Pregnancy category **C**

Action: Stimulates adrenal
cortex to produce, secrete
corticosterone, cortisol; suppresses adrenal function
(chronic use); potent mineralocorticoid

➔**Therapeutic Outcome:** Increased production of adrenal
steroids in adrenal insufficiency

Uses: Testing adrenocortical
function, treatment of adrenal
insufficiency caused by administration of corticosteroids
(long term), multiple sclerosis,
🅿 infantile spasms

Dosage and routes
*Testing of adrenocortical
function*
Adult: IM/SC up to 80 U in
divided doses; **IV** 10-25 U in
500 ml D₅W given over 8 hr

Inflammation
Adult: SC/IM 40 U in 4
divided doses (aqueous) or 40
U q12-24h (gel/repository
form)

🅿 *Infantile spasms*
Infant: IM gel 20 U/day ×2
wk, increase if needed

Available forms: Inj 25, 40
U/vial; repository inj 40,
80/ml

Adverse effects
CNS: **Convulsions,** dizziness,
euphoria, insomnia, headache,
mood swings, behavioral
changes, depression, psychosis,
increasing intracranial pressure, papilledema
CV: **Necrotizing angiitis,
shock, heart failure,** hypertension
EENT: Cataracts, glaucoma
ENDO: Cushingoid symp-
toms, diabetes mellitus, antibody formation, growth retar-
🅿 dation in children, menstrual
irregularities
GI: Nausea, vomiting, **peptic
ulcer perforation,** pancreatitis,
distention, ulcerative esophagitis
GU: Water, sodium retention,
hypokalemia
*INTEG: Impaired wound
healing,* rash, urticaria, hirsutism, petechiae, ecchymoses,
sweating, acne, hyperpigmentation
MS: Weakness, osteoporosis,
compression fractures, muscle
atrophy, steroid myopathy,
myalgia, arthralgia

Contraindications: Hypersensitivity, scleroderma, osteoporosis, CHF, peptic ulcer disease, hypertension, systemic
fungal infections, smallpox
vaccination, recent surgery,
ocular herpes simplex, primary
adrenocortical insufficiency/
hyperfunction

Precautions: Pregnancy **C,**
lactation, latent TB, hepatic
disease, hypothyroiditis,
childbearing-age women,
psychiatric diagnosis, myasthenia gravis, acute gouty arthritis,
thromboembolic disorders

Pharmacokinetics	
Absorption	Rapidly absorbed (IM, SC)
Distribution	Widely distributed to tissues
Metabolism	Unknown
Excretion	Unknown
Half-life	<20 min

Pharmacodynamics

	IM (gelatin repository)	IV
Onset	Unknown	Unknown
Peak	3-12 hr	1 hr
Duration	Up to 3 days	Unknown

Interactions
Individual drugs
Amphotericin B: ↑ hypokalemia

Insulin: ↑ need for insulin

Mezlocillin: ↑ hypokalemia

Phenobarbital: ↓ corticotropin effect

Phenytoin: ↓ corticotropin effect

Piperacillin: ↑ hypokalemia

Rifampin: ↓ corticotropin effect

Ticarcillin: ↑ hypokalemia

Drug classifications
Anticoagulants, oral: Altered prothrombin time

Anticonvulsants: ↓ corticotropin effect

Barbiturates: ↓ corticotropin effect

Diuretics, potassium depleting: ↑ hypokalemia

Estrogens: ↑ corticotropin effect

Hypoglycemics, oral: ↑ need for hypoglycemic

Live virus vaccines: ↓ antibody reactions

NSAIDs: ↑ risk of ulceration

Oral contraceptive: Blocked metabolism of corticotropin

NURSING CONSIDERATIONS
Assessment
• Monitor I&O ratio, weight weekly; report gain over 5 lb/wk

• Obtain 2-hr postprandial chest x-ray, serum potassium, 17-KS, 17-OHCS, cortisol, during long-term treatment

• Assess for dependent edema, moon face, pulmonary edema, cerebral edema; monitor baseline ECG, B/P, chest x-ray, GTT, pulse

• Assess for increased stress in patient's life that may require increased corticosteroids; assess for infection which drug may mask

• Assess for mental status: affect, mood, increased aggressiveness, irritability; a change in mental status may require decreased steroids; changes can be extreme

P • Identify growth rate of child; growth suppression may occur frequently

• Identify hypoadrenalism in P neonates if drug was given during pregnancy

• Identify allergic reaction: rash, urticaria, fever, nausea, vomiting, dyspnea; drug should be discontinued immediately; administer epinephrine 1:1000

Nursing diagnoses
☑ Infection, risk for (adverse reactions)

☑ Injury, risk for (adverse reactions)

☑ Knowledge deficit (teaching)

Implementation
• Give diet with decreased sodium, increased potassium for dependent edema; increase protein in diet for nitrogen loss before giving; give deep IM using 21 G needle, massage, rotate sites; injection is painful

• Store unused portion in refrigerator; use within 24 hr

IV IV route
• Give by direct **IV**: give over 2 min; dilute 25 U/1 ml sterile water or normal saline or 40 U/2 ml

• Give by intermittent inf: dilute 10-25 U/500 ml D_5W, 0.9% NaCl, D_5/0.9% NaCl, or

---

LR; give over 8 hr; or 40
U/12-48 hr
• Store unused portion in
refrigerator; use within 24 hr

Additive compatibilities:
Calcium gluconate, chloramphenicol, cytarabine, dimenhydrinate, erythromycin
gluceptate, heparin, hydrocortisone, methicillin, norepinephrine, oxytetracycline,
penicillin G potassium, potassium chloride, tetracycline,
vancomycin

Additive incompatibilities:
Aminophylline, sodium bicarbonate

Patient/family education
• Caution patient to avoid
vaccinations during drug
treatment; tell patient to notify
anyone involved in medical or
dental care that this drug is
being taken
• Teach patient to maintain
adequate hydration up to 2
L/day unless contraindicated
• Advise patient to avoid OTC
products: salicylates, products
with alcohol
• Teach patient not to discontinue medication abruptly;
adrenal crisis may occur; drug
should be tapered off over
several wk; teach patient that
drug does not cure condition,
only decreases symptoms
• Teach patient to wear Medic
Alert ID specifying steroid
therapy
• Instruct patient to notify
prescriber of infection: increased temp, sore throat,
muscular pain

Evaluation
Positive therapeutic outcome
• Absence of inflammation,
pain

• Increased muscle strength in
multiple sclerosis

---

cortisone ⚷ (R)
(kor'ti-sone)
Cortone Acetate
Func. class.: Corticoste-
roid, synthetic
Chem. class.: Short-acting
glucocorticoid
Pregnancy category   C

Action: Decreases inflammation by suppression of migration of polymorphonuclear
leukocytes, fibroblasts, reversal
of increased capillary permeability, and lysosomal stabilization; suppresses adrenal
function with long-term use

▶**Therapeutic Outcome:** Replacement of cortisol in adrenal
insufficiency

Uses: Inflammation, severe
allergy, adrenal insufficiency,
collagen disorders, respiratory
and dermatologic disorders

Dosage and routes
Adult: PO/IM 25-300 mg qd
or q2 days, titrated to patient
response
P *Child:* PO 2.5-10 mg/kg/day;
IM 1-5 mg/kg/day

Available forms: Tabs 5, 10,
25 mg; inj 50 mg/ml

Adverse effects
*CNS: Depression, flushing,
sweating,* headache, mood
changes
CV: Hypertension, **circulatory
collapse, thrombophlebitis,
embolism,** tachycardia, **necrotizing angiitis, CHF,** edema
EENT: Fungal infections,
increased intraocular pressure,
blurred vision

GI: Diarrhea, nausea, abdominal distention, **GI hemorrhage,** increased appetite, **pancreatitis**
HEMA: **Thrombocytopenia**
INTEG: Acne, poor wound healing, ecchymosis, bruising, petechiae
MS: Fractures, osteoporosis, weakness

Contraindications: Psychosis, hypersensitivity, idiopathic thrombocytopenia, acute glomerulonephritis, amebiasis, fungal infections, nonasthmatic **P** bronchial disease, child <2 yr, AIDS, TB

Precautions: Pregnancy **C,** diabetes mellitus, glaucoma, osteoporosis, seizure disorders, ulcerative colitis, CHF, myasthenia gravis, renal disease, esophagitis, peptic ulcer

Pharmacokinetics	
Absorption	Slowly IM
Distribution	Widely, crosses placenta
Metabolism	Liver
Excretion	Unknown
Half-life	½ hr

Pharmacodynamics		
	PO	IM
Onset	Unknown	Unknown
Peak	2 hr	20-48 hr
Duration	1½ days	1½ days

Interactions
Individual drugs
Amphotericin B: ↑ hypokalemia
Insulin: ↑ need for insulin
Mezlocillin: ↑ hypokalemia
Phenobarbital: ↓ effectiveness of cortisone
Phenytoin: ↓ effectiveness of cortisone
Drug classifications
Contraceptives, oral: blocked metabolism of cortisone

Diuretics, potassium-wasting: ↑ side effects
NSAIDs: ↑ GI symptoms
Salicylates: ↑ GI symptoms
☑ *Herb/drug*
Aloe: ↑ potassium deficiency
Buckthorn bark/berry: ↑ potassium deficiency
Cascara sagrada bark: ↑ potassium deficiency, chronic use
Rhubarb root: ↑ potassium deficiency
Senna leaf/fruits: ↑ potassium deficiency
Lab test interferences
↑ Cholesterol, ↑ sodium, ↑ blood glucose, ↑ uric acid, ↑ calcium, ↑ urine glucose
↓ Calcium, ↓ potassium, ↓ T_4, ↓ T_3, ↓ thyroid ^{131}I uptake test, ↓ urine 17-OHCS, ↓ 17-KS, ↓ PBI
False negative: Skin allergy tests

NURSING CONSIDERATIONS
Assessment
• Assess for adrenal insufficiency symptoms: weakness, nausea, vomiting, confusion, anxiety, restlessness, decreased B/P, weight loss; check before and during treatment
• Monitor potassium, blood sugar, urine glucose for patient on long-term therapy; hypokalemia and hyperglycemia can occur
• Check B/P, pulse q4h; notify prescriber if chest pain occurs
• Monitor I&O ratio and weight daily; be alert for decreasing urinary output and increasing edema with bilateral rales, dyspnea, weight gain
• Monitor plasma cortisol levels during long-term therapy (normal level: 138-635 nmol/L if drawn at 8 AM)

- Assess for symptoms of infection: increased temp, WBC even after withdrawal of medication; drug masks symptoms of infection
- Monitor for potassium depletion: paresthesias, fatigue, nausea, vomiting, depression, polyuria, dysrhythmias, weakness, edema, hypertension, cardiac symptoms, weight daily; notify prescriber of weekly gain >5 lb
- Assess for mental changes: affect, mood, behavioral changes, aggression; depression, psychoses may occur

Nursing diagnoses

☑ Infection, risk for (adverse reactions)
☑ Injury, risk for (adverse reactions)
☑ Knowledge deficit (teaching)

Implementation

IM route
- Give after shaking susp (parenteral); titrate dose; use lowest effective dosage
- Give IM inj deep in large muscle mass; rotate sites; avoid deltoid; use a 21 G needle
- Administer in 1 dose in AM to prevent adrenal suppression; avoid SC administration; damage may be done to tissue; do not give **IV**

PO route
- Administer with food or milk to decrease GI symptoms

Patient/family education
- Advise patient that ID as steroid user should be carried at all times
- Instruct patient to notify prescriber if therapeutic response decreases; dosage adjustment may be needed; teach not to discontinue this medication abruptly or adrenal crisis

can result; teach all aspects of drug usage, including cushingoid symptoms
- Caution patient to avoid OTC products: salicylates, potassium, alcohol in cough products, cold preparations unless directed by prescriber
- Teach patient symptoms of adrenal insufficiency: nausea, anorexia, fatigue, dizziness, dyspnea, weakness, joint pain, tarry stools, bruising, blurred vision
- Advise patient to avoid persons with known infections; report probable infection rapidly; drug masks infection
- Caution patient that diet modification is necessary if on long-term treatment: increased calcium, potassium, and protein; also low sodium and carbohydrates

Evaluation

Positive therapeutic outcome
- Ease of respirations, decreased inflammation

---

cyclobenzaprine (℞)
(sye-kloe-ben′za-preen)
cyclobenzaprine HCl, Flexeril
Func. class.: Skeletal muscle relaxant, central acting
Chem. class.: Tricyclic amine salt
Pregnancy category   B

Action: Unknown; may be related to antidepressant effects
Therapeutic Outcome: Relaxation of skeletal muscle
Uses: Adjunct for relief of muscle spasm and pain in musculoskeletal conditions

---

Adverse effects: *italic* = common; **bold** = life-threatening

Dosage and routes
Adult: PO 10 mg tid × 1 wk, not to exceed 60 mg/day × 3 wk

P *Child:* 20-40 mg/kg/day in 2-4 divided doses

Available forms: Tabs 10 mg

Adverse effects
CNS: Dizziness, weakness, drowsiness, headache, tremor, depression, insomnia, confusion, paresthesia
CV: Postural hypotension, tachycardia, **dysrhythmias**
EENT: Diplopia, temporary loss of vision
GI: Nausea, vomiting, hiccups, dry mouth, constipation
GU: Urinary retention, frequency, change in libido
INTEG: Rash, pruritus, fever, facial flushing, sweating

Contraindications: Acute recovery phase of MI, dysrhythmias, heart block, CHF, **P** hypersensitivity, child <12 yr, intermittent porphyria, thyroid disease

Precautions: Renal disease, hepatic disease, addictive per- **G** sonality, pregnancy **B,** elderly

◼ Do Not Confuse:

cyclobenzaprine/cyproheptadine

Pharmacokinetics

Distribution	Well
Metabolism	Liver, partially
Excretion	Kidney (unchanged)
Half-life	1-3 days

Pharmacodynamics

Onset	1 hr
Peak	3-8 hr
Duration	12-24 hr

Interactions
Individual drugs

Alcohol: ↑ CNS depression
Drug classifications

Antidepressants, tricyclic: ↑ CNS depression
Antihistamines: ↑ CNS depression
Barbiturates: ↑ CNS depression
MAOI: Do not use within 14 days
Opiates: ↑ CNS depression
Sedative/hypnotics: ↑ CNS depression
⬚ Herb/drug

Kava: ↑ CNS depression

NURSING CONSIDERATIONS
Assessment
• Monitor ECG in epileptic patients; poor seizure control has occurred in patients taking this drug
• Check for allergic reactions: rash, fever, respiratory distress
• Check for severe weakness, numbness, in extremities
• Assess for CNS depression: dizziness, drowsiness, psychiatric symptoms

Nursing diagnoses
✓ Physical mobility, impaired uses
✓ Injury, risk for (adverse reactions)
✓ Knowledge deficit (teaching)

Implementation
• Give with meals for GI symptoms
• Store in airtight container at room temp

Patient/family education
• Teach patient not to discontinue medication quickly; insomnia, nausea, headache, spasticity, tachycardia will occur; drug should be tapered off over 1-2 wk

---

- Caution patient not to take with alcohol, other CNS depressants
- Advise to avoid altering activities while taking this drug
- Caution patient to avoid hazardous activities if drowsiness/dizziness occurs
- Caution patient to avoid using OTC medication: cough preparations, antihistamines, unless directed by prescriber
- Teach patient to use gum, frequent sips of water for dry mouth

Evaluation

Positive therapeutic outcome
- Decreased pain, spasticity; muscle spasms of acute, painful musculoskeletal conditions are generally short term; long-term therapy is seldom warranted

Treatment of overdose:

Empty stomach with emesis, gastric lavage, then administer activated charcoal; use anticonvulsants if indicated; monitor cardiac function

---

cyclophosphamide
✏ (℞)
(sye-kloe-foss'fa-mide)
Cytoxan, Neosar, Procytox ✦
Func. class.: Antineoplastic alkylating agent
Chem. class.: Nitrogen mustard
Pregnancy category **D**

Action: Alkylates DNA, RNA; inhibits enzymes that allow synthesis of amino acids in proteins; is also responsible for cross-linking DNA strands; activity is not cell cycle phase specific

▶**Therapeutic Outcome:** Prevention of rapidly growing malignant cells

Uses: Hodgkin's disease, lymphomas, leukemia, multiple myeloma, neuroblastoma, retinoblastoma, Ewing's sarcoma, cancer of female reproductive tract, lung, prostate

Dosage and routes

Adult: PO initially 1-5 mg/ kg over 2-5 days; maintenance 1-5 mg/kg; **IV** initially 40-50 mg/kg in divided doses over 2-5 days; maintenance 10-15 mg/kg q7-10 days, or 3-5 mg/kg q3 days

Child: PO/**IV** 2-8 mg/kg or 60-250 mg/m^2 in divided doses × 6 or more days; maintenance **IV** 10-15 mg/kg q7-10 days or 30 mg/kg q3-4 wk; or PO 2-5 mg/kg 2×/wk dose should be reduced by half when bone marrow suppression occurs

Renal dose

CrCl 25-50 ml/min 50% of dose; CrCL <25 ml/min avoid use

Available forms: Powder for inj **IV** 100, 200, 500 mg, 1, 2 g; tabs 25, 50 mg

Adverse effects

CNS: Headache, dizziness
CV: **Cardiotoxicity** (high doses)
ENDO: Syndrome of inappropriate antidiuretic hormone (SIADH)
GI: Nausea, vomiting, diarrhea, weight loss, colitis, **hepatotoxicity**
GU: **Hemorrhagic cystitis, hematuria, neoplasms, amenorrhea, azoospermia, sterility, ovarian fibrosis**
HEMA: **Thrombocytopenia,**

Adverse effects: *italic* = common; **bold** = life-threatening

leukopenia, pancytopenia, myelosuppression
INTEG: Alopecia, dermatitis
RESP: Fibrosis
Contraindications: Lactation, pregnancy **D**
Precautions: Radiation therapy

⊠ **Do Not Confuse:**
cyclophosphamide/cyclosporine, Cytoxan/Cytosar, Cytoxan/Cytotec

Pharmacokinetics

Absorption	Well absorbed (PO)
Distribution	Widely distributed; crosses placenta, blood-brain barrier (50%)
Metabolism	Liver to active drug
Excretion	Kidneys, unchanged (30%)
Half-life	4-6½ hr

Pharmacodynamics

Unknown

Interactions
Individual drugs

Allopurinol: ↑ bone marrow suppression
Chloramphenicol: ↓ cyclophosphamide
Doxorubicin: ↑ cardiotoxicity
Phenobarbital: ↑ toxicity
Radiation: ↑ toxicity, bone marrow suppression
Rifampin: ↑ toxicity, bone marrow suppression
Succinylcholine: ↑ neuromuscular blockade
Drug classifications

Aminoglycosides: ↑ nephrotoxicity
Anticoagulants, oral: ↑ bleeding
Antineoplastics: ↑ toxicity, bone marrow suppression
Bone marrow–suppressing drugs: ↑ bone marrow suppression

Corticosteroids: ↓ cyclophosphamide effect
Diuretics, loop: ↑ ototoxicity
Live virus vaccines: ↓ antibody reaction
Salicylates: ↑ risk of bleeding
Lab test interferences

↑ Uric acid
False positive: Pap test
False negative: PPD, mumps trichophytin, *Candida*
↓ Pseudocholinesterase

NURSING CONSIDERATIONS
Assessment

⚠ • Assess symptoms indicating severe allergic reaction: rash, pruritus, urticaria, purpuric skin lesions, itching, flushing
• Assess for tachypnea, ECG changes, dyspnea, edema, fatigue
• Monitor CBC, differential, platelet count weekly; withhold drug if WBC count is <4000/mm^3 or platelet count is <75,000/mm^3; notify prescriber of results
• Monitor renal function studies: BUN, creatinine, serum uric acid, urine CrCl before and during therapy; I&O ratio; report fall in urine output to <30 ml/hr
• Monitor temp q4h (may indicate beginning of infection)
• Monitor liver function tests before and during therapy (bilirubin, AST, ALT, LDH) as needed or monthly; note jaundice of skin or sclera, dark urine, clay-colored stools, itchy skin, abdominal pain, fever, diarrhea
• Assess for bleeding: hematuria, stool guaiac, bruising or petechiae, mucosa or orifices q8h

---

- Identify dyspnea, rales, unproductive cough, chest pain, tachypnea
- Identify effects of alopecia on body image; discuss feelings about body changes
- Identify edema in feet, joint pain, stomach pain, shaking; prescriber should be notified
- Identify inflammation of mucosa, breaks in skin

Nursing diagnoses

☑ Injury, risk for (adverse reactions)

☑ Body image disturbance (adverse reactions)

☑ Infection, risk for (adverse reactions)

☑ Knowledge deficit (teaching)

Implementation

- Give fluids **IV** or PO before chemotherapy to hydrate patient
- Give antacid before oral agent, pc PM, before hs; antiemetic 30-60 min before giving drug to prevent vomiting, and prn; antibiotics for prophylaxis of infection
- Give top or syst analgesics for pain; give in AM so drug can be eliminated before hs

IV **IV route**

- Give **IV** after diluting 100 mg/5 ml of sterile or bacteriostatic water; shake; let stand until clear; may be further diluted in up to 250 ml D$_5$ 0.9% NaCl, D$_5$/0.9% NaCl, 0.45% NaCl, LR, Ringer's; give 100 mg or less/min through 3-way stopcock of glucose or saline inf
- Use 21, 23, 25 G needle; check site for irritation, phlebitis

Syringe compatibilities:
Bleomycin, cisplatin, doxapram, doxorubicin, droperidol, fluorouracil, furosemide, heparin, leucovorin, methotrexate, metoclopramide, mitomycin, mitoxantrone, vinblastine, vincristine

Y-site compatibilities:
Amifostine, amikacin, ampicillin, azlocillin, aztreonam, bleomycin, cefamandole, cefazolin, cefepime, cefoperazone, cefotaxime, cefoxitin, cefuroxime, cephalothin, cephapirin, chloramphenicol, chlorpromazine, cimetidine, cisplatin, cladribine, clindamycin, dexamethasone, diphenhydramine, doxorubicin, doxycycline, droperidol, erythromycin, famotidine, filgrastim, fludarabine, fluorouracil, furosemide, gallium, ganciclovir, gentamicin, granisetron, heparin, hydromorphone, idarubicin, kanamycin, leucovorin, lorazepam, melphalan, methotrexate, methylprednisolone, metoclopramide, metronidazole, mezlocillin, minocycline, mitomycin, moxalactam, nafcillin, ondansetron, oxacillin, paclitaxel, penicillin G potassium, piperacillin, piperacillin/tazobactam, prochlorperazine, promethazine, propofol, ranitidine, sargramostim, sodium bicarbonate, teniposide, tetracycline, thiotepa, ticarcillin, ticarcillin-clavulanate, tobramycin, trimethoprim-sulfamethoxazole, vancomycin, vinblastine, vincristine, vinorelbine

Additive compatibilities:
Cisplatin with etoposide, hydroxyzine, methotrexate, methotrexate with fluorouracil, mitoxantrone, ondansetron

Solution compatibilities:
Amino acids 4.25%/D$_{25}$, D$_5$/0.9% NaCl, D$_5$W, 0.9% NaCl

Patient/family education
- Teach patient to avoid use of products containing aspirin or ibuprofen, razors, commercial mouthwash, since bleeding may occur; to report symptoms of bleeding (hematuria, tarry stools)
- Instruct patient to report signs of anemia (fatigue, headache, irritability, faintness, shortness of breath)
- Teach patient to report any changes in breathing or coughing even several months after treatment
- Advise patient that hair may be lost during treatment; a wig or hair piece may make patient feel better; new hair may be different in color, texture
- Teach patient not to have any vaccinations without the advice of the prescriber; serious reactions can occur
- Advise patient contraception is needed during treatment and for several months after the completion of therapy

Evaluation
Positive therapeutic outcome
- Prevention of rapid division of malignant cells
- Increased appetite, increased weight

---

cyclosporine (℞)
(sye-kloe-spor'een)
Neoral, Sandimmune, SangCya
Func. class.: Immunosuppressant
Chem. class.: Fungus-derived peptide

Pregnancy category C

Action: Produces immunosuppression by inhibiting T lymphocytes

Therapeutic Outcome: Absence of transplant rejection

Uses: Organ transplants to prevent rejection, rheumatoid arthritis, psoriasis

Investigational uses: Pancreas, bone marrow, heart/lung transplantation

Dosage and routes
P *Adult and child:* PO 15 mg/kg several hours before surgery, daily for 2 wk; reduce dosage by 2.5 mg/kg/wk to 5-10 mg/kg/day; **IV** 5-6 mg/kg several hours before surgery; daily, switch to PO form as soon as possible

Available forms: Oral sol 100 mg/ml; inj 50 mg/ml; soft gelatin caps 25, 50, 100 mg

Adverse effects
CNS: Tremors, headache
GI: Nausea, vomiting, diarrhea, *oral Candida, gum hyperplasia,* **hepatotoxicity,** pancreatitis
GU: **Albuminuria, hematuria, proteinuria, renal failure**
INTEG: Rash, acne, *hirsutism*

Contraindications: Hypersensitivity

Precautions: Severe renal disease, severe hepatic disease, pregnancy **C**

Do Not Confuse:
cyclosporine/Cycloserine,
cyclosporine/
cyclophosphamide

Pharmacokinetics

Absorption	Poorly absorbed (PO)
Distribution	Crosses placenta
Metabolism	Liver to mercaptopurine
Excretion	Kidney, minimal
Half-life	Biphasic 1.2 hr, 25 hr

Pharmacodynamics

	PO
Onset	Unknown
Peak	4 hr
Duration	Unknown

Interactions
Individual drugs
Amphotericin B: ↑ cyclosporine action
Carvedilol: ↑ carvedilol level
Cimetidine: ↑ cyclosporine action
Digoxin: ↑ digoxin level
Etoposide: ↑ etoposide level
Ketoconazole: ↑ cyclosporine action
Phenytoin: ↓ cyclosporine action
Rifampin: ↓ cyclosporine action
Drug classifications:
Androgens: ↑ cyclosporine levels
Antifungals, azole: ↑ cyclosporine level
Calcium channel blockers: ↑ cyclosporine levels
Corticosteroids: ↑ cyclosporine level
Macrolides: ↑ cyclosporine level
Oral contraceptives: ↑ cyclosporine level
Rifamycins: ↓ cyclosporine levels
Food/drug
Grapefruit: ↑ CNS side effects

NURSING CONSIDERATIONS
Assessment
• Monitor renal studies: BUN, creatinine at least monthly during treatment, 3 mo after treatment
• Monitor liver function studies: alk phosphatase, AST, ALT, bilirubin
• Monitor drug blood levels during treatment
• Assess for hepatotoxicity: dark urine, jaundice, itching, light-colored stools; drug should be discontinued
• Assess for nephrotoxicity: 6 wks postop, CyA trough level >200 ng/ml, intracapsular pressure <40 mm Hg, rise in creatinine 0.15 mg/dl/day

Nursing diagnoses
☑ Mobility, impaired (uses)
☑ Infection, risk for (uses)
☑ Knowledge deficit (teaching)

Implementation
PO route
• Give with meals for GI upset or drug placed in chocolate milk
🚫• Do not crush, chew caps
• Give with oral antifungal for *Candida* infections
IV route
• Give **IV** after diluting each 50 mg/20-100 ml of normal saline or D₅W; run over 2-6 hr; use an infusion pump, glass inf bottles only

Additive compatibilities:
Ciprofloxacin

Y-site compatibility:
Cefmetazole, propofol, sargramostim

Sol compatibilities:
D₅W, NaCl 0.9%
• Give for several days before transplant surgery
• Give with corticosteroids

Patient/family education
• Advise patient to report fever, rash, severe diarrhea, chills, sore throat, fatigue, since serious infections may occur; also to report clay-colored stools, cramping (may indicate hepatotoxicity)
• Caution patient to use contraceptive measures during treatment and for 12 wk after ending therapy; drug is teratogenic
• Caution patient to avoid crowds and persons with known infections to reduce risk of infection

Evaluation
Positive therapeutic outcome
• Absence of graft rejection

---

cyproheptadine (℞)
(si-proe-hep′ta-deen)
cyproheptadine HCl,
Periactin
Func. class.: Antihistamine, H$_1$-receptor antagonist
Chem. class.: Piperidine
Pregnancy category   B

Action: Acts on blood vessels, GI, respiratory system by competing with histamine for H$_1$-receptor site; decreases allergic response by blocking histamine; blocks serotonin to increase appetite and relieve vascular headaches

Therapeutic Outcome: Absence of allergy symptoms and rhinitis

Uses: Allergy symptoms, rhinitis, pruritus, cold urticaria

Investigational uses: Appetite stimulant, management of vascular headache

Dosage and routes
Adult: PO 4 mg tid-qid, not to exceed 0.5 mg/kg/day
P *Child 7-14 yr:* PO 4 mg bid-tid, not to exceed 16 mg/day
P *Child 2-6 yr:* PO 2 mg bid-tid, not to exceed 12 mg/day
Available forms: Tabs 4 mg; syr 2 mg/5 ml

Adverse effects
CNS: Dizziness, drowsiness, poor coordination, fatigue, anxiety, euphoria, confusion, paresthesia, neuritis
CV: Hypotension, palpitations, tachycardia
EENT: Blurred vision, dilated pupils; tinnitus; nasal stuffiness; dry nose, throat, mouth
GI: Constipation, dry mouth, nausea, vomiting, anorexia, diarrhea, weight gain
GU: Retention, dysuria, frequency, increased appetite
HEMA: **Hemolytic anemia, leukopenia, thrombocytosis, agranulocytosis**
INTEG: Rash, urticaria, photosensitivity
MISC: **Anaphylaxis**
RESP: Increased thick secretions, wheezing, chest tightness

Contraindications: Hypersensitivity to H$_1$-receptor antagonist, acute asthma attack, lower respiratory tract disease

Precautions: Increased intraocular pressure, renal disease, cardiac disease, hypertension, bronchial asthma, seizure disorder, stenosed peptic ulcers, hyperthyroidism, prostatic hypertrophy, bladder neck obstruction, pregnancy **B**,
G elderly

☑ Herb/drug ◯ Do Not Crush ◆ Alert ⟶ Key Drug G Geriatric P Pediatric

Do Not Confuse:
cyproheptadine/cyclobenza-
prine

Pharmacokinetics
Absorption	Well absorbed
Distribution	Unknown
Metabolism	Liver, complete
Excretion	Kidneys
Half-life	Unknown

Pharmacodynamics
Onset	15-60 min
Peak	1-2 hr
Duration	8 hr

Interactions
Individual drugs
Alcohol: ↑ CNS depression

Drug classifications
CNS depressants: ↑ CNS
depression
MAOIs: ↑ anticholinergic
effect
Opiates: ↑ CNS depression
Sedative/hypnotics: ↑ CNS
depression

Herb/drug
Henbane leaf: ↑ anticholiner-
gic effect
Kava: ↑ CNS depression

Lab test interferences
False negative: Skin allergy
tests (discontinue antihistamine
3 days before testing)

NURSING CONSIDERATIONS
Assessment
• Assess respiratory status:
rate, rhythm, increase in bronchial secretions, wheezing,
chest tightness; provide fluids
to 2 L/ day to decrease secretion thickness
• Monitor I&O ratio: be alert
for urinary retention, frequency, dysuria, especially
elderly; drug should be discontinued if these occur; monitor
food intake, weight if using as
an appetite stimulant

Nursing diagnoses
✓ Airway clearance, ineffective
(uses)
✓ Injury, risk for (side effects)
✓ Knowledge deficit (teaching)
✓ Noncompliance (teaching,
overuse)

Implementation
• May give with food to decrease GI upset
• Syrup may be used for patients with difficulty swallowing or children
• Store in tight, light-resistant
container

Patient/family education
• Teach all aspects of drug
uses; tell patient to notify
prescriber if confusion, sedation, hypotension occur; to
avoid driving and other hazardous activity if drowsiness
occurs; to avoid alcohol and
other CNS depressants that
may potentiate effect
• Caution patient not to exceed recommended dosage;
dysrhythmias may occur
• Teach patient hard candy,
gum, frequent rinsing of
mouth may be used for dryness

Evaluation
Positive therapeutic outcome
• Absence of running or con-
gested nose, rashes

Treatment of overdose:
Administer ipecac syrup or
lavage, diazepam, vasopressors,
barbiturates (short acting)

cytarabine ℞
(sye-tare'a-been)
Ara-C, Cytosar ✦, Cytosar-U, cytosine arabinoside, Depo Cyt, Tarabine PFS
Func. class.: Antineoplastic, antimetabolite
Chem. class.: Pyrimidine nucleoside

Pregnancy category   D

Action: Competes with physiologic substrate of DNA synthesis, thus interfering with cell replication in the S phase of the cell cycle (before mitosis)

⇒Therapeutic Outcome: Prevention of rapidly growing malignant cells

Uses: Acute myelocytic leukemia, acute lymphocytic leukemia, chronic myelocytic leukemia, and in combination for non-Hodgkin's lymphomas in Ⓟ children

Dosage and routes
Acute myelocytic leukemia
Adult: **IV** inf 200 mg/m²/day × 5 days; IT 30 mg/m² q4 days, then another dose every 1-4 days × 4 days; SC 1 mg/kg Ⓟ 1-2 ×/wk (maintenance)

Lymphomatous meningitis
Liposomal (DepoCyt):
Adult: Intrathecally: 50 mg q14 days × 2 doses (wk 1, 3) then 50 mg q14 days × 3 doses (wk 5, 7, 9) followed by 1 dose wk 13; then 50 mg q28 day × 4 doses (wk 17, 21, 25, 29); reduce dose to 25 mg for subsequent doses, if neurotoxicity occurs

In combination
Ⓟ *Child:* **IV** inf 100 mg/m²/day × 5-10 days

Available forms: Inj 100, 500 mg, 1, 2 g; inj 20 mg/ml; liposomal 10 mg/ml

Adverse effects
CNS: Neuritis, dizziness, headache, personality changes, ataxia, mechanical dysphasia, **coma**
CV: Chest pain, **cardiopathy**
CYTARABINE SYNDROME: Fever, myalgia, bone pain, chest pain, rash, conjunctivitis, malaise (6-12 hr after administration)
EENT: Sore throat, conjunctivitis
GI: Nausea, vomiting, anorexia, diarrhea, stomatitis, **hepatotoxicity,** abdominal pain, hematemesis, **GI hemorrhage**
GU: Urinary retention, **renal failure, hyperuricemia**
HEMA: **Thrombophlebitis, bleeding, thrombocytopenia, leukopenia, myelosuppression, anemia**
INTEG: Rash, fever, freckling, cellulitis
RESP: **Pneumonia,** dyspnea

Contraindications: Hypersensitivity, infants, pregnancy **D**

Precautions: Renal disease, hepatic disease

◼ Do Not Confuse:
Cytosar/Cytoxan, Cytosar/Cytovene

Pharmacokinetics	
Absorption	Complete
Distribution	Widely distributed; crosses blood-brain barrier, placenta
Metabolism	Liver, extensively
Excretion	Kidneys
Half-life	1-3 hr

Pharmacodynamics	
Unknown	

Interactions
Individual drugs
Cyclophosphamide: ↑ cardiotoxicity, CHF
Radiation: ↑ toxicity, bone marrow suppression

Drug classifications
Antineoplastics: ↑ toxicity, bone marrow suppression

NURSING CONSIDERATIONS
Assessment
• Assess buccal cavity q8h for dryness, sores or ulceration, white patches, pain, bleeding, dysphagia; obtain prescription for viscous lidocaine (Xylocaine)
• Assess symptoms indicating severe allergic reaction: rash, pruritus, urticaria, purpuric skin lesions, itching, flushing
• Assess tachypnea, dyspnea, edema, fatigue; identify dyspnea, rales, unproductive cough, chest pain, tachypnea
◆• Assess for cytarabine syndrome 6-12 hr after inf: fever, myalgia, bone pain, chest pain, rash, conjunctivitis, malaise; corticosteroid may be ordered
• Monitor CBC, differential, platelet count weekly; withhold drug if WBC count is <4000/mm³ or platelet count is <75,000/mm³
• Assess for increased uric acid levels, swelling, joint pain primarily in extremities; patient should be well hydrated to prevent urate deposits
• Monitor renal function studies: BUN, creatinine, serum uric acid, urine CrCl before and during therapy; I&O ratio; report fall in urine output to <30 ml/hr
• Monitor temp q4h (may indicate beginning of infection)

• Monitor liver function tests before and during therapy (bilirubin, AST, ALT, LDH) as needed or monthly; note yellowing of skin or sclera, dark urine, clay-colored stools, itchy skin, abdominal pain, fever, diarrhea
• Assess for bleeding: hematuria, stool guaiac, bruising or petechiae, mucosa or orifices q8h
• Identify edema in feet, joint pain, stomach pain, shaking; prescriber should be notified
• Identify inflammation of mucosa, breaks in skin

Nursing diagnoses
☑ Injury, risk for (adverse reactions)
☑ Body image disturbance (adverse reactions)
☑ Infection, risk for (adverse reactions)
☑ Knowledge deficit (teaching)

Implementation
• Avoid contact with skin; very irritating; wash completely to remove
• Give fluids **IV** or PO before chemotherapy to hydrate patient
• Give antiemetic 30-60 min before giving drug to prevent vomiting, and prn; antibiotics for prophylaxis of infection
• Give top or syst analgesics for pain
• Give in AM so drug can be eliminated before hs
• Provide liquid diet: carbonated beverages; gelatin may be added if patient is not nauseated or vomiting
• Provide rinsing of mouth tid-qid with water, club soda; brushing of teeth bid-qid with soft brush or cotton-tipped applicators for stomatitis; use unwaxed dental floss

C

• Give **IV** direct after diluting 100 mg/5 ml of sterile water for inj; give by direct **IV** over 1-3 min through free-flowing tubing

IV **IV inf**
• May be further diluted in 50-100 ml normal saline or D_5W and given over 30 min to 24 hr depending on dosage

Syringe compatibilities:
Metoclopramide

Y-site compatibilities:
Amifostine, amsacrine, aztreonam, cefepime, chlorpromazine, cimetidine, cladribine, dexamethasone, diphenhydramine, droperidol, famotidine, filgrastim, fludarabine, gentamicin, granisetron, heparin, hydrocortisone, hydromorphone, idarubicin, lorazepam, melphalan, methotrexate, methylprednisolone, metoclopramide, morphine, ondansetron, paclitaxel, piperacillin/tazobactam, prochlorperazine, promethazine, propofol, ranitidine, sargramostim, sodium bicarbonate, teniposide, thiotepa, vinorelbine

Additive incompatibilities:
Carbenicillin, fluorouracil, heparin, regular insulin, nafcillin, oxacillin, penicillin G sodium

Additive compatibilities:
Corticotropin, daunorubicin with etoposide, etoposide, hydroxyzine, lincomycin, mitoxantrone, potassium chloride, prednisolone, ondansetron, sodium bicarbonate, vincristine

Solution compatibilities:
Amino acids, 4.25%/D_{25}, D_5/LR, D_5/0.2% NaCl, D_5/0.9% NaCl, D_{10}/0.9% NaCl, D_5W, invert sugar 10% in electrolyte #1, Ringer's LR, 0.9% NaCl, sodium lactate 1/6 mol/L, TPN #57

Intrathecal route
• Reconstitute with 0.9% NaCl (preservative free) or other compatible sol; to prevent contamination use immediately; discard unused portions if any

SC/IM route
• Reconstitute 100 mg/5 ml or 500 mg/10 ml with bacteriostatic water for inj with benzyl alcohol 0.9%; do not use sol with precipitate; stable for 48 hr

Patient/family education
• Advise patient that contraceptive measures are recommended during therapy
• Teach patient to avoid use of products containing aspirin or ibuprofen, razors, commercial mouthwash, since bleeding may occur; to report symptoms of bleeding (hematuria, tarry stools)
• Advise patient to report signs of anemia (fatigue, headache, irritability, faintness, shortness of breath)
• Instruct patient to report any changes in breathing or coughing even several months after treatment; to avoid crowds and persons with respiratory tract or other infections; neurotoxicity
• Caution patient not to have any vaccinations without the advice of the prescriber; serious reactions can occur

Evaluation
Positive therapeutic outcome
• Prevention of rapid division of malignant cells

---

dacarbazine (R)
(da-kar′ba-zeen)
dacarbazine, DTIC ✤, DTIC-Dome
Func. class.: Antineoplastic misc agent
Chem. class.: Imidazole
Pregnancy category C

Action: Alkylates DNA, RNA; inhibits enzymes that allow synthesis of amino acids in proteins; also responsible for cross-linking DNA strands; activity is not cell cycle phase specific

➡ **Therapeutic Outcome:** Prevention of rapidly growing malignant cells

Uses: Hodgkin's disease, sarcomas, neuroblastoma, malignant melanoma

Investigational uses: Metastatic sarcoma

Dosage and routes
Malignant melanoma
Adult: **IV** 2-4.5 mg/kg or 70-160 mg/m² qd × 10 days; repeat q4 wk depending on response or 250 mg/m² qd × 5 days; repeat q3 wk

Hodgkin's Disease
Adult: **IV** 150 mg/m² qd × 5 days with other agents, repeat q4 wk or 375 mg/m² on day 1 when given in combination, repeat q15 days

Available forms: Inj 100, 200 mg

Adverse effects
CNS: Facial paresthesia, flushing, fever, malaise
GI: Nausea, anorexia, vomiting, **hepatotoxicity** (rare)
HEMA: **Thrombocytopenia, leukopenia,** anemia
INTEG: Alopecia, dermatitis, pain at inj site

Contraindications: Lactation
Precautions: Radiation therapy, pregnancy (1st trimester) **C**

Pharmacokinetics

Absorption	Complete bioavailability (**IV**)
Distribution	Widely distributed; concentrates in liver
Metabolism	Liver (50%, 5% protein bound)
Excretion	Kidneys, unchanged (50%)
Half-life	Initial 35 min, terminal 5 hr

Pharmacodynamics

Unknown

Interactions
Individual drugs
Phenobarbital: ↑ toxicity
Phenytoin: ↑ metabolism, ↓ effect
Radiation: ↑ toxicity, bone marrow suppression
Drug classifications
Aminoglycosides: ↑ nephrotoxicity
Anticoagulants: ↑ risk of bleeding
Antineoplastics: ↑ toxicity, bone marrow suppression
Bone marrow–suppressing drugs: ↑ bone marrow suppression, toxicity
Diuretics, loop: ↑ ototoxicity
Live vaccines: ↑ adverse reactions, ↓ antibody reaction
Salicylates: ↑ risk of bleeding

NURSING CONSIDERATIONS
Assessment
• Assess symptoms indicating severe allergic reaction: rash, pruritus, urticaria, purpuric skin lesions, itching, flushing; drug should be discontinued

• Monitor CBC, differential, platelet count weekly; withhold drug if WBC count is <4000/mm³ or platelet count is <100,000/mm³

• Monitor renal function studies: BUN, creatinine, urine CrCl before and during therapy; I&O ratio; report fall in urine output to <30 ml/hr

• Monitor temp q4h (may indicate beginning of infection)

• Monitor liver function tests before and during therapy (bilirubin, AST, ALT, LDH) as needed or monthly; note jaundice of skin or sclera, dark urine, clay-colored stools, itchy skin, abdominal pain, fever, diarrhea; hepatoxicity can be serious and fatal

• Assess for bleeding: hematuria, stool guaiac, bruising or petechiae, mucosa or orifices q8h; check for inflammation of mucosa, breaks in skin

• Identify effects of alopecia on body image; discuss feelings about body changes

Nursing diagnoses
☑ Injury, risk for (adverse reactions)
☑ Body image disturbance (adverse reactions)
☑ Infection, risk for (adverse reactions)
☑ Knowledge deficit (teaching)

Implementation
• Give fluids **IV** or PO before chemotherapy to hydrate patient

• Give antiemetic 30-60 min before giving drug to prevent vomiting, and prn; antibiotics for prophylaxis of infection

• Provide liquid diet: carbonated beverages; gelatin may be added if patient is not nauseated or vomiting

• After diluting 100 mg/9.9 ml of sterile water for inj (10 mg/ml), give by direct **IV** over 1 min through Y-tube or 3-way stopcock

• May be further diluted in 50-250 ml of D₅W or normal saline for inj and given over 30 min

• Watch for extravasation; give 3-5 ml of mixture of 4 ml sodium thiosulfate 10% plus 5 ml sterile water SC as prescribed

Y-site compatibilities:
Amifostine, aztreonam, filgrastim, fludarabine, granisetron, melphalan, ondansetron, paclitaxel, sargramostim, teniposide, thiotepa, vinorelbine

Additive incompatibilities:
Hydrocortisone sodium succinate, cysteine

Additive compatibilities:
Bleomycin, carmustine, cyclophosphamide, cytarabine, dactinomycin, doxorubicin, fluorouracil, mercaptopurine, methotrexate, ondansetron, vinblastine

Patient/family education
• Teach patient to avoid use of products containing aspirin or ibuprofen, razors, commercial mouthwash, since bleeding may occur; to report symptoms of bleeding (hematuria, tarry stools)

• Instruct patient to report signs of anemia (fatigue, headache, irritability, faintness, shortness of breath)

• Advise patient that hair may be lost during treatment; a wig or hair piece may make patient feel better; new hair may be different in color, texture

• Caution patient not to have any vaccinations without the

advice of prescriber; serious reactions can occur

• Advise patient contraception is needed during treatment and for several months after the completion of therapy; drug has teratogenic properties

Evaluation
Positive therapeutic outcome
• Prevention of rapid division of malignant cells

daclizumab (R)
(dah-kliz′uh-mab)
Zenapax
Func. class.: Immunosuppressive
Chem class.: Humanized IgGl monoclonal antibody
Pregnancy category   C

Action: Binds to the IL-2 (Interleukin-2) receptor antagonist

Therapeutic Outcome: Prevention of graft rejection

Uses: Acute allograft rejection in renal transplant patients

Dosage and routes
Adult: IV 1 mg/kg as part of a regimen that includes cyclosporine and corticosteroids, mix calculated vol with 50 ml of 0.9% NaCl and give via peripheral/central vein over 15 min

Available forms: Inj 25 mg/ml

Adverse effects
CNS: Chills, tremors, headache, prickly sensation
CV: Hypertension, **tachycardia, thrombosis, bleeding**
GI: Vomiting, nausea, diarrhea, constipation, abdominal pain, pyrosis
GU: Oliguria, dysuria, **renal**

tubular necrosis, renal damage, hydronephrosis
INTEG: Impaired wound healing
RESP: Dyspnea, wheezing, **pulmonary edema,** coughing, atelectasis, congestion, hypoxia

Contraindications: Hypersensitivity

Precautions: Pregnancy **C**, child <2 yr, lactation, elderly

Pharmacokinetics
Unknown

Pharmacodynamics
Unknown

Interactions
Unknown

NURSING CONSIDERATIONS
Assessment
• Monitor blood studies: Hgb, WBC, platelets during treatment qmo; if leukocytes are <3000/mm³, drug should be discontinued
• Monitor liver function studies: alk phosphatase, AST, ALT, bilirubin
• Assess for hepatotoxicity: dark urine, jaundice, itching, light-colored stools; drug should be discontinued
• Assess for anaphylaxis: have corticosteroids, epinephrine available

Nursing diagnoses
☑ Injury, risk for (uses)
☑ Knowledge deficit (teaching)

Implementation
• Give all other medications PO if possible; avoid IM injection, since infection may occur

IV route
• Solution compatibilities 0.9% NaCl
• Protect undiluted sol from

direct light; should be used with drugs for immunosuppression

Patient/family education
• Teach patient to report fever, chills, sore throat, fatigue, since serious infection may occur
• Instruct patient to use contraception (women), before, during and for 4 mo after treatment
• Advise patient to avoid vaccinations during treatment
• Advise patient to drink fluids during treatment

Evaluation
Positive therapeutic outcome
• Absence of graft rejection

---

dactinomycin (℞)
(dak-ti-noe-mye'sin)
actinomycin D, Cosmegen
Func. class.: Antineoplastic, antibiotic
Pregnancy category   C

Action: Inhibits DNA, RNA, protein synthesis; derived from *Streptomyces parvulus;* replication is decreased by binding to DNA, which causes strand splitting; cell cycle nonspecific; a vesicant

▶**Therapeutic Outcome:** Prevention of rapidly growing malignant cells, immunosuppression

Uses: Sarcomas, melanomas, trophoblastic tumors in women, testicular cancer, Wilms' tumor, rhabdomyosarcoma

Dosage and routes
Adult: **IV** 500 µg/m²/day × 5 days; stop drug for 2-4 wk; then repeat cycle

P *Child:* **IV** 15 µg/kg/day × 5 days, not to exceed 500 µg/day; stop drug until bone marrow recovery, then repeat cycle

Available forms: Inj 0.5 mg/vial

Adverse effects
CNS: Malaise, fatigue, lethargy, fever
EENT: Cheilitis, dysphagia, esophagitis
GI: Nausea, vomiting, anorexia, stomatitis, **hepatotoxicity,** abdominal pain, diarrhea
HEMA: **Thrombocytopenia, leukopenia, aplastic anemia**
INTEG: Rash, alopecia, pain at inj site, folliculitis, acne, desquamation, *extravasation*
MS: Myalgia

Contraindications: Hypersensitivity, herpes infections, child <6 months

Precautions: Renal disease, hepatic disease, pregnancy **C**, lactation, bone marrow suppression

Pharmacokinetics	
Absorption	Complete bioavailability
Distribution	Widely distributed; crosses placenta
Metabolism	Unknown
Excretion	Bile; feces, unchanged (50%); kidneys (10%)
Half-life	36 hr

Pharmacodynamics
Unknown

Interactions
Individual drugs
Radiation: ↑ toxicity, bone marrow suppression
Drug classifications
Antineoplastics: ↑ toxicity, bone marrow suppression

Bone marrow–suppressing drugs: ↑ bone marrow suppression

Live virus vaccines: ↓ antibody reaction

Lab test interferences
↑ Uric acid

NURSING CONSIDERATIONS
Assessment
• Assess buccal cavity q8h for dryness, sores or ulceration, white patches, pain, bleeding, dysphagia; obtain prescription for viscous lidocaine (Xylocaine)

❗• Assess symptoms indicating severe allergic reaction: rash, pruritus, urticaria, purpuric skin lesions, itching, flushing; drug should be discontinued

• Monitor CBC, differential, platelet count weekly; withhold drug if WBC count is <4000/mm^3 or platelet count is <100,000/mm^3; notify prescriber of results if WBC <20,000/mm^3, platelets <150,000/mm^3

• Monitor renal function studies: BUN, creatinine, serum uric acid, urine CrCl before and during therapy; I&O ratio; report fall in urine output to <30 ml/hr

• Monitor temp q4h (may indicate beginning of infection)

• Monitor liver function tests before and during therapy (bilirubin, AST, ALT, LDH) as needed or monthly; note jaundice of skin or sclera, dark urine, clay-colored stools, itchy skin, abdominal pain, fever, diarrhea

• Assess for bleeding: hematuria, stool guaiac, bruising or petechiae, mucosa or orifices q8h; check for inflammation of mucosa, breaks in skin

• Identify effects of alopecia on body image; discuss feelings about body changes

Nursing diagnoses
☑ Injury, risk for (adverse reactions)
☑ Body image disturbance (adverse reactions)
☑ Oral mucous membranes, altered (adverse reactions)
☑ Infection, risk for (adverse reactions)
☑ Knowledge deficit (teaching)

Implementation
• Provide antacid before oral agent; give drug pc PM, before hs; antiemetic 30-60 mins before giving drug to prevent vomiting, and prn; antibiotics for prophylaxis of infection

• Provide liquid diet: carbonated beverages; gelatin may be added if patient is not nauseated or vomiting

• Help patient rinse mouth tid-qid with water, club soda, brush teeth bid-qid with soft brush or cotton-tipped applicators for stomatitis, use unwaxed dental floss

• Drug should be prepared by experienced personnel using proper precautions

• Give after diluting 0.5 mg/1.1 ml of sterile water for inj without preservative; use 2.2 ml (0.25 mg/ml), give by direct **IV** at 0.5 mg or less/min through Y-tube or 3 way stopcock of inf in progress

Intermittent inf
• May be further diluted in 50 ml D$_5$W or normal saline for inf; run over 10-15 min

• Give hydrocortisone, sodium thiosulfate to infiltration area, and ice compress after stopping inf

• Store in darkness in cool environment

Y-site compatibilities:
Allopurinol, amifostine, aztreonam, cefepime, fludarabine, granisetron, melphalan, ondansetron, sargramostim, teniposide, thiotepa, vinorelbine

Patient/family education
• Teach patient to avoid use of products containing aspirin or ibuprofen, razors, commercial mouthwash, since bleeding may occur; to report symptoms of bleeding (hematuria, tarry stools)
• Instruct patient to report signs of anemia (fatigue, headache, irritability, faintness, shortness of breath)
• Advise patient that hair may be lost during treatment; a wig or hair piece may make patient feel better; new hair may be different in color, texture
• Caution patient not to have any vaccinations without the advice of the prescriber, serious reactions can occur
• Advise patient that contraception is needed during treatment and for several months after the completion of therapy

Evaluation
Positive therapeutic outcome
• Prevention of rapid division of malignant cells

---

dalteparin (℞)
(dahl'ta-pear-in)
Fragmin
Func. class.: Anticoagulant
Chem. class.: Low molecular weight heparin

Pregnancy category   B

Action: Prevents conversion of fibrinogen to fibrin and prothrombin to thrombin by enhancing inhibitory effects of antithrombin III

▣**Therapeutic Outcome:**
Absence of deep vein thrombosis

Uses: Unstable angina/non-Q-wave MI; prevention of deep vein thrombosis in abdominal surgery patients

Investigational uses: Systemic anticoagulation in venous/arterial thromboembolic complications

Dosage and routes
Adult: SC 2500 IU each day starting 1-2 hr prior to surgery and repeat qd × 5-10 days postoperatively; to be used SC only

Unstable angina/non-Q-wave MI
SC 120 IU/kg, do not exceed 10,000 IU g12h with concurrent aspirin, continue until stable

Systemic anticoagulation
Adult: SC 200 IU/kg qd or 100 IU/kg bid

Available forms: Prefilled syringes, 2500, 5000 IU/0.2 ml; 10,000 IU multidose vials

Adverse effects
CNS: **Intracranial bleeding**
HEMA: **Thrombocytopenia**
INTEG: Pruritus, superficial wound infection
SYST: Hypersensitivity, **hemorrhage, anaphylaxis** possible

Contraindications: Hypersensitivity to this drug, heparin, or other anticoagulants; hemophilia, leukemia with bleeding, thrombocytopenic purpura, cerebrovascular hemorrhage, cerebral aneurysm, severe hypertension, other severe cardiac disease

---

G Precautions: Elderly, pregnancy **B**, hepatic disease, severe renal disease, blood dyscrasias, subacute bacterial endocarditis, **P** acute nephritis, lactation, child, recent childbirth, peptic ulcer disease, pericarditis, pericardial effusion, recent lumbar puncture, vasculitis, other diseases where bleeding is possible

Pharmacokinetics	
Absorption	Unknown
Distribution	Unknown
Metabolism	Liver
Excretion	Kidney
Half-life	2 hr

Pharmacodynamics	
Onset	Unknown
Peak	4 hr
Duration	Unknown

Interactions
Drug classifications
Anticoagulants: ↑ risk of bleeding
Platelet inhibitors: ↑ risk of bleeding
Salicylates: ↑ risk of bleeding
☒ Herb/drug
Bromelain, cinchona: ↑ risk of bleeding

NURSING CONSIDERATIONS
Assessment
• Assess for blood studies (Hct, occult blood in stools) during treatment since bleeding can occur
◑• Assess for bleeding gums, petechiae, ecchymosis, black tarry stools, hematuria, epistaxis, decrease in Hct, B/P; may indicate bleeding, possible hemorrhage; notify prescriber immediately, drug should be discontinued
• Assess for hypersensitivity: fever, skin rash, urticaria; notify prescriber immediately

• Assess for needed dosage change q1-2wk; dose may need to be decreased if bleeding occurs

Nursing diagnoses
☑ Injury, risk for (uses, adverse reactions)
☑ Tissue perfusion (uses) altered
☑ Knowledge deficit (teaching)

D

Implementation
SC route
• Do not give IM or **IV** drug route; approved is SC only; do not mix with other inj or sol
• Give by SC only; have patient sit or lie down; SC inj may be 2 in from umbilicus in a U-shape, upper outer side or high or upper outer quadrangle of the buttocks; rotate inj sites
• Changing needles is not recommended

Patient/family education
• Advise patient to avoid OTC preparations that contain aspirin; other anticoagulants, serious drug interaction may occur
• Advise patient to use soft-bristle toothbrush to avoid bleeding gums, avoid contact sports, use electric razor, avoid IM injection
• Instruct patient to report any signs of bleeding: gums, under skin, urine, stools; unusual bruising

Evaluation
Positive therapeutic outcome
• Absence of deep vein thrombosis

Treatment of overdose:
Protamine sulfate 1% given **IV**; 1 mg protamine/100 anti-Xa IU of dalteparin given

---

♣ Canada Only   Adverse effects: *italic* = common; **bold** = life-threatening

danaparoid (℞)
(dan-a-pair'oid)
orgaran
Func. class.: Anticoagulant
Chem. class.: Low molecular weight heparin

Pregnancy category B

Action: Prevents conversion of fibrinogen to fibrin and prothrombin to thrombin by enhancing inhibitory effects of antithrombin III

Therapeutic Outcome: Absence of deep vein thrombosis

Uses: Prevention of vein thrombosis in hemodialysis, stroke, elective surgery for malignancy or total hip replacement, hip fracture surgery

Dosage and routes
Prevention of venous thrombosis
Adult: SC 750 anti-Xa units bid × 7-10 days

Hemodialysis
Adult: **IV** 2400-4800 anti-Xa units given predialysis

Available forms: Inj 750 anti-Xa units in 0.6 ml H_2O for injection

Adverse effects
SYST: Hypersensitivity, **hemorrhage**
HEMA: **Thrombocytopenia**
INTEG: Rash

Contraindications: Hypersensitivity to this drug, sulfites, pork; hemophilia, leukemia with bleeding; thrombocytopenia purpura; cerebrovascular hemorrhage, cerebral aneurysm, severe hypertension, other severe cardiac disease

Precautions: Hypersensitivity to heparin, elderly, pregnancy **B**, hepatic disease, severe renal disease, blood dyscrasias, subacute bacterial endocarditis, acute nephritis, lactation, child, recent childbirth, peptic ulcer disease, pericarditis, pericardial effusion, recent lumbar puncture, vasculitis, other diseases where bleeding is possible

Pharmacokinetics	
Absorption	Unknown
Distribution	Unknown
Metabolism	Unknown
Excretion	Kidneys
Half-life	2-3 hr

Pharmacodynamics	
Onset	Unknown
Peak	4 hr
Duration	Unknown

Interactions
Individual drugs
Aspirin: ↑ risk of bleeding

Drug classifications
Anticoagulants, oral: ↑ risk of bleeding
Platelet inhibitors: ↑ risk of bleeding
Salicylates: ↑ risk of bleeding

Herb/drug
Bromelain: ↑ risk of bleeding
Cinchona bark: ↑ risk of bleeding

NURSING CONSIDERATIONS
Assessment
• Monitor blood studies (Hct, occult blood in stools) during treatment since bleeding can occur; aPTT, ACT, antifactor Xa test, platelets
• Assess for bleeding gums, petechiae, ecchymosis, black tarry stools, hematuria, epistaxis, decrease in Hct, B/P; may indicate bleeding, possible hemorrhage; notify prescriber immediately, drug should be discontinued

- Assess for hypersensitivity: fever, skin rash, urticaria; notify prescriber immediately
- Assess for needed dosage change q1-2wk; dose may need to be decreased if bleeding occurs

Nursing diagnoses
☑ Tissue perfusion, altered (uses)
☑ Injury, risk for (adverse reactions)
☑ Knowledge deficit (teaching)

Implementation
SC route
- Have patient sit or lie down; SC inj may be around the navel in a U-shape, upper outer side of thigh or upper outer quadrangle of the buttocks; rotate inj sites
- Changing needles is not recommended

Patient/family education
- Advise to avoid OTC preparations that may cause serious drug interactions unless directed by prescriber; may contain aspirin, other anticoagulants
- Advise to use soft-bristle toothbrush to avoid bleeding gums, avoid contact sports, use electric razor, avoid IM injection
- Advise to report any signs of bleeding: gums, under skin, urine, stools; unusual bruising

Evaluation
Positive therapeutic outcome
- Absence of deep vein thrombosis

Treatment of overdose:
Protamine sulfate 1% given **IV**; 1 mg protamine/100 anti-Xa IU of Fragmin given

---

danazol (℞)
(da′na-zole)
Cyclomen ✤, danazol, Danocrine
Func. class.: Androgen, hormone
Chem. class.: α-Ethinyl testosterone derivative
Pregnancy category   X

Action: Atrophy of endometrial tissue; decreases FSH, LH, which are controlled by pituitary; this leads to amenorrhea/anovulation; has weak androgen, anabolic activity

▶ **Therapeutic Outcome:** Decreased pain and nodules/fibrocystic breast disease; correction in hereditary angioedema; atrophy of endometrial tissue (ectopic)

Uses: Endometriosis, prevention of hereditary angioedema, fibrocystic breast disease

Dosage and routes
Endometriosis
Adult: PO 100-500 mg bid, uninterrupted for 3-9 mo
Fibrocystic breast disease
Adult: PO 100-400 mg qd in 2 divided doses × 2-6 mo
Hereditary angioedema prevention
Adult: PO 200 mg bid-tid until desired response, then decrease dose to 100 mg at 1-3 mo intervals

Available forms: Caps 50, 100, 200 mg

Adverse effects
CNS: Dizziness, headache, fatigue, tremors, paresthesias, flushing, sweating, anxiety, lability, insomnia, carpal tunnel syndrome
CV: Increased B/P

EENT: Conjunctival edema, nasal congestion
ENDO: Abnormal GTT
GI: Nausea, vomiting, constipation, weight gain, **cholestatic jaundice**
GU: Hematuria, amenorrhea, atrophic vaginitis, decreased libido, decreased breast size, clitoral hypertrophy, testicular atrophy
INTEG: Rash, acneiform lesions, oily hair and skin, flushing, sweating, acne vulgaris, alopecia, hirsutism
MS: Cramps, spasms

Contraindications: Severe renal disease, severe cardiac disease, severe hepatic disease, hypersensitivity, genital bleeding (abnormal), pregnancy **X**

Precautions: Migraine headaches, seizure disorders

▧ Do Not Confuse:
danazol/Dantrium

Pharmacokinetics

Absorption	GI absorption
Distribution	Unknown
Metabolism	Liver
Excretion	Kidneys
Half-life	4½ hr

Pharmacodynamics
Unknown

Interactions
Individual drugs
Cyclosporine: ↑ risk of nephrotoxicity
Carbamazepine: ↑ carbamazepine level
Drug classifications
Anticoagulants: ↑ pro-time
Lab test interferences
↑ Cholesterol, ↓ cholesterol, ↓ T_4, ↓ T_3, ↓ thyroid ^{131}I uptake test, ↓ 17-KS, ↓ PBI
Interferences: GTT

NURSING CONSIDERATIONS
Assessment
• Assess for lower abdominal (endometrial) pain before and throughout treatment to identify if treatment is effective
• Monitor potassium, blood sugar, urine glucose while patient is on long-term therapy
• Assess breast for fibrocystic nodules; check for pain, tenderness before therapy and throughout to identify if treatment is effective
• Monitor weight daily; notify prescriber if weekly weight gain is >5 lb; I&O ratio; be alert for decreasing urinary output, increasing edema, hypertension, cardiac symptoms, jaundice
• Assess for mental status: affect, mood, behavioral changes, aggression, sleep disorders, depression; change may be extreme
• Assess for signs of virilization: deepening of voice, decreased libido, facial hair (may not be reversible)

Nursing diagnoses
☑ Infection, risk for (adverse reactions)
☑ Injury, risk for (adverse reactions)
☑ Knowledge deficit (teaching)

Implementation
• Store in airtight container at room temp
• Provide ROM exercise for patients who are immobile
• Give with food or milk to decrease GI symptoms
🚫• Do not crush, chew caps

Patient/family education
• Teach patient to notify prescriber if therapeutic response decreases; advise that endometriosis tends to recur after drug is discontinued; not to discon-

---

☑ Herb/drug 🚫 Do Not Crush ◆ Alert ⊶ Key Drug **G** Geriatric **P** Pediatric

tinue medication abruptly but to taper over several weeks

• Advise patient that alternate contraceptive measures are needed during treatment; amenorrhea may occur with higher dosages

• Teach patient to report menstrual irregularities; that amenorrhea usually occurs but menstruation resumes 2-3 mo after termination of therapy; that drug should induce anovulation; reversible within 60-90 days after drug is discontinued

• Teach patient about routine breast self-exam technique, to report any increase in nodule size

• Instruct patient to report masculinization: deepening voice, facial hair growth, body hair growth

Evaluation

Positive therapeutic outcome

• Decreased pain in endometriosis

• Decreased size, pain in fibrocystic breast disease

• Decreased signs of angioedema (hereditary)

---

dantrolene (℞)

(dan'troe-leen)

Dantrium, Dantrium Intravenous

Func. class.: Skeletal muscle relaxant, direct acting
Chem. class.: Hydantoin

Pregnancy category   C

Action: Interferes with intracellular release from the sarcoplasmic reticulum of calcium necessary to initiate contraction; slows catabolism in malignant hyperthermia

▶**Therapeutic Outcome:** Decreased muscle spasticity; absence of malignant hyperthermia

Uses: Spasticity in multiple sclerosis, stroke, spinal cord injury, cerebral palsy, prevention and treatment of malignant hyperthermia

Dosage and routes
Spasticity
Adult: PO 25 mg/day; may increase by 25-100 mg bid-qid, not to exceed 400 mg/day × 1 wk

▣ *Child:* PO 1 mg/kg/day given in divided doses bid-tid; may increase gradually, not to exceed 100 mg qid

Malignant hyperthermia
▣ *Adult and child:* **IV** 1 mg/kg; may repeat to total dose of 10 mg/kg; PO 4-8 mg/kg/day in 4 divided doses × 3 days to prevent further hyperthermia; postcrisis follow-up 4-8 mg/kg/day for 1-3 days

Prevention of malignant hyperthermia
▣ *Adult and child:* PO 4-8 mg/kg/day in 3-4 divided doses × 1-2 days before procedures; give last dose 4 hr preoperatively; **IV** 2.5 mg/kg prior to anesthesia

Available forms: Caps 25, 50, 100 mg; powder for inj 20 mg/vial

Adverse effects
CNS: Dizziness, weakness, fatigue, drowsiness, headache, disorientation, insomnia, paresthesias, tremors, **seizures**
CV: Hypotension, chest pain, palpitations
EENT: Nasal congestion, blurred vision, mydriasis
GI: **Hepatic injury,** *nausea,*

D

---

constipation, vomiting, increased AST and alkaline phosphatase, abdominal pain, dry mouth, anorexia, hepatitis
GU: Urinary frequency, nocturia, impotence, crystalluria
HEMA: Eosinophilia
INTEG: Rash, pruritus, photosensitivity

Contraindications: Hypersensitivity, compromised pulmonary function, active hepatic disease, impaired myocardial function

Precautions: Peptic ulcer disease, renal disease, hepatic disease, stroke, seizure disorder, diabetes mellitus, pregnancy **C,** elderly

🅖 nancy **C,** elderly

🅝 **Do Not Confuse:**
Dantrium/danazol

Pharmacokinetics	
Absorption	PO (30%-35%)
Distribution	Unknown
Metabolism	Liver, extensively
Excretion	Kidney
Half-life	9 hr

Pharmacodynamics		
	PO	IV
Onset	Unknown	Immediate
Peak	5 hr	5 hr
Duration	Dose related	Dose related

Interactions
Individual drugs
Alcohol: ↑ CNS depression
Clofibrate: ↑ action of dantrolene
Verapamil IV: ↑ hyperkalemia
Warfarin: ↑ action of dantrolene
Drug classifications
Antidepressants, tricyclic: ↑ CNS depression
Antihistamines: ↑ CNS depression
Barbiturates: ↑ CNS depression

Estrogens: ↑ hepatotoxicity
Opiates: ↑ CNS depression
Sedative/hypnotics: ↑ CNS depression

NURSING CONSIDERATIONS
Assessment
• Monitor I&O ratio; check for urinary retention, frequency, hesitancy, especially
🅖 elderly
• Monitor ECG in epileptic patients; poor seizure control has occurred with patients taking this drug; assess for increased seizure activity in epilepsy patient
• Monitor hepatic function by frequent determination of AST, ALT, renal function studies, CBC
• Assess for allergic reactions: rash, fever, respiratory distress
• Monitor for severe weakness, numbness in extremities
• Assess for CNS depression: dizziness, drowsiness, psychiatric symptoms
◆• Assess for signs of hepatotoxicity: jaundice, yellow sclera, pain in abdomen, nausea, fever; drug should be discontinued if these signs and symptoms occur

Nursing diagnoses
☑ Pain, chronic (uses)
☑ Physical mobility, impaired (uses)
☑ Injury, risk for (adverse reactions)
☑ Knowledge deficit (teaching)

Implementation
PO route
• Give with meals for GI symptoms; capsules may be opened and mixed with liquid; patient should drink after mixing
• Store in airtight container at room temp

☑ Herb/drug　🅢 Do Not Crush　◆ Alert　☮ Key Drug　🅖 Geriatric　🅟 Pediatric

IV route

- Administer **IV** after reconstituting 20 mg/60 ml sterile water for inj without bacteriostatic agent (333 µg/ml); shake until clear; give by rapid **IV** push through Y-tube or 3-way stopcock; follow by prescribed doses immediately; assess site for extravasation, phlebitis
- Protect diluted sol from light; use reconstituted sol within 6 hr

Patient/family education

- Notify prescriber of abdominal pain, jaundiced sclera, clay-colored stools, change in color of urine, rash, itching
- Caution patient not to take with alcohol, other CNS depressants; severe CNS depression can occur; avoid using OTC medication: cough preparations, antihistamines, unless directed by prescriber
- Tell patient that if improvement does not occur within 6 wk, prescriber may discontinue
- Caution patient to avoid hazardous activities if drowsiness, dizziness, blurred vision occurs; wait several days to identify patient response to medication
- Teach patient to use sunscreen, protective clothing for photosensitivity
- Instruct patient to take medication as prescribed; do not double doses; take dose if missed within 1 hr of scheduled time

Evaluation

Positive therapeutic outcome
- Decreased pain, spasticity
- Absence or decreased symptoms of malignant hyperthermia

Treatment of overdose:

Induce emesis of conscious patient; lavage, dialysis

---

daunorubicin ℞
(daw-noe-roo'bi-sin)
Cerubidine
Func. class.: Antineoplastic, antibiotic
Chem. class.: Anthracycline glycoside
Pregnancy category   D

D

Action: Inhibits DNA synthesis, primarily; derived from *Streptomyces coeruleorubidus;* replication is decreased by binding to DNA, which causes strand splitting; cell cycle specific (S phase); a vesicant

Therapeutic Outcome: Prevention of rapidly growing malignant cells; immunosuppression

Uses: Myelogenous, monocytic leukemia, acute nonlymphocytic leukemia, Ewing's sarcoma, Wilms' tumor, neuroblastoma, rhabdomyosarcoma

Dosage and routes
Single agent
Adult: **IV** 60 mg/m²/day × 3-5 day q4 wk
In combination
Adult: **IV** 45 mg/m²/day × 3 days, then 2 days of subsequent courses with cytosine arabinoside
Child: **IV** 25-60 mg/m² depending on cycle

Available forms: Inj 20 mg powder/vial

Adverse effects

CNS: Fever, chills
CV: **Dysrhythmias, CHF,**

pericarditis, myocarditis, peripheral edema
GI: Nausea, vomiting, anorexia, mucositis, **hepatotoxicity**
GU: Impotence, sterility, amenorrhea, gynecomastia, hyperuricemia
HEMA: **Thrombocytopenia, leukopenia, anemia**
INTEG: Rash, extravasation, dermatitis, reversible alopecia, cellulitis, thrombophlebitis at inj site
OTHER: Anaphylaxis
Contraindications: Hypersensitivity, pregnancy **D,** lactation, syst infections, cardiac disease
Precautions: Renal, hepatic disease, gout, bone marrow suppression
 Do Not Confuse:

daunorubicin/doxorubicin

Pharmacokinetics

Absorption	Complete
Distribution	Widely distributed; crosses placenta
Metabolism	Liver, extensively
Excretion	Biliary (40%-50%)
Half-life	18½ hr

Pharmacodynamics

Unknown

Interactions
Individual drugs

Cyclophosphamide: ↑ cardiotoxicity, CHF
Radiation: ↑ toxicity, bone marrow suppression
Drug classifications

Antineoplastics: ↑ toxicity, bone marrow suppression
Lab test interferences

↑ Uric acid

NURSING CONSIDERATIONS
Assessment

• Assess buccal cavity q8h for dryness, sores or ulceration, white patches, pain, bleeding, dysphagia; obtain prescription for viscous lidocaine (Xylocaine)
• Assess symptoms indicating severe allergic reaction: rash, pruritus, urticaria, purpuric skin lesions, itching, flushing; drug should be discontinued
• Assess tachypnea, ECG changes, dyspnea, edema, fatigue
• Monitor CBC, differential, platelet count weekly; withhold drug if WBC count is <4000/mm^3 or platelet count is <100,000/mm^3; notify prescriber of results if WBC <20,000/mm^3, platelets <150,000/mm^3
• Assess for increased uric acid levels, swelling, joint pain primarily in extremities; patient should be well hydrated to prevent urate deposits
• Monitor renal function studies: BUN, creatinine, serum uric acid, urine CrCl before and during therapy; I&O ratio; report fall in urine output to <30 ml/hr
• Monitor temp q4h (may indicate beginning of infection)
• Monitor liver function tests before and during therapy (bilirubin, AST, ALT, LDH) as needed or monthly; note jaundice of skin or sclera, dark urine, clay-colored stools, itchy skin, abdominal pain, fever, diarrhea; hepatoxicity can be severe
• Assess for bleeding: hematuria, stool guaiac, bruising or petechiae, mucosa or orifices

---

q8h; check for inflammation of mucosa, breaks in skin
• Identify effects of alopecia on body image; discuss feelings about body changes

Nursing diagnoses

☑Injury, risk for (adverse reactions)
☑Cardiac output, decreased (adverse reactions)
☑Body image disturbance (adverse reactions)
☑Infection, risk for (adverse reactions)
☑Knowledge deficit (teaching)

Implementation

• Avoid contact with skin; very irritating; wash completely to remove
• Give fluids **IV** or PO before chemotherapy to hydrate patient; give antiemetic 30-60 min before giving drug to prevent vomiting, and prn; antibiotics for prophylaxis of infection
• Provide liquid diet: carbonated beverages; gelatin may be added if patient is not nauseated or vomiting
• Help patient rinse mouth tid-qid with water, club soda, brush teeth bid-qid with soft brush or cotton-tipped applicators for stomatitis, use unwaxed dental floss
• Drug should be prepared by experienced personnel using proper precautions
• Give **IV** after diluting 20 mg/4 ml sterile water for inj (5 mg/ml); rotate; further dilute in 10-15 ml normal saline; give over 3-5 min by direct **IV** through Y-tube or 3-way stopcock of inf of D_5W or 0.9% NaCl

Intermittent inf route
• Dilute further in 50-100 ml 0.9% NaCl, LR, D_5W; give over 15 min (50 ml), 30 min (100 ml)

Y-site incompatibilities:

Fludarabine

Y-site compatibilities:

Amifostine, filgrastim, granisetron, melphalan, methotrexate, ondansetron, sodium bicarbonate, teniposide, thiotepa, vinorelbine

Additive incompatibilities:

Dexamethasone, heparin

Additive compatibilities:

Cytarabine with etoposide, hydrocortisone; not recommended for admixing

Solution compatibilities:

$D_{3.3}/0.3\%$ NaCl, D_5W, Normosol R, Ringer's, 0.9% NaCl

Patient/family education

• Teach patient to avoid use of products containing aspirin or ibuprofen, razors, commercial mouthwash, since bleeding may occur; to report symptoms of bleeding (hematuria, tarry stools)
• Instruct patient to report signs of anemia (fatigue, headache, irritability, faintness, shortness of breath); signs of infection; bleeding, bruising
• Advise patient that hair may be lost during treatment; a wig or hair piece may make patient feel better; new hair may be different in color, texture
• Caution patient not to have any vaccinations without the advice of the prescriber; serious reactions can occur
• Advise patient that contraception is needed during treatment and for several months after the completion of therapy

Evaluation

Positive therapeutic outcome
• Prevention of rapid division of malignant cells

---

deferoxamine (℞)

(de-fer-ox'a-meen)

Desferal

Func. class.: Heavy metal antagonist

Chem. class.: Chelating agent

Pregnancy category C

Action: Binds iron ions (ferric ions) to form water-soluble complex that is removed by kidneys

➡ Therapeutic Outcome: Excretion of excess iron and aluminum

Uses: Acute, chronic iron intoxication, hemochromatosis, hemosiderosis

Dosage and routes
Acute iron toxicity
P *Adult and child:* IM/**IV** 1 g; then 500 mg q4h × 2 doses; then 500 mg q4-12h × 2 doses, not to exceed 15 mg/kg/hr or 6 g/24 hr

Chronic iron toxicity
P *Adult and child:* IM 500 mg-1 g/day plus **IV** inf 2 g given by separate line with each blood transfusion, not to exceed 15 mg/kg/hr or 6 g/24 hr; SC 1-2 g over 8-24 hr by SC infusion pump

Available forms: Powder for inj 500 mg/vial

Adverse effects

CNS: Flushing, **shock following rapid IV administration**
CV: Hypotension, tachycardia

EENT: Blurred vision, cataracts, decreased healing, *ototoxicity*
GI: Diarrhea, abdominal cramps
GU: Dysuria, pyelonephritis, red urine
INTEG: Urticaria, erythema, pruritus, pain at inj site, fever
MS: Leg cramps
SYST: **Anaphylaxis**

Contraindications: Hypersensitivity, anuria, severe renal disease

Precautions: Pregnancy C,
P lactation, child <3 yr

◨ Do Not Confuse:
deferoxamine/cefuroxime

Pharmacokinetics	
Absorption	Well absorbed (IM, SC); completely absorbed (**IV**)
Distribution	Widely distributed
Metabolism	Plasma enzymes
Excretion	Kidneys, unchanged; chelated, excess iron removed by feces and bile (33%-35%)
Half-life	1 hr

Pharmacodynamics
Unknown

Interactions: None

NURSING CONSIDERATIONS
Assessment

• Assess for poisoning: type of iron agent, time, amount ingested, acute or chronic
◆ • Assess for acute iron toxicity: acute early symptoms (nausea, vomiting, abdominal cramping, bloody diarrhea); acute late symptoms (metabolic acidosis, coma, shock)
• Assess vision and hearing periodically; ototoxicity may occur

---

- Check VS during **IV** administration; watch for dropping B/P, urine color (urine may turn red), rash, urticaria; if these occur, drug should be discontinued; resuscitation equipment should be available for anaphylaxis
- Monitor I&O, renal function studies: BUN, creatinine, CrCl, serum iron levels

Nursing diagnoses
☑ Poisoning (uses)
☑ Knowledge deficit (teaching)

Implementation
IV IV route
- Give **IV** (used for shock) after diluting 500 mg/2 ml water for inj; when dissolved, must be further diluted with D₅W, LR, or 0.9% NaCl; run at <15 mg/kg/hr; 2 g/1000 ml usually given over 24 hr; to be used only for short time; IM is preferred route
- Administer only when epinephrine 1:1000 is available for anaphylaxis

IM route
- Give IM after diluting with 2 ml sterile water for inj per 500 mg of drug; rotate inj sites; give deep in large muscle mass; rotate sites

SC route
- Use abdominal SC tissue by inf pump for 8-24 hr/treatment; use only for chronic iron toxicity

Patient/family education
- Teach patient that urine may turn red; this is not blood but iron excretion
- Caution patient to avoid vitamin C preparations including multivitamins unless approved by prescriber
- Instruct patient that tests are required after treatment for chronic iron toxicity including

blood, hearing, and eye tests; stress the importance of follow-up

Evaluation
Positive therapeutic outcome
- Decreased symptoms of heavy metal intoxication

D

---

delavirdine (℞)
(de-la-veer′din)
Rescriptor
Func. class.: Nonnucleoside reverse transcriptase inhibitor (NNRII)
Pregnancy category   C

Action: Binds directly to reverse transcriptase and blocks RNA, DNA causing a disruption of the enzyme's site

➡ **Therapeutic Outcome:** Improvement of HIV-1 infection

Uses: HIV-1 in combination with zidovudine or didanosine

Dosage and routes
P *Adult and child ≥16 yr:* 400 mg tid

Available forms: Tabs 100 mg

Adverse effects
CNS: Headache, fatigue
GI: Diarrhea, abdominal pain, nausea, vomiting, dyspepsia, **hepatotoxicity**
GU: **Nephrotoxicity**
HEMA: **Neutropenia, leukopenia, thrombocytopenia, anemia, granulocytopenia**
INTEG: Rash
MS: Pain myalgia

Contraindications: Hypersensitivity to this drug or atevirdine

Precautions: Liver disease,
P pregnancy **C,** lactation, chil-

---

dren, renal disease, myelosuppression

Pharmacokinetics	
Absorption	Well
Distribution	Highly protein bound
Metabolism	Liver
Excretion	Kidneys, feces
Half-life	6 hr

Pharmacodynamics

Unknown

Interactions
Drug classifications
Alprazolam: ↑ level of alpra-
zolam
Antacids: ↓ delavirdine levels
Anticonvulsants: ↓ delavirdine
levels
Astemizole: ↑ level of astemi-
zole
Cisapride: ↑ level if cisapride
Clarithromycin: ↑ level of
clarithromycin or ↑ level of
delavirdine
Dapsone: ↑ level of dapsone
Ergots: ↑ ergotism
Felodipine: ↑ level of felo-
dipine
Fluoxetine: ↑ level of delavir-
dine
Indinavir: ↑ level of indinavir
Ketoconazole: ↑ level of
delavirdine
Midazolam: ↑ level of mida-
zolam
Nifidepine: ↑ level of nifide-
pine
Oral contraceptives: ↓ action
Protease inhibitors: ↓ action
of protease inhibitors
Quinidine and warfarin: ↑
level of both quinidine and
warfarin
Rifamycins: ↓ delavirdine
levels

NURSING CONSIDERATIONS
Assessment
• Assess signs of infection,
anemia
• Assess liver studies: ALT,
AST; renal studies
• Assess C&S before drug
therapy; drug may be taken as
soon as culture is taken; repeat
C&S after treatment; determine the presence of other
sexually transmitted disease
• Assess bowel pattern before,
during teatment; if severe
abdominal pain with bleeding
occurs, drug should be
discontinued; monitor hydration
• Assess skin eruptions; rash,
urticaria, itching
• Assess allergies before treatment, reaction to each
medication; place allergies
on chart
• Assess plasma delavirdine
concentrations (trough 10
micromolar)
• Assess CBC, blood chemistry, plasma HIV RNA, absolute
CD4+/CD8+/cell counts/%,
serum β-2 microglobulin,
serum ICD+24 antigen levels
• Assess for signs of delavirdine
toxicity: severe nausea, vomiting, maculopapular rash

Nursing diagnoses
☑ Infection (risk for uses)
☑ Diarrhea (side effects)
☑ Knowledge deficit (teaching)

Patient/family education
• Advise patient to take as
prescribed; if dose is missed,
take as soon as remembered up
to 1 hr before next dose; do
not double dose
• Advise patient that drug
must be taken in equal intervals around the clock to maintain blood levels for duration
of therapy

☑ Herb/drug   Ⓢ Do Not Crush   ◆ Alert   ☞ Key Drug   Ⓖ Geriatric   Ⓟ Pediatric

- Advise patient that tabs may be dissolved, drink right away, rinse cup with water, and drink that to get all medication
- Instruct patient to make sure health care provider knows of all the medications being taken
- Advise patient that if severe rash, mouth sores, swelling, aching muscles/joints, or eye redness occur, stop taking and notify health care provider
- Advise patient not to breast-feed if taking this drug

denileukin diftitox
See Appendix A,
Selected New Drugs

desmopressin (℞)
(des-moe-press'in)
DDAVP, Stimate
Func. class.: Pituitary hormone
Chem. class.: Synthetic antidiuretic hormone

Pregnancy category   B

Action: Promotes reabsorption of water by action on renal tubular epithelium in the kidney; causes smooth muscle constriction and increase in plasma factor VIII levels, which increases platelet aggregation resulting in vasopressor effect; similar to vasopressor

▶ **Therapeutic Outcome:** Prevention of nocturnal enuresis, decreased bleeding in hemophilia A, von Willebrand's disease type 1, control and stabilization of water in diabetes insipidus

Uses: Hemophilia A, von Willebrand's disease type 1, nonnephrogenic diabetes insipidus, symptoms of polyuria/polydipsia caused by pituitary dysfunction, nocturnal enuresis

Dosage and routes
Primary nocturnal enuresis
P *Child ≥6 yr:* Intranasal 20 μg (10 μg in each nostril) hs, may increase to 40 μg; PO 0.2 mg hs, may be increased to max 0.6 mg hs

Diabetes insipidus
Adult: Intranasal 0.1-0.4 ml qd in divided doses (1-4 sprays with pump); **IV**/SC 0.5-1 ml qd in two divided doses

P *Child 3 mo to 12 yr:* Intranasal 0.05-0.3 ml qd or in divided doses bid

Hemophilia/von Willebrand's disease
P *Adult and child:* **IV** 0.3 μg/kg in NaCl over 15-30 min; may repeat if needed

Available forms: Intranasal 0.01 mg/ml; inj 4 μg/ml; tabs 0.1, 0.2 mg; rhinal tube delivery 2.5 mg/vial

Adverse effects
CNS: Drowsiness, headache, lethargy, flushing
CV: Increased B/P
EENT: Nasal irritation, congestion, rhinitis
GI: Nausea, heartburn, cramps
GU: Vulval pain
SYST: **Anaphylaxis IV**

Contraindications: Hypersensitivity, nephrogenic diabetes insipidus

Precautions: Pregnancy **B,** CAD, lactation, hypertension

Pharmacokinetics

Absorption	Nasal (up to 20%)
Distribution	Unknown
Metabolism	Unknown
Excretion	Unknown; breast milk
Half-life	8 min (initial), 76 min (terminal)

Pharmacodynamics

	INTRANASAL	IV/SC
Onset	1 hr	Rapid
Peak	1-2 hr	15-30 min
Duration	8-20 hr	3 hr

Interactions
Individual drugs
Alcohol: ↑ adverse reactions
Carbamazepine: ↑ response of desmopressin
Chlorpropamide: ↑ response of desmopressin
Clofibrate: ↑ response of desmopressin
Demeclocycline: ↑ adverse reactions
Epinephrine (large doses): ↑ adverse reactions
Heparin: ↑ adverse reactions
Lithium: ↑ adverse reactions
Norepinephrine: ↑ adverse reactions

NURSING CONSIDERATIONS
Assessment
• Monitor I&O ratio, urine osmolality, sp gr, weight daily; check for edema in extremities; if water retention is severe, diuretic may be prescribed; check pulse, B/P when giving drug **IV** or SC
• Assess for water intoxication: lethargy, behavioral changes, disorientation, neuromuscular excitability, dehydration, poor skin turgor, severe thirst, dry skin, tachycardia
• Assess intranasal use: nausea, congestion, cramps, headache; usually decreased with decreased dosage
• Monitor for enuresis during treatment (nocturnal enuresis)
• Assess for allergic reaction including anaphylaxsis (**IV** route)
• Assess for nasal mucosa changes: congestion, edema, discharge, scarring (nasal route)
• Monitor urine volume osmolality and plasma osmolality (diabetes insipidus)
• Monitor factor VIII coagulant activity before using for hemostasis

Nursing diagnoses
☑ Fluid volume deficit (uses)
☑ Fluid volume excess (side effects)
☑ Knowledge deficit (teaching)

Implementation
• Store in refrigerator or cool environment
IV **IV route**
Direct IV
• Give undiluted over 1 min in diabetes insipidus or **IV** for hemophilia
Intermittent inf
• Give single dose diluted in 50 ml of 0.9% NaCl (adult and **P** child >10 kg); a single dose/10 ml as an **IV** inf over 15-30 min in von Willebrand's disease or hemophilia A

Patient/family education
• Use demonstration, return demonstration to teach technique for nasal instillation: draw medication into tube, insert tube into nostril to instill drug and blow on other end to deliver sol into nasal cavity; rinse after use
• Teach patient to notify prescriber of dyspnea, vomiting, cramping, drowsiness, headache, nasal congestion
• Caution patient to avoid OTC products (cough, hay

fever), since these preparations may contain epinephrine and decrease drug response; do not use with alcohol

• Advise patient to wear Medic Alert ID or other identification specifying disease and medication used

• Advise patient if dose is missed, take when remembered up to 1 hr before next dose; do not double doses

Evaluation

Positive therapeutic outcome

• Absence of severe thirst

• Decreased urine output, osmolality

• Absence of bleeding (hemophilia)

---

dexamethasone (℞)
(dex-ah-meth'ah-sone)
Decadron, Deronil ✦, Dexasone ✦, Dexon, Hexadrol, Mymethasone
dexamethasone acetate (℞)
Dalalone DP, Dalalone LA, Decadron-LA, Decaject-LA, Dexacen LA-8, Dexasone-LA, Dexone LA, Solurex-LA
dexamethasone sodium phosphate (℞)
Dalalone, Decadron Phosphate, Decaject, Dexacen-4, Dexone, Hexadrol Phosphate, Solurex
Func. class.: Corticosteroid
Chem. class.: Glucocorticoid, long-acting
Pregnancy category C

Action: Decreases inflammation by suppression of migration of polymorphonuclear leukocytes, fibroblasts, reversal

of increased capillary permeability and lysosomal stabilization

Uses: Inflammation, allergies, neoplasms, cerebral edema, septic shock, collagen disorders

Dosage and routes
Inflammation
Adult: PO 0.75-9 mg/day or phosphate IM 0.5-9 mg/day; or acetate IM 4-16 mg into joint of tissue q1-3wk

▣ *Child:* PO 0.08-0.3 mg/kg/day in divided doses q6-12h

Shock (Phosphate)
Adult: **IV** single dose 1-6 mg/kg or **IV** 40 mg q2-6h as needed up to 72 hr

Cerebral edema (Phosphate)
Adult: **IV** 10 mg, then 4-6 mg IM q6h × 2-4 days, then taper over 1 wk

▣ *Child:* PO 0.2 mg/kg/day in divided doses

Adrenocortical Insufficiency
▣ *Child:* 23.3 μg/kg/day in 3 divided doses

Available forms: Dexamethasone: tabs 0.25, 0.5, 0.75, 1, 1.5, 2, 4, 6 mg; 20, 24 phosphate; elix 0.5 mg/5 ml; oral sol 0.5 mg/5 ml, 0.5 mg/1 ml; inj acetate 8, 16 mg/ml; inj phosphate 4, 10 mg/ml

Adverse effects
CNS: Depression, flushing, sweating, headache, mood changes, euphoria, psychosis, **seizures**
CV: Hypertension, **circulatory collapse, thrombophlebitis, embolism,** tachycardia, edema
EENT: Fungal infections, increased intraocular pressure, blurred vision
ENDO: HPA suppression
GI: Diarrhea, nausea, abdomi-

nal distention, **GI hemor-rhage,** *increased appetite,* **pancreatitis**
HEMA: **Thrombocytopenia**
INTEG: Acne, poor wound healing, ecchymosis, petechiae
META: Hypokalemia
MS: Fractures, osteoporosis, weakness

Contraindications: Psychosis, hypersensitivity, idiopathic thrombocytopenia, acute glomerulonephritis, amebiasis, fungal infections, nonasthmatic bronchial disease, child <2 yr, AIDS, TB **P**

Precautions: Pregnancy **C,** lactation, diabetes mellitus, glaucoma, osteoporosis, seizure disorders, ulcerative colitis, CHF, myasthenia gravis, renal disease, peptic ulcer, esophagitis

Do Not Confuse: **N**
Decadron/Percodan

Pharmacokinetics

Absorption	Unknown
Distribution	Unknown
Metabolism	Liver
Excretion	Kidneys
Half-life	3-4½ hr

Pharmacodynamics

	PO	IM
Onset	1 hr	Unknown
Peak	1-2 hr	8 hr
Duration	2½ days	6 days

Interactions
Individual drugs
Alcohol: ↑ side effects
Amphotericin B: ↑ side effects
Cholestyramine: ↓ action of dexamethasone
Colestipol: ↓ action of dexamethasone
Cyclosporine: ↑ side effects
Digoxin: ↑ side effects

Ephedrine: ↓ action of dexamethasone
Indomethacin: ↑ side effects
Isoniazid: ↓ effects of isoniazid
Ketoconazole: ↑ side effects
Neostigmine: ↓ effects of neostigmine
Phenytoin: ↓ action of dexamethasone
Rifampin: ↓ action of dexamethasone
Sometrem: ↓ effects of sometrem
Theophylline: ↓ action of dexamethasone

Drug classifications
Antacids: ↓ action of dexamethasone
Antibiotics, macrolide: ↑ action of dexamethasone
Anticholinesterases: ↓ effects of anticholinesterases
Anticoagulants: ↓ effects of anticoagulants
Anticonvulsants: ↓ effects of anticonvulsants
Antidiabetics: ↓ effects of antidiabetics
Barbiturates: ↓ action of dexamethasone
Contraceptives, oral: ↑ action of dexamethasone
Diuretics: ↑ side effects
Estrogens: ↑ action of dexamethasone
Salicylates: ↓ effects of salicylates
Toxoids/Vaccines: ↓ effects of toxoids/vaccines
Herb/drug
Aloe: ↑ hypokalemia
Buckthorn bark/berry: ↑ hypokalemia
Cascara sagrada: ↑ hypokalemia
Ephedra: ↑ hypokalemia
Senna pod/leaf: ↑ hypokalemia

D

Lab test interferences
↑ Cholesterol, ↑ Na, ↑ blood glucose, ↑ uric acid, ↑ Ca, ↑ urine glucose

↓ Ca, ↓ K, ↓ T_4, ↓ T_3, ↓ thyroid ^{131}I uptake test, ↓ urine 17-OHCS, ↓ 17-KS, ↓ PBI

False negative: Skin allergy tests

NURSING CONSIDERATIONS
Assessment
• Monitor K, blood sugar, urine glucose while on long-term therapy; hypokalemia and hyperglycemia
• Monitor weight daily; notify prescriber of weekly gain >5 lb
• Monitor B/P q4h, pulse; notify prescriber of chest pain
• Monitor I&O ratio; be alert for decreasing urinary output, increasing edema
• Monitor plasma cortisol levels during long-term therapy (normal: 138-635 nmol/L SI units when drawn at 8 AM)
• Assess infection: fever, WBC even after withdrawal of medication; drug masks infection
• Assess potassium depletion: paresthesias, fatigue, nausea, vomiting, depression, polyuria, dysrhythmias, weakness
• Assess edema, hypertension, cardiac symptoms
• Assess mental status: affect, mood, behavioral changes, aggression

Nursing diagnoses
☑ Infection, risk for (adverse reaction)
☑ Knowledge deficit (teaching)
☑ Mobility, impaired (uses)

Implementation
☑ **IV route**
• **IV** undiluted direct over 1 min or less or diluted with NS or D_5W and give as an **IV** inf at prescribed rate
• After shaking suspension (parenteral); do not give suspension **IV**
• Titrated dose; use lowest effective dose

Syringe compatibilities:
Granisetron, metoclopramide, ranitidine, sufentanil

Y-site compatibilities:
Acyclovir, allopurinol, amifostine, amikacin, amphotericin B cholesteryl, amsacrine, aztreonam, cefepime, cisatracurium, cisplatin, cladribine, cyclophosphamide, cytarabine, doxorubicin, doxorubicin liposome, famotidine, filgrastim, fluconazole, fludarabine, foscarnet, heparin, melphalan, meperidine, meropenem, morphine, ondansetron, paclitaxel, piperacillin/tazobactam, potassium chloride, propofol, remifentanil, sargramostim, sodium bicarbonate, sufentanil, tacrolimus, teniposide, theophylline, vinorelbine, vit B/C, zidovudine

Additive compatibilities:
Aminophylline, bleomycin, cimetidine, floxacillin, furosemide, lidocaine, meropenem, nafcillin, netilmicin, ondansetron, prochlorperazine, ranitidine, verapamil

IM route
• IM inj deeply in large muscle mass; rotate sites; avoid deltoid; use 21G needle
• In one dose in AM to prevent adrenal suppression; avoid SC administration, may damage tissue

PO route
• Give with food or milk to decrease GI symptoms
• Provide assistance with ambulation in patient with bone

---

tissue disease to prevent fractures

Patient/family education
• Advise that ID as steroid user should be carried
• Teach to notify prescriber if therapeutic response decreases; dosage adjustment may be needed
• Teach not to discontinue abruptly or adrenal crisis can result
• Teach to avoid OTC products: salicylates, alcohol in cough products, cold preparations unless directed by prescriber
• Teach patient all aspects of drug usage, including cushingoid symptoms
• Instruct patient to notify health care provider of infection
• Teach symptoms of adrenal insufficiency: nausea, anorexia, fatigue, dizziness, dyspnea, weakness, joint pain

Evaluation
Positive therapeutic outcome
Ease of respirations, decreased inflammation

---

dexmedetomidine
See Appendix A,
Selected New Drugs

---

dextroamphetamine
(R)
(dex-troe-am-fet′a-meen)
Dexedrine, Dexedrine Spansules, dextroamphetamine sulfate, Ferndex
Func. class.: Cerebral stimulant
Chem. class.: Amphetamine
Pregnancy category C
Controlled substance schedule II

Action: Increases release of norepinephrine, dopamine in cerebral cortex to reticular activating system

⬧**Therapeutic Outcome:** Increased alertness, decreased fatigue, ability to stay awake (narcolepsy); increased attention span, decreased hyperactivity (ADHD)

Uses: Narcolepsy, attention deficit disorder with hyperactivity

Dosage and routes
Narcolepsy
Adult: PO 5-60 mg qd in divided doses
P *Child >12 yr:* PO 10 mg qd increasing by 10 mg/day at weekly intervals
P *Child 6-12 yr:* PO 5 mg qd increasing by 5 mg/wk (max 60 mg/day)
ADHD
P *Child >6 yr:* PO 5 mg qd-bid increasing by 5 mg/day at weekly intervals
P *Child 3-6 yr:* PO 2.5 mg qd increasing by 2.5 mg/day at weekly intervals

---

☑ Herb/drug 🚫 Do Not Crush ◆ Alert ☛ Key Drug G Geriatric P Pediatric

Available forms: Tabs 5, 10 mg; sus rel caps 5, 10, 15 mg

Adverse effects

CNS: Hyperactivity, insomnia, restlessness, talkativeness, dizziness, headache, chills, stimulation, dysphoria, irritability, aggressiveness, tremor, dependence, addiction

CV: Palpitations, **tachycardia,** hypertension, decrease in heart rate, **dysrhythmias**

GI: Anorexia, dry mouth, diarrhea, constipation, weight loss, metallic taste

GU: Impotence, change in libido

INTEG: Urticaria

Contraindications: Hypersensitivity to sympathomimetic amines, hyperthyroidism, hypertension, glaucoma, severe arteriosclerosis, drug abuse, cardiovascular disease, anxiety

Precautions: Gilles de la Tourette's disorder, pregnancy **C,** **P** lactation, child <3 yr

Pharmacokinetics

Absorption	Well absorbed
Distribution	Widely distributed; crosses placenta
Metabolism	Liver
Excretion	Kidneys, pH dependent: increased pH, increased reabsorption
Half-life	10-30 hr; increased when urine is alkaline

Pharmacodynamics

Onset	½ hr
Peak	1-3 hr
Duration	4-10 hr

Interactions
Individual drugs
Acetazolamide: ↓ excretion, ↑ effect
Ammonium chloride: ↓ effect
Ascorbic acid: ↓ effect
Haloperidol: ↑ CNS effect

Meperidine: Hypertensive crisis
Sodium bicarbonate: ↓ excretion, ↑ effect
Thyroid: ↑ effects
Drug classifications
Adrenergic blockers: ↓ adrenergic blocking effect
Antidepressants, tricyclics: ↑ dysrhythmias
Antidiabetics: ↓ antidiabetic effect
β-Adrenergic blockers: ↑ hypertension
Barbiturates: ↓ absorption of barbiturate
Cardiac glycosides: ↑ dysrhythmias
MAOI: Hypertensive crisis
Phenothiazines: ↑ CNS effect
Sympathomimetics: ↑ effect
Food/drug
Caffeine: ↑ amine effect

NURSING CONSIDERATIONS
Assessment
• Monitor VS, B/P, since this drug may reverse antihypertensives; check patients with cardiac disease more often for increased B/P
• Monitor CBC, urinalysis; for diabetic patients monitor blood sugar, urine sugar; insulin changes may be required, since eating will decrease
• Monitor height and weight q3 mo since growth rate in **P** children may be decreased; appetite is suppressed so weight loss is common during the first few months of treatment
• Monitor mental status: mood, sensorium, affect, stimulation, insomnia; aggressiveness may occur; depression with crying spells may occur after drug has worn off
• Assess for physical dependency; should not be

D

Adverse effects: *italic* = common; **bold** = life-threatening

used for extended time except in ADHD; dosage should be decreased gradually to prevent withdrawal symptoms

• Assess for narcoleptic symptoms before medication and after; ability to stay awake should increase significantly

P • In children or adults with ADHD, monitor for improved organizational skills, attention span, attending to tasks, impulse control, socialization, and ability to get along better with others

• Assess for withdrawal symptoms: headache, nausea, vomiting, muscle pain, weakness; drug tolerance develops after long-term use; dosage should not be increased if tolerance develops; this medication has a high abuse potential

Nursing diagnoses

☑ Thought processes, altered (uses, adverse reactions)
☑ Coping, impaired individual (uses)
☑ Family coping, impaired individual (uses)
☑ Knowledge deficit (teaching)

Implementation

• Give at least 6 hr before hs to avoid sleeplessness; titrate to patient's response; lowest dosage should be used to control symptoms

• Give gum, hard candy, frequent sips of water for dry mouth at beginning of treatment; these symptoms tend to lessen with time

🚫 • Do not crush, chew sus rel forms

Patient/family education

• Advise patient to decrease caffeine consumption (coffee, tea, cola, chocolate), which may increase irritability and stimulation; to avoid OTC preparations unless approved by prescriber; to avoid alcohol ingestion; these may cause serious drug interactions

• Caution patient to taper off drug over several weeks, or depression, increased sleeping, lethargy may occur

• Caution patient to avoid hazardous activities until patient is stabilized on medication

• Instruct patient not to double doses if medication is missed; prescriber may suggest drug holidays (ADHD) during the school year to assess progress and determine continued drug necessity

• Instruct patient/family to notify prescriber if significant side effects occur: tremors, insomnia, palpitations, restlessness, drug changes may be needed

• Inform patient that if dry mouth occurs to use frequent sips of water, sugarless gum, hard candy during beginning therapy; dry mouth lessens with continued treatment

• Advise patient to get needed rest; patients will feel more tired at end of day; to give last dose at least 6 hr before hs to avoid insomnia

Evaluation

Positive therapeutic outcome

• Decreased activity in ADHD
• Absence of sleeping during day in narcolepsy

Treatment of overdose:

Administer fluids, hemodialysis, peritoneal dialysis, antihypertensives for increased B/P; ammonium chloride for increased excretion

---

dextromethorphan (OTC)

(dex-troe-meth-or'fan)
Balminil DM ✤, Benylin DM,
Broncho-Grippol-DM ✤,
Children's Hold, Delsym,
Dextromethorphan, DM
Syrup ✤, Hold DM,
Koffex ✤, Neo-DM ✤,
Ornex-DM ✤, Pertussin,
Pertussin ES, Robidex ✤,
Robitussin Cough Calmers,
Robitussin Pediatric,
Sedatuss ✤, St. Joseph
Cough Suppressant, Sucrets
Cough Control, Suppress,
Trocal, Vicks Formula 44
Func. class.: Antitussive,
nonnarcotic
Chem. class.: Levorphanol
derivative

Pregnancy category C

Action: Depresses cough
center in medulla by direct
effect related to levorphanol

➡**Therapeutic Outcome:** Absence of cough

Uses: Nonproductive cough
carried by minor respiratory
tract infections or irritants that
might be inhaled

Dosage and routes
Adult: PO 10-20 mg q4h, or
30 mg q6-8h, not to exceed
120 mg/day; sus rel liq 60 mg
bid, not to exceed 120 mg/
day

P *Child 6-12 yr:* PO 5-10 mg
q4h; sus rel liq 30 mg bid, not
to exceed 60 mg/day

P *Child 2-6 yr:* PO 2.5-5 mg
q4h, or 7.5 mg q6-8h, not to
exceed 30 mg/day

Available forms: Loz 5, 7.5
mg; sol 3.5. 5, 7.5, 10, 15

mg/5 ml; syr 15 mg/15 ml,
12.5 mg/5 ml; sus action liq
30 mg/5 ml

Adverse effects
CNS: Dizziness
GI: Nausea

Contraindications: Hypersensitivity, asthma/emphysema,
productive cough

Precautions: Nausea/
vomiting, increased temp,
persistent headache, pregnancy **C**

Pharmacokinetics

Absorption	Rapid (PO); slow (sus rel)
Distribution	Unknown
Metabolism	Liver
Excretion	Kidneys
Half-life	Unknown

Pharmacodynamics

	PO	PO-SUS
Onset	15-30 min	Unknown
Peak	Unknown	Unknown
Duration	3-6 hr	12 hr

Interactions
Individual drugs
Alcohol: ↑ CNS depression
Selegiline: ↑ confusion,
coma
Drug classifications
Analgesics: ↑ CNS depression
Antihistamines: ↑ CNS de-
pression
Antidepressants: ↑ CNS
depression
MAOI: ↑ hypotension, hyper-
pyrexia

NURSING CONSIDERATIONS
Assessment
• Assess cough: type, frequency, character including
sputum; provide adequate
hydration to 2 L/day to
decrease viscosity of secretions

Nursing diagnoses
☑ Airway clearance, ineffective (uses)
☑ Knowledge deficit (teaching)

Implementation
G • Administer decreased dosage to elderly patients; their metabolism may be slowed; do not provide water within 30 min of administration because it dilutes drug
• Shake susp before administration

Patient/family education
• Caution patient to avoid driving or other hazardous activities until stabilized on this medication; may cause drowsiness, dizziness in some individuals
• Advise patient to avoid smoking, smoke-filled rooms, perfumes, dust, environmental pollutants, cleaners, which increase cough; may use gum, hard candy to prevent dry mouth
• Advise patient to avoid alcohol or other CNS depressants while taking this medication; drowsiness will be increased
• Caution patient that any cough lasting over a few days should be assessed by prescriber

Evaluation
Positive therapeutic outcome
• Absence of dry, irritating cough

**dextrose
(D-glucose) (℞)**
Glucose, Glutose, Insta-Glucose, Insulin Reaction
Func. class.: Caloric agent

Pregnancy category   D

Action: Needed for adequate utilization of amino acids; decreases protein, nitrogen loss; prevents ketosis

➔**Therapeutic Outcome:** Provides calories, prevents severe hypoglycemia

Uses: Increases intake of calories; increases fluids in patients unable to take adequate fluids, calories orally; 2.5%-11.5% forms provide calories, increased hydration; 20%-70% forms used to treat severe hypoglycemia

Dosage and routes
P *Adult and child:* **IV**, depends on individual requirements

Available forms: Inj **IV** 2.5%, 5%, 10%, 20%, 40%, 50%, 60%, 70%; oral gel 40%; chewable tabs 5 g

Adverse effects
CNS: Confusion, **loss of consciousness,** dizziness
CV: Hypertension, **CHF, pulmonary edema**
ENDO: Hyperglycemia, rebound hypoglycemia, hyperosmolar syndrome, hyperglycemic nonketolytic syndrome
GU: Glycosuria, osmotic diuresis
INTEG: Chills, flushing, warm feeling, rash, urticaria, extravasation necrosis

Contraindications: Hyperglycemia, delirium tremens, hemorrhage (cranial/spinal), CHF, pregnancy **D**

Precautions: Renal, liver, cardiac disease, diabetes mellitus

Pharmacokinetics	
Absorption	Well absorbed (PO); completely absorbed (**IV**)
Distribution	Widely distributed
Metabolism	Unknown
Excretion	Unknown
Half-life	Unknown

Pharmacodynamics		
	IV	PO
Onset	Immediate	Rapid
Peak	Immediate	Rapid
Duration	Immediate	Rapid

Interactions
Individual drugs
Insulin: ↑ need for insulin
Drug classifications
Corticosteroids: ↑ fluid retention/electrolyte excretion
Hypoglycemics, oral: ↑ need for hypoglycemic

NURSING CONSIDERATIONS
Assessment
• Assess I&O, skin turgor, edema, electrolytes (potassium, sodium, calcium, chloride, magnesium), blood glucose, ammonia, phosphate
• Monitor inj site for extravasation: redness along vein, edema at site, necrosis, pain, hard tender area; site should be changed immediately
• Monitor temp q4h for increased fever, indicating infection; if infection suspected, inf is discontinued and tubing, bottle, catheter tip cultured
• Monitor serum glucose in patients receiving hypertonic glucose 5% and over
• Assess nutritional status: calorie count by dietician; GI system function

Nursing diagnoses
☑ Nutrition: less than body requirements (uses)
☑ Fluid volume excess (adverse reactions)
☑ Knowledge deficit (teaching)

Implementation
PO route
• Oral glucose preparations (gel, chewable tabs) are to be used for conscious patients only; serum blood glucose should be monitored after first oral dose; if glucose has not increased by 20 mg/100 ml in 20-30 min, dose should be repeated and serum glucose checked again

IV route
• Give only protein (4%) and dextrose (up to 12.5%) via peripheral vein; stronger sol requires central **IV** administration
• May be given undiluted via prepared sol; give 10% sol (5 ml/15 sec), 20% sol (1000 ml/3 hr or more), 50% sol (500 ml/30-60 min); too rapid **IV** administration may cause fluid overload and hyperglycemia
• After changing **IV** catheter, change dressing q24h with aseptic technique

Patient/family education
• Teach patient reason for dextrose infusion
• Provide literature and information on when and how to use oral products for hypoglycemia
• Review hypoglycemia/hyperglycemia symptoms
• Review blood glucose monitoring procedure

Evaluation
Positive therapeutic outcome
• Increased weight
• Blood glucose level at normal limits for patient
• Adequate hydration

D

---

dezocine (℞)
(dez'oh-seen)
Dalgan
Func. class.: Narcotic agonist-antagonist analgesic
Chem. class.: Opioid, synthetic
Pregnancy category　C

Action: Inhibits ascending pain pathways in limbic system, thalamus, midbrain, hypothalamus by binding to opiate receptor sites, which alters pain perception and response

Therapeutic Outcome: Relief of moderate, severe pain

Uses: Moderate to severe pain

Dosage and routes
Adult: IM 5-20 mg q3-6h, not to exceed 120 mg/day; **IV** 2.5-10 mg q2-4h

Available forms: Inj 5, 10, 15 mg single-dose vials, multiple dose 10 mg/ml

Adverse effects
CNS: Drowsiness, dizziness, confusion, sedation, anxiety, headache, depression, delirium, sleep disturbances, dependency
CV: Hypotension, pulse irregularity, hypertension, chest pain, pallor, edema, thrombophlebitis
EENT: Blurred vision, slurred speech, diplopia
GI: Nausea, vomiting, anorexia, constipation, cramps, abdominal pain, dry mouth, diarrhea
GU: Urinary frequency, hesitancy, retention
INTEG: Inj site reactions, pruritus, rash, swelling, chills
RESP: Respiratory depression, hiccups

Contraindications: Hypersensitivity

Precautions: Addictive personality, pregnancy C, lactation, increased intracranial pressure, respiratory depression, hepatic disease, renal **P** disease, child <18 yr, elderly, **G** biliary surgery, COPD, sulfite sensitivity

Pharmacokinetics

Absorption	Completely absorbed (IM, **IV**)
Distribution	Not known
Metabolism	Liver, extensively
Excretion	Kidneys
Half-life	1½-7 hr

Pharmacodynamics

	IM	IV
Onset	½ hr	10 min
Peak	1-2 hr	30 min
Duration	2-4 hr	2-4 hr

Interactions
Individual drugs
Alcohol: ↑ respiratory depression, hypotension, sedation
Cimetidine: ↑ recovery
Erythromycin: ↑ recovery
Nalbuphine: ↓ analgesia
Pentazocine: ↓ analgesia
Drug classifications
Antihistamines: ↑ respiratory depression, hypotension
CNS depressants: ↑ respiratory depression, hypotension
MAOI: Do not use 2 wk before dezocine
Phenothiazines: ↑ respiratory depression, hypotension
Sedative/hypnotics: ↑ respiratory depression, hypotension

NURSING CONSIDERATIONS
Assessment
• Assess respiratory status: respiratory depression, character, rate, rhythm; notify prescriber if respirations are

---

<12/min; note CV status, bradycardia, syncope; monitor ECG continuously
• Assess pain: location, intensity, duration, alleviating factors

Nursing diagnoses
☑ Pain (uses)
☑ Sensory-perceptual alteration: visual, auditory (adverse reactions)
☑ Breathing pattern, ineffective (adverse reactions)
☑ Knowledge deficit (teaching) (preoperatively)

Implementation
IM route
• Give deeply in large muscle mass; rotate sites; do not give SC
IV IV route
• Give undiluted ≤5 mg over 2-3 min

Patient/family education
• Caution patients to avoid CNS depressants: alcohol, sedative/hypnotics for at least 24 hr after taking this drug
• Discuss with patient that dizziness, drowsiness, and confusion are common; to avoid getting up without assistance
• Advise patient to make position changes to lessen orthostatic hypotension

Evaluation
Positive therapeutic outcome
• Decreased pain perception

Treatment of overdose: Narcan 0.2-0.8 **IV**, O_2, **IV** fluids, vasopressors

diazepam ⚷ (℞)
(dye-az′e-pam)
Apo-Diazepam ✦, diazepam, Novo-Diapam ✦, PMS-Diazepam ✦, Valium, Valrelease, Vivol ✦, Zetran
Func. class.: Antianxiety
Chem. class.: Benzodiazepine

Pregnancy category D
Controlled substance schedule IV

Action: Potentiates the actions of GABA, especially in limbic system, reticular formation; enhances presympathetic inhibition, inhibits spinal polysynaptic afferent paths

▶**Therapeutic Outcome:** Decreased anxiety, restlessness, insomnia

Uses: Anxiety, acute alcohol withdrawal, adjunct in seizure disorders; preoperative skeletal muscle relaxation; rectally for acute repetitive seizures

Investigational uses: Panic attacks

Dosage and routes
Anxiety/convulsive disorders
Adult: PO 2-10 mg tid-qid; ext rel 15-30 mg qd

🄶 **Elderly:** PO 1-2 mg qd bid, increase slowly as needed

🄿 **Child >6 mo:** PO 1-2.5 mg tid-qid

Muscle relaxation
🄶 **Elderly:** PO 2-5 mg bid-qid

Tetanic muscle spasms
🄿 **Child <5 yr:** IM/**IV** 5-10 mg q3-4h prn

🄿 **Infants >30 days:** IM/**IV** 1-2 mg q3-4h prn

✦ Canada Only   Adverse effects: *italic* = common; **bold** = life-threatening

Status epilepticus
Adult: IV bol 5-20 mg, 2 mg/min; may repeat q5-10 min, not to exceed 60 mg; may repeat in 30 min if seizures reappear

P *Child:* **IV** bol 0.1-0.3 mg/kg (1 mg/min over 3 min); may repeat q15 min × 2 doses

Adult: RECT 0.2 mg/kg, may repeat 4-12 hr later

P *Child 6-11 yr:* RECT 0.3 mg/kg, may repeat 4-12 hr later

P *Child 2-5 yr:* RECT 0.5 mg/kg, may repeat 4-12 hr later

Available forms: Tabs 2, 5, 10 mg; ext rel caps 15 mg; inj, emulsified 5 mg/ml; oral sol 5 mg/5 ml, 5 mg/ml; gel, rectal delivery system 10, 15, 20 mg, twin packs

Adverse effects
CNS: Dizziness, drowsiness, confusion, headache, anxiety, tremors, stimulation, fatigue, depression, insomnia, hallucinations
CV: Orthostatic hypotension, **ECG changes, tachycardia,** hypotension
EENT: Blurred vision, tinnitus, mydriasis
GI: Constipation, dry mouth, nausea, vomiting, anorexia, diarrhea
HEMA: **Neutropenia**
INTEG: Rash, dermatitis, itching
RESP: **Respiratory depression**

Contraindications: Hypersensitivity to benzodiazepines, narrow-angle glaucoma, psychosis, pregnancy **D**

G **Precautions:** Elderly, debilitated, hepatic disease, renal disease

N **Do Not Confuse:**
diazepam/Ditropan

Pharmacokinetics	
Absorption	Rapid (PO); erratic (IM)
Distribution	Widely distributed; crosses blood-brain barrier, placenta
Metabolism	Liver, extensively
Excretion	Kidneys, breast milk
Half-life	20-80 hr

Pharmacodynamics			
	PO	IM	IV
Onset	½ hr	15 min	5 min
Peak	1-2 hr	½-1½ hr	15 min
Duration	2-3 hr	1-1½ hr	15 min

Interactions
Individual drugs
Alcohol: ↑ CNS depression
Cimetidine: ↑ adverse reactions
Digoxin: ↑ digoxin level
Disulfiram: ↓ effect of diazepam
Isoniazid: ↓ effect of diazepam
Propranolol: ↓ effect of diazepam
Rifampin: ↓ effect of diazepam
Valproic acid: ↓ effect of diazepam
Drug classifications
Barbiturates: ↑ effect of both drugs
CNS depressants: ↑ CNS depression
Opiates: ↓ diazepam effects
Oral contraceptives: ↓ diazepam effects
Smoking: ↓ diazepam effect
☑ *Herb/drug*
Kava: ↑ diazepam effect
Lab test interferences
↑ AST/ALT, ↑ serum bilirubin
False ↑ 17-OHCS
↓ RAIU

☑ Herb/drug   ◉ Do Not Crush   ◆ Alert   ⛬ Key Drug   **G** Geriatric   **P** Pediatric

NURSING CONSIDERATIONS
Assessment

- Assess degree of anxiety; what precipitates anxiety and whether drug controls symptoms; other signs of anxiety: dilated pupils, inability to sleep, restlessness, inability to focus
- Assess for alcohol withdrawal symptoms, including hallucinations (visual, auditory), delirium, irritability, agitation, fine to coarse tremors
- Monitor B/P (with patient lying, standing), pulse, respiratory rate; if systolic B/P drops 20 mm Hg, hold drug, notify prescriber; monitor respirations q5-15 min if given **IV**
- Monitor blood studies: CBC during long-term therapy; blood dyscrasias have occurred (rarely)
- Monitor for seizure control; type, duration, and intensity of convulsions; what precipitates seizures
- Monitor hepatic studies: AST, ALT, bilirubin, creatinine, LDH, alkaline phosphatase
- Assess mental status: mood, sensorium, affect, sleeping pattern, drowsiness, dizziness, suicidal tendencies, and ability of drug to control these symptoms; check for tolerance, withdrawal symptoms: headache, nausea, vomiting, muscle pain, weakness after long-term use

Nursing diagnoses

- ✓ Anxiety (uses)
- ✓ Injury, risk of (uses, adverse reactions)
- ✓ Coping, ineffective individual (uses)
- ✓ Knowledge deficit (teaching)
- ✓ Noncompliance (teaching)

Implementation
PO route

- Give with food or milk for GI symptoms; crush tab if patient is unable to swallow medication whole; do not crush ext rel caps; use sugarless gum, hard candy, frequent sips of water for dry mouth
- Reduce narcotic dosage by ⅓ if given concomitantly with diazepam
- Check to see PO medication has been swallowed

IV IV route

- Administer **IV** into large vein; do not dilute or mix with any other drug; give **IV** 5 mg or less/1 min or total dose over 3 min or more (children, infants); cont inf is not recommended
- Check **IV** site for thrombosis or phlebitis, which may occur rapidly

Syringe compatibilities:
Cimetidine

Syringe incompatibilities:
Benzquinamide, doxapram, glycopyrrolate, heparin, nalbuphine

Y-site compatibilities:
Cefmetazole, dobutamine, nafcillin, quinidine, sufentanil

Y-site incompatibilities:
Hydromorphone, fluconazole, foscarnet, heparin, pancuronium, potassium chloride, vecuronium, vitamin B with C

Additive compatibilities:
Netilmicin, verapamil

Patient/family education

- Advise patient that drug may be taken with food; that drug is not to be used for everyday stress or used longer than 4 mo unless directed by prescriber; take no more than prescribed amount; may be habit forming

---

♣ Canada Only   Adverse effects: *italic* = common; **bold** = life-threatening

• Caution patient to avoid OTC preparations unless approved by a prescriber; to avoid alcohol, other psychotropic medications unless prescribed; that smoking may decrease diazepam effect; not to discontinue medication abruptly after long-term use
• Inform patient to avoid driving, activities that require alertness; drowsiness may occur; to rise slowly or fainting 🄶 may occur, especially in elderly
• Advise patient not to become pregnant while using this drug
• Inform patient that drowsiness may worsen at beginning of treatment

Evaluation

Positive therapeutic outcome
• Decreased anxiety, restlessness, insomnia

Treatment of overdose:
Lavage, VS, supportive care, flumazenil

---

diazoxide (R)
(dye-az-ox′ide)
Hyperstat IV, Proglycem
Func. class.: Antihypertensive
Chem. class.: Vasodilator
Pregnancy category   C

Action: Decreases release of insulin from β-cells in pancreas, resulting in an increase in blood glucose; relaxes vascular smooth muscle (peripheral arterioles)

▸**Therapeutic Outcome:** Decreased B/P, increased blood glucose

Uses: Hypoglycemia caused by hyperinsulinism; emergency treatment of hypertension

Dosage and routes
Hypoglycemia
🄿*Adult and child:* PO 3-8 mg/kg/day in 2-3 divided doses q8-12h
🄿*Infants and neonates:* PO 8-15 mg/kg/day in 2-3 divided doses 8-12h
Hypertension
🄿*Adult and child:* IV 1-3 mg/kg q5-15 min, max 150 mg/dose

Available forms: Caps 50 mg; oral susp 50 mg/ml; inj 15 mg/ml, 300 mg/20 ml

Adverse effects

CNS: Headache, weakness, malaise, anxiety, dizziness, insomnia, paresthesia, **seizures, cerebral ischemia, paralysis**
CV: **Tachycardia,** palpitations, hypotension, transient hypertension, **shock, MI**
EENT: Diplopia, cataracts, ring scotoma, subconjunctival hemorrhage, lacrimation
GI: Nausea, vomiting, anorexia, abdominal pain, transient loss of taste, diarrhea
GU: Reversible nephrotic syndrome, decreased urinary output, hematuria
HEMA: **Thrombocytopenia, leukopenia,** eosinophilia, decreased Hgb, Hct
INTEG: Increased hair growth or loss of scalp hair, rash, dermatitis, herpes
META: Hyperuricemia, sodium/fluid retention, ketoacidosis, hyperglycemia, azotemia

Contraindications: Hypersensitivity to this drug or thiazides, functional hypoglycemia

Precautions: Pregnancy C, lactation, renal disease, diabetes mellitus, CV disease, gout

---

Pharmacokinetics

Absorption	Well absorbed (PO); completely absorbed (**IV**)
Distribution	Crosses blood-brain barrier, placenta
Metabolism	Liver (50%)
Excretion	Kidney, unchanged (50%)
Half-life	20-36 hr

Pharmacodynamics

	PO	IV
Onset	1 hr	1-2 min
Peak	8-12 hr	5 min
Duration	8 hr	3-12 hr

Interactions
Individual drugs
Coumadin: ↑ effects
Drug classifications
Diuretics, thiazides: ↑ hyperglycemia

Hydantoins: ↓ anticonvulsant effect

Sulfonylureas: ↑ hyperglycemia

NURSING CONSIDERATIONS
Assessment

• Assess for allergies to sulfonamide; cross-sensitivity may occur
• Assess B/P q5 min until stabilized
• Monitor electrolytes, blood studies: potassium, sodium, chloride, carbon dioxide, CBC, serum glucose
• Monitor weight daily, I&O; edema in feet, legs daily; check skin turgor, dryness of mucous membranes for hydration status
• Assess for rales, dyspnea, orthopnea; peripheral edema, fatigue, weight gain, jugular vein distention (congestive heart failure)
• Assess for signs of hyperglycemia: acetone breath, increased urinary output, severe thirst, lethargy, dizziness

Nursing diagnoses
☑ Cardiac output, decreased (adverse reactions)
☑ Injury, risk for (side effects)
☑ Knowledge deficit (teaching)

Implementation
PO route
• Shake susp before using
• Store protected from light and heat
IV IV route
• Give by direct **IV** over 30 sec or less; may repeat q5-15 min until desired response; do not administer dark solution
• Give to patient in recumbent position; keep in that position for 1 hr after

Syringe compatibility:
Heparin
Y-site incompatibilities:
Hydralazine, propranolol

Evaluation
Positive therapeutic outcome
• Decreased B/P in hypertension

Treatment of overdose:
Administer levarterenol, dopamine, or norepinephrine for hypotension, dialysis

---

diclofenac (℞)
(dye-kloe′fen-ak)
Cataflam, diclofenac, Voltaren, Voltaren Rapide ✦, Voltaren SR ✦, Voltaren XR
Func. class.: Nonsteroidal antiinflammatory
Chem. class.: Phenylacetic acid
Pregnancy category   B

Action: Inhibits prostaglandin synthesis by decreasing enzyme needed for biosynthesis; anal-

---

gesic, antiinflammatory, antipyretic properties

⇒**Therapeutic Outcome:** Decreased pain, inflammation

Uses: Acute, chronic rheumatoid arthritis, osteoarthritis, ankylosing spondylitis, analgesia, primary dysmenorrhea, ophthalmic: to decrease inflammation after cataract extraction

Dosage and routes
Osteoarthritis
Adult: PO 100-125 mg/day in 2-3 divided doses; after therapeutic response occurs, decrease to least amount to control symptoms

Rheumatoid arthritis
Adult: PO 150-200 mg/day in 2-4 divided doses; after therapeutic response decrease to lowest amount to control symptoms

Ankylosing spondylitis
Adult: PO 100-125 mg/day in 4-5 divided doses; give 25 mg qid and 25 mg hs if needed

Analgesia/primary dysmenorrhea
Adult: PO 50 mg tid, max 150 mg/day (cataflam)

After cataract surgery
Adult: Ophth ȋ gtt qid × 2 wk beginning 24 hr after surgery

Available forms: Enteric coated tabs 25, 50, 75, 100 mg; tabs ext rel 100 mg; tabs 50 mg potassium; ophth sol 1%; suppositories 50 mg ❀, 100 mg ❀

Adverse effects
CNS: Dizziness, drowsiness, fatigue, tremors, confusion, insomnia, anxiety, depression, nervousness, paresthesia, muscle weakness
CV: **CHF,** tachycardia, peripheral edema, palpitations, dysrhythmias, hypotension, hypertension, fluid retention
EENT: Tinnitus, hearing loss, blurred vision
GI: Nausea, anorexia, vomiting, diarrhea, jaundice, **cholestatic hepatitis,** constipation, flatulence, cramps, dry mouth, peptic ulcer, GI bleeding
GU: **Nephrotoxicity: dysuria, hematuria, oliguria, azotemia, cystitis, UTI**
HEMA: **Blood dyscrasias,** epistaxis, bruising
INTEG: Purpura, rash, pruritus, sweating, erythema, petechiae, photosensitivity, alopecia
RESP: Dyspnea, hemoptysis, pharyngitis, **bronchospasm, laryngeal edema,** rhinitis, shortness of breath

Contraindications: Hypersensitivity to aspirin, iodides, other NSAIDs, asthma

Precautions: Pregnancy **B,**
P lactation, children, bleeding disorders, GI disorders, cardiac disorders, hypersensitivity to other antiinflammatory agents, CrCl <30 ml/min

◪ **Do Not Confuse:**
Cataflam/Catapres

Pharmacokinetics	
Absorption	Well absorbed (PO, ophth)
Distribution	Crosses placenta; 90% bound to plasma proteins
Metabolism	Liver (50%)
Excretion	Breast milk
Half-life	1-2 hr

Pharmacodynamics		
	PO	OPHTH
Onset	Unknown	Unknown
Peak	2-3 hr	Unknown
Duration	Unknown	Unknown

Interactions
Individual drugs
Acetaminophen (long-term use): ↑ renal reactions
Alcohol: ↑ adverse reactions, ↑ GI side effects
Aspirin: ↓ effectiveness, ↑ adverse reactions, ↑ GI side effects
Colchicine: ↑ GI side effects
Cyclosporine: ↑ toxicity
Digoxin: ↑ toxicity, ↑ levels
Insulin: ↓ insulin effect
Lithium: ↑ toxicity
Methotrexate: ↑ toxicity
Phenytoin: ↑ toxicity
Drug classifications
Anticoagulants: ↑ risk of bleeding
Antidiabetics: ↑ need for dosage adjustment
Antihypertensives: ↓ effect of antihypertensives
Antineoplastics: ↑ risk of hematologic toxicity
β-Adrenergic blockers: ↑ antihypertension
Cephalosporins: ↑ risk of bleeding
Diuretics: ↓ effectiveness of diuretics
Glucocorticoids: ↑ adverse reactions
NSAIDs: ↑ adverse reactions
Potassium supplements: ↑ adverse reactions
Radiation: ↑ risk of hematologic toxicity

NURSING CONSIDERATIONS
Assessment
• Assess for pain of rheumatoid arthritis, osteoarthritis, ankylosing spondylitis; check ROM, inflammation of joints, characteristics of pain
• Assess ophth patients for pain, inflammation, redness, swelling
⬇• Monitor blood counts during therapy; watch for decreasing platelets; if low, therapy may need to be discontinued, restarted after hematologic recovery; and for blood dyscrasias (thrombocytopenia): bruising, fatigue, bleeding, poor healing
• Assess LFTs and uric acid periodically

Nursing diagnoses
☑ Pain (uses)
☑ Mobility, impaired physical (uses)
☑ Injury, risk for (side effects)
☑ Knowledge deficit (teaching)

Implementation
PO route
• Administer with food or milk to decrease gastric symptoms;
🚫• Do not crush, dissolve, or chew enteric coated or sus rel caps
Ophth route
• Administer with patient recumbent or tilting head back; pull down on lower lid; when conjunctival sac is exposed, instill 1 drop; wait a few minutes before instilling other drops

Patient/family education
• Teach patient that drug must be continued for prescribed time to be effective; to avoid aspirin, alcoholic beverages
• Caution patient to report bleeding, bruising, fatigue, malaise, since blood dyscrasias do occur
• Advise patient to report hepatotoxicity: flu symptoms, nausea, vomiting, jaundice, pruritus, lethargy
• Instruct patient to use sunscreen to prevent photosensitivity
• Teach patient to avoid use in 3rd trimester of pregnancy
• Instruct patient to use caution when driving; drowsiness, dizziness may occur

- Teach patient to take with a full glass of water to enhance absorption; do not crush, break, or chew

Evaluation
Positive therapeutic outcome
- Decreased pain in arthritic conditions
- Decreased inflammation in arthritic conditions
- Decreased ocular irritation

---

dicloxacillin (℞)
(dye-klox-a-sill'in)
dicloxacillin sodium, Dycill, Dynapen, Pathocil
Func. class.: Antiinfective
Chem. class.: Penicillinase-resistant penicillin
Pregnancy category   B

Action: Interferes with cell wall replication of susceptible organisms; osmotically unstable cell wall swells, bursts from osmotic pressure

Therapeutic Outcome: Bactericidal effects for the following: gram-positive cocci *Staphylococcus aureus, Streptococcus pyogenes, S. viridans, S. faecalis, S. bovis, S. pneumoniae;* infections caused by penicillinase-producing *Staphylococcus* organisms

Uses: Penicillinase-producing staphylococci, streptococci; respiratory tract, skin, skin structure infections; sinusitis

Dosage and routes
Adult: PO 0.5-4 g/day in divided doses q6h
Child: PO 12.5-50 mg/kg in divided doses q6h, max 4 g/d

Available forms: Caps 125, 250, 500 mg; powder for oral susp 62.5 mg/5 ml

Adverse effects
CNS: Lethargy, hallucinations, anxiety, depression, twitching, **coma, convulsions**
GI: Nausea, vomiting, diarrhea, increased AST, ALT, abdominal pain, glossitis, pseudomembranous colitis
GU: Oliguria, proteinuria, hematuria, vaginitis, **moniliasis, glomerulonephritis**
HEMA: Anemia, increased bleeding time, **bone marrow depression, granulocytopenia**
SYST: **Anaphylaxis**

Contraindications: Hypersensitivity to penicillins; neonates

Precautions: Hypersensitivity to cephalosporins, pregnancy **B**, severe renal or hepatic disease

Do Not Confuse:
Pathocil/Bactocil

Pharmacokinetics
Absorption	Rapid, incomplete (35%-75%)
Distribution	Widely distributed; crosses placenta
Metabolism	Liver (6%-10%)
Excretion	Kidneys, unchanged (60%); breast milk
Half-life	½-1 hr, increased in hepatic renal disease

Pharmacodynamics
Onset	½ hr
Peak	½-2 hr

Interactions
Individual drugs
Aspirin: ↑ dicloxacillin concentrations
Disulfiram: ↑ dicloxacillin concentrations
Probenecid: ↑ dicloxacillin levels, ↓ renal excretion
Drug classifications
Oral anticoagulants: ↑ anticoagulant effects

Oral contraceptives: ↓ action of oral contraceptives

Food/drug

Food, carbonated drinks, citrus fruit juices: ↓ absorption

Herb/drug

Khat: ↓ absorption

Lab test interferences

False positive: Urine glucose, urine protein

NURSING CONSIDERATIONS
Assessment

• Assess patient for previous sensitivity reaction to penicillins or other cephalosporins; cross-sensitivity between penicillins and cephalosporins is common

• Assess patient for signs and symptoms of infection including characteristics of wounds, sputum, urine, stool, WBC >10,000, fever; obtain baseline information and during treatment

• Obtain C&S before beginning drug therapy to identify if correct treatment has been initiated

• Assess for allergic reactions: rash, urticaria, pruritus, chills, fever, joint pain may occur a few days after therapy begins; epinephrine and resuscitation equipment should be available for anaphylactic reaction

◆• Identify urine output; if decreasing, notify prescriber (may indicate nephrotoxicity); check for increased BUN, creatinine

• Monitor blood studies: AST, ALT, CBC, Hct, bilirubin, LDH, alkaline phosphatase, Coombs' test monthly if patient is on long-term therapy

• Monitor electrolytes: potassium, sodium, chloride

monthly if patient is on long-term therapy

• Assess bowel pattern qd; if severe diarrhea occurs, drug should be discontinued; may indicate pseudomembranous colitis

• Monitor for bleeding: ecchymosis, bleeding gums, hematuria, stool guaiac daily if on long-term therapy

• Assess for overgrowth of infection: perineal itching, fever, malaise, redness, pain, swelling, drainage, rash, diarrhea, change in cough, sputum

Nursing diagnoses

☑ Infection, risk for (uses)
☑ Diarrhea (side effects)
☑ Knowledge deficit (teaching)
☑ Noncompliance (teaching)
☑ Injury, risk for (side effects)

Implementation

• Give in even doses around the clock; if GI upset occurs, give with food; drug must be given for 10-14 days to ensure organism death and prevent superinfection; store in airtight container

🚫• Do not crush, chew caps

• Shake susp well before each dose; store in refrigerator for 2 wk or 1 wk at room temp

Patient/family education

• Teach patient to report sore throat, bruising, bleeding, joint pain; may indicate blood dyscrasias (rare)

• Advise patient to contact prescriber if vaginal itching, loose, foul-smelling stools, furry tongue occur; may indicate superinfection

• Instruct patient to take all medication prescribed for the length of time ordered

• Advise patient to notify prescriber of diarrhea with

blood or pus, which may indicate pseudomembranous colitis

Evaluation
Positive therapeutic outcome
• Absence of signs/symptoms of infection (WBC <10,000, temp WNL, absence of red draining wounds)
• Reported improvement in symptoms of infection

Treatment of anaphylaxis: Withdraw drug, maintain airway, administer epinephrine, aminophylline, O_2, **IV** corticosteroids

---

didanosine (℞)
(dye-dan'oh-seen)
Videx, DDL, dideoxyinosine
Func. class.: Antiviral
Chem. class.: Synthetic purine nucleoside of deoxyadenosine

Pregnancy category B

Action: Nucleoside analog incorporating into cellular DNA by viral reverse transcriptase, thereby terminating the cellular DNA chain that prevents viral replication

➯**Therapeutic Outcome:** Antiviral against the retroviruses, primarily HIV

Uses: Advanced HIV, or AIDS, infections in adults and [P] children who have been unable to use zidovudine or who have not responded to treatment

Dosage and routes
Adult >75 kg: PO 300 mg tabs or 375 mg buffered powder bid

Adult 50-74 kg: PO 200 mg tabs or 250 mg buffered powder bid

Adult 35-49 kg: PO 125 mg tabs or 167 mg buffered powder bid

Renal dose
Reduce dosage if CrCl <60 ml/min

[P] *Child:* PO tabs 90-120 mg/m² q12 hr; buffered powder packets 112.5-150 mg/m² q12hr

[P] *Child:* BSA 1.1-1.4 m² PO tabs 100 mg q8-12hr; reconstituted pedi powder 125 mg q8-12hr

[P] *Child:* BSA 0.8-1 m² PO tabs 75 mg q8-12hr; reconstituted pedi powder 94 mg q8-12hr

[P] *Child:* BSA 0.5-0.7 m² PO tabs 50 mg q8-12 hr; reconstituted pedi powder 62 mg q8-12hr

[P] *Child:* BSA <0.4 m² PO tabs 25 mg q8-12hr; reconstituted pedi powder 31 mg q8-12hr

Available forms: Buffered chewable/dispersable tabs 25, 50, 100, 150 mg; buffered powder for oral sol 100, 167, 250, 375 mg; pedi powder for oral sol 2, 4 g

Adverse effects
CNS: **Peripheral neuropathy, seizures,** confusion, *anxiety,* hypertonia, abnormal thinking, asthenia, *insomnia, CNS depression,* pain, dizziness, chills, fever
CV: Hypertension, vasodilatation, **dysrhythmia,** syncope, **CHF,** palpitations
EENT: Ear pain, otitis, photophobia, visual impairment, retinal depigmentation
GI: **Pancreatitis,** *diarrhea, nausea,* vomiting, *abdominal pain,* constipation, stomatitis, dyspepsia, liver abnormalities, flatulence, taste perversion, dry

---

mouth, oral thrush, melena, increased ALT, AST, alkaline phosphatase, amylase, **hepatic failure**

GU: Increased bilirubin, uric acid

HEMA: **Leukopenia, granulocytopenia, thrombocytopenia, anemia**

INTEG: Rash, pruritus, alopecia, ecchymosis, hemorrhage, petechiae, sweating

MS: Myalgia, arthritis, myopathy, muscular atrophy

RESP: Cough, pneumonia, dyspnea, asthma, epistaxis, hypoventilation, sinusitis

Contraindications: Hypersensitivity

Precautions: Renal, hepatic disease, pregnancy **B,** lactation, children, sodium-restricted diets, elevated amylase, preexistent peripheral neuropathy, phenylketonuria, hyperuricemia

Pharmacokinetics	
Absorption	Rapidly absorbed (up to 40%)
Distribution	Unknown
Metabolism	Not metabolized
Excretion	Kidneys (55%)
Half-life	0.8-1.6 hr, shorter in children

Pharmacodynamics	
Onset	Unknown
Peak	Up to 1 hr
Duration	Unknown

Interactions
Individual drugs
Atropine: ↑ anticholinergic effects
Dapsone: ↓ absorption of dapsone
Disopyramide: ↑ anticholinergic effects
Itraconazole: ↓ absorption of itraconazole

Ketoconazole: ↓ absorption of ketoconazole
Quinidine: ↑ anticholinergic effects
Drug classifications
Antacids, magnesium, aluminum: ↑ side effects
Antidepressants, tricyclic: ↑ anticholinergic effects
Antihistamines: ↑ anticholinergic effects
Fluoroquinolones: ↓ absorption of fluoroquinolones
Phenothiazines: ↑ anticholinergic effects
Tetracyclines: ↓ absorption of tetracyclines
Food/drug
↓ absorption

NURSING CONSIDERATIONS
Assessment
• Assess for peripheral neuropathy: tingling or pain in hands and feet, distal numbness; if these occur during therapy, drug may be decreased or discontinued
• Assess for pancreatitis: abdominal pain, nausea, vomiting, elevated liver enzymes; drug should be discontinued, since condition can be fatal
• Assess children by dilated retinal examination q6mo to rule out retinal depigmentation
• Monitor CBC, differential, platelet count monthly; withhold drug if WBC is <4000 or platelet count is <75,000; notify prescriber of results
• Monitor renal function studies: BUN, serum uric acid, urine CrCl before, during therapy; these may be elevated throughout treatment
• Monitor temp q4h; may indicate beginning infection
• Monitor liver function tests before, during therapy (bilirubin, AST, ALT, amylase, alka-

line phosphatase) as needed or monthly

Nursing diagnoses

☑ Infection, risk for (uses)

☑ Injury, risk for (adverse reactions)

☑ Knowledge deficit (teaching)

Implementation

• Give on empty stomach, 1 hr ac or 2 hr pc, q12h; food decreases effectiveness of drug

• Patient should chew tabs; may be crushed and mixed with water

• Pedi powder for oral sol should be prepared in the pharmacy; shake before using

• Packets for oral sol must be mixed with ½ glass of water; stir until dissolved

Patient/family education

• Advise patient to take on empty stomach; not to take dapsone at same time as DDL; not to mix powder with fruit juice; to chew tab or crush and dissolve in water; to drink powder immediately after mixing; to use exactly as prescribed

• Instruct patient to report signs of infection: increased temp, sore throat, flu symptoms; to avoid crowds and those with known infections

• Instruct patient to report signs of anemia: fatigue, headache, faintness, shortness of breath, irritability

• Instruct patient to report bleeding; avoid use of razors and commercial mouthwash

• Advise patient that hair may be lost during therapy; a wig or hair piece may make patient feel better

• Caution patient to avoid OTC products and other medications without approval of prescriber

• Teach patient not to have any sexual contact without use of a condom; needles should not be shared; blood from infected individual should not come in contact with another's mucous membranes

Evaluation

Positive therapeutic outcome

• Absence of opportunistic infection, symptoms of HIV

---

diethylstilbestrol
(dye-eth-il-stil-bess'trole)
(stilboestrol) (℞)
DES
diethylstilbestrol diphosphate (℞)
DES, Honvol ✦, Stilphostrol
Func. class.: Estrogen
Chem. class.: Nonsteroidal synthetic estrogen
Pregnancy category   X

Action: Needed for adequate functioning of female reproductive system; it affects release of pituitary gonadotropins, inhibits ovulation, promotes adequate calcium use in bone structures; responsible for maintenance of water and secondary sex characteristics; lowers cholesterol, retention of water and sodium

▶**Therapeutic Outcome:** Decreased vaginal, vulval itching, dryness, redness, inflammation; decreased spread of malignant cells

Uses: Postmenopausal breast cancer, prostatic cancer, vasomotor symptoms of menopause

---

Dosage and routes
Prostatic cancer
Adult: PO 1-3 mg qd, then 1 mg qd; PO 50-200 mg tid (diphosphate); IM 5 mg 2 times/wk, then 4 mg 2 times/wk; **IV** 0.25-1 g qd × 5 days, then 1-2 times/wk

Breast cancer (post-menopausal)
Adult: PO 15 mg qd

Available forms:
Diethylstilbestrol: tabs 1, 5 mg; diethylstilbestrol diphosphate: tabs 50 mg; inj 0.25 g

Adverse effects
CNS: Dizziness, headache, migraines, depression
CV: Hypotension, thrombophlebitis, edema, **thromboembolism, stroke, pulmonary embolism, MI**
EENT: Contact lens intolerance, increased myopia, astigmatism
GI: Nausea, vomiting, diarrhea, anorexia, pancreatitis, cramps, constipation, increased appetite, increased weight, **cholestatic jaundice**
GU: Amenorrhea, cervical erosion, breakthrough bleeding, dysmenorrhea, vaginal candidiasis, breast changes, *gynecomastia, testicular atrophy, impotence,* **hepatic adenoma, increased risk of breast/endometrial cancer**
INTEG: Rash, urticaria, acne, hirsutism, alopecia, oily skin, seborrhea, purpura, melasma
META: Folic acid deficiency, hypercalcemia, hyperglycemia

Contraindications: Breast cancer, thromboembolic disorders, reproductive cancer, genital bleeding (abnormal, undiagnosed), pregnancy **X**

Precautions: Hypertension, asthma, blood dyscrasias, gallbladder disease, CHF, diabetes mellitus, bone disease–blocking agents, MI

Pharmacokinetics	
Absorption	Well absorbed
Distribution	Widely distributed; crosses placenta
Metabolism	Liver
Excretion	Kidneys
Half-life	Unknown

Pharmacodynamics
Unknown

Interactions
Individual drugs
Cyclosporine: ↑ toxicity
Dantrolene: ↑ toxicity
Rifampin: ↓ action of diethylstilbestrol
Tamoxifen: ↓ tamoxifen action
Drug classifications
Anticoagulants: ↓ action of anticoagulants
Antidepressants, tricyclic: ↑ toxicity
Barbiturates: ↓ action of diethylstilbestrol
Corticosteroids: ↑ action of diethylstilbestrol
Hepatotoxics: ↑ toxicity
Oral hypoglycemics: ↓ action of hypoglycemics
Food/drug
• ↑ caffeine level
Smoking
• ↑ CV reactions
Lab test interferences
↑ BSP retention test, ↑ PBI, ↑ T_4, ↑ serum sodium, ↑ platelet aggregation, ↑ thyroxine-binding globulin (TBG), ↑ prothrombin, ↑ factors VII, VIII, IX, X, ↑ triglycerides
↓ Serum folate, ↓ serum triglyceride, ↓ T_3 resin uptake

test, ↓ GTT, ↓ antithrombin III, ↓ metyrapone test
False positive: LE prep, ANA

NURSING CONSIDERATIONS
Assessment
• Monitor blood glucose in patient with diabetes; increased urine glucose may occur; if female patient has an intact uterus, check weight daily; notify prescriber if weekly weight gain is >5 lb; if increased, diuretic may be ordered; monitor I&O ratio; be alert for decreasing urinary output and increasing edema
• Monitor B/P; watch for increase caused by water and sodium retention; check liver function studies, including AST, ALT, bilirubin, alkaline phosphatase
• Assess edema, hypertension, cardiac symptoms, jaundice
• Assess mental status: affect, mood, behavioral changes, aggression

Nursing diagnoses
☑Sexual dysfunction (uses)
☑Injury, risk for physical (teaching)

Implementation
• Administer with a progesterone for 10-13 days/mo for female patients with an intact uterus
PO route
• Give titrated dosage; provide food or milk to decrease GI symptoms
• Give in one dose in AM for prostatic cancer
IV IV route
• Give **IV** after diluting in 300 mg of dextrose or saline inj; give at a rate of 1-2 ml/min × 15 min; may increase rate to complete inf 1 hr after starting

Patient/family education
• Instruct patient to weigh weekly, report gain >5 lb
• Teach female patient to report immediately breast lumps, vaginal bleeding, edema, jaundice, dark urine, clay-colored stools, dyspnea, headache, blurred vision, abdominal pain, numbness, stiffness, or pain in legs, chest pain; male to report impotence or gynecomastia
• Advise patient to check with prescriber before using OTC drugs; to take medication as prescribed; do not double doses; if dose is missed take as soon as remembered
• Advise patient to use non-hormonal contraception during treatment
• Inform diabetic patients that medication may need to be adjusted

Evaluation
Positive therapeutic outcome
• Decrease in tumor size in prostatic cancer, breast cancer

---

digitoxin (℞)
(di-ji-tox′in)
Crystodigin, digitoxin
Func. class.: Antidysrhythmic, cardiac glycoside, cardiotonic
Chem. class.: Digitalis preparation
Pregnancy category   C

Action: Inhibits sodium-potassium ATPase, which makes more calcium available for contractile proteins, resulting in increased cardiac output
➡**Therapeutic Outcome:** Positive inotropic and negative chronotropic effect

---

☑ Herb/drug   ⓢ Do Not Crush   ◆ Alert   ⦿ Key Drug   ⓖ Geriatric   ⓟ Pediatric

Uses: Rapid digitalization in CHF, atrial fibrillation, atrial flutter, atrial tachycardia

Dosage and routes

🅟 *Adult and child >12 yr:* PO 1.2-1.6 mg initially; give in divided doses over 24 hr; then 150 µg qd; rapid loading dose 0.6 mg, then 0.4 mg, then 0.2 mg q4-6h; slow loading dose 0.2 mg bid x 4 days, then maintenance

Maintenance dose: 0.05-0.3 mg/qd, usual 0.15 mg qd

🅟 *Child <1 yr:* 0.045 mg/kg

🅟 *Child 1-2 yr:* 0.04 mg/kg

🅟 *Child >2 yr:* 0.03 mg/kg (0.75 mg/m^2)

Maintenance: 10% of digitalizing dose

Available forms: Tabs 100 µg (0.1 mg), 200 µg (0.2 mg)

Adverse effects

CNS: Headache, drowsiness, apathy, confusion, disorientation, fatigue, depression, hallucinations

CV: Dysrhythmias, hypotension, bradycardia, AV block

EENT: Blurred vision, yellow-green halos, photophobia, diplopia

GI: Nausea, vomiting, anorexia, abdominal pain, diarrhea

MS: Muscular weakness

Contraindications: Hypersensitivity to digitalis, ventricular fibrillation, ventricular tachycardia, carotid sinus syndrome, 2nd- or 3rd-degree heart block

Precautions: Hepatic disease, acute MI, AV block, hypokalemia, hypomagnesemia, sinus node disease, lactation, severe respiratory disease, hypothyroidism, elderly, pregnancy **C** 🅖

Pharmacokinetics	
Absorption	Complete
Distribution	Widely distributed, 90-97% protein binding
Metabolism	Liver
Excretion	Kidneys
Half-life	5-7 days

Pharmacodynamics	
Onset	1-4 hr
Peak	4-12 hr
Duration	14-21 days

Interactions

Individual drugs

Amiodarone: ↑ levels of digitoxin

Colestipol: ↓ effects digitoxin

Cholestyramine: ↓ effects digitoxin

Diltiazem: ↑ levels of digitoxin

Piperacillin: ↑ hypokalemia

Quinidine: ↑ toxicity digitoxin

Rifampin: ↓ effects digitoxin

Spironolactone: ↑↓ blood levels

Succinylcholine: ↑ toxicity

Thyroid: ↓ level of digitoxin

Ticarcillin: ↑ hypokalemia

Drug classifications

Adrenergics: ↑ toxicity

Barbiturates: ↓ effects digitoxin

Diuretics, thiazide: ↑ hypokalemia, hypomagnasemia

Hydantoins: ↓ effects digitoxin

Thioamines: ↑ toxicity digitoxin

Herb/drug

Aloe: ↑ action

Buckthorn bark/berry: ↑ action

Cascara sagrada bark: ↑ action

Ephedra: ↑dysrhythymias

Ginseng, Siberian: ↑ action

Hawthorn: ↑ cardiac toxicity

Licorice: ↑ toxicity

Psyllium: ↓ absorption
Quinine: ↑ action
Lab test interferences
↑ CPK

NURSING CONSIDERATIONS
Assessment
• Check apical pulse for 1 min before giving drug; if pulse <60 in adult or <90 in an **P**infant, take again in 1 hr; if <60 in adult, call prescriber; note rate, rhythm, character
• Monitor electrolytes: potassium, sodium, chloride, magnesium, calcium; renal function studies: BUN, creatinine; blood studies: ALT, AST, bilirubin, Hct, Hgb before initiating treatment and periodically thereafter
• Monitor I&O ratio, daily weight; check skin turgor, lung sounds, peripheral edema
• Monitor drug levels (therapeutic level 9-25 ng/ml)

Nursing diagnoses
☑ Cardiac output, decreased (uses)
☑ Impaired gas exchange (adverse reactions)
☑ Knowledge deficit (teaching)

Implementation
• Give PO with or without food; tabs may be crushed and mixed with food/fluids for swallowing difficulty
• Give potassium supplements if ordered for potassium levels <3 mEq/L, or give foods high in potassium: bananas, orange juice

Patient/family education
• Instruct patient not to stop drug abruptly; teach all aspects of drug; to take exactly as ordered; to keep tabs in container protected from light
• Teach patient to avoid OTC medications, since many adverse drug interactions may occur; do not take antacid or cold products at same time
• Emphasize the importance of notifying prescriber of any loss of appetite, lower stomach pain, diarrhea, weakness, drowsiness, headache, blurred or yellow vision, rash, depression, toxicity
• Teach patient toxic symptoms of this drug and when to notify prescriber
• Advise patient to report shortness of breath, difficulty breathing, weight gain, edema, persistent cough
• Advise patient to carry ID with diagnosis and medication used

Evaluation
Positive therapeutic outcome
• Decreased weight, edema, pulse, respiration, rales
• Increased urine output
• Serum digitoxin level (9-25 ng/ml)

Treatment of overdose:
Discontinue drug; administer potassium; monitor ECG, administer an adrenergic blocking agent, digoxin immune Fab

---

digoxin ⚷ (℞)
(di-jox'in)
digoxin, Lanoxicaps, Lanoxin, Novo-Digoxin ✤
Func. class.: Inotropic antidysrhythmic, cardiac glycoside
Chem. class.: Digitalis preparation
Pregnancy category   C

Action: Inhibits sodium-potassium ATPase, which makes more calcium available

---

for contractile proteins, resulting in increased cardiac output

→ **Therapeutic Outcome:** Decreased edema, pulse, respiration, rales

Uses: Rapid digitalization in CHF, atrial fibrillation, atrial flutter, atrial tachycardia; cardiogenic shock, paroxysmal atrial tachycardia

Dosage and routes
Adult: **IV** *digitalizing dose* 0.6-1.0 mg given as 50% of the dose initially, additional fractions given at 4-8 hr intervals; PO *digitalizing dose* 0.75-1.25 mg given as 50% of the dose initially, additional fractions given at 4-8 hr intervals; *maintenance* 0.063-0.5 mg/day (tabs), or 0.350-0.5 mg/day (gelatin cap)

P *Child >10 yr:* **IV** *digitalizing dose* 8-12 μg/kg given as 50% of the dose initially, additional fractions given at 4-8 hr intervals; PO *digitalizing dose* 0.01-0.015 mg/kg given as 50% of the dose initially, additional fractions given at 6-8 hr intervals; maintenance 25%-35% of the loading dose qd as a single dose

P *Child 5-10 yr:* **IV** *digitalizing dose* 0.015-0.03 mg/kg given as 50% of the dose initially, additional fractions given at 4-8 hr intervals; PO *digitalizing dose* 0.02-0.035 mg/kg given as 50% of the dose initially, additional fractions given at 6-8 hr intervals; *maintenance* 25%-35% of the loading dose qd in 2 divided doses

P *Child 2-5 yr:* **IV** *digitalizing dose* 0.025-0.035 mg/kg given as 50% of the dose initially, additional fractions given at

4-8 hr intervals; PO *digitalizing dose* 0.03-0.04 mg/kg given as 50% of the dose initially, additional fractions given at 6-8 hr intervals; *maintenance* 25%-35% of the loading dose qd in 2 divided doses

P *Child 1-2 yr:* **IV** *digitalizing dose* 0.03-0.05 mg/kg given as 50% of the dose initially, additional fractions given at 4-8 hr intervals; PO *digitalizing dose* 0.035-0.06 mg/kg given as 50% of the dose initially, additional fractions given at 4-8 hr intervals; *maintenance* 25%-35% of the loading dose qd in 2 divided doses

P *Infants:* **IV** *digitalizing dose* 0.02-0.03 mg/kg given as 50% of the dose initially, additional fractions given at 4-8 hr intervals; PO *digitalizing dose* 0.025-0.035 mg/kg given as 50% of the dose initially, additional fractions given at 6-8 hr intervals; *maintenance* 25%-35% of the loading dose qd in 2 divided doses

P *Infants, premature:* **IV** *digitalizing dose* 0.015-0.025 mg/kg given as 50% of the dose initially, additional fractions given at 4-8 hr intervals; PO *digitalizing dose* 0.02-0.03 mg/kg given as 50% of the dose initially, additional fractions given at 6-8 hr intervals; *maintenance* 20%-30% of the loading dose qd in 2 divided doses

Available forms: Caps 0.05, 0.1, 0.2 mg; elix 0.05 mg/ml; tabs 0.125, 0.25, 0.5 mg; inj 0.05 ✤, 0.25 mg/ml; pedi inj 0.01 mg/ml

Adverse effects
CNS: Headache, drowsiness, apathy, confusion, disorienta-

---

tion, fatigue, depression, hallucinations

CV: **Dysrhythmias, hypotension,** bradycardia, **AV block**

EENT: Blurred vision, yellow-green halos, photophobia, diplopia

GI: Nausea, vomiting, anorexia, abdominal pain, diarrhea

Contraindications: Hypersensitivity to digitalis, ventricular fibrillation, ventricular tachycardia, carotid sinus syndrome, 2nd- or 3rd-degree heart block

Precautions: Renal disease, acute MI, AV block, severe respiratory disease, hypothyroidism, elderly, pregnancy **C,** sinus nodal disease, lactation, hypokalemia

🖎 Do Not Confuse:

Lanoxin/Lasix,
Lanoxin/Lomotil,
Lanoxin/Xanax

Pharmacokinetics

Absorption	Unknown
Distribution	Widely distributed; 20%-25% protein bound
Metabolism	Liver, small amount; also intestinal bacteria
Excretion	Urine
Half-life	1½ days

Pharmacodynamics

	PO	IV
Onset	½-1½ hr	5-30 min
Peak	2-6 hr	1-5 hr
Duration	After steady state	6-8 days

Interactions
Individual drugs

Amiodarone: ↑ digoxin levels, bradycardia

Amphotericin B: ↑ hypokalemia, toxicity

Calcium IV: ↑ risk of fatal dysrhythmias, digoxin toxicity

Carbenicillin: ↑ hypokalemia

Charcoal: ↓ levels of digoxin by absorption

Cholestyramine: ↓ digoxin level

Colestipol: ↓ digoxin level

Diltiazem: ↑ blood levels

Kaolin/pectin: ↓ absorption

Metoclopramide: ↓ digoxin level

Propafenone: ↑ digoxin levels, toxicity

Rifampin: ↓ digoxin effects

Thyroid: ↓ level of digoxin

Ticarcillin: ↑ hypokalemia

Verapamil: ↑ blood levels of digoxin, ↓ positive inotropic effect

Drug classifications

Antacids: ↓ digoxin absorption

Antidysrhythmics: ↑ bradycardia

Barbiturates: ↓ effects of digoxin

β-Adrenergic blockers: ↑ bradycardia

Calcium channel blockers: ↑ digoxin levels, toxicity

Diuretics, thiazide: ↑ hypokalemia, toxicity

Hydantoins: ↓ effects of digoxin

🗹 Herb/drug

Aloe: ↑ action

Buckthorn bark/berry: ↑ action

Cascara sagrada bark: ↑ action

Ephedra: ↑ dysrhythmias

Ginseng, Siberian: ↑ action

Hawthorn: ↑ cardiac toxicity

Indian snakeroot: ↑ bradycardia

Licorice: ↑ digoxin toxicity

Phyllium: ↓ absorption

Quinine: ↑ action

Lab test interferences
↑ CPK

NURSING CONSIDERATIONS
Assessment
• Assess and document apical pulse for 1 min before giving drug; if pulse <60 in adult or <90 in an infant or is significantly different, take again in 1 hr; if <60 in adult, call prescriber; note rate, rhythm, character

• Monitor electrolytes: potassium, sodium, chloride, magnesium, calcium; renal function studies: BUN, creatinine; other blood studies: ALT, AST, bilirubin, Hct, Hgb, drug levels (therapeutic level 0.5-2 ng/ml) before initiating treatment and periodically thereafter

• Monitor I&O ratio, daily weights; monitor turgor, lung sounds, edema

• Monitor cardiac status: apical pulse, character, rate, rhythm; resolution of atrial dysrhythmias by ECG; if tachydysrhythmia develops, hold drug; delay cardioversion while drug levels are determined

• Monitor ECG continuously during parenteral loading doses and for patients with suspected toxicity; provide hemodynamic monitoring for patients with heart failure or administer multiple cardiac drugs

Nursing diagnoses
☑Cardiac output, decreased (uses)
☑Impaired gas exchange (adverse reactions)
☑Knowledge deficit (teaching)

Implementation
• Do not give at same time as antacids or other drugs that decrease absorption

PO route
• Give PO with or without food; may crush tabs
• Give potassium supplements if ordered for potassium levels <3, or give foods high in potassium: bananas, orange juice

IV IV route
• Give **IV** undiluted or 1 ml of drug/4 ml sterile water, D_5, or NS; give over >5 min through Y-tube or 3-way stopcock; during digitalization close monitoring is necessary
• Store protected from light

Syringe compatibilities:
Heparin, milrinone

Syringe incompatibility:
Doxapram

Y-site compatibilities:
Amrinone, cefmetazole, ciprofloxacin, cisatracurium, diltiazem, famotidine, meperidine, meropenem, midazolam, milrinone, morphine, potassium chloride, propofol, remifentanil, tacrolimus, vit B/C

Y-site incompatibilities:
Fluconazole, foscarnet

Additive compatibilities:
Bretylium, cimetidine, floxacillin, furosemide, lidocaine, ranitidine, verapamil

Additive incompatibility:
Dobutamine

Patient/family education
• Caution patient to avoid OTC medications including cough, cold, allergy preparations, antacids, since many adverse drug interactions may occur; do not take antacid at same time
• Instruct patient to notify prescriber of any loss of appetite, lower stomach pain, diarrhea, weakness, drowsiness, headache, blurred or yellow-

green vision, rash, depression; teach toxic symptoms of this drug and when to notify prescriber
• Advise patient to maintain a sodium-restricted diet as ordered; to take potassium supplements as ordered to prevent toxicity
• Instruct patient to report shortness of breath, difficulty breathing, weight gain, edema, persistent cough
• Teach patient purpose of drug is to regulate the heart's functioning
• Teach patient that as outpatient to check and record pulse for 1 min before taking dose; if there is a change of >15 bpm from usual pulse, prescriber should be notified
• Teach patient to take medication at the same time each day, take missed doses within 12 hr; do not double doses; notify prescriber if doses are missed for 2 days or more
• Advise patient to carry ID describing dosage and reason for digoxin

Evaluation
Positive therapeutic outcome
• Decreased weight, edema, pulse, respiration, rales
• Increased urine output
• Serum digoxin level 0.5-2 ng/ml

Treatment of overdose: Discontinue drug, administer potassium, monitor ECG, administer an adrenergic blocking agent, digoxin immune Fab

---

digoxin immune Fab (ovine) ⚯ (R)
(di-jox'in)
Digibind
Func. class.: Antidote, digoxin specific

Pregnancy category   C

Action: Antibody fragments bind to free digoxin to reverse digoxin or digitoxin toxicity by not allowing digoxin or digitoxin to bind to sites of action

▶**Therapeutic Outcome:** Correction of digoxin toxicity

Uses: Reversal of life-threatening digoxin or digitoxin toxicity, including severe bradycardia, ventricular tachycardia/fibrillation, severe hypertension

Dosage and routes
Digoxin toxicity
Adult: **IV** dose (mg) = dose ingested (mg) × serum digoxin conc × 5.6 × wt in kg ÷ 1000; if ingested amount is unknown, give 800 mg **IV**; if digoxin liquid caps, **IV** or digoxin used, do not multiply ingested dose by 0.8; Digitoxin body load in mg = serum digitoxin conc × 0.56 × wt in kg ÷ 1000

Available forms: Inj 38 mg/vial (binds 0.5 mg digoxin or digitoxin)

Adverse effects
CV: **Worsening of CHF,** *ventricular rate increase,* **atrial fibrillation,** *low cardiac output*
INTEG: Hypersensitivity, allergic reactions, facial swelling, redness
META: Hypokalemia
RESP: **Impaired respiratory function, rapid respiratory rate**

Contraindications: Mild digoxin toxicity, hypersensitivity

P Precautions: Children, lactation, cardiac disease, renal disease, pregnancy **C,** allergy to ovine proteins

Pharmacokinetics

Absorption	Complete
Distribution	Widely distributed into plasma, interstitial fluids
Metabolism	Unknown
Excretion	Kidneys
Half-life	Biphasic (14-20 hr); increased in renal disease

Pharmacodynamics

Onset	30 mins (variable)
Peak	Unknown
Duration	Unknown

Interactions
Individual drugs
Digitoxin: ↓ effect of digitoxin
Digoxin: ↓ effect of digoxin
Lanatoside C: ↓ effect of lanatoside
Lab test interferences
Interference: Immunoassay (digoxin)

NURSING CONSIDERATIONS
Assessment
• Assess for hypokalemia: ST depression, flat T waves, presence of U wave, ventricular dysrhythmias
• Obtain information on previous allergies: previous exposure to sheep (ovine) proteins; scratch test may be performed before use of this product; hypersensitive reactions are more common in persons with previous exposure
• Monitor vital signs before, throughout, and after infusion

• Monitor heart rate, B/P q10 min during inf and after it is complete until stabilized; hemodynamic monitoring is used for unstable or hypotensive patients; check potassium levels until toxicity is resolved
• Assess for oxygen or perfusion deficit: hypotension, chest pain, dizziness, loss of consciousness
• Assess respiratory status: auscultate lung fields for bibasilar crackles in patients with advanced CHF

Nursing diagnoses
✓ Injury, risk for (uses)
✓ Knowledge deficit (teaching)

Implementation
• Give after diluting 40 mg/4 ml of sterile water (10 mg/ml), mix gently; may be further diluted with 0.9% NaCl; sol should be clear, colorless
• Give by bol if cardiac arrest is imminent or **IV** over 30 min using a 0.22 μm filter
• Store reconstituted sol for up to 4 hr in refrigerator

Patient/family education
• Teach that purpose of medication is to bind excess digoxin and reduce high blood levels
• Instruct patients to report fever, chills, itching, sweating, dyspnea
• Advise other prescribers that this medication has been used previously

Evaluation
Positive therapeutic outcome
• Correction of digoxin toxicity
• Digoxin blood levels 0.5-2 ng/ml
• Digitoxin blood level 9-25 ng/ml

dihydrotachysterol (℞)
(dye-hye-droh-tak-iss'ter-ole)
DHT Intensol ✿, Hytakerol
Func. class.: Parathyroid agent (calcium regulator)
Chem. class.: Vitamin D analog

Pregnancy category C

Action: Increases intestinal absorption of calcium, increases renal tubular absorption of phosphorus; is able to regulate calcium levels by regulation of calcitonin, parathyroid hormone

▶**Therapeutic Outcome:** Prevention of continued calcium loss in bones

Uses: Renal osteodystrophy, hypoparathyroidism, pseudohypoparathyroidism, familial hypophosphatemia, postoperative tetany

Investigational uses: Renal osteodystrophy

Dosage and routes
Hypophosphatemia
🅟*Adult and child:* PO 0.5-2 mg qd; maintenance 0.3-1.5 mg qd

Hypoparathyroidism/pseudohypoparathyroidism
Adult: PO 0.8-2.4 mg qd × 4 days, maintenance 0.2-2 mg qd regulated by serum calcium levels

🅟*Child:* PO 1-5 mg qd 1 wk, maintenance 0.2-1 mg qd regulated by serum calcium levels

Renal osteodystrophy
Adult: PO 0.1-0.25 mg qd, then 0.2-1 mg/day

Available forms: Tab 0.125, 0.2, 0.4 mg; cap 0.125 mg;

oral sol 0.2, 0.25 mg/5 ml, 0.2 mg/ml ✿ (Intensol)

Adverse effects
CNS: Drowsiness, headache, vertigo, fever, lethargy
CV: **Dysrhythmias,** hypertension
EENT: Tinnitus
GI: Nausea, diarrhea, vomiting, jaundice, anorexia, dry mouth, constipation, cramps, metallic taste
GU: **Polyuria,** hypercalciuria, hyperphosphatemia, **hematuria**
MS: Myalgia, arthralgia, decreased bone development

Contraindications: Hypersensitivity, renal disease, hyperphosphatemia, hypercalcemia

Precautions: Pregnancy **C,** renal calculi, lactation, CV disease

Pharmacokinetics	
Absorption	Well absorbed
Distribution	Liver, fat
Metabolism	Liver
Excretion	Feces (inactive, active metabolites)
Half-life	Unknown

Pharmacodynamics	
Onset	2 wk
Peak	2 wk
Duration	2 wk

Interactions
Individual drugs
Cholestyramine: ↓ absorption of dihydrotachysterol
Colestipol: ↓ absorption of dihydrotachysterol
Mineral oil: ↓ absorption of dihydrotachysterol
Phenytoin: ↓ effect of dihydrotachysterol
Verapamil: ↑ dysrhythmias

🌣 Herb/drug 🚫 Do Not Crush ◆ Alert 🔑 Key Drug 🅖 Geriatric 🅟 Pediatric

Drug classifications

Barbiturates: ↓ effect of dihydrotachysterol

Calcium supplements: ↑ hypercalcemia

Cardiac glycosides: ↑ dysrhythmias

Corticosteroids: ↓ effect of dihydrotachysterol

Diuretics, thiazide: ↑ hypercalcemia

Lab test interferences

False ↑ cholesterol

NURSING CONSIDERATIONS
Assessment

• Monitor BUN, urinary calcium, AST, ALT, cholesterol, alkaline phosphatase, creatinine, uric acid, chloride, magnesium, electrolytes, urine pH, phosphate; may increase calcium; should be kept at 9-10 mg/dl; keep vitamin D at 50-135 IU/dl, phosphate at 70 mg/dl; these tests should be checked before and throughout treatment

• Monitor for increased blood level, since toxic reaction may occur rapidly

• Monitor for dry mouth, metallic taste, polyuria, bone pain, muscle weakness, headache, fatigue, tinnitus, change in LOC, irregular pulse, dysrhythmias, increased respirations, anorexia, nausea, vomiting, cramps, diarrhea, constipation; may indicate hypercalcemia; if these occur, discontinue drug, give laxatives, low-calcium diet

• Monitor renal status: decreased urinary output (oliguria, anuria), edema in extremities, weight gain >5 lb, periorbital edema

• Assess nutritional status; check diet for sources of vitamin D (milk, some seafood), calcium (dairy products, dark green vegetables); phosphates (dairy products) must be avoided

Nursing diagnoses

☑ Nutrition: Less than body requirements (uses)

☑ Knowledge deficit (teaching)

Implementation

◎• Do not crush, chew caps

• May be increased q4 wk depending on blood level; give with meals for GI symptoms

• Store in tight, light-resistant containers at room temp

• Restrict sodium, potassium if required

• Restriction of fluids may be required for chronic renal failure

Patient/family education

• Teach symptoms of hypercalcemia and when to report symptoms to prescriber

• Teach patient about foods rich in calcium, vitamin D; provide list of calcium-rich foods; renal failure patients are given a renal diet

• Caution patient not to double doses, take exactly as prescribed

Evaluation

Positive therapeutic outcome

• Prevention of bone deficiencies

• Calcium, phosphorus at normal levels

D

diltiazem (℞)
(dil-tye′a-zem)
Apo-Diltiaz ♣, Cardizem, Cardizem SR, Cardizem CD, diltiazem, Dilacor-XR, Tiazac
Func. class.: Calcium channel blocker, anti-anginal
Chem. class.: Benzothiazepine
Pregnancy category   C

Action: Inhibits calcium ion influx across cell membrane during cardiac depolarization, produces relaxation of coronary vascular smooth muscle, dilates coronary arteries, slows SA/AV node conduction times, dilates peripheral arteries

➡ **Therapeutic Outcome:** Decreased angina pectoris, dysrhythmias, B/P

Uses
Oral: Angina pectoris due to coronary insufficiency, hypertension, vasospasm
Parenteral: Atrial fibrillation, flutter
Investigational use:
Raynaud's syndrome

Dosage and routes
Adult: PO 30 mg qid, increasing dose gradually to 180-360 mg/day in divided doses or 60-120 mg bid; may increase to 240-360 mg/day

Adult IV: 0.25 mg/kg as a bolus over 2 min initially, then 0.35 mg/kg may be given after 15 min; if no response, may give cont inf 5-15 mg/hr for up to 24 hr

Adult: PO 180-240 mg (Cardizem CD) qd

Available forms: Tab 30, 60, 90, 120 mg; tab ext rel 120, 180, 240 mg; cap sus rel 60, 90, 120, 180, 240 mg; caps ext rel 120, 180, 240, 300, 360 mg; inj **IV** 5 mg/ml (5, 10 ml)

Adverse effects
CNS: Headache, fatigue, drowsiness, dizziness, depression, weakness, insomnia, tremor, paresthesia
CV: **Dysrhythmia,** *edema*
CHF: Bradycardia, hypotension, palpitations, **heart block,** peripheral edema, angina
GI: Nausea, vomiting, diarrhea, gastric upset, *constipation,* increased liver function studies
GU: Nocturia, polyuria, **acute renal failure**
INTEG: Rash, pruritus, flushing, photosensitivity

Contraindications: Sick sinus syndrome, 2nd- or 3rd-degree heart block, hypotension less than 90 mm Hg systolic, acute MI, pulmonary congestion

Precautions: CHF, hypotension, hepatic injury, pregnancy ▣ **C,** lactation, children, renal disease

▧ **Do Not Confuse:**
Cardizem CD/Cardizem SR, Cardizem/Cardene, Cardizem SR/Cardene SR

Pharmacokinetics

Absorption	Well absorbed
Distribution	Not known
Metabolism	Liver, extensively
Excretion	Metabolites (96%)
Half-life	3½-9 hr

Pharmacodynamics

	PO	PO-SUS REL	IV
Onset	½ hr	Unknown	Unknown
Peak	2-3 hr	Unknown	Unknown
Duration	6-8 hr	12 hr	Unknown

Interactions
Individual drugs
Alcohol: ↑ hypotension
Carbamazepine: ↑ toxicity
Cyclosporine: ↑ cyclosporine effect
Digoxin: ↑ digoxin levels, bradycardia, CHF
Phenobarbital: ↓ effectiveness
Phenytoin: ↓ effectiveness
Propranolol: ↑ toxicity
Drug classifications
Antihypertensives: ↑ hypotension
β-Adrenergic blockers: ↑ bradycardia, CHF, ↑ beta blocker effect
Nitrates: ↑ nitrates
Food/drug
Grapefruit: ↑ hypotension

NURSING CONSIDERATIONS
Assessment
• Assess fluid volume status: I&O ratio and record, weight, distended red veins, crackles in lung, color, quality, and sp gr of urine, skin turgor, adequacy of pulses, moist mucous membranes, bilateral lung sounds, peripheral pitting edema; dehydration symptoms of decreasing output, thirst, hypotension, dry mouth and mucous membranes should be reported
• Monitor B/P and pulse, respiration, ECG and intervals (PR, QRS QT); PCWP, CVP often during infusion; if B/P drops 30 mm Hg, stop inf and call prescriber

• Monitor ALT, AST, bilirubin daily; if these are elevated, hepatotoxicity is suspected
• If platelets are <150,000/mm^3, drug is usually discontinued and another drug started
• Assess for extravasation: change site q48h
Nursing diagnoses
☑Cardiac output, decreased (uses)
☑Knowledge deficit (teaching)
Implementation
PO route
• Give with meals for GI symptoms; may be crushed and mixed with food/fluids for swallowing difficulty
🚫• Do not chew or crush sus rel caps
• Store in airtight container at room temp
IV route
• Give direct **IV** undiluted over 2 min
• For continuous inf dilute 125 mg/100 ml (1.25 mg/ml) or 250 mg/250 ml (1 mg/ml) or 250 mg/500 ml (0.5 mg/ml) of D$_5$W, 0.9% NaCl, D$_5$/0.45% NaCl; give 10 mg/hr; may increase by 5 mg/hr to 15 mg/hr; may continue inf up to 24 hr
Y-site compatibilities:
Albumin, amikacin, amphotericin B, aztreonam, bretylium, bumetanide, cefazolin, cefotaxime, cefotetan, cefoxitin, ceftazidime, ceftriaxone, cefuroxime, cimetidine, ciprofloxacin, clindamycin, digoxin, dobutamine, dopamine, doxycycline, epinephrine, erythromycin, esmolol, fentanyl, fluconazole, gentamicin, hetastarch, hydromorphone, imipenem-cilastatin, labetalol, lidocaine, lorazepam, meperidine, metoclopramide,

metronidazole, midazolam, milrinone, morphine, multivitamins, nicardipine, nitroglycerin, norepinephrine, oxacillin, penicillin G potassium, pentamidine, piperacillin, potassium chloride, potassium phosphates, ranitidine, sodium nitroprusside, theophylline, ticarcillin, ticarcillin/clavulanate, tobramycin, trimethoprim-sulfamethoxazole, vancomycin, vecuronium

Patient/family education

• Caution patient to avoid hazardous activities until stabilized on drug and dizziness is no longer a problem
• Instruct patient to limit caffeine consumption; to avoid alcohol and OTC drugs unless directed by prescriber
• Tell patient to comply in all areas of medical regimen; diet, exercise, stress reduction, drug therapy; to notify prescriber of irregular heart beat, shortness of breath, swelling of feet and hands, pronounced dizziness, constipation, nausea, hypotension
• Teach patient to use as directed even if feeling better; may be taken with other cardiovascular drugs (nitrates, β-blockers)

Evaluation

Positive therapeutic outcome
• Decreased anginal pain
• Decreased B/P
• Absence of dysrhythmias

Treatment of overdose:

Defibrillation, atropine for AV block, vasopressor for hypotension

---

dimenhydrinate
(OTC, ℞)(OTC, ℞)
(dye-men-hye'dri-nate)
Apo-Dimenhydrinate ✤, Calm-X, Children's Dramamine, dimenhydrinate, Dimentabs, Dinate, Dramamine, Dramanate, Dymenate, Gravol ✤, Gravol L/A ✤, Hydrate, Nauseatol ✤, Novo-Dimenate ✤, PMS-Dimenhydrinate ✤, Travamine ✤, Triptone Caplets
Func. class.: Antiemetic, antihistamine, anticholinergic
Chem. class.: H_1-receptor antagonist, ethanolamine derivative
Pregnancy category **B**

Action: Vestibular stimulator is decreased; anticholinergic, antiemetic, antihistamine response

Therapeutic Outcome: Absence of motion sickness

Uses: Motion sickness, nausea, vomiting

Dosage and routes
Adult: PO 50-100 mg q4h; IM/**IV** 50 mg as needed

P *Child:* IM/PO 5 mg/kg divided in 4 equal doses

Available forms: Tab 50 mg; inj 50 mg/ml; elixir 15 mg/5 ml ✤, chew tab 50 mg

Adverse effects

CNS: Drowsiness, restlessness, headache, dizziness, insomnia, confusion, nervousness, tingling, vertigo; hallucinations and **convulsions** in young **P** children

CV: Hypertension, *hypotension,* palpitations

EENT: Dry mouth, blurred vision, diplopia, nasal congestion, photosensitivity
GI: Nausea, anorexia, vomiting, *constipation*
INTEG: Rash, urticaria, fever, chills, flushing
MISC: Anaphylaxis

Contraindications: Hypersensitivity to narcotics, shock

P **Precautions:** Children, cardiac
G dysrhythmias, elderly, asthma, pregnancy **B,** prostatic hypertrophy, bladder neck obstruction, narrow-angle glaucoma, stenosing peptic ulcer, pyloroduodenal obstruction

D

CNS depressants: ↑ CNS depression
MAOIs: ↑ anticholinergic effect
Opiates: ↑ CNS depression
Phenothiazines: ↑ anticholinergic reactions
Sedative/hypnotics: ↑ CNS depression

Herb/drug
Henbane leaf: ↑ anticholinergic effect
Lab test interferences
False negative: Skin allergy tests (discontinue antihistamines 3 days before testing)

Pharmacokinetics	
Absorption	Well absorbed (PO, IM)
Distribution	Unknown; crosses placenta
Metabolism	Liver
Excretion	Kidneys, breast milk
Half-life	Unknown

Pharmacodynamics			
	PO	IM	IV
Onset	15-60 min	30 min	Immediate
Peak	1-2 hr	1-2 hr	Unknown
Duration	4-6 hr	4-6 hr	4-6 hr

Interactions
Individual drugs
Alcohol: ↑ CNS depression
Atropine: ↑ anticholinergic reactions
Disopyramide: ↑ anticholinergic reactions
Haloperidol: ↑ anticholinergic reactions
Quinidine: ↑ anticholinergic reactions
Drug classifications
Antidepressants: ↑ anticholinergic reactions
Antihistamines: ↑ anticholinergic reactions

NURSING CONSIDERATIONS
Assessment
• Assess for signs of toxicity to other drugs or masking of symptoms of disease (brain tumor, intestinal obstruction); monitor GI symptoms including nausea, vomiting, abdominal pain, increased bowel sounds
• Monitor VS, B/P; check patients with cardiac disease more often
• Monitor I&O; check for dehydration (poor skin turgor, increased sp gr, tachycardia, severe thirst) especially in the
G elderly

Nursing diagnoses
✓ Injury, risk for (side effects)
✓ Knowledge deficit (teaching)

Implementation
PO route
• Tab may be swallowed whole, chewed, or allowed to dissolve; give 1-2 hr before activity that may cause motion sickness; use measuring device for liq for correct dosing
IM route
• Give IM injection in large muscle mass; aspirate to avoid IV administration; massage

---

♣ Canada Only   Adverse effects: *italic* = common; **bold** = life-threatening

IV **IV route**

• Give **IV** directly after diluting 50 mg/10 ml or NaCl inj; give 50 mg or less over 2 min

Syringe incompatibilities:
Butorphanol, chlorpromazine, glycopyrrolate, hydroxyzine, midazolam, pentobarbital, prochlorperazine, promazine, promethazine, thiopental

Syringe compatibilities:
Atropine, diphenhydramine, droperidol, fentanyl, heparin, hydromorphone, meperidine, metoclopramide, morphine, pentazocine, perphenazine, ranitidine, scopolamine

Y-site compatibilities:
Acyclovir

Y-site incompatibilities:
Aminophylline, heparin, hydrocortisone sodium succinate, hydroxyzine, phenobarbital, phenytoin, prednisolone, prochlorperazine, promazine, promethazine

Additive compatibilities:
Amikacin, calcium gluconate, chloramphenicol, corticotropin, erythromycin, heparin, hydroxyzine, methicillin, norepinephrine, penicillin G potassium, pentobarbital, phenobarbital, potassium chloride, prochlorperazine, vancomycin, vit B/C

Additive incompatibilities:
Tetracycline, thiopental

Patient/family education

• Teach all aspects of drug uses; to notify prescriber if confusion, sedation, hypotension occur; to avoid driving and other hazardous activity if drowsiness occurs; to avoid alcohol and other CNS depressants that may potentiate effect

• Tell patient not to exceed recommended dosage

• Inform patient hard candy, gum, frequent rinsing of mouth may be used for dryness

• Advise patient that a false negative result may occur with skin testing; these procedures should not be scheduled until 4 days after discontinuing use

• Caution patient to avoid hazardous activities, activities requiring alertness; dizziness may occur; instruct patient to request assistance with ambulation

• Caution patient to avoid alcohol, other CNS depressants when taking this medication; response will be increased

Evaluation

Positive therapeutic outcome

• Absence of motion sickness

• Absence of nausea, vomiting

dinoprostone (℞)
(dye-noe-prost'one)
Prepidil, Prostin E₂
Func. class.: Oxytocic, abortifacient
Chem. class.: Prostaglandin E₂

Pregnancy category   C

Action: Stimulates uterine contractions similar to labor by myometrium stimulation, causing abortion; acts within 30 hr for complete abortion; GI smooth muscle stimulation, effacement, dilatation of the cervix

▶**Therapeutic Outcome:** Beginning of labor, fetal expulsion

Uses: Abortion during 2nd trimester, benign hydatidiform mole, expulsion of uterine contents in fetal deaths to 28 wk, missed abortion, cervical effacement and dilatation in term pregnancy when they have not occurred spontaneously

Dosage and routes
Adult: Vag supp 20 mg; repeat q3-5h until abortion occurs; max dose is 240 mg

Adult: Gel; warm to room temperature; choose correct length shielded catheter (10 or 20 mm), fill catheter by pushing plunger; patient remain recumbent for 15-30 min

Available forms: Vag supp 20 mg; gel 0.5 mg/3 g (prefilled syringe); gel 0.5 mg

Adverse effects
CNS: Headache, dizziness, chills, fever
CV: Hypotension, **dysrhythmias**
EENT: Blurred vision
GI: Nausea, vomiting, diarrhea
GU: Vaginitis, vaginal pain, vulvitis, vaginismus
INTEG: Rash, skin color changes
MS: Leg cramps, joint swelling, weakness
Insert: Uterine hyperstimulation, fever, nausea, vomiting, diarrhea, abdominal pain
Gel: Uterine contractile abnormality, GI side effects, back pain, fever; **fetal: bradycardia, late deceleration**

Contraindications: Hypersensitivity, uterine fibrosis, cervical stenosis, pelvic surgery, pelvic inflammatory disease (PID), respiratory disease

Precautions: Hepatic disease, renal disease, cardiac disease, asthma, anemia, jaundice, diabetes mellitus, convulsive disorders, hypertension, hypotension, pregnancy **C**

▧ Do Not Confuse:
Prepidil/bepridil

Pharmacokinetics	
Absorption	Rapidly absorbed
Distribution	Unknown
Metabolism	Enzymes
Excretion	Kidneys
Half-life	Unknown

D

Pharmacodynamics		
	GEL	SUPP
Onset	Rapid	10 min
Peak	30-45 min	Unknown
Duration	Unknown	2-3 hr

Interactions
Individual drugs
Alcohol: ↓ oxytoxic effect
Oxytocin: ↑ effect

NURSING CONSIDERATIONS
Assessment
• Assess dilatation and effacement of the cervix, uterine contractions, fetal heart tones; watch for contractions lasting over 1 min, hypertonus, fetal distress; drug should be slowed or discontinued
• Assess for fever that occurs approximately 30 min following supp insertion (abortion)
• Monitor for nausea, vomiting, diarrhea; these may require medication
• Assess for hypersensitive reaction: dyspnea, rash, chest discomfort
• Assess respiratory rate, rhythm, depth; notify prescriber of abnormalities, in pulse, B/P
• Check vaginal discharge; itching, irritation indicates vaginal infection

Nursing diagnoses
☑ Injury, high risk for (side effects)
☑ Knowledge deficit (teaching)

Implementation

Supp route

• Warm suppository by running warm water over package; insert high in vagina, wear gloves to prevent absorption; have patient recumbent for at least 10 min

Gel route

• Do not allow to come in contact with skin; use soap and water to wash after use
• Gel should be at room temp
• Place patient in dorsal or lithotomy position to insert gel into cervical canal; remove catheter; discard all items after use; keep supine 15-30 min

Patient/family education

• Teach patient all aspects of treatment including purpose of medication and expected results
• Tell patient that gel may produce warmth in her vagina
• Caution patient that if contractions are longer than 1 min to notify nurse or prescriber
• Advise patient to notify prescriber of cramping, pain, increased bleeding, chills, increased temp, or foul-smelling discharge; these symptoms may indicate uterine infection

Evaluation

Positive therapeutic outcome

• Progression of labor
• Abortion

---

diphenhydramine ⚷
(OTC, ℞)
(dye-fen-hye′dra-meen)
Allerdryl ✦, AllerMax, Allermed, Banophen, Beldin, Belix, Bena-D 10, Bena-D 50, Benadryl, Benadryl 25, Benadryl Kapseals, Benahist 10, Benahist 50, Ben-Allergin-50, Benoject-10, Benoject-50, Benylin Cough, Bydramine, Compoz, Diphenacen-50, Diphenadryl, Diphen Cough, Diphenhist, diphenhydramine HCl, Dormarex 2, Dormin, Fynex, Gen-D-Phen, Genahist, Hydramine, Hydramyn, Hydril, Hyrexin-50, Insomnal ✦, Nervine, Nidryl, Nighttime Sleep Aid, Nordryl, Nordryl Cough, Nytol, Phendry, Sleep-Eze 3, Sominex 2, Tusstat, Twilite, Uni-Bent Cough, Wehdryl
Func. class.: Antihistamine, antitussive
Chem. class.: Ethanolamine derivative, H_1-receptor antagonist
Pregnancy category **B**

Action: Acts on blood vessels, GI, respiratory system by competing with histamine for H_1-receptor site; decreases allergic response by blocking histamine; causes increased heart rate, vasodilatation, secretions

▷**Therapeutic Outcome:** Absence of allergy symptoms and rhinitis, decreased dystonic symptoms, absence of motion sickness, absence of cough, ability to sleep

Uses: Allergy symptoms, rhinitis, motion sickness, antiparkinsonism, nighttime sedation,

---

infant colic, nonproductive cough, anaphylaxis, nasal allergies, allergic dermatoses, dystonic reactions

Dosage and routes
Adult: PO 25-50 mg q4-6h, not to exceed 400 mg/day; IM/**IV** 10-50 mg, not to exceed 400 mg/day

P *Child >12 kg:* PO/IM/**IV** 5 mg/kg/day in 4 divided doses, not to exceed 300 mg/day

Renal dose
CrCl 10-50 ml/min dose q6-12h; CrCl <10 ml/min dose q12-18h

Available forms: Caps 25, 50 mg; tabs 25, 50 mg; elix 12.5 mg/5 ml; syr 12.5 mg/5 ml; liquid 6.25 mg/5 ml; inj 10, 50 mg/ml

Adverse effects
CNS: Dizziness, drowsiness, poor coordination, fatigue, anxiety, euphoria, confusion, paresthesia, neuritis, **seizures**
EENT: Blurred vision, dilated pupils, tinnitus, nasal stuffiness, dry nose, throat, mouth
GI: Dry mouth, nausea, anorexia, diarrhea
GU: Retention, dysuria, frequency
HEMA: **Thrombocytopenia, agranulocytosis, hemolytic anemia**
INTEG: Photosensitivity
RESP: Increased thick secretions, wheezing, chest tightness
MISC: **Anaphylaxis**

Contraindications: Hypersensitivity to H_1-receptor antagonist, acute asthma attack, lower respiratory tract disease

Precautions: Increased intraocular pressure, renal disease, cardiac disease, hypertension, bronchial asthma, seizure disorder, stenosed peptic ulcers, hyperthyroidism, prostatic hypertrophy, bladder neck obstruction, pregnancy **B**

N Do Not Confuse:
diphenhydramine/dicyclomine

D

Pharmacokinetics
Absorption	Well absorbed (PO, IM); minimally absorbed (top); completely absorbed (**IV**)
Distribution	Widely distributed; crosses placenta
Metabolism	Liver (95%)
Excretion	Kidneys, breast milk
Half-life	2½-7 hr

Pharmacodynamics
	PO	IM	IV
Onset	15-60 min	30 min	Immediate
Peak	1-4 hr	1-4 hr	Unknown
Duration	4-8 hr	4-8 hr	4-8 hr

Interactions
Individual drugs
Alcohol: ↑ CNS depression
Disopyramide: ↑ anticholinergic response
Quinidine: ↑ anticholinergic response
Drug classifications
Antidepressants, tricyclic: ↑ anticholinergic response
CNS depressants: ↑ CNS depression
MAOIs: ↑ anticholinergic effect
Opiates: ↑ CNS depression
Sedative/hypnotics: ↑ CNS depression
Herb/drug
Henbane leaf: ↑ anticholinergic effect

Lab test interferences

False negative: Skin allergy tests (discontinue antihistamines 3 days before testing)

NURSING CONSIDERATIONS
Assessment

• Assess respiratory status: rate, rhythm, increase in bronchial secretions, wheezing, chest tightness; provide fluids to 2 L/day to decrease secretion thickness

• Monitor I&O ratio: be alert for urinary retention, frequency, dysuria, especially 🅖 elderly; drug should be discontinued if these occur

• Monitor CBC during long-term therapy; blood dyscrasias may occur but are rare

• If giving for dystonic reactions, assess type of involuntary movements and evaluate response to this medication

• Assess cough characteristics including type, frequency, thickness of secretions, and evaluate response to this medication if using for cough

Nursing diagnoses

☑ Injury, risk for (side effects)
☑ Sleep pattern disturbance (uses)
☑ Knowledge deficit (teaching)

Implementation

• Give 20 min before hs if using for sleep aid

PO route

• Give with meals if GI symptoms occur; absorption may be slightly decreased; cap may be opened and drug mixed with food/fluids for patients with swallowing difficulties

IM route

• Give IM injection in large muscle mass; aspirate to avoid **IV** administration; rotate sites

🔳 **IV route**

• Give **IV** undiluted 25 mg/min; may be diluted with 0.9% NaCl, D_5W, $D_{10}W$, 0.45% NaCl, D_5/0.9% NaCl, D_5/0.45% NaCl, D_5/0.25% NaCl, LR, Ringer's, give 25 mg/min or less

Syringe incompatibilities:
Pentobarbital, phenytoin, thiopental

Syringe compatibilities:
Atropine, butorphanol, chlorpromazine, cimetidine, cisatracurium, dimenhydrinate, doxorubicin liposome, droperidol, fentanyl, fluphenazine, glycopyrrolate, hydromorphone, hydroxyzine, meperidine, metoclopramide, midazolam, morphine, nalbuphine, pentazocine, perphenazine, prochlorperazine, promazine, promethazine, ranitidine, remifentanil, scopolamine, sufentanil, thiothixene

Y-site compatibilities:
Acyclovir, aldesleukin, amifostine, amsacrine, aztreonam, ciprofloxacin, cisplatin, cladribine, cyclophosphamide, cytarabine, doxorubicin, famotidine, filgrastim, fluconazole, fludarabine, gallium, granisetron, heparin, hydrocortisone, idarubicin, melphalan, meperidine, meropenem, methotrexate, ondansetron, paclitaxel, piperacillin/tazobactam, potassium chloride, propofol, sargramostim, sufentanil, tacrolimus, teniposide, thiotepa, vinorelbine, vit B/C

Y-site incompatibilities:
Foscarnet

Additive compatibilities:
Amikacin, aminophylline, ascorbic acid, bleomycin, cephapirin, erythromycin,

---

☑ Herb/drug 🔘 Do Not Crush ◆ Alert ⟳ Key Drug 🅖 Geriatric 🅟 Pediatric hydrocortisone, lidocaine, methicillin, methyldopate, nafcillin, netilmicin, penicillin G potassium, penicillin G sodium, polymyxin B, vit B/C

Additive incompatibilities: Amobarbital, cephalothin, thiopental

Patient/family education
• Tell patient that a false-negative result may occur with skin testing; these procedures should not be scheduled until 3 days after discontinuing use
• Caution patient to avoid hazardous activities and activities requiring alertness, since dizziness may occur; instruct patient to request assistance with ambulation
• Teach patient to use sunscreen to prevent photosensitivity
• Advise patient to avoid alcohol, other depressants; CNS depression may occur
• Teach all aspects of drug uses; to notify prescriber if confusion, sedation, hypotension occur; to avoid driving and other hazardous activity if drowsiness occurs; to avoid alcohol or other CNS depressants that may potentiate effect
• Teach patient hard candy, gum, frequent rinsing of mouth may be used for dryness

Evaluation
Positive therapeutic outcome
• Absence of motion sickness
• Absence of nausea, vomiting
• Ability to sleep
• Absence of cough
• Decrease in involuntary movements

Treatment of overdose:
• Administer ipecac syrup or lavage, diazepam, vasopressors, barbiturates (short acting)

diphenoxylate with atropine/difenoxin with atropine (℞)
(dye-fen-ox′i-late)
Diphenatol, Lofene, Logen, Lomanate, Lomotil, Lonox, Lo-Trop, Motofen, Nor-mil
Func. class.: Antidiarrheal
Chem. class.: Phenylpiperidine derivative, opiate agonist

Pregnancy category C
Controlled substance schedule V (diphenoxylate/atropine); IV (difenoxin/atropine)

Action: Inhibits gastric motility by acting on mucosal receptors responsible for peristalsis; related to narcotic analgesics as adjunct

▶**Therapeutic Outcome:** Decreased loose stools

Uses: Diarrhea (cause undetermined)

Dosage and routes
Adult: PO 2.5-5 mg qid, titrated to patient response
▣ *Child 2-12 yr:* PO 0.3-0.4 mg/kg/day in divided doses

Available forms: Tab 2.5 mg diphenoxylate/0.025 mg atropine; tab 1 mg difenoxin/0.025 mg atropine; liq 2.5 mg diphenoxylate/0.025 mg atropine/5 ml

Adverse effects
CNS: Drowsiness, headache, sedation, depression, weakness,

lethargy, flushing, **hyperthermia**

CV: Tachycardia

EENT: Blurred vision, nystagmus, mydriasis

GI: Nausea, vomiting, abdominal pain, glossitis, colitis

GU: Urine retention

INTEG: Rash, urticaria, pruritus, **angioneurotic edema**

Contraindications: Hypersensitivity, severe liver disease, pseudomembranous enterocolitis, glaucoma, child <2 yr, electrolyte imbalances

Precautions: Hepatic disease, renal disease, ulcerative colitis, pregnancy C, lactation, elderly

🚫 **Do Not Confuse:**
Diphenatol/diphenidol, Lomotil/Lamictal, Lomotil/Lanoxin, Lomotil/Lasix

Pharmacokinetics	
Absorption	Well absorbed
Distribution	Unknown
Metabolism	Liver, active metabolite
Excretion	Kidneys
Half-life	2½ hr

Pharmacodynamics	
Onset	45-60 min
Peak	2 hr
Duration	3-4 hr

Interactions
Individual drugs
Alcohol: ↑ action of alcohol
Disopyramide: ↑ anticholinergic effect
Drug classifications
Anticholinergics: ↑ anticholinergic effect
Antidepressants, tricyclic: ↑ anticholinergic effect
Antihistamines: ↑ CNS depression
Barbiturates: ↑ action of barbiturates

CNS depressants: ↑ action of CNS depressants
MAOIs: Hypertensive crisis; do not use together
Opiates: ↑ action of narcotics
Sedative/hypnotics: ↑ CNS depression

NURSING CONSIDERATIONS
Assessment
• Monitor electrolytes (potassium, sodium, chloride) if on long-term therapy; fluid status, skin turgor
• Assess bowel pattern before, during treatment; check for rebound constipation after termination of medication; check bowel sounds
• Check response after 48 hr; if no response, drug should be discontinued and other treatment initiated
• Assess for abdominal distention and toxic megacolon, which may occur in ulcerative colitis

Nursing diagnoses
☑ Diarrhea (uses)
☑ Constipation (adverse reactions)
☑ Knowledge deficit (teaching)
☑ Noncompliance (teaching)

Implementation
• Give for 48 hr only; tabs may be given with food, crushed and mixed with fluids; liq should be measured accurately

Patient/family education
• Advise patient to avoid alcohol and OTC products unless directed by prescriber; may cause increased CNS depression
• Caution patient not to exceed recommended dosage; that drug may be habit forming
• Advise patient that drug may cause drowsiness; to avoid

hazardous activities until response to drug is determined
• Teach patient that dry mouth can be decreased by frequent sips of water, hard candy, sugarless gum

Evaluation
Positive therapeutic outcome
• Decreased diarrhea

dipyridamole (℞)
(dye-peer-id'a-mole)
Apo-Dipyridamole ✦,
dipyridamole, Novo-
Dipiradol ✦, Persantine,
Persantine IV
Func. class.: Coronary vasodilator, antiplatelet agent
Chem. class.: Nonnitrate
Pregnancy category B

Action: Inhibits adenosine uptake, which produces coronary vasodilatation; increases oxygen saturation in coronary tissues, coronary blood flow; acts on small vessels with little effect on vascular resistance; may increase development of collateral circulation; decreased platelet aggregation by the inhibition of phosphodiesterases (enzymes)

Therapeutic Outcome: Inhibition of platelet aggregation; absence of ischemic attacks, reinfarction

Uses: Prevention of transient ischemic attacks, inhibition of platelet adhesion to prevent myocardial reinfarction, thromboembolism, with warfarin in prosthetic heart valves, prevention of coronary bypass graft occlusion with aspirin; possibly effective for long-term therapy of chronic angina pectoris

Dosage and routes
Transient ischemic attacks
Adult: PO 50 mg tid, 1 hr ac, not to exceed 400 mg qd
Inhibition of platelet adhesion
Adult: PO 50-75 mg qid in combination with aspirin or warfarin

Available forms: Tabs 25, 50, 75 mg; inj 10 mg/2 ml

Adverse effects
CNS: Headache, dizziness, weakness, fainting, syncope
CV: Postural hypotension
GI: Nausea, vomiting, anorexia, diarrhea
INTEG: Rash, flushing

Contraindications: Hypersensitivity, hypotension

Precautions: Pregnancy **B**

Pharmacokinetics

Absorption	30%-50% (PO)
Distribution	Widely distributed; crosses placenta
Metabolism	Liver
Excretion	Bile, undergoes enterohepatic recirculation; enters breast milk
Half-life	10 hr

Pharmacodynamics

	PO	IV
Onset	Unknown	Unknown
Peak	2½ hr	6 min
Duration	6 hr	½ hr
Therapeutic effect	Several mo	

Interactions
Individual drugs
Aspirin: ↑ antiplatelet effect
Theophylline: ↓ effects of disopyramide (thallium)
Drug classifications
Anticoagulants: ↑ risk of bleeding

NSAIDs: ↑ risk of bleeding
Thrombolytics: ↑ risk of bleeding

NURSING CONSIDERATIONS
Assessment
• Monitor B/P, pulse baseline and during treatment until stable; take B/P with patient lying, standing; orthostatic hypotension is common
• Assess cardiac status: chest pain, what aggravates or ameliorates condition
• If using by **IV** route, monitor vital signs before, during, and after infusion; monitor for chest pain, bronchospasm; use ECG for identifying dysrhythmias; use aminophylline up to 250 mg **IV** for bronchospasm and chest pain if chest pain is unrelieved with the 250 mg dose of aminophylline; give SL dose of nitroglycerin

Nursing diagnoses
☑ Cardiac output, decreased (uses)
☑ Pain (uses)
☑ Knowledge deficit (teaching)

Implementation
PO route
• Give with 8 oz of water; to improve absorption give on an empty stomach; if GI symptoms occur may give with meals
• Tabs may be crushed, mixed with food or fluids for swallowing difficulty or swallowed whole
• Store at room temp
IV Intermittent inf
• Give by **IV** after diluting each 5 mg/2 ml or more in D₅W, 0.45% NaCl, or 0.9% NaCl; 20-50 ml should be given; give over 4 min; do not give undiluted

Patient/family education
• Teach patient that this medication is not a cure; that drug may have to be taken continuously in evenly spaced doses only as directed; if a dose is missed, take one when remembered up to 4 hr; do not double doses
• Inform patient that it is necessary to quit smoking to prevent excessive vasoconstriction
• Advise patient to rise slowly from sitting or lying down to prevent orthostatic hypotension
• Caution patient not to use alcohol or OTC medication unless approved by prescriber
• Caution patient to avoid hazardous activities until stabilized on medication; dizziness may occur

Evaluation
Positive therapeutic outcome
• Absence of reinfarction, ischemic attacks

Treatment of overdose: Administer **IV** phenylephrine

---

dirithromycin (℞)
(die-rith-roe-mie′sin)
Dynabac
Func. class.: Antibacterial
Chem. class.: Macrolide

Pregnancy category   C

Action: Binds to 50S ribosomal subunits of susceptible bacteria; suppresses protein synthesis

Therapeutic Outcome: Bactericidal action against *Moraxella catarrhalis, Streptococcus pneumoniae, S. pyogenes, Legionella pneumophilia, Mycoplasma pneumoniae, Staphylo-*

---

*coccus aureus, S. agalactiae,
Streptococcus* sp., *S. viridans,
Bordetella pertussis, Propioni-
bacterium acnes*

Uses: Infections of upper and
lower respiratory tract

Dosage and routes
Adult: PO 500 mg qd, given
for 7-14 days depending on
infections

Available forms: Tab, enteric
coated 250 mg

Adverse effects
*GI: Abdominal pain, nausea,
diarrhea, vomiting, dyspepsia,*
GI disorders, flatulence, abnormal stools, anorexia, constipation, **pseudomembranous
colitis**
*CNS: Headache, dizziness,
insomnia*
HEMA: Increased platelet
count, increased eosinophils
RESP: Cough, dyspnea
INTEG: Pruritus, urticaria

Contraindications: Hypersensitivity to this drug or any
other macrolide, or erythromycin, bacteremias

Precautions: Pregnancy **C**,
lactation, children, hepatic,
renal disease

Pharmacokinetics	
Absorption	Rapidly absorbed
Distribution	Widely distributed
Metabolism	No hepatic metabo-lism
Excretion	Bile, feces (up to 97%)
Half-life	Plasma half-life 8 hr, terminal 44 hr

Pharmacodynamics	
Unknown	

Interactions
Drug classifications
Antacids: Slightly enhanced
absorption of dirithromycin
H₂ antagonists: Slightly enhanced absorption of dirithromycin
Xanthines: May alter effect of
xanthine
Food/drug
↑ absorption

NURSING CONSIDERATIONS
Assessment
• Assess I&O ratio; report
hematuria, oliguria in renal
disease
• Monitor liver function
studies: AST, ALT if on long-
term therapy
• Monitor renal studies: Urinalysis, protein, blood
• Monitor C&S before drug
therapy; drug may be given as
soon as culture is taken; C&S
may be repeated after treatment
• Assess bowel pattern before,
during treatment; pseudomembranous colitis may occur
• Assess for skin eruptions,
itching
• Assess respiratory status:
rate, character, wheezing,
tightness in chest; discontinue
drug
• Identify allergies before
treatment, reaction of each
medication; place allergies on
chart, notify all people giving
drugs
Nursing diagnoses
✓ Infection, risk for (uses)
✓ Diarrhea (side effects)
✓ Knowledge deficit (teaching)
✓ Noncompliance (teaching)

Implementation
• Give adequate intake of
fluids (2 L) during diarrhea
episodes

🚫 • Administer whole; do not cut, crush, chew tablets
• Give with food or within 1 hr of food at same time each day
• Store at room temperature in tight container

Patient/family education
• Teach patient to take with full glass of water; give with food
• Instruct patient to report sore throat, fever, fatigue; may indicate superinfection
• Teach patient to notify nurse of diarrhea stools, dark urine, pale stools, yellow discoloration of eyes or skin, severe abdominal pain
• Instruct patient to take at evenly spaced intervals; complete dosage regimen

Evaluation
Positive therapeutic outcome
• C&S negative for infection

Treatment of hypersensitivity: Withdraw drug, maintain airway, administer epinephrine, aminophylline, O₂, **IV** corticosteroids

---

disopyramide (℞)
(dye-soe-peer'a-mide)
disopyramide, Norpace, Norpace CR, Rhythmodan
Func. class.: Antidysrhythmic (class IA)
Chem. class.: Nonnitrate
Pregnancy category   **C**

Action: Prolongs action potential duration and effective refractory period; reduces disparity in refractory between normal and infarcted myocardium; prevents increased myocardial excitability and conduction contractility

➡**Therapeutic Outcome:** Suppression of supraventricular dysrhythmias

Uses: PVCs, ventricular tachycardia, supraventricular tachycardia, atrial flutter, fibrillation

Investigational uses: Supraventricular tachycardia (prevention, treatment)

Dosage and routes
Adult: PO 100-200 mg q6h; in renal dysfunction 100 mg q6h; sus rel cap 200 mg q12h

P *Child 12-18 yr:* PO 6-15 mg/kg/day, in divided doses q6h

P *Child 4-12 yr:* PO 10-15 mg/kg/day in divided doses q6h

P *Child 1-4 yr:* PO 10-20 mg/kg/day in divided doses q6h

P *Child <1 yr:* PO 10-30 mg/kg/day, in divided doses q6h

Renal dose
CrCl 30-40 ml/min dose q8h; CrCl 15-30 ml/min dose q12h; CrCl <15 ml/min dose q24h

Available forms: Caps 100, 150 mg (as phosphate); cont rel caps 100, 150 mg; tabs, sus rel 250 mg ♣

Adverse effects
CNS: Headache, dizziness, psychosis, fatigue, depression, paresthesias, anxiety, insomnia
CV: Hypotension, bradycardia, angina, PVCs, tachycardia, increases in QRS and QT segments, **cardiac arrest,** edema, weight gain, AV block, **CHF,** syncope, chest pain
EENT: Blurred vision, dry nose, throat, eyes, narrow-angle glaucoma
GI: Dry mouth, constipation,

nausea, anorexia, flatulence, diarrhea, vomiting
GU: Retention, hesitancy, impotence
HEMA: **Thrombocytopenia, agranulocytosis,** anemia (rare), decreased Hgb, Hct
INTEG: Rash, pruritus, urticaria
META: Hypoglycemia
MS: Weakness, pain in extremities

Contraindications: Hypersensitivity, 2nd- or 3rd-degree heart block, cardiogenic shock, CHF (uncompensated), sick sinus syndrome, QT prolongation

Precautions: Pregnancy **C,** lactation, diabetes mellitus, renal disease, children, hepatic disease, myasthenia gravis, narrow-angle glaucoma, cardiomyopathy, conduction abnormalities

Pharmacokinetics

Absorption	Well absorbed
Distribution	Widely distributed
Metabolism	Liver
Excretion	Kidneys
Half-life	4-10 hr

Pharmacodynamics

	PO	PO-SUS REL
Onset	½-3½ hr	Unknown
Peak	2 hr	Unknown
Duration	1½-8 hr	12 hr

Interactions
Individual drugs
Erythromycin: ↑ effects of disopyramide
Flecainide: ↑ levels, toxicity
Lidocaine: Bradycardia, arrest
Mexiletine: ↑ levels, toxicity
Phenobarbital: ↓ effects of disopyramide
Phenytoin: ↑ blood levels, toxicity

Procainamide: ↑ levels, toxicity
Quinidine: ↑ levels, toxicity
Rifampin: ↓ disopyramide levels
Warfarin: ↑ level, bleeding
Drug classifications
Anticoagulants: ↓ prothrombin time
Antidysrhythmics: Widening of QRS or QRT
β-adrenergic Blockers: ↑ dysrhythmias, arrest
Lab test interferences
↑ CPK

NURSING CONSIDERATIONS
Assessment
• Assess respiratory status: auscultate lung fields for bibasilar crackles in patients with advanced CHF
• Monitor I&O ratio and electrolytes: potassium, sodium, chloride; watch for decreasing urinary output, possible retention
• Monitor liver function studies: AST, ALT, bilirubin, alkaline phosphatase
• Monitor ECG to determine drug effectiveness, measure PR, QRS, QT intervals; check for PVCs, other dysrhythmias; monitor B/P for hypotension; check for prolonged widening QT intervals, QRS complex; if QT or QRS increase by 50% or more, withhold next dose, notify prescriber
• Monitor for dehydration or hypovolemia
• Monitor for CNS symptoms: psychosis, numbness, depression; if these occur, drug should be discontinued

Nursing diagnoses
✓ Cardiac output, decreased (uses)
✓ Knowledge deficit (teaching)

Implementation
🚫 • Do not crush or break sus rel caps
• Give 1 hr ac or 2 hr pc
• If changing from regular release to sus rel cap, give sus rel 6 hr after last dose of regular release

Patient/family education
• Teach patient to report side effects immediately to prescriber; to take exactly as prescribed; if dose is missed take when remembered if within 3-4 hr of next dose; do not double doses
• Teach patient to complete follow-up appointment with prescriber including pulmonary function studies, chest x-ray
• Instruct patient that dry mouth may be relieved by frequent sips of water, hard candy, sugarless gum
• Caution patient to make position changes from lying to standing slowly to prevent orthostatic hypotension

Evaluation
Positive therapeutic outcome
• Decreased PVCs, ventricular tachycardia

Treatment of overdose: Administer O_2, artificial ventilation, ECG; administer dopamine for circulatory depression; administer diazepam or thiopental for convulsions, isoproterenol

dobutamine (℞)
(doe-byoo′ta-meen)
dobutamine, Dobutrex
Func. class.: Adrenergic direct-acting β_1-agonist, inotropic agent
Chem. class.: Catecholamine

Pregnancy category B

Action: Causes increased contractility, increased coronary blood flow and heart rate by acting on β_1-receptors in heart; minor alpha/beta$_2$ effects

➤**Therapeutic Outcome:** Cardiac output increased with decreased fatigue and dyspnea

Uses: Cardiac surgery, refractory heart failure, cardiac decompensation

Investigational uses: Cardiogenic shock in children, congenital heart disease in children undergoing cardiac cath

Dosage and routes
Adult: **IV** inf 2.5-10 µg/kg/ min; may increase to 40 µg/ kg/min if needed

P *Child:* **IV** inf 5-20 µg/kg/min over 10 min for cardiac cath

Available forms: Inj 12.5 mg/ml

Adverse effects
CNS: Anxiety, headache, dizziness
CV: Palpitations, tachycardia, hypertension, PVCs, angina
GI: Heartburn, nausea, vomiting
MS: Muscle cramps (leg)

Contraindications: Hypersensitivity, idiopathic hypertrophic subaortic stenosis

---

Precautions: Pregnancy **B**, lactation, children, hypertension

Do Not Confuse:
dobutamine/dopamine, Dobutrex/Diamox

Pharmacokinetics

Absorption	Complete
Distribution	Unknown
Metabolism	Liver
Excretion	Kidney
Half-life	2 min

Pharmacodynamics

Onset	1-5 min
Peak	10 min
Duration	<10 min

Interactions
Individual drugs
Bretylium: ↑ dysrhythmias
Disopyramide: ↑ hypotension
Guanethidine: ↑ pressor response
Oxytocin: ↑ dysrhythmias
Phenytoin: ↑ hypotension, bradycardia
Drug classifications
Anesthetics: ↑ dysrhythmias
Antidepressants, tricyclic: ↑ pressor response
Antihypertensives: ↑ hypotension
β-adrenergic Blockers: ↑ pressor response
Cardiac glycosides: ↑ inotropic effect
MAOIs: ↑ dysrhythmias

NURSING CONSIDERATIONS
Assessment
• Assess for hypovolemia; if present, correct before beginning treatment with dobutamine; avoid use in patients with atrial fibrillation before digitalization
• Monitor ECG for dysrhythmias, ischemia during treatment; some patients may not need continuous ECG monitoring; also monitor PCWP, CVP, CO_2, urinary output; notify prescriber if <30 ml hr
• Assess for heart failure: bibasilar crackles, S_3 gallop, dyspnea, neck vein distention in patients with cardiomyopathy or CHF
• Assess for oxygenation or perfusion deficit: decreased B/P, chest pain, dizziness, loss of consciousness
• Monitor B/P and pulse q5 min during inf; if B/P drops 30 mm Hg, stop inf and call prescriber
• Monitor ALT, AST, bilirubin daily
• Monitor for sulfite sensitivity, which may be life threatening

Nursing diagnoses
☑ Cardiac output, decreased (uses)
☑ Knowledge deficit (teaching)

Implementation
IV route
• Reconstitute 250 mg/10 ml of D_5W or sterile water for inj; may add another 10 ml to dissolve completely if needed, then dilute in 50 ml or more D_5W, 0.9% NaCl, 0.45% NaCl, D_5/0.45% NaCl, D_5/0.9% NaCl, D_5/LR, LR; titrate to patient response; use inf pump for correct dose
• Use a CVP catheter or large peripheral vein, use infusion pump, titrate to patient response
• Change **IV** site q48hrs

Syringe compatibilities:
Heparin, ranitidine

Syringe incompatibility:
Doxapram

Y-site compatibilities:
Amifostine, amrinone, atracurium, aztreonam, bretylium,

calcium chloride, calcium gluconate, ciprofloxacin, cladribine, diazepam, diltiazem, dopamine, enalaprilat, epinephrine, famotidine, fentanyl, fluconazole, granisetron, haloperidol, hydromorphone, regular insulin, labetalol, lidocaine, lorazepam, magnesium sulfate, meperidine, milrinone, morphine, nicardipine, nitroglycerin, norepinephrine, pancuronium, potassium chloride, propofol, ranitidine, sodium nitroprusside, streptokinase, tacrolimus, theophylline, thiotepa, tolazoline, vecuronium, verapamil, zidovudine

Y-site incompatibilities:
Acyclovir, alteplase, aminophylline, foscarnet, phytonadione

Additive compatibilities:
Amiodarone, atracurium, atropine, dopamine, enalaprilat, epinephrine, flumazenil, hydralazine, isoproterenol, lidocaine, meperidine, meropenem, metaraminol, morphine, nitroglycerin, norepinephrine, phentolamine, phenylephrine, procainamide, propranolol, ranitidine, verapamil

Additive incompatibilities:
Acyclovir, aminophylline, bumetanide, calcium gluconate, diazepam, digoxin, furosemide, insulin, magnesium sulfate, phenytoin, potassium phosphate, sodium bicarbonate

Patient/family education
• Teach patient reason for medication and expected results, reason for all monitoring and procedures
• Advise patient to report dyspnea, headache, **IV** site discomfort

Evaluation
Positive therapeutic outcome
• Increased cardiac output
• Decreased PCWP, adequate CVP
• Decreased dyspnea, fatigue, edema, ECG
• Increased urine output

Treatment of overdose:
Discontinue drug, support circulation

docusate calcium (OTC)
(dok'yoo-sate)
DC Softgels, Pro-Cal-Sof, Sulfalax Calcium, Surfak
docusate sodium (OTC)
Colace, Coloxyl, Diocto, Dioeze, Diosuccin, Disonate, Di-Sosal, DOS, Doxinate, D-S-S, Duosol, Modane, Pro-Sof, Regulex SS, Regulex ✦, Regutol
Func. class.: Laxative, emollient
Chem. class.: Anionic surfactant

Pregnancy category **C**

Action: Increases water, fat penetration in intestine; allows for easier passage of stool; increases electrolyte, water secretion in colon

▶**Therapeutic Outcome:** Passage of softened stool, absence of constipation

Uses: To soften stools, prevent constipation, soften fecal impaction (rec route)

Dosage and routes
Adult: PO 50-300 mg qd (docusate sodium) or 240 mg (docusate calcium or docusate potassium) prn; enema 5 ml (docusate sodium)

P *Child >12 yr:* Enema 2 ml
(docusate sodium)

P *Child 6-12 yr:* PO 40-120 mg
qd (docusate sodium)

P *Child 3-6 yr:* PO 20-60 mg qd
(docusate sodium)

P *Child <3 yr:* PO 10-40 mg qd
(docusate sodium)

Available forms: Caps 50,
100, 240, 250, 300 mg; tabs
50, 100 mg; oral sol 10, 50
mg/ml, 16.7, 20 mg/ml;
enema conc 18 g/100 ml
Docusate calcium: Caps 50,
240 mg
Docusate sodium: Caps 50,
100, 240, 250 mg; tabs 50,
100 mg; syr 50, 60 mg/15 ml;
liq 150 mg/15 ml; oral sol 10,
50 mg/ml; enema 283 mg/
3.9 g cap

Adverse effects

EENT: Bitter taste, throat
irritation
GI: Nausea, anorexia, cramps,
diarrhea
INTEG: Rash

Contraindications: Hypersensitivity, obstruction, fecal impaction, nausea/vomiting

Precautions: Pregnancy **C**

Pharmacokinetics

Absorption	Minimal (PO)
Distribution	Unknown
Metabolism	Not metabolized
Excretion	Bile
Half-life	Unknown

Pharmacodynamics

	PO	REC
Onset	24-72 hr	4-6 hr
Peak	Unknown	Unknown
Duration	Unknown	Unknown

Interactions: None

NURSING CONSIDERATIONS
Assessment

• Assess cramping, rectal
bleeding, nausea, vomiting; if
these symptoms occur, drug
should be discontinued; identify cause of constipation;
identify whether fluids, bulk,
or exercise is missing from
lifestyle

Nursing diagnoses

☑ Bowel elimination, altered:
constipation (uses)
☑ Bowel elimination, altered:
diarrhea (side effects)
☑ Knowledge deficit (teaching)
☑ Noncompliance (teaching)

Implementation
PO route

• Dilute oral sol in juice or
other fluid to disguise taste
• Give tabs or caps with 8 oz
of liq; give on empty stomach
for increased absorption, results

Patient/family education

• Discuss with patient that
adequate fluid consumption is
as necessary as bulk, exercise
for adequate bowel function
• Teach patient that normal
bowel movements do not
always occur daily
• Advise patient not to use in
presence of abdominal pain,
nausea, vomiting; tell patient
to notify prescriber if unrelieved constipation or if symptoms of electrolyte imbalance
occur: muscle cramps, pain,
weakness, dizziness, excessive
thirst
• Advise patient that drug may
take up to 3 days to soften
stools
• Caution patients with heart
disease to avoid using the
Valsalva maneuver to expedite
evacuation

D

Evaluation
Positive therapeutic outcome
• Decreased constipation within 3 days

dofetilide
See Appendix A, Selected New Drugs

dolasetron (℞)
(do-la'se-tron)
Anzemet
Func. class.: Antiemetic
Chem. class.: 5-HT receptor antagonist
Pregnancy category **C**

Action Prevents nausea, vomiting by blocking serotonin peripherally, centrally, and in the small intestine

➡**Therapeutic Outcome:** Control of nausea, vomiting

Uses: Prevention of nausea, vomiting associated with cancer chemotherapy and prevention of postoperative nausea, vomiting

Investigational uses: Radiotherapy-induced nausea/vomiting

Dosage and routes
Prevention of nausea/ vomiting associated with cancer chemotherapy
Adult: **IV** 1.8 mg/kg as a single dose ½ hr prior to chemotherapy

P *Child 2-16 yr:* PO 1.8 mg/kg 1 hr prior to chemotherapy

Prevention of postoperative nausea/vomiting
Adult: **IV** 12.5 mg as a single dose 15 min before cessation of anesthesia; PO 100 mg 2 hr before surgery (prevention only)

P *Child 2-16 yr:* **IV** 0.35 mg/kg as a single dose 15 min before cessation of anesthesia; PO 1.2 mg/kg within 2 hr before surgery (prevention only)

Available forms: Tabs 50, 100 mg; inj 20 mg/ml (12.5 mg/0.625 ml)

Adverse effects
CNS: **Headache,** dizziness, fatigue, drowsiness
CV: **Dysrhythmias,** ECG changes, hypotension, tachycardia, hypertension
GI: **Diarrhea,** constipation, increased AST, ALT, abdominal pain, anorexia
GU: Urinary retention, oliguria
MISC: Rash, **bronchospasm**

Contraindications: Hypersensitivity

P **Precautions:** Pregnancy **B,**
G lactation, children, elderly

Pharmacokinetics
Absorption	Completely absorbed
Distribution	Unknown
Metabolism	Liver, extensively
Excretion	Kidneys
Half-life	Unknown

Pharmacodynamics
Unknown

Interactions
Individual drugs
Cimetidine: ↑ dolasetron levels
Rifampin: ↓ dolasetron levels
Drug classifications
Antidysrhythmics: ↑ dysrhythmias

NURSING CONSIDERATIONS
Assessment
- Assess for absence of nausea, vomiting during chemotherapy
- Assess for hypersensitivity reaction: rash, bronchospasm
- Assess for cardiac conditions, electrolyte imbalances or dysrhythmias

Nursing diagnoses
☑ Knowledge deficit (teaching)
☑ Noncompliance (teaching)

Implementation
Ⅳ IV route
- Administer by injection 100 mg/30 sec or less or diluted in 50 ml compatible sol; give over 15 sec
- Store at room temp for 24 hr after dilution

Patient/family education
- Instruct patient to report diarrhea, constipation, rash, or changes in respirations
- Teach patient reason for medication and expected results

Evaluation
Positive therapeutic outcome
- Absence of nausea, vomiting during cancer chemotherapy

---

donepezil (℞)
(don-ep-ee′zill)
Aricept
Func. class.: Reversible cholinesterase
Pregnancy category   C

Action: Elevates acetylcholine concentrations (cerebral cortex) by slowing degradation of acetylcholine released in cholinergic neurons; does not alter underlying dementia

➡ **Therapeutic Outcome:** Decreased symptoms of Alzheimer's disease

Uses: Treatment of mild to moderate dementia in Alzheimer's disease

Dosage and routes
Adult: PO 5-10 mg qd; may increase to 10 mg qd after 4-6 wk

Available forms: Tabs 5, 10 mg

Adverse effects
CNS: Dizziness, insomnia, somnolence, headache, fatigue, abnormal dreams, syncope, **seizures**
CV: **Atrial fibrillation,** hypotension or hypertension
GI: *Nausea, vomiting,* anorexia, *diarrhea*
GU: Frequency, UTI, incontinence
INTEG: Rash, flushing
MS: Cramps, arthritis
RESP: Rhinitis, URI, cough, pharyngitis

Contraindications: Hypersensitivity to this drug or piperidine derivatives

Precautions: Sick sinus syndrome, history of ulcers, GI bleeding, hepatic disease, bladder obstruction, asthma, pregnancy **C,** lactation, children, seizures, asthma, COPD

Pharmacokinetics
Absorption	Well
Distribution	Unknown
Metabolism	Liver to metabolites
Excretion	Unknown
Half-life	10 hr (single dose)

Pharmacodynamics
Unknown

Interactions
Individual drugs
Carbamazepine: ↓ donepezil effect

Dexamethasone: ↓ donepezil effect

Phenytoin: ↓ donepezil effect

Phenobarbital: ↓ donepezil effect

Rifampin: ↓ donepezil effect

Drug classification
Anticholinergics: ↓ activity

Cholinergic agonists: synergistic effects

Cholinesterase inhibitors: synergistic effects

NSAIDs: ↑ gastric acid secretions

NURSING CONSIDERATIONS
Assessment
• Monitor B/P: hypotension, hypertension
• Assess mental status: affect, mood, behavioral changes, depression, complete suicide assessment
• Assess GI status: nausea, vomiting, anorexia, diarrhea
• Assess GU status: urinary frequency, incontinence

Nursing diagnoses
☑Confusion, chronic (uses)
☑Memory, impaired (uses)

Implementation
• Give between meals; may be given with meals for GI symptoms
• Administer dosage adjusted to response no more than q6wk
• Provide assistance with ambulation during beginning therapy; dizziness, ataxia may occur

Patient/family education
• Advise to report side effects: twitching, nausea, vomiting, sweating; indicates overdose
• Advise to use drug exactly as prescribed; at regular intervals, preferably between meals; may be taken with meals for GI upset
• Advise to notify prescriber of nausea, vomiting, diarrhea (dose increase or beginning treatment), or rash
• Advise not to increase or abruptly decrease dose, serious consequences may result
• Instruct patient that drug is not a cure

Evaluation
Positive therapeutic outcome
• Decrease in confusion; improved mood

Treatment of overdose: Withdraw drug, administer tertiary anticholinergics, provide supportive care

---

dopamine (℞)
(doe'pa-meen)
dopamine HCl, Intropin, Revimine ✦
Func. class.: Agonist, vasopressor, inotropic agent
Chem. class.: Catecholamine

Pregnancy category C

Action: Causes increased cardiac output; acts on β_1- and α-receptors, causing vasoconstriction in blood vessels; when low doses are administered, causes renal and mesenteric vasodilatation; β_1 stimulation produces inotropic effects with ↑ cardiac output

⇨**Therapeutic Outcome:** Increased B/P, cardiac output

Uses: Shock; to increase perfusion; hypotension

Investigational uses: COPD,
RDS in infants
Dosage and routes
Adult: **IV** inf 2-5 µg/kg/min,
not to exceed 50 µg/kg/min;
titrate to patient's response
Child: **IV** 5-20 µg/kg/min
adjust depending on response
COPD
Adult: **IV** 4 µg/kg/min
CHF
Adult: **IV** 2-5 µg/kg/min
RDS
Infants: **IV** 5 µg/kg/min
Available forms: Inj 40, 160
mg/ml; conc for **IV** inf 0.8,
1.6, 3.2 mg/ml in D_5W
Adverse effects
CNS: Headache
CV: Palpitations, **tachycardia**,
hypertension, **ectopic beats**,
angina, **wide QRS complex**,
peripheral vasoconstriction
GI: Nausea, vomiting, diarrhea
INTEG: Necrosis, tissue
sloughing with extravasation,
gangrene
RESP: Dyspnea
Contraindications: Hypersensitivity, ventricular fibrillation,
tachydysrhythmias, pheochromocytoma
Precautions: Pregnancy C,
lactation, arterial embolism,
peripheral vascular disease
Do Not Confuse:
dopamine/dobutamine

Pharmacokinetics

Absorption	Complete
Distribution	Widely
Metabolism	Liver
Excretion	Kidney, plasma
Half-life	2 min

Pharmacodynamics

Onset	2-5 min
Peak	Unknown
Duration	<10 min

Interactions
Individual drugs
Phenytoin: ↑ hypotension,
bradycardia
Drug classifications
α-Adrenergic blockers: ↓
action of dopamine
Anesthetics: ↑ dysrhythmias
Antidepressants, tricyclic:
↑ pressor response
β-Adrenergic blockers: ↓
cardiac response
Cardiac glycosides: ↑ inotropic effect
Ergots: Severe hypertension
MAOIs: ↑ hypertension (severe)

NURSING CONSIDERATIONS
Assessment
• Monitor ECG for dysrhythmias, ischemia during
treatment; some patients may
not need continuous ECG
monitoring; also monitor
PCWP, CVP, CO_2, urinary
output; notify prescriber if <30
ml/hr
• Assess for heart failure:
bibasilar crackles, S_3 gallop,
dyspnea, neck vein distention
in patients with cardiomyopathy or CHF
• Assess for oxygenation or
perfusion deficit: decreased
B/P, chest pain, dizziness, loss
of consciousness
• Monitor B/P and pulse q5
min during inf; if B/P drops
30 mm Hg, stop inf and call
prescriber
• Check for extravasation:
change site q48h

Nursing diagnoses

☑ Cardiac output, decreased (uses)
☑ Tissue perfusion, altered (uses)
☑ Fluid volume excess (uses)
☑ Knowledge deficit (teaching)

Implementation

• Give by continuous inf; dilute 200-400 mg/250-500 ml D_5W, 0.9% NaCl, D_5/LR, D_5/0.45% NaCl, D_5/0.9% NaCl, LR; do not use discolored sol; sol is stable for 24 hr; give 0.5-5 µg/kg/min; may increase by 1-4 µg/kg/min q15-30 min until desired patient response; use inf pump

Additive compatibilities:

Aminophylline, atracurium, bretylium, calcium chloride, cephalothin, chloramphenicol, dobutamine, enalaprilat, flumazenil, heparin, hydrocortisone, kanamycin, lidocaine, meropenem, methylprednisolone, nitroglycerin, oxacillin, potassium chloride, ranitidine, verapamil

Syringe compatibilities:

Doxapram, heparin, ranitidine

Y-site compatibilities:

Aldesleukin, amifostine, amiodarone, amrinone, atracurium, aztreonam, cefmetazole, cefpirome, ciprofloxacin, cladribine, diltiazem, dobutamine, enalaprilat, epinephrine, esmolol, famotidine, fentanyl, fluconazole, foscarnet, granisetron, haloperidol, heparin, hydrocortisone, hydromorphone, labetalol, lidocaine, lorazepam, meperidine, methylprednisolone, metronidazole, midazolam, milrinone, morphine, nicardipine, nitroglycerin, norepinephrine, ondansetron, pancuronium, piperacillin/tazobactam, potassium chloride, propofol, raniti-dine, sargramostim, sodium nitroprusside, streptokinase, tacrolimus, theophylline, thiotepa, tolazoline, vecuronium, verapamil, vit B/C, warfarin, zidovudine

Patient/family education

• Teach patient reason for medication, expected results, reason for all monitoring, and procedures
• Advise patient to report all side effects

Evaluation

Positive therapeutic outcome
• Increased cardiac output

Treatment of overdose: Discontinue drug, support circulation; give a short-acting α-blocker

---

doxacurium (R)

(dox'a-cure-ee-yum)
Nuromax
Func. class.: Neuromuscular blocker (nondepolarizing)

Pregnancy category   C

Action: Inhibits transmission of nerve impulses by binding with cholinergic receptor sites, antagonizing action of acetylcholine; no analgesic response

➡**Therapeutic Outcome:** Paralysis of all skeletal muscles

Uses: Facilitation of endotracheal intubation, skeletal muscle relaxation during mechanical ventilation, surgery, or general anesthesia

Dosage and routes

Adult: **IV** 0.05 mg/kg; 0.08 mg/kg is used for prolonged neuromuscular blockade; maintenance 0.025 mg/kg

---

P *Child 2-12 yr:* **IV** 0.03-0.05 mg/kg; may decrease for maintenance dose

Available forms: Inj 1 mg/ml

Adverse effects

CV: Decreased B/P, **ventricular fibrillation, MI, cardiovascular accident**

EENT: Diplopia

INTEG: Rash, urticaria

RESP: **Prolonged apnea, bronchospasm,** *wheezing,* **respiratory depression**

MS: Weakness, prolonged skeletal muscle relaxation, *paralysis*

Contraindications: Hypersensitivity

Precautions: Pregnancy **C,** renal, hepatic disease, lactation, **P** children <3 mo, fluid and electrolyte imbalances, neuro-muscular disease, respiratory **G** disease, obesity, elderly, severe burns

Pharmacokinetics	
Absorption	Complete
Distribution	Unknown
Metabolism	Unknown
Excretion	Kidneys, bile, unchanged
Half-life	½-2 hr; increased in renal transplant patient

Pharmacodynamics	
Onset	Up to 5 min
Peak	Unknown
Duration	1½ hr

Interactions
Individual drugs

Clindamycin: ↑ paralysis length and intensity

Colistin: ↑ paralysis length and intensity

Lidocaine: ↑ paralysis length and intensity

Lithium: ↑ paralysis length and intensity

Magnesium: ↑ paralysis length and intensity

Polymyxin B: ↑ paralysis length and intensity

Procainamide: ↑ paralysis length and intensity

Quinidine: ↑ paralysis length and intensity

Succinylcholine: ↑ paralysis length and intensity

Drug classifications

Aminoglycosides: ↑ paralysis length and intensity

β-adrenergic Blockers: ↑ paralysis length and intensity

Diuretics, potassium-losing: ↑ paralysis length and intensity

General anesthesia: ↑ paralysis length and intensity

NURSING CONSIDERATIONS
Assessment

• Monitor for electrolyte imbalances (potassium, magnesium) before drug is used; electrolyte imbalances may lead to increased action of this drug

• Monitor vital signs (B/P, pulse, respirations, airway) until fully recovered; rate, depth, pattern of respirations, strength of hand grip; patient should be intubated before use

• Monitor recovery: decreased paralysis of face, diaphragm, leg, arm, rest of body; residual weakness and respiratory problems may occur during recovery period

• Monitor allergic reactions: rash, fever, respiratory distress, pruritus; drug should be discontinued

Nursing diagnoses

☑ Breathing pattern, ineffective (uses)

☑ Communication, impaired verbal (adverse reactions)

☑ Anxiety (adverse reactions)
☑ Knowledge deficit (teaching)

Implementation

• Anesthesiologist uses peripheral nerve stimulator to determine neuromuscular blockade; deep tendon reflexes should be monitored during extended periods

• Give direct **IV** undiluted over 1 min, or diluted in 1050 ml of D_5W, ½ NaCl or NS and give as an infusion at prescribed rate (only by qualified person, usually an anesthesiologist); do not administer IM

• Further dilute in D_5W, 0.9% NaCl, D_5/0.9% NaCl q15-25 min (intermittent inf)

• Maintenance is given q20-45 min after 1st dose (cont inf); titrate to patient response

• Store in light-resistant area

Y-site compatibilities:
Etomidate, thiopental

Solution compatibilities:
LR, D_5/LR, D_5/0.9% NaCl

Patient/family education

• Provide reassurance if communication is difficult during recovery from neuromuscular blockade

• Provide explanation to patients regarding all procedures or treatments; patient will remain conscious if anesthesia is not given also

Evaluation

Positive therapeutic outcome

• Paralysis of jaw, eyelid, head, neck, rest of body as evaluated by peripheral nerve stimulator

Treatment of overdose:
Administer edrophonium or neostigmine, atropine; monitor VS; may require mechanical ventilation

---

doxapram (℞)
(dox'a-pram)
Dopram
Func. class.: Analeptic (respiratory/cerebral stimulant)
Pregnancy category **B**

Action: Respiratory stimulation through activation of peripheral carotid chemoreceptor in low dosages; with higher dosages medullary respiratory centers are stimulated, producing general CNS stimulation

Therapeutic Outcome: Ease of breathing, ABGs at normal limits

Uses: COPD, postanesthesia CNS and respiratory stimulation, prevention of acute hypercapnia, drug-induced CNS depression

Dosage and routes
Postanesthesia stimulation
Adult: **IV** inj 0.5-1 mg/kg, not to exceed 1.5 mg/kg total as a single inj; **IV** inf 250 mg in 250 ml sol, not to exceed 4 mg/kg; run at 1-3 mg/min
Drug-induced CNS depression
Adult: **IV** priming **IV** dose of 2 mg/kg, repeated in 5 min; repeat q1-2h until patient awakens; **IV** inf priming dose 2 mg/kg at 1-3 mg/min, not to exceed 3 g/day
COPD (hypercapnia)
Adult: **IV** inf 1-2 mg/min, not to exceed 3 mg/min for no longer than 2 hr
Apnea of premature infant
P *Infant:* 2.5-3 mg/kg loading dose followed by infusion of 1 mg/kg/hr

---

Available forms: Inj **IV** 20 mg/ml

Adverse effects
CNS: **Convulsions** (clonus/generalized), *headache,* restlessness, dizziness, confusion, paresthesias, flushing, sweating, bilateral Babinski's sign, rigidity, depression
CV: *Chest pain, hypertension, change in heart rate,* lowered T waves, tachycardia, arrhythmias
EENT: Pupil dilation, sneezing
GI: Nausea, vomiting, diarrhea, hiccups
GU: Retention, incontinence
INTEG: Pruritus, irritation at inj site
RESP: **Laryngospasm, bronchospasm,** rebound hypoventilation, dyspnea, cough, tachypnea, hiccups

Contraindications: Hypersensitivity, seizure disorders, severe hypertension, severe bronchial asthma, severe dyspnea, severe cardiac disorders, pneumothorax, pulmonary embolism, severe respiratory disease

Precautions: Bronchial asthma, pheochromocytoma, severe tachycardia, dysrhythmias, pregnancy **B,** hypertension, lactation, children

Pharmacokinetics	
Absorption	Complete
Distribution	Unknown
Metabolism	Liver
Excretion	Kidneys, metabolites
Half-life	2.5-4 hr

Pharmacodynamics	
Onset	20-40 sec
Peak	1-2 min
Duration	5-10 min

Interactions
Individual drugs
Enflurane: ↑ dysrhythmias
Halothane: ↑ dysrhythmias
Drug classifications
MAOI: ↑ hypertension
Skeletal muscle relaxants: May mask the effects of skeletal muscle relaxants
Sympathomimetics: Synergistic pressor effect

NURSING CONSIDERATIONS
Assessment
• Monitor B/P, heart rate, deep tendon reflexes, level of consciousness, ABGs before administration q30 min; check for Po_2, Pco_2, O_2 saturation during treatment
• Monitor ECG; watch for hypertension, increased pulse, increased pulmonary artery pressures
• Monitor for hypertension: dysrhythmias, tachycardia, dyspnea, skeletal muscle hyperactivity; may indicate overdosage; discontinue if these occur
• Assess for respiratory stimulation: increased respiratory rate, depth, abnormal rhythm; check for patent airway; elevate head of bed to 45 degrees or higher, position patient on side
• Check for extravasation: redness, inflammation, pain; may cause phlebitis; change **IV** site q48h

Nursing diagnoses
✓Breathing pattern, ineffective (uses)
✓Impaired gas exchange (uses)
✓Knowledge deficit (teaching)

Implementation
• May give by **IV** diluted with equal parts of sterile water for inj; may be diluted 250 mg/

250 ml (1 mg/ml) of D_5W, $D_{10}W$ (dilute 400 mg/180 ml of compatible IV sol [2 mg/ml] and run as inf over 2 hr
• Give **IV** undiluted over 5 min; **IV** inf at 1-3 mg/min; adjust for desired respiratory response, using inf pump **IV**; if an inf is used after initial dose, start at 1-3 mg/min; adjust for desired respiratory response, using inf pump **IV**; if an inf is used after initial dose, start at 1-3 mg/min depending on patient response; D/C after 2 hr; wait 1-2 hr and repeat
• Give only after adequate airway is established; ensure O_2, **IV** barbiturates, resuscitative equipment available
• Discontinue inf if side effects occur; narrow margin of safety

Syringe compatibilities:
Amikacin, bumetadine, chlorpromazine, cimetidine, cisplatin, cyclophosphamide, dopamine, doxycycline, epinephrine, hydroxyzine, imipramine, isoniazid, lincomycin, methotrexate, netilmicin, phytonadione, pyridoxine, terbutaline, thiamine, tobramycin, vincristine

Syringe incompatibilities:
Aminophylline, ascorbic acid, cefoperazone, cefotaxime, cefotetan, cefuroxime, dexamethasone, diazepam, digoxin, dobutamine, folic acid, furosemide, hydrocortisone, ketamine, methylprednisolone, minocycline, thiopental, ticarcillin

Patient/family education
• Teach all aspects of drug, purpose, expected reactions
• Caution patient if difficulty breathing or shortness of breath occurs to notify nurse or prescriber

Evaluation
Positive therapeutic outcome
• Increased breathing capacity
• ABGs WNL for patient
Treatment of overdose:
Lavage, activated charcoal; monitor electrolytes, VS; diazepam for seizures; discontinue inf

doxazosin (℞)
(dox-ay′zoe-sin)
Cardura
Func. class.: Peripheral α-adrenergic blocker, antihypertensive
Chem. class.: Quinazoline
Pregnancy category **B**

Action: Peripheral blood vessels are dilated, peripheral resistance lowered; reduction in B/P results from α-adrenergic receptors being blocked

Therapeutic Outcome: Decreased B/P, decreased symptoms of BPH

Uses: Hypertension alone or as an adjunct, urinary outflow obstruction, symptoms of benign prostatic hyperplasia
Investigational uses: CHF with digoxin and diuretics
Dosage and routes
BPH
Adult: PO 1 mg qd, increase in stepwise manner to 2, 4, 8 mg qd as needed, max 8 mg
Hypertension
Adult: PO 1 mg qd, increasing up to 16 mg qd if required; usual range 4-16 mg/day
G *Elderly:* PO 0.5 mg qhs, gradually increase

Available forms: Tabs 1, 2, 4, 8 mg

Adverse effects

CNS: Dizziness, headache, drowsiness, anxiety, depression, vertigo, weakness, fatigue, asthenia

CV: Palpitations, *orthostatic hypotension,* **tachycardia,** edema, **dysrhythmias,** chest pain

EENT: Epistaxis, tinnitus, dry mouth, red sclera, pharyngitis, rhinitis

GI: Nausea, vomiting, diarrhea, constipation, abdominal pain

GU: Incontinence, polyuria

Contraindications: Hypersensitivity to quinazolines

Precautions: Pregnancy **B,** children, lactation, hepatic disease

Do Not Confuse:
Cardura/Coumadin,
Cardura/Ridaura

Pharmacokinetics

Absorption	Well absorbed
Distribution	Not known; 98% plasma protein bound
Metabolism	Liver, extensively (<63%)
Excretion	Kidneys
Half-life	22 hr

Pharmacodynamics

Onset	2 hr
Peak	2-6 hr
Duration	6-12 hr

Interactions
Individual drugs
Clonidine: ↓ effects of clonidine
Indomethacin: ↓ hypotensive effects
Verapamil: ↑ hypotensive effects

Drug classifications
β-Adrenergic blockers: ↑ postural hypotension
NSAIDs: ↓ hypotensive effects
Herb/drug
Angelica: ↑ doxazosin effect
Lab test interferences
False positive: Urine acetone

NURSING CONSIDERATIONS
Assessment
• Monitor B/P (lying, standing) and pulse, syncope; check for edema in feet, legs daily; I&O; monitor for weight daily; notify prescriber of changes
• Assess skin turgor, dryness of mucous membranes for hydration status
• Assess for orthostatic hypotension; tell patient to rise slowly from sitting or lying position; assess pulse, jugular venous distention q4h, rales, dyspnea, orthopnea with B/P

Nursing diagnoses
✓ Cardiac output, decreased (uses)
✓ Injury, potential for physical (side effects)
✓ Knowledge deficit (teaching)
✓ Noncompliance (teaching)

Implementation
• Store in tight container at 86° F (30° C) or less
• May be used in combination with other antihypertensives
• May be given with food to prevent GI symptoms

Patient/family education
• Teach patient not to discontinue drug abruptly; emphasize the importance of complying with dosage schedule, even if feeling better; if dose is missed take as soon as remembered; take at same time each day
• Instruct patient to take 1st

dose at hs to decrease orthostatic B/P changes
• Teach patient not to use OTC products (cough, cold, allergy) unless directed by prescriber; also to avoid large amounts of caffeine
• Emphasize the need to rise slowly to sitting or standing position to minimize orthostatic hypotension
• Teach patient to notify prescriber of mouth sores, sore throat, fever, swelling of hands or feet, irregular heartbeat, chest pain
• Caution patient to report excessive perspiration, dehydration, vomiting, diarrhea; may lead to fall in B/P
• Caution patient that drug may cause dizziness, fainting, lightheadedness; may occur during 1st few days of therapy; to avoid hazardous activities
• Teach patient how to take B/P, and normal readings for age group; to take B/P q7 days

Evaluation
Positive therapeutic outcome
• Decreased B/P in hypertension; decreased symptoms of BPH
• Decreased symptoms in BP

Treatment of overdose:
Administer volume expanders or vasopressors; discontinue drug; place in supine position

doxepin (℞)
(dox'e-pin)
Adepin, doxepin HCl, Novo-Doxepin ✦, Sinequan, Sinequan Concentrate, Triadapin ✦, Zonolon Topical Cream
Func. class.: Antidepressant, tricyclic; antianxiety
Chem. class.: Dibenzoxepin, tertiary amine
Pregnancy category   C

Action: Blocks reuptake of norepinephrine, serotonin into nerve endings, increasing action of norepinephrine, serotonin in nerve cells; has anticholinergic effects

Therapeutic Outcome: Decreased symptoms of depression after 2-3 wk

Uses: Major depression, anxiety; topical-pruritus

Investigational uses: Chronic pain management

Dosage and routes
Oral conc should be diluted with 120 ml of water, milk, or orange, grapefuit, tomato, prune, pineapple juice. Do not mix with grape juice.

Adult: PO 75 mg/day, may increase to 300 mg/day for severely ill

Elderly: PO 10-25 mg hs, increase qwk by 10-25 mg to desired dose

Available forms: Caps 10, 25, 50, 75, 100, 150 mg; oral conc 10 mg/ml; cream 5%

Adverse effects
CNS: Dizziness, drowsiness, confusion, headache, anxiety, tremors, stimulation, weakness, insomnia, nightmares, extrapyramidal symptoms

---

☑ Herb/drug ⬙ Do Not Crush ◆ Alert ⟿ Key Drug Ⓖ Geriatric ⓅPediatric

(elderly), increased psychiatric symptoms, paresthesia
***CV:** Orthostatic hypotension, ECG changes,* **tachycardia, hypertension,** palpitations
***EENT:** Blurred vision,* tinnitus, mydriasis, ophthalmoplegia, glossitis
***GI:** Diarrhea, dry mouth,* nausea, vomiting, **paralytic ileus,** increased appetite, cramps, epigastric distress, jaundice, **hepatitis,** stomatitis, constipation
***GU:** Retention,* **acute renal failure**
HEMA: **Agranulocytosis, thrombocytopenia, eosinophilia, leukopenia**
INTEG: Rash, urticaria, sweating, pruritus, photosensitivity

Contraindications: Hypersensitivity to tricyclic antidepressants, urinary retention, narrow-angle glaucoma, prostatic hypertrophy

Precautions: Suidical patients, elderly, pregnancy **C** (topical), PO (unknown)

Do Not Confuse:
Sinequan/Serentil

Pharmacokinetics
Absorption	Well absorbed
Distribution	Widely distributed; crosses placenta
Metabolism	Liver, extensively
Excretion	Kidneys, breast milk
Half-life	8-24 hr

Pharmacodynamics
Unknown

Interactions
Individual drugs
Alcohol: ↑ CNS depression
Cimetidine: ↑ levels, toxicity
Clonidine: Severe hypotension; avoid use

Disulfiram: Organic brain syndrome
Fluoxetine: ↑ levels, toxicity
Guanethidine: ↓ effects of guanethidine
Sertraline: ↑ doxepin effect
Drug classifications
Analgesics: ↑ CNS depression
Anticholinergics: ↑ side effects
Antihistamines: ↑ CNS depression
Antihypertensives: May block antihypertensive effect
Barbiturates: ↑ CNS depression
Benzodiazepines: ↑ CNS depression
CNS depressants: ↑ CNS depression
MAOIs: Hypertensive crisis, convulsions
Oral contraceptives: ↑ effects, toxicity
Phenothiazines: ↑ toxicity
Sedative/hypnotics: ↑ CNS depression
Sympathomimetics, indirect acting: ↓ effects
Smoking
↑ metabolism, ↓ effects
Lab test interferences
↑ Serum bilirubin, ↑ blood glucose, ↑ alkaline phosphatase, ↓ blood glucose

NURSING CONSIDERATIONS
Assessment
• Monitor B/P (with patient lying, standing), pulse q4h; if systolic B/P drops 20 mm Hg, hold drug, notify prescriber; take Vs q4h in patients with cardiovascular disease
• Monitor blood studies: CBC, leukocytes, differential, cardiac enzymes if patient is receiving long-term therapy
• Monitor hepatic studies: AST, ALT, bilirubin
• Check weight weekly; appe-

tite may increase with drug
• Assess ECG for flattening of T wave, bundle branch block, AV block, dysrhythmias in cardiac patients; drug should be discontinued gradually several days before surgery
• Assess for extrapyramidal
G symptoms primarily in elderly: rigidity, dystonia, akathisia
• Assess mental status: mood, sensorium, affect, suicidal tendencies; increase in psychiatric symptoms: depression, panic
• Monitor urinary retention, constipation; constipation is
P more likely to occur in children
G or elderly
• Assess for withdrawal symptoms: headache, nausea, vomiting, muscle pain, weakness; do not usually occur unless drug was discontinued abruptly
• Identify alcohol consumption; if alcohol is consumed, hold dose until AM

Nursing diagnoses
☑ Coping, ineffective individual (uses)
☑ Injury, risk for (side effects)
☑ Knowledge deficit (teaching)

Implementation
• Give with food or milk for GI symptoms; do not give with carbonated beverages
• Give dosage hs if oversedation occurs during day; may
G take entire dose hs; elderly may not tolerate once/day dosing
• Store at room temp; do not freeze
• Provide safety measures,
G primarily for elderly

Patient/family education
• Tell patient that therapeutic effects may take 2-3 wk; to use caution in driving and other activities requiring alertness because of drowsiness, dizziness, blurred vision
• Advise patient to avoid rising quickly from sitting to stand-
G ing, especially elderly
• Teach patient to avoid alcohol ingestion, other CNS depressants; not to discontinue medication quickly after long-term use: may cause nausea, headache, malaise
• Teach patient to wear sunscreen or large hat, since photosensitivity occurs
• Teach patient to increase fluids, bulk in diet if constipa-
G tion occurs, especially elderly; to take gum, hard sugarless candy, or frequent sips of water for dry mouth

Evaluation
Positive therapeutic outcome
• Decrease in depression
• Absence of suicidal thoughts

Treatment of overdose:
ECG monitoring, induce emesis, lavage, activated charcoal, administer anticonvulsant

---

doxercalciferol
See Appendix A, Selected New Drugs

---

doxorubicin (℞)
(dox-oh-roo'bi-sin)
Adriamycin PFS, Adriamycin RDF, Rubex

doxorubicin liposome (℞)
Doxil

Func. class.: Antineoplastic, antibiotic
Chem. class.: Anthracycline glycoside

Pregnancy category **D**

Action: Inhibits DNA synthesis primarily; derived from *Streptomyces peucetius;* replication is decreased by binding to DNA, which causes strand splitting; active throughout entire cell cycle; a vesicant

▶**Therapeutic Outcome:** Prevention of rapidly growing malignant cells

Uses: Wilms' tumor; bladder, breast, cervical, head, neck, liver, lung, ovarian, prostatic, stomach, testicular, thyroid cancer; Hodgkin's disease; acute lymphoblastic leukemia; myeloblastic leukemia; neuroblastomas; lymphomas; sarcomas

Dosage and routes
Doxorubicin
Adult: **IV** 60-75 mg/m^2 q3 wk, or 30 mg/m^2 on days 1-3 of 4-wk cycle, not to exceed 550 mg/m^2 cumulative dose

P *Child:* **IV** 30 mg/m^2/day × 3 days, may repeat q4 wk

Doxorubicin liposome
Adult: **IV** 20 mg/m^2 q3wk

Available forms: Inj 10, 20, 50 mg

Adverse effects
CV: Increased B/P, **sinus tachycardia, PVCs,** chest pain, **bradycardia, extrasystole**
GI: Nausea, vomiting, anorexia, mucositis, **hepatotoxicity**
GU: Impotence, sterility, amenorrhea, gynecomastia, hyperuricemia
HEMA: **Thrombocytopenia, leukopenia, anemia**
INTEG: Rash, necrosis at inj site, dermatitis, reversible alopecia, cellulitis, thrombophlebitis at inj site

Contraindications: Hypersensitivity, pregnancy (1st trimester) **D**, lactation, systemic infections

Precautions: Renal, hepatic, cardiac disease, gout, bone marrow suppression (severe)

Do Not Confuse:
Adriamycin/Aredia,
Adriamycin/Idamycin,
doxorubicin/idarubicin,
doxorubicin/daunorubicin

Pharmacokinetics	
Absorption	Complete bioavailability
Distribution	Widely distributed; crosses placenta
Metabolism	Liver, extensively
Excretion	Bile (40%-50%)
Half-life	12 min; 3½ hr; 29⅔ hr

Pharmacodynamics
Unknown

Interactions
Individual drugs
Cyclophosphamide: ↑ cardiotoxicity, CHF
Mercaptopurine: ↑ liver disorders, hepatitis
Radiation: ↑ toxicity, bone marrow suppression

Drug classifications
Antineoplastics: ↑ toxicity, bone marrow suppression
Live virus vaccines: ↑ adverse reactions, ↓ antibody response
Lab test interferences
↑ Uric acid

NURSING CONSIDERATIONS
Assessment
• Monitor ECG; watch for ST-T wave changes, low QRS and T; possible dysrhythmias (sinus tachycardia, heart block, PVCs) may occur
• Assess buccal cavity q8h for dryness, sores or ulceration, white patches, pain, bleeding, dysphagia; obtain prescription for viscous lidocaine (Xylocaine)
• Assess symptoms indicating severe allergic reaction: rash, pruritus, urticaria, purpuric skin lesions, itching, flushing; drug should be discontinued
• Assess tachypnea, ECG changes, dyspnea, edema, fatigue
• Monitor CBC, differential, platelet count weekly; withhold drug if WBC count is <4000/mm^3 or platelet count is <100,000/mm^3; notify prescriber of results if WBC <20,000/mm^3, platelets <150,000/mm^3
• Assess for increased uric acid levels, swelling, joint pain, primarily extremities; patient should be well hydrated to prevent urate deposits
• Monitor renal function studies: BUN, creatinine, serum uric acid, urine CrCl before and during therapy; I&O ratio; report fall in urine output to <30 ml/hr
• Monitor temp q4h (may indicate beginning of infection)

• Monitor liver function tests before and during therapy (bilirubin, AST, ALT, LDH) as needed or monthly; note jaundice of skin or sclera, dark urine, clay-colored stools, itchy skin, abdominal pain, fever, diarrhea
• Assess for bleeding: hematuria, stool guaiac, bruising or petechiae, mucosa or orifices q8h; inflammation of mucosa, breaks in skin
• Identify effects of alopecia on body image; discuss feelings about body changes

Nursing diagnoses
☑ Injury, risk for (adverse reactions)
☑ Body image disturbance (adverse reactions)
☑ Infection, risk for (adverse reactions)
☑ Knowledge deficit (teaching)

Implementation
• Avoid contact with skin; very irritating; wash completely to remove; give fluids **IV** or PO before chemotherapy to hydrate patient
• Give antiemetic 30-60 min before giving drug to prevent vomiting and prn; give antibiotics for prophylaxis of infection
• Provide liq diet: carbonated beverages; gelatin may be added if patient is not nauseated or vomiting
• Help patient to rinse mouth tid-qid with water or club soda, brush teeth bid-qid with soft brush or cotton-tipped applicators for stomatitis, use unwaxed dental floss
• Drug should be prepared by experienced personnel using proper precautions

---

- Do not interchange doxorubicin with doxorubicin liposome
- Give **IV** after diluting 10 mg/5 ml of NaCl for inj; another 5 ml of diluent/10 mg is recommended; shake; give over 3-5 min; give through Y-tube or 3-way stopcock through free-flowing D_5 inf or NS
- **IV** Liposome Inj (Doxil): dilute dose up to 90 mg/250 ml D_5W, give over ½ hr; do not admix with other solution medications
- Use hydrocortisone, dexamethasone, or sodium bicarbonate (1 mEq/1 ml) for extravasation: apply ice compress

Syringe compatibilities:
Bleomycin, cisplatin, cyclophosphamide, droperidol, fluorouracil, leucovorin, methotrexate, metoclopramide, mitomycin, vincristine

Syringe incompatibilities:
Furosemide, heparin

Y-site compatibilities:
Amifostine, aztreonam, bleomycin, chlorpromazine, cimetidine, cisplatin, cladribine, cyclophosphamide, dexamethasone, diphenhydramine, droperidol, famotidine, filgrastim, fludarabine, fluorouracil, granisetron, hydromorphone, leucovorin calcium, lorazepam, melphalan, methotrexate, methylprednisolone, metoclopramide, mitomycin, morphine, ondansetron, paclitaxel, prochlorperazine, promethazine, propofol, ranitidine, sargramostim, sodium bicarbonate, teniposide, thiotepa, vinblastine, vincristine, vinorelbine

Y-site incompatibilities:
Furosemide, heparin

Additive incompatibilities:
Aminophylline, cephalothin, dexamethasone, diazepam, fluorouracil, hydrocortisone

Additive compatibilities:
Ondansetron

D

Patient/family education
- Tell patient that urine and other body fluids may be red-orange for 48 hr; contraceptive measures are recommended during therapy; drug is teratogenic to fetus
- Advise patient to avoid use of products containing aspirin or ibuprofen, razors, commercial mouthwash, since bleeding may occur; to report symptoms of bleeding (hematuria, tarry stools)
- Instruct patient to report signs of anemia (fatigue, headache, irritability, faintness, shortness of breath)
- Inform patient that hair may be lost during treatment; a wig or hair piece may make patient feel better; new hair may be different in color, texture
- Caution patient not to have any vaccinations without the advice of the prescriber; serious reactions can occur

Evaluation
Positive therapeutic outcome
- Prevention of rapid division of malignant cells

doxycycline ℞
(dox-i-sye′kleen)
Apo-Doxy ✦, Doryx, Doxy,
Doxy-Caps, Doxycin ✦,
doxycycline, Monodox,
Novodoxyclin ✦,
Vibramycin, Vibramycin **IV**,
Vibra-Tabs
Func. class.: Antiinfective
Chem. class.: Tetracycline

Pregnancy category   D

Action: Inhibits protein synthesis, phosphorylation in microorganisms by binding to 30S ribosomal subunits, reversibly binding to 50S ribosomal subunits; bacteriostatic

▶**Therapeutic Outcome:** Bactericidal action against the following: gram-positive pathogens *Bacillus anthracis, Clostridium perfringens, C. tetani, Listeria monocytogenes, Nocardia, Propionibacterium acnes, Actinomyces israelii;* gram-negative pathogens *Haemophilus influenzae, Legionella pneumophila, Versinia enterocolitica, V. pestis, Neisseria gonorrhoeae, N. meningitidis, Mycoplasma, Chlamydia, Rickettsia*

Uses: Syphilis, gonorrhea, *Chlamydia,* lymphogranuloma venereum, uncommon gram-negative or positive organisms, malaria prophylaxis, acne

Investigational uses: Traveler's diarrhea, Lyme disease, prevention of chronic bronchitis

Dosage and routes
Adult: PO/**IV** 100 mg q12h on day 1, then 100 mg/day; **IV** 200 mg in 1-2 inf on day 1, then 100-200 mg/day

P *Child >8 yr (>45 kg):* PO/**IV** 2.2-4.4 mg/kg/day in divided doses q12h

Gonorrhea (Patients allergic to penicillin)
Adult: Uncomplicated, PO 200 mg, then 100 mg hs and 100 mg bid × 3 days or 300 mg, then 300 mg in 1 hr; disseminated, 100 mg PO bid × at least 7 days

Chlamydia trachomatis
Adult: PO 100 mg bid × 7days

Syphilis
Adult: PO 300 mg/day in divided doses × 10 days

Available forms: Tabs 50, 100 mg; caps 50, 100 mg; syr 50 mg/ml; powder for inj 100, 200 mg; powder for oral susp 25 mg/5 ml

Adverse effects
CNS: Fever
CV: Pericarditis
EENT: Dysphagia, glossitis, decreased calcification of deciduous teeth, oral candidiasis
GI: Nausea, abdominal pain, vomiting, diarrhea, anorexia, enterocolitis, **hepatotoxicity,** flatulence, abdominal cramps, gastric burning, stomatitis
GU: Increased BUN
HEMA: **Eosinophilia, neutropenia, thrombocytopenia, hemolytic anemia**
INTEG: Rash, urticaria, photosensitivity, increased pigmentation, **exfoliative dermatitis,** pruritus, **angioedema**

Contraindications: Hypersensitivity to tetracyclines, children <8 yr, pregnancy **D**

Precautions: Hepatic disease, lactation

☑ Herb/drug ⬓ Do Not Crush ◆ Alert ⟳ᴨ Key Drug **G** Geriatric **P** Pediatric

Pharmacokinetics

Absorption	Well absorbed
Distribution	Widely distributed, crosses placenta
Metabolism	Some hepatic recycling
Excretion	Bile, feces; kidneys unchanged (20%-40%)
Half-life	15-22 hr; increased in severe renal disease

Pharmacodynamics

	PO	IV
Onset	1½-4 hr	Immediate
Peak	1½-4 hr	Infusion's end

Interactions
Individual drugs
Calcium: Forms chelates, ↓ absorption
Carbamazepine: ↑ effect of carbamazepine
Cholestyramine: ↓ doxycycline effect
Colestipol: ↓ doxycycline effect
Iron: Forms chelates, ↓ absorption
Magnesium: Forms chelates, ↓ absorption
Phenytoin: ↓ effect of doxycycline
Sucralfate: ↓ doxycycline effect
Warfarin: ↑ effect of warfarin
Drug classifications
Anticoagulants, oral: ↑ effect of anticoagulants
Barbiturates: ↓ effect of doxycycline
Contraceptives, oral: ↓ effect of oral contraceptive
Food/drug
↓ absorption with dairy products
Lab test interferences
False ↑ Urinary catecholamines, false ↑ ALT, false ↑ AST

NURSING CONSIDERATIONS
Assessment
• Assess patient for previous sensitivity reaction
• Assess patient for signs and symptoms of infection including characteristics of wounds, sputum, urine, stool, WBC >10,000, fever; obtain baseline information before and during treatment
• Obtain C&S before beginning drug therapy to identify if correct treatment has been initiated
• Assess for allergic reactions: rash, urticaria, pruritus, chills, fever, joint pain; angioedema may occur a few days after therapy begins
• Assess bowel pattern daily; if severe diarrhea occurs, drug should be discontinued
• Monitor for bleeding: ecchymosis, bleeding gums, hematuria, stool guaiac daily if on long-term therapy; blood dyscrasias may occur
• Assess for overgrowth of infection: perineal itching, fever, malaise, redness, pain, swelling, drainage, rash, diarrhea, change in cough, sputum

Nursing diagnoses
☑ Infection, risk for (uses)
☑ Diarrhea (side effects)
☑ Injury, risk for (side effects)
☑ Knowledge deficit (teaching)
☑ Noncompliance (teaching)

Implementation
PO route
🚫• Do not crush, chew caps
• Give around the clock to maintain proper blood levels; give with food to increase absorption of drug; do not give within 3 hr of other agents; drug reactions may occur

---

• Give with 8 oz of water, 1 hr before hs to prevent ulceration
• Shake liq preparation well before giving; use calibrated device for proper dosing
• Do not give with iron, calcium, magnesium products or antacids, which decrease absorption and form insoluble chelate

IV IV route
• Check for irritation, extravasation, phlebitis daily; change site q72h
• For intermittent inf, dilute each 100 mg/10 ml 0.9% NaCl, sterile water for inj; further dilute in at least 100 ml 0.9% NaCl, D_5W, Ringer's, LR, D_5/LR; protect from direct light; give over 1-4 hr

Syringe compatibilities:
Doxapram

Y-site compatibilities:
Acyclovir, amifostine, amiodarone, aztreonam, cyclophosphamide, diltiazem, filgrastim, fludarabine, granisetron, hydromorphone, magnesium sulfate, melphalan, meperidine, morphine, ondansetron, perphenazine, propofol, sargramostim, tacrolimus, teniposide, theophylline, thiotepa, vinorelbine

Y-site incompatibilities:
Hetastarch

Additive compatibilities:
Ranitidine

Patient/family education
• Teach patient to report sore throat, bruising, bleeding, joint pain; may indicate blood dyscrasias (rare)
• Advise patient to contact prescriber if vaginal itching, loose, foul-smelling stools, furry tongue occur; may indicate superinfection; report itching, rash, pruritus, urticaria
• Instruct patient to take all medication prescribed for the length of time ordered; drug must be taken around the clock to maintain blood levels; do not give medication to others
• Advise patient to notify prescriber of diarrhea with blood or pus

Evaluation
Positive therapeutic outcome
• Absence of signs/symptoms of infection (WBC <10,000, temp WNL, absence of red draining wounds)
• Reported improvement in symptoms of infection

droperidol (℞)
(droe-per'i-dole)
droperidol, Inapsine
Func. class.: Neuroleptic, tranquilizer, antiemetic
Chem. class.: Butyrophenone derivative

Pregnancy category   C

Action: Acts on CNS at subcortical levels, producing tranquilization, sleep; antiemetic

Therapeutic Outcome: Maintenance of anesthesia

Uses: Premedication for surgery; induction, maintenance in general anesthesia; postoperatively for nausea and vomiting

Dosage and routes
Induction
Adult: **IV**/IM 0.22-0.275 mg/kg given with analgesic or general anesthetic; may give 1.25-2.5 mg additionally

---

P *Child 2-12 yr:* **IV**/IM 88-165 µg/kg, titrated to response needed

Premedication
Adult: IM/**IV** 2.5-10 mg ½-1 hr before surgery

P *Child 2-12 yr:* IM/**IV** 88-165 µg/kg

Maintaining general anesthesia
Adult: **IV** 1.25-2.5 mg

Regional anesthesia adjunct
Adult: IM/**IV** 2.5-5 mg

Diagnostic procedures without general anesthesia
Adult: IM 2.5-10 mg ½-1 hr before procedure; 1.25-2.5 mg may be needed additionally

Available forms: Inj 2.5 mg/ml

Adverse effects
CNS: Dystonia, akathisia, flexion of arms, fine tremors, dizziness, anxiety, drowsiness, restlessness, hallucinations, depression
CV: **Tachycardia,** *hypotension*
EENT: Upward rotation of eyes, oculogyric crisis
INTEG: *Chills, facial sweating, shivering*
RESP: **Laryngospasm, bronchospasm**

Contraindications: Hyper-
P sensitivity, child <2 yr

G **Precautions:** Elderly, cardiovascular disease (hypotension, bradydysrhythmias), renal disease, liver disease, Parkinson's disease, pregnancy **C**

Pharmacokinetics	
Absorption	Well absorbed (IM)
Distribution	Crosses blood-brain barrier, placenta
Metabolism	Liver
Excretion	Kidneys, unchanged (10%)
Half-life	2-3 hr

Pharmacodynamics	
	IM/IV
Onset	3-10 min
Peak	30 min
Duration	3-6 hr

Interactions
Individual drugs
Alcohol: ↑ CNS depression
Lithium: ↑ side effects of lithium
Drug classifications
Amphetamines: ↓ effects of amphetamines
Anticholinergics: ↓ effects of anticholinergics
Anticoagulants: ↓ effects of anticoagulants
Anticonvulsants: ↓ effects of anticonvulsants
Antihypertensives: ↑ hypotension
Antiparkinsonian agents: ↓ effects of antiparkinsonian agents
Antipsychotics: ↑ CNS depression
Barbiturates: ↑ CNS depression
CNS depressants: ↑ CNS depression
Nitrates: ↑ hypotension
Opiates: ↑ CNS depression
Herb/drug
Kava: ↑ action

NURSING CONSIDERATIONS
Assessment
◆• Check VS q10 min during **IV** administration, q30 min after IM dose; for increasing heart rate or decreasing B/P,

---

notify prescriber at once; do not place patient in Trendelenburg's position, or sympathetic blockade may occur, causing respiratory arrest
• Assess extrapyramidal reactions: dystonia, akathisia, extended neck, restlessness, tremors; if these occur, an anticholinergic should be given
• If given for nausea or vomiting, monitor for significant loss of fluids, bowel sounds before and during administration

Nursing diagnoses
☑ Injury, risk for (adverse reactions)
☑ Knowledge deficit (teaching)

Implementation
IM route
• Give deeply in large muscle mass

IV IV route
• Give direct **IV** undiluted; give through Y-tube or 3-way stopcock at 10 mg or less/min; titrate to patient response
• Intermittent inf may be given by adding dose to 250 ml LR, D_5W, 0.9% NaCl; give slowly
• Give anticholinergics (benztropine, diphenhydramine) for extrapyramidal reaction
• Give only with crash cart, resuscitative equipment nearby

Syringe compatibilities:
Atropine, bleomycin, butorphanol, chlorpromazine, cimetidine, cisplatin, cyclophosphamide, dimenhydrinate, diphenhydramine, doxorubicin, fentanyl, glycopyrrolate, hydroxyzine, meperidine, metoclopramide, midazolam, mitomycin, morphine, nalbuphine, pentazocine, perphenazine, prochlorperazine, promazine, promethazine, scopolamine, vinblastine, vincristine

Syringe incompatibilities:
Fluorouracil, furosemide, heparin, methotrexate, pentobarbital

Y-site compatibilities:
Amifostine, aztreonam, bleomycin, cisatracurium, cisplatin, cladribine, cyclophosphamide, cytarabine, doxorubicin, doxorubicin liposome, famotidine, filgrastim, fluconazole, fludarabine, granisetron, hydrocortisone sodium succinate, idarubicin, melphalen, meperidine, metoclopramide, mitomycin, ondansetron, paclitaxel, potassium chloride, propofol, remifentanil, sargramostim, teniposide, thiotepa, vinblastine, vincristine, vinorelbine, vit B/C

Y-site incompatibilities:
Fluorouracil, foscarnet, furosemide, leucovorin, methotrexate, nafcillin

Additive incompatibilities:
Barbiturates

Patient/family education
• Advise patient that orthostatic hypotension is common; to rise from lying or sitting position slowly
• Caution patient that drowsiness may occur; to call for assistance for ambulation

Evaluation
Positive therapeutic outcome
• Decreased anxiety
• Absence of vomiting during and after surgery

---

dyphylline (℞)
(dye'fi-lin)
Dilor, Dyflex-200, Dylline,
dyphylline, Lufyllin,
Neothylline
Func. class.: Bronchodilator, phosphodiesterase
inhibitor
Chem. class.: Xanthine,
ethylenediamide
Pregnancy category **B**

Action: Relaxes smooth muscle of respiratory system by
blocking phosphodiesterase,
which increases cyclic AMP;
cyclic AMP results in positive
inotropic, chronotropic effects,
bronchodilatation, stimulation
of CNS

➔**Therapeutic Outcome:** Bronchodilatation with ease of
breathing

Uses: Bronchial asthma, bronchospasm in chronic bronchitis, COPD

Dosage and routes
Adult: PO 200-800 mg q6h;
IM 250-500 mg q6h injected
slowly

Available forms: Tabs 200,
400 mg; elix 33.3, 53.3 mg/5
ml; inj 250 mg/ml

Adverse effects
*CNS: Anxiety, restlessness,
insomnia, dizziness,* **convulsions,** headache, lightheadedness, muscle twitching
*CV: Palpitations, sinus tachy-
cardia,* hypotension, flushing,
dysrhythmias
*GI: Nausea, vomiting, an-
orexia,* dyspepsia, epigastric
pain
INTEG: Flushing, urticaria
OTHER: Fever, dehydration,
albuminuria, hyperglycemia
RESP: Tachypnea

Contraindications: Hypersensitivity to xanthines, tachydysrhythmias

ᴳ Precautions: Elderly, CHF,
cor pulmonale, hepatic disease,
active peptic ulcer disease,
diabetes mellitus, hyperthy-
ᴾroidism, hypertension, children, renal disease, pregnancy
B, glaucoma

D

Pharmacokinetics

Absorption	Well absorbed (PO)
Distribution	Unknown
Metabolism	Liver
Excretion	Kidneys (85%)
Half-life	2 hr; increased in renal disease

Pharmacodynamics

	PO	IM
Onset	Unknown	Unknown
Peak	1 hr	Unknown
Duration	6 hr	Unknown

Interactions
Individual drugs
Cimetidine: ↓ metabolism,
↑ toxicity
Ketamine: Do not use
together; seizures may occur
Drug classifications
Barbiturates: ↓ effect of dy-
phylline
β-Adrenergic blockers: ↓ me-
tabolism, ↑ toxicity
Benzodiazepines: ↓ sedative
effect
Sympathomimetics: ↑ CNS,
CV adverse reactions
Smoking
↑ metabolism, ↓ effect
Food/drug
**Caffeinated foods (cola,
coffee, tea, chocolate):**
↑ CNS, CV, adverse reactions

NURSING CONSIDERATIONS
Assessment
• Monitor dyphylline blood
levels (therapeutic level is <20

μg/ml); toxicity may occur with small increase above 20 G μg/ml, especially elderly; determine whether theophylline was given recently (24 hr)

• Monitor I&O; an increase in diuresis occurs; dehydration G may result in elderly or P children

• Assess respiratory rate, rhythm, depth; before and during treatment auscultate lung fields bilaterally; notify prescriber of abnormalities

• Assess for allergic reactions: rash, urticaria; if these occur, drug should be discontinued

Nursing diagnoses
☑ Injury, high risk for (uses, adverse reactions)
☑ Airway clearance, ineffective (uses)
☑ Activity intolerance (uses)
☑ Knowledge deficit (teaching)

Implementation
PO route
• Give 1 hr ac and 2 hr pc to increase absorption; elix should be measured accurately
IM route
• Inject slowly; do not give by **IV** route; do not administer if cloudy or a precipitate occurs

Patient/family education
• Teach patient to take doses as prescribed, not to skip doses or double dose; patient should check OTC medications and current prescription medications for ephedrine, which increases CNS stimulation; tell patient not to drink alcohol or caffeine products (tea, coffee, chocolate, colas) or cardiovascular effects may occur

• Advise patient to avoid hazardous activities; dizziness may occur

• Caution patient if GI upset occurs, to take drug with 8 oz water; avoid food, since absorption may be decreased

• Teach patient to notify prescriber of change in smoking habit; a change in dosage may be required

• Instruct patient to report nausea, vomiting, insomnia, tachycardia, dysrhythmias, convulsions, or restlessness; can indicate toxicity

• Teach patient to increase fluids to 2 L/day to decrease viscosity of secretions

Evaluation
Positive therapeutic outcome
• Decreased dyspnea
• Clear lung fields bilaterally

---

edrophonium (℞)
(ed-roe-fone'ee-yum)
Enlon, Reversol, Tensilon
Func. class.: Cholinergics, anticholinesterase
Chem. class.: Quaternary ammonium compound
Pregnancy category   C

Action: Inhibits destruction of acetylcholine, which increases concentration at sites where acetylcholine is released; this facilitates transmission of impulses across myoneural junction

Therapeutic Outcome: Reversal of nondepolarizing neuromuscular blockers; absence of difficulty with muscular function in myasthenia gravis

Uses: Diagnosis of myasthenia gravis; curare antagonist; differentiation of myasthenic crisis from cholinergic crisis; reversal of nondepolarizing neuromuscular blockers

---

☑ Herb/drug   ◎ Do Not Crush   ◆ Alert   ⟜ Key Drug   G Geriatric   P Pediatric

Dosage and routes
Tensilon test (myasthenia gravis diagnosis)
Adult: **IV** 1-2 mg over 15-30 sec, then 8 mg if no response; IM: 10 mg; if cholinergic reaction occurs, retest after ½ hr with 2 mg IM

P *Child >34 kg:* **IV** 2 mg; if no response in 45 sec, then 1 mg q45 sec, not to exceed 10 mg; IM 5 mg

P *Child <34 kg:* **IV** 1 mg; if no response in 45 sec, then 1 mg q45 sec, not to exceed 5 mg; IM 2 mg

P *Infant:* **IV** 0.5 mg

Reversal of nondepolarizing neuromuscular blockers
Adult: **IV** 10 mg over 30-45 sec, may repeat, not to exceed 40 mg

Differentiation of myasthenic crisis from cholinergic crisis
Adult: **IV** 1 mg, if no response in 1 min, may repeat

Available forms: Inj 10 mg/ml

Adverse effects
CNS: Dizziness, headache, sweating, weakness, **convulsions,** uncoordination, **paralysis,** drowsiness, **loss of consciousness**
CV: Dysrhythmias, bradycardia, hypotension, **AV block,** ECG changes, **cardiac arrest,** syncope
EENT: Miosis, blurred vision, lacrimation, visual changes
GI: Nausea, diarrhea, vomiting, cramps, increased salivary and gastric secretions, dysphagia, increased peristalsis
GU: Frequency, incontinence, urgency
INTEG: Rash, urticaria

RESP: **Respiratory depression, bronchospasm, constriction, laryngospasm, respiratory arrest,** dyspnea, increased bronchial secretions

Contraindications: Obstruction of intestine, renal system, hypersensitivity

Precautions: Seizure disorders, bronchial asthma, coronary occlusion, hyperthyroidism, dysrhythmias, peptic ulcer, megacolon, poor GI motility, pregnancy **C,** bradycardia, hypotension

E

Pharmacokinetics

Absorption	Unknown
Distribution	Unknown
Metabolism	Unknown
Excretion	Unknown
Half-life	Unknown

Pharmacodynamics

	IM	IV
Onset	2-10 min	30-60 sec
Peak	Unknown	Unknown
Duration	12-45 min	6-25 min

Interactions
Individual drugs
Atropine: ↓ action of edrophonium
Digitalis: ↑ bradycardia
Magnesium: ↓ action of edrophonium
Polymixin: ↓ action of edrophonium
Procainamide: ↓ action of edrophonium
Quinidine: ↓ action of edrophonium
Drug classifications
Anesthetics: ↓ action of edrophonium
Anticholinergics: ↓ effect of edrophonium
Antidysrhythmics: ↓ action of edrophonium

✦ Canada Only   Adverse effects: *italic* = common; **bold** = life-threatening

Antihistamines: ↓ action of edrophonium

Corticosteroids: ↓ action of edrophonium

Muscle relaxants, depolarizing: ↑ action of muscle relaxant

Phenothiazines: ↓ edrophonium action

NURSING CONSIDERATIONS
Assessment
• Assess vital signs, respiration during test
• Monitor diabetic patient carefully—this drug lowers blood glucose

Nursing diagnoses
☑ Breathing pattern, ineffective (uses)
☑ Knowledge deficit (teaching)

Implementation
IV route
• Administer undiluted 2 mg or less over 15-30 sec, or give as continuous inf in myasthenia crisis
◆• Give only after ensuring that atropine sulfate is available for cholinergic crisis
• Give only after all other cholinergics have been discontinued
• Store at room temp

Y-site compatibilities:
Heparin, hydrocortisone, potassium chloride, vit B/C

Patient/family education
• Instruct patient to wear Medic Alert ID specifying myasthenia gravis and drugs taken

Evaluation
Positive therapeutic outcome
• Increased muscle strength, hand grasp; improved gait; absence of labored breathing (if severe)

Treatment of overdose:
Respiratory support, atropine 1-4 mg (**IV**)

---

efavirenz (℞)
(ef-ah-veer'enz)
Sustiva
Func. class.: Antiviral
Chem. class.: Nonnucleoside reverse transcriptase inhibitor (NNRTI)

Pregnancy category   C

Action: Binds directly to reverse transcriptase and blocks RNA, DNA causing a disruption of the enzyme's site

Therapeutic Outcome: Improvement of HIV-1 infection

Uses: HIV-1 in combination with other antiretrovirals

Dosage and routes
Given in combination with protease inhibitor or nucleoside analog reverse transcriptase inhibitors (NRTIs)

Adult: PO 600 mg qd hs

P *Child:*
10-<15 kg: PO 200 mg qd hs
15-<20 kg: PO 250 mg qd hs
20-<25 kg: PO 300 mg qd hs
25-<32.5 kg: PO 350 mg qd hs
32.5-<40 kg: PO 400 mg qd hs
≥40 kg: Adult dose

Available forms: Caps 50, 100, 200 mg

Adverse effects
CNS: Headache, dizziness, fatigue, impaired concentration, insomnia, abnormal dreams, depression
GI: Diarrhea, abdominal pain, *nausea*

☑ Herb/drug   Ⓢ Do Not Crush   ◆ Alert   Key Drug   Ⓖ Geriatric   Ⓟ Pediatric

INTEG: Rash, erythema multiforme, **Stevens-Johnson Syndrome, toxic epidermal necrolysis**
GU: Hematuria, kidney stones

Contraindiations Hypersensitivity

Precautions: Liver disease, ℗ pregnancy **C,** lactation, children <3 yr, renal disease, myelosuppression

Pharmacokinetics	
Absorption	Well
Distribution	Highly protein bound
Metabolism	Liver
Excretion	Kidneys, feces
Half-life	Terminal 52-76 hr

Pharmacodynamics
Unknown

Interactions
Individual drugs
Indinavir: ↑ level of indinavir
Midazolam: Do not give together
Ritonavir: ↑ levels of both drugs
Saquinavir: ↓ level of saquinavir
Triazolam: Do not give together
Warfarin: ↑ level of warfarin
Drug classifications
Benzodiazepines: Do not give together
Ergots: Do not give together
Estrogens: ↑ levels of both drugs
Food/drug
↑ absorption of high fat foods

NURSING CONSIDERATIONS
Assessment
• Assess signs of infection, anemia
• Assess liver studies: ALT, AST; renal studies

• Assess C&S before drug therapy; drug may be taken as soon as culture is taken; repeat C&S after treatment; determine the presence of other sexually transmitted disease
• Assess bowel pattern before, during treatment; if severe abdominal pain with bleeding occurs, drug should be discontinued; monitor hydration
• Assess skin eruptions; rash, urticaria, itching
• Assess allergies before treatment, reaction to each medication; place allergies on chart
• Assess CBC, blood chemistry, plasma HIV RNA, absolute CD4+/CD8+/cell counts/%, serum β-2 microglobulin, serum ICD+24 antigen levels, cholesterol, hepatic enzymes
• Assess for signs of toxicity: severe nausea/vomiting, maculopapular rash

Nursing diagnoses
☑ Infection, risk for (uses)
☑ Diarrhea (side effects)
☑ Knowledge deficit (teaching)

Implementation
• Give hs to decrease CNS side effects

Patient/family education
• Advise patient to take as prescribed; if dose is missed, take as soon as remembered; do not double dose, take with water/juice; may be taken with or without food
• Instruct patient to make sure health care provider knows of all the medications being taken

• Advise patient that if severe rash occurs, stop taking and notify health care provider

• Advise patient not to breast-feed or become pregnant if taking this drug

• Advise patient that adverse reactions: rash, dizziness, abnormal dreams, insomnia, lessen after a month

• Teach patient to avoid hazardous activities if dizziness, drowsiness occurs

Evaluation

Positive therapeutic outcome
• Improvement in symptoms of HIV-1 infection

---

enalapril/ enalaprilat (℞)
(e-nal'april/e-nal'a-pril-at)
Vasotec, Vasotec IV
Func. class.: Antihypertensive
Chem. class.: Angiotensin-converting enzyme inhibitor

Pregnancy category **D** (2nd/3rd trimesters), **C** (1st trimester)

Action: Selectively suppresses renin-angiotensin-aldosterone system; inhibits ACE; prevents conversion of angiotensin I to angiotensin II, resulting in dilatation of arterial and venous vessels

➡ **Therapeutic Outcome:** Decreased B/P in hypertension; decreased preload, afterload in CHF

Uses: Hypertension, systolic CHF, diabetic neuropathy, post MI, left ventricular dysfunction

Dosage and routes
Adult: PO 5 mg/day, may increase or decrease to desired response; range 10-40 mg/day

Hypertension
Adult: **IV** 1.25 mg q6h over 5 min

P *Child:* PO 0.1 mg/kg/day in 1-2 divided doses, max 0.5 mg/kg/day

P *Child:* **IV** 5-10 μg/kg/dose q8-24h

Patients on diuretics
Adult: **IV** 0.625 mg over 5 min, may give additional doses of 1.25 mg q6h

Renal dose
Adult: PO 2.5 mg qd (CrCl <30 ml/min) increase gradually; **IV** CrCl >30 ml/min 1.25 mg q6h; CrCl <30 ml/min 0.625 mg as one-time dose, increase as per B/P

CHF
Adult: PO 5-20 mg/day in 2 divided doses

Available forms: Tabs 2.5, 5, 10, 20 mg; inj 1.25 mg/ml

Adverse effects
CNS: Insomnia, dizziness, paresthesias, headache, fatigue, anxiety
CV: Hypotension, chest pain, tachycardia, **dysrhythmias,** syncope
EENT: Tinnitus, visual changes, sore throat, double vision, dry burning eyes
GI: Nausea, vomiting, colitis, cramps, diarrhea, constipation, flatulence, dry mouth, loss of taste
GU: **Proteinuria, renal failure,** increased frequency of polyuria or oliguria
HEMA: **Agranulocytosis, neutropenia**

INTEG: Rash, purpura, alopecia, hyperhidrosis
META: Hyperkalemia
RESP: Dyspnea, dry cough, rales, angioedema

Contraindications: Hypersensitivity, history of angioedema, pregnancy **D** (2nd/3rd trimesters), lactation

Precautions: Renal disease, hyperkalemia, hepatic failure, dehydration, bilateral renal artery stenosis, pregnancy **C** (1st trimester)

Do Not Confuse:
enalapril/ramipril, enalapril/Eldepryl

Pharmacokinetics

Absorption	Well absorbed (PO), complete (**IV**)
Distribution	Unknown
Metabolism	Liver (active metabolite—enalaprilat)
Excretion	Kidneys (60%—enalaprilat, 20%—enalapril)
Half-life	Enalaprilat 11 hr, increased in renal disease

Pharmacodynamics

	PO	IV
Onset	1 hr	15 min
Peak	4-6 hr	1-4 hr
Duration	24 hr	6 hr

Interactions
Individual drugs
Alcohol: ↑ hypotension (large amounts)
Allopurinol: ↑ hypersensitivity
Digoxin: ↑ serum levels
Hydralazine: ↑ toxicity
Indomethacin: ↓ antihypertensive effect
Lithium: ↑ serum levels
Prazosin: ↑ toxicity
Drug classifications
α-Adrenergic blockers: ↑ hypotension
Antacids: ↓ absorption

Antihypertensives: ↑ hypotension
Diuretics: ↑ hypotension
Diuretics, potassium-sparing: ↑ toxicity
Ganglionic blockers: ↑ hypotension
Potassium supplements: ↑ toxicity
Sympathomimetics: ↑ toxicity
Lab test interferences
Interferences: Glucose/insulin tolerance tests

NURSING CONSIDERATIONS
Assessment
• Monitor blood studies: neutrophils, decreased platelets
• Monitor B/P, orthostatic hypotension, syncope; if changes occur dosage change may be required
• Monitor electrolytes: K, Na, Cl during 1st 2 wk of therapy
• Monitor renal studies: protein, BUN, creatinine; increased levels may indicate nephrotic syndrome and renal failure
• Monitor renal symptoms: polyuria, oliguria, frequency, dysuria
• Establish baselines in renal, liver function tests before therapy begins and 1 wk into therapy
• Check potassium levels throughout treatment, although hyperkalemia rarely occurs
• Check for edema in feet, legs daily
• Assess for allergic reactions: rash, fever, pruritus, urticaria; drug should be discontinued if antihistamines fail to help

Nursing diagnoses
✓ Cardiac output, decreased (uses)
✓ Injury, potential for (adverse reactions)

✅ Knowledge deficit (teaching)
✅ Noncompliance (teaching)

Implementation

PO route

• Store in air-tight container at 86° F (30° C) or less
• Severe hypotension may occur after 1st dose of this medication; decreased hypotension may be prevented by reducing or discontinuing diuretic therapy 3 days before beginning benazepril therapy
• Give by **IV** inf of 0.9% NaCl (as ordered) to expand fluid volume if severe hypotension occurs

IV route

• Give **IV** direct over 5 min
• Dilute in 50 ml 0.9% NaCl, D_5W, $D_5/0.9\%$ NaCl, D_5/LR; diluted solution may be used for 24 hr

Y-site compatibilities:

Allopurinol, amifostine, amikacin, aminophylline, ampicillin, ampicillin/sulbactam, aztreonam, butorphanol, calcium gluconate, cefazolin, cefoperazone, ceftazidime, ceftizoxime, chloramphenicol, cimetidine, cladribine, clindamycin, dextran 40, dobutamine, dopamine, erythromycin lactobionate, esmolol, famotidine, fentanyl, filgrastim, ganciclovir, gentamicin, granisetron, heparin, hetastarch, hydrocortisone, labetalol, lidocaine, magnesium sulfate, melphalan, meropenem, methylprednisolone, metronidazole, morphine, nafcillin, nicardipine, penicillin G potassium, phenobarbital, piperacillin, piperacillin/tazobactam, potassium chloride, potassium phosphate, propofol, ranitidine, teniposide, thiotepa, tobramycin, trimethoprim/sulfameth-oxazole, vancomycin, vinorelbine

Y-site incompatibilities:

Amphotericin B, phenytoin

Additive compatibilities:

Dobutamine, dopamine, heparin, meropenem, nitroglycerin, nitroprusside, potassium chloride

Patient/family education

• Advise patient not to discontinue drug abruptly; advise patient to tell all persons associated with health care
• Teach patient not to use OTC products (cough, cold, allergy medications) unless directed by physician, to avoid salt substitutes; serious side effects can occur; xanthines, such as coffee, tea, chocolate, cola can prevent action of drug
• Instruct patient on the importance of complying with dosage schedule, even if feeling better; to continue with medical regimen to decrease B/P: exercise, cessation of smoking, decreasing stress, diet modifications
• Emphasize the need to rise slowly to sitting or standing position to minimize orthostatic hypotension; not to exercise in hot weather, which can cause increased hypotension
• Advise patient to notify prescriber of mouth sores, sore throat, fever, swelling of hands or feet, irregular heartbeat, chest pain, coughing, shortness of breath
• Caution patient to report excessive perspiration, dehydration, vomiting, diarrhea; may lead to fall in B/P
• Caution patient that drug may cause skin rash or impaired perspiration; that angio-

edema may occur and to D/C if it occurs

• Caution patient that drug may cause dizziness, fainting, light-headedness; may occur during 1st few days of therapy; to avoid activities that may be hazardous

• Teach patient how to take B/P, and normal readings for age group

Evaluation

Positive therapeutic outcome
• Decreased B/P in hypertension

Treatment of overdose:
Lavage, **IV** atropine for bradycardia; **IV** theophylline for bronchospasm, digitalis, O_2; diuretic for cardiac failure, hemodialysis

---

enoxacin (℞)
(en-ox'a-sin)
Penetrex
Func. class.: Antiinfective
Chem. class.: Fluoroquinolone
Pregnancy category C

Action: Interferes with conversion of intermediate DNA fragments into high–molecular-weight DNA in bacteria; DNA gyrase inhibitor

Therapeutic Outcome: Bactericidal against the following organisms: staphylococci, *Enterobacter* sp, *Escherichia coli, Klebsiella* sp, *Neisseria gonorrhea, Pseudomonas aeruginosa*

Uses: Uncomplicated urethral or cervical gonorrhea, uncomplicated and complicated urinary tract infections (UTI)

Dosage and routes
Gonorrhea
Adult: PO 400 mg as a single dose
Uncomplicated UTI
Adult: PO 200 mg q12h × 7 days
Complicated UTI
Adult: PO 400 mg q12h × 14 days
Renal dose
CrCl <30 ml/min give initial dose, then give 50% of dose q12h

Available forms: Tabs 200, 400 mg

Adverse effects
CNS: Dizziness, headache, fatigue, somnolence, depression, insomnia, anxiety, **seizures**
EENT: Visual disturbances, dizziness
GI: Diarrhea, nausea, vomiting, anorexia, flatulence, heartburn, dry mouth, increased AST, ALT
INTEG: Rash, pruritus, photosensitivity

Contraindications: Hypersensitivity to quinolones

P Precautions: Pregnancy **C**,
G lactation, children, elderly, renal disease, seizure disorders

Do Not Confuse:
enoxacin/enoxaparin

Pharmacokinetics	
Absorption	Well absorbed
Distribution	Widely
Metabolism	Liver 20%
Excretion	Kidneys 50%-80%
Half-life	3-6 hr, increased in renal disease

Pharmacodynamics	
Onset	Unknown
Peak	Unknown

Adverse effects: *italic* = common; **bold** = life-threatening

Interactions
Individual drugs
Aminophylline: ↑ level of aminophylline

Bismuth subsalicylate: ↓ enoxacin level, ↓ effects of enoxacin

Caffeine: ↓ effect of enoxacin

Cyclosporine: ↑ nephrotoxicity

Digoxin: ↑ digoxin levels

Nitrofurantoin: ↓ effectiveness

Probenecid: ↑ blood levels

Sucralfate: ↓ absorption of enoxacin

Theophylline: ↑ toxicity

Warfarin: ↑ warfarin effect, ↑ toxicity

Zinc sulfate: ↓ absorption of enoxacin, ↓ effects of enoxacin

Food/drug
↓ absorption

NURSING CONSIDERATIONS
Assessment
• Assess patient for previous sensitivity reaction to quinolones

• Assess patient for signs and symptoms of infection including WBC >10,000, hematuria, foul-smelling urine; obtain baseline information before and during treatment

• Complete C&S testing before beginning drug therapy; this will identify if correct treatment has been initiated

• Assess for allergic reactions: rash, urticaria, pruritus

• Identify urine output; also monitor increases in BUN, creatinine

• Monitor blood studies: AST, ALT

Nursing diagnoses
☑ Infection, risk for (uses)
☑ Diarrhea (adverse reactions)
☑ Knowledge deficit (teaching)
☑ Noncompliance (teaching)

Implementation
• Give 1 hr ac or 2 hr pc to maintain proper blood levels

• Give with 8 oz of water, 1 hr before hs to prevent ulceration

• Do not give 4 hr before or 2 hr after medication

• Give 2 hr before or 2 hr after antacids, zinc, iron, or calcium

Patient/family education
• Instruct patient to increase fluids to 3L/day to prevent crystallization in the kidney

• Instruct patient to report itching, rash, pruritus, urticaria

• Instruct patient to contact prescriber if adverse reactions occur or if inflammation or pain of tendon occurs

• Instruct patient to take all medication prescribed for the length of time ordered; drug must be taken as ordered

• Advise patient to limit intake of alkaline foods and drugs: milk, dairy products, peanuts, vegetables, alkaline antacids, sodium bicarbonate

Evaluation
Positive therapeutic outcome
• Reported improvement in symptoms of infection

• Negative C&S test results

---

enoxaparin (℞)
(ee-nox′a-par-in)
Lovenox
Func. class.: Anticoagulant
Chem. class.: Unfractionated porcine heparin (low-molecular heparin)
Pregnancy category   B

Action: Prevents conversion of fibrinogen to fibrin and prothrombin to thrombin by enhancing inhibitory effects of antithrombin III; produces

---

higher ratio of anti-factor Xa to anti-factor IIa

→ **Therapeutic Outcome:** Prevention of deep vein thrombosis

Uses: Prevention of deep vein thrombosis, pulmonary emboli in hip and knee replacement

Dosage and routes
Hip/knee replacement
Adult: SC 30 mg bid given 12-24 hr post-op for 7-10 day, provided that hemostasis has been established

Abdominal surgery
Adult: SC 40 mg qd × 7-10 days to prevent thromboembolic complications

Prevention of ischemic complications in unstable angina/non-Q-wave MI with aspirin
Adult: SC 1 mg/kg q12h until stable with aspirin 100-325 mg qd

Available forms: Inj 30 mg/0.3 ml, 40 mg/0.4 ml, 60 mg/0.6 ml, 80 mg/0.8 ml, 100 mg/1 ml

Adverse effects
CNS: Fever, confusion
CV: **Cardiac toxicity**
GI: Nausea
GU: Edema, peripheral edema
HEMA: **Hypochromic anemia, thrombocytopenia,** bleeding
INTEG: Ecchymosis

Contraindications: Hypersensitivity to this drug, heparin, or pork; hemophilia; leukemia with bleeding; peptic ulcer disease; thrombocytopenic purpura, heparin-induced thrombocytoparia

Precautions: Alcoholism, elderly, pregnancy **B**, hepatic disease (severe), renal disease

(severe), blood dyscrasias, severe hypertension, subacute bacterial endocarditis, acute nephritis, lactation, children

Do Not Confuse:
enoxaparin/enoxacin

E

Pharmacokinetics	
Absorption	Well absorbed
Distribution	Unknown
Metabolism	Unknown
Excretion	Unknown
Half-life	4½ hr

Pharmacodynamics	
Onset	Unknown
Peak	3-5 hr
Duration	Unknown

Interactions
Drug classifications
Anticoagulants: ↑ bleeding
Antiplatelets: ↑ bleeding
NSAIDs: ↑ bleeding
Salicylates: ↑ bleeding
Herb/drug
Bromelain: ↑ risk of bleeding
Cinchona bark: ↑ risk of bleeding
Lab test interferences
↑ T_3 uptake, AST/ALT
↓ Uric acid, platelets

NURSING CONSIDERATIONS
Assessment
• Monitor blood studies (Hct, occult blood in stools), anti-Xa levels q3mo; platelet count q2-3 days; thrombocytopenia may occur
• Assess patient for bleeding gums, petechiae, ecchymosis, black tarry stools, hematuria, epistaxis, decrease in B/P; indicate bleeding and possible hemorrhage; notify prescriber immediately
• Assess for neurosymptoms in patients that have received spinal anesthesia

Nursing diagnoses
☑ Injury, risk for (uses, adverse reactions)
☑ Tissue perfusion, altered (uses)
☑ Knowledge deficit (teaching)

Implementation
• Give at same time each day to maintain steady blood levels
• Administer SC deeply; do not give IM; sol is clear to yellow; do not use sol with precipitate; apply gentle pressure for 1 min
• Give to recumbent patient, rotate sites (left/right anterolateral, left/right posterolateral abdominal wall)

Patient/family education
• Warn patient to avoid OTC preparations unless directed by prescriber because they could cause serious drug interactions
• Instruct patient to use soft-bristled toothbrush to avoid bleeding gums; to avoid contact sports; to use electric razor; to avoid IM inj
• Advise patient to report any signs of bleeding, bruising: gums, under skin, urine, stools

Evaluation
Positive therapeutic outcome
• Absence of deep vein thrombosis

---

entacapone
See Appendix A,
Selected New Drugs

---

ephedrine (℞, OTC)
(e-fed′rin)
ephedrine, ephedrine sulfate, Neorespin, Kondon's Nasal Jelly, Pretz-D, Vicks Vatronel
Func. class.: Bronchodilator, adrenergic, mixed direct and indirect effects; bronchodilator, nasal decongestant, vasopressor
Chem. class.: Phenylisopropylamine

Pregnancy category   C

Action: Increases contractility and heart rate by acting on β-receptors in the heart; also acts on α-receptors, causing vasoconstriction in blood vessels

➡Therapeutic Outcome: Decreased nasal congestion, bronchodilatation, stimulation, increased B/P

Uses: Shock; increased perfusion; hypotension, bronchodilatation; nasal congestion; orthostatic hypotension, depression, narcolepsy; vasopressor

Dosage and routes
Adult: IM/SC 25-50 mg, not to exceed 150 mg/24 hr; **IV** 10-25 mg, not to exceed 150 mg/24 hr
ℙ *Child:* SC/**IV** 3 mg/kg/day or 100 mg/m^2/day in divided doses q4-6h

Bronchodilator
Adult: PO 25-50 mg bid-qid, not to exceed 400 mg/day; IM/SC 12½-25 mg
ℙ *Child 6-12 yr:* 6.25-12.5 mg q4h, max 75 mg/24 hr

☑ Herb/drug ⓢ Do Not Crush ◆ Alert ⊶ Key Drug Ⓖ Geriatric ℙ Pediatric

P *Child >2 yr:* PO 2-3 mg/kg/day or 100 mg/m^2/day in 4-6 divided doses

Nasal decongestant
P *Adult and child >6 yr:* Nasal i-ii sprays in each nostril prn q4hr for <3-4 days

Stimulation
Adult: PO 25-50 mg q3-4hr prn

P *Child:* PO 3 mg/kg/day or 100 mg/m^2/day in 4-6 divided doses

Orthostatic hypotension
Adult: PO 25 mg qd-qid

P *Child:* PO 3 mg/kg/day in 4-6 divided doses

Labor
Adult: Administer dose to maintain B/P at or <130/80 mm Hg

Available forms: Inj 25, 30, 50 mg/ml; caps 25, 50 mg; nasal spray 0.25% nasal drops 0.5%; nasal jelly 1%

Adverse effects
CNS: Tremors, anxiety, insomnia, headache, dizziness, confusion, hallucinations, **convulsions, CNS depression, cerebral hemorrhage**
CV: Palpitations, tachycardia, hypertension, chest pain, **dysrhythmias**
EENT: Rebound congestion (nasal)
GI: Anorexia, nausea, vomiting
GU: Dysuria, urinary retention
RESP: Dyspnea

Contraindications: Hypersensitivity to sympathomimetics, angle-closure glaucoma, nonanaphylactic shock during general anesthesia

Precautions: Pregnancy **C,** cardiac disorders, hyperthyroidism, diabetes mellitus, prostatic hypertrophy

Pharmacokinetics

Absorption	Well absorbed (PO/IM/SC) complete (**IV**)
Distribution	Unknown
Metabolism	Liver
Excretion	Kidneys—unchanged
Half-life	3-5 hr

Pharmacodynamics

	PO	SC	IM	IV	NASAL
Onset	¼-1 hr	Unkn	15-30 min	5 min	Unkn
Peak	Unkn	Unkn	Unkn	Unkn	Unkn
Duration	2-4 hr	1 hr	1 hr	2 hr	6 hr

Interactions
Drug classifications
α-Adrenergic blockers: ↓ effect of ephedrine
Anesthetics, halothane: Increased dysrhythmias
Antidepressants, tricyclics: ↓ effect of vasopressor
β-Adrenergic blockers: Blocks therapeutic effect
Bronchodilators, aerosol: ↑ action of bronchodilator
Cardiac glycosides: ↑ dysrhythmia
Diuretics: ↓ effect of ephedrine
MAOIs: ↑ chance of hypertensive crisis
Oxytoxics: ↑ severe hypertension
Sympathomimetics: ↑ adrenergic side effects

NURSING CONSIDERATIONS
Assessment
• Monitor respiratory function: vital capacity, forced expiratory volume, ABGs, lung sounds, heart rate, baseline rhythm (bronchodilator)

E

• Monitor for evidence of allergic reactions; paradoxical bronchospasm; withhold dose; notify prescriber
• Monitor ECG, B/P, pulse, q5 min when using **IV** route (shock)
• Assess for paresthesias and coldness of extremities; peripheral blood flow may decrease; long term use may produce pseudo anxiety state requiring sedatives, increased lactic acid with severe metabolic acidosis
• Assess nasal congestion to identify factors contributing to ongoing congestion (nasal use)
• Assess mental status and sleeping patterns; mood, sensorium, ability to stay awake

Nursing diagnoses
☑ Airway clearance, ineffective (uses)
☑ Gas exchange impaired (uses)
☑ Sleep pattern disturbance (uses)
☑ Knowledge deficit (teaching)

Implementation
PO route
• Administer several hr (up to 6 hr) before hs to prevent sleeplessness
IV IV route
• Give **IV** directly undiluted using 3-way stopcock or Y-site; give 10-25 mg slowly, may repeat in 5-10 min
• Use clear sol without precipitate; unused sol should be discarded

Additive compatibilities:
Chloramphenicol, lidocaine, metaraminol, nafcillin, penicillin G potassium

Syringe compatibilities:
Pentobarbital

Y-site compatibilities:
Etomidate, propofol

Solution compatibilities:
0.9% NaCl, 0.45% NaCl, D5W, D10W, Ringers, LR

Patient/family education
• Advise patient to avoid use of OTC medications—extra stimulation may occur, and not to use alcohol

Evaluation
Positive therapeutic outcome
• Increased B/P (vasopressor)
• Ability to stay awake (absence of narcolepsy) or improved mood (absence of depression)
• Absence of bronchospasm
• Decreased nasal congestion

---

epinephrine 🔑
(℞, OTC)
(ep-i-nef′rin)
Adrenalin Chloride, Ana-Guard, AsthmaHaler, AsthmaNefrin, Bronitin Mist, Bronkaid Mist, Dysne-Inhal, epinephrine, Epinal, Epitrate, Eppy/N, Glaucon, epinephrine HCl, Epinephrine Pediatric, EpiPen Jr., Medihaler-Epi, microNefrin, Nephron Inhalant, Primatene Mist, S-2 Inhalant, Sus-Phrine, Vaponefrin
Func. class.: Bronchodilator, adrenergic, cardiac stimulant
Chem. class.: Catecholamine

Pregnancy category   **C**

Action: β_1- and β_2-agonist causing increased levels of cyclic AMP producing bronchodilatation, cardiac, and CNS stimulation; large doses cause vasoconstriction; small doses can cause vasodilation via β_2-vascular receptors

---

☑ Herb/drug   Ⓢ Do Not Crush   ◆ Alert   🔑 Key Drug   Ⓖ Geriatric   Ⓟ Pediatric

➡️**Therapeutic Outcome:** Vasoconstrictor, cardiac stimulator, bronchodilator, decreased aqueous humor

Uses: Acute asthmatic attacks, hemostasis, bronchospasm, anaphylaxis, allergic reactions, cardiac arrest, adjunct in anesthesia

Dosage and routes
Asthma
🅿️**Adult and child:** Inh 1-2 puffs of 1:100 or 2.25% racemic q15 min

Bronchodilator (parenteral epinephrine solution)
Adult: SC 0.2-0.5 mg, q20 min-4 hr max 1 mg/dose

Anaphylactic shock/ vasopressor
Adult: SC/IM 0.5 mg, repeat q5 min if needed, then **IV** 0.1-0.25 mg, repeat q5-15 min or infusion 1 mg/min, increase to 4 mg/min

🅿️**Child:** SC/IM/**IV** 10 µg/ kg, repeat q5-15 min, up to 0.3 mg

Anaphylactic reaction/ asthma
Adult: SC/IM 0.2-0.5 mg, repeat q10-15 min, not to exceed 1 mg/dose; epinephrine susp 0.5 mg SC, may repeat 0.5-1.5 mg q6h

🅿️**Child:** SC 0.01 mg/kg, repeat q15min × 2 doses, then q4h as needed, up to 0.5 mg/dose; epinephrine susp 0.025 mg/kg SC, may repeat q6h, max 0.75 mg in child ≤30 kg

Bronchodilator
🅿️**Adult and child:** Inh 1-2 inh of 1:100 or 2.25% racepineprine—0.2 mg/dose, may repeat q3h

Adult: Ophth: 1 gtt qd or bid

Cardiac arrest
Adult: IC, **IV**, endotracheal 0.1-1 mg repeat q5 min prn

🅿️**Child:** IC, **IV**, endotracheal 5-10 µg q5 min, may use 0.1 µg/kg/min **IV** inf after initial dose

Available forms: Aerosol 0.16 mg/spray, 0.2 mg/spray, 0.25 mg/spray, inj 1:1000 (1 mg/ml), 1:200 (5 mg/ml), 0.01 mg/ml (1:100,000), 0.1 mg/ml (1:10,000), 0.5 mg/ml (1:2,000); IM, **IV**, SC; sol for nebulization 1:100, 1.25% 2.25% (base)

Adverse effects
CNS: Tremors, anxiety, insomnia, headache, dizziness, weakness, drowsiness, headache, confusion, hallucinations, **cerebral hemorrhage**
CV: Palpitations, tachycardia, hypertension, *dysrhythmias,* increased T wave
GI: Anorexia, nausea, vomiting
RESP: Dyspnea

Contraindications: Hypersensitivity to sympathomimetics, narrow-angle glaucoma, nonanaphylactic shock during general anesthesia, OBS, cardiac dilatation, coronary insufficiency, cerebral arteriosclerosis, organic heart disease

Precautions: Pregnancy **C,** cardiac disorders, hyperthyroidism, diabetes mellitus, prostatic hypertrophy, elderly, lactation

Pharmacokinetics	
Absorption	Well absorbed (PO), complete (**IV**)
Distribution	Unknown, crosses placenta
Metabolism	Liver
Excretion	Breast milk
Half-life	Unknown

Pharmacodynamics			
	SC	IM	IV	INH
Onset	3-5 min	5-10 min	Imme-diate	1 min
Peak	Un-known	Un-known	Un-known	Un-known
Dura-tion	1-4 hr	1-4 hr	Un-known	1-4 hr

Interactions
Individual drugs
Insulin: ↑ need for insulin in diabetics
Lithium: ↓ effect of epineph-rine
Methyldopa: ↑ pressor response
Drug classifications
α-Adrenergic blockers: ↓ hy-pertensive effects
Anesthetics, general: ↑ dys-rythmias
Antidepressants, tricyclics: ↑ pressor response
Antihistamines: ↑ pressor response
β-Adrenergic blockers: Block therapeutic effect
Bronchodilators, aerosol: ↑ action of bronchodilator
Cardiac glycosides: ↑ dys-rhythmias
Diuretics: ↓ vascular response
Ergots: ↓ vascular response
MAOIs: ↑ chance of hyperten-sive crisis
Other sympathomimetics: ↑ adrenergic side effects, addi-tive effects
Phenothiazines: ↓ vascular response

NURSING CONSIDERATIONS
Assessment
• Monitor respiratory function: vital capacity, forced expiratory volume, ABGs, lung sounds, heart rate, rhythm (baseline); amount, color of sputum

• Monitor ECG during admin-istration continuously; if B/P increases, drug should be decreased; check B/P, pulse q5min after parenteral route; CVP, PCWP, SVR; inadvertent high arterial B/P can result in angina, aortic rupture, cerebral hemorrhage
• Check inj site for tissue sloughing; if this occurs, ad-minister phentolamine mixed with 0.9% NaCl
• Monitor for evidence of allergic reactions, paradoxical bronchospasm, withhold dose, notify prescriber; sulfite sensi-tivity, which may be life threat-ening

Nursing diagnoses
☑ Airway clearance, ineffective (uses)
☑ Gas exchange impaired (uses)
☑ Cardiac output, decreased (uses)
☑ Sensory-perceptual alteration, visual (uses) (ophth)
☑ Knowledge deficit (teaching)

Implementation
IV route
• Give after diluting 1 mg of 1:1000 sol/10 ml or more; 0.9% NaCl yields 1:10,000 sol, give 1 mg/min
• Give by continuous inf after further diluting in 0.9% NaCl, D5W, D10W, D5/LR, LR—give via 3-way stopcock; for Y-site, use inf pump; ↑ dose of insulin in diabetic patients

Syringe compatibilities:
Doxapram, heparin, milrinone

Y-site compatibilities:
Amrinone, atracurium, calcium chloride, calcium gluconate, diltiazem, dobutamine, dopa-mine, famotidine, fentanyl, furosemide, heparin, hydrocor-tisone sodium succinate, hy-

dromorphone, labetalol, lorazepam, midazolam, milrinone,
morphine, nicardipine, nitroglycerin, norepinephrine, pancuronium, phytonadione,
potassium chloride, propofol,
ranitidine, vecuronium, vit
B/C

Y-site incompatibilities:
Ampicillin

Additive compatibilities:
Amikacin, cimetidine, dobutamine, floxacillin, furosemide, metaraminol, ranitidine,
verapamil

Additive incompatibilities:
Aminophylline, mephenter-
mine, sodium bicarbonate,
warfarin

SC/IM route
• Rotate inj sites, massage
well, do not use gluteal (IM)
site
• Shake suspension before
using

Inh route
• Use 2.25% sol diluted in
nebulizer/respirator
• 10 gtt of a 1% sol should be
placed in nebulizer

Endotracheal route
• Only used in intubated
patient; use **IV** dose that
should be injected by endotracheal tube into bronchi

Patient/family education
• Tell patient not to use OTC
medications; extra stimulation
may occur; to use this medication before other medications
and allow at least 5 min between each, to prevent overstimulation
• Teach patient that paradoxical bronchospasm may occur
and to stop drug immediately
and notify health care provider;
to limit caffeine products such

as chocolate, coffee, tea, and
colas
• Patient should rinse mouth
after inh
• Patient should report blurred
vision, irritation with ophth
preparations

Evaluation
Positive therapeutic outcome
• Absence of dyspnea, wheez-
ing
• Improved airway exchange,
improved ABGs
• Decreased aqueous humor
• Stabilization of heart rate
and cardiac output

Treatment of overdose:
Administer a B_2-adrenergic
blocker, vasodilators, α-blocker

epirubicin
*See Appendix A,
Selected New Drugs*

epoetin (℞)
(ee-poe′e-tin)
Epogen, rHU-EPO, Eprex ✦,
Erythropoietin, Procrit
Func. class.: Biologic
modifier, hormone
Chem. class.: Amino acid
polypeptide

Pregnancy category   C

Action: Erythropoietin is one
factor controlling rate of red
cell production; drug is developed by recombinant DNA
technology

Therapeutic Outcome: Decreased anemia with increased
RBCs

Uses: Anemia caused by reduced endogenous erythropoietin production, primarily

end-stage renal disease; to correct hemostatic defect in uremia; anemia caused by AZT (zidovudine) treatment in HIV-positive patients; anemia caused by chemotherapy; reduction of allogeneic blood transfusion in surgery patients

Dosage and routes
Anemia secondary to chemotherapy
Adult: SC 150 U/kg 3×/wk, may increase after 2 mo up to 300 U/kg 3×/wk

Anemia in chronic renal failure
Adult: SC/**IV** 50-100 U/kg 3×/wk, then adjust dose by 25 U/kg/dose to maintain appropriate HCT; maintenance 12.5-25 U/kg, titrate to target HCT

Anemia secondary to zidovudine treatment
Adult: SC/**IV** 100 U/kg 3×/wk × 2 mo; may increase by 50-100 U/kg q1-2 mo, up to 300 U/kg 3×/wk

Available forms: Inj 2000, 3000, 4000, 10,000, 20,000 U/ml

Adverse effects
CNS: **Seizures,** coldness, sweating, headache
CV: *Hypertension,* **hypertensive encephalopathy**
MS: Bone pain

Contraindications: Hypersensitivity to mammalian cell-derived products, or human albumin, severe hypertension, erythropoietin levels of >200 mU/ml

Precautions: Seizure disorder, uncontrolled hypertension, porphyria, pregnancy **C**

Pharmacokinetics

Absorption	Well absorbed (SC), completely absorbed (**IV**)
Distribution	Unknown
Metabolism	Unknown
Excretion	Unknown
Half-life	5-14 hr

Pharmacodynamics

	SC/IV
Onset	Unknown
Peak	Unknown
Duration	Unknown
Increased RBC count	1-6 wk

Interactions: None

NURSING CONSIDERATIONS
Assessment
• Monitor renal studies: urinalysis, protein, blood, BUN, creatinine; I&O; report drop in output to <50 ml/hr
• Monitor blood studies: ferritin, transferrin monthly, transferrin sat ≥20%; ferritin ≥100 ng/ml; HCT 2×/wk until stabilized in target range (30%-33%) then at regular intervals; those with endogenous erythropoietin levels of <500 U/L respond to this agent; check for symptoms of anemia: fatigue, pallor, dyspnea
• Assess for CNS symptoms: coldness, sweating, pain in long bones
• Assess CV status: B/P before and during treatment; hypertension may occur rapidly leading to hypertension encephalopathy
• Assess patient during hemodialysis for bruits, thrills or shunts; drug prevents severe anemia in chronic renal failure; clotting may need to be treated with increased anticoagulant
• Monitor serum iron levels, ferritin, transferrin levels; iron

---

therapy may be needed to prevent recurring anemia
• Monitor B/P, check for rising B/P as HCT rises
• Monitor blood studies: BUN, creatinine, uric acid, platelets, WBC, phosphorus, potassium, bleeding time. Hct, Hgb, RBCs, reticulocytes should be checked in chronic renal failure

Nursing diagnoses
☑ Fatigue (uses)
☑ Activity intolerance (uses)
☑ Knowledge deficit (teaching)

Implementation

IV IV route
• Administer by direct route at end of dialysis by venous line, do not shake
• If HCT increases by 4% in 2 wk, decrease dose by 25 U/kg
• Give additional heparin to lower chance of clots

Solution compatibilities: NaCl 0.9%, $D_{10}W$, $D_{10}W$/ Albumin, sterile water for inj, TPN

SC route
• Give by SC route in patients not using dialysis

Patient/family education
• Teach patient how to take B/P
• Advise patients to take iron supplements, vit B_{12}, folic acid as directed
• Teach patient to avoid driving or hazardous activity during treatment
• Teach patients with renal disease to include high-iron and low-potassium foods in their diets (meat, dark green leafy vegetables, eggs, enriched breads)
• Teach patient the reason for treatment, expected results

• Advise patient to use contraception (pregnancy may occur)

Evaluation

Positive therapeutic outcome
• Increased appetite
• Enhanced sense of well-being
• Increase in reticulocyte count in 1-2 wk, Hgb, HCT

E

---

eptifibatide (℞)
(ep-tih-fib'ah-tide)
Integrilin
Func. class.: Antiplatelet agent
Chem. class.: Glycoprotein IIb/IIIa inhibitor
Pregnancy category   B

Action: Platelet glycoprotein antagonist. This agent reversibly prevents fibrinogen, von Willebrand's factor from binding to the glycoprotein IIb/IIIa receptor, inhibiting platelet aggregation

➔ **Therapeutic Outcome:** Decreased platelets

Uses: Acute coronary syndrome including those with PCI (percutaneous coronary intervention)

Dosage and routes
Acute coronary syndrome
Adult: **IV** BOL 180 µg/kg as soon as diagnosed, then **IV** CONT 2 µg/kg/min until discharge or CABG up to 72 hr; may decrease inf rate to 0.5 µg/kg/min if undergoing PCI; continue inf for 20-24 hr postprocedure, allowing up to 96 hr of treatment

---

PCI in patients without acute coronary syndrome
Adult: IV BOL 135 µg/kg given immediately before PCI; then 0.5 µg/kg/min × 20-24 hr

Available forms: 2 mg/ml (10 ml), 0.75 mg/ml (100 ml)

Adverse effects
CV: **Stroke,** hypotension
SYST: **Bleeding**

Contraindications: Hypersensitivity, active internal bleeding; history of bleeding, stroke within 1 mo; major surgery with severe trauma, severe hypotension, history of intracranial bleeding, intracranial neoplasm, arteriovenous malformation/aneurysm, aortic dissection, dependence on renal dialysis

Precautions: Bleeding, pregnancy **B,** lactation, children, elderly, renal function impairment

Pharmacokinetics	
Absorption	Unknown
Distribution	Unknown
Metabolism	Limited
Excretion	Kidneys
Half-life	2.5 hr

Pharmacodynamics	
Onset	Unknown
Peak	Unknown
Duration	Unknown

Interactions
Individual drugs
Aspirin: ↑ bleeding
Clopidogrel: ↑ bleeding
Dipyridamole: ↑ bleeding
Heparin: ↑ bleeding
Ticlopidine: ↑ bleeding
Drug classifications
Anticoagulants: ↑ bleeding
NSAIDs: ↑ bleeding

Platelet Receptor Inhibitors IIb, IIIa: Do not give together
Thrombolytics: ↑ bleeding

NURSING CONSIDERATIONS
Assessment
• Monitor platelets, Hgb, Hct, creatinine, PT/APTT baseline, INR, within 6 hr of loading dose and qd thereafter; patients undergoing PCI should have ACT monitored; maintain APTT 50-70 sec unless PCI is to be performed; during PCI, ACT should be 300-350 sec; if platelets drop <100,000/mm³, obtain additional platelet counts; if thrombocytopenia is confirmed, discontinue drug; also draw Hct, Hgb, serum creatinine
• Monitor ECG continuously

Nursing diagnoses
☑ Tissue perfusion, altered (uses)
☑ Knowledge deficit (teaching)

Implementation
IV IV route
• After withdrawing the bolus dose from 10 ml vial, give **IV** push over 1-2 min; follow bolus dose with continuous inf using inf pump, give drug undiluted directly from the 100 ml vial, spike the 100 ml vial with a vented infusion set, use caution when centering the spike on the circle of the stopper top

Solution compatibilities: 0.9% NaCl, D₅
• Discontinuing drug prior to CABG
• Give all medications PO if possible, avoid IM inj and catheters

Patient/family education
• Teach patient to report bruising, bleeding, chest pain

☒ Herb/drug Ⓢ Do Not Crush ◆ Alert ⊶ Key Drug Ⓖ Geriatric Ⓟ Pediatric

Evaluation
Positive therapeutic outcome
• Decreased platelets

---

ergonovine (℞)
(er-goe-noe′veen)
Ergometrine, ergotrate
maleate
Func. class.: Oxytocic
Chem. class.: Ergot alkaloid

Pregnancy category   N/A

Action: Stimulates uterine and vascular smooth muscle contractions, decreases bleeding

➧**Therapeutic Outcome:** Uterine contraction, decreases bleeding

Uses: Treatment of postpartum or postabortion hemorrhage

Investigational uses: To induce a coronary artery spasm

Dosage and routes
Oxytoxic
Adult: IM 0.2 mg q2-4h, not to exceed 5 doses; **IV** 0.2 mg given over 1 min

Induced coronary artery spasm
Adult: **IV** 50 mg q5 min up to 400 µg or until chest pain occurs

Available forms: Inj 0.2 mg/ml

Adverse effects
CNS: Headache, dizziness, fainting
CV: Hypertension, chest pain
EENT: Tinnitus
GI: Nausea, vomiting
GU: Cramping
INTEG: Sweating
RESP: Dyspnea

Contraindications: Hypersensitivity to ergot medication, augmentation of labor, before delivery of placenta, spontaneous abortion (threatened), pelvic inflammatory disease (PID)

Precautions: Hepatic disease, renal disease, cardiac disease, asthma, anemia, convulsive disorders, hypertension, glaucoma, obliterative vascular disease

E

Pharmacokinetics

Absorption	Well absorbed (IM), completely absorbed (IV)
Distribution	Unknown
Metabolism	Liver
Excretion	Kidneys
Half-life	Unknown

Pharmacodynamics

	IM	IV
Onset	2-5 min	Immediate
Peak	Unknown	Unknown
Duration	3 hr	45 min

Interactions
Drug classifications
Ergots: ↑ hypertension
Sympathomimetics: ↑ hypertension

NURSING CONSIDERATIONS
Assessment
• Monitor B/P, pulse; watch for change that may indicate hemorrhage; check respiratory rate, rhythm, depth; notify prescriber of abnormalities
• Assess fundal tone, nonphasic contractions; check for relaxation or severe cramping
• Assess for ergotism or overdose: nausea, vomiting, weakness, muscular pain, insensitivity to cold, paresthesia of extremities; drug should be decreased or inf discontinued

---

♣ Canada Only   Adverse effects: *italic* = common; **bold** = life-threatening

• Before administering ergonovine, calcium levels should be checked; if hypocalcemia is present, correction should be made to increase effectiveness of this drug

• Monitor prolactin levels and decreased breast milk production

Nursing diagnoses

☑ Tissue perfusion, decreased (uses)

☑ Injury, risk for (adverse reactions)

☑ Knowledge deficit (teaching)

Implementation

IM route

• Contractions begin in 2-5 min, drug is given q2-4h for contractions to continue; give deeply in large muscle mass; rotate inj sites if additional doses are given

IV IV route

• Give **IV** directly after dilution with 5 ml of 0.9% NaCl, give over >1 min through Y-site of free-running **IV** of 0.9% NaCl or D₅W

Additive compatibilities: Amikacin, cephapirin, sodium bicarbonate

Patient/family education

• Advise patient to report increased blood loss, increased temp or foul-smelling lochia

• Inform patient that cramping is normal—pad count should be done to determine amount of bleeding

• Tell patient not to smoke during treatment to prevent excessive vasoconstriction

Evaluation

Positive therapeutic outcome

• Absence of severe bleeding

Treatment of overdose: Stop drug; give vasodilators, heparin, dextran

---

ergotamine (℞)
(er-got′a-meen)
Ergostat, Ergomar ✦, Gynergen, Medihaler Ergotamine
Func. class.: α-Adrenergic blocker, vascular headache suppressant
Chem. class.: Ergot alkaloid-amino acid
Pregnancy category   X

Action: Constricts smooth muscle in peripheral, cranial blood vessels, relaxes uterine muscle; blocks serotonin release

➲**Therapeutic Outcome:** Absence of headache

Uses: Vascular headache (migraine, histamine, cluster)

Dosage and routes
Adult: 2 mg, then 1-2 mg qh or q½h for SL, not to exceed 6 mg/day or 10 mg/wk; inh 1 puff, may repeat in 5 min, not to exceed 6/24 hr

Available forms: SL tab 2 mg; tab 1 mg; oral inh 360 µg/dose

Adverse effects
CNS: Numbness in fingers, toes, headache, weakness
CV: Transient tachycardia, chest pain, bradycardia, edema, claudication, increase or decrease in B/P
GI: Nausea, vomiting
MS: Muscle pain

Contraindications: Hypersensitivity to ergot preparations, occlusion (peripheral, vascular), CAD, hepatic disease, renal disease, peptic ulcer, hypertension, Raynaud's disease, peripheral vascular dis-

---

☑ Herb/drug   Ⓢ Do Not Crush   ◆ Alert   ⊶ Key Drug   🄶 Geriatric   🄿 Pediatric ease, intermittent claudication, pregnancy **X**

G Precautions: Lactation, elderly,
P children, anemia

Pharmacokinetics

Absorption	Erratic (PO), poor (SL), rapidly (SC, IM)
Distribution	Crosses blood-brain barrier
Metabolism	Liver—extensively
Excretion	Kidneys (metabolites)
Half-life	Biphasic 2.7 hr, 21 hr

Pharmacodynamics

	PO	SL
Onset	1-2 hr	Unknown
Peak	½-3 hr	Unknown
Duration	Unknown	Unknown

Interactions
Individual drugs
Methysergide: ↑ effect
Sumatriptan: ↑ vasoconstriction
Drug classifications
Antiinfectives (macrolide): ↑ vasoconstriction, ↑ ergot toxicity
Ergots: ↑ hypertension
Oral contraceptives: ↑ vasoconstriction
Sympathomimetics: ↑ hypertension

NURSING CONSIDERATIONS
Assessment
• Assess characteristics of pain: duration, intensity, location, frequency, alleviating factors; also identify if halos, nausea, vomiting, blurred vision occur with headache. Assess before and during treatment
• Assess for ergotism or overdose: nausea, vomiting, weakness, muscular pain, insensitivity to cold, paresthesia of extremities; drug should be decreased or infusion discontinued

• Check for hypertension: B/P, pulse, monitor all peripheral pulses; if hypertension occurs, notify prescriber; also check for tachycardia or bradycardia

Nursing diagnoses
✓ Pain, acute (uses)
✓ Injury, risk for (adverse reactions)
✓ Knowledge deficit (teaching)

Implementation
SL route
• Have patient place tab under tongue; patient should not chew, crush, or swallow SL tab
• Patient should not drink, eat, or smoke until tab has dissolved
Inh route
• Teach patient how to use inhaler, protect ampules from heat/light

Patient/family education
• Caution patient not to smoke during treatment to prevent excessive vasoconstriction
• Advise patient to avoid alcohol or OTC medications unless approved by prescriber
• Tell patient to inform prescriber if pregnancy occurs

Treatment of overdose: Stop drug, give vasodilators, heparin, dextran

E

---

erythromycin base (℞)
(eh-rith-roh-my'sin)
Apo Erythro ✦, E-Mycin, Eramycin, Erybid ✦, Ery C, Erythromid ✦, Erythromycin Base Filmtab, Erythromycin Delayed-Release, Novo-Rythro Encap ✦, PCE Dispertab, Robimycin
erythromycin estolate (℞)
Ilosone, Ilosone Pulvules, Novo-Rythro ✦
erythromycin ethylsuccinate (℞)
Apo-Erythro-ES ✦, EES, Ery Ped, Novo-Rythro ✦
erythromycin gluceptate (℞)
Iiotycin Gluceptate
erythromycin lactobionate (℞)
Erythrocin, erythromycin lactobionate
erythromycin stearate (℞)
Apo-Erythro-s ✦, erythromycin stearate, Novo-Rythro ✦
Func. class.: Antiinfective
Chem. class.: Macrolide

Pregnancy category C

Action: Binds to 50S ribosomal subunits of susceptible bacteria and suppresses protein synthesis

➡**Therapeutic Outcome:** Bactericidal action against the following organisms: *Neisseria gonorrhoeae, Streptococcus pneumoniae, Mycoplasma pneumoniae, Corynebacterium diphtheriae, Bordetella pertussis, Borrelia burgdorferi, Listeria monocytogenes;* syphilis, Legionnaire's disease; streptococci; staphylocci; gram-positive bacilli: *Clostridium, Corynebacterium;* gram-negative pathogens: *Neisseria, Haemophilus influenzae, Legionella pneumophila, Mycoplasma,* and *Chlamydia trachomatis, Entamoeba histolytica*

Uses: Mild to moderate respiratory tract, skin, soft tissue infections

Dosage and routes
Soft tissue infections
Adult: PO 250-500 mg q6h (base, estolate, stearate); PO 400-800 mg q6h (ethylsuccinate); **IV** inf 15-20 mg/kg/day (lactobionate) divided q6h

🄿*Child:* PO 30-50 mg/kg/day in divided doses q6h (salts); **IV** 20-40 mg/kg/day in divided doses q6h (lactobionate)

N. gonorrhoeae/PID
Adult: IV 500 mg q6h × 3 days (gluceptate, lactobionate), then PO 250 mg (base, estolate, stearate) or 400 mg (ethylsuccinate) q6h × 1 wk

Syphilis
Adult: PO 20 g in divided doses over 15 days (base, estolate, stearate)

Chlamydia
Adult: PO 500 mg q6h × 1 wk or 250 mg qid × 2 wk

🄿*Infant:* PO 50 mg/kg/day in 4 divided doses × 3 wk or more

🄿*Newborn:* PO 50 mg/kg/day in 4 divided doses × 2 wk or more

Intestinal amebiasis
Adult: PO 250 mg q6h × 10-14 days (base, estolate, stearate)

P **Child:** PO 30-50 mg/kg/day in divided doses q6h × 10-14 days (base, estolate, stearate)

Available forms: Base: tab, enteric-coated 250, 333, 500 mg; tabs, film-coated 250, 500 mg; caps, enteric-coated 125, 250 mg; estolate: tabs, chewable 125, 250 mg; tab 500 mg; caps 125, 250 mg; drops 100 mg/ml; susp 125, 250 mg/5 ml; stearate: tabs, film-coated 250, 500 mg; ethylsuccinate: tabs, chewable 200, 100 mg/2.5 ml, 200, 400 mg/5 ml; susp 200, 400 mg; powder for susp 100 mg/2.5 ml, 200 and 400 mg/ 5 ml powder for inj; 500 mg and 1 g (lactobionate); 250 mg, 500 mg, 1 g (as gluceptate)

Adverse effects
CV: **Dysrhythmias**
EENT: Hearing loss, tinnitus
GI: Nausea, vomiting, diarrhea, hepatotoxicity, abdominal pain, stomatitis, heartburn, anorexia, pruritus ani
GU: Vaginitis, moniliasis
INTEG: Rash, urticaria, pruritus, thrombophlebitis (**IV** site)
SYST: **Anaphylaxis**

Contraindications: Hypersensitivity, preexisting liver disease (estolate), hepatic disease

Precautions: Pregnancy **B,** hepatic disease, lactation

Pharmacokinetics	
Absorption	Well absorbed (PO), minimally absorbed (top, ophth)
Distribution	Widely distributed; minimally distributed (CSF); crosses placenta
Metabolism	Liver, partially
Excretion	Bile, unchanged; kidneys (minimal), unchanged
Half-life	1-3 hr

Pharmacodynamics		
	PO	IV
Onset	1 hr	Rapid
Peak	4 hr	Infusion's end

E

Interactions
Individual drugs
Alfentanil: ↑ toxicity
Bromocriptine: ↑ toxicity
Carbamazepine: ↑ toxicity, from ↑ levels
Clindamycin: ↑ action of clindamycin
Cyclosporine: ↑ toxicity
Digoxin: ↑ blood levels of digoxin, ↑ action of digoxin
Dihydropyridine: ↑ action of dihydropyridine
Disopyramide: ↑ toxicity
Lovastatin: ↑ action of lovastatin
Methylprednisolone: ↑ toxicity
Midazolam: ↑ action of midazolam
Simvastatin: ↑ action of simvastatin
Theophylline: ↑ toxicity from ↑ levels
Triazolam: ↑ effects of triazolam

Drug classifications
Antihistamines: ↑ levels of antihistamine
Calcium antagonists: ↑ action of calcium antagonists
Ergots: ↑ ergotism
Oral anticoagulants: ↑ effects of oral anticoagulants
Penicillins: ↑ or ↓ action of penicillins

Lab test interferences
False ↑ 17-OHCS/17-KS, false ↑ AST/ALT
↓ Folate assay

NURSING CONSIDERATIONS
Assessment
• Assess patient for previous sensitivity reaction

- Assess patient for signs and symptoms of infection including characteristics of wounds, sputum, urine, stool, WBC >10,000, earache, fever; obtain baseline information before and during treatment

- Obtain C&S test results before beginning drug therapy to identify if correct treatment has been initiated

- Assess for allergic reactions: rash, urticaria may occur a few days after therapy begins

- Identify urine output; if decreasing, notify prescriber (may indicate nephrotoxicity); also monitor increases in BUN, creatinine

- Monitor blood studies: AST, ALT, CBC, Hct, bilirubin, LDH, alk phosphatase, Coombs' test monthly if patient is on long-term therapy

- Monitor electrolytes: potassium, sodium, chloride monthly if patient is on long-term therapy

- Assess bowel pattern qd; if severe diarrhea occurs, drug should be discontinued

- Assess for overgrowth of infection: perineal itching, fever, malaise, redness, pain, swelling, drainage, rash, diarrhea, change in cough, sputum

Nursing diagnoses
☑ Infection, risk for (uses)
☑ Diarrhea (adverse reactions)
☑ Knowledge deficit (teaching)
☑ Noncompliance (teaching)
☑ Injury, risk for (adverse reactions)

Implementation
PO route
- Give around the clock on an empty stomach, at least 1 hr ac or 2 hr pc; may be taken with food if GI upset occurs; do not take with juices; take dose with a full glass of water: use calibrated measuring device for drops or susp; shake well

- Store susp in refrigerator

- Chewable tab may be crushed or chewed, not swallowed whole

- Do not open, crush, or chew time-release cap or tab, enteric-coated tab may be given

IV IV route
- Add 10 ml of sterile water for inj without preservatives to 250- or 500-mg vials and 20 ml to 1-g vial; sol is stable for 1 wk after reconstitution if refrigerated

- Intermittent inf: dilute further in 100-250 ml of 0.9% NaCl or D₅W

- Give over 20-60 min to avoid phlebitis; assess for pain along vein; slow inf if pain occurs; apply ice to site and notify prescriber if unable to relieve pain

- Continuous inf: may also be administered as an infusion in a dilution of 1 g/L of 0.9% NaCl, D₅W, over 4 hr

Additive compatibilities:
Calcium gluconate, corticotropin, dimenhydrinate, heparin, hydrocortisone, lidocaine, methicillin, penicillin G potassium, potassium chloride, sodium bicarbonate

Additive incompatibilities:
Aminophylline, cephapirin, pentobarbital, secobarbital, streptomycin, tetracycline

Syringe incompatibilities:
Heparin

Erythromycin lactobionate
Additive incompatibilities:
Cephalothin, colistimethate, floxacillin, furosemide, heparin, metaraminol, metoclopramide, tetracycline, vit B/C

Additive compatibilities:
Aminophylline, ampicillin, cimetidine, diphenhydramine, hydrocortisone, lidocaine, methicillin, penicillin G potassium, penicillin G sodium, pentobarbital, polymyxin B, potassium chloride, prednisolone, prochlorperazine, promazine, ranitidine, sodium bicarbonate, verapamil

Syringe incompatibilities:
Ampicillin, heparin

Syringe compatibilities:
Methicillin

Y-site incompatibilities:
Fluconazole

Y-site compatibilities:
Acyclovir, amiodarone, cyclophosphamide, enalaprilat, esmolol, famotidine, foscarnet, hydromorphone, idarubicin, labetalol, lorazepam, magnesium sulfate, merperidine, midazolam, morphine, multivitamins, perphenazine, vit B/C, zidovudine

Patient/family education
• Teach patient to report sore throat, bruising, bleeding, joint pain—may indicate blood dyscrasias (rare)
• Advise patient to contact prescriber if vaginal itching, loose, foul-smelling stools, furry tongue occur—may indicate superimposed infection
• Instruct patient to take all medication prescribed for the length of time ordered

Evaluation
Positive therapeutic outcome
• Absence of signs/symptoms of infection (WBC <10,000, temp WNL, absence of red, draining wounds, earache)
• Reported improvement in symptoms of infection

Treatment of overdose:
Withdraw drug, maintain airway, administer epinephrine, aminophylline, O_2, **IV** corticosteroids

esmolol (℞)
(ez'moe-lole)
Brevibloc
Func. class.: β-Adrenergic blocker (antidysrhythmic II)
Pregnancy category C

Action: Competitively blocks stimulation of β_1-adrenergic receptors in the myocardium; produces negative chronotropic, inotropic activity (decreases rate of SA node discharge, increases recovery time), slows conduction of AV node, decreases heart rate, decreases O_2 consumption in myocardium; also decreases renin-aldosterone-angiotensin system at high doses; inhibits β_2-receptors in bronchial system slightly

Therapeutic Outcome: Decreased supraventricular tachycardia

Uses: Supraventricular tachycardias, noncompensatory tachycardia, hypertensive crisis

Dosage and routes
Adult: **IV** loading dose— 500 μg/kg/min over 1 min; maintenance—50 μg/kg/min for 4 min; may repeat q5 min, increasing maintenance inf by 50 μg/kg/min (max of 200 μg/kg/min); titrate to patient response

Available forms: Inj 10 mg, 250 mg/ml

Adverse effects

CNS: Confusion, light-headedness, paresthesia, somnolence, fever, dizziness, fatigue, headache, depression, anxiety, **seizures**

CV: Hypotension, bradycardia, chest pain, peripheral ischemia, shortness of breath, CHF, conduction disturbances

GI: Nausea, vomiting, anorexia, gastric pain, flatulence, constipation, heartburn, bloating

GU: Urinary retention, impotence, dysuria

INTEG: Induration, inflammation at site, discoloration, edema, erythema, burning pallor, flushing, rash, pruritus, dry skin, alopecia

RESP: **Bronchospasm,** dyspnea, cough, wheezing, nasal stuffiness

Contraindications: 2nd- or 3rd-degree heart block, cardiogenic shock, CHF, cardiac failure, hypersensitivity

Precautions: Hypotension, pregnancy **C,** peripheral vascular disease, diabetes, hypoglycemia, thyrotoxicosis, renal disease, lactation

▧ **Do Not Confuse:**
Brevibloc/Brevital

Pharmacokinetics

Absorption	Complete
Distribution	Unknown
Metabolism	Liver
Excretion	Kidneys
Half-life	9 min

Pharmacodynamics

Onset	Rapid
Peak	Unknown
Duration	1-2 min

Interactions

Individual drugs

Alcohol: ↑ hypotension (large amounts)

Epinephrine: α-Adrenergic stimulation

Hydralazine: ↑ hypotension, bradycardia

Prazosin: ↑ hypotension, bradycardia

Thyroid: ↓ effect of esmolol

Verapamil: ↑ myocardial depression

Drug classifications

Antihypertensives: ↑ hypertension

β₂-Agonists: ↓ bronchodilation

Cardiac glycosides: ↑ bradycardia

Nitrates: ↑ hypotension

Theophyllines: ↓ bronchodilatation

Smoking
↑ tachycardia

▧ *Herb/drug*

Aloe: ↑ hypokalemia

Buckthorn bark/berry: ↑ hypokalemia

Cascara sagrada bark: ↑ hypokalemia

Senna pod/leaf: ↑ hypokalemia

Lab test interferences
↑ Liver function tests

NURSING CONSIDERATIONS
Assessment

• Monitor B/P during beginning treatment, periodically thereafter; pulse q4h; note rate, rhythm, quality; apical/radial pulse before administration; notify prescriber of any significant changes (pulse <50 bpm)

• Check for baselines in renal, liver function tests before therapy begins

• Assess for edema in feet, legs daily, monitor I&O, daily

weight; check for jugular vein distention, rales bilaterally, dyspnea (CHF)

• Monitor skin turgor, dryness of mucous membranes for hydration status, especially **G** elderly

Nursing diagnoses

✓ Cardiac output, decreased (uses)

✓ Injury, risk for (adverse reactions)

✓ Knowledge deficit (teaching)

✓ Noncompliance (teaching)

Implementation

• Give by intermittent inf after diluting 5 g/500 ml D_5W, 0.9% NaCl, D_5/0.45% NaCl, D_5/LR, D_5/0.9% NaCl, 0.45% NaCl, LR, (10 mg/ml)

• Give loading dose over 1 min, then maintenance dose over 4 min, may repeat loading dose q5 min with increased maintenance dose; maintenance should not be >200 μg/kg/min and be administered up to 48 hr; dosage should be tapered at a rate of 25 μg/kg/min

• Store at room temp for 24 hr; sol should be clear

Y-site compatibilities:
Amikacin, aminophylline, ampicillin, amiodarone, atracurium, butorphanol, calcium chloride, cefazolin, cefmetazole, cefoperazone, ceftazidime, ceftizoxime, chloramphenicol, cimetidine, cisatracurium, clindamycin, diltiazem, dopamine, enalaprilat, erythromycin, famotidine, fentanyl, gentamicin, heparin, hydrocortisone, regular insulin, labetalol, magnesium sulfate, methyldopa, metronidazole, midazolam, morphine, nafcillin, nitroglycerin, norepinephrine, nitroprusside, pancuronium, penicillin G potassium, phenytoin, piperacillin, polymyxin B, potassium chloride, potassium phosphate, propofol, ranitidine, remifentanil, streptomycin, tacrolimus, tobramycin, trimethoprim-sulfamethoxazole, vancomycin, vecuronium

Y-site incompatibilities:
Furosemide

Additive compatibilities:
Aminophylline, atracurium, bretylium, heparin

Additive incompatibilities:
Diazepam, procainamide, sodium bicarbonate, thiopental

Patient/family education
• Teach patient need for medication and expected results
• Caution patient to rise slowly to prevent orthostatic hypotension
• Advise patient to notify if pain, swelling occurs at **IV** site

Evaluation

Positive therapeutic outcome
• Absence of dysrhythmias

Treatment of overdose:
Defibrillation, vasopressor for hypotension

---

estazolam (℞)
(ess-taz′oh-lam)
ProSom
Func. class.: Sedative-hypnotic
Chem. class.: Benzodiazepine derivative
Pregnancy category X
Controlled substance schedule IV

Action: Produces CNS depression at the limbic, thalamic, hypothalamic levels of the

---

Adverse effects: *italic* = common; **bold** = life-threatening

CNS; may be mediated by neurotransmitter γ-aminobutyric acid (GABA); results are sedation, hypnosis, skeletal muscle relaxation, anxiolytic action

▶ **Therapeutic Outcome:** Ability to sleep, relaxation

Uses: Insomnia (short-term)

Dosage and routes
Adult: PO 1-2 mg hs

G *Elderly:* PO 0.5-1 mg hs

Available forms: Tabs 1, 2 mg

Adverse effects
CNS: Lethargy, drowsiness, daytime sedation, dizziness, confusion, light-headedness, headache, anxiety, irritability, weakness, tremors, depression, lack of coordination
CV: Chest pain, pulse changes, palpitations, tachycardia
GI: Nausea, vomiting, diarrhea, heartburn, abdominal pain, constipation, anorexia, taste alteration
HEMA: **Leukopenia, granulocytopenia (rare)**
INTEG: Dermatitis, allergy, sweating, flushing, pruritus
MISC: Joint pain, respiratory congestion, dependency

Contraindications: Hypersensitivity to benzodiazepines, pregnancy **X**, sleep apnea

Precautions: Hepatic disease, renal disease, suicidal individu-
G als, drug abuse, elderly, psycho-
P sis, child <18, lactation, depression, **pulmonary insufficiency**

◥ **Do Not Confuse:**
ProSom/Proscar,
ProSom/Prozac

Pharmacokinetics

Absorption	Well absorbed
Distribution	Crosses blood-brain barrier, placenta
Metabolism	Liver
Excretion	Kidneys, feces, breast milk
Half-life	10-24 hr

Pharmacodynamics

Onset	15-45 min
Peak	1½-2 hr
Duration	7-8 hr

Interactions
Individual drugs
Alcohol: ↑ CNS depression
Cimetidine: ↑ action
Digoxin: ↑ digoxin action
Disulfiram: ↑ action
Isoniazid: ↑ action
Ketoconazole: ↑ action
Levodopa: ↓ action of levodopa
Metoprolol: ↑ action
Phenytoin: ↑ phenytoin action
Propoxyphene: ↑ action
Propranolol: ↑ action
Rifampin: ↓ action of chlordiazepoxide
Theophylline: ↓ sedative effects
Valproic acid: ↑ action
Drug classifications
Analgesics, opioid: ↑ CNS depression
Antidepressants: ↑ CNS depression
Antihistamines: ↑ CNS depression
Barbiturates: ↓ effect of chlordiazepoxide
Contraceptives: ↑ effect
MAOIs: ↑ CNS depression
▨ *Herb/drug*
Kava: ↑ CNS depression

NURSING CONSIDERATIONS
Assessment
• Assess patient's sleep pattern and note physical circumstances that interrupt sleep

---

▨ Herb/drug ◨ Do Not Crush ◆ Alert ⊶ Key Drug G Geriatric P Pediatric (sleep apnea, obstructed air-way, pain/discomfort, urinary frequency) and psychologic (fear, anxiety); patient's bed-time routine, pre-sleep cues/props

• Identify potential for abuse; this drug may lead to physical and psychologic dependency; amount of drug should be limited

• Monitor blood studies: Hct, Hgb, RBCs, serum folate (if on long-term therapy), pro-time in patients receiving anti-coagulants because action of anticoagulant may be increased

• Assess patient's mental status: mood, sensorium, af-fect, memory (long-term, short-term); for physical dependency: more frequent requests for medication, shakes, anxiety, pinpoint pupils

Nursing diagnoses

✓ Sleep pattern disturbance
✓ Knowledge deficit (teaching)
✓ Noncompliance (teaching)

Implementation

• Give ½-1 hr before hs for sleeplessness; on empty stom-ach for fast onset, but may be taken with food if GI symp-toms occur

• Store in air-tight container in cool environment

Patient/family education

• Advise patient to avoid driv-ing or other activities requiring alertness; to avoid alcohol ingestion or CNS depressants; serious CNS depression may result plus tachycardia, flush-ing, headache, hypotension

• Provide patient with alter-nate measures to improve sleep (reading, exercise several hr before hs, warm bath, warm milk, TV, self-hypnosis, deep breathing)

• Inform patient that hangover **G** is common in elderly but less common than with barbitu-rates

• Teach patient symptoms of withdrawal: nausea, vomiting, anxiety, hallucinations, insom-nia, tachycardia, fever, cramps, tremors, seizures

• Advise patient to watch for allergic reaction (rash) and to discontinue drug if rash occurs

• Advise patient to notify prescriber if pregnancy is sus-pected

• Teach patient not to discon-tinue drug abruptly, taper over 1-2 wk

Evaluation

Positive therapeutic outcome

• Ability to sleep at night
• Decreased amount of early AM awakenings

E

estradiol/estradiol cypionate/estradiol valerate/estradiol transdermal system (R)

(ess-tra-dye'ole)

Alora, Cypionate, depGynogen, Depo Estradiol, Depogen, Dura-Estrin, Estra-D, Estradiol Cypionate, Estro-Cyp, Estroject-L.A., Estronol-LA/ Estrace, Esaderm/Deladiol-40, Delestrogen, Dioval 40, Dioval XX, Duragen-10, Duragen-20, Duragen-40, Estradiol Valerate, Estra-L 20, Estra-L 40, FemPatch, Gynogen L.A. "10", Gynogen L.A. "20", Gynogen L.A. "40", L.A.E. 20, Valergen 10, Valergen 20, Valergen 40/ Estrace, Estraderm TTS

Func. class.: Estrogen
Chem. class.: Nonsteroidal synthetic estrogen

Pregnancy category   X

Action: Needed for adequate functioning of female reproductive system; affects release of pituitary gonadatropins, inhibits ovulation, promotes adequate calcium use in bone structure

▶Therapeutic Outcome: Decreased tumor size in prostatic cancer; increased estrogen levels in menopause, female hypogonadism

Uses: Menopause, breast cancer, prostatic cancer, atrophic vaginitis, kraurosis vulvae, hypogonadism, castration, primary ovarian failure, prevention of osteoporosis

Dosage and routes
Menopause/hypogonadism/ castration/ovarian failure
Adult: PO 1-2 mg qd 3 wk on, 1 wk off or 5 days on, 2 days off; IM 1-5 mg q3-4wk (cypionate), 10-20 mg q4wk (valerate); TOP Estraderm 0.05 mg/24h applied 2×/wk, Climera 0.05 mg/hr applied 1×/wk in a cyclic regimen, women with hysterectomy may use continuously

Prostatic cancer
Adult: PO 1-2 mg qd 3 wk on, 1 wk off or 5 days on, 2 days off; IM 0.2-1 mg qwk

Breast cancer
Adult: PO 10 mg tid × 3 mo or longer

Atropic vaginitis/Kraurosis vulvae
Adult: Vag cream 2-4 g qd × 1-2 wk, then 1 g 1-3 ×/wk cycled

Available forms: Estradiol tabs 0.5, 1, 2 mg; cypionate inj IM 5 mg/ml; valerate inj IM 10, 20, 40 mg/ml; transderm 0.1 mg/24-hr release rate; vag cream 100 µg/g

Adverse effects
CNS: Dizziness, headache, migraine, depression, **seizures**
CV: Hypotension, thrombophlebitis, edema, **thromboembolism, stroke, pulmonary embolism, myocardial infarction**
EENT: Contact lens intolerance, increased myopia, astigmatism
GI: Nausea, vomiting, diarrhea, anorexia, pancreatitis, cramps, constipation, increased appetite, increased weight, **cholestatic jaundice, hepatic adenoma**

GU: Amenorrhea, cervical erosion, breakthrough bleeding, dysmenorrhea, vaginal candidiasis, breast changes, *gynecomastia, testicular atrophy, impotence,* **increased risk of breast, endometrial cancer**
INTEG: Rash, urticaria, acne, hirsutism, alopecia, oily skin, seborrhea, purpura, melasma
META: Folic acid deficiency, hypercalcemia, hyperglycemia

Contraindications: Breast cancer, thromboembolic disorders, reproductive cancer, genital bleeding (abnormal, undiagnosed), pregnancy **X**

Precautions: Hypertension, asthma, blood dyscrasias, gallbladder disease, CHF, diabetes mellitus, bone disease, depression, migraine headache, convulsive disorders, hepatic disease, renal disease, family history of cancer of breast or reproductive tract

Pharmacokinetics

Absorption	Well absorbed
Distribution	Widely distributed, crosses placenta
Metabolism	Unknown
Excretion	Unknown
Half-life	Unknown

Pharmacodynamics

	PO	IM	IV
Onset	Rapid	Slow	Rapid
Peak	Unknown	Unknown	Unknown
Duration	Unknown	Unknown	Unknown

Interactions
Individual drugs
Cyclosporine: ↑ toxicity
Dantrolene: ↑ toxicity
Tamoxifen: ↓ tamoxifen action

Drug classifications
Anticoagulants: ↓ action of anticoagulants
Antidepressants, tricyclics: ↑ toxicity
Barbiturates: ↓ action of chlorotrianisene
Corticosteroids: ↑ action of corticosteroids
Oral hypoglycemics: ↓ action of hypoglycemics
Food/drug
Grapefruit: ↑ estrogen level
Lab test interferences
↑ BSP retention test; ↑ PBI; ↑ T$_4$; ↑ serum sodium; ↑ platelet aggregation; ↑ thyroxine-binding globulin (TBS); ↑ prothrombin; ↑ factors VII, VIII, IX, X; ↑ triglycerides
↓ Serum folate, ↓ serum triglyceride, ↓ T$_3$ resin uptake test, ↓ glucose tolerance test, ↓ antithrombin III, ↓ pregnanediol, ↓ metyrapone test
False positive: LE prep, antinuclear antibodies

NURSING CONSIDERATIONS
Assessment
• Monitor blood glucose in patient with diabetes; increased urine glucose may occur
• Monitor B/P q4h; watch for increase caused by water and sodium retention
• Monitor I&O ratio; be alert for decreasing urinary output and increasing edema; monitor weight daily; notify prescriber if weekly weight gain is >5 lb; if increased, diuretic may be ordered
• Obtain liver function studies, including AST, ALT, bilirubin, alk phosphatase
• Assess edema, hypertension, cardiac symptoms, jaundice
• Assess mental status: affect, mood, behavioral changes, aggression; depression may

occur, drug may need to be discontinued

• Assess female patient for intact uterus, if so, progesterone should be added to estrogen therapy to decrease risk of endometrial cancer

Nursing diagnoses

☑ Sexual dysfunction (uses)
☑ Injury, risk for (adverse reactions)

Implementation

PO route

• Give titrated dose, use lowest effective dose
• Give with food or milk to decrease GI symptoms

IM route

• Administer deeply in large muscle mass; drug is painful
• Rotate syringe to mix oil and medication

Trans route

• Apply to area free of hair to ensure adhesion
• Start trans dose 7 days before last PO dose if routes are to be changed

Vag route

• Place cream in applicator by attaching tube to applicator; squeeze cream into tube to mark; insert with patient reclining
• Applicator should be washed after each use

Patient/family education

• Tell patient to take exactly as prescribed; do not double doses
◆• Advise patient that increased weight gain and symptoms of fluid retention should be reported to prescriber: edema of feet, ankles, sacral area; abnormal vaginal bleeding; breast lumps; hepatic disease (dark urine, clay-colored stools, jaundice of skin, sclera, pruritus)

◆• Caution patient that thromboembolic symptoms should be reported: tenderness in legs, chest pain, dyspnea, headaches, blurred vision

• Inform patient to use sunscreen and protective clothing because sunburns may occur

• Advise patient to stop smoking—smokers have a greater chance of thromboembolic disorder

• Tell patient to use a nonhormonal birth control, and to notify prescriber if pregnancy is suspected

Evaluation

Positive therapeutic outcome

• Reversal of menopausal symptoms
• Decrease in tumor size in prostatic or breast cancer
• Decrease in itching, inflammation of vagina
• Absence of symptoms of osteoporosis

---

estramustine (℞)
(ess-tra-muss'teen)
Emcyt
Func. class.: Antineoplastic
Chem. class.: Hormone, alkylating agent
Pregnancy category　D

Action: Combination drug consisting of nitrogen mustard/estrogen; estrogen is a carrier for the nitrogen mustard into estrogen-dependent tissue; acts like a weak alkylating agent; decreases serum testosterone levels

➡**Therapeutic Outcome:** Prevention of rapidly growing malignant cells

Uses: Metastatic prostate cancer (palliative treatment only)

☑ Herb/drug　◎ Do Not Crush　◆ Alert　◆ᴛ Key Drug　◐ Geriatric　ℙ Pediatric

Dosage and routes
Adult: PO 10-16 mg/kg in 3-4 divided doses/day; treatment may continue for 3 mo; 600 mg/m²/day in 3 divided doses

Available forms: Cap 140 mg

Adverse effects
CNS: Headache, anxiety, seizures, insomnia, mood swings
CV: **Myocardial infarction,** hypertension, **CHF, CVA**
GI: Nausea, vomiting, anorexia, **hepatotoxicity**
GU: **Renal failure,** impotence, gynecomastia
HEMA: Anemia, thrombocytopenia, leukopenia
INTEG: Rash, urticaria, pruritus, flushing, alopecia
RESP: Dyspnea, **emboli,** hoarseness

Contraindications: Hypersensitivity to estradiol, thromboembolic disorders, pregnancy **D**

Precautions: Edema, hepatic disease, CVA, MI, seizures, hypertension, diabetes mellitus

Pharmacokinetics	
Absorption	Well absorbed
Distribution	Prostatic area
Metabolism	Liver
Excretion	Bile, feces
Half-life	20 hr (terminal)

Pharmacodynamics	
Onset	1-2 hr
Peak	1-2 hr
Duration	1-2 hr

Interactions
Drug classifications
Calcium supplements:
Blocked absorption
Live virus vaccines: ↑ adverse reactions

Food/drug
Calcium (dairy foods):
Blocked absorption
Smoking
↑ cardiotoxicity

NURSING CONSIDERATIONS
Assessment
• Assess symptoms indicating severe allergic reaction: rash, pruritus, urticaria, purpuric skin lesions, itching, flushing
• Monitor temp q4h (may indicate beginning of infection)
• Monitor liver function tests before and during therapy (bilirubin, AST, ALT, LDH) as needed or monthly; yellowing of skin, sclera, dark urine, clay-colored stools, itchy skin, abdominal pain, fever, diarrhea; renal function studies: BUN, urine CrCl, electrolytes before and during therapy
• Assess patient for bleeding: hematuria, stool guaiac, bruising or petechiae, mucosa or orifices q8h; inflammation of mucosa, breaks in skin

Nursing diagnoses
✓ Injury, risk for (adverse reactions)
✓ Body image disturbance (adverse reactions)
✓ Infection, risk for (adverse reactions)
✓ Knowledge deficit (teaching)

Implementation
• Give in divided doses over 1-3 mo; administer with water 1 hr ac or 2 hr pc; give antiemetic if nausea, vomiting, or anorexia become severe; do not give with calcium-rich products or antacids with calcium
🚫• Do not crush, chew caps

Patient/family education
• Teach patient to avoid use of products containing aspirin or ibuprofen, razors, commercial mouthwash—bleeding may occur; to report symptoms of bleeding (hematuria, tarry stools)
• Instruct patient to report signs of anemia, (fatigue, headache, irritability, faintness, shortness of breath)
• Caution patient that contraception is needed during treatment and several mo after
• Teach patient to watch for pain, swelling, redness, tenderness, change in vision and chest pain; should be reported immediately to prescriber (thromboembolic disorders)

Evaluation
Positive therapeutic outcome
• Prevention of rapid division of malignant cells

---

estrogenic substances, conjugated ⊶ (℞)
C.E.S ✹, conjugated estrogens, Premarin, Premarin Intravenous
Func. class.: Estrogen hormone
Chem. class.: Nonsteroidal synthetic estrogen
Pregnancy category **X**

Action: Needed for adequate functioning of female reproductive system; affects release of pituitary gonadotropins; inhibits ovulation; promotes adequate calcium use in bone structures
▸**Therapeutic Outcome:** Decreased tumor size in prostatic cancer; increased estrogen levels in menopause, female hypogonadism

Uses: Menopause, breast cancer, prostatic cancer, abnormal uterine bleeding, hypogonadism, castration, primary ovarian failure, osteoporosis

Dosage and routes
Menopause
Adult: PO 0.3-1.25 mg qd 3 wk on, 1 wk off
Osteoporosis
Adult: PO 0.625 mg qd or in a cycle
Atrophic vaginitis
Adult: Vag 2-4g cream qd × 21 days, off 7 days, repeat
Prostatic cancer
Adult: PO 1.25-2.5 mg tid
Breast cancer
Adult: PO 10 mg tid × 3 mo or longer
Abnormal uterine bleeding
Adult: **IV**/IM 25 mg, repeat in 6-12 hr
Ovariectomy/primary ovarian failure
Adult: PO 1.25 mg qd 3 wk on, 1 wk off
Hypogonadism
Adult: PO 2.5 mg bid-tid × 20 days/mo

Available forms: Tabs 0.3, 0.625, 0.9, 1.25, 2.5 mg; inj 25 mg/vial; vag cream 0.625 mg/g

Adverse effects
CNS: Dizziness, headache, migraine, depression, **seizures**
CV: Hypotension, thrombophlebitis, edema, **thromboembolism, stroke, pulmonary embolism, MI**
EENT: Contact lens intolerance, increased myopia, astigmatism
GI: Nausea, vomiting, diar-

rhea, anorexia, pancreatitis, cramps, constipation, increased appetite, increased weight, **cholestatic jaundice, hepatic adenoma**

GU: Amenorrhea, cervical erosion, breakthrough bleeding, dysmenorrhea, vaginal candidiasis, breast changes, *gynecomastia, testicular atrophy, impotence,* **increased risk of breast, endometrial cancer**

INTEG: Rash, urticaria, acne, hirsutism, alopecia, oily skin, seborrhea, purpura, melasma

META: Folic acid deficiency, hypercalcemia, hyperglycemia

Contraindications: Breast cancer, thromboembolic disorders, reproductive cancer, genital bleeding (abnormal, undiagnosed), pregnancy **X**, lactation

Precautions: Hypertension, asthma, blood dyscrasias, gallbladder disease, CHF, diabetes mellitus, bone disease, depression, migraine headache, convulsive disorders, hepatic disease, renal disease, family history of cancer of breast or reproductive tract

◤ Do Not Confuse:
Premarin/Provera

Pharmacokinetics

Absorption	Well absorbed (PO), completely absorbed **(IV)**	
Distribution	Widely distributed, crosses placenta	
Metabolism	Liver—exclusively; hepatic recirculation	
Excretion	Kidney	
Half-life	Unknown	

Pharmacodynamics

	PO	IM	IV
Onset	Rapid	Slow	Immediate
Peak	Unknown	Unknown	Unknown
Duration	Unknown	Unknown	Unknown

E

Interactions
Individual drugs
Cyclosporine: ↑ toxicity
Dantrolene: ↑ toxicity
Phenylbutazone: ↓ action of phenylbutazone
Rifampin: ↓ action of phenylbutazone
Tamoxifen: ↓ tamoxifen action
Drug classifications
Anticoagulants: ↓ action of anticoagulants
Anticonvulsants: ↓ action of chlorotrianisene
Antidepressants, tricyclics: ↑ toxicity
Barbiturates: ↓ action of chlorotrianisene
Corticosteroids: ↑ action of corticosteroids
Oral hypoglycemics: ↓ action of hypoglycemics
Food/drug
Grapefruit: ↑ estrogen level
Lab test interferences
↑ BSP retention test; ↑ PBI, ↑ T_4; ↑ serum sodium; ↑ platelet aggressability; ↑ thyroxine-binding globulin (TBG); ↑ prothrombin; ↑ factors VII, VIII, IX, X; ↑ triglycerides
↓ Serum folate, ↓ serum triglyceride, ↓ T_3 resin uptake test, ↓ glucose tolerance test, ↓ antithrombin III, ↓ pregnanediol, ↓ metyrapone test
False positive: LE prep, antinuclear antibodies

NURSING CONSIDERATIONS
Assessment
- Monitor blood glucose in patient with diabetes; increased urine glucose may occur
- Monitor B/P q4h; watch for increase caused by water and sodium retention
- Monitor I&O ratio; be alert for decreasing urinary output and increasing edema; monitor weight daily; notify prescriber if weekly weight gain is >5 lb; if increased, diuretic may be ordered
- Obtain liver function studies, including AST, ALT, bilirubin, alk phosphatase
- Assess edema, hypertension, cardiac symptoms, jaundice
- Assess mental status: affect, mood, behavioral changes, aggression; depression may occur, drug may need to be discontinued
- Assess female patient for intact uterus, if so, progesterone should be added to estrogen therapy to decrease risk of endometrial cancer

Nursing diagnoses
- ☑ Sexual dysfunction (uses)
- ☑ Injury, risk for (adverse reactions)

Implementation
PO route
- Give titrated dose, use lowest effective dose
- Give in one dose in AM for prostatic cancer, vaginitis, hypogonadism
- Give with food or milk to decrease GI symptoms

IM route
- Reconstitute after withdrawing at least 5 ml of air from container and inject sterile diluent on vial side, rotate to dissolve
- Give IM injection deeply in large muscle

IV route
- Direct IV: Reconstitute as for IM, inject into distal port of running IV line of D_5W, 0.9% NaCl, LR, at a rate of 5 mg/min or less

Y-site compatibilities: Heparin/hydrocortisone, potassium chloride, vit B/C

Vag route
- Place cream in applicator by attaching tube to applicator, squeeze cream into tube to mark, insert with patient recumbent
- Applicator should be washed after each use

Patient/family education
- Caution patient to take exactly as prescribed and not to double doses
- Advise patient that increased weight gain and symptoms of fluid retention should be reported to prescriber: edema of feet, ankles, sacral area; abnormal vaginal bleeding; breast lumps; hepatic disease (dark urine, clay-colored stools, jaundice of skin, sclera, pruritus)
- Caution patient that thromboembolic symptoms should be reported: tenderness in legs, chest pain, dyspnea, headaches, blurred vision
- Inform patient that sunburns may occur and to use sunscreen and protective clothing
- Advise patient to stop smoking because smoking increases the chance of developing a thromboembolic disorder
- Tell patient to use a nonhormonal birth control, and to notify prescriber if pregnancy is suspected

---

Evaluation
Positive therapeutic outcome
• Reversal of menopause symptoms
• Decrease in tumor size in prostatic, breast cancer
• Decrease in itching, inflammation of vagina
• Absence of symptoms of osteoporosis

etanercept (R)
(eh-tan'er-sept)
Enbrel
Func. class.: Biological
Pregnancy category   B

Action: Binds to tumor necrosis factor (TNF), which decreases inflammation and immune response

Therapeutic Outcome: Decreased pain, inflammation

Uses: Acute, chronic rheumatoid arthritis that has not responded to other treatments

Dosage and routes
Osteoarthritis
Adult: SC 25 mg 2×/wk, may be given with other drugs for rheumatoid arthritis
P *Child 4-17 yr:* SC 0.4 mg/kg, max 25 mg, 2×/wk

Available forms: Powder for inj: 25 mg

Adverse effects
CNS: Headache, asthenia, dizziness
GI: Abdominal pain, dyspepsia
INTEG: Rash, *inj site reaction*
RESP: Pharyngitis, rhinitis, *cough, URI*, non-URI sinusitis

Contraindications: Hypersensitivity, sepsis

Precautions: Pregnancy **B**,
P lactation, children <4 yr

Pharmacokinetics
Absorption	Rapidly
Distribution	Unknown
Metabolism	Unknown
Excretion	Unknown
Half-life	115 hr

Pharmacodynamics
Onset	Unknown
Peak	Unknown
Duration	Unknown

Interactions
Drug classifications
Immunizations: Do not give concurrently
Vaccines: Do not give concurrently

NURSING CONSIDERATIONS
Assessment
• Assess for pain of rheumatoid arthritis; check ROM, inflammation of joints, characteristics of pain

Nursing diagnoses
☑ Pain (uses)
☑ Mobility, impaired physical (uses)
☑ Injury, risk for (side effects)
☑ Knowledge deficit (teaching)

Implementation
SC route
• Administer after reconstituting 1 ml of supplied diluent, slowly inject diluent into vial, swirl contents, do not shake, sol should be clear/colorless, do not use if cloudy or discolored
• Do not admix with other sol or medications; do not use filter

Patient/family education
• Teach patient that drug must be continued for prescribed time to be effective; to avoid aspirin, alcoholic beverages

---

• Instruct patient to use caution when driving; dizziness may occur
• Teach patient about self-administration, if appropriate: inj should be made in thigh, abdomen, upper arm; rotate sites at least 1 in from old site

Evaluation

Positive therapeutic outcome
• Decreased pain in arthritic conditions
• Decreased inflammation in arthritic conditions

---

ethambutol (℞)

(e-tham'byoo-tole)
Etibi ✿, Myambutol
Func. class.: Antitubercular
Chem. class.: Diisopropyl-ethylene diamide derivative

Pregnancy category   C

Action: Inhibits RNA synthesis, decreases tubercle bacilli replication

⇒ **Therapeutic Outcome:** Resolution of TB infection

Uses: Pulmonary tuberculosis, as an adjunct, other mycobacterial infections

Dosage and routes
P *Adult and child >13 yr:* PO 15-25 mg/kg/day as a single dose

Renal dose
CrCl 10-50 ml/min dose q24-36h; CrCl <10 ml/min dose q48h

Retreatment
Adult: PO 25 mg/kg/day as single dose × 2 mo with at least 1 other drug, then decrease to 15 mg/kg/day as single dose, max 2.5 g/day

P *Child:* 15 mg/kg/day

Available forms: Tabs 100, 400 mg

Adverse effects
CNS: Headache, confusion, fever, malaise, dizziness, *disorientation,* hallucinations
EENT: Blurred vision, optic neuritis, photophobia, decreased visual acuity
GI: Abdominal distress, anorexia, nausea, vomiting
INTEG: Dermatitis, pruritus, **toxic epidermal necrolysis**
META: Elevated uric acid, acute gout, liver function impairment
MISC: **Thrombocytopenia,** joint pain, bloody sputum, **anaphylaxis**

Contraindications: Hypersensitivity, optic neuritis, child <13 yr

Precautions: Renal disease, diabetic retinopathy, cataracts, ocular defects, hepatic and hematopoietic disorders, pregnancy C

Pharmacokinetics

Absorption	Rapidly absorbed
Distribution	Widely distributed, crosses blood-brain barrier, placenta
Metabolism	Liver
Excretion	Kidneys— unchanged
Half-life	3 hr, increased in liver, kidney disease

Pharmacodynamics

Onset	Rapid
Peak	2-4 hr

Interactions
Individual drugs
Cisplatin: ↑ renal toxicity
Drug classifications
Antacids, aluminum: ↓ absorption

NURSING CONSIDERATIONS
Assessment

• Obtain C&S tests including sputum tests before initiating treatment; monitor q mo to detect resistance

• Monitor liver studies qwk: ALT, AST, bilirubin; renal studies: before, qmo: BUN, creatinine, output, specific gravity, urinalysis, uric acid

• Assess patient's mental status often: affect, mood, behavioral changes; psychosis may occur with hallucinations, confusion

• Assess patient's hepatic status: decreased appetite, jaundice, dark urine, fatigue

• Assess patient for visual disturbance that may indicate optic neuritis: blurred vision, change in color perception may lead to blindness

Nursing diagnoses

☑ Infection, risk for (uses)
☑ Diarrhea (adverse reactions)
☑ Sensory-perceptual alterations (adverse reactions)
☑ Knowledge deficit (teaching)
☑ Noncompliance (teaching)

Implementation

• Give with meals to decrease GI symptoms, at same time each day to maintain blood level

• Give 2 hr before antacids

• Give antiemetic if vomiting occurs

Patient/family education

• Advise patient that compliance with dosage schedule and duration is necessary to eradicate disease; to keep scheduled appointments including ophthalmic appointments or relapse may occur

• Caution patient to report weakness, fatigue, loss of appetite, nausea, vomiting, yellowing of skin or eyes, tingling/numbness of hands/feet, weight gain, or decreased urine output

• Instruct patient to report any visual changes or rash to physician

• Caution patient to inform prescriber if pregnancy is suspected

Evaluation
Positive therapeutic outcome

• Decreased symptoms of TB

E

---

ethosuximide (℞)

(eth-oh-sux′i-mide)
Zarontin
Func. class.: Anticonvulsant
Chem. class.: Succinimide
Pregnancy category   C

Action: Inhibits spike and wave formation in absence seizures (petit mal); decreases amplitude, frequency, duration, spread of discharge in minor motor seizures

Therapeutic Outcome: Decreased seizure activity

Uses: Absence seizures, partial seizures, tonic-clonic seizures

Dosage and routes

Adult and child >6 yr: PO 250 mg bid initially; may increase by 250 mg q4-7d, not to exceed 1.5 g/day

Child 3-6 yr: PO 250 mg/day or 125 mg bid; may increase by 250 mg q4-7d, not to exceed 1.5 g/day

Available forms: Cap 250 mg; syr 250 mg/5 ml

Adverse effects

CNS: Drowsiness, dizziness, fatigue, euphoria, lethargy, anxiety, aggressiveness, irrita-

---

bility, depression, insomnia, headache
EENT: Myopia, blurred vision
GI: Nausea, vomiting, heartburn, anorexia, diarrhea, abdominal pain, cramps, constipation, hiccups, weight loss, gum hypertrophy, tongue swelling
GU: Vaginal bleeding; pink, brown urine
HEMA: **Agranulocytosis, aplastic anemia, thrombocytopenia, leukocytosis, eosinophilia, pancytopenia**
INTEG: Urticaria, pruritic erythema, hirsutism, **Stevens-Johnson syndrome**

Contraindications: Hypersensitivity to succinimide derivatives

Precautions: Lactation, pregnancy **C**, hepatic disease, renal disease

Pharmacokinetics

Absorption	Rapidly, completely absorbed
Distribution	Body water
Metabolism	Liver
Excretion	Kidneys, 10% unchanged
Half-life	Adult—60 hr; **P** child—24-30 hr

Pharmacodynamics

Onset	Several hr, days
Peak	1-7 days
Duration	Days
Steady state	4-7 days

Interactions
Individual drugs
Alcohol: ↑ CNS depression
Phenytoin: ↑ metabolism, ↓ effectiveness
Valproic acid: ↑ or ↓ valproic acid levels

Drug classifications
Antidepressants: ↑ CNS depression, decreased seizure threshold
Antihistamines: ↑ CNS depression
MAOIs: ↓ seizure threshold
Opiates: ↑ CNS depression
Phenothiazines: ↓ seizure threshold
Sedative/hypnotics: ↑ CNS depression

NURSING CONSIDERATIONS
Assessment
• Monitor drug level: therapeutic level 30-50 µg/ml
• Assess blood studies; CBC platelets q2 wk until stabilized, then qmo × 12, then q3 mo
• Assess mental status: mood, sensorium, affect, memory (long, short)
• Assess respiratory depression: rate, depth, character
• Assess blood dyscrasias: fever, sore throat, bruising, rash, jaundice

Nursing diagnoses
✓ Injury, risk for (adverse reactions)
✓ Knowledge deficit (teaching)

Implementation
• Administer on empty stomach for best absorption

Patient/family education
• Teach patient to carry ID card or Medic-Alert bracelet stating patient's name, drugs taken, condition, prescriber's name, phone number
• Caution patient to avoid driving, other activities that require alertness; to avoid alcohol ingestion and CNS depressants because increased sedation may occur
• Advise patient not to discontinue medication abruptly after

---

long-term use; absence seizures may occur
• Inform patient that drug must be taken as prescribed; not to double doses because serious reactions may occur; may take drug within 4 hr if missed
• Advise patient to notify prescriber of hepatic symptoms, blood dyscrasia (fatigue, fever, sore throat, bruises, rash)
• Inform patient about symptoms of thrombocytopenia, leukopenia; instruct to notify prescriber if these occur
• Caution patient to notify prescriber if pregnancy is anticipated or suspected
• Inform patient that urine may become pink or brown
🚫 • Do not chew, crush caps

Evaluation
Positive therapeutic outcome
• Decreased seizure activity

Treatment of overdose:
Lavage, activated charcoal, warming blanket, vital signs; monitor electrolytes

---

etidronate (℞)
(eh-tih-droe'nate)
Didronel, Didronel IV
Func. class.: Parathyroid agent (calcium regulator)
Chem. class.: Diphosphate
Pregnancy category **C**

Action: Decreases bone resorption and new bone development (accretion)

→**Therapeutic Outcome:** Decreased bone reabsorption, calcium levels WNL

Uses: Paget's disease, heterotopic ossification, hypercalcemia of malignancy

Dosage and routes
Paget's disease
Adult: PO 5-10 mg/kg/day 2 hr ac with water, not to exceed 20 mg/kg/day, max 6 mo or 11-20 mg/kg/day for max of 3 mo

Heterotopic ossification
Adult: PO 20 mg/kg qd × 2 wk, then 10 mg/kg/day for 10 wk, total 12 wk

Hypercalcemia
Adult: **IV** 7.5 mg/kg/day × 3 days, then 20 mg/kg/day (PO)

Heterotopic ossification/hip replacement
Adult: PO 20 mg/kg/day × 4 wk before and 3 mo after surgery

Available forms: Tabs 200, 400 mg; inj 300 mg/6 ml

Adverse effects
CNS: **Seizures**
GI: *Nausea, diarrhea*
GU: **Nephrotoxicity**
MS: *Bone pain,* hypocalcemia, decreased mineralization of nonaffected bones

Contraindications: Pathologic fractures, children, colitis, severe renal disease with creatinine >5 mg/dl

Precautions: Pregnancy **C**, renal disease, lactation, restricted vit D/Ca

Do Not Confuse:
etidronate/etretinate, etidronate/etomidate

E

P

Pharmacokinetics

Absorption	Poorly absorbed (PO), completely absorbed (**IV**)
Distribution	50% bond to crystals in osteogenesis
Metabolism	None
Excretion	Feces (unabsorbed), kidney (unchanged)
Half-life	5-7 hr; in bone >3 mo

Pharmacodynamics

	PO	IV
Onset	4 wk	24 hr
Peak	Unknown	3-4 days
Duration	Up to 1 yr	10-12 days

Interactions
Individual drugs
Didanosine: ↓ absorption of etidronate
Calcitonin: ↑ effect of calcitonin
Drug classifications
Antacids: ↓ absorption of etidronate
Mineral supplements with magnesium, calcium, or aluminum: ↓ absorption of etidronate
Food/drug
Dairy products: ↓ absorption of etidronate

NURSING CONSIDERATIONS
Assessment
• Assess for GI symptoms, polyuria, flushing, head swelling, tingling, headache—may indicate hypercalcemia; nervousness, irritability, twitching, seizures, spasm, paresthesia indicates hypocalcemia at start of treatment
• Identify nutritional status; evaluate diet for sources of vitamin D (milk, some seafood), calcium (dairy products, dark green vegetables), phosphates
• Monitor BUN, creatinine, uric acid, chloride, electrolytes, urine pH, urinary calcium, magnesium, phosphate, urinalysis (calcium should be kept at 9-10 mg/dl), albumin, alk phosphatase baseline and q3-6 mo; check urine sediment for casts throughout treatment
• Assess for increased drug level—toxic reactions occur rapidly; have calcium chloride or gluconate on hand if calcium level drops too low; check for tetany

Nursing diagnoses
☑ Injury, risk for (adverse reactions)
☑ Pain, chronic (uses)
☑ Knowledge deficit (teaching)

Implementation
PO route
• Administer on empty stomach to improve absorption (2 hr ac)
IV IV route
• Used in hypercalcemias—give by intermittent inf after diluting 300 mg/250 ml or more 0.9% NaCl; run over 2-3 hr

Patient/family education
• Teach method of inj if patient will be responsible for self-medication
• Caution patient to notify prescriber of hypercalcemic relapse: renal calculi, nausea, vomiting, thirst, lethargy, deep bone or flank pain
• Teach patient that warmth and flushing occur and last 1 hr
• Teach patient to follow a low-calcium diet as prescribed (Paget's disease, hypercalcemia)
• Advise patient to notify prescriber of diarrhea, nausea; dose may be divided to lessen these symptoms

• Inform patient that metallic taste may occur with **IV** dosing

Evaluation
Positive therapeutic outcome
• Calcium levels 9-10 mg/dl
• Decreasing symptoms of Paget's disease including pain
• Decreased bone loss in osteoporosis

---

etodolac (℞)
(ee-toe-doe′lak)
Lodine, Lodine XL
Func. class.: Nonsteroidal antiinflammatory, non-opioid analgesic
Pregnancy category C

Action: Inhibits prostaglandin synthesis by decreasing enzyme needed for biosynthesis; analgesic, antiinflammatory properties

➔**Therapeutic Outcome:** Decreased pain, inflammation

Uses: Mild to moderate pain, osteoarthritis

Dosage and routes
Osteoarthritis
Adult: PO 800-1200 mg/day in divided doses q6-8h initially, then adjust to 600-1200 mg/day in divided doses; do not exceed 1200 mg/day; patients <60 kg not to exceed 20 mg/kg

Analgesia
Adult: PO 200-400 mg q6-8h prn for acute pain; do not exceed 1200 mg/day; patients <60 kg, not to exceed 20 mg/kg

Available forms: Caps 200, 300 mg; tabs 400, 500 mg; ext rel 400, 600 mg

Adverse effects
CNS: Dizziness, headache, drowsiness, fatigue, tremors, confusion, insomnia, anxiety, depression, light-headedness, vertigo
CV: Tachycardia, peripheral edema, fluid retention, palpitations, dysrhythmias, CHF
EENT: Tinnitus, hearing loss, blurred vision, photophobia
GI: Nausea, anorexia, vomiting, diarrhea, jaundice, **cholestatic hepatitis,** constipation, flatulence, cramps, dry mouth, peptic ulcer, dyspepsia, **GI bleeding**
GU: **Nephrotoxicity: dysuria, hematuria, oliguria, azotemia, cystitis,** UTI
HEMA: **Blood dyscrasias,** epistaxis, bruising
INTEG: Erythema, urticaria, purpura, rash, pruritus, sweating, **Steven-Johnson syndrome**

Contraindications: Hypersensitivity; patients in whom aspirin, iodides, or other NSAIDs have produced asthma, rhinitis, urticaria, nasal polyps, angioedema, bronchospasm

Precautions: Pregnancy **C**, lactation, children, bleeding, GI, cardiac disorders, elderly; renal, hepatic disorders

Do Not Confuse: Lodine/codeine

Pharmacokinetics	
Absorption	Well absorbed
Distribution	Highly bound to plasma protein
Metabolism	Unknown
Excretion	Unknown
Half-life	7 hr

Pharmacodynamics	
Onset	½ hr
Peak	1-2 hr
Duration	4-12 hr

Interactions
Individual drugs

Acetaminophen (long-term use): ↑ renal reactions
Alcohol: ↑ adverse reactions
Aspirin: ↓ effectiveness, ↑ adverse reactions
Coumadin: ↑ anticoagulant effects
Cyclosporine: ↑ toxicity
Digoxin: ↑ toxicity, ↑ levels
Insulin: ↓ insulin effect
Lithium: ↑ toxicity
Methotrexate: ↑ toxicity
Phenytoin: ↑ toxicity
Probenecid: ↑ toxicity
Sulfonylurea: ↑ toxicity
Drug classifications

Antacids: ↓ etodolac effect
Anticoagulants: ↑ risk of bleeding
Antihypertensives: ↓ effect of antihypertensives
Antineoplastics: ↑ risk of hematologic toxicity
β-Adrenergic blockers: ↓ effect
Cephalosporins: ↑ risk of bleeding
Diuretics: ↓ effectiveness of diuretics, ↓ antihypertensive effects
Glucocorticoids: ↑ adverse reactions
Hypoglycemics: ↓ hypoglycemic effect
Nonsteroidal antiinflammatories: ↑ adverse reactions
Potassium supplements: ↑ adverse reactions
Radiation: ↑ risk of hematologic toxicity
Sulfonamides: ↑ toxicity

NURSING CONSIDERATIONS
Assessment
• Assess pain: location, frequency, characteristics; relief after med
• Assess for GI bleeding: black stools, hematemesis
• Assess for asthma, aspirin hypersensitivity, nasal polyps that may be hypersensitive to etodolac
• Monitor blood counts during therapy; watch for decreasing platelets; if low, therapy may need to be discontinued, then restarted after hematologic recovery; watch for blood dyscrasia (thrombocytopenia): bruising, fatigue, bleeding, poor healing

Nursing diagnoses
☑ Pain (uses)
☑ Mobility, impaired physical (uses)
☑ Knowledge deficit (teaching)
☑ Injury, risk for (adverse reactions)

Implementation
• Administer with food or milk to decrease gastric symptoms; food will slow absorption slightly, will not decrease absorption.
🚫• Do not crush, chew ext rel tabs

Patient / family education
• Inform patient that drug must be continued for prescribed time to be effective; to avoid aspirin, alcoholic beverages
• Caution patient to report bleeding, bruising, fatigue, malaise because blood dyscrasias can occur
• Instruct patient to use caution when driving; drowsiness, dizziness may occur
• Teach patient to take with a full glass of water to enhance

---

absorption; do not crush, break, or chew medication

Evaluation
Positive therapeutic outcome
• Decreased pain
• Decreased inflammation
• Increased mobility

---

etoposide (VP-16) (℞)
(e-toe'poe-side)
Etopophos, VePesid
Func. class.: Antineoplastic
—misc.
Chem. class.: Semisynthetic
podophyllotoxin
Pregnancy category **D**

Action: Inhibits mitotic activity through metaphase to mitosis; also inhibits cells from entering mitosis, depresses DNA, RNA synthesis

Therapeutic Outcome: Prevention of rapid growth of malignant cells

Uses: Leukemias, lung, testicular cancer, lymphomas, neuroblastoma, melanoma, ovarian cancer; being investigated for use in leukemia, lymphoma

Dosage and routes
Adult: **IV** 45-75 mg/m²/day × 3-5 days given q3-5 wk or 200-250 mg/m²/wk, or 125-140 mg/m²/day 3 × wk, q5 wk

Adult: **PO** 70 mg/m²/day × 4 days, repeated q3-4 wk up to 100 mg/m²/day × 5 days q3-4 wk

Available forms: Inj 20 mg/ml; 113.6 etoposide phosphate = 100 etoposide; caps 50 mg

Adverse effects
CNS: Headache, *fever*
CV: **Hypotension**
GI: Nausea, *vomiting, anorexia,* **hepatotoxicity**
GU: **Nephrotoxicity**
HEMA: **Thrombocytopenia, leukopenia, myelosuppression, anemia**
INTEG: *Rash, alopecia,* phlebitis at **IV** site
RESP: **Bronchospasm**
SYST: **Anaphylaxis**

Contraindications: Hypersensitivity, bone marrow depression, severe hepatic disease, severe renal disease, bacterial infection, pregnancy **D**

Precautions: Renal disease, hepatic disease, lactation, children, gout

Do Not Confuse:
VePesid/Versed

Pharmacokinetics	
Absorption	Variably absorbed
Distribution	Rapidly absorbed, 97% protein binding, crosses placenta
Metabolism	Liver—some
Excretion	Kidneys, unchanged 50%, breast milk
Half-life	3 hr initially, 15 hr terminally

Pharmacodynamics
Unknown

Interactions
Individual drugs
Radiation: ↑ toxicity, bone marrow suppression
Drug classifications
Antineoplastics: ↑ toxicity, bone marrow suppression
Live virus vaccines: ↑ adverse reactions

NURSING CONSIDERATIONS
Assessment
• Monitor B/P, (baseline and q15 min) during administration
• Monitor CBC, differential, platelet count weekly; withhold drug if WBC is <4000 or platelet count is <75,000; notify prescriber of results—recovery will take 3 wk
• Monitor renal function studies: BUN, urine CrCl before, during therapy; I&O ratio; report fall in urine output of 30 ml/hr; for decreased hyperuricemia
• Monitor for cold, fever, sore throat (may indicate beginning infection); notify prescriber if these occur
• Assess for bleeding: hematuria, guaiac, bruising or petechiae, mucosa or orifices q8h: no rectal temp; avoid IM inj; use pressure to venipuncture sites
• Identify nutritional status: an antiemetic may need to be prescribed
• Assess for symptoms indicating severe allergic reactions: rash, pruritus, urticaria, itching, flushing, bronchospasm, hypotension; epinephrine and crash cart should be nearby

Nursing diagnoses
☑ Injury, risk for (adverse reactions)
☑ Body image disturbance (adverse reactions)
☑ Infection, risk for (adverse reactions)
☑ Knowledge deficit (teaching)

Implementation
PO route
• Caps need to be refrigerated

IV route
• Give by intermittent inf
• Sol should be prepared by qualified personnel and only under controlled conditions
• Use Luer Loc tubing to prevent leakage; do not let sol come in contact with skin—if contact occurs, wash well with soap and water
• Give after diluting 100 mg/250 ml or more D_5W or NaCl to a concentration of 0.2-0.4 mg/ml; infuse over 30-60 min; phosphate may be given over 5 min-3½ hr; may dilute further to 0.1 mg/ml in 0.9% NaCl, D_5W
• Give hyaluronidase 150 U/ml to 1 ml NaCl to infiltration area; ice compress for treatment of vesicant activity

Y-site compatibilities:
Allopurinol, amifostine, aztreonam, cladribine, fludarabine, granisetron, melphalan, ondansetron, paclitaxel, piperacillin/tazobactam, sargramostim, sodium bicarbonate, teniposide, thiotepa, vinorelbine

Y-site incompatibility:
Idarubicin

Additive compatibilities:
Carboplatin, cisplatin, cytarabine, floxuridine, fluorouracil, hydroxyzine, ifosfamide, ondansetron

Patient/family education
• Teach patient to avoid use of products containing aspirin or ibuprofen, razors, commercial mouthwash because bleeding may occur; to report symptoms of bleeding (hematuria, tarry stools)
• Instruct patient to report signs of anemia (fatigue, head-

ache, irritability, faintness, shortness of breath)
• Teach patient to report any changes in breathing or coughing even several months after treatment
• Advise patient that contraception will be necessary during treatment because teratogenesis may occur
• Caution patient that hair loss may occur during treatment; a wig or hairpiece may make patient feel better; new hair will be different in color, texture
• Advise patient to avoid vaccinations during treatment because serious reactions may occur
• Teach patient to report signs/symptoms of infection; fever, chills, sore throat; patient should avoid crowds and persons with known infections

Evaluation
Positive therapeutic outcome
• Decreased spread of malignant, leukemic cells

exemestane
See Appendix A,
Selected New Drugs

factor IX complex (human)/factor IX (℞)
Konyne 80, Proplex T, Proplex SX-T, Profilnine Heat-Treated/Alphanine, Alpha Nine SD, Mononine
Func. class.: Hemostatic
Chem. class.: Factors II, VII, IX, X

Pregnancy category **C**

Action: Causes an increase in blood levels of clotting factors II, VII, IX, X; factor IX (human) has IX activity only

Therapeutic Outcome: Replacement of factors II, VII, IX, X

Uses: Hemophilia B (Christmas disease), factor IX deficiency, anticoagulant reversal, control of bleeding in patients with factor VIII inhibitors; reversal of overdose of anticoagulants in emergencies

Dosage and routes
Bleeding in hemophilia A and inhibitors of factor VIII
Adult and child: 75 U/kg, repeat in 12 hr

Bleeding in hemophilia B
Adult and child: Give to establish 25% of normal factor IX activity or 60-75 U/kg/day then 10-20 U/kg/day × 1 wk

Prophylaxis of bleeding in hemophilia B
Adult and child: 10-20 U/kg/day × 1 wk

Reversal of oral anticoagulant
Adult and child: 15 U/kg

F

Factor VII deficiency (use Proplex T)
P *Adult and child:* 0.5 U/kg × body weight (kg) × desired factor IX increase (in % of normal); repeat q4-6h if needed

Factor IX AlphaNine, AlphaNine SD (minor to moderate hemorrhage)
P *Adult and child:* Give amount to increase plasma factor IX level to 20%-30%

Serious hemorrhage
P *Adult and child:* Give amount to increase plasma factor IX level to 30%-50% given as daily inf

Mononine
Minor hemorrhage
P *Adult and child:* Give amount to increase plasma factor IX level to 15%-25% (20-30 U/kg), may repeat in 24 hr

Major trauma
P *Adult and child:* Give amount to increase plasma factor IX level to 25%-50% (75 U/kg) q1830 h for up to 10 days

Available forms: Inj (number of units noted on label)

Adverse effects
CNS: Headache, dizziness, malaise, paresthesia, *lethargy, chills, fever, flushing*
CV: Hypotension, tachycardia, **MI, venous thrombosis, pulmonary embolism**
EENT: Tinnitus, eyelid swelling
GI: Nausea, vomiting, abdominal cramps, jaundice, **viral hepatitis**
HEMA: **Thrombosis, hemolysis, AIDS, DIC**
INTEG: Rash, flushing, *urticaria*
RESP: Bronchospasm

Contraindications: Hypersensitivity, hepatic disease, DIC, elective surgery, mild factor IX deficiency

Precautions: Neonates/
P infants, pregnancy **C**

Pharmacokinetics	
Absorption	40% (PO), complete (**IV**)
Distribution	Unknown
Metabolism	Rapidly cleared from plasma, liver 30%
Excretion	70% unchanged—kidneys
Half-life	24 hr

Pharmacodynamics
Unknown

Interactions
Individual drugs
Aminocaproic acid: ↑ risk of thrombosis; do not use together

NURSING CONSIDERATIONS
Assesment
• Monitor blood studies (coagulation factor assays by % normal: 5% prevents spontaneous hemorrhage, 30%-50% for surgery, 80%-100% for severe hemorrhage); check for bleeding q15-30 min, immobilize and apply ice to affected joints
• Monitor for increased B/P, pulse
• Monitor I&O; if urine becomes orange or red, notify prescriber
• Assess for allergic or pyrogenic reaction: fever, chills, rash, itching; slow inf rate if not severe
◆• Assess for DIC: bleeding, ecchymosis, hypersensitivity, changes in coagulation tests

---

Nursing diagnoses
✓ Injury, risk for (uses)
✓ Tissue perfusion, altered (uses)
✓ Knowledge deficit (teaching)

Implementation

IV **IV route**
• Give hepatitis B vaccine before administration
• Give **IV** after warming to room temp 3 ml/min or less, with plastic syringe only; do not admix
• Give after dilution with provided diluent, 50 U/ml or 25 U/ml; give so as not to exceed 10 ml/min; decrease rate if fever, headache, flushing, tingling occur
• Give after crossmatch is completed if patient has blood type A, B, AB, to determine incompatibility with factor
• Store reconstituted sol for 3 hr at room temp or up to 2 yr if refrigerated (powder); check expiration date

Patient/family education
• Advise patient to report any signs of bleeding: gums, under skin, urine, stools, emesis
• Caution patient about risk of viral hepatitis, AIDS; that immunization for hepatitis B may be given first; to be tested q2-3 mo for HIV, even though the risk is low
• Tell patient to carry ID identifying disease and treatment; avoid, salicylates, to inform other health professionals about condition

Evaluation
Positive therapeutic outcome
• Prevention of hemorrhage

famciclovir (℞)
(fam-sye-klo'vir)
Famvir
Func. class.: Antiviral
Chem. class.: Guanosine nucleoside

Pregnancy category **B**

Action: Inhibits DNA polymerase and viral DNA synthesis by the conversion of this guanosine nucleoside to penciclovir

➔**Therapeutic Outcome:** Decreasing size and number of lesions

Uses: Treatment of acute herpes zoster, genital herpes, recurrent herpes in HIV patients

Dosage and routes
Adult: PO 500 mg q8h

Renal dose
If CrCl ≥ 60 ml/min, 500 mg q8h; if 40-59 ml/min, 500 mg q12h; if 20-39 ml/min, 500 mg q24h

Recurrent mucocutaneous herpes simplex
Adult: PO 500 mg bid × 1 wk

Available forms: Tabs 125, 250, 500 mg

Adverse effects
CNS: Headache, fatigue, dizziness, paresthesia, somnolence, fever
GI: Nausea, vomiting, diarrhea, constipation, *abdominal pain, anorexia*
GU: Decreased sperm count
INTEG: Pruritis
MS: Back pain, arthralgia
RESP: Pharyngitis, sinusitis

Contraindications: Hypersensitivity to this drug or penciclovir

F

Precautions: Renal disease, pregnancy **B,** hypersensitivity to acyclovir, ganciclovir

Pharmacokinetics

Absorption	Well absorbed
Distribution	Unknown
Metabolism	Intestinal tissue, blood, liver
Excretion	Breast milk, kidney, bile
Half-life	3 hr

Pharmacodynamics

Onset	Unknown
Peak	1 hr
Duration	8 hr

Interactions
Individual drugs
Cimetidine: ↓ metabolism
Digoxin: ↓ renal excretion
Probenecid: ↓ renal excretion
Theophylline: ↓ renal excretion

NURSING CONSIDERATIONS
Assessment
• Assess amount and distribution of lesions; also burning, itching, or pain (early symptoms of herpes infection)
• Monitor renal function studies: urine CrCl, BUN before and during treatment if patient has decreased renal function; dose may need to be lowered
• Monitor bowel pattern before, during treatment; diarrhea may occur

Nursing diagnoses
☑ Infection, risk for (uses)
☑ Knowledge deficit (teaching)

Implementation
• Give with or without meals; absorption does not appear to be lowered when taken with food

• Give within 72 hr of the appearance of rash in herpes zoster

Patient/family education
• Teach patient how to recognize signs of beginning infection
• Teach patient how to prevent the spread of infection to others
• Teach patient reason for medication and expected results

Evaluation
Positive therapeutic outcome
• Decreased size and spread of lesions

---

famotidine (℞, OTC)
(fa-moe'to-deen)
Pepcid AC acid controller, Pepcid, Pepcid IV
Func. class.: H_2-Histamine receptor antagonist, antiulcer agent

Pregnancy category   B

Action: Inhibits histamine at H_2-receptor site in gastric parietal cells, which inhibits gastric acid secretion

⇒**Therapeutic Outcome:** Healing of duodenal ulcers or gastric ulcers; prevention of duodenal ulcers; decreases symptoms of GERD or Zollinger-Ellison syndrome, heartburn

Uses: Short-term treatment of active duodenal ulcer, maintenance therapy for duodenal ulcer, Zollinger-Ellison syndrome, multiple endocrine adenomas, gastric ulcers, heartburn

---

Dosage and routes
Renal dose
CrCl <10 ml/min 20 mg hs or dose q36-48hr

Duodenal ulcer
Adult: PO 40 mg qd hs × 4-8 wk, then 20 mg qd hs if needed (maintenance); **IV** 20 mg q12h if unable to take PO

Hypersecretory conditions
Adult: PO 20 mg q6h; may give 160 mg q6h if needed; **IV** 20 mg q12h if unable to take PO

Heartburn relief/prevention
Adult: 10 mg with water or 1 hr before eating

Available forms: Tabs 10 (OTC), 20, 40 mg; powder for oral susp 40 mg/5 ml; inj 10 mg/ml, 20 mg/50 ml 0.9% NaCl

Adverse effects
CNS: Headache, dizziness, paresthesia, **seizure,** depression, anxiety, somnolence, insomnia, fever
EENT: Taste change, tinnitus, orbital edema
GI: Constipation, nausea, vomiting, anorexia, cramps, abnormal liver enzymes
HEMA: **Thrombocytopenia**
INTEG: Rash
MS: Myalgia, arthralgia
RESP: **Bronchospasm**

Contraindications: Hypersensitivity

Precautions: Pregnancy **B,** lactation, children <12 yr, severe renal disease, severe hepatic function, elderly

Pharmacokinetics

Absorption	50% absorbed (PO)
Distribution	Plasma, protein binding (15%-20%)
Metabolism	Liver (30% active metabolizing)
Excretion	Kidneys (70%)
Half-life	2½-3½ hr

Pharmacodynamics

	PO	IV
Onset	30-60 min	Immediate
Peak	1-3 hr	½-3 hr
Duration	6-12 hr	6-12 hr

F

Interactions
Individual drugs
Ketoconazole: ↓ absorption of ketoconazole
Drug classifications
Antacids: ↓ absorption of famotidine

NURSING CONSIDERATIONS
Assessment
• Assess patient with ulcers or suspected ulcers: epigastric, abdominal pain, hematemesis, occult blood in stools, blood in gastric, aspirate prior to treatment—throughout treatment, monitor gastric pH (5 should be maintained)
• Monitor I&O ratio, BUN, creatinine, CBC with differential monthly

Nursing diagnoses
☑ Pain (uses)
☑ Knowledge deficit (teaching)

Implementation
PO route
• Give antacids 1 hr before or 2 hr after famotidine; may be given with foods or liq
• Administer oral susp after shaking well; discard unused sol after 1 mo
IV IV route
• Give **IV** direct after diluting 2 ml of drug (10 mg/ml) in 0.9% NaCl to total volume of

5-10 ml; inject over 2 min to prevent hypotension
• Administer **IV** intermittent inf after diluting 20 mg of drug in 100 ml of LR, 0.9% NaCl, D_5W, $D_{10}W$; run over 15-30 min
• Store in cool environment (oral); **IV** solution is stable for 48 hr at room temp; do not use discolored sol

Y-site compatibilities:

Acyclovir, allopurinol, amifostine, aminophylline, amphotericin, ampicillin, ampicillin/sulbactam, amrinone, amsacrine, atropine, aztreonam, bretylium, calcium gluconate, cefazolin, cefoperazone, cefotaxime, cefotetan, cefoxitin, ceftazidime, ceftizoxime, ceftriaxone, cefuroxime, cephalothin, cephapirin, chlorpromazine, cisplatin, cladribine, cyclophosphamide, cytarabine, dexamethasone, dextran 40, digoxin, diphenhydramine, dobutamine, dopamine, doxorubicin, droperidol, enalaprilat, epinephrine, erythromycin lactobionate, esmolol, filgrastim, fluconazole, fludarabine, folic acid, gentamicin, granisetron, haloperidol, heparin, hydrocortisone, hydromorphone, hydroxyzine, imipenem/cilastatin, regular insulin, isoproterenol, labetalol, lidocaine, lorazepam, magnesium sulfate, melphalan, meperidine, methotrexate, methylprednisolone, metoclopramide, mezlocillin, midazolam, morphine, nafcillin, nitroglycerin, nitroprusside, norepinephrine, ondansetron, oxacillin, paclitaxel, perphenazine, phenylephrine, phenytoin, phytonadione, piperacillin, potassium chloride, potassium phosphate, procainamide, propofol, sargramostim, sodium bicarbonate, teniposide, theophylline, thiamine, thiotepa, ticarcillin, ticarcillin/clavulanate, verapamil, vinorelbine

Additive compatibilities:

Cefazolin, cefmetazole, flumazenil

Patient/family education

• Caution patient to avoid driving, other hazardous activities until stabilized on this medication; dizziness may occur
• Advise patient to avoid black pepper, caffeine, alcohol, harsh spices, extremes in temperature of food; tell patient to avoid OTC preparations: aspirin, cough, cold preparations; condition may worsen
• Tell patient that smoking decreases the effectiveness of the drug; that smoking cessation should be considered
• Instruct patient that drug must be continued for prescribed time to be effective and taken exactly as prescribed; doses are not to be doubled; to take missed dose when remembered up to 1 hr before next dose
• Tell patient to report bruising, fatigue, malaise; blood dyscrasias may occur
• Tell patient to report diarrhea, black tarry stools, sore throat, rash, dizziness, confusion, rash, or delirium to prescriber immediately

Evaluation

Positive therapeutic outcome
• Decreased pain in abdomen
• Healing of ulcers

---

fat emulsions (R)
(fat ee-mul'shuns)
Intralipid 10%, Intralipid
20%, Liposyn II 10%, Liposyn
II 20%, Liposyn III 10%,
Liposyn III 20%, Soyacal 20%
Func. class.: Caloric
Chem. class.: Fatty acid,
long chain
Pregnancy category   C

Action: Needed for energy,
heat production; consists of
neutral triglycerides, primarily
unsaturated fatty acids

Therapeutic Outcome: Increased available calories and
fatty acids

Uses: Increase calorie intake,
prevent fatty acid deficiency

Dosage and routes
Deficiency
Adult and child: **IV** 8%-10%
of required calorie intake (intralipid)

Adjunct to TPN
Adult: **IV** 1 ml/min over
15-30 min (10%) or 0.5 ml/
min over 15-30 min (20%);
may increase to 500 ml over
4-8 hr if no adverse reactions
occur; not to exceed 2.5 g/kg

Child: **IV** 0.1 ml/min over
10-15 min (10%) or 0.05 ml/
min over 10-15 min (20%);
may increase to 1 g/kg over 4
hr if no adverse reactions
occur; not to exceed 4 g/kg

Prevention of deficiency
Adult: **IV** 500 ml 2 × wk
(10%), given 1 ml/min for 30
min, not to exceed 500 ml
over 6 hr

Child: **IV** 5-10 ml/kg/day
(10%), given 0.1 ml/min for
30 min, not to exceed 100
ml/hr

Available forms: 10% (50,
100, 200, 250, 500 ml), 20%
(50, 100, 200, 250, 500 ml)

Adverse effects
CNS: Dizziness, headache,
drowsiness, focal seizures
CV: **Shock**
GI: Nausea, vomiting, **hepatomegaly**
HEMA: **Hyperlipemia, hypercoagulation, thrombocytopenia, leukopenia, leukocytosis**
RESP: Dyspnea, **fat in lung
tissue**

Contraindications: Hypersensitivity, hyperlipemia, lipid
necrosis, acute pancreatitis
accompanied by hyperlipemia,
hyperbilirubinemia of the
newborn

Precautions: Severe liver
disease, diabetes mellitus,
thrombocytopenia, gastric
ulcers, premature, term
newborns, pregnancy **C,** sepsis

Pharmacokinetics

Absorption	Completely absorbed
Distribution	Intravascular space
Metabolism	Conversion to triglycerides, to free fatty acids
Excretion	Unknown
Half-life	Unknown

Pharmacodynamics

Unknown

Interactions: None

NURSING CONSIDERATIONS
Assessment
• Monitor triglycerides, free
fatty acid levels, platelet counts
daily to prevent fat overload,
thrombocytopenia
• Monitor liver function
studies: AST, ALT, Hct,

F

Hgb—notify prescriber if abnormal
• Assess nutritional status: calorie count by dietician; monitor weight daily

Nursing diagnoses
☑ Nutrition, less than body requirements (uses)
☑ Knowledge deficit (teaching)

Implementation
• Administer using inf pump at prescribed rate; do not use in-line filter sized for lipid emulsion; clogging will occur
• Do not use mixed sol that look oily or are not separated; discard unused sol
• Change **IV** tubing at each inf: infection may occur with old tubing
• Give by intermittent inf at a rate of 10% sol (1 ml/min); 20% sol (0.5 ml/min) initially for 15-30 min; may be increased to 10% sol (120 ml/hr) or 20% (62.5 ml/hr) if no adverse reactions occur; do not give more than 500 ml
P during the first day; children should be given 10% (0.1 mg/ml) or 20% (0.05 ml/min) initially for 15-30 min, may be increased 1 g/kg/4hr, do not give more than 10% (100 ml/hr) or 20% (50 ml/hr)

Y-site compatibilities:
Ampicillin, cefamandole, cefazolin, cefoxitin, cephapirin, clindamycin, digoxin, dopamine, erythromycin, furosemide, gentamicin, IL-2, isoproterenol, lidocaine, kanamycin, norepinephrine, oxacillin, penicillin G potassium, ticarcillin, tobramycin

Y-site incompatibilities:
Amikacin, tetracycline

Additive compatibilities:
Cefamandole, chloramphenicol, cimetidine, cyclosporine, diphenhydramine, famotidine, heparin, hydrocortisone, multivitamins, nizatidine, penicillin G potassium

Patient/family education
• Teach patient reason for use of lipids and expected results

Evaluation
Positive therapeutic outcome
• Increased weight
• Fatty acids at adequate levels

---

felodipine (℞)
(fell-oh'di-peen)
Plendil, Renedil ✤
Func. class.: Calcium-channel blocker, antihypertensive
Chem. class.: Dihydropyridine
Pregnancy category C

Action: Inhibits calcium ion influx across cell membrane, resulting in dilation of peripheral arteries

Therapeutic Outcome: Decreased B/P in hypertension

Uses: Essential hypertension, alone or with other antihypertensives

Dosage and routes
Adult: PO 5 mg qd initially, usual range 5-10 mg qd; do not exceed 20 mg qd; do not adjust dosage at intervals of <2 wk
G *Elderly:* PO 2.5 mg qd
Hepatic disease
PO 2.5-5 mg qd, max 10 mg/day

Available forms: Ext rel tabs 2.5, 5, 10 mg

☑ Herb/drug   ◎ Do Not Crush   ✤ Alert   ☛ Key Drug   G Geriatric   P Pediatric

Adverse effects

CNS: Headache, fatigue, drowsiness, dizziness, anxiety, depression, nervousness, insomnia, light-headedness, paresthesia, tinnitus, psychosis, somnolence

CV: **Dysrhythmias,** edema, **CHF,** hypotension, palpitations, **MI, pulmonary edema,** tachycardia, syncope, AV block, angina

GI: Nausea, vomiting, diarrhea, gastric upset, constipation, increased liver function studies, dry mouth

HEMA: Anemia

INTEG: Rash, pruritus

MISC: Flushing, sexual difficulties, cough, nasal congestion, shortness of breath, wheezing, epistaxis, respiratory infection, chest pain

Contraindications: Hypersensitivity, sick sinus syndrome, 2nd- or 3rd-degree heart block

Precautions: CHF, hypotension <90 mm Hg systolic, hepatic injury, pregnancy **C,** lactation, children, renal disease, elderly

Do Not Confuse:
Plendil/pindolol,
Plendil/Prinivil

Pharmacokinetics

Absorption	Well absorbed
Distribution	Unknown; protein binding >99%
Metabolism	Liver, extensively
Excretion	Kidneys
Half-life	11-16 hr

Pharmacodynamics

Onset	2-3 hr
Peak	2½-5 hr
Duration	<24 hr

Interactions

Individual drugs

Alcohol: ↑ hypotension
Carbamazepine: ↑ toxicity
Digoxin: ↑ digoxin levels, ↑ bradycardia, CHF
Phenobarbital: ↓ effectiveness
Phenytoin: ↓ effectiveness
Propranolol: ↑ toxicity
Theophylline: ↓ theophylline level

Drug classifications

Antihypertensives: ↑ hypotension
β-Adrenergic blockers: ↑ bradycardia, CHF
Nitrates: ↑ nitrates

Food/drug

Grapefruit: ↑ felodipine level

NURSING CONSIDERATIONS

Assessment

• Assess fluid volume status: I&O ratio and record; weight; skin turgor; adequacy of pulses; moist mucous membranes; bilateral lung sounds; peripheral pitting edema—dehydration symptoms of decreasing output, thirst, hypotension, dry mouth, and mucous membranes should be reported

• Monitor ALT, AST, bilirubin daily if these are elevated

• Monitor cardiac status: B/P, pulse, respiration, ECG

Nursing diagnoses

☑ Cardiac output, decreased (uses)

☑ Knowledge deficit (teaching)

Implementation

• Give once a day, with food for GI symptoms

Ⓢ• Do not crush, chew tabs

Patient/family education

• Caution patient to avoid hazardous activities until stabilized on drug, and dizziness is no longer a problem

• Instruct patient to limit caffeine consumption; to avoid alcohol and OTC drugs unless directed by prescriber

• Urge patient to comply in all areas of medical regimen: diet, exercise, stress reduction, drug therapy; to notify prescriber of irregular heart beat, shortness of breath, swelling of feet and hands, pronounced dizziness, constipation, nausea, hypotension

• Teach patient to use as directed even if feeling better; may be taken with other cardiovascular drugs (nitrates, beta blockers)

Evaluation

Positive therapeutic outcome
• Decreased B/P

fenofibrate (micronized) (℞)
(fen-oh-fee′ brate)
Tricor
Func. class.: Antilipemic
Chem. class.: Aryloxisobu-tyric acid derivative
Pregnancy category   C

Action: Inhibits biosynthesis of low-density and very low-density lipoproteins, which are responsible for triglyceride development; mobilizes triglycerides from tissue; increases excretion of neutral sterols

Therapeutic Outcome: Decreasing cholesterol levels and low-density lipoproteins, decreased pruritus

Uses: Types IV, V hyperlipidemia that do not respond to other treatment

Dosage and routes
Adult: PO 67 mg/day

Available forms: Cap 67 mg

Adverse effects
CNS: Fatigue, weakness, drowsiness, dizziness
CV: Angina, **dysrhythmias**
GI: Nausea, vomiting, dyspepsia, increased liver enzymes, flatulence, hepatomegaly, gastritis
GU: Dysuria, proteinuria, oliguria
INTEG: Rash, urticaria, pruritus
MISC: Polyphagia, weight gain
MS: Myalgias, arthralgias

Contraindications: Severe hepatic disease, severe renal disease, primary biliary cirrhosis

Precautions: Peptic ulcer, pregnancy **C,** lactation, pancreatitis

Pharmacokinetics	
Absorption	Unknown
Distribution	Unknown
Metabolism	Unknown
Excretion	Unknown
Half-life	Unknown

Pharmacodynamics	
Peak	6-8 hr

Interactions
Drug classifications
Anticoagulants, oral: ↑ effect of anticoagulants
Bile acid sequestrants: ↓ absorption
Diuretics, thiazide: ↓ action of fenofibrate
Estrogens: ↓ action of fenofibrate
HMG-CoA reductase inhibitors: Do not use together

⬚ Herb/drug   ◙ Do Not Crush   ◆ Alert   ☞ Key Drug   Ⓖ Geriatric   Ⓟ Pediatric

Immunosuppressants: ↓ fenofibrate elimination
Nephrotoxics: ↓ fenofibrate elimination
Food/drug
↓ absorption

NURSING CONSIDERATIONS
Assessment
• Assess lipid levels, liver function tests, baseline and periodically during treatment
• Assess for pancreatitis, renal failure, rhabdomyolysis, myositis, drug should be discontinued
• Assess nutrition: fat, protein, carbohydrates, nutritional analysis should be completed by dietician
• Assess skin integrity after patient has been receiving drug; itching, pruritus often occur from bile deposits on skin
• Monitor cardiac glycoside level if both drugs are being administered—cardiac glycoside levels will be decreased
• Monitor for signs of vit A, D, K deficiency; serum cholesterol, triglyceride levels, electrolytes if on extended therapy
• Monitor bowel pattern daily; increase bulk, water in diet if constipation develops
Nursing diagnoses
✓ Knowledge deficit (teaching)
✓ Noncompliance (teaching)
Implementation
• Give with evening meal; if dose is increased, take with breakfast and evening meal
🚫• Do not chew, crush caps
• Store in cool environment in tight, light-resistant container
Patient/family education
• Inform patient that compliance is needed because toxicity may result if doses are missed

• Teach patient that risk factors—high-fat diet, smoking, alcohol consumption, absence of exercise—should be decreased
• Caution patient to practice birth control while on this drug
• Teach patient to notify prescriber if the GI symptoms of diarrhea, abdominal or epigastric pain, nausea, or vomiting occur
• Instruct patient to report GU symptoms: dysuria, proteinuria, oliguria, decreased libido, impotence
Evaluation
Positive therapeutic outcome
• Decrease in cholesterol to desired level after 8 wk

---

fenoldopam (℞)
(fen-nahl'doh-pam)
Corlopam
Func. class.: Antihypertensive
Chem class.: Vasodilator
Pregnancy category B

Action: Antagonizes D_1-like dopamine receptors; binds to α_2-adrenoreceptors; increases renal blood flow

➡ **Therapeutic Outcome:** B/P, decreased

Uses: Hypertensive crisis when urgent decrease of pressure required; including malignant hypertension
Dosage and routes
Adult: CONT **IV** titrate initial dose upward or downward no more frequently than q15 min; increments should range between 0.05-0.1 μg/kg/min; initial doses of 0.03-0.1 μg/

---

kg/min titrated slowly result in less reflex tachycardia

Available forms: Inj conc 10 mg/ml

Adverse effects

CNS: Headache, anxiety, dizziness

CV: Hypotension, ST-T-wave changes, angina pectoris, palpitations, **MI, ischemic heart disease**

GI: Nausea, vomiting, constipation, diarrhea

HEMA: **Leukocytosis, bleeding**

META: Increased BUN, glucose, LDH, creatinine, hypokalemia

Contraindications: Hypersensitivity, sulfite sensitivity

Precautions: Tachycardia, **P** pregnancy **B**, lactation, children, intraocular pressure, hypokalemia

Pharmacokinetics	
Absorption	Unknown
Distribution	Steady state 20 min
Metabolism	Unknown
Excretion	Unknown
Half-life	5 min (elimination)

Pharmacodynamics	
Onset	Unknown
Peak	Unknown
Duration	Unknown

Interactions

Drug classifications

β-Adrenergic blockers: ↑ hypotension

NURSING CONSIDERATIONS

Assessment

• Monitor B/P q5 min until stabilized, then q1h ×2 hr, then q4h

• Monitor pulse, jugular venous distention q4h

• Monitor electrolytes, blood studies: K, Na, Cl, CO_2, CBC, serum glucose

• Monitor weight daily, I&O

• Assess edema in feet, legs daily

• Assess skin turgor, dryness of mucous membranes for hydration status

• Assess rales, dyspnea, orthopnea

• Assess **IV** site for extravasation, rate

• Assess postural hypotension, take B/P sitting, standing

Nursing diagnoses

☑ Tissue perfusion, altered (uses)

☑ Knowledge deficit (teaching)

☑ Noncompliance (teaching)

Implementation

IV **IV route**

• Administer after diluting contents of ampules in 0.9% NaCl, or 5% dextrose inj (40 µg/ml); then add 4 ml of conc. (40 mg of drug/1000 ml); 2 ml of conc. (20 mg of drug/500 ml); 1 ml of conc. (10 mg of drug/250 ml)

• Give to patient in recumbent position; keep in that position for 1 hr after administration

• Diluted sol is stable in normal light/temp for 24 hr

Patient/family education

• Advise patient to change positions slowly, to prevent orthostatic hypotension

• Instruct patient to report dyspnea, chest pain, bleeding

Evaluation

Positive therapeutic outcome

• Decreased B/P

fenoprofen (℞)
(fen-oh-proe'fen)
fenoprofen, Nalfon
Func. class.: Nonsteroidal antiinflammatory, non-opioid analgesic
Chem. class.: Propionic acid derivative

Pregnancy category **B**

Action: Inhibits prostaglandin synthesis by decreasing enzyme needed for biosynthesis; analgesic, antiinflammatory, antipyretic

Therapeutic Outcome: Decreased pain, inflammation

Uses: Mild to moderate pain, osteoarthritis, rheumatoid arthritis, acute gout, arthritis, ankylosing spondylitis, inflammation, dysmenorrhea

Dosage and routes
Pain
Adult: PO 200 mg q4-6h as needed

Arthritis
Adult: PO 300-600 mg qid, not to exceed 3.2 g/day

Available forms: Caps 200, 300 mg; tab 600 mg

Adverse effects
CNS: Dizziness, headache, drowsiness, fatigue, tremors, confusion, insomnia, anxiety, depression
CV: Tachycardia, peripheral edema, palpitations, **dysrhythmias**
EENT: Tinnitus, hearing loss, blurred vision
GI: Nausea, anorexia, vomiting, diarrhea, jaundice, **cholestatic hepatitis**, constipation, flatulence, cramps, dry mouth, peptic ulcer

GU: Nephrotoxicity: dysuria, hematuria, oliguria, azotemia
HEMA: Blood dyscrasias
INTEG: Purpura, rash, pruritus, sweating

Contraindications: Hypersensitivity, asthma, severe renal disease, severe hepatic disease

Precautions: Pregnancy **B**, (1st and 2nd trimesters), lactation, children, bleeding disorders, GI disorders, cardiac disorders, hypersensitivity to other antiinflammatory agents, elderly, CrCl <30 ml/min, hypertension

Pharmacokinetics	
Absorption	Well absorbed
Distribution	Does not cross placenta
Metabolism	Extensively—liver
Excretion	Unchanged—kidneys
Half-life	2-4 hr

Pharmacodynamics	
Onset	15-30 min
Peak	2 hr
Duration	4-6 hr

Interactions
Individual drugs
Alcohol: ↑ GI reactions
Furosemide: ↑ toxic effects
Insulin: ↑ effects
Methotrexate: ↑ effects
Phenytoin: ↑ effects
Plicamycin: ↑ bleeding
Probenecid: ↓ effects
Spironolactone: ↓ effects
Sulfinpyrazone: ↓ effects
Valproic acid: ↑ effects, ↑ bleeding
Vancomycin: ↑ ototoxicity
Drug classifications
Antacids: ↓ effects of fenoprofen
Anticoagulants: ↑ effects
Barbiturates: ↓ fenoprofen effect

Carbonic anhydrase inhibitors: ↑ toxic effects
Corticosteroids: ↑ GI reactions
NSAIDs: ↑ gastric ulcers
Salicylates: ↑ GI toxicity
Steroids: ↓ effects of fenoprofen, ↑ gastric ulcers
Sulfonylamides: ↑ effects of sulfonylamides

NURSING CONSIDERATIONS
Assessment
• Monitor liver function; renal function, other blood studies: AST, ALT, bilirubin, creatinine, BUN, CBC, Hct, Hgb, pro-time if patient is on long-term therapy
• Check I&O ratio; decreasing output may indicate renal failure (long-term therapy)
• Assess for allergic reactions: rash, urticaria; if these occur, drug may have to be discontinued
• Assess for ototoxicity: tinnitus, ringing, roaring in ears; audiometric testing needed before, after long-term therapy
• Assess for visual changes: blurring, halos; corneal, retinal damage
• Check edema in feet, ankles, legs
• Identify prior drug history; there are many drug interactions
• Monitor pain: location, duration, type, intensity, prior to dose and 1 hr after; ROM prior to dose and after

Nursing diagnoses
☑ Pain (uses)
☑ Mobility, impaired (uses)
☑ Knowledge deficit (teaching)
☑ Injury, risk for (adverse reactions)

Implementation
• Administer to patient crushed or whole; chewable tab may be chewed (do not crush enteric product)
• Give with food or milk to decrease gastric symptoms; absorption may be slowed; give 30 min ac or 2 hr pc

Patient/family education
• Teach patient to report any symptoms of renal toxicity, visual changes, ototoxicity, allergic reactions, bleeding (long-term therapy)
• Advise patient to take with 8 oz of water and sit upright for ½ hr after dose to prevent ulceration
• Caution patient not to exceed recommended dosage— acute poisoning may result— and to take as prescribed, do not double dose
• Instruct patient to read label on other OTC drugs; many contain other antiinflammatories
• Inform patient that the therapeutic response takes up to 1 mo (arthritis)
• Teach patient to report tinnitus, confusion, diarrhea, sweating, hyperventilation, blurred vision, fever, joint aches
• Caution patient to avoid alcohol ingestion; GI bleeding may occur

Evaluation
Positive therapeutic outcome
• Decreased pain
• Decreased inflammation
• Increased mobility

---

fentanyl (R)
(fen'ta-nill)
fentanyl, Sublimaze,
Fentanyl Oralet, Actiq
Func. class.: Narcotic
analgesic
Chem. class.: Opiate,
synthetic phenylpiperidine
derivative

Pregnancy category C

**Controlled substance
schedule II**

Action: Inhibits ascending
pain pathways in CNS, in-
creases pain threshold, alters
pain perception by binding to
opiate receptors

Therapeutic Outcome: Relief
of pain, supplement to anesthesia

Uses: Preoperatively, postoperatively; adjunct to general
anesthetic, when combined
with droperidol; Fentanyl
Oralet-anesthesia as premedication, conscious sedation; Actiq-
breakthrough cancer pain

Dosage and routes
Anesthetic
Adult: **IV** 0.05-0.1 mg q2-3
min prn

Preoperatively
Adult: IM 0.05-0.1 mg
q30-60 min before surgery

Postoperatively
Adult: IM 0.05-0.1 mg q1-
2hr prn

P *Child:* IM 0.02-0.03 mg/9 kg

Fentanyl oralet
Adult transmucosal: 5 μg/
kg = fentanyl IM 0.75-1.25
μg/kg, do not exceed 5 μg/kg

P *Child transmucosal:* May
need doses of 5-15 μg/kg;

must be watched continuously
for hypoventilation

Actiq
Adult transmucosal: 200 μg,
redose if needed 15 min after
completion of 1st dose, do not
give more than 2 doses during
titration period. When a successful dose is found, have
patient consume ≤4 doses/day

Available forms: Inj 0.05
mg/ml; lozenges 100, 200,
300, 400 μg; lozenges on a
stick 200, 400, 600, 800,
1200, 1600 μg

Adverse effects
CNS: Dizziness, delirium,
euphoria, light-headedness,
sedation, dysphoria, agitation,
anxiety
CV: **Bradycardia, cardiac
arrest,** hypotension or hypertension, facial flushing, chills
EENT: Blurred vision, miosis
GI: Nausea, vomiting, diarrhea, cramps
MS: Muscle rigidity
RESP: **Respiratory depression, arrest, laryngospasm**

Contraindications: Hypersensitivity to opiates, myasthenia
gravis

G Precautions: Elderly, respiratory depression, increased
intracranial pressure, seizure
disorders, severe respiratory
disorders, cardiac dysrhythmias, pregnancy **C**

Pharmacokinetics	
Absorption	Well absorbed (IM), completely absorbed (**IV**)
Distribution	Unknown, crosses placenta
Metabolism	Extensively—liver, 80% bound to plasma proteins

Excretion	Kidneys—up to 25% unchanged, breast milk
Half-life	1½-6 hr

Pharmacodynamics

	IM	IV
Onset	7-8 min	Rapid
Peak	30 min	3-5 min
Duration	1-2 hr	½-1 hr

Interactions
Individual drugs
Alcohol: ↑ respiratory depression, hypotension, ↑ sedation
Cimetidine: ↑ recovery
Erythromycin: ↑ recovery
Nalbuphine: ↓ analgesia
Pentazocine: ↓ analgesia
Drug classifications
Antihistamines: ↑ respiratory depression, hypotension
CNS depressants: ↑ respiratory depression, hypotension
MAOIs: Do not use 2 wk before fentanyl
Phenothiazines: ↑ respiratory depression, hypotension
Sedative/hypnotics: ↑ respiratory depression, hypotension
☑ Herb/drug
Kava: ↑ fentanyl action
Lab test interferences
↑ Amylase, ↑ lipase

NURSING CONSIDERATIONS
Assessment
• Monitor vital signs after parenteral route (B/P, pulse, respiration); note muscle rigidity; take drug history before administering drug; check liver, kidney function tests; assess for respiratory dysfunction: respiratory depression, character, rate, rhythm; notify prescriber if respirations are <10/min
• Monitor CNS changes: dizziness, drowsiness, hallucinations, euphoria, LOC, pupil reaction
• Monitor allergic reactions: rash, urticaria; drug should be discontinued
• Assess for pain: intensity, location, duration, type, before and 15 min after IM route or 3-5 min after **IV** route

Nursing diagnoses
☑ Pain (uses)
☑ Sensory-perceptual alteration: visual, auditory (adverse reactions)
☑ Breathing pattern, ineffective (adverse reactions)
☑ Knowledge deficit (teaching)

Implementation
• Give by inj (IM, **IV**), only with resuscitative equipment available; give slowly to prevent rigidity
• Give **IV** undiluted by anesthesiologist or diluted with 5 ml or more sterile water or 0.9% NcCl given through Y-tube or 3-way stopcock given at 0.1 mg or less/ 1.2 min
• Store in light-resistant area at room temp

Transmucosal
• Remove foil just before administration, instruct patient to place under tongue and suck, not chew (Oralet); place between cheek and lower gum, moving it back and forth and suck, not chew (Actiq); all products not used or partially used should be flushed down the toilet

Syringe compatibilities:
Atracurium, atropine, bupivacaine/ketamine, butorphanol, chlorpromazine, cimetidine, clonidine/lidocaine, dimenhydrinate, diphenhydramine, droperidol, heparin,

---

hydromorphone, hydroxyzine, meperidine, metoclopramide, midazolam, morphine, pentazocine, perphenazine, prochlorperazine, promazine, promethazine, ranitidine, scopolamine

Syringe incompatibilities:
Pentobarbital

Y-site compatibilities:
Amphotericin B cholesteryl, atracurium, cisatracurium, diltiazem, dobutamine, dopamine, enalaprilat, epinephrine, esmolol, etomidate, furosemide, heparin, hydrocortisone, hydromorphone, labetalol, lorazepam, midazolam, milrinone, morphine, nafcillin, nicardipine, nitroglycerin, norepinephrine, pancuronium, potassium chloride, propofol, ranitidine, remifentanil, sargramostim, thiopental, vecuronium, vit B/C

Additive compatibilities:
Bupivacaine, sodium bicarbonate

Additive incompatibilities:
Methohexital, pentobarbital, thiopental

Solution compatibilities:
D_5W, 0.9% NaCl

Patient/family education
• Advise patient to report any symptoms of CNS changes, allergic reactions
• Instruct patient to avoid CNS depressants: alcohol, sedative/hypnotics for at least 24 hr after taking this drug
• Teach patient that dizziness, drowsiness, confusion are common, and to avoid getting up without assistance
• Discuss in detail with patient all aspects of the drug

Evaluation
Positive therapeutic outcome
• Maintenance of anesthesia
• Decreased pain

Treatment of overdose:
Narcan 0.2-0.8 **IV**, O_2, **IV** fluids, vasopressors

fentanyl transdermal (℞)
(fen'ta-nill)
Duragesic-25, Duragesic-50, Duragesic-75, Duragesic-100
Func. class.: Narcotic, analgesic
Chem. class.: Opiate, synthetic phenylpiperidine

Pregnancy category **C**
Controlled substance schedule **II**

Action: Inhibits ascending pain pathways in CNS, increases pain threshold, alters pain perception by binding to opiate receptors

Therapeutic Outcome: Relief of chronic pain

Uses: Management of chronic pain for those requiring opioid analgesia

Dosage and routes
Adult: 25 µg/hr; may increase until pain relief occurs; apply patch to flat surface on upper torso and wear for 72 hr; apply new patch on different site for continued relief

Available forms: Patches 2.5, 5, 7.5, 10 mg

Adverse effects
CNS: Dizziness, delirium, euphoria, light-headedness, sedation, dysphoria, agitation, anxiety

CV: Bradycardia, **cardiac arrest,** hypotension or hypertension, facial flushing, chills
EENT: Blurred vision, miosis
GI: Nausea, vomiting, diarrhea, cramps
RESP: **Respiratory depression, laryngospasm, bronchospasm;** depresses cough; hypoventilation

Contraindications: Hypersensitivity to opiates, myasthenia gravis

G Precautions: Elderly, respiratory depression, increased intracranial pressure, seizure disorders, severe respiratory disorders, cardiac dysrhythmias, pregnancy **C,** fever

Pharmacokinetics	
Absorption	92% (skin), continuously for 72 hr
Distribution	Crosses placenta
Metabolism	Extensively—liver
Excretion	Up to 25%—kidneys unchanged
Half-life	17 hr after removal of patch

Pharmacodynamics	
Onset	6 hr
Peak	12-24 hr
Duration	72 hr

Interactions
Individual drugs
Alcohol: ↑ respiratory depression, hypotension, ↑ sedation
Cimetidine: ↑ recovery
Erythromycin: ↑ recovery
Nalbuphine: ↓ analgesia
Pentazocine: ↓ analgesia
Drug classifications
Antihistamines: ↑ respiratory depression, hypotension
CNS depressants: ↑ respiratory depression, hypotension
MAOIs: Do not use 2 wk before fentanyl

Phenothiazines: ↑ respiratory depression, hypotension
Sedative/hypnotics: ↑ respiratory depression, hypotension
☑ Herb/drug
Kava: ↑ fentanyl level
Lab test interferences
↑ Amylase, ↑ lipase

NURSING CONSIDERATIONS
Assessment
• Assess for respiratory dysfunction: respiratory depression, character, rate, rhythm; notify prescriber if respirations are <10/min
• Monitor CNS changes: dizziness, drowsiness, hallucinations, euphoria, LOC, pupil reaction
• Monitor allergic reactions: rash, urticaria; drug should be discontinued
• Assess for pain: intensity, location, duration, type—before and after administration

Nursing diagnoses
☑ Pain (uses)
☑ Sensory-perceptual alteration: visual, auditory (adverse reactions)
☑ Breathing pattern, ineffective (adverse reactions)
☑ Knowledge deficit (teaching)

Implementation
• Narcotic analgesics should be used to control pain until relief is obtained with transdermal patch; patients may continue to require other narcotics for breakthrough pain; if >100 µg/hr is required, use multiple systems
• Apply patch to chest on a flat area with skin intact; for skin preparation, use clear water with no soap; clip hair, skin should be dry before applying patch; apply immediately after removing from package and

---

press firmly in place with palm of hand; flush old patch down toilet immediately upon removal

Use pain dosing
• Dosage is titrated based on patient's report of pain; dosage is determined by calculating the previous 24-hr requirement and converting to equianalgesic morphine dose
• To convert to another narcotic analgesic, remove transdermal patch and begin treatment with half the equal pain controlling dose of the new analgesic in 12-18 hr
• Medication should be tapered gradually after long-term use to prevent withdrawal symptoms

Patient/family education
• Advise patient to report any symptoms of CNS changes, allergic reactions
• Instruct patients to avoid CNS depressants: alcohol, sedative/hypnotics for at least 24 hr after this drug
• Discuss with patient that dizziness, drowsiness, and confusion are common and to avoid getting up without assistance
• Discuss all aspects of the drug in detail

Evaluation
Positive therapeutic outcome
• Decreased pain

Treatment of overdose: Narcan 0.2-0.8 **IV**, O_2, **IV** fluids, vasopressors

---

ferrous fumarate (℞, OTC)
(fer'us)
Femiron, Feostat, Feostat Drops, Hemocyte, Ircon, Nephro-Fer, Novofumar ♣, Palafer ♣, Span-FF
ferrous gluconate (℞, OTC)
Fergon, Fertinic ♣, Novoferrogluc ♣
ferrous sulfate (℞, OTC)
Apo-Ferrous Sulfate ♣, Feosol, Fer-gen-sol, Fer-Iron Drops, Fero-Grad, Mol-Iron
ferrous sulfate, dried (℞, OTC)
Fe^{50}, Feosol, Feratab, Novoferrosulfa ♣, PMS-Ferrous Sulfate, Slow Fe
ferric gluconate complex (℞, OTC)
Ferrlecit
Func. class.: Hematinic
Chem. class.: Iron preparation

Pregnancy category   A

Action: Replaces iron stores needed for red blood cell development, energy and O_2 transport, utilization; fumarate contains 33% elemental iron; gluconate, 12%; sulfate, 20%; iron, 30%; ferrous sulfate exsiccated

➡ **Therapeutic Outcome:** Prevention and correction of iron deficiency

Uses: Iron deficiency anemia, prophylaxis for iron deficiency in pregnancy

Dosage and routes
Fumarate
Adult: PO 200 mg tid-qid

P *Child 2-12 yr:* PO 3 mg/kg/ day (elemental iron) tid-qid

P *Child 6 mo-2 yr:* PO up to 6 mg/kg/day (elemental iron) tid-qid

P *Child 6 mo-2 yr:* PO 6 mg/ kg/day in 3-4 divided doses

P *Infants:* PO 10-25 mg/day (elemental iron) in 3-4 divided doses

Gluconate
Adult: PO 200-600 mg tid

P *Child 6-12 yr:* PO 300-900 mg qd

P *Child <6 yr:* PO 100-300 mg qd

Sulfate
Adult: PO 0.750-1.5 g/day in divided doses tid

P *Child 6-12 yr:* 600 mg/day in divided doses

Pregnancy
Adult: PO 300-600 mg/day in divided doses

Complex
Adult: **IV** inf (125 mg) 10 ml/100 ml of NaCl for inj given over 1 hr

Available forms
Fumarate: Tabs 63, 195, 200, 324, 325 mg; tab, chewable 100 mg; tab, controlled-release 300 mg; oral susp 100 mg/5 ml, 45 mg/0.6 ml

Gluconate: Tabs 300, 320, 325, mg; caps 86, 325, 435 mg; tab, film-coated 300 mg; elix 300 mg/5 ml

Sulfate: Tabs 195, 300, 325, mg; tab, enteric-coated 325 mg; tab, extended-release, time-release cap 525 mg

Dried: Tabs, 200 mg; tabs ext rel 160 mg; caplets ext rel 160 mg

Complex: Inj 62.5 mg/5 ml (12.5 mg/ml)

Adverse effects
GI: Nausea, constipation, epigastric pain, black and red tarry stools, vomiting, diarrhea
INTEG: Temporarily discolored tooth enamel and eyes

Contraindications: Hypersensitivity, ulcerative colitis/ regional enteritis, hemosiderosis/ hemochromatosis, peptic ulcer disease, hemolytic anemia, cirrhosis

Precautions: Anemia (long-term), pregnancy **A**

Pharmacokinetics	
Absorption	Up to 30%
Distribution	Bound to transferrin, crosses placenta
Metabolism	Recycled
Excretion	Feces, urine, skin, breast milk
Half-life	Unknown

Pharmacodynamics
Unknown

Interactions
Individual drugs
Chloramphenicol: ↑ absorption of iron products
Cholestyramine: ↓ absorption of iron
Cimetidine: ↓ absorption of iron
L-thyroxine: ↓ L-thyroxine absorption
Levodopa: ↓ absorption of levodopa
Methyldopa: ↓ absorption of methyldopa
Penicillamine: ↓ absorption of penicillamine
Quinolone: ↓ absorption of quinolone
Tetracycline: ↓ absorption of iron products

☑ Herb/drug 🚫 Do Not Crush ◆ Alert ⊶ Key Drug **G** Geriatric **P** Pediatric

Vitamin C: ↑ absorption of iron products
Drug classifications
Fluoroquinolones: ↓ absorption of fluoroquinolone
Food/drug
Caffeine: ↓ absorption
Dairy products: ↓ absorption
Lab test interferences
False positive: Occult blood

NURSING CONSIDERATIONS
Assessment
• Monitor blood studies: Hct, Hgb, reticulocytes, bilirubin before treatment, at least monthly
• Assess for toxicity: nausea, vomiting, diarrhea (green, then tarry stools,) hematemesis, pallor, cyanosis, shock, coma
• Assess bowel elimination; if constipation occurs, increase water, bulk, activity before laxatives are required
• Assess nutrition: amount of iron in diet (meat, dark green leafy vegetables, dried beans, dried fruits, eggs); provide referral to dietician if indicated
• Identify cause of iron loss or anemia, including salicylates, sulfonamides, antimalarials, quinidine

Nursing diagnoses
☑ Nutrition, less than body requirements (uses)
☑ Fatigue (uses)
☑ Knowledge deficit (teaching)

Implementation
• Give between meals for best absorption; may give with juice; do not give with antacids or milk, delay at least 1 hr; if GI symptoms occur, give PC even if absorption is decreased; eggs, milk products, chocolate, caffeine interfere with absorption
🚫 • Do not crush, chew tabs

• Give liq preparations through plastic straw to avoid discoloration of tooth enamel; dilute thoroughly
• Give at least 1 hr before bedtime because corrosion may occur in stomach
• Give for <6 mo for anemia
• Store in air-tight, light-resistant container

Patient/family education
• Advise patient that iron will make stools black or dark green; that iron poisoning may occur if increased beyond recommended level
• Tell patient not to crush; swallow tab whole; to keep out of reach of children
• Caution patient not to substitute one iron salt for another; elemental iron content differs (e.g., 300 mg ferrous fumarate contains about 100 mg elemental iron, whereas 300 mg ferrous gluconate contains only about 30 mg elemental iron)
• Caution patient to avoid reclining position for 15-30 min after taking drug to avoid esophageal corrosion; to follow diet high in iron

Evaluation
Positive therapeutic outcome
• Decreased fatigue, weakness
• Improvement in Hct, Hgb, reticulocytes

Treatment of overdose:
Induce vomiting; give eggs, milk until lavage can be done

fexofenadine (℞)
(fex-oh-fin′a-deen)
Allegra
Func. class.: H_1 histamine antagonist
Chem. class: Piperidine, peripherally selective

Pregnancy category C

Action: Acts on blood vessels, GI, respiratory system by competing with histamine for H_1-receptor site; decreases allergic response by blocking pharmacologic effects of histamine; less sedation rate than with other antihistamines; causes increased heart rate, vasodilation, increased secretions

➡ **Therapeutic Outcome:** Absence of allergy symptoms and rhinitis

Uses: Rhinitis, allergy symptoms, chronic idiopathic urticaria

Dosage and routes
P *Adult and child >12 yr:* 60 mg bid

Renal dose
CrCl <80 ml/min
60 mg qd

Available forms: Cap 60 mg

Adverse effects
CNS: Headache, stimulation, drowsiness, sedation, fatigue, confusion, blurred vision, tinnitus, restlessness, tremors, P paradoxical excitation in chilG dren or elderly
CV: Hypotension, palpitations, bradycardia, tachycardia, **dysrhythmias (rare)**
GI: Nausea, diarrhea, abdominal pain, vomiting, constipation
GU: Frequency, dysuria, urinary retention, impotence

HEMA: Hemolytic anemia, thrombocytopenia, leukopenia, agranulocytosis, pancytopenia
INTEG: Rash, eczema, photosensitivity, urticaria
RESP: Thickening of bronchial secretions; dry nose, throat

Contraindications: HypersenP sitivity, newborn or premature infants, lactation, severe hepatic disease

Precautions: Pregnancy **C**,
G elderly, children, respiratory
P disease, narrow-angle glaucoma, prostatic hypertrophy, bladder neck obstruction, asthma

Pharmacokinetics	
Absorption	Well absorbed
Distribution	Unknown
Metabolism	Liver
Excretion	Kidneys

Pharmacodynamics	
Onset	15-30 min
Peak	1-2 hr
Duration	8-12 hr

Interactions
Individual drugs
Alcohol: ↑ CNS depression
Procarbazine: ↑ CNS depression
Drug classifications
Anticoagulants, oral: ↓ action
CNS depressants: ↑ CNS depression
MAOIs: ↑ anticholinergic effect
Opiates: ↑ CNS depression
Sedative/hypnotics: ↑ CNS depression
Food/drug
↓ absorption
Lab test interferences
False negative: Skin allergy tests (discontinue antihistamine 3 days before testing)

▨ Herb/drug Ⓢ Do Not Crush ◆ Alert ⟳ Key Drug G Geriatric P Pediatric

NURSING CONSIDERATIONS
Assessment
• Assess respiratory status: rate, rhythm, increase in bronchial secretions, wheezing, chest tightness; provide fluids to 2 L/day to decrease secretion thickness
• Monitor I&O ratio: be alert for urinary retention, frequency, dysuria, especially elderly; drug should be discontinued if these occur

Nursing diagnoses
✓ Airway clearance, ineffective (uses)
✓ Injury, risk for (side effects)
✓ Knowledge deficit (teaching)
✓ Noncompliance (teaching, overuse)

Implementation
• Give on an empty stomach 1 hr before or 2 hr pc to facilitate absorption
• Store in tight, light-resistant container

Patient/family education
• Teach all aspects of drug uses; to notify prescriber if confusion, sedation, hypotension occur; to avoid driving or other hazardous activity if drowsiness occurs; to avoid alcohol or other CNS depressants that may potentiate effect
• Instruct patient to take 1 hr before or 2 hr pc to facilitate absorption
• Instruct patient not to exceed recommended dose; dysrhythmias may occur
• Teach patient that hard candy, gum, frequent rinsing of mouth may be used for dryness

Evaluation
Positive therapeutic outcome
• Absence of running or congested nose, rashes

Treatment of overdose: Administer ipecac syrup or lavage, diazepam, vasopressors, barbiturates (short acting)

fibrinolysin/ desoxyribonuclease
(Ph)
(fye-brin-oe-lye'sin/dez-ox-ee-rye-boe-nuke'lee-ase)
Elase
Func. class.: Enzyme
Chem. class.: Proteolytic-bovine

Pregnancy category C

Action: Dissolves fibrin in clots and fibrinous exudates, attacks DNA in areas of disintegrating cells

Therapeutic Outcome: A clean wound

Uses: Debridement of wounds, vaginitis, cervicitis, ulcerative colitis, 2nd-, 3rd-degree burns; irrigating wounds, topically

Dosage and routes
Debridement/intravaginally
Adult: Oint 5 g × 5 applications

Irrigating
Adult: Irrig dilution depends on type of wound

Available forms: Fibrinolysin with desoxyribonuclease 666.6 U/g; powder for reconstitution fibrinolysin 25 U/desoxyribonuclease 15,000 U

Adverse effects
INTEG: Hyperemia

Contraindications: Hypersensitivity to bovine or mercury products, hematoma

Precautions: Pregnancy **C**

Pharmacokinetics

Absorption	Not absorbed
Distribution	Unknown
Metabolism	Unknown
Excretion	Unknown
Half-life	Unknown

Pharmacodynamics

Unknown

Interactions: None

NURSING CONSIDERATIONS
Assessment
• Assess for signs of irritation and inflammation around wound; drug should be discontinued
• Assess wound for drainage, color, odor, size, depth before and during therapy

Nursing diagnoses
☑ Skin integrity, altered (uses)
☑ Knowledge deficit (teaching)

Implementation
Top route
• Apply after reconstituting top sol with 10-50 ml sterile NaCl sol; use only fresh sol; reconstituted sol is stable for 24 hr; remove necrotic debris, dry eschar
• Saturate gauze with sol; pack area; remove in 6-8 hr and clean; repeat tid-qid
• Apply top oint after flushing wound with saline, water or, let dry or pat dry, then apply a small amount of oint to area and cover with a nonadhesive dressing; change qd or bid
Vag route
• Place 5 ml in applicator, apply with patient recumbent

Patient/family education
• Teach patient reason for treatment and expected results

Evaluation
Positive therapeutic outcome
• Decrease in wound scarring, tissue necrosis

filgrastim (℞)
(fill-gras'stim)
Neupogen
Func. class.: Biologic modifier
Chem. class.: Granulocyte colony-stimulating factor

Pregnancy category C

Action: Stimulates proliferation and differentiation of neutrophils; a glycoprotein

➡ **Therapeutic Outcome:** Absence of infection

Uses: To decrease infection in patients receiving antineoplastics that are myelosuppressive; to increase WBC in patients with drug-induced neutropenia

Dosage and routes
🅿 *Adult and child:* **IV**/SC 5 µg/kg/day in a single dose; may increase by 5 µg/kg in each chemotherapy cycle; give qd for up to 2 wk until the absolute neutrophil count (ANC) has reached 10,000/mm^3; response to G-CSF is much greater with SC than **IV** therapy

Available forms: Inj 300 µg/ml

Adverse effects
CNS: Fever
GI: Nausea, vomiting, diarrhea, mucositis, anorexia
HEMA: **Thrombocytopenia**
INTEG: Alopecia, exacerbation of skin conditions
MS: Osteoporosis, skeletal pain
RESP: **Respiratory distress syndrome**

🖉 Herb/drug 🅢 Do Not Crush ◆ Alert ⟲π Key Drug 🅖 Geriatric 🅿 Pediatric

Contraindications: Hypersensitivity to proteins of *E. coli*

Precautions: Pregnancy **C**, lactation, cardiac conditions, ▣ children, myeloid malignancies

Pharmacokinetics

Absorption	Well absorbed (SC), completely absorbed (**IV**)
Distribution	Unknown
Metabolism	Unknown
Excretion	Unknown
Half-life	Unknown

Pharmacodynamics

	IV	SC
Onset	5-60 min	5-60 min
Peak	24 hr	2-8 hr
Duration	up to 1 wk	up to 1 wk

Interactions
Drug classifications
Antineoplastics: ↑ neutrophils, do not use together 24 hr before or after antineoplastics

Lab test interferences
↑ Uric acid, ↑ lactate dehydrogenase, ↑ alk phosphatase

NURSING CONSIDERATIONS
Assessment
• Monitor blood studies: CBC, platelet count before treatment and twice weekly; neutrophil counts (ANC) may be increased for 2 days after therapy, but treatment should continue until ANC >10,000/mm^3
• Assess for bone pain: frequency, intensity, duration; analgesics may be given; opiates should not be used
• Check B/P, heart rate, respiration, baseline and during treatment

Nursing diagnoses
☑ Infection, risk for (uses)
☑ Pain, acute (adverse reaction)
☑ Knowledge deficit (teaching)

Implementation
Ⅳ IV route
• Give 300 μg/ml or 480 μg/1.6 ml; allow to warm to room temp; give single dose over 1 min or less through Y-tube or medport
• Use single-use vials; after dose is withdrawn, do not reenter vial
• Give for 2 wk or until ANC is 10,000/mm^3 after the expected chemotherapy neutrophil nadir
• Store in refrigerator; do not freeze; may store at room temp for up to 6 hr; avoid shaking

Y-site compatibilities:
Acyclovir, allopurinol, amikacin, aminophylline, ampicillin, ampicillin/sulbactam, aztreonam, bleomycin, bumetanide, buprenorphine, butorphanol, calcium gluconate, carboplatin, carmustine, cefazolin, cefotetan, ceftazidime, chlorpromazine, cimetidine, cisplatin, cyclophosphamide, cytarabine, dacarbazine, daunorubicin, dexamethasone, diphenhydramine, doxorubicin, doxycycline, droperidol, enalaprilat, famotidine, floxuridine, fluconazole, fludarabine, gallium, ganciclovir, granisetron, haloperidol, hydrocortisone, hydromorphone, hydroxyzine, idarubicin, ifosfamide, leucovorin, lorazepam, mechlorethamine, melphalan, meperidine, mesna, methotrexate, metoclopramide, miconazole, minocycline, mitoxantrone, morphine, nalbuphine, netilmicin, ondansetron, plicamycin, potas-

F

sium chloride, promethazine, ranitidine, sodium bicarbonate, streptozocin, ticarcillin, ticarcillin/clavulanate, tobramycin, trimethoprim-sulfamethoxazole, vancomycin, vinblastine, vincristine, vinorelbine, zidovudine

Patient/family education
• Teach patient technique for self-administration: dose, side effects, disposal of containers and needles; provide instruction sheet

Evaluation
Positive therapeutic outcome
• Absence of infection

---

finasteride (R)
(fin-ass'te-ride)
Proscar, Propecia
Func. class.: Androgen hormone inhibitor
Chem. class.: 5-α-reductase inhibitor

Pregnancy category X

Action: Inhibits 5-α-reductase and reduction in DHT; DHT induces androgenic effects by binding to androgen receptors in the cell nuclei of the prostate gland, liver, skin; prevents development of benign prostatic hypertrophy (BPH)

Therapeutic Outcome: Reduced prostate size

Uses: Symptomatic benign prostatic hyperplasia; male-pattern baldness (Propecia)

Dosage and routes
Proscar
Adult: PO 5 mg qd × 6-12 mo

Propecia
Adult: PO 1 mg qd

Available forms: Tabs 1, 5 mg

Adverse effects
GU: Impotence, decreased libido, decreased volume of ejaculate

Contraindications: Hypersensitivity, pregnancy **X**, children, women who are pregnant or may become pregnant should not handle tablets

Precautions: Large residual urinary volume, severely diminished urinary flow, liver function abnormalities

Do Not Confuse:
Proscar/Prosom,
Proscar/Prozac

Pharmacokinetics	
Absorption	(63%)
Distribution	Plasma protein binding, crosses blood-brain barrier
Metabolism	Liver
Excretion	Kidneys—metabolites (39%), feces (57%)
Half-life	6-15 hr

Pharmacodynamics	
Onset	Immediate
Peak	1-2 hr
Duration	14 days

Interactions
Drug classifications
Anticholinergics: ↓ effect of finasteride
Bronchodilators, adrenergic: ↓ effect of finasteride
Theophylline: ↓ effect of finasteride

NURSING CONSIDERATIONS
Assessment
• Assess urinary patterns, residual urinary volume, severely diminished urinary flow; PSA levels and digital rectal exam before initiating therapy and periodically thereafter

---

• Monitor liver function studies before initiating treatment; extensively metabolized in liver

Nursing diagnoses
☑ Urinary elimination, altered (uses)
☑ Knowledge deficit (teaching)

Implementation
• Administer without regard to meals; give for a minimum of 6 mo; not all patients will respond
• Store at temp <86° F (30° C); protect from light; keep container tightly closed

Patient/family education
• Advise patient that pregnant women or women who may become pregnant should not touch crushed tab or come into contact with semen of a patient taking this drug; may adversely affect development of male fetus
• Inform patient that volume of ejaculate may be decreased during treatment; impotence and decreased libido may also occur
• Inform patient that Propecia results may not occur for 3 mo
• Inform patient that Proscar results may not occur for 6-12 mo

Evaluation
Positive therapeutic outcome
• Decreased postvoiding dribbling, frequency, nocturia
• Increased urinary flow

---

flecainide (℞)
(flek'a-nide)
Tambocor
Func. class.: Antidysrhythmic (Class IC)

Pregnancy category   C

Action: Decreases conduction in all parts of the heart, with greatest effect on the His-Purkinje system, which stabilizes the cardiac membrane

▶ **Therapeutic Outcome:** Absence of dysrhythmias

Uses: Life-threatening ventricular dysrhythmias, sustained ventricular tachycardia; supraventricular tachydysrhythmias

Dosage and routes
Adult: PO 50-100 mg q12h; may increase every 4 days by 50 mg q12h to desired response, not to exceed 400 mg/day

Renal dose
CrCl <35 ml/min dose 50%-75%

Available forms: Tabs 50, 100, 150 mg

Adverse effects
CNS: Headache, dizziness, involuntary movement, confusion, psychosis, restlessness, irritability, paresthesias, ataxia, flushing, somnolence, depression, anxiety, malaise
CV: Hypotension, **bradycardia,** angina, PVCs, **heart block, cardiovascular collapse, arrest, dysrhythmias, CHF, fatal ventricular tachycardia**
EENT: Tinnitus, *blurred vision,* hearing loss
GI: Nausea, vomiting, anorexia, constipation, abdominal pain, flatulence, change in taste

F

GU: Impotence, decreased libido, polyuria, urinary retention

HEMA: **Leukopenia, thrombocytopenia**

INTEG: Rash, urticaria, edema, swelling

RESP: Dyspnea, **respiratory depression**

Contraindications: Hypersensitivity, severe heart block, cardiogenic shock, nonsustained ventricular dysrhythmias, frequent PVCs, non–life-threatening dysrhythmias

Precautions: Pregnancy **C,** **P** lactation, children, renal disease, liver disease, CHF, respiratory depression, myasthenia gravis

Pharmacokinetics	
Absorption	Well absorbed
Distribution	Widely distributed
Metabolism	Liver
Excretion	30% kidneys, unchanged
Half-life	14 hr

Pharmacodynamics	
Onset	Unknown
Peak	3 hr
Duration	Unknown

Interactions
Individual drugs
Amiodarone: ↑ blood levels, ↑ toxicity
Digoxin: ↑ blood levels, ↑ toxicity
Disopyramide: ↑ levels, ↑ toxicity
Flecainide: ↑ levels, ↑ toxicity
Lidocaine: Bradycardia, arrest
Mexiletine: ↑ levels, ↑ toxicity
Phenytoin: ↑ blood levels
Procainamide: ↑ levels, ↑ toxicity
Quinidine: ↑ levels, ↑ toxicity
Warfarin: ↑ level, ↑ bleeding

Drug classifications
β-Adrenergic blockers: ↑ dysrhythmias, arrest
Calcium channel blockers: ↑ dysrhythmias, arrest

NURSING CONSIDERATIONS
Assessment
• Monitor ECG continuously to determine drug effectiveness; measure PR, QRS, QT intervals; check for PVCs, other dysrhythmias; monitor B/P continuously for hypotension, hypertension, and rebound hypertension (after 1-2 hr); check for dehydration or hypovolemia
• Monitor I&O ratio; electrolytes: [K (potassium), Na (sodium)], Cl (chloride); check weight daily and for signs of CHG or pulmonary toxicity: dyspnea, fatigue, cough, fever, chest pain; if these occur, drug should be discontinued
• Monitor liver function studies: AST, ALT, bilirubin, alk phosphatase
• Assess patient for CNS symptoms: confusion, psychosis, numbness, depression, involuntary movements; if these occur, drug should be discontinued
• Assess patient for hyperthyroidism: lethargy, dizziness, constipation, enlarged thyroid gland, edema of extremities, cool, pale skin; assess patient for hyperthyroidism: restlessness; tachycardia; eyelid puffiness; weight loss; frequent urination; menstrual irregularities; dyspnea; warm, moist skin
• Monitor cardiac rate, respiration: rate, rhythm, char-

---

acter, chest pain; watch for ventricular tachycardia, supraventricular tachycardia, or fibrillation

Nursing diagnoses
☑ Cardiac output, decreased (uses)
☑ Knowledge deficit (teaching)

Implementation
• Give reduced dosage slowly with ECG monitoring; do not increase dose fewer than 4 days apart
• Give with meals if GI upset occurs

Patient/family education
• Instruct patient to report side effects immediately to health care provider
• Instruct patient to complete follow-up appointment with health care provider including pulmonary function studies, chest x-ray

Evaluation
Positive therapeutic outcome
• Absence of dysrhythmias

---

fluconazole (℞)
(floo-kon'a-zole)
Diflucan
Func. class.: Antifungal
Pregnancy category **C**

Action: Inhibits ergosterol biosynthesis, causes direct damage to membrane phospholipids in the cell wall of fungi

▷ **Therapeutic Outcome:** Fungistatic fungicidal against the following susceptible organisms: *Candida, Cryptococcus neoformans*

Uses: Oropharyngeal esophageal candidiasis in AIDS patients, chronic mucocutaneous candidiasis, urinary candidiasis, cryptococcal meningitis, peritonitis

Dosage and routes
Renal dose
CrCl 11-50 ml/min dose 50%
Vaginal candidiasis
Adult: PO 150 mg as a single dose
Serious fungal infections
Adult: PO/**IV** 50-400 mg initially, then 200 mg once daily for 4 wk
🅿 *Child:* 6-12 mg/kg/day
Oropharyngeal candidiasis in AIDS patients
Adult: PO 200 mg initially, then 100 mg daily for at least 2 wk
🅿 *Child:* 3 mg/kg/day

Available forms: Tabs 50, 100, 150, 200 mg; inj 200, 400 mg; powder for oral susp 10 mg, 40 mg/ml

Adverse effects
CNS: Headache
GI: Nausea, vomiting, diarrhea, cramping, flatus, increased AST, ALT, **hepatotoxicity**
INTEG: **Stevens-Johnson syndrome**

Contraindications: Hypersensitivity

Precautions: Renal disease, pregnancy **C**

🚫 **Do Not Confuse:**
Diflucan/Diprivan

Pharmacokinetics	
Absorption	Well absorbed (PO)
Distribution	Widely distributed (peritoneum, cerebrospinal fluid)
Metabolism	<10%—liver
Excretion	80% kidneys (unchanged)
Half-life	30 hr, increased in renal disease

Pharmacodynamics		
	PO	IV
Onset	Unknown	Immediate
Peak	2-4 hr	Infusion's end
Duration	Unknown	Unknown

Interactions
Individual drugs
Cimetidine: ↓ effect of fluconazole
Cyclosporine: ↑ effect
Phenytoin: ↑ effect
Rifampin: ↓ effect of fluconazole
Theophylline: ↑ effect
Warfarin: ↑ anticoagulation
Zidovudine: ↑ effect
Drug classification
Cyclosporines: ↑ renal dysfunction
Oral contraceptives: ↓ effect
Sulfonylureas: ↑ effect

NURSING CONSIDERATIONS
Assessment
• Assess for signs and symptoms of infection
• Obtain cultures for C&S before beginning treatment; therapy may be started after culture is taken
◆• Monitor for renal toxicity: increasing BUN, serum creatinine; if BUN is >40 mg/dl or if serum creatinine is >3 mg/dl, drug may be discontinued or dosage reduced
• Monitor for hepatotoxicity: increased AST, ALT, alk phosphatase, bilirubin; drug will be discontinued if hepatotoxicity occurs
Nursing diagnoses
☑ Infection, risk for (uses)
☑ Injury, risk for (adverse reactions)
☑ Knowledge deficit (teaching)

Implementation
ⅣV route
• Give after diluting according to package directions; run at 200 mg/hr or less; do not use plastic containers in connections
• Do not admix
• Administer **IV** using an in-line filter, using distal veins; check for extravasation and necrosis q2h
• Give drug only after C&S confirms organism, drug needed to treat condition
• Store protected from moisture and light, diluted sol is stable for 24 hr

Y-site compatibilities:
Acyclovir, aldesleukin, allopurinol, amifostine, amikacin, aminophylline, ampicillin/sulbactam, aztreonam, benztropine, cefazolin, cefepime, cefotetan, cefoxitin, chlorpromazine, cimetidine, dexamethasone, diphenhydramine, dobutamine, dopamine, droperidol, famotidine, filgrastim, fludarabine, foscarnet, gallium, ganciclovir, gentamicin, granisetron, heparin, hydrocortisone, immune globulin, leucovorin, lorazepam, melphalan, meperidine, meropenem, metoclopramide, metronidazole, midazolam, morphine, nafcillin, nitroglycerin, ondansetron, oxacillin, paclitaxel, pancuronium, penicillin G, potassium, phenytoin, piperacillin/tazobactam, prochlorperazine, promethazine, propofol, ranitidine, sargramostim, sulfamethoxazole, tacrolimus, teniposide, theophylline, thiotepa, ticarcillin/clavulanate, tobramycin, vancomycin, vecuronium, vinorelbine, zidovudine

---

☑ Herb/drug   🚫 Do Not Crush   ◆ Alert   ⚫ᴛ Key Drug   🅖 Geriatric   🅟 Pediatric

Y-*site incompatibilities:*
Amphotericin B, ampicillin, calcium gluconate, cefotaxime, ceftriaxone, ceftazidime, cefuroxime, chloramphenicol, clindamycin, diazepam, digoxin, erythromycin lactobionate, furosemide, haloperidol, hydroxyzine, imipenem/cilastatin, pentamidine, ticarcillin, trimethoprim/sulfamethoxazole

Additive compatibilities:
Acyclovir, amikacin, amphotericin B, cefazolin, ceftazidime, clindamycin, gentamicin, heparin, meropenem, metronidazole, morphine, piperacillin, potassium chloride, theophylline

Patient/family education
• Caution patient that long-term therapy may be needed to clear infection; to take entire course of medication; take in equal intervals (PO)
• Teach patient the signs and symptoms of hepatotoxicity: nausea, vomiting, clay-colored stools, dark urine, anorexia, fatigue, jaundice—health care prescriber should be notified immediately
• Inform patient that medication may be taken with food to reduce GI effects
• Advise patient to consider using alternative contraception if using oral contraceptives

Evaluation
Positive therapeutic outcome
• Decreasing oral candidiasis, fever, malaise, rash
• Negative C&S for infecting organism

flucytosine (℞)
(floo-sye′toe-seen)
Ancobon, Ancotil ✦, 5-FC
Func. class.: Antifungal
Chem. class.: Pyrimidine (fluorinated)
Pregnancy category   C

Action: Converted to fluorouracil after entering fungi; inhibits RNA, DNA synthesis; synergism action when used with amphotericin B in some infections

Therapeutic Outcome: Fungicidal against the following susceptible organisms: *Candida, Cryptococcus*

Uses: *Candida* infections (septicemia, endocarditis, pulmonary, urinary tract infections), *Cryptococcus* (meningitis, pulmonary, urinary tract infections)

Dosage and routes
Adult and child >50 kg: PO 50-150 mg/kg/day q6h
Adult and child <50 kg: PO 1.5-4.5 g/m²/day or 50-100 mg/kg/day in 4 divided doses
Renal dose
CrCl 10-50 ml/min give q16h; CrCl <10 ml/min give q24h
Available forms: Caps 250, 500 mg

Adverse effects
CNS: Headache, confusion, dizziness, sedation, vertigo
GI: Nausea, vomiting, anorexia, diarrhea, abdominal distention, cramps, enterocolitis, increased AST, ALT, alk phosphatase, **bowel perforation (rare)**
GU: Increased BUN, creatinine

HEMA: **Thrombocytopenia, agranulocytosis, anemia, leukopenia, pancytopenia**
INTEG: Rash

Contraindications: Hypersensitivity

Precautions: Renal disease, impaired hepatic function, bone marrow depression, blood dyscrasias, radiation/chemotherapy, pregnancy **C**

Do Not Confuse:
flucytosine/fluorouracil

Pharmacokinetics

Absorption	Well absorbed
Distribution	Widely distributed, crosses blood-brain barrier, crosses placenta
Metabolism	Unknown
Excretion	90% kidneys—unchanged
Half-life	3-6 hr, increased in renal disease

Pharmacodynamics

Onset	Rapid
Peak	2½-6 hr
Duration	6 hr

Interactions
Individual drugs
Amphotericin B: ↑ toxicity
Cytarabine: ↓ antifungal action
Drug classifications
Antineoplastics: ↑ bone marrow depression
Radiation: ↑ bone marrow depression
Lab test interferences
False: ↑ Creatinine

NURSING CONSIDERATIONS
Assessment
• Assess patient for signs and symptoms of infection before beginning treatment and during therapy

• Obtain cultures for C&S before initiating treatment; therapy may be started after culture is taken
• Monitor renal toxicity: increasing BUN, serum creatinine; if BUN is >40 mg/dl or if serum creatinine is >3 mg/dl, drug may be discontinued or dosage reduced
• Monitor for hepatotoxicity: increased AST, ALT, alk phosphatase, bilirubin; drug will be discontinued if hepatotoxicity occurs

Nursing diagnoses
☑ Infection, risk for (uses)
☑ Diarrhea (adverse reactions)
☑ Knowledge deficit (teaching)

Implementation
• Give a few caps at a time with food to decrease nausea, vomiting over 15 min; store in tight, light-resistant containers at room temp
⊘ • Do not crush, chew caps
• Use symptomatic treatment as ordered for adverse reactions: aspirin, antihistamines, antiemetics, antispasmodics

Patient/family education
• Advise patient that medication may cause dizziness, drowsiness, and confusion; to avoid hazardous activities until side effects are determined
• Instruct patient to notify prescriber if rash, fever, sore throat, fatigue, muscle weakness, diarrhea, bruising, bleeding occur
• Caution patient to take medication exactly as prescribed; not to double doses—missed doses should be taken when remembered within 1 hr of next dose

---

Evaluation

Positive therapeutic outcome
• Decreasing oral candidiasis, fever, malaise, rash
• Negative C&S for infection organism

---

fludrocortisone (℞)

(floo-droe-kor′ti-sone)

Florinef

Func. class.: Corticosteroid

Chem. class.: Mineralocorticoid

Pregnancy category **C**

Action: Promotes increased reabsorption of sodium and loss of potassium, water, hydrogen from the distal renal tubules

→ **Therapeutic Outcome:** Treatment of adrenal insufficiency symptoms

Uses: Adrenal insufficiency, salt-losing adrenogenital syndrome

Dosage and routes
Adult: PO 0.1-0.2 mg qd

℗ *Child:* PO 0.05-0.1 mg/day

Available forms: Tab 0.1 mg

Adverse effects

CNS: Flushing, sweating, headache
CV: Hypertension, **circulatory collapse, thrombophlebitis, embolism,** tachycardia
MS: Fractures, osteoporosis, weakness

Contraindications: Hypersensitivity, acute glomerulonephritis, amebiasis

Precautions: Pregnancy **C**, osteoporosis, CHF, lactation

Pharmacokinetics

Absorption	Well absorbed
Distribution	Widely
Metabolism	Liver
Excretion	Kidneys, breast milk
Half-life	3½ hr

Pharmacodynamics
Unknown

Interactions
Individual drugs
Amphotericin B: ↑ hypokalemia
Mezlocillin: ↑ hypokalemia
Phenobarbital: ↓ effect of fludrocortisone
Piperacillin: ↑ hypokalemia
Rifampin: ↓ effect of fludrocortisone
Drug classifications
Diuretics: ↑ hypokalemia
Nondepolarizing neuromuscular blocking agents: ↑ neuromuscular blockade
Food/drug
↑ **salt/sodium ingestion:** ↑ hypokalemia, ↑ hypernatremia
Herb/drug
Aloe: ↑ hypokalemia
Buckthorn: ↑ hypokalemia
Cascara sagrada: ↑ hypokalemia
Senna: ↑ hypokalemia
Lab test interferences
↑ Potassium, ↑ chloride
↓ Hematocrit

NURSING CONSIDERATIONS
Assessment
• Monitor patient for fluid retention: weigh daily, notify prescriber of weekly gain >5 lb; B/P q4h, pulse; notify prescriber if chest pain occurs: I&O ratio; be alert for decreasing urinary output and increasing edema

F

• Check for potassium depletion: paresthesias, fatigue, nausea, vomiting, depression, polyuria, dysrhythmias, weakness

Nursing diagnoses

☑ Fluid volume deficit (uses)
☑ Fluid volume excess (adverse reactions)
☑ Knowledge deficit (teaching)

Implementation

• Administer titrated dose; use lowest effective dose; scored tab may be broken if lower dose is necessary
• Give with food or milk to decrease GI symptoms

Patient/family education

• Advise patient to carry ID as steroid user at all times during diagnosis and treatment
• Caution patient not to discontinue this medication abruptly—Addisonian crisis may occur
• Counsel patient to follow dietary regimen recommended by prescriber—should include high potassium and, possibly, low sodium
• Advise patient to report weight gain >5 lbs; edema in legs, hands; abdominal cramping; muscle cramps; nausea; vomiting; anorexia; dizziness or weakness

Evaluation

Positive therapeutic outcome

• Correction of adrenal insufficiency
• Electrolytes and fluids in normal range

---

flumazenil (℞)

(flu-maz'e-nil)
Mazicon, Ronazicon
Func. class.: Benzodiazepine receptor antagonist
Chem. class.: Imidazobenzodiazepine derivative

Pregnancy category   C

Action: Antagonizes the actions of benzodiazepines on the CNS, competitively inhibits the activity at the benzodiazepine receptor complex

Therapeutic Outcome: Reversed benzodiazepine toxic effects

Uses: Reversal of the sedative effects of benzodiazepines

Dosage and routes
Reversal of conscious sedation or in general anesthesia
Adult: **IV** 0.2 mg (2 ml) given over 15 sec; wait 45 sec, then give 0.2 mg (2 ml) if consciousness does not occur; may be repeated at 60-sec intervals as needed, up to 4 additional times (max total dose 1 mg); dose is to be individualized

Management of suspected benzodiazepine overdose
Adult: **IV** 0.2 mg (2 ml) given over 30 sec; wait 30 sec, then give 0.3 mg (3 ml) over 30 sec if consciousness does not occur; further doses of 0.5 mg (5 ml) can be given over 30 sec at intervals of 1 min up to cumulative dose of 3 mg

Available forms: Inj 0.1 mg/ml

Adverse effects

CNS: Dizziness, agitation, emotional lability, confusion, **convulsions,** somnolence

---

CV: Hypertension, palpitations, cutaneous vasodilation, **dysrhythmias,** bradycardia, tachycardia, chest pain
EENT: Abnormal vision, blurred vision, tinnitus
GI: Nausea, vomiting, hiccups
SYST: Headache, injection site pain, increased sweating, fatigue, rigors

Contraindications: Hypersensitivity to this drug or benzodiazepines, serous tricyclic antidepressant overdose, patients given benzodiazepine for control of life-threatening condition

Precautions: Pregnancy **C,** lactation, children, elderly, renal disease, seizures, head injury, labor and delivery, hepatic disease, hypoventilation, panic disorder, drug and alcohol dependency, ambulatory patients

Do Not Confuse:
Mazicon/Mivacron

Pharmacokinetics

Absorption	Complete
Distribution	Unknown
Metabolism	Liver
Excretion	Unknown
Half-life	41-79 min

Pharmacodynamics

Onset	1 min
Peak	10 min
Duration	Unknown

Interactions: None

NURSING CONSIDERATIONS
Assessment
• Assess cardiac status using continuous monitoring
• Assess for seizures; protect patient from injury
• Assess for GI symptoms: nausea, vomiting; place in side-lying position to prevent aspiration
• Assess for allergic reactions: flushing, rash, urticaria, pruritus

Nursing diagnoses
☑ Injury, risk for (uses)
☑ Poisoning (uses)

Implementation
• Give directly undiluted or diluted in 0.9% NaCl, D_5W, or LR; give over 15 sec
• Check airway and **IV** access before administration

Additive compatibilities:
Aminophylline, cimetidine, dobutamine, dopamine, famotidine, heparin, lidocaine, procainamide, ranitidine

Patient/family education
• Caution patient that amnesia may continue
• Instruct patient to avoid any hazardous activities for 18-24 hr after discharge
• Inform patient not to take any alcohol or nonprescription drugs for 18-24 hr—serious reactions may occur

Evaluation
Positive therapeutic outcome
• Decreased sedation, respiratory depression
• Absence of toxicity

fluorouracil
(5-fluorouracil) (℞)
(flure-oh-yoor'a-sil)
Adrucil, 5-FU
Func. class.: Antineoplastic, antimetabolite
Chem. class.: Pyrimidine antagonist
Pregnancy category D

Action: Inhibits DNA synthesis; interferes with cell

replication by competitively inhibiting thymidylate synthesis, S phase of cell cycle-specific vesicant

→**Therapeutic Outcome:** Prevention of rapidly growing malignant cells

Uses: Cancer of breast, colon, rectum, stomach, pancreas; multiple active keratoses; basal cell carcinoma (top)

Dosage and routes
Adult: **IV** 12 mg/kg/day × 4 days, not to exceed 800 mg/day; may repeat with 6 mg/kg on day 6, 8, 10, 12; maintenance is 10-15 mg/kg/wk as a single dose, not to exceed 1 g/wk

Adult: Top 1, 2% sol apply to lesion on head, neck, or on other areas 5% bid

Available forms: Inj 50 mg/ml; cream 1, 5%; sol 1, 2, 5%

Adverse effects
CNS: Lethargy, malaise, weakness
CV: Myocardial ischemia, angina
EENT: Epistaxis
GI: *Anorexia, stomatitis,* diarrhea, nausea, vomiting, **hemorrhage, enteritis glossitis**
GU: Renal failure
HEMA: **Thrombocytopenia, leukopenia, myelosuppression, anemia, agranulocytosis**
INTEG: Rash, fever

Contraindications: Hypersensitivity, myelosuppression, pregnancy **D,** poor nutritional status, serious infections

Precautions: Renal disease, hepatic disease, bone marrow depression, angina, lactation, **P** children

❑ Do Not Confuse:
fluorouracil/flucytosine

Pharmacokinetics	
Absorption	Completely bioavailable (**IV**), minimal (Top)
Distribution	Widely distributed, concentration in tumor
Metabolism	Liver—converted to active metabolite
Excretion	Lungs (60%-80%), kidneys (up to 15%)
Half-life	20 hr terminal

Pharmacodynamics	
Unknown	

Interactions
Individual drugs
Radiation: ↑ toxicity, bone marrow suppression
Drug classifications
Antineoplastics: ↑ toxicity bone marrow suppression
Lab test interferences
↑ Liver function studies, ↑ 6-HIAA
↓ Albumin

NURSING CONSIDERATIONS
Assessment
• Monitor ECG; watch for ST-T wave changes, low QRS and T, possible dysrhythmias (sinus tachycardia, heart block, PVCs)
• Assess buccal cavity q8h for dryness, sores or ulceration, white patches, oral pain, bleeding, dysphagia; obtain prescription for viscous lidocaine (Xylocaine)
• Assess symptoms indicating severe allergic reaction: rash, pruritus, urticaria, purpuric skin lesions, itching, flushing
• Assess tachypnea, ECG changes, dyspnea, edema, fatigue; identify dyspnea, rales, unproductive cough, chest pain, tachypnea
• Monitor CBC, differential, platelet count weekly; withhold

drug if WBC count is <4000/ mm³ or platelet count is <100,000/mm³; notify prescriber of results if WBC <20,000/mm³, platelets <50,000/mm³
- Monitor renal function studies: BUN, creatinine, serum uric acid, urine CrCl before and during therapy; I&O ratio; report fall in urine output to <30 ml/hr
- Monitor temp q4h (may indicate beginning of infection)
- Monitor liver function tests before and during therapy (bilirubin, AST, ALT, LDH) as needed or monthly; jaundice of skin, sclera, dark urine, clay-colored stools, itchy skin, abdominal pain, fever, diarrhea
- Assess for bleeding: hematuria, stool guaiac, bruising or petechiae, mucosa or orifices q8h; inflammation of mucosa, breaks in skin

Nursing diagnoses
☑ Injury, risk for (adverse reactions)
☑ Body image disturbance (adverse reactions)
☑ Infection, risk for (adverse reactions)
☑ Knowledge deficit (teaching)

Implementation
- Avoid contact with skin (very irritating); wash completely to remove
- Give fluids **IV** or PO before chemotherapy to hydrate patient
- Give antiemetic 30-60 min before giving drug to prevent vomiting, and prn for several days thereafter; antibiotics for prophylaxis of infection
- Provide liq diet: carbonated beverages; gelatin may be added if patient is not nauseated or vomiting
- Provide rinsing of mouth tid-qid with water, club soda; brushing of teeth bid-qid with soft brush or cotton-tipped applicators for stomatitis; use unwaxed dental floss

IV **IV route**
- **IV** undiluted; may inject through Y-tube or 3-way stopcock; give over 1-3 min
- May be diluted in NS, D₅W, given over 2-8 hr as an **IV** inf

Top route
- Wear gloves when applying; may use with a loose dressing

Syringe compatibilities:
Bleomycin, cisplatin, cyclophosphamide, furosemide, heparin, leucovorin, methotrexate, metoclopramide, mitomycin, vinblastine, vincristine

Syringe incompatibilities:
Droperidol

Y-site compatibilities:
Allopurinol, amifostine, aztreonam, bleomycin, cefepime, cisplatin, cyclophosphamide, doxorubicin, fludarabine, furosemide, granisetron, heparin, hydrocortisone, leucovorin, mannitol, melphalan, methotrexate, metoclopramide, mitomycin, paclitaxel, piperacillin/tazobactam, potassium chloride, propofol, sargramostin, thiotepa, thiposide, vinblastine, vincristine, vit B/C

Y-site incompatibilities:
Droperidol, vinorelbine

Additive compatibilities:
Bleomycin, cephalothin, etoposides, floxuridine, hydromorphone, ifosfamide, leucovorin, methotrexate, mitoxantrone, prednisolone, vincristine, cyclophosphamide, mitoxantrone

---

Additive incompatibilities:
Carboplatin, cisplatin, cytarabine, diazepam, doxorubicin

Solution compatibilities:
Amino acids 4.25%/D_{25}, D_5/LR, $D_{3.3}$/0.3 NaCl, D_5W, 0.9% NaCl, TPN #23

Patient/family education

• Caution patient that contraceptive measures are recommended during therapy

• Teach patient to avoid using aspirin- or ibuprofen-containing products, razors, commercial mouthwash because bleeding may occur; to report symptoms of bleeding (hematuria, tarry stools)

• Instruct patient to report signs of anemia (fatigue, headache, irritability, faintness, shortness of breath)

Evaluation

Positive therapeutic outcome

• Prevention of rapid division of malignant cells

---

fluoxetine (R)

(floo-ox'uh-teen)
Prozac
Func. class.: Antidepressant, SSRI

Pregnancy category　B

Action: Inhibits CNS neuron uptake of serotonin, but not of norepinephrine

▣ **Therapeutic Outcome:** Decreased symptoms of depression after 2-3 wk

Uses: Major depressive disorder, obsessive-compulsive disorder (OCD), bulimia nervosa

Investigational uses: Alcoholism, anorexia nervosa, ADHD, bipolar II affective disorder, borderline personality disorder, cataplexy, narcolepsy, kleptomania, migraine, obesity, post-traumatic stress disorder, schizophrenia, Tourette's syndrome, trichotillomania, levodopa-induced dyskinesia, social phobia

Dosage and routes

Depression/OCD
Adult: PO 20 mg qd AM; after 4 wk if no clinical improvement is noted, dose may be increased to 20 mg bid in AM, afternoon, not to exceed 80 mg/day

🄶 **Elderly:** PO 10 mg/day, increase as needed

🄿 **Child 5-18 yr:** PO 5-10 mg/kg/day, max 20 mg/day

Bulimia Nervosa
Adult: PO 60 mg/day in AM

Available forms: Pulvules 10, 20 mg; liq 20 mg/5 ml

Adverse effects

CNS: Headache, nervousness, insomnia, drowsiness, anxiety, tremor, dizziness, fatigue, sedation, poor concentration, abnormal dreams, agitation, **convulsions**

CV: Hot flashes, palpitations, angina pectoris, **hemorrhage,** hypertension, first-degree tachycardia

EENT: Visual changes, ear/eye pain, photophobia, tinnitus

GI: Nausea, diarrhea, dry mouth, anorexia, dyspepsia, constipation, cramps, vomiting, taste changes, flatulence, decreased appetite

GU: Dysmenorrhea, decreased libido, urinary frequency, urinary tract infection, amenorrhea, cystitis, impotence

INTEG: Sweating, rash, pruritus, acne, alopecia, urticaria

MS: Pain, arthritis, twitching

RESP: *Infection, pharyngitis, nasal congestion, sinus headache, sinusitis, cough dyspnea, bronchitis, asthma, hyperventilation, pneumonia*
SYST: *Asthenia, viral infection, fever, allergy, chills*

Contraindications: Hypersensitivity

P Precautions: Pregnancy **B**, **G** lactation, children, elderly

Do Not Confuse:
Prozac/Proscar, Prozac/Prosom, Prozac/Prilosec

Pharmacokinetics

Absorption	Well absorbed
Distribution	Crosses blood-brain barrier
Metabolism	Liver, extensively to norfluoxetine
Excretion	Kidneys, unchanged (12%), metabolite (7%); steady state 28-35 days, protein binding 94%
Half-life	1-3 days metabolite up to 1 wk

Pharmacodynamics

Onset	Unknown
Peak	6-8 hr
Duration	Unknown

Interactions
Individual drugs

Alcohol: ↑ CNS depression
Buspirone: ↑ worsening of OCD
Carbamazepine: ↑ toxicity
Clozapine: ↑ clozapine levels
Dextromethorphan: ↑ hallucinations
Digoxin: ↑ toxicity
Haloperidol: ↑ haloperidol effect
Lithium: ↑ toxicity
L-tryptophan: ↑ toxicity
Phenytoin: ↑ hydantoin levels

Drug classifications

Barbiturates: ↑ CNS depression
Benzodiazepines: ↑ CNS depression
CNS depressants: ↑ CNS depression
MAOIs: Hypertensive crisis, convulsions
Oral anticoagulants: ↑ effects, toxicity
Sedative/hypnotics: ↑ CNS depression

Herb/drug

Kava: ↑ action
St. John's Wort: Do not use together

Lab test interferences

↑ Serum bilirubin, ↑ blood glucose, ↑ alk phosphatase
↓ VMA, ↓ 5-HIAA, ↓ blood glucose
False: ↑ Urinary catecholamines

NURSING CONSIDERATIONS
Assessment

• Monitor B/P (lying, standing), pulse q4h; if systolic B/P drops 20 mm hg, hold drug and notify prescriber; take vital signs q4h in patients with cardiovascular disease
• Monitor blood studies: CBC, leukocytes, differential, cardiac enzymes if patient is receiving long-term therapy; check platelets, bleeding can occur
• Monitor hepatic studies: AST, ALT, bilirubin
• Check weight qwk; appetite may increase with drug
• Assess ECG for flattening of T wave, bundle branch block, AV block, dysrhythmias in cardiac patients
• Assess mental status: mood, sensorium, affect, suicidal tendencies; increase in psychi-

F

---

atric symptoms: depression, panic
• Monitor urinary retention, constipation; constipation is **P** **G** more likely to occur in children or elderly
• Identify patient's alcohol consumption; if alcohol is consumed, hold dose until AM

Nursing diagnoses

☑ Coping, ineffective individual (uses)
☑ Injury, risk for (side effects)
☑ Knowledge deficit (teaching)
☑ Noncompliance (teaching)

Implementation

• Give with food or milk for GI symptoms
• Give dosage hs if oversedation occurs during day; may **G** take entire dose hs; elderly may not tolerate once/day dosing
• Store at room temp; do not freeze

Patient/family education

• Teach patient that therapeutic effects may take 1-4 wk
• Instruct patient to use caution in driving or other activities requiring alertness because of drowsiness, dizziness, blurred vision; to avoid rising quickly from sitting to stand- **G** ing, especially elderly; to use sunscreen to prevent photosensitivity
• Caution patient to avoid alcohol ingestion, other CNS depressants
• Advise patient not to discontinue medication quickly after long-term use: may cause nausea, headache, malaise
• Instruct patient to increase fluids, bulk in diet if constipation, urinary retention occur, **G** especially elderly
• Advise patient to take gum, hard sugarless candy, or fre-quent sips of water for dry mouth

Evaluation

Positive therapeutic outcome
• Decrease in depression
• Absence of suicidal thoughts
• Decreased symptoms of OCD

---

fluphenazine decanoate (℞)
(floo-fen'ah-zeen)
Modecate Concentrate, Prolixin Decanoate
fluphenazine enanthate (℞)
Moditen Enanthate ✦, Prolixin Enanthate
fluphenazine hydrochloride (℞)
Apo-Fluphenazine ✦, Moditen HCL ✦, Moditen HCl-H.P. ✦, Permitil ✦, Prolixin
Func. class.: Antipsychotic/neuroleptic
Chem. class.: Phenothiazine, piperazine
Pregnancy category   **C**

Action: Depresses cerebral cortex, hypothalamus, limbic system, which control activity and aggression; blocks neurotransmission produced by dopamine at synapse; exhibits strong α-adrenergic and anticholinergic blocking action; mechanism for antipsychotic effects is unclear

Therapeutic Outcome: Decreased signs and symptoms of psychosis

Uses: Psychotic disorders, schizophrenia

Dosage and routes
Enanthate, decanoate
🅿 *Adult and child >12 yr:* IM 12.5-25 mg q1-3 wk
HCl
Adult: PO 2.5-10 mg, in divided doses q6-8h, not to exceed 20 mg qd; IM initially 1.25 mg then 2.5-10 mg in divided doses q6-8h
🅿 *Child:* PO 0.25-3.5 mg qd in divided doses q4-6h, max 10 mg/qd

Available forms: HCl tabs 1, 2.5, 5, 10 mg; elix 2.5 mg/5 ml; conc 5 mg/ml; inj 2.5 mg/ml, enanthate, decanoate depot inj 25 mg/ml

Adverse effects
CNS: Extrapyramidal symptoms: pseudoparkinsonism, akathisia, dystonia, tardive dyskinesia, drowsiness, headache, **seizures, neuroleptic malignant syndrome**
CV: Orthostatic hypotension, hypertension, **cardiac arrest,** ECG changes, **tachycardia**
EENT: Blurred vision, glaucoma, dry eyes
GI: Dry mouth, nausea, vomiting, anorexia, constipation, diarrhea, jaundice, weight gain, **paralytic ileus, hepatitis**
GU: Urinary retention, urinary frequency, enuresis, impotence, amenorrhea, gynecomastia
HEMA: Anemia, **leukopenia, leukocytosis, agranulocytosis, aplastic anemia, thrombocytopenia**
INTEG: Rash, photosensitivity, dermatitis
RESP: **Laryngospasm,** dyspnea, **respiratory depression**

Contraindications: Hypersensitivity, circulatory collapse, liver damage, cerebral arteriosclerosis, coronary disease, severe hypertension/hypotension, blood dyscrasias,
🅿 coma, child <12 yr, brain damage, bone marrow depression, alcohol and barbiturate withdrawal

Precautions: Pregnancy **C,** lactation, seizure disorders, hypertension, hepatic disease,
🅖 cardiac disease, elderly

🆖 **Do Not Confuse:**
Prolixin/Proloid

Pharmacokinetics

Absorption	Well absorbed (PO, IM)
Distribution	Widely absorbed, crosses blood-brain barrier, placenta
Metabolism	Liver, extensively
Excretion	Kidneys (metabolites)
Half-life	HCl-4.7-15.3 hr, enanthate 3½-4 days, decanoate 6.8-14.3 days

Pharmacodynamics

	PO/IM	IM	IM
	HCl	Enanthate	Decanoate
Onset	1 hr	1-2 days	1-3 days
Peak	1½-2 hr	2-3 days	1-2 days
Duration	6-8 hr	1-3 wk	>4 wk

Interactions
Individual drugs
Alcohol: ↑ effects of both drugs, oversedation
Bromocriptine: ↓ antiparkinson activity
Disopyramide: ↑ anticholinergic effects
Epinephrine: ↑ toxicity
Guanethidine: ↓ antihypertensive response
Levodopa: ↓ antiparkinson activity
Lithium: ↓ fluphenazine levels, ↑ extrapyramidal symptoms, masking of lithium toxicity

Magnesium hydroxide: ↓ absorption of fluphenazine
Norepinephrine: ↓ vasoresponse, ↑ toxicity

Drug classifications
Antacids: ↓ absorption of fluphenazine
Anticholinergics: ↑ anticholinergic effects
Antidepressants: ↑ CNS depression
Antidiarrheals, adsorbent: ↓ absorption
Antihistamines: ↑ CNS depression
Antihypertensives: ↑ hypotension
Antithyroid agents: ↑ agranulocytosis
Barbiturates: ↑ CNS depression
β-Adrenergic blockers: ↑ effects of both drugs
General anesthetics: ↑ CNS depression
MAOIs: ↑ CNS depression
Opiates: ↑ CNS depression
Sedative/hypnotics: ↑ CNS depression

Lab test interferences
↑ liver function tests, ↑ cardiac enzymes, ↑ cholesterol, ↑ blood glucose, ↑ prolactin, ↑ bilirubin, ↑ PBI, ↑ cholinesterase I, ↑ alk phosphatase, ↑ leukocytes, ↑ granulocytes, ↑ platelets
↓ hormones (blood and urine)
False positive: Pregnancy tests, PKU, urine bilirubin
False negative: Urinary steroids, 17-OHCS

NURSING CONSIDERATIONS
Assessment
• Assess mental status: orientation, mood, behavior, presence of hallucinations, and type before initial administration and monthly; this drug should significantly reduce psychotic behavior
• Check for swallowing of PO medication; check for hoarding or giving of medication to other patients
• Monitor I&O ratio, palpate bladder if low urinary output occurs, especially in elderly; urinalysis recommended before, during prolonged therapy
• Monitor bilirubin, CBC, liver function studies monthly
• Assess affect, orientation, LOC, reflexes, gait, coordination, sleep pattern disturbances
• Monitor B/P with patient sitting, standing, and lying down; take pulse and respirations q4h during initial treatment; establish baseline before starting treatment; report drops of 30 mm Hg; obtain baseline ECG, Q-wave and T-wave changes
• Check for dizziness, faintness, palpitations, tachycardia on rising; severe orthostatic hypotension is common
• Identify for neuroleptic malignant syndrome: hyperpyrexia, muscle rigidity, increased CPK, altered mental status; drug should be discontinued
• Assess for extrapyramidal symptoms including akathisia (inability to sit still, no pattern to movements), tardive dyskinesia (bizarre movements of the jaw, mouth, tongue, extremities), pseudoparkinsonism (rigidity, tremors, pill rolling, shuffling gate), an antiparkinson drug should be prescribed
• Assess for constipation, urinary retention daily; if these occur, increase bulk, water in diet

---

Nursing diagnoses
- ☑ Thought processes, altered (uses)
- ☑ Coping, ineffective individual (uses)
- ☑ Knowledge deficit (teaching)
- ☑ Noncompliance (teaching)

Implementation
PO route
- Give drug in liq form mixed in glass of juice or cola if hoarding is suspected; do not mix in caffeine drinks, tannics, or pectinates; decrease dose in ☰ elderly
- Give PO with full glass of water, milk; or give with food to decrease GI upset
- Store in tight, light-resistant container, oral sol in amber bottle

SC route
- May be given by this route; however, it is painful

IM route
- Inject in deep muscle mass, use a 21-G needle into dorsal gluteal site, keep patient recumbent for ½ hr—prevents orthostatic hypotension

Syringe compatibilities:
Benztropine, diphenhydramine, hydroxyzine

Patient/family education
- Teach patient to use good oral hygiene; frequent rinsing of mouth, sugarless gum for dry mouth
- Caution patient to avoid hazardous activities until drug response is determined; dizziness, blurred vision may occur
- Inform patient that orthostatic hypotension occurs often and to rise from sitting or lying position gradually, to remain lying down after IM inj for at least 30 min; tell patient to avoid hot tubs, hot showers, tub baths because hypotension may occur; tell patient that in hot weather, heat stroke may occur—extra precautions are necessary to stay cool
- Instruct patient to avoid abrupt withdrawal of this drug, or extrapyramidal symptoms may result; drug should be withdrawn slowly
- Teach patient to avoid OTC preparations (cough, hayfever, cold) unless approved by physician because serious drug interactions may occur; avoid use with alcohol, CNS depressants; increased drowsiness may occur
- Instruct patient to use a sunscreen and sunglasses to prevent burns
- Teach patient about extrapyramidal symptoms and necessity of meticulous oral hygiene beause oral candidiasis may occur
- Instruct patient to take antacids 2 hr before or after this drug
- Advise patient to report sore throat, malaise, fever, bleeding, mouth sores; if these occur, CBC should be drawn and drug discontinued

Evaluation
Positive therapeutic outcome
- Decrease in emotional excitement, hallucinations, delusions, paranoia
- Reorganization of patterns of thought, speech

Treatment of overdose:
Lavage if orally ingested; provide airway; *do not induce vomiting or use epinephrine*

---

flurazepam (℞)
(flure-az'e-pam)
Apo-flurazepam ✦,
Dalmane, Durapam,
flurazepam, Novo-
Flupam ✦, Somnol ✦,
Som-Pam ✦
Func. class.: Sedative-
hypnotic
Chem. class.: Benzodiaze-
pine derivative

Pregnancy category　X
**Controlled substance
schedule　IV** (USA),
schedule　F (Canada)

Action: Produces CNS depression at the limbic, thalamic,
hypothalamic levels of CNS;
may be mediated by neuro-
transmitter γ-aminobutyric acid
(GABA); results are sedation,
hypnosis, skeletal muscle relaxation, anticonvulsant activity,
anxiolytic action

➡**Therapeutic Outcome:** Ability to sleep, relaxation

Uses: Insomnia

Dosage and routes
Adult: PO 15-30 mg hs; may
repeat dose once if needed
G *Geriatric:* PO 15 mg hs; may
increase if needed

Available forms: Caps 15,
30 mg

Adverse effects
*CNS: Lethargy, drowsiness,
daytime sedation,* dizziness,
confusion, light-headedness,
headache, anxiety, irritability
CV: Chest pain, pulse changes
GI: Nausea, vomiting, diarrhea, heartburn, abdominal
pain, constipation
HEMA: Leukopenia, granulocytopenia (rare)

Contraindications: Hypersensitivity to benzodiazepines,
pregnancy **X**, lactation, intermittent porphyria, uncon-
trolled pain

Precautions: Anemia, hepatic
disease, renal disease, suicidal
G individuals, drug abuse, elderly,
P psychosis, child <15 yr

Pharmacokinetics

Absorption	Well absorbed
Distribution	Widely absorbed, crosses blood-brain barrier, crosses placenta
Metabolism	Liver to active, inactive metabolites
Excretion	Kidneys, breast milk
Half-life	2½ hr, 30-200 hr active metabolites

Pharmacodynamics

Onset	15-30 min
Peak	½-1 hr
Duration	7-8 hr

Interactions
Individual drugs
Alcohol: ↑ CNS depression
Cimetidine: ↑ action of fluraz-
epam
Disulfiram: ↑ action of fluraz-
epam
Fluoxetine: ↑ action of fluraz-
epam
Isoniazid: ↑ action of fluraze-
pam
Ketoconazole: ↑ action of
flurazepam
Levodopa: ↓ action of levo-
dopa
Metoprolol: ↑ action of flur-
azepam
Propoxyphene: ↑ action of
flurazepam
Propranolol: ↑ action of
flurazepam
Rifampin: ↓ action of fluraze-
pam

Theophylline: ↓ sedative effects
Valproic acid: ↑ action of flurazepam
Drug classifications
Analgesics, opioid: ↑ CNS depression
Antidepressants: ↑ CNS depression
Antihistamines: ↑ CNS depression
Barbiturates: ↓ effect of flurazepam
Contraceptives: ↑ effect
Herb/drug
Kava: ↑ effect
Lab test interferences
↑ AST/ALT, ↑ serum bilirubin
False: ↑ urinary 17-OHCS, ↓ RAI uptake

NURSING CONSIDERATIONS
Assessment
• Assess anxiety reaction: inability to sleep, apprehension, dread, foreboding, or uneasiness related to unidentified source of danger
• Assess for previous drug dependence or tolerance; if drug dependent or tolerant, amount of medication should be restricted
• Monitor B/P (lying, standing), pulse; if systolic B/P drops 20 mm Hg, hold drug, notify prescriber; I&O, may indicate renal dysfunction
• Monitor blood studies: CBC during long-term therapy; blood dyscrasias have occurred rarely
• Monitor hepatic studies: AST, ALT, bilirubin, creatinine, LDH, alk phosphatase
• Monitor patient's mental status: mood, sensorium, affect, sleeping patterns, drowsiness, dizziness, suicidal tendencies

Nursing diagnoses
☑ Sleep pattern disturbance (uses)
☑ Knowledge deficit (teaching)
☑ Noncompliance (teaching)

Implementation
• Give after removing cigarettes to prevent fires
• Give after trying conservative measures for insomnia
• Give ½-1 hr before hs for sleeplessness; give on empty stomach with full glass of water or juice for best absorption and to decrease corrosion (do not chew); give pc to decrease GI symptoms if used for sedation
• Provide assistance with ambulation after receiving dose
• Provide safety measures: nightlight, call bell within easy reach
• Check to see if PO medication has been swallowed
• Store in tight container in cool environment

Patient/family education
• Inform patient that drug may be taken with food; if dose is missed take as soon as remembered; do not double doses
• Advise patient to avoid OTC preparations unless approved by a physician, to avoid alcohol ingestion or other psychotropic medications unless prescribed by a health care provider, that 1-2 wk of therapy may be required before therapeutic effects occur
• Caution patient to avoid driving, activities requiring alertness—drowsiness may occur; until medication response is known, tell patient that drowsiness may worsen at beginning of treatment

F

- Instruct patient not to discontinue medication abruptly after long-term use
- Caution patient to rise slowly or fainting may occur, especially in elderly [G]
- Inform patient that hangover is common in elderly [G]

Evaluation
Positive therapeutic outcome
- Increased well-being
- Decreased anxiety, restlessness, sleeplessness, dread

Treatment of overdose: Lavage, activated charcoal; monitor electrolytes, vital signs

---

flurbiprofen (R)
(flure-bi′proe-fen)
Ansaid, Froben ✤, Ocufen
Func. class.: Nonsteroidal antiinflammatory
Chem. class.: Phenylalkanoic acid
Pregnancy category C

Action: Inhibits prostaglandin synthesis by decreasing enzyme needed for biosynthesis; analgesic, antiinflammatory, antipyretic; inhibits enzyme system necessary for biosynthesis of prostaglandins; inhibits miosis

➡ **Therapeutic Outcome:** Decreased pain, inflammation

Uses: Mild-to-moderate pain, osteoarthritis, rheumatoid arthritis, acute gout, arthritis, ankylosing spondylitis, inflammation, dysmenorrhea; inhibition of intraoperative miosis, corneal edema

Dosage and routes
Adult: PO 200-300 mg qd in 2-4 divided doses, max 300 mg/day or 100 mg/dose;

ophth 1 gtt q½-2h before surgery (4 gtt total)

Available forms: Sol 0.03%; tabs 50, 100 mg

Adverse effects
CNS: Depression, flushing, sweating, headache, mood changes
CV: Hypertension, **circulatory collapse,** thrombophlebitis, embolism, tachycardia, edema
EENT: Burning, stinging in the eye, irritation, bleeding or redness; fungal infections, increased intraocular pressure, blurred vision
GI: Diarrhea, nausea, abdominal distention, **GI hemorrhage,** increased appetite, pancreatitis
INTEG: Acne, poor wound healing, ecchymosis, petechiae
MS: Fractures, osteoporosis, weakness

Contraindications: Hypersensitivity, epithelial herpes simplex keratitis

Precautions: Pregnancy **C,** lactation, child, aspirin or NSAID hypersensitivity, allergy, bleeding disorder [P]

▧ **Do Not Confuse:**
Ansaid/Asacol, Ocufen/Ocuflox, Ocufen/Ocupress

Pharmacokinetics	
Absorption	Well absorbed (PO)
Distribution	Widely distributed (PO)
Metabolism	Liver—extensively
Excretion	Kidneys
Half-life	3-6 hr

Pharmacodynamics
Unknown

Interactions
Individual drugs
Alcohol: ↑ GI upset
Aspirin: ↓ effect of flurbiprofen
Carbachol: ↓ effect when used with other ophthalmics
Epinephrine: ↓ effect of epinephrine
Heparin: ↑ bleeding
Radiation: ↑ effects
Drug classifications
Antihypertensives: ↓ antihypertensive effect
Cephalosporins: ↑ bleeding
Hypoglycemics, oral: ↑ hypoglycemic effect
NSAIDs: ↑ GI upset

NURSING CONSIDERATIONS
Assessment
• Assess for pain: joint pain (duration, intensity, ROM); baseline and during treatment

Implementation
Ophth route
• Excess sol must be wiped away promptly to prevent its flow into lacrimal system, producing systemic symptoms
• Protect sol from sun
PO route
• Give ½ hr ac or 2 hr pc

Patient/family education
• Advise patient to report change in vision, blurring, or loss of sight during miosis; rash, tinnitus, black stools, headache, chills, fever (systemic)
• Caution patient not to use for any other condition than prescribed
• Inform patient to avoid use with OTC medications for pain or with alcohol unless approved by prescriber
• Advise patient to avoid hazardous activities because dizziness or drowsiness occurs

Evaluation
Positive therapeutic outcome
• Absence of corneal edema, intraoperative miosis (ophth)
• Decreased pain, inflammation

---

flutamide (℞)
(floo′ta-mide)
Euflex ✤, Eulexin
Func. class.: Antineoplastic hormone
Chem. class.: Antiandrogen

Pregnancy category   D

Action: Interferes with testosterone uptake in the nucleus or testosterone activity in target tissues; arrests tumor growth in androgen-sensitive tissue, i.e., prostate gland

Therapeutic Outcome: Prevention of rapidly growing malignant cells

Uses: Metastatic prostatic carcinoma, stage D2 in combination with LHRH agonistic analogs (leuprolide)

Dosage and routes
Adult: PO 250 mg q8h tid, for a daily dosage of 750 mg

Available forms: Cap 125, 250 ✤ mg

Adverse effects
CNS: Hot flashes, drowsiness, confusion, depression, anxiety, paresthesia
GI: Diarrhea, nausea, vomiting, increased liver function studies, **hepatitis,** anorexia
GU: Decreased libido, impotence, gynecomastia
HEMA: Leukopenia, thrombocytopenia, hemolytic anemia
INTEG: Irritation at site, rash, photosensitivity

MISC: Edema, neuromuscular and pulmonary symptoms, hypertension

🔲 **Do Not Confuse:**
Eulexin/Edecrin

Contraindications: Hypersensitivity, pregnancy **D**

Pharmacokinetics	
Absorption	Well absorbed
Distribution	Unknown
Metabolism	Liver
Excretion	Unknown
Half-life	6 hr

Pharmacodynamics
Unknown

Interactions
Individual drugs
Leuprolide: ↑ synergistic effect

NURSING CONSIDERATIONS
Assessment
• Monitor CBC, bilirubin, creatinine, AST, ALT, alk phosphatase, which may be elevated
• Identify CNS symptoms: drowsiness, confusion, depression, anxiety

Nursing diagnoses
☑ Injury, risk for (adverse reactions)
☑ Sexual dysfunction (adverse reactions)
☑ Body image disturbance (adverse reactions)
☑ Infection, risk for (adverse reactions)
☑ Knowledge deficit (teaching)

Implementation
• Used in combination with LHRH agonist (leuprolide)
• May be given with food or fluids

Patient/family education
• Tell the patient to report side effects: decreased libido, impotence, breast enlargement, hot flashes, diarrhea, which occur when the two drugs are given together
• Inform patient that this drug is taken with leuprolide for medical castration

Evaluation
Positive therapeutic outcome
• Prevention of rapid division of malignant cells

fluvastatin (℞)
(flu'vah-stay-tin)
Lescol
Func. class.: Antilipidemic
Chem. class.: Synthetically derived fermentation product
Pregnancy category   **X**

Action: Inhibits HMG-CoA reductase enzyme, which reduces cholesterol synthesis

⬛ **Therapeutic Outcome:** Decreased cholsterol levels and LDLs, increased HDLs

Uses: As an adjunct in primary hypercholesterolemia (types Ia, Iib), coronary atherosclerosis in CAD

Dosage and routes
Adult: PO 20-40 mg qd in PM initially, usual range 20-80, not to exceed 80 mg; should be given in 2 doses (40 mg AM, 40 mg PM); dosage adjustments may be made in 4 wk intervals or more

Available forms: Caps 20, 40 mg

Adverse effects
CNS: Headache, dizziness, insomnia

EENT: Lens opacities
GI: Nausea, constipation, diarrhea, dyspepsia, flatus, liver dysfunction, pancreatitis
HEMA: **Thrombocytopenia, hemolytic anemia, leukopenia**
INTEG: Rash, pruritus
MISC: Fatigue, influenza
MS: Myalgia, myositis, rhabdomyolysis
RESP: Upper respiratory infection, rhinitis, cough, pharyngitis, sinusitis

Contraindications: Hypersensitivity, pregnancy **X**, lactation, active liver disease

Precautions: Past liver disease, alcoholism, severe acute infections, trauma, hypotension, uncontrolled seizure disorders, severe metabolic disorders, electrolyte imbalance

Pharmacokinetics	
Absorption	Unknown
Distribution	Unknown
Metabolism	Liver
Excretion	Feces, kidneys
Half-life	14 hr

Pharmacodynamics
Unknown

Interactions
Individual drugs
Bile acid sequestrants: ↓ effects of fluvastin
Cholestyramine: ↓ action of fluvastin
Colestipol: ↓ action of fluvastin
Cyclosporine: ↑ risk of myopathy
Digoxin: ↑ action
Erthyromycin: ↑ risk of myopathy
Gemfibrozil: ↑ risk of myopathy
Niacin: ↑ risk of myopathy

Rifampin: ↓ effects of fluvastin
Warfarin: ↑ action

NURSING CONSIDERATIONS
Assessment
• Assess nutrition: fat, protein, carbohydrates; nutritional analysis should be completed by dietician before treatment
• Monitor bowel pattern daily; diarrhea may be a problem
• Assess fasting lipid profile (cholesterol, LDL, HDL, TG) q8 wk, then q3-6 mo when stable
• Monitor liver function studies q1-2mo during the first 1½ yr of treatment; AST, ALT, liver function tests may be increased
• Monitor renal studies in patients with compromised renal system: BUN, I&O ratio, creatinine
• Monitor eyes with slit lamp before, 1 mo after treatment begins, annually; lens opacities may occur

Nursing diagnoses
☑ Diarrhea (adverse reactions)
☑ Knowledge deficit (teaching)
☑ Noncompliance (teaching)

Implementation
• Give with evening meal; if dosage is increased, take with breakfast and evening meal
• Store in cool environment in airtight, light-resistant container

Patient/family education
• Inform patient that compliance is needed for positive results to occur, not to double doses
• Teach patient that risk factors should be decreased: high-fat diet, smoking, alcohol consumption, absence of exercise

- Advise patient to notify prescriber if the GI symptoms of diarrhea, abdominal or epigastric pain, nausea, vomiting, or if chills, fever, sore throat occur
- Advise patient that treatment is chronic
- Advise patient that blood work and eye exam will be necessary during treatment
- Instruct patient to report suspected pregnancy, not to use during pregnancy

Evaluation
Positive therapeutic outcome
- Decreased cholesterol levels, serum triglyceride
- Improved ratio of HDLs

---

folic acid (vitamin B₉)
(PO, OTC; IM/IV, Ph)
(foe-lik a'sid)
Apo-Folic ✦, Folate, Folvite, Novofolacid ✦, Vitamin B₉
Func. class.: Vitamin B-complex group
Chem. class.: Supplement

Pregnancy category　A

Action: Needed for erythropoiesis; increases RBC, WBC, and platelet formation in megaloblastic anemias

▶Therapeutic Outcome: Absence of macrocytic, megaloblastic anemias

Uses: Megaloblastic or macrocytic anemia caused by folic acid deficiency; liver disease; alcoholism; hemolysis; intestinal obstruction; pregnancy

Dosage and routes
Supplement
Adult: PO/IM/SC/**IV** 0.1 mg qd
ⓟ *Child:* PO/IM/SC/**IV** 0.05 mg qd

Megaloblastic/macrocytic anemia
ⓟ *Adult and child >4 yr:* PO/SC/IM/**IV** 1 mg qd × 4-5 days
ⓟ *Child <4 yr:* PO/SC/IM/**IV** 0.3 mg or less qd
Pregnancy/lactation: PO/SC/IM/**IV** 0.8 mg qd

Prevention of megaloblastic/macrocytic anemia
Pregnancy: PO/SC/IM/**IV** 1 mg qd

Available forms: Tabs 0.4, 0.8, 1 mg; inj 5 mg/ml

Adverse effects
INTEG: Flushing
RESP: Bronchospasm

Contraindications: Hypersensitivity, anemias other than megaloblastic/macrocytic anemia, vit B₁₂ deficiency anemia, uncorrected pernicious anemia

Precautions: Pregnancy **A**

Pharmacokinetics
Absorption	Well absorbed
Distribution	Liver, crosses placenta
Metabolism	Liver (converted to active metabolite)
Excretion	Kidneys (unchanged)
Half-life	Unknown

Pharmacodynamics
Onset	Unknown
Peak	½-1 hr
Duration	Unknown

Interactions
Individual drugs
Aspirin: ↓ folate level
Methotrexate: ↓ action of folic acid
Phenytoin: ↑ need for folic acid
Sulfasalazine: ↓ action of folic acid

🔲 Herb/drug　🚫 Do Not Crush　◆ Alert　◑ᴛ Key Drug　ⒼGeriatric　ⓟ Pediatric

Triamterene: ↓ action of folic acid

Drug classifications

Estrogens: ↑ need for folic acid

Glucocorticoids: ↑ need for folic acid

Sulfonamides: ↓ action of folic acid

NURSING CONSIDERATIONS

Assessment

• Assess patient for fatigue, dyspnea, weakness, shortness of breath, activity intolerance (signs of megaloblastic anemia)

• Monitor Hgb, Hct, and reticulocyte count; folate levels: 6-15 μg/ml baseline and throughout treatment

• Assess nutritional status: bran, yeast, dried beans, nuts, fruits, fresh vegetables, asparagus; if high folic acid foods are missing from the diet, a referral to a dietician may be indicated

• Identify drugs currently taken: alcohol, oral contraceptives, hydantoins, trimethoprim; these drugs may cause increased folic acid use by the body and contribute to deficiency

Nursing diagnoses

✓ Nutrition, less than body requirements (uses)

✓ Fatigue (uses)

✓ Activity intolerance (uses)

✓ Knowledge deficit (teaching)

Implementation

IV **IV route**

• Give **IV** directly, undiluted 5 mg or less/min—or may be added to most **IV** sol or TPN

• Store in light-resistant container

Y-site compatibilities:

Famotidine

Solution compatibilities:

$D_{20}W$

Solution incompatibilities:

$D_{40}W$, $D_{50}W$, calcium gluconate

Patient/family education

• Advise patient to take drug exactly as prescribed; not to double doses, toxicity may occur

• Instruct patient to notify prescriber of side effects—rash or fever may indicate hypersensitivity

• Advise patient that urine may become more yellow

• Instruct patient to increase intake of foods rich in folic acid in diet as recommended by dietician or health care provider

Evaluation

Positive therapeutic outcome

• Absence of fatigue, weakness, dyspnea

• Absence of symptoms of megaloblastic anemia

**follitropin alfa/
follitropin beta** (℞)

(fol'ee-tro-pin)

Gonal-F/Follistim

Func. class.: Ovulation stimulant

Chem. class.: Gonadotropin

Pregnancy category   **X**

Action: Stimulates ovarian follicular growth in primary ovarian failure

➡ **Therapeutic Outcome:** Pregnancy

Uses: Induction of ovulation, assisted reproductive technologies (in vitro fertilization)

Dosage and routes
Adult:
Ovulation induction
SC 75 IU, may increase by 37.5 IU after 2 wks, may increase again after 1 wk by 37.5 IU; treatment should not exceed 35 days unless a serum estradiol rise indicates imminent follicular development

Follicle stimulation
SC 150 IU/day on day 2 or 3 of the follicular phase, should not exceed 10 days

Available forms: Gonal-F powder for injection 75 IU, 150 IU; Follistim powder for inj 75 IU

Adverse effects
CNS: Malaise
GI: Nausea, vomiting, constipation, increased appetite, abdominal pain
GU: Polyuria, frequency, birth defects, spontaneous abortions, multiple ovulation, breast pain
INTEG: Rash, dermatitis, urticaria, alopecia

Contraindications: Hypersensitivity, pregnancy **X,** undiagnosed vaginal bleeding, intracranial lesion, ovarian cyst not caused by polycystic ovarian disease

Precautions: Lactation, arterial thromboembolism

Pharmacokinetics	
Absorption	Unknown
Distribution	Unknown
Metabolism	Unknown
Excretion	Feces
Half-life	Unknown

NURSING CONSIDERATIONS
Implementation
• Give immediately after dissolving contents of ampule in 1-2 ml of sterile saline, discard unused portion
• Administer drug at same time qd to maintain drug level

Patient/family education
• Teach patient that multiple births are common after taking this drug
• Teach patient to notify prescriber of low abdominal pain; may indicate ovarian cyst, cyst rupture
• Teach patient method of taking, recording basal body temp to determine whether ovulation has occurred
• Teach patient that if ovulation can be determined (there is a slight decrease, then a sharp increase for ovulation), to attempt coitus 3 days before and qod until after ovulation
• Teach patient to notify prescriber immediately if pregnancy is suspected

Evaluation
• Ovulation, pregnancy

foscarnet (℞)
(foss-kar′net)
Foscavir
Func. class.: Antiviral
Chem. class.: Inorganic pyrophosphate organic analog

Pregnancy category   C

Action: Antiviral activity is produced by selective inhibition at the pyrophosphate binding site on virus-specific DNA polymerases and reverse transcriptases at concentrations that do not affect cellular DNA polymerases

→ **Therapeutic Outcome:** Virostatic agents against CMV retinitis

Uses: Treatment of CMV (cytomegalovirus), retinitis, HSV infections; used with ganciclovir for relapsing patients

Dosage and routes
Adult: **IV** inf 60 mg/kg given over at least 1 hr, q8h × 2-3 wk initially, then 90-120 mg/kg/day over 2 hr, usually give with at least 750-1000 ml 0.9% NaCl qd

Renal dose
Adult: **IV**
Male:

$$\frac{\text{weight (kg)} \times (140 - \text{age})}{72 \times \text{serum creatinine (mg/dl)}} = \text{Ccr}$$

Female: 0.85 × above value; dose based on table provided in package insert

Available forms: Inj 24 mg/ml

Adverse effects
CNS: Fever, dizziness, *headache,* **seizures,** *fatigue,* neuropathy, tremor, ataxia, dementia, stupor, EEG abnormalities, vertigo, **coma,** abnormal gait, hypertonia, extrapyramidal disorders, hemiparesis, **paralysis,** hyperreflexia, paraplegia, **tetany,** hyporeflexia, neuralgia, neuritis, celebral edema, *paresthesia,* depression, *confusion, anxiety,* insomnia, somnolence, amnesia, hallucinations, agitation
CV: Hypertension, palpitations, ECG abnormalities, 1st degree AV block, nonspecific ST-T segment changes, hypotension, cerebrovascular disorder, cardiomyopathy, **cardiac arrest,** bradycardia, **dysrhythmias**
EENT: Visual field defects, vocal cord paralysis, speech disorders, taste perversion, eye pain, conjunctivitis, tinnitus, otitis
GI: Nausea, vomiting, diarrhea, anorexia, abdominal pain, constipation, dysphagia, rectal hemorrhage, dry mouth, melena, flatulence, ulcerative stomatitis, pancreatitis, enteritis, enterocolitis, glossitis, proctitis, stomatitis, increased amylases, gastroenteritis, **pseudomembranous colitis,** duodenal ulcer, **paralytic ileus, esophageal ulceration,** abnormal A-G ratio, increased AST, ALT, cholecystitis, **hepatitis,** dyspepsia, tenesmus, hepatosplenomegaly, jaundice
GU: **Acute renal failure,** decreased CrCl and increased serum creatinine, **glomerulonephritis, toxic nephropathy, nephrosis, renal tubular disorders, pyelonephritis,** uremia, **hematuria, albuminuria,** dysuria, polyuria
HEMA: Anemia, *granulocytopenia, leukopenia, thrombocytopenia,* platelet abnormalities, **thrombosis, pulmonary embolism, coagulation disorders, decreased prothrombin, hypochromic anemia, pancytopenia, hemolysis, leukocytosis,** lymphadenopathy, epistaxis, lymphopenia
INTEG: **Rash,** sweating, pruritus, skin ulceration, seborrhea, skin discoloration, alopecia, acne, dermatitis, pain/inflammation at injection site, facial edema, dry skin, urticaria
MS: Arthralgia, myalgia
RESP: Coughing, dyspnea, pneumonia, sinusitis, pharyngitis, **pulmonary infiltration,**

F

stridor, **pneumothorax, hemoptysis, bronchospasm,** bronchitis, **respiratory depression, pleural effusion, pulmonary hemorrhage,** rhinitis
SYST: Hypokalemia, hypocalcemia, hypomagnesemia, increased alk phosphatase, LDH, BUN, acidosis, hypophosphatemia, hyperphosphatemia, dehydration, glycosuria, increased creatine phosphokinase, hypervolemia, infection, **sepsis, death, ascites,** hyponatremia, hypochloremia, hypercalcemia

Contraindications: Hypersensitivity, CrCl <0.4 ml/kg

Precautions: Pregnancy **C**, **P** lactation, children, elderly, **G** renal disease, seizure disorders, electrolyte/mineral imbalances, severe anemia

Pharmacokinetics

Absorption	Complete (**IV**)
Distribution	14%-17% plasma protein binding
Metabolism	Not metabolized
Excretion	Kidneys (90%) unchanged, breast milk
Half-life	2-8 hr; ↑ in renal disease

Pharmacodynamics

Onset	48 hr
Peak	2 wk
Duration	Unknown

Interactions
Individual drugs
Amphotericin B: ↑ nephrotoxicity
Ciprofloxacin: Seizures
Pentamide: ↑ nephrotoxicity
Zidovudine: ↑ anemia
Drug classification
Aminoglycosides: ↑ nephrotoxicity

NURSING CONSIDERATIONS
Assessment
• Culture should be done before treatment with foscarnet is begun; cultures of blood, urine, and throat may all be taken; CMV is not confirmed by this method; the diagnosis is made by an ophth exam
• Assess kidney and liver function; increased hemopoietic studies: BUN, serum creatinine, creatitinine clearance, AST, ALT, A-G ratio, baseline and during treatment; blood counts should be done q2wk; watch for decreasing granulocytes, Hgb; if low, therapy may have to be discontinued and restarted after hematologic recovery; blood transfusions may be required
• Assess for GI symptoms: severe nausea, vomiting, diarrhea; severe symptoms may necessitate discontinuing drug
• Monitor electrolytes and minerals: calcium, phosphorous, magnesium, sodium, potassium; watch closely for tetany during first administration
◆• Assess for symptoms of blood dyscrasias (anemia, granulocytopenia); bruising, fatigue, bleeding, poor healing
• Assess for symptoms of allergic reactions: flushing, rash, urticaria, pruritus

Nursing diagnoses
☑ Infection, risk for (uses)
☑ Injury, risk for (adverse reactions)
☑ Knowledge deficit (teaching)

Implementation
IV **IV route**
• Administer increased fluids before and during drug administration to induce diuresis and minimize renal toxicity

---

☑ Herb/drug   ◎ Do Not Crush   ◆ Alert   ✜ Key Drug   **G** Geriatric   **P** Pediatric

• Administer via inf pump, at no more than 1 mg/kg/min; do not give by rapid or bolus **IV**; give by central venous line or peripheral vein; standard 24 mg/ml sol may be used without dilution if using by central line; dilute the 24 mg/ml sol to 12 mg/ml with D_5W or 0.9% NaCl if using peripheral vein

• Monitor patient closely during therapy; if tingling, numbness, paresthesias occur, stop inf and obtain lab sample for electrolytes

Y-site compatibilities:
Aldesleukin, aminophylline, amikacin, ampicillin, aztreonam, benzquinamide, cefazolin, cefoperazone, cefoxitin, ceftazidime, ceftizoxime, ceftriaxone, cefuroxime, chloramphenicol, cimetidine, clindamycin, dexamethasone, dopamine, erythromycin, fluconazole, flucytosine, furosemide, gentamicin, heparin, hydrocortisone, hydromorphone, hydroxyzine, imipenem-cilastatin, metoclopramide, metronidazole, miconazole, morphine, nafcillin, oxacillin, penicillin G potassium, phenytoin, piperacillin, ranitidine, ticarcillin/clavulanate, tobramycin

Y-site incompatibilities:
Acyclovir, amphotericin B, calcium, co-trimoxazole, diazepam, digoxin, gancyclovir, haloperidol, leucovorin, midazolam, pentamidine, phenytoin, prochlorperazine, vancomycin

Patient/family education
• Advise patient to notify prescriber if sore throat, swollen lymph nodes, malaise, fever occur—may indicate presence of other infections

• Advise patient to report perioral tingling, numbness in extremities, and paresthesias; inf should be stopped and electrolytes should be requested

• Caution patient that serious drug interactions may occur if OTC products are ingested; check first with prescriber

• Inform patient that drug is not a cure, but will control symptoms

• Advise patient that ophth exams must be continued

Evaluation
Positive therapeutic outcome
• Improvement in CMV retinitis

---

fosfomycin (℞)
(foss-foe-mye′sin)
Monurol
Func. class.: Urinary anti-infective

Pregnancy category B

Action: Interferes with protein synthesis in bacterial cell by binding to ribosomal subunit, causing misreading of genetic code; inaccurate peptide sequence forms in protein chain, causing bacterial death

Therapeutic Outcome: Bactericidal effects for the following organisms *E. faecalis, E. coli*

Uses: Urinary tract infections

Dosage and routes
Adult >18 yr: 1 sachet with or without food, always mix with water before ingesting

Available forms: Single-dose sachet (3 g fosfomycin), orange flavored

---

Adverse effects: *italic* = common; **bold** = life-threatening

Adverse effects
CNS: Headache, dizziness, fever, insomnia, somnolence, migraine, asthenia, nervousness
GI: Nausea, vomiting, anorexia, constipation, dry mouth, flatulence, increased SGPT; *diarrhea,* dyspepsia
GU: Vaginitis, dysuria, hematuria, menstrual disorder
INTEG: Rash, pruritus

Contraindications: Hypersensitivity

Precautions: Pregnancy **B,** child <12 yrs, lactation, renal disease

Pharmacokinetics	
Absorption	Well absorbed
Distribution	Unknown
Metabolism	Liver
Excretion	Mostly unchanged in kidneys, feces
Half-life	4-8 hr

Pharmacodynamics
Unknown

Interactions
Individual drugs
Calcium: ↓ absorption of fosfomycin
Metoclopramide: ↑ urinary excretion of fosfomycin
Drug classifications
Antacids: ↓ absorption of fosfomycin
Food/drug
↓ absorption

NURSING CONSIDERATIONS
Assessment
• Assess patient for signs and symptoms of infection including characteristics of urine, WBC >10,000, fever; obtain baseline information and during treatment
• Complete culture and sensitivity before beginning drug therapy; this will ensure that correct treatment has been initiated
• Assess for overgrowth of infection: perineal itching, fever, pain
• Assess urine pH; urine should be kept alkaline

Nursing diagnoses
☑ Infection, risk for (uses)
☑ Diarrhea (side effects)
☑ Knowledge deficit (teaching)
☑ Noncompliance (teaching)
☑ Injury, risk for (side effects)

Implementation
• Pour contents of sachet into 3-4 oz (½ cup) of water, stir to dissolve, use cold water, take immediately
• Only a single dose is necessary
• Give 1 hr ac or 2 hr pc antacids or calcium
• Give adequate fluids of 2-3 L/day, unless contraindicated
• Store at 59-86° F

Patient/family education
• Give patient directions to dissolve sachet, caution patient not to take in dry form
• Instruct patient not to take with antacids or calcium products

Evaluation
Positive therapeutic outcome
• Absence of signs/symptoms of infection (WBC <10,000, temp WNL)
• Reported improvement in symptoms of infection
• Negative C&S

fosinopril (℞)

(foss-in-o'pril)

Monopril

Func. class.: Antihypertensive

Chem. class.: Angiotensin-converting enzyme (ACE) inhibitor

Pregnancy category C (1st trimester), D (2nd/3rd trimesters)

Action: Selectively suppresses renin-angiotensin-aldosterone system; inhibits ACE; prevents conversion of angiotensin I to angiotensin II; results in dilation of arterial, venous vessels

Therapeutic Outcome: Decreased B/P in hypertension

Uses: Hypertension, alone or in combination with thiazide diuretics, systolic CHF

Dosage and routes

Adult: PO 10 mg qd initially, then 20-40 mg/day divided bid or qd

Renal dose

5 mg qd

Available forms: Tabs 10, 20, 40 mg

Adverse effects

CNS: Insomnia, paresthesia, headache, dizziness, fatigue, memory disturbance, tremor, mood change

CV: Hypotension, chest pain, palpitations, angina, orthostatic hypotension

GI: Nausea, constipation, vomiting, diarrhea

GU: **Proteinuria,** increased BUN, creatinine, decreased libido

HEMA: Decreased Hct, Hgb, **eosinophilia, leukopenia, neutropenia**

INTEG: **Angioedema,** rash, flushing, sweating, photosensitivity, pruritus

META: Hyperkalemia

MS: Arthralgia, myalgia

RESP: Cough, sinusitis, dyspnea, **bronchospasm**

Contraindications: Hypersensitivity to ACE inhibitors, lactation, children, pregnancy **D** (2nd/3rd trimesters)

Precautions: Impaired liver function, hypovolemia, blood dyscrasias, CHF, COPD, asthma, elderly, pregnancy **C** (1st trimester)

Do Not Confuse:
Monopril/minoxidil

Pharmacokinetics

Absorption	30%
Distribution	Crosses placenta
Metabolism	Liver—converted to fosinoprilate
Excretion	50% kidneys (metabolities), 50% feces
Half-life	12 hr—fosinoprilat

Pharmacodynamics

Onset	1 hr
Peak	2-6 hr
Duration	24 hr

Interactions

Individual drugs

Alcohol: ↑ hypotension (large amounts)

Allopurinol: ↑ hypersensitivity

Digoxin: ↑ serum levels

Hydralazine: ↑ toxicity

Indomethacin: ↓ antihypertensive effect

Lithium: ↑ serum levels

Prazosin: ↑ toxicity

Drug classifications

Adrenergic blockers: ↑ hypotension

Antacids: ↓ absorption

Antihypertensives: ↑ hypotension

Diuretics: ↑ hypotension
Diuretics, potassium sparing: ↑ toxicity
Ganglionic blockers: ↑ hypotension
Potassium supplements: ↑ toxicity
Sympathomimetics: ↑ toxicity

Lab test interferences
False positive: Urine acetone

NURSING CONSIDERATIONS
Assessment
• Monitor blood studies: neutrophils, decreased platelets
• Monitor B/P, check for orthostatic hypotension, syncope; if changes occur, dosage change may be required
• Monitor renal studies: protein, BUN, creatinine; watch for increased levels that may indicate nephrotic syndrome and renal failure; monitor urine daily for protein; monitor renal symptoms: polyuria, oliguria, frequency, dysuria
• Establish baselines in renal, liver function tests before therapy begins
• Check potassium levels throughout treatment although hyperkalemia rarely occurs
• Check for edema in feet, legs daily, monitor weight daily
• Assess for allergic reactions: rash, fever, pruritus, urticaria; drug should be discontinued if antihistamines fail to help

Nursing diagnoses
✓ Cardiac output, decreased (uses)
✓ Injury, risk for (side effects)
✓ Knowledge deficit (teaching)
✓ Noncompliance (teaching)

Implementation
• Store in air-tight container at 86° F (30° C) or less
• Severe hypotension may occur after 1st dose of this

medication; ↓ hypotension may be prevented by reducing or discontinuing diuretic therapy 3 days before beginning benzapril therapy

Patient/family education
• Advise patient not to discontinue drug abruptly—warn patient to tell all persons associated with his care
• Teach patient not to use OTC products (cough, cold, allergy) unless directed by prescriber because serious side effects can occur; xanthines such as coffee, tea, chocolate, cola can prevent action of drug
• Teach patient the importance of complying with dosage schedule, even if feeling better; to continue with medical regimen to decrease B/P: exercise, smoking cessation, decreasing stress, diet modifications
• Emphasize the need to rise slowly to sitting or standing position to minimize orthostatic hypotension; not to exercise in hot weather or increased hypotension can occur
• Teach patient to notify prescriber of mouth sores, sore throat, fever, swelling of hands or feet, irregular heartbeat, chest pain, coughing, shortness of breath
• Instruct patient to report excessive perspiration, dehydration, vomiting, diarrhea; may lead to fall in B/P
• Caution patient that drug may cause dizziness, fainting, light-headedness; may occur during 1st few days of therapy; to avoid activities that may be hazardous
• Teach patient how to take B/P, and normal readings for age group

---

Evaluation
Positive therapeutic outcome
• Decreased B/P in hypertension

Treatment of overdose: 0.9% NaCl **IV** inf, hemodialysis

---

fosphenytoin (℞)
(foss-fen′i-toy-in)
Cerebyx
Func. class.: Anticonvulsant
Chem. class.: Hydantoin
Pregnancy category   D

Action: Inhibits spread of seizure activity in motor cortex by altering ion transport; increases AV conduction

➔**Therapeutic Outcome:** Decreased seizures, absence of dysrhythmias

Uses: Generalized tonic-clonic seizures, status epilepticus

Dosage and routes
Status epilepticus
🅟 *Adult and child:* **IV** loading dose 15-20 mg PE/kg given at 100-150 mg PE/min
Nonemergent/maintenance dosing
🅟 *Adult and child:* IM/**IV** loading dose 10-20 mg PE/kg; maintenance dosing 4-6 mg PE/kg/day given at a rate of <150 mg PE/min

Available forms: Inj 150 mg (100 mg phenytoin), 750 mg (500 mg phenytoin)

Adverse effects
CNS: Drowsiness, dizziness, insomnia, paresthesias, depression, suicidal tendencies, aggression, headache, confusion
CV: Hypotension, **ventricular fibrillation**

EENT: Nystagmus, diplopia, blurred vision
GI: Nausea, vomiting, constipation, anorexia, weight loss, hepatitis, jaundice, gingival hyperplasia
GU: **Nephritis,** urine discoloration
HEMA: **Agranulocytosis, leukopenia, aplastic anemia, thrombocytopenia, megaloblastic anemia**
INTEG: Rash, lupus erythematosus, *Stevens-Johnson syndrome,* hirsutism
SYST: Hypocalcemia

Contraindications: Hypersensitivity, psychiatric conditions, pregnancy **D,** bradycardia, SA and AV block, Stokes-Adams syndrome

Precautions: Allergies, hepatic disease, renal disease

Pharmacokinetics

Absorption	Unknown
Distribution	Unknown
Metabolism	Liver
Excretion	Kidneys
Half-life	Unknown

Pharmacodynamics
Unknown

Interactions
Individual drugs
Alcohol: ↑ CNS depression
Amiodarone: ↑ fosphenytoin level
Carbamazepine: ↓ effectiveness
Chloramphenicol: ↑ fosphenytoin level
Cimetidine: ↑ fosphenytoin level
Isoniazid: ↓ metabolism, ↑ action
Valproic acid: ↑ seizures

Drug classifications
Anticonvulsants: ↑ CNS depression
Antidepressants: ↑ CNS depression
Antihistamines: ↑ CNS depression
Barbiturates: ↑ CNS depression, ↓ effect of fosphonytoin
Benzodiazepines: ↑ blood levels
Estrogens: ↑ fosphenytoin level
General anesthetics: ↑ CNS depression
H₂ Antagonists: ↑ fosphenytoin level
Hypnotics: ↑ CNS depression
Opiates: ↑ CNS depression
Phenothiazines: ↑ fosphenytoin level
Salicylates: ↑ fosphenytoin level
Sedatives: ↑ CNS depression
Sulfonamides: ↑ fosphenytoin level

Lab test interferences
↓ Dexamethasone,
↓ metyrapone test serum,
↓ PBI, ↓ urinary steroids
↑ Glucose, ↑ alkaline phosphatase, ↑ BSP

NURSING CONSIDERATIONS
Assessment
• Assess seizure activity including type, location, duration, and character; provide seizure precaution
• Assess renal studies: urinalysis, BUN, urine creatinine
• Monitor hepatic studies: ALT, AST, bilirubin, creatinine
• Assess allergic reaction: red raised rash; if this occurs, drug should be discontinued
• Monitor for toxicity: bone marrow depression, nausea, vomiting, ataxia, diplopia, cardiovascular collapse, slurred speech, confusion
• Assess drug level: toxic level 30-50 μg/ml
◆ Assess for rash, discontinue as soon as rash develops, serious adverse reactions such as Stevens-Johnson syndrome can occur
• Assess mental status: mood, sensorium, affect, memory
G (long, short), especially elderly
• Assess for blood dyscrasias: fever, sore throat, bruising, rash, jaundice, epistaxis (long-term treatment only)
• Monitor blood studies: RBC, Hct, Hgb, reticulocyte counts weekly for 4 wk then monthly; also check thyroid function tests, serum calcium

Nursing diagnoses
☑ Injury, risk for (uses, adverse reactions)
☑ Knowledge deficit (teaching)
☑ Noncompliance (teaching)

Implementation
Ⓜ **IV route**
• Administer by direct **IV** after diluting with D₅ or 0.9% NaCl 1.5-25 mg PE/ml

Solution compatibilities:
D₅W, D₁₀W, amino acid inj 10%, D₅LR, D₅/0.9% NaCl, Plasmalyte A, LR, per sterile water for inj

Additive compatibilities:
potassium chloride

Patient/family education
• Teach patient the reason for and expected outcome of treatment
• Instruct patient not to use machinery or engage in hazardous activity; drowsiness, dizziness may occur

---

☑ Herb/drug Ⓢ Do Not Crush ◆ Alert ☛ Key Drug G Geriatric P Pediatric

• Advise patient to carry medical ID identifying drug used
• Advise patient to notify prescriber of rash, bleeding, bruising, slurred speech, jaundice of skin or eyes, joint pain, nausea, vomiting, severe headache
• Advise patient to keep all medical appointments, including lab work, physical assessment

Evaluation
Positive therapeutic outcome
• Decreased seizure activity

---

furosemide ⚥ (℞)
(fur-oh′se-mide)
Apo-Furosemide ✚, Fumide, Furomide M.D., Furosemide, Furoside, Lasix, Lasix Special ✚, Luramide, Myrosemide, Novosemide ✚, Uritol ✚
Func. class.: Loop diuretic
Chem. class.: Sulfonamide derivative

Pregnancy category   C

Action: Acts on the ascending loop of Henle in the kidney, inhibiting the reabsorption of the electrolytes sodium and chloride, causing excretion of sodium, calcium, magnesium, chloride, water, and some potassium; decreases reabsorption of sodium and chloride and increases the excretion of potassium in the distal tubule of the kidney; responsible for slight antihypertensive effect and peripheral vasodilation

▶**Therapeutic Outcome:** Decreased edema in lung tissue, peripherally; decreased B/P

Uses: Edema in congestive heart failure, nephrotic syndrome, ascites, caused by hepatic disease, hepatic cirrhosis; may be used alone or as adjunct with antihypertensives such as spironolactone, triamterene; should not be used with ethacrynic acid

Investigational uses: Hypercalcemia in malignancy

Dosage and routes
Adult: PO 20-80 mg/day in AM, may give another dose in 6 hrs, up to 600 mg/day; IM/**IV** 20-40 mg, increased by 20 mg q2h until desired response

▣ *Child:* PO/IM/**IV** 2 mg/kg, may increase by 1-2 mg/kg/q6-8h up to 6 mg/kg

Pulmonary edema
Adult: **IV** 40 mg given over several min, repeated in 1 hr; increase to 80 mg if needed

Available forms: Tabs 20, 40, 80 mg; oral sol 10 mg/ml, 40 mg/5 ml; inj IM, **IV** 10 mg/ml

Adverse effects
CNS: Headache, fatigue, weakness, vertigo, paresthesias
CV: Orthostatic hypotension, chest pain, ECG changes, **circulatory collapse**
EENT: Loss of hearing, ear pain, tinnitus, blurred vision
ELECT: Hypokalemia, hypochloremic alkalosis, hypomagnesemia, hyperuricemia, hypocalcemia, hyponatremia, metabolic alkalosis
GI: Nausea, diarrhea, dry mouth, vomiting, anorexia, cramps, oral or gastric irritations, pancreatitis

---

GU: Polyuria, **renal failure,** *glycosuria*
HEMA: Thrombocytopenia, agranulocytosis, leukopenia neutropenia, anemia
INTEG: Rash, pruritus, purpura, **Stevens-Johnson syndrome,** sweating, photosensitivity, urticaria
MS: Cramps, stiffness

Contraindications: Hypersensitivity to sulfonamides, anuria, **P** hypovolemia, infants, lactation, electrolyte depletion

Precautions: Diabetes mellitus, dehydration, severe renal disease, pregnancy **C,** cirrhosis, ascites

⬛ Do Not Confuse:
furosemide/torsemide,
Lasix/Lomotil, Lasix/Luvox,
Lasix/Lanoxin

Pharmacokinetics			
	PO		
Absorption	GI tract (60%-70%)		
	PO/IM/**IV**		
Distribution	Crosses placenta		
Metabolism	Liver (30%-40%)		
Excretion	Breast milk, urine, feces		
Half-life	½-1 hr		

Pharmacodynamics			
	PO	IM	IV
Onset	1 hr	½ hr	5 mins
Peak	1-2 hrs	Unknown	½ hr
Duration	6-8 hrs	4-8 hrs	2 hrs

Interactions
Individual drugs
Alcohol: ↑ orthostatic hypotension
Chloral hydrate: ↑ sweating, flushing when given with **IV** furosemide
Cisplatin: ↑ risk of ototoxicity
Clofibrate: ↑ furosemide effects

Ethacrynic acid: Combination with furosemide may cause ↑ chance of dysrhythmias (do not use together)
Indomethacin: ↓ diuretic
Lithium: ↓ renal clearance, causing increased toxicity
Phenytoin: ↓ diuretic effect caused by ↓ absorption
Probenecid: ↓ effects of furosemide
Succinylcholine: Action of succinylcholine is ↑ by low doses and ↓ by high doses of furosemide
Theophylline: May ↑ or ↓ the effect of theophylline
Vancomycin: ↑ risk of ototoxicity
Drug classifications
Adrenergic blockers: ↑ effects
Aminoglycosides: ↑ ototoxicity, nephrotoxicity
Anticoagulants: ↑ anticoagulant effect caused by ↓ plasma protein binding
Antidiabetics: ↓ hypoglycemic effect
Antihypertensives: ↑ antihypertensive effect
Cephalosporins: ↑ nephrotoxicity
Corticosteroids: ↑ potassium loss caused by potassium depletion effects of both drugs
Digitalis glycosides: ↑ potassium and magnesium loss with relating dysrhythmias
Opiates: ↑ orthostatic hypotension
Salicylates: ↓ diuretic effect
Food/drug
↓ diuresis

NURSING CONSIDERATIONS
Assessment
• Assess patient for tinnitus, hearing loss, ear pain; periodic

---

testing of hearing is needed when high doses of this drug are given by **IV** route

• Monitor for renal, cardiac, neurologic, GI, pulmonary manifestations of hypokalemia: acidic urine, reduced urine osmolality, nocturia, polyuria and polydipsia; hypotension, broad T-wave, U-wave, ectopy, tachycardia, weak pulse; muscle weakness, altered LOC, drowsiness, apathy, lethargy, confusion, depression; anorexia, nausea, cramps, constipation, distension, paralyticileus; hypoventilation, respiratory muscle weakness

• Monitor for CNS, GI, cardiovascular, integumentary, neurologic manifestations of hypocalcemia: personality changes, anxiety, disturbances, depression and psychosis; nausea, vomiting, constipation, abdominal pain from muscle spasm; decreased contractility, decreased cardiac output, hypotension, lengthened ST segment, prolonged QT interval; scaling eczema, alopecia, hyperpigmentation; tetany, muscle twitching, cramping grimacing, seizure, altered deep tendon reflexes, spasm

• Monitor for CNS, neuromuscular, GI, cardiac manifestations of hypomagnesemia, agitation; muscle twitching, paresthesias, hyperactive reflexes, positive Babinski reflex, dysphagia, nystagmus seizures, tetany; nausea, vomiting, diarrhea, anorexia, abdominal distention; ectopy, tachycardia, broad, flat or inverted T-waves, depressed ST segment, prolonged OT, decreased cardiac output, hypotension

• Monitor for CV, GI, neurologic manifestations of

hyponatremia: ↑ B/P, cold, clammy skin, hypovolemia or hypervolemia; anorexia, nausea, vomiting, diarrhea, abdominal cramps; lethargy, increased ICP, confusion headache, seizures, coma, fatigue, tremors, hyperreflexia

• Monitor for neurologic, respiratory manifestations of hyperchloremia: weakness, lethargy, coma; deep rapid breathing

• Assess fluid volume status: I&O ratios and record, count or weigh diapers as appropriate, weight, distended red veins, crackles in lung, color, quality and sp gr of urine, skin turgor, adequacy of pulses, moist mucous membranes, bilateral lung sounds, peripheral pitting edema; dehydration symptoms of decreasing output, thirst, hypotension, dry mouth and mucous membranes should be reported

• Monitor electrolytes: potassium, sodium, calcium, magnesium; also include BUN, blood pH, ABGs, uric acid, CBC, blood sugar

• Assess B/P before and during therapy lying, standing and sitting as appropriate; orthostatic hypotension can occur rapidly

Nursing diagnoses
☑ Fluid volume deficit (side effects)
☑ Fluid volume excess (uses)
☑ Knowledge deficit (teaching)

Implementation
• Give in AM to avoid interference with sleep
• Potassium replacement if potassium level is <3.0 whole,

or use oral sol slightly, drug may be crushed if patient is unable to swallow

PO route
• With food, if nausea occurs, absorption may be reduced

IV IV route
• Do not use sol that is yellow, or has a precipitate, or crystals

Implementation

IV Direct IV
• Give undiluted through Y-tube on 3-way stopcock; give 20 mg or less/min

Int Inf
• May be added to NS, D_5W, $D_{10}W$, $D_{20}W$; invert sugar 10% in electrolyte #1, LR, sodium lactate y_6m, use within 24 hr to assure compatibility; give through Y-tube or 3-way stopcock; give at 4 mg/min or less, use inf pump

Syringe compatibilities:
Bleomycin, cisplatin, cyclophosphamide, fluorouracil, heparin, leucovorin, methotrexate, mitomycin

Syringe incompatibilities:
Doxapram, doxorubicin, droperidol, metaclopramide, milrinone

Y-site compatibilities:
Allopurinol, amifostine, amikacin, aztrenom, bleomycin, cefepime, cefmetazole, cisplatin, cladribine, cyclophosphamide, cytarabine, dexamethasone, epinephrine, fentanyl, fludarabine, fluorouracil, foscarnet, gallium, granisetron, heparin, hydrocortisone, hydromorphone, indomethacin, kanamycin, leucovorin, lorazepam, melphalan, meropenem, methotrexate, mitomycin, morphine, nitroglycerin, norepinephrine, paclitaxel, piperacillin/tazobactam, potassium chloride, propofol, ranitidine, sargramostim, tacrolimus, teniposide, thiotepa, tobramycin, tolazoline, vitamin B complex with C

Y-site incompatibilities:
Amsacrine, bleomycin, doxorubicin, droperidol, esmolol, fluconazole, gentamicin, idarubicin, metoclopramide, milrinone, netilmicin, ondansetron, quinidine, vinblastine, vincristine

Additive compatibilities:
Amikacin, aminophylline, ampicillin, atropine, bumetanide, calcium gluconate, cefamandole, cefoperazone, cefuroxime, cimetidine, cloxacillin, dexamethasone, diamorphine, digoxin, epinephrine, heparin, isosorbide, kanamycin, lidocaine, meropenem, morphine, nitroglycerin, penicillin G, potassium chloride, ranitidine, scopolamine, sodium bicarbonate, theophylline, tobramycin, verapamil

Additive incompatibilities:
Bleomycin, dobutamine, gentamicin, chlorpromazine, diazepam, erythromycin, isoproterenol, meperidine, metoclopramide, netilmicin, opium alkaloids, prochlorperazine, tetracycline

Patient/family education

General
• Teach patient to take the medication early in the day to prevent nocturia
• Instruct the patient to take with food or milk if GI symptoms of nausea and anorexia occur
• Teach patient to maintain a record of weight on a weekly basis and notify physician of weight loss of >5 lbs

---

- Caution the patient that this drug causes a loss of potassium, that food rich in potassium should be added to the diet; refer to a dietician for assistance in planning
- Caution the patient not to exercise in hot weather or stand for prolonged periods of time because orthostatic hypotension will be enhanced
- Advise patient to wear protective clothing and sunscreen to prevent photosensitivity
- Teach patient not to use alcohol or any over-the-counter medications without physician's approval, serious drug reactions may occur
- Emphasize the need to contact physician immediately if muscle cramps, weakness, nausea, dizziness, or numbness occurs
- Teach patient to take and record own B/P and pulse
- Caution the patient that orthostatic hypotension may occur and patient should rise slowly from sitting or reclining positions and lie down if dizziness occurs
- Teach patient to continue taking medication even if feeling better, this drug controls symptoms but does not cure the condition
- Advise the patient with hypertension to continue other medical treatment (exercise, weight loss, relaxation techniques, cessation of smoking)

Evaluation

Positive therapeutic outcome
- Decreased edema
- Decreased B/P
- Lowered calcium level in malignancy
- Increased diuresis

gabapentin (R)
(gab'a-pen-tin)
Neurontin
Func. class.: Anticonvulsant
Pregnancy category **C**

Action: Mechanism unknown; may increase seizure threshold; structurally similar to GABA; gabapentin binding sites in neocortex, hippocampus

Therapeutic Outcome: Decreased seizure activity

Uses: Adjunct treatment of partial seizures, with or without generalization in adults

Investigational uses: Chronic pain

Dosage and routes
Adult: PO 900-1800 mg/day in 3 divided doses; may titrate by giving 300 mg on the first day, 300 mg bid on second day, 300 mg tid on third day; may increase to 1800 mg/day by adding 300 mg on subsequent days

Available forms: Caps 100, 300, 400 mg

Adverse effects
CNS: Dizziness, fatigue, anxiety, somnolence, ataxia, amnesia, abnormal thinking, unsteady gait, depression
CV: Vasodilation
EENT: Dry mouth, blurred vision, diplopia
GI: Constipation, increased appetite, dental abnormalities
GU: Impotence, bleeding, *UTI*
HEMA: **Leukopenia,** decreased WBC

G

INTEG: Pruritus, abrasion
MS: Myalgia
RESP: Rhinitis, pharyngitis, coughing
Contraindications: Hypersensitivity to this drug
Precautions: Hepatic disease, renal disease, pregnancy **C**, lactation, child <12 yr, elderly

Pharmacokinetics

Absorption	Unknown
Distribution	Unknown
Metabolism	None
Excretion	Urine unchanged
Half-life	5-7 hr

Pharmacodynamics

Onset	Unknown
Peak	Unknown
Duration	Unknown

Interactions
Drug classifications
Antacids: ↓ gabapentin levels

NURSING CONSIDERATIONS
• Assess renal studies: urinalysis, BUN, urine creatinine q3mo
• Hepatic studies: ALT, AST, bilirubin
• Assess description of seizures
• Assess mental status: mood, sensorium, affect, behavioral changes; if mental status changes, notify prescriber
• Assess eye problems, need for ophthalmic examinations before, during, after treatment (slit lamp, fundoscopy, tonometry)
• Monitor for allergic reaction: purpura, red raised rash; if these occur, drug should be discontinued

Nursing diagnoses
☑ Knowledge deficit (teaching)
☑ Noncompliance (teaching)

Implementation
• Give at least 2 hr pc with antacids
• Store at room temp away from heat and light
• Give hard candy, frequent rinsing of mouth, gum for dry mouth
• Provide assistance with ambulation during early part of treatment; dizziness occurs
• Provide seizure precautions: padded side rails; move objects that may harm patient
• Provide increased fluids, bulk in diet for constipation

Evaluation
Positive therapeutic outcome
• Decreased seizure activity; document on patient's chart

Patient/family education
• Advise patient to carry Medic Alert ID stating patient's name, drugs taken, condition, prescriber's name and phone number
• Teach patient to avoid driving, other activities that require alertness
• Teach patient not to discontinue medication quickly after long-term use
• Teach patient not to break, crush, or chew caps

Treatment of overdose: Lavage, VS

---

gallamine (℞)
(gal'a-meen)
Flaxedil
Func. class.: Neuromuscular blocker (nondepolarizing)
Pregnancy category　C

Action: Inhibits transmission of nerve impulses by binding with cholinergic receptor sites,

  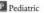

antagonizing action of acetylcholine; no analgesic response

→ **Therapeutic Outcome:** Paralysis of all skeletal muscles

Uses: Facilitation of endotracheal intubation, skeletal muscle relaxation during mechanical ventilation, surgery, or general anesthesia

Dosage and routes

Adult and child >1 mo: **IV** 1 mg/kg, not to exceed 100 mg, then 0.5-1 mg/kg q30-40 min

Child <1 mo, >5 kg: **IV** 0.25-0.75 mg/kg, then 0.01-0.05 mg/kg q30-40 min

Available forms: Inj 20 mg/ml

Adverse effects

CNS: **Malignant hyperthermia**

CV: Bradycardia, tachycardia, increased, decreased B/P

EENT: Increased secretions

GI: Decreased motility

INTEG: Rash, flushing, pruritus, urticaria

RESP: **Prolonged apnea, bronchospasm, cyanosis, respiratory depression**

Contraindications: Hypersensitivity to iodides

Precautions: Pregnancy C, thyroid disease, collagen disease, cardiac disease, lactation, children <2 yr, electrolyte imbalances, dehydration, neuromuscular disease (myasthenia gravis), respiratory disease, renal disease

Pharmacokinetics	
Absorption	Complete bioavailability
Distribution	Extracellular space, crosses placenta
Metabolism	Plasma
Excretion	Kidneys—unchanged
Half-life	2½ hr

Pharmacodynamics	
Onset	2 min
Peak	5 min
Duration	30 min

Interactions

Individual drugs

Clindamycin: ↑ paralysis, length, and intensity

Colistin: ↑ paralysis, length, and intensity

Lidocaine: ↑ paralysis, length, and intensity

Lithium: ↑ paralysis, length, and intensity

Magnesium: ↑ paralysis, length, and intensity

Polymyxin B: ↑ paralysis, length, and intensity

Procainamide: ↑ paralysis, length, and intensity

Quinidine: ↑ paralysis, length, and intensity

Succinylcholine: ↑ paralysis, length, and intensity

Drug classifications

Aminoglycosides: ↑ paralysis, length, and intensity

β-Adrenergic blockers: ↑ paralysis, length, and intensity

Diuretics, potassium-losing: ↑ paralysis, length, and intensity

General anesthetics: ↑ paralysis, length, and intensity

NURSING CONSIDERATIONS

Assessment

• Monitor for electrolyte imbalances (potassium, magnesium), before drug is used; electrolyte imbalances may lead to increased action of this drug

• Monitor vital signs (B/P, pulse, respirations, airway) until fully recovered; rate, depth, pattern of respirations, strength of hand grip; patient should be intubated before use

• Monitor recovery: decreased paralysis of face, diaphragm, leg, arm, rest of body; residual weakness and respiratory problems may occur during recovery period

• Monitor allergic reactions: rash, fever, respiratory distress, pruritus; if present, drug should be discontinued

Nursing diagnoses
☑ Breathing pattern, ineffective (uses)
☑ Communication, impaired verbal (adverse reactions)
☑ Fear (adverse reactions)
☑ Knowledge deficit (teaching)

Implementation
• Use peripheral nerve stimulator by anesthesiologist to determine neuromuscular blockade; deep tendon reflexes should be monitored during extended use

• Give **IV** undiluted by direct **IV** over 1 min, or diluted in 10-50 ml of D_5W, ½ NaCl or NS and give as an infusion at prescribed rate (only by qualified person, usually an anesthesiologist); do not administer IM

• Further dilute in D_5W, 0.9% NaCl, D_5/0.9% NaCl q15-25 min (intermittent infusion)

• Maintenance dose is given q20-45 min after 1st dose (continuous infusion); titrate to patient response

• Store in light-resistant area

Patient/family education
• Provide reassurance if communication is difficult during recovery from neuromuscular blockade

• Provide explanation regarding all procedures or treatments; patient will remain conscious if anesthetic is not given also

Evaluation
Positive therapeutic outcome
• Paralysis of jaw, eyelid, head, neck, rest of body as evaluated by peripheral nerve stimulator

Treatment of overdose: Administer edrophonium or neostigmine, atropine—monitor VS; may require mechanical ventilation

gallium (℞)
(gal'ee-yum)
Ganite
Func. class.: Electrolyte modifier
Chem. class.: Hypocalcemic drug
Pregnancy category   C

Action: Lowers serum calcium levels by inhibiting calcium resorption from bone

➲**Therapeutic Outcome:** Decrease calcium level to 5-9 mg/dl

Uses: Cancer-related hypercalcemia

Dosage and routes
Adult: **IV** 100-200 mg/m² qd × 5 days; inf over 24 hr

Available forms: Inj 25 mg/ml

☑ Herb/drug   🚫 Do Not Crush   ◆ Alert   ☞ Key Drug   G Geriatric   P Pediatric

Adverse effects
CV: Tachycardia
EENT: Blurred vision, optic neuritis, hearing loss
GU: **Nephrotoxicity,** increased BUN, creatinine
HEMA: **Anemia, leukopenia**
META: *Hypophosphatemia,* hypocalcemia, decreased serum bicarbonate

Contraindications: Hypersensitivity, severe renal disease

Precautions: Pregnancy **C,** lactation, children, mild renal disease

Pharmacokinetics
Absorption	Completely absorbed
Distribution	Unknown
Metabolism	Unknown
Excretion	Kidneys (unchanged)
Half-life	Unknown

Pharmacodynamics
Onset	12-24 hr
Peak	Unknown
Duration	Unknown

Interactions
Individual drugs
Amphotericin B: ↑ nephrotoxicity
Drug classifications
Aminoglycosides: ↑ nephrotoxicity

NURSING CONSIDERATIONS
Assessment
• Renal status: BUN, creatinine, urine output; if creatinine level is 2.5 mg/dl or more, drug should be discontinued
• Monitor calcium, phosphate, bicarbonate—all levels may be decreased and supplements of phosphate may be needed; calcium daily, phosphate 2-3 ×/wk
• Assess for hypercalcemia: nausea, vomiting, fatigue, weakness, thirst, dehydration, dysrhythmias, headache, confusion, coma, decreased reflexes
• For hypocalcemia: dysrhythmias, hypotension, paresthesia; twitching, colic, laryngospasm; hypercalcemia: poor coordination, myalgia, hypotonia, shortened ST segment and QT interval, prolonged PR interval, cone-shaped T wave, sinus bradycardia; Trousseau's, Chvostek's sign: tremors, tetany, cramping, grimacing, seizures, altered deep tendon reflexes and spasms, personality changes including irritability, depression, psychosis
• Monitor for indications of hypophosphatemia: weakness, malaise, tremors, memory loss, inattention, confusion, decreased reflexes, aching bone pain, joint stiffness, rapid, shallow respiration, decreased tidal volume, nausea, vomiting, anorexia, portal hypertension

Nursing diagnoses
☑ Injury, risk for (uses)
☑ Knowledge deficit (teaching)

Implementation
• Provide adequate hydration with **IV** saline, 2 L/day during treatment; saline increases the extracellular calcium
• Give by continuous **IV** inf after dilution of dose/1 L 0.9% NaCl or D$_5$W, run over 24 hr, use inf pump
• Store solution for 48 hr at room temp or 1 wk in refrigerator

Y-site compatibilities:
Acyclovir, allopurinol, aminophylline, ampicillin/sulbactam, amifostine, aztreonam, cefazolin, ceftazidime, ceftriaxone, cimetidine, ciprofloxacin, cladribine, cyclophosphamide, dexamethasone,

diphenhydramine, filgrastim, fluconazole, furosemide, granisetron, heparin, hydrocortisone, fosfimide, magnesium sulfate, mannitol, melphalan, meperidine, mesna, methotrexate, metoclopramide, ondansetron, piperacillin, piperacillin/tazobactam, potassium chloride, ranitidine, sodium bicarbonate, teniposide, thiotepa, ticarcillin/clavulanate, trimethoprim, sulfamethoxazole, vancomycin, vinorelbine

Patient/family education

• Instruct patient to follow dietary guidelines given by prescriber, including adequate calcium (dietary products, broccoli) and vit D (fortified milk, grain products, fish oil)
• Explain purpose of drug and expected results

Evaluation

Positive therapeutic outcome

• Decreased serum calcium levels to 5-9 mg/dl

---

ganciclovir (DHPG) (R)

(gan-sye′kloe-vir)
Cytovene, Vitrasert
Func. class.: Antiviral
Chem. class.: Synthetic nucleoside analog
Pregnancy category   C

Action: Inhibits replication of herpes viruses in vitro, in vivo by selective inhibition of the human CMV DNA polymerase and by direct incorporation into viral DNA

▶**Therapeutic Outcome:** Decreased proliferation of virus responsible for CMV retinitis

Uses: Cytomegalovirus (CMV) retinitis in immunocompromised persons, including those with AIDS, after indirect ophthalmoscopy confirms diagnosis

Dosage and routes
Induction treatment
Adult: IV 5 mg/kg given over 1 hr q12h × 2-3 wk

Maintenance treatment
Adult: IV inf 5 mg/kg given over 1 hr, qd × 7 days/wk; or 6 mg/kg qd × 5 days/wk; dosage must be reduced in renal impairment; intravenous **IV** 200 μg every week

Prevention of CMV
Adult: IV 5 mg/kg q12h × 1-2 wks, then 5 mg/kg/day or 6 mg/kg × 5 day of each week

Renal dose
Reduce dose in renal disease CrCl <70 ml/min

Available forms: Powder 500 mg/vial, caps 250, 500 mg; implant, intraviteral 4.5 mg per 5-8 wk

Adverse effects
CNS: Fever, chills, **coma,** *confusion,* abnormal thoughts, dizziness, bizarre dreams, *headache,* psychosis, tremors, somnolence, *paresthesia, weakness,* **seizures**
CV: Dysrhythmia, hypertension/hypotension
EENT: Retinal detachment in CMV retinitis
GI: Abnormal LFTs, nausea, vomiting, anorexia, diarrhea, abdominal pain, **hemorrhage**
GU: **Hematuria,** increased creatinine, BUN
HEMA: **Granulocytopenia, thrombocytopenia, irreversible neutropenia, anemia, eosinophilia**

INTEG: *Rash,* alopecia, *pruritus,* urticaria, pain at inj site, phlebitis
RESP: Dyspnea

Contraindications: Hypersensitivity to acyclovir or ganciclovir, absolute neutrophil count <500, platelet count <25,000

Precautions: Preexisting cytopenias, renal function impairment, pregnancy **C,** lactation, children <6 mo, elderly

Do Not Confuse:
Cytovene/Cytosar

Pharmacokinetics

Absorption	Completely absorbed
Distribution	Crosses blood-brain barrier, CSF
Metabolism	Not metabolized
Excretion	Kidneys (90%) unchanged, breast milk
Half-life	3 hr

Pharmacodynamics

Unknown

Interactions
Individual drugs
Cyclosporine: ↑ toxicity
Imipenem with cilastatin:
↑ chance of seizures
Probenecid: ↑ toxicity
Radiation: ↑ bone marrow depression
Zidovudine: ↑ bone marrow depression
Drug classifications
Antineoplastics: ↑ bone marrow depression

NURSING CONSIDERATIONS
Assessment
• Culture should be done before treatment with ganciclovir is initiated; cultures of blood, urine, and throat may all be taken; CMV is not confirmed by this method; the diagnosis is made by an ophth exam
• Assess kidney, liver function; increased hemopoietic studies: BUN, serum creatinine, AST creatinine clearance, ALT, A-G ratio, baseline, and drip treatment; blood counts should be done q2wk; watch for decreasing granulocytes, Hgb; if low, therapy may have to be discontinued and restarted after hematologic recovery; blood transfusions may be required
• Assess for GI symptoms: severe nausea, vomiting, diarrhea; severe symptoms may necessitate discontinuing drug
• Monitor electrolytes and minerals: calcium, phosphorous, magnesium, sodium, potassium; watch closely for tetany during 1st administration
• Assess for symptoms of blood dyscrasias (anemia, granulocytopenia); bruising, fatigue, bleeding, poor healing
• Assess for symptoms of allergic reactions: flushing, rash, urticaria, pruritus
• Monitor for leukopenia/neutropenia/thrombocytopenia: WBCs, platelets q2day during 2 ×/day dosing and q1wk thereafter; check for leukopenia with qd WBC count in patients with prior leukopenia with other nucleoside analogs or for whom leukopenia counts are <1000 cells/mm^3 at start of treatment
• Monitor serum creatinine or creatinine clearance at least q2wk

Nursing diagnoses
☑ Infection, risk for (uses)
☑ Injury, risk for (uses, adverse reactions)

G

☑ Knowledge deficit (teaching)

Implementation
PO route
• Give with food

IV route
• Medicine should be mixed under strict aseptic conditions using gloves, gown, and mask, and using precautions for antineoplastics
• Administer **IV** after diluting 500 mg/10 ml sterile water for inj (50 mg/ml); shake; further dilute in 100 ml D_5W, 0.9% NaCl, LR and run over 1 hr; use inf pump
• Give slowly; do not give by bolus **IV**, IM, SC inj
• Use diluted sol within 12 hr, do not refrigerate or freeze; do not use sol with particulate matter or discoloration, fludarabine, sargramostim

Y-site compatibilities:
Allopurinol, cisplatin, cyclophosphamide, enalaprilat, filgrastim, fluconazole, granisetron, melphalan, methotrexate, paclitaxel, propofol, tacrolimus, teniposide, thiotepa

Y-site incompatibilities:
Amsacrine, fludarabine, foscarnet, ondansetron, sargramostim, vinorelbine

Patient/family education
• Advise patient to notify prescriber if sore throat, swollen lymph nodes, malaise, fever occur—may indicate other infections
• Advise patient to report perioral tingling, numbness in extremities, and paresthesias
• Caution patient that serious drug interactions may occur if OTC products are ingested; check first with prescriber
• Inform patient that drug is not a cure, but will control symptoms
• Advise patient that regular ophth exams must be continued
• Inform patient that major toxicities may necessitate discontinuing drug
• Instruct patient to use contraception during treatment and that infertility may occur; men should use barrier contraception for 90 days after treatment
• Teach patient to take PO with food
• Teach patient to report infection: fever, chills, sore throat; blood dyscrasias: bruising, bleeding, petechiae
• Tell patient to avoid crowds, persons with respiratory infection
• Advise patient to use sunscreen to prevent burns

Evaluation
Positive therapeutic outcome
• Decreased symptoms of CMV

---

ganirelex
See Appendix A, Selected New Drugs

---

gatifloxacin
See Appendix A, Selected New Drugs

---

gemcitabine (Ŗ)
(gem-sit′a-been)
Gemzar
Func. class.: Misc. antineoplastic
Chem. class.: Nucleoside analog
Pregnancy category **D**

Action: Exhibits antitumor activity by killing cells undergoing DNA synthesis (S phase) and blocking GL/S-phase boundary

⇒Therapeutic Outcome: Prevention of growth of tumor

Uses: Adenocarcinoma of the pancreas: nonresectable stage II, III, or metastatic stage IV; in combination with cisplatin for inoperable, advanced, or metastatic non-small cell lung cancer

Dosage and routes
Adult: **IV** 100 mg/m² given over ½ hr qwk × 7 wk, then 1 wk rest period; subsequent cycles should be infused once qwk × 3 wk out of every 4 wk

3 wk schedule
Adult: **IV** 1250 mg/m² given over ½ hr on days 1, 8 of each 21-day cycle; give cisplatin 100 mg/m² after the inf of gemcitabine on day 1

Non-small-cell lung cancer 4 wk schedule
Adult: **IV** 1000 mg/m² given over ½ hr on days 1, 8, 15 of each 28-day cycle. Give cisplatin **IV** 100 mg/m² on day 1 after gemcitabine

Available forms: Lyophilized powder 20 mg/ml

Adverse effects
GI: Diarrhea, nausea, vomiting, anorexia, constipation, stomatitis
HEMA: Leukopenia, anemia, neutropenia, thrombocytopenia
INTEG: Irritation at site, rash, alopecia
OTHER: Dyspnea, fever, ***hemorrhage,*** infection

Contraindications: Hypersensitivity, pregnancy **D**

Ⓟ Precautions: Lactation, children, elderly, myelosuppression, irradiation
Ⓖ

G

Pharmacokinetics	
Absorption	Unknown
Distribution	Unknown
Metabolism	Unknown
Excretion	Unknown
Half-life	42-79 min

Pharmacodynamics
Unknown

Interactions
Drug classifications
Antineoplastics: ↑ myelosuppression, diarrhea
NSAIDs: ↑ bleeding
Salicylates: ↑ bleeding
Radiation: ↑ myelosuppression

NURSING CONSIDERATIONS
Assessment
• Monitor CBC, differential, platelet count weekly; withhold drug if WBC is <3500/mm³, or platelet count <100,000/mm³; notify prescriber of these results; drug should be discontinued
• Assess for blood dyscrasias, bruising, bleeding, petechiae
• Monitor I&O, nutritional intake
• Monitor hepatic/renal studies

- Assess food preferences: list likes, dislikes
- Assess buccal cavity q8h for dryness, sores or ulceration, white patches, oral pain, bleeding, dysphagia
- Assess GI symptoms: frequency of stools; cramping
- Assess signs of dehydration: rapid respirations, poor skin turgor, decreased urine output, dry skin, restlessness, weakness

Nursing diagnoses
☑ Infection, risk for (adverse reactions)
☑ Nutrition, altered: less than body requirements (adverse reaction)

Implementation
- Provide for rinsing of mouth tid-qid with water, club soda; brushing of teeth bid-tid with soft brush or cotton-tipped applicator for stomatitis; use unwaxed dental floss
- Give nutritious diet with iron, vitamin supplement, low fiber, few dairy products
- Give increased fluid intake to 2-3 L/day to prevent dehydration, unless contraindicated

ⅣIV route
- After reconstituting with 0.9% NaCl 5 ml/200 mg vial of drug or 25 ml/1 gm of drug, shake (40 mg/ml) may be further diluted with 0.9% NaCl to concentrate as low as 0.1 mg/ml
- Change **IV** site q48h

Patient/family education
- Advise to avoid foods with citric acid or hot or rough texture if stomatitis is present; to drink adequate fluids
- Advise to report stomatitis; any bleeding, white spots, ulcerations in mouth; tell patient to examine mouth qd, report symptoms

- Advise to report signs of anemia: fatigue, headache, faintness, shortness of breath, irritability
- Advise to use contraception during therapy
- Instruct patient to avoid use with NSAIDs, salicylates, alcohol

Evaluation
Positive therapeutic outcome
- Decrease in tumor size, decrease in spread of cancer

Treatment of overdose:
Induce vomiting, provide supportive care

---

gemfibrozil (℞)
(gem-fye′broe-zil)
Lopid
Func. class.: Antilipemic
Chem. class.: Aryloxisobutyric acid derivative

Pregnancy category   C

Action: Inhibits biosynthesis of VLDL, decreases triglycerides, increased HDLs

Therapeutic Outcome: Decreased hepatic triglyceride production, VLDL; accelerates removal of cholesterol from liver

Uses: Type II, III, IV, V hyperlipidemia as adjunct with diet therapy

Dosage and routes
Adult: PO 1200 mg in divided doses bid 30 min ac

Available forms: Caps 300 mg 🍁, Tabs 600 mg

Adverse effects
CNS: Dizziness, blurred vision
GI: Nausea, vomiting, dyspepsia, diarrhea, abdominal pain

☑ Herb/drug   Ⓢ Do Not Crush   ⬥ Alert   ⛬ Key Drug   Ⓖ Geriatric   Ⓟ Pediatric

HEMA: Leukopenia, anemia, eosinophilia, thrombocytopenia
INTEG: Rash, urticaria, pruritus
MISC: Task perversion

Contraindications: Severe hepatic disease, preexisting gallbladder disease, severe renal disease, primary biliary cirrhosis, hypersensitivity

Precautions: Monitor hematologic and hepatic function, pregnancy **C**, lactation

Pharmacokinetics

Absorption	Well absorbed
Distribution	Unknown, plasma protein binding >90%
Metabolism	Liver—minimal
Excretion	Kidney—unchanged (70%), feces (6%)
Half-life	1½ hr

Pharmacodynamics

Onset	1-2 hr
Peak	1-2 hr
Duration	2-4 months

Interactions
Individual drugs
Lovastatin: ↑ rhabdomyolysis
Simivastatin: ↑ rhabdomyolysis
Drug classifications
Anticoagulants, oral: ↑ effect of anticoagulants
Lab test interferences
↑ Liver function studies, ↑ CPK, ↑ BSP, ↑ thymol turbidity, ↑ glucose
↓ Hgb, ↓ Hct, ↓ WBC

NURSING CONSIDERATIONS
Assessment
• Assess nutrition: fat, protein, carbohydrates—nutritional analysis should be performed by dietician before treatment is initiated
• Assess renal studies, LFTs, CBC if patient is on long-term therapy; if LFTs increase, drug should be discontinued
• Monitor bowel pattern daily; diarrhea may be a problem
• Monitor triglycerides, cholesterol baseline and throughout treatment; LDL and VLDL should be watched closely and if increased, drug should be discontinued

Nursing diagnoses
☑ Diarrhea (adverse reactions)
☑ Knowledge deficit (teaching)
☑ Noncompliance (teaching)

Implementation
• Give 30 min before AM and PM meals
⊘ • Do not crush, chew caps

Patient/family education
• Inform patient that compliance is needed for positive results to occur; not to double doses
• Caution patient to decrease risk factors: high-fat diet, smoking, alcohol consumption, lack of exercise
• Advise patient to notify health care prescriber if the GI symptoms of diarrhea, abdominal or epigastric pain, nausea, vomiting occur; or if chills, fever, sore throat, occur

Evaluation
Positive therapeutic outcome
• Decreased cholesterol levels, serum triglyceride and improved ratio with high-density lipoproteins (HDLs)

gentamicin (℞)
(jen-ta-mye′sin)
Alcomicin ✤, Apogen,
Cidomycin ✤, Garamycin,
Garamycin Intrathecal,
Garamycin **IV** Piggyback,
Garamycin Pediatric,
Gentamicin Sulfate,
gentamicin sulfate
IV Piggyback, Jenamicin,
Pediatric Gentamicin Sulfate
Func. class.: Antiinfective
Chem. class.: Aminoglyco-
side

Pregnancy category   C

Action: Interferes with protein synthesis in bacterial cell by binding to ribosomal subunit, causing misreading of genetic code; inaccurate peptide sequence forms in protein chain, causing bacterial death

➔**Therapeutic Outcome:** Bactericidal effects for the following organisms *Proteus aeruginosa, Proteus, Klebsiella, Serratia, Escherichia coli, Enterobacter, Citrobacter, Staphylococcus, Shigella, Salmonella, Acinetobacter*

Uses: Severe systemic infections of CNS; respiratory, GI, and urinary tracts; acute PID; bone; skin; soft tissues caused by susceptible strains

Dosage and routes
Severe systemic infections
Adult: **IV** inf 3-5 mg/kg/day in 3 divided doses q8h; dilute in 50-200 ml NS or D_5W given over 30 min-1 hr; IM 3 mg/kg/day in divided doses q8h

Adult: Intrathec 4-8 mg qd

🅿 *Child:* **IV**/IM 2-2.5 mg/ kg q8h

🅿 *Neonates and infants:*
IV/IM 2.5 mg/kg q8-12h

🅿 *Neonates <1 wk:* 2.5 mg/kg q12-24h

🅿 *Infants and child >3 mo:*
Intrathec 1-2 mg qd
Once-daily dosing/extended interval dosing

Adult: **IV** 5-7 mg/kg/dose, adjust according to levels

Dental/respiratory procedures/GI/GU surgery (prophylaxis endocarditis)
Adult: IM 1.5 mg/kg ½-1 hr before procedure with ampicillin

Top
🅿 *Adult, child:* Apply to cleansed area 3-4 times daily

Ophth
🅿 *Adult, child:* 1-2 drops of ophth sol q2-4h or ophth oint 2-3 times daily

🅿 *Child:* IM 2.5 mg/kg ½-1 hr before procedure with ampicillin

Available forms: Inj 10, 40, 60, 80, 100 mg; intrathec 2 mg/ml; ophth sol 0.3%, ophth oint 0.3%, top oint 0.1%, top cream 0.1%

Adverse effects
CNS: Confusion, depression, numbness, tremors, **convulsions,** muscle twitching, **neurotoxicity,** dizziness, vertigo
CV: Hypotension, hypertension, palpitations
EENT: Ototoxicity, deafness, visual disturbances, tinnitus
GI: Nausea, vomiting, anorexia, increased ALT, AST, bilirubin, hepatomegaly, **hepatic necrosis,** splenomegaly
GU: **Oliguria, hematuria, renal damage, azotemia, renal failure, nephrotoxicity**

☑ Herb/drug   🚫 Do Not Crush   ◆ Alert   �ળ Key Drug   🅖 Geriatric   🅿 Pediatric

HEMA: **Agranulocytosis, thrombocytopenia, leukopenia, eosinophilia,** anemia
INTEG: Rash, burning, urticaria, dermatitis, alopecia

Contraindications: Severe renal disease, hypersensitivity

P **Precautions:** Neonates, mild renal disease, pregnancy **C,** hearing deficits, myasthenia
G gravis, lactation, elderly, Parkinson's disease

N **Do Not Confuse:**
Garamycin/kanamycin

Pharmacokinetics

Absorption	Well absorbed (IM)
Distribution	Distributed in extracellular fluids, poorly distributed in CSF; crosses placenta
Metabolism	Liver, minimal
Excretion	Mostly unchanged (79%) kidneys
Half-life	1-2 hr, infants 6-7 hr, increased in renal disease

Pharmacodynamics

	IM	IV
Onset	Rapid	Rapid
Peak	½-1½ hr	Infusion's end

Interactions
Individual drugs
Amphotericin B: ↑ ototoxicity, neurotoxicity, nephrotoxicity
Cisplatin: ↑ ototoxicity, neurotoxicity, nephrotoxicity
Ethacrynic acid: ↑ ototoxicity, neurotoxicity, nephrotoxicity
Furosemide: ↑ ototoxicity, neurotoxicity, nephrotoxicity
Mannitol: ↑ ototoxicity, neurotoxicity, nephrotoxicity
Methoxyflurane: ↑ ototoxicity, neurotoxicity, nephrotoxicity

Polymyxin: ↑ ototoxicity, neurotoxicity, nephrotoxicity
Succinylcholine: ↑ neuromuscular blockade, respiratory depression
Vancomycin: ↑ ototoxicity, neurotoxicity, nephrotoxicity
Drug classifications
Anesthetics: ↑ neuromuscular blockade, respiratory depression
Aminoglycosides: ↑ ototoxicity, neurotoxicity
Nondepolarizing neuromuscular blockers: ↑ neuromuscular blockade, respiratory depression
Penicillins: ↑ ototoxicity, neurotoxicity, nephrotoxicity

G

NURSING CONSIDERATIONS
Assessment
• Assess patient for previous sensitivity reaction
• Assess patient for signs and symptoms of infection including characteristics of wounds, sputum, urine, stool, WBC >10,000, fever; obtain baseline information and during treatment
• Complete culture and sensitivity before beginning drug therapy; this will ensure that correct treatment has been initiated
• Assess for allergic reactions: rash, urticaria, pruritus, chills, fever, joint pain may occur a few days after therapy begins
• Identify urine output; if decreasing, notify prescriber (may indicate nephrotoxicity); also, increased BUN, creatinine, urine CrCl <80 ml/min
• Monitor blood studies: AST, ALT, CBC, Hct, bilirubin, LDH, alk phosphatase, Coombs' test monthly if patient is on long-term therapy

---

• Monitor electrolytes: potassium, sodium, chloride, magnesium monthly if patient is on long-term therapy

• Monitor for bleeding: ecchymosis, bleeding gums, hematuria; assess stool guaiac daily if on long-term therapy

• Assess for overgrowth of infection: perineal itching, fever, malaise, redness, pain, swelling, drainage, rash, diarrhea, change in cough, sputum

• Obtain weight before treatment; calculation of dosage is usually based on ideal body weight, but may be calculated on actual body weight

• Monitor I&O ratio; urinalysis daily for proteinuria, cells, casts; report sudden change in urine output

• Monitor VS during inf, watch for hypotension, change in pulse

• Assess **IV** site for thrombophlebitis including pain, redness, swelling q30 min, change site if needed; apply warm compresses to discontinued site

• Obtain serum peak, drawn at 30-60 min after **IV** inf or 60 min after IM inj, trough level drawn just before next dose; blood level should be 2-4 times bacteriostatic level

• Assess urine pH if drug is used for UTI; urine should be kept alkaline

• Assess for deafness by audiometric testing, ringing, roaring in ears, vertigo; assess hearing before, during, after treatment

• Assess for dehydration: high sp gr, decrease in skin turgor, dry mucous membranes, dark urine

Nursing diagnoses
☑ Infection, risk for (uses)
☑ Diarrhea (side effects)
☑ Knowledge deficit (teaching)
☑ Noncompliance (teaching)
☑ Injury, risk for (side effects)

Implementation
IM route
• Give deeply in large muscle mass; rotate sites

Top route
• Wash hands, wear gloves, clean skin before applying

Ⅳ IV route
• Give in even doses around the clock; drug must be given for 10-14 days to ensure organism death and prevent superimposed infection

• Give by INT inf over ½-1 hr, flush with 0.9% NaCl or D_5W after inf

• Separate aminoglycosides and penicillins by ≥1 hr

• Store in tight container

Syringe compatibilities:
Clindamycin, methicillin, penicillin G sodium

Y-site compatibilities:
Acyclovir, amifostine, amiodarone, amsacrine, atracurium, aztreonam, cefpirome, ciprofloxacin, cyclophosphamide, cytarabine, diltiazem, enalaprilat, esmolol, famotidine, fluconazole, fludarabine, foscarnet, granisetron, hydromorphone, IL-2, insulin, labetalol, lorazepam, magnesium sulfate, melphalan, meperidine, meropenem, midazolam, morphine, multivitamins, ondansetron, paclitaxel, pancuronium, perphenazine, sargramostim, tacrolimus, teniposide, theophylline, thiotepa, tolazine, vecuronium, vinorelbine, vitamin B with C, zidovudine

Y-site incompatibilities:
Idarubicin, indomethacin, zidovudine

Additive compatibilities:
Atracurium, aztreonam, bleomycin, cefoxitin, cimetidine, ciprofloxacin, fluconazole, meropenem, methicillin, metronidazole, ofloxacin, penicillin G sodium, ranitidine, verapamil

Patient/family education
• Teach patient to report sore throat, bruising, bleeding, joint pain—may indicate blood dyscrasias (rare)
• Advise patient to contact prescriber if vaginal itching, loose, foul-smelling stools, furry tongue occur—may indicate superimposed infection

Evaluation
Positive therapeutic outcome
• Absence of signs/symptoms of infection (WBC <10,000, temp WNL, absence of red, draining wounds)
• Reported improvement in symptoms of infection

Treatment of overdose:
Withdraw drug, hemodialysis

glatiramer (R)
(glah-teer´a-mer)
Copaxone
Func. class.: Multiple sclerosis agent
Pregnancy category   B

Action: Unknown; may modify the immune responses responsible for multiple sclerosis
Therapeutic outcome: Decreased symptoms of multiple sclerosis

Uses: Reduction of the frequency of relapses in patients with relapsing-remitting multiple sclerosis

Dosage and routes
Adult: SC 20 mg/day
Available forms: Inj 20 mg/ml
Adverse effects
CNS: Anxiety, hypertonia, tremor, vertigo, speech disorder, agitation, confusion
CV: Migraine, palpitations, syncope, tachycardia, vasodilation
EENT: Ear pain
GI: Nausea, vomiting, diarrhea, anorexia, gastroenteritis
GU: Urgency, dysmenorrhea, vaginal moniliasis
HEMA: Ecchymosis, lymphadenopathy
INTEG: Pruritus, rash, sweating, urticaria, erythema
META: Edema, weight gain
MS: Arthralgia
RESP: Bronchitis, dyspnea

Contraindications: Hypersensitivity to this drug or mannitol
Precautions: Immune disorders, renal disease, pregnancy **B**, lactation

Pharmacokinetics	
Absorption	Unknown
Distribution	Unknown
Metabolism	Unknown
Excretion	Unknown
Half-life	Unknown

Pharmacodynamics
Unknown

NURSING CONSIDERATIONS
Assessment
• Monitor blood, renal, hepatic studies; prior to treatment
• Assess for CNS symptoms: anxiety, confusion, vertigo
• Assess GI status: diarrhea, vomiting, abdominal pain, gastroenteritis

• Assess cardiac status: tachycardia, palpitations, vasodilation, chest pain

Nursing diagnoses

☑ Knowledge deficit (teaching)
☑ Noncompliance (teaching)

Implementation

SC route

• Use a sterile syringe/needle to transfer the supplied diluent into the vial, rotate vial gently, do not shake; withdraw medication using a syringe with 27G needle; administer SC into hip, thigh, arm; discard unused portion

• Use SC route only; do not give IM or **IV**

• Do not use sol that contains precipitate or is discolored

Patient/family education

• Give written, detailed instructions about the drug; provide initial and return demonstrations on inj procedure; give information on use and disposal of drug

• Advise that blurred vision, sweating may occur

• Advise that irregular menses, dysmenorrhea, or metorrhagia as well as breast pain may occur; use contraception during treatment

• Advise that if pregnancy is suspected or if nursing notify prescriber

• Advise not to change dosing or to stop taking drug without advice of prescriber

Evaluation

Positive therapeutic outcome

• Decreased symptoms of multiple sclerosis

---

glipizide (℞)
(glip-i′zide)
Glucotrol, Glucotrol XL
glimepiride (℞)
(gly-meh′pih-ride)
Amaride
Func. class.: Antidiabetic
Chem. class.: Sulfonylurea
(2nd generation)
Pregnancy category   C

Action: Causes functioning β-cells in pancreas to release insulin, leading to drop in blood glucose levels; may improve insulin binding to insulin receptors or increase the number of insulin receptors with prolonged administration; may also reduce basal hepatic glucose secretion; not effective if patient lacks functioning β-cells

➡ **Therapeutic Outcome:** Decrease in polyuria, polydipsia, polyphagia, clear sensorium, absence of dizziness, stable gait

Uses: Stable adult-onset diabetes mellitus (type II) NIDDM

Dosage and routes
glipizide
Adult: PO 5 mg initially, then increase to desired response; max 40 mg/day in divided doses or 15 mg/dose

🄶 *Elderly/hepatic disease:* PO 2.5 mg initially, then increase to desired response; max 40 mg/day in divided doses or 15 mg/dose

glimepiride
Adult: PO 1-2 mg qd, then increase q1-2wk up to 8 mg/day

Renal dose
Adult: PO 1 mg qd with breakfast, may titrate upward as needed

Available forms: glipizide: tabs 5, 10 mg scored; ext rel tab 10 mg; glimepiride: tabs 1, 2, 4 mg

Adverse effects
CNS: Headache, weakness, dizziness, drowsiness, tinnitus, fatigue, vertigo
ENDO: **Hypoglycemia**
GI: **Hepatotoxicity, cholestatic jaundice,** nausea, vomiting, diarrhea, heartburn
HEMA: **Leukopenia, thrombocytopenia, agranulocytosis, aplastic anemia,** increased AST, ALT, alk phosphatase, **pancytopenia, hemolytic anemia**
INTEG: Rash, allergic reactions, pruritus, urticaria, eczema, photosensitivity, erythema

Contraindications: Hypersensitivity to sulfonylureas, juvenile or brittle diabetes

Precautions: Pregnancy **C**, elderly, cardiac disease, severe renal disease, severe hepatic disease, thyroid disease

Do Not Confuse:
Glucotrol/glyburide

Pharmacokinetics	
Absorption	Completely absorbed GI tract
Distribution	Unknown
Metabolism	Liver
Excretion	Via kidneys
Half-life	2-4 hr

Pharmacodynamics	
Onset	1-1½ hr
Peak	1-3 hr
Duration	10-24 hr

Interactions
Individual drugs
Alcohol: Disulfiram-like reaction
Chloramphenicol: ↑ hypoglycemia
Cimetidine: ↑ hypoglycemia
Diazoxide: Both drugs may have action decreased
Digoxin: ↓ action of glipizide
Guanethidine: ↑ hypoglycemia
Insulin: ↑ hypoglycemia
Isoniazid: Possible ↓ action of glipizide
Methyldopa: ↑ hypoglycemia
Phenobarbital: Possible ↓ action of glipizide
Phenytoin: Possible ↓ action of glipizide
Probenecid: ↑ hypoglycemia
Rifampin: Possible ↓ action of glipizide
Drug classifications
Anticoagulants: ↑ hypoglycemia
Calcium channel blockers: Possible ↓ action of glipizide
Contraceptives, oral: Possible ↓ action of glipizide
Corticosteroids: Possible ↓ action of glipizide
Diuretics, thiazide: Possible ↓ action of glipizide
Estrogens: Possible ↓ action of glipizide
MAOIs: ↑ hypoglycemia
NSAIDs: ↑ hypoglycemia
Phenothiazine: Possible ↓ action of glipizide
Salicylates: ↑ hypoglycemia
Sympathomimetics: Possible ↓ action of glipizide
Thyroid preparations: Possible ↓ action of glipizide
Herb/drug
Broom: ↓ hyperglycemic effect
Buchu: ↓ hyperglycemic effect
Chromium: ↑ or ↓ hypoglycemic effect

Dandelion: ↓ hyperglycemic effect
Fenugreek: ↑ or ↓ hypoglycemic effect
Ginseng: ↑ or ↓ hypoglycemic effect
Karela: ↑ glucose tolerance
Juniper: ↓ hyperglycemic effect

NURSING CONSIDERATIONS
Assessment
• Assess for hypoglycemic/hyperglycemic reactions that can occur soon pc; hypoglycemic reactions (sweating, weakness, dizziness, anxiety, tremors, hunger); hyperglycemic reactions
• Monitor CBC (baseline, q3mo) during treatment; check liver function tests periodically AST, LDH, and renal studies: BUN, creatinine during treatment

Nursing diagnoses
☑ Nutrition, altered: more than body requirements (uses)
☑ Nutrition altered: less than body requirements (adverse reactions)
☑ Injury, risk for (adverse reactions)
☑ Knowledge deficit (teaching)
☑ Noncompliance (teaching)

Implementation
• Convert from other oral hypoglycemic agents or insulin dosage of <40 U/day; change may be made without gradual dosage change.
• Convert patients taking >40 U/day of insulin gradually by receiving oral hypoglycemic and 50% of previous insulin dosage for 3-5 days
• Monitor serum or urine glucose and ketones 3 times/day during conversion

• Give drug 30 min before breakfast—if large dose is required, may be divided into two; give with meals to decrease GI upset and provide best absorption
• Give tab crushed and mixed with meal or fluids for patients with difficulty swallowing
• Store in tight container in cool environment

Patient/family education
• Teach patient to check for symptoms of cholestatic jaundice: dark urine, pruritus, yellow sclera; if these occur, prescriber should be notified
• Teach patient to use capillary blood glucose test or Chemstrip 3 ×/day
• Teach patient symptoms of hypo/hyperglycemia, what to do about each
• Instruct patient that drug must be continued on daily basis; explain consequence of discontinuing drug abruptly
• Teach patient to take drug in AM to prevent hypoglycemic reactions at night
• Caution patient to avoid OTC medications unless prescribed by a prescriber
• Teach patient that diabetes is lifelong illness; that this drug is not a cure
• Instruct patient that all food included in diet plan must be eaten to prevent hypoglycemia
• Advise patient to carry Medic-Alert ID and a glucagon emergency kit for emergency purposes

Evaluation
Positive therapeutic outcome
• Decrease in polyuria, polydipsia, polyphagia, clear sensorium, absence of dizziness, stable gait

---

glyburide (℞)
(glye′byoor-ide)
DiaBeta ✳, Euglucon ✳,
Glynase PresTab, Micronase
Func. class.: Antidiabetic
Chem. class.: Sulfonylurea
(2nd generation)
Pregnancy category **B**

Action: Causes functioning
β-cells in pancreas to release
insulin, leading to drop in
blood glucose levels; may
improve insulin binding to
insulin receptors and increase
number of insulin receptors
with prolonged administration;
may also reduce basal hepatic
glucose secretion; not effective
if patient lacks functioning
β-cells

Therapeutic Outcome: Decrease in polyuria, polydipsia,
polyphagia, clear sensorium,
absence of dizziness, stable gait

Uses: Stable adult-onset diabetes mellitus (type II) NIDDM

Dosage and routes
DiaBeta/micronase
Adult: PO 2.5-5 mg initially,
then increased to desired response
G *Elderly:* PO 1.25 mg initially,
then increased to desired
response; max 20 mg/day,
maintenance 1.25-20 mg/qd

Glynase PresTab
Adult: PO 1.5-3 mg/day
initially, may increase by 1.5
mg/wk
G *Elderly:* PO 0.75-3 mg/day,
may increase by 1.5 mg/wk

Available forms: Tabs 1.25,
2.5, 5 mg; tabs micronized
(Glynase PresTab) 1.5, 3, 6 mg

Adverse effects
CNS: Headache, weakness,
paresthesia, tinnitus, fatigue,
vertigo
ENDO: **Hypoglycemia**
GI: Nausea, fullness, heartburn, **hepatoxicity, cholestatic
jaundice,** vomiting, diarrhea
HEMA: **Leukopenia, thrombocytopenia, agranulocytosis, aplastic anemia,** increased
AST, ALT, alk phosphatase
INTEG: Rash, allergic reactions, pruritus, urticaria, eczema, photosensitivity, erythema
MS: Joint pains

Contraindications: Hypersensitivity to sulfonylureas, juvenile or brittle diabetes

Precautions: Pregnancy **B**,
G elderly, cardiac disease, severe
renal disease, severe hepatic
disease, thyroid disease, severe
hypoglycemic reactions

Do Not Confuse:
glyburide/Glucotrol, DiaBeta/
Zebeta

Pharmacokinetics	
Absorption	Completely absorbed GI tract
Distribution	90%-95% plasma protein binding
Metabolism	Liver
Excretion	Urine, feces (me-tabolites), crosses placenta
Half-life	10 hr

Pharmacodynamics	
Onset	2-4 hr
Peak	4 hr
Duration	24 hr

Interactions
Individual drugs
Alcohol: Disulfiram-like reac-
tion
Charcoal: ↓ glyburide action

G

Chloramphenicol: ↑ hypoglycemia
Cholestyramine: ↓ glyburide action
Diazoxide: Both drugs may have action decreased
Digoxin: ↓ digoxin level
Fenfluramine: ↑ glyburide action
Gemfibrozil: ↑ glyburide
Guanethidine: ↑ hypoglycemia
Insulin: ↑ hypoglycemia
Isoniazid: ↓ action of glyburide
Methyldopa: ↑ hypoglycemia
Phenobarbital: ↓ action of glyburide
Phenylbutazone: ↑ glyburide
Phenytoin: ↓ action of glyburide
Probenecid: ↑ hypoglycemia
Rifampin: ↓ action of glyburide
Sulfinpyrazone: ↑ glyburide
Drug classifications
Androgens: ↑ glyburide action
Anticoagulants: ↑ hypoglycemia
Antidepressants, tricyclics: ↑ glyburide action
β-Adrenergic blockers: ↓ glyburide acid
Diuretics, thiazide: ↓ action of glyburide
Estrogens: ↓ action of glyburide
Histamine H₂ antagonists: ↑ glyburide action
Magnesium salts: ↑ glyburide action
MAOIs: ↑ hypoglycemia
NSAIDs: ↑ hypoglycemia
Salicylates: ↑ hypoglycemia
Sulfonamides: ↑ glyburide action
Urinary acidifers: ↑ glyburide acid
Urinary alkalinizers: ↓ glyburide action

☑ *Herb/drug*
Broom: ↓ glyburide action
Buchu: ↓ glyburide action
Chromium: ↑ or ↓ glyburide effect
Dandelion: ↓ glyburide action
Fenugreek: ↑ or ↓ glyburide effect
Ginseng: ↑ or ↓ glyburide effect
Karela: ↑ glucose tolerance
Juniper: ↓ glyburide action

NURSING CONSIDERATIONS
Assessment
• Assess for hypoglycemic/hyperglycemic reactions that can occur soon pc; hypoglycemic reactions (sweating, weakness, dizziness, anxiety, tremors, hunger); hyperglycemic reactions
• Monitor CBC (baseline, q3mo) during treatment; check liver function tests periodically AST, LDH and renal studies: BUN, creatinine during treatment

Nursing diagnoses
☑ Nutrition, altered: more than body requirements (uses)
☑ Nutrition altered: less than body requirements (adverse reactions)
☑ Injury, risk for (adverse reactions)
☑ Knowledge deficit (teaching)
☑ Noncompliance (teaching)

Implementation
• Conversion from other oral hypoglycemic agents or insulin dosage of <40 U/day; change may be made without gradual dosage change
• Patients taking >40 U/day of insulin convert gradually by receiving oral hypoglycemic and 50% of previous insulin dosage for 3-5 days

---

☑ Herb/drug   ☒ Do Not Crush   ✦ Alert   ☞ Key Drug   🄶 Geriatric   🄿 Pediatric

• Monitor serum or urine glucose and ketones 3 times/day during conversion

• Give drug 30 min before breakfast—if large dose is required, may be divided into two; give with meals to decrease GI upset and provide best absorption

• Give tab crushed and mixed with meal or fluids for patients with difficulty swallowing

• Store in tight container in cool environment

Patient/family education

• Teach patient to check for symptoms of cholestatic jaundice: dark urine, pruritus, yellow sclera; if these occur, prescriber should be notified

• Teach patient to use capillary blood glucose test or Chemstrip 3 ×/day

• Teach patient symptoms of hypo/hyperglycemia, what to do about each

• Instruct patient that drug must be continued on daily basis; explain consequence of discontinuing drug abruptly

• Teach patient to take drug in AM to prevent hypoglycemic reactions at night

• Caution patient to avoid OTC medications unless prescribed by a prescriber

• Teach patient that diabetes is lifelong illness; that this drug is not a cure

• Instruct patient that all food included in diet plan must be eaten to prevent hypoglycemia

• Advise patient to carry Medic Alert ID and a glucagon emergency kit for emergency purposes

Evaluation

Positive therapeutic outcome

• Decrease in polyuria, polydipsia, polyphagia, clear sensorium, absence of dizziness, stable gait

glycerin (OTC)
(gli′ser-in)
Fleet Babylax, glycerin USP, Glycerol, Ophthalgan, Osmoglyn, Sani-Supp
Func. class.: Laxative, hyperosmotic, antiglaucoma agent
Chem. class.: Trihydric alcohol
Pregnancy category **C**

Action: Increases osmotic pressure by drawing fluid into colon lumen from extravascular spaces to intravascular

Therapeutic Outcome: Absence of constipation, intraocular pressure, intracranial pressure, absence of edema in the cornea

Uses: Constipation, intraocular pressure in glaucoma; intracranial pressure, edema in the superficial layers of the cornea

Dosage and routes

Adult and child >6 yr: Rec supp 3 g; enema 5-15 ml

Child <6 yr: Rec supp 1-1.5 g; enema 2-5 ml

Corneal edema
Adult: Ophth 1-2 gtt q3-4 h

Intraocular pressure reduction
Adult: PO 1-1.5 g/kg once, then 500 mg/kg q6h

Child: PO 1-1.5 g/kg qd once, then 500 mg/kg 4-8 hr after first dose

Available forms: Rec sol 4 ml/applicator; supp; oral sol 0.6/ml; ophth sol 7.5 ml/container

G

Adverse effects
CNS: Headache, confusion, **convulsions**
GI: Nausea, vomiting, diarrhea
META: Dehydration

Contraindications: Hypersensitivity

Precautions: Pregnancy **C**

Pharmacokinetics	
Absorption	Well absorbed (PO), not absorbed (rectal)
Distribution	To intravascular space
Metabolism	Liver—80%, kidneys—20%
Excretion	Kidneys
Half-life	30 min

Pharmacodynamics			
	PO	REC	OPHTH
Onset	10-30 min	Unknown	Unknown
Peak	30-120 min	30 min	Unknown
Duration	6-8 hr	Unknown	Up to 4 hr

Interactions
Drug classifications
Diuretics: ↓ effect of glycerin (ophth)

NURSING CONSIDERATIONS
Assessment
• Assess patient for cause of constipation; identify whether fluids, bulk, or exercise is missing from lifestyle; check for distention, bowel sounds
• After administration, check for cramping, rec bleeding, nausea, vomiting; if these symptoms occur, drug should be discontinued
• Identify stool characteristics: consistency, color, amount, shape, volume

Nursing diagnoses
✓ Constipation (uses)
✓ Knowledge deficit (teaching)

Implementation
Rec route
• Insert glycerin supp after removing wrapper; may cause evacuation in ½ hr
• For evening use 4-ml applications of fluid, have patient in side-lying position, have patient retain for a few min
Ophth route
• Instill 1-2 gtt in one or both eyes by pulling down on conjunctival sac
• Do not use ophth sol that is discolored, has a precipitate, or is cloudy
PO route
• Pour over cracked ice and sip through a straw
• To prevent severe cerebral dehydration headache have patient recumbent during and after administration
• Give by mixing 50% glycerin sol with 0.9% NaCl with flavoring, or use oral sol that is already flavored—flavoring improves taste and prevents GI symptoms
• Storage in cool environment; do not freeze

Patient/family education
• Caution patient not to use laxatives for long-term therapy; normal bowel tone will be lost; that normal bowel movements do not always occur daily
• Advise patient not to use in presence of abdominal pain, nausea, vomiting
• Instruct patient to notify prescriber if constipation is unrelieved or if weakness, dizziness, excessive thirst occur

Evaluation
Positive therapeutic outcome
• Decreased constipation
• Decreased intraocular pressure

---

glycopyrrolate (℞)
(glye-koe-pye'roe-late)
glycopyrrolate, Robinul,
Robinul Forte
Func. class.: Cholinergic
blocker
Chem. class.: Quaternary
ammonium compound
Pregnancy category **B**

Action: Inhibits action of
acetylcholine at receptor sites
in autonomic nervous system,
which controls secretions, free
acids in stomach

Therapeutic Outcome: Decreased secretions in the respiratory tract, GI system

Uses: Decreased secretions
before surgery, reversal of
neuromuscular blockade, peptic ulcer disease, irritable bowel
syndrome

Dosage and routes
Preoperatively
Adult: IM 0.002 mg/lb ½-1
hr before surgery

P *Child 2-12 yr:* IM 0.002-
0.004 mg/lb

P *Child <2 yr:* IM 0.004 mg/lb

*Reversal of neuromuscular
blockage*
P *Adult and child:* IV 0.2 mg
for each mg of neostigmine or
5 mg **IV** of pyridostigmine
simultaneously

GI disorders
Adult: PO 1-2 mg bid-tid;
IM/IV 0.1-0.2 mg tid-qid,
titrated to patient response

Available forms: Tabs 1, 2
mg; inj 0.2 mg/ml

Adverse effects
CNS: Confusion, anxiety,
restlessness, irritability, delusions, hallucinations, headache,
sedation, depression, incoherence, dizziness, lethargy, flushing, weakness
CV: Palpitations, tachycardia,
postural hypotension, paradoxical bradycardia
EENT: Blurred vision, photophobia, dilated pupils, difficulty swallowing, increased
intraocular pressure, mydriasis,
cycloplegia
*GI: Dryness of mouth, constipa-
tion,* nausea, vomiting, abdominal distress, paralytic ileus,
altered taste perception
GU: Hesitancy, retention,
impotence
INTEG: Urticaria, allergic
reactions
MISC: Suppression of lactation, nasal congestion, decreased sweating, **anaphylaxis**

Contraindications: Hypersensitivity, narrow-angle glaucoma, myasthenia gravis,
P GI/GU obstruction, child <3
yr, tachycardia, myocardial
ischemia, hepatic disease, ulcerative colitis, toxic megacolon

Precautions: Pregnancy **B,**
elderly, lactation, prostatic
hypertrophy, renal disease,
CHF, pulmonary disease,
hyperthyroidism

Pharmacokinetics	
Absorption	Well absorbed (PO, SC, IM)
Distribution	Unknown
Metabolism	Not metabolized
Excretion	Unchanged feces
Half-life	2 hr

Adverse effects: *italic* = common; **bold** = life-threatening

Pharmacodynamics			
	PO	IM	IV
Onset	Un-known	15-30 min	Immediate
Peak	1 hr	30-45 min	10-15 min
Duration	8-12 hr	2-7 hr	2-7 hr

Interactions
Individual drugs
Amantadine: ↑ anticholinergic effect
Disopyramide: ↑ anticholinergic effect
Potassium chloride, oral: ↑ GI lesions
Quinidine: ↑ anticholinergic effect
Drug classifications
Antacids: ↓ absorption of glycopyrrolate
Anticholinergics: ↑ anticholinergic effect
Antidepressants, tricyclic: ↑ anticholinergic effect
Antidiarrheals: ↓ absorption of glycopyrrolate
Antihistamines: ↑ anticholinergic effect

NURSING CONSIDERATIONS
Assessment
• Monitor I&O ratio; retention commonly causes decreased urinary output; check for urinary hesitation; palpate bladder if retention occurs
• Monitor ECG for ectopic ventricular beats, PVC, tachycardia
• Monitor for bowel sounds; check for constipation; increase fluids, bulk, exercise if constipation occurs
• Assess for tolerance over long-term therapy; dose may have to be increased or changed
• Assess mental status: affect, mood, CNS depression, worsening of psychiatric symptoms during early therapy

Nursing diagnoses
✓ Knowledge deficit (teaching)

Implementation
IV **IV route**
• Administer **IV** undiluted, give at a rate of 0.2 mg or less over 1-2 min through Y-tube or 3-way stopcock; do not add to **IV** sol
• Administer parenteral dose with patient recumbent to prevent postural hypotension
Syringe compatibilities:
Atropine, benzquinamide, chlorpromazine, cimetidine, codeine, diphenhydramine, droperidol, droperidol/fentanyl, hydromorphone, hydroxyzine, levorphanol, lidocaine, meperidine, meperidine/promethazine, midazolam, morphine, nalbuphine, neostigmine, oxymorphone, procaine, prochlorperazine, promazine, promethazine, pyridostigmine, ranitidine, scopolamine, triflupromazine, trimethobenzamide
Y-site compatibilities:
Propofol
PO route
• Give PO with or after meals to prevent GI upset; may give with fluids other than water
IM route
• Give IM deeply in large muscle mass

Patient/family education
• Caution patient not to operate machinery or engage in hazardous activities if drowsiness occurs
• Advise patient not to take OTC products, cough, cold preparations with alcohol, antihistamines without approval of prescriber

---

🌿 Herb/drug 🚫 Do Not Crush ◆ Alert ⚘ Key Drug 🅖 Geriatric 🅟 Pediatric

• Caution patient not to discontinue this drug abruptly—tapering should be done over 1 wk

Evaluation

Positive therapeutic outcome

• Decreased secretions, bronchial, GI

goserelin (R)
(goe'se-rel-lin)

Zoladex

Func. class.: Gonadotropin-releasing hormone, antineoplastic

Chem. class.: Synthetic decapeptide analog of LHRH

Pregnancy category   X

Action: Inhibitor of pituitary gonadotropin secretion; initially increases LH and FSH, with increases in testosterone, reduction in sex steroid levels

Therapeutic Outcome: Decrease in tumor size and spread of malignant cells

Uses: Advanced prostate cancer (10.8 mg); endometriosis, advanced breast cancer, endometrial thinning (3.6 mg)

Dosage and routes

Adult: SC 3.6 mg q28 days (implant)

Available forms: Depot inj 3.6, 10.8 mg

Adverse effects

CNS: Headaches, **spinal cord compression,** anxiety, depression

CV: **Dysrhythmia, cerebrovascular accident,** hypertension, **MI,** chest pain

ENDO: Gynecomastia, breast tenderness, hot flashes

GI: Nausea, vomiting, constipation, diarrhea, ulcer

GU: Spotting, breakthrough bleeding, decreased libido, renal insufficiency, urinary obstruction, urinary tract infection

INTEG: Rash, pain on inj

MS: Osteoneuralgia

Contraindications: Hypersensitivity to LHRH, LHRH-agonist analogs, lactation, nondiagnosed vaginal bleeding, pregnancy **X,** breast cancer **(D)**

Precautions: Children, lactation

Pharmacokinetics

Absorption	Well absorbed
Distribution	Unknown
Metabolism	Unknown
Excretion	Unknown
Half-life	4½ hr

Pharmacodynamics

Onset	Unknown
Peak	14-28 days
Duration	Treatment length

Interactions: None

Lab test interferences

↑ Alk phosphatase, ↑ estradiol, ↑ FSH, ↑ LH, ↑ testosterone levels

↓ Testosterone levels, ↓ progesterone

NURSING CONSIDERATIONS

Assessment

• Assess for relief of bone pain (back pain)

• Monitor I&O ratios, palpate bladder for distention (urinary obstruction) at beginning of treatment—renal insufficiency and obstruction may occur

Nursing diagnoses

☑ Sexual dysfunction (uses)

☑ Knowledge deficit (teaching)

Implementation
• Administer via implant inserted by qualified persons into upper subcutaneous tissue in abdominal wall q28 days or q12 wk (10.8 mg)

Patient/family education
• Caution patient that gynecomastia and postmenopausal symptoms may occur but will decrease after treatment is discontinued
• Teach patient to contact prescriber if difficulty urinating occurs during treatment

Evaluation
Positive therapeutic outcome
• More normal levels of prostate-specific antigen, acid phosphatase, alk phosphatase; testosterone level of <25 mg/dl

---

granisetron (℞)
(grane-iss'e-tron)
Kytril
Func. class.: Antiemetic
Chem. class.: 5-HT₃ receptor antagonist
Pregnancy category   C

Action: Prevents nausea, vomiting by blocking serotinin peripherally, centrally, and in the small intestine

▷**Therapeutic Outcome:** Absence of nausea and vomiting

Uses: Prevention of nausea, vomiting associated with cancer chemotherapy including high-dose cisplatin

Dosage and routes
P *Adult and child:* **IV** 10 µg/kg over 5 min, 30 min before the start of cancer chemotherapy; *adult:* PO 1 mg bid, give 1st dose 1 hr before chemotherapy and next dose 12 hr after 1st

Available forms: Inj 1 mg/ml; tab 1 mg

Adverse effects
CNS: Headache, asthenia, anxiety, dizziness
CV: Hypertension
GI: Diarrhea, *constipation,* increased AST, ALT, *nausea*
HEMA: **Leukopenia,** anemia, **thrombocytopenia**
MISC: Rash, **bronchospasm**

Contraindications: Hypersensitivity

P **Precautions:** Pregnancy **C,**
G lactation, children, elderly

Pharmacokinetics	
Absorption	Unknown
Distribution	Unknown
Metabolism	Liver
Excretion	Unknown
Half-life	10-12 hr

Pharmacodynamics
Unknown

Interactions: None

NURSING CONSIDERATIONS
Assessment
• Assess patient for absence of nausea, vomiting during chemotherapy
• Assess patient for hypersensitive reaction: rash, bronchospasm

Nursing diagnoses
☑ Fluid deficit (uses)
☑ Knowledge deficit (teaching)

Implementation
• Administer **IV**
• Dilute in 0.9% NaCl for inj or D₅W (20-50 ml), give ≥5 min
• Store at room temp for 24-hr dilution

Additive compatibilities:
Dexamethasone, methylprednisolone

Y-site incompatibilities:
Fluorouracil, furosemide, sodium bicarbonate

Y-site compatibilities:
Acyclovir, allopurinol, amifostine, amikacin, aminophylline, amphotericin B cholesteryl, ampicillin, ampicillin/sulbactam, amsacrine, aztreonam, bleomycin, bumetanide, buprenorphine, butorphanol, calcium gluconate, carboplatin, carmustine, cefazolin, cefepime, cefonicid, cefoperazone, cefotaxime, cefotetan, cefoxitin, ceftazidime, ceftizoxime, ceftriaxone, cefuroxime, chlorpromazine, cimetidine, ciprofloxacin, cisplatin, cladribine, clindamycin, cyclophosphamide, cytarabine, dacarbazine, dactinomycin, daunorubicin, dexamethasone, diphenhydramine, dobutamine, dopamine, doxorubicin, doxorubicin liposome, doxycycline, droperidol, enalaprilat, etoposide, famotidine, filgrastim, floxuridine, fluconazole, fluorouracil, fludarabine, furosemide, gallium, ganciclovir, gentamicin, haloperidol, heparin, hydrocortisone, hydromorphone, hydroxyzine, idarubicin, ifosfamide, imipenem-cilastatin, leucovorin, lorazepam, magnesium sulfate, melphalan, meperidine, mesna, methotrexate, methylprednisolone, metoclopramide, metronidazole, mezlocillin, miconazole, minocycline, mitomycin, mitoxantrone, morphine, nalbuphine, netilmicin, ofloxacin, paclitaxel, piperacillin, piperacillin/tazobactam, plica-mycin, potassium chloride, prochlorperazine, promethazine, propofol, ranitidine, sargramostim, sodium bicarbonate, streptozocin, teniposide, thiotepa, ticarcillin, ticarcillin/clavulanate, tobramycin, trimethoprim-sulfamethoxazole, vancomycin, vinblastine, vincristine, vinorelbine, zidovudine

Solution compatibilities:
D_5W, 0.9% NaCl

Patient/family education
• Advise patient to report diarrhea, constipation, rash, or changes in respirations

Evaluation
Positive therapeutic outcome
• Absence of nausea, vomiting during cancer chemotherapy

G

---

griseofulvin microsize (℞)
(gris-ee-oh-ful'vin)
Fulvicin-U/F, Grifulvin V, Grisactin, Grisovin-FP ✦
griseofulvin ultramicrosize (℞)
Fulvicin-P/G, Grisactin Ultra, Gris-PEG
Func. class.: Antifungal
Chem. class.: Penicillium griseofulvum derivative
Pregnancy category   C

Action: Arrests fungal cell division at metaphase (mitosis); binds to human keratin, making it resistant to disease

➧**Therapeutic Outcome:** Absence of fungicidal infection

Uses: Mycotic infections: *Tinea corporis, T. pedis, T. cruris, T. barbae, T. capitis, T. unguium* if caused by *Epider-*

---

mophyton, Microsporum, Trichophyton

Dosage and routes
Adult: PO 500-1000 mg qd in single or divided doses (microsize), 125-165 mg bid (ultramicrosize) or 250-330 mg qd; may need 500-660 mg in divided doses for severe infections

P *Child:* PO 10 mg/kg/day or 30 mg/m²/day (microsize) or 5 mg/kg/day (ultramicrosize)

Available forms: Microcaps 125, 250 mg; tabs 250, 500 mg; oral susp 125 mg/5 ml; ultratabs 125, 165, 250, 330 mg

Adverse effects
CNS: Headache, peripheral neuritis, paresthesias, confusion, dizziness, fatigue
EENT: Transient hearing loss
GU: Proteinuria, cylinduria, precipitate porphyria, increased thirst
GI: Nausea, vomiting, anorexia, diarrhea, cramps, dry mouth, flatulence, **bleeding**
HEMA: **Leukopenia, granulocytopenia, neutropenia, monocytosis**
INTEG: Rash, urticaria, photosensitivity, lichen planus

Contraindications: Hypersensitivity, porphyria, hepatic disease, lupus erythematosus

Precautions: Penicillin sensitivity, pregnancy **C**

Pharmacokinetics	
Absorption	Ultra products (completely absorbed), others (variably absorbed)
Distribution	Keratin in skin; liver, muscle, fat
Metabolism	Liver
Excretion	Feces
Half-life	10-24 hr

Pharmacodynamics	
Onset	4 hr
Peak	1 day
Duration	2 day

Interactions
Individual drugs
Alcohol: ↑ CNS depression, tachycardia
Cyclosporine: ↓ action of warfarin
Phenobarbital: ↓ action of griseofulvin
Drug classifications
Contraceptives, oral: ↓ effect of contraceptive
Salicylates: ↓ action of warfarin
Food/drug
Fat (meat, dairy products): ↑ absorption

NURSING CONSIDERATIONS
Assessment
• Assess patient's skin for fungal infections: peeling, dryness, itching before and throughout treatment
• Monitor blood studies: leukocytes, CBC, platelets, although blood dyscrasias are rare
◆• Monitor for renal toxicity: increased BUN, serum creatinine—if serum creatinine >1.7 mg/100 dl, dosage may be reduced (rare)
• Monitor for hepatotoxicity: increasing AST, ALT, alk phosphatase
• Monitor for allergic reaction: dermatitis, rash; drug should be discontinued, give antihistamines for mild reaction or epinephrine for severe reaction; if patient is allergic to penicillin a cross-sensitivity may exist with this medication

---

Nursing diagnoses
- ☑ Skin integrity, impaired (uses)
- ☑ Infection, risk for (uses)
- ☑ Knowledge deficit (teaching)

Implementation
- Give with meals (fatty) to prevent GI upset
- Administer drug carefully, making sure there is no confusion with dosage form (microsize vs ultrasize); with meals to decrease GI symptoms; store in tight, light-resistant container at room temp
- Administer drug until three separate cultures are negative for infective organism; use PO only when topical drug is ineffective

Patient/family education
- Teach patient that long-term therapy may be needed to clear infection (2 wk-6 mo depending on organism); compliance is needed even after feeling better
- Instruct patient in proper hygiene: hand-washing technique, nail care, use of concomitant top agents if prescribed to clear infection
- Advise patient to avoid alcohol because nausea, vomiting, hypertension may occur
- Advise patient to use sunscreen or avoid direct sunlight to prevent photosensitivity
- Caution patient to notify prescriber of sore throat, fever, skin rash, which may indicate overgrowth of organisms
- Advise patient to use a nonhormonal form of contraception during treatment and to notify prescriber if pregnancy is anticipated

Evaluation
Positive therapeutic outcome
- Decrease in itching, peeling, dryness

guaifenesin (℞, OTC)
(gwye-fen′e-sin)
Amonidrin, Anti-tuss, Balminil ✦, Breonesin, Fenesin, Gee-Gee, Genatuss, GG-Cen, Glyate, Glycotuss, Glytuss, Guaifenesin, Guiatuss, Halotussin, Humibid, Humibid L.A., Hytuss, Hytuss 2X, Malotuss, Monafed, Mytussin, Naldecon Senior EX, Resyl ✦, Robitussin, Scot-Tussin Expectorant, Sinumist-SR, Uni-Tussin
Func. class.: Expectorant

Pregnancy category C

Action: Acts as an expectorant by stimulating a gastric mucosal reflex to increase the production of lung mucus

➡ **Therapeutic Outcome:** Decreased cough

Uses: Dry, nonproductive cough

Dosage and routes
Adult: PO 100-400 mg q4-6h, or 600-1200 mg q12h (ext-rel) not to exceed 2.4 g/day

🅿 *Child 6-12 yr:* PO 100-200 mg q4h or 600 mg q12h (ext rel); not to exceed 1.2 g/day

🅿 *Child 2-6 yr:* PO: 50-100 mg q4h; not to exceed 600 mg/day

Available forms: Tabs 100, 200 mg; tab, ext rel 600 mg; cap 200 mg; syr 100 mg, 200/5 ml; liq 200 mg/5 ml; ext-rel cap 300 mg

Adverse effects
CNS: Drowsiness
GI: Nausea, anorexia, vomiting

G

Contraindications: Hypersensitivity, persistent cough

Precautions: Pregnancy **C**

Pharmacokinetics

Absorption	Well absorbed
Distribution	Unknown
Metabolism	Unknown
Excretion	Unknown
Half-life	Unknown

Pharmacodynamics

	PO	PO ER
Onset	½ hr	Unknown
Peak	Unknown	Unknown
Duration	4-6 hr	12 hr

Interactions: None

NURSING CONSIDERATIONS
Assessment
• Assess cough: type, frequency, character, including characteristics of sputum; lung sounds bilaterally; fluids should be increased to 2 L/day to decrease secretion viscosity (thickness)

Nursing diagnoses
☑ Airway clearance, ineffective (uses)
☑ Knowledge deficit (teaching)

Implementation
• Store at room temp; provide room humidification to assist with liquefying secretions
• Avoid fluids for ½ hr after administration

Patient/family education
• Caution patient to avoid driving, other hazardous activities if drowsiness occurs (rare)
• Advise patient to avoid smoking, smoke-filled rooms, perfumes, dust, environmental pollutants, cleansers
• Instruct patient to notify prescriber if dry, nonproductive cough lasts over 7 days

Evaluation
Positive therapeutic outcome
• Absence of dry cough
• Thinner, more productive cough that raises secretions

---

guanabenz (℞)
(gwan′a-benz)
Wytensin
Func. class.: Antihypertensive
Chem. class.: Central α_2-adrenergic agonist
Pregnancy category   C

Action: Stimulates central α_2-adrenergic receptors in the CNS, resulting in decreased sympathetic outflow from brain with decreased peripheral resistance

➡ **Therapeutic Outcome:** Decreased B/P in hypertension

Uses: Hypertension

Dosage and routes
Adult: PO 4 mg bid, increasing in increments of 4-8 mg/day q1-2 wk, not to exceed 32 mg bid

Available forms: Tabs 4, 8 mg

Adverse effects
CNS: Drowsiness, dizziness, sedation, headache, depression, weakness
CV: Severe rebound hypertension, chest pain, dysrhythmias, palpitations, hypotension
EENT: Nasal congestion, blurred vision, miosis
GI: Nausea, diarrhea, constipation, dry mouth, anorexia, abnormal taste
GU: Impotence, frequency, gynecomastia
MS: Backache, extremity pain
RESP: Dyspnea

Contraindications: Hypersensitivity to guanabenz

Precautions: Pregnancy **C**, lactation, children <12 yr, severe coronary insufficiency, recent MI, cerebrovascular disease, severe hepatic or renal failure, elderly

Pharmacokinetics	
Absorption	70%-80%
Distribution	Widely distributed
Metabolism	Liver, extensively
Excretion	Kidneys
Half-life	6 hr

Pharmacodynamics	
Onset	1 hr
Peak	2-4 hr
Duration	12 hr

Interactions
Individual drugs
Alcohol: ↑ hypotension
Ephedrine: Blocked antihypertensive effect
Levodopa: ↑ hypotension
Norepinephrine: ↑ pressor, mydriatic effects
Phenylephrine: ↑ pressor, mydriatic effects
Drug classifications
Amphetamines: ↑ pressor, mydriatic effect
Antidepressants, tricyclic: Blocked effect of guanadrel
Antihypertensive: ↑ hypotension
MAOIs: Blocked antihypertensive effect
Nitrates: ↑ hypotension
Lab test interferences
False positive: Urine acetone

NURSING CONSIDERATIONS
Assessment
• Monitor blood studies: neutrophils, decreased platelets
• Monitor renal studies: protein, BUN, creatinine; watch for increased levels that may

indicate nephrotic syndrome; polyuria, oliguria, frequency
• Obtain baselines in renal, liver function tests before therapy begins; potassium levels, although hyperkalemia rarely occurs
• Monitor B/P, pulse if the drug is being used for hypertension; notify prescriber of change
• Watch for allergic reaction: rash, fever, pruritus, urticaria; drug should be discontinued if antihistamines fail to help
• Watch for symptoms of CHF: edema, dyspnea, wet rales, B/P, weight gain

Nursing diagnoses
✓ Cardiac output, decreased (uses)
✓ Injury, risk for (side effects)
✓ Knowledge deficit (teaching)
✓ Noncompliance (teaching)

Implementation
• Give in AM and at bedtime
• Store in air-tight container at room temp

Patient/family education
• Instruct patient not to discontinue drug abruptly—withdrawal symptoms may occur: anxiety, increased B/P, headache, insomnia, increased pulse, tremors, nausea, sweating
• Advise patient not to use OTC cough, cold, or allergy products unless directed by prescriber
• Teach patient to comply with dosage schedule even if feeling better; drug controls symptoms, does not cure
• Caution patient to rise slowly to sitting or standing position to minimize orthostatic hypotension, especially in the elderly

• Teach patient that excessive perspiration, dehydration, vomiting may occur; diarrhea may lead to fall in blood pressure; consult prescriber if these occur

• Inform patient that drug may cause dizziness, fainting; light-headedness may occur during first few days of therapy; drug may cause dry mouth—use hard candy, saliva product, or frequent rinsing of mouth; that compliance is necessary; not to skip or stop drug unless directed by prescriber; that drug may cause skin rash or impaired perspiration

• Teach patient to avoid hazardous activities because drug may cause drowsiness, dizziness

Evaluation
Positive therapeutic outcome
• Decreased B/P

Treatment of overdose: Vasopressor for hypotension, discontinue drug

---

guanadrel (Ⓡ)
(gwahn′a-drel)
Hylorel
Func. class.: Antihypertensive
Chem. class.: Adrenergic blocker, (peripheral guanethidine derivative)

Pregnancy category   **B**

Action: Inhibits sympathetic vasoconstriction by inhibiting release of norepinephrine; depletes norepinephrine stores in adrenergic nerve endings and the adrenal medulla

➡**Therapeutic Outcome:** Decreased B/P in hypertension

Uses: Hypertension (moderate to severe) as an adjunct

Dosage and routes
Adult: PO 5 mg bid, adjusted to desired response weekly or monthly; may need 20-75 mg/day in divided doses, higher doses are given tid or qid

Ⓖ*Elderly:* PO 5 mg/day; titrate as needed

Renal dose
CrCl 10-150 ml/min dose q12-24h; CrCl <10 ml/min dose q24-48h

Available forms: Tabs 10, 25 mg

Adverse effects
CNS: Drowsiness, fatigue, weakness, feeling of faintness, insomnia, dizziness, mental changes, memory loss, hallucinations, *depression,* anxiety, *confusion, paresthesia, headache*
CV: Orthostatic hypotension, bradycardia, **CHF,** palpitations, chest pain, tachycardia, dysrhythmias
EENT: Nasal stuffiness, tinnitus, visual changes, sore throat, double vision, dry burning eyes
GI: Nausea, cramps, diarrhea, constipation, dry mouth, anorexia, indigestion
GU: Ejaculation failure, impotence, dysuria, nocturia, urinary frequency
INTEG: Rash, purpura, alopecia
MS: Leg cramps, aching, pain, inflammation
RESP: Bronchospasm, dyspnea, cough, rales, SOB

Contraindications: Hypersensitivity, pheochromocytoma, Ⓟlactation, CHF, child <18 yr

---

G **Precautions:** Elderly, bronchial asthma, peptic ulcer, electrolyte imbalances, vascular disease, pregnancy **B**

Pharmacokinetics	
Absorption	Well absorbed
Distribution	Widely distributed, minimally distributed in the CNS
Metabolism	Liver (50%)
Excretion	Kidneys, unchanged (50%)
Half-life	10-12 hr

Pharmacodynamics	
Onset	½-2 hr
Peak	4-6 hr
Duration	4-14 hr

Interactions
Individual drugs
Alcohol: ↑ hypotension
Ephedrine: Blocked antihypertensive effect
Levodopa: ↑ hypotension
Norepinephrine: ↑ pressor, mydriatic effects
Phenylephrine: ↑ pressor, mydriatic effects
Drug classifications
Amphetamines: ↑ pressor, mydriatic effect
Antidepressants, tricyclic: Blocked effect of guanadrel
Antihypertensive: ↑ hypotension
MAOIs: Blocked antihypertensive effect
Nitrates: ↑ hypotension
Lab test interferences
False positive: Urine acetone

NURSING CONSIDERATIONS
Assessment
• Monitor blood studies: neutrophils, decreased platelets
• Monitor renal studies: protein, BUN, creatinine; watch for increased levels that may indicate nephrotic syndrome; polyuria, oliguria, urinary frequency
• Obtain baselines in renal, liver function tests before therapy begins; potassium levels, although hyperkalemia rarely occurs
• Monitor B/P, pulse if the drug is being used for hypertension; notify prescriber of changes
• Assess for allergic reaction: rash, fever, pruritus, urticaria; drug should be discontinued if antihistamines fail to help
• Symptoms of CHF: edema, dyspnea, wet rales, increased B/P, weight gain

Nursing diagnoses
✓ Cardiac output, decreased (uses)
✓ Injury, risk of physical (side effects)
✓ Knowledge deficit (teaching)
✓ Noncompliance (teaching)

Implementation
• Usually given as adjunct with other cardiovascular drugs (diuretics) to decrease edema
• Store in air-tight container at 86° F (30° C) or less

Patient/family education
• Instruct patient not to discontinue drug abruptly, or withdrawal symptoms may occur: anxiety, increased B/P, headache, insomnia, increased pulse, tremors, nausea, sweating
• Advise patient not to use OTC (cough, cold, or allergy) products unless directed by prescriber
• Teach patient to comply with dosage schedule even if feeling better; drug controls symptoms, does not cure
• Caution patient to change position slowly, to rise slowly to sitting or standing position

G

to minimize orthostatic hypotension, especially in the **G** elderly

• Caution patient that drug may cause dizziness, fainting; light-headedness may occur during first few days of therapy; that drug may cause dry mouth—use hard candy, saliva product, or frequent rinsing of mouth
• Instruct patient that compliance is necessary; not to skip or stop drug unless directed by prescriber
• Inform patient that drug may cause skin rash
• Teach patient to avoid hazardous activities because drug may cause drowsiness, dizziness

Evaluation
Positive therapeutic outcome
• Decreased B/P

---

guanethidine (℞)
(gwahn-eth-i′deen)
Apo-Guanethidine ✦,
guanethidine sulfate,
Ismelin
Func. class.: Antihypertensive
Chem. class.: Adrenergic blocker, (peripheral guanethidine derivative)
Pregnancy category   C

Action: Inhibits sympathetic vasoconstriction by inhibiting release of norepinephrine, depletes norepinephrine stores in adrenergic nerve endings and the adrenal medulla

➡**Therapeutic Outcome:** Decreased B/P

Uses: Moderate to severe hypertension

Dosage and routes
Adult: PO 10 mg qd, increase by 10-12.5 mg qwk; may require 25-50 mg qd
Adult: (hospitalized) 25-50 mg; may increase by 25-50 mg/day or qod
P *Child:* PO 0.2 mg/kg/day (6 mg/m²/day); increase q 7-10 day 0.2 mg/kg or 6 mg/m²/day

Available forms: Tabs 10, 25 mg

Adverse effects
CNS: Depression, anxiety, drowsiness, fatigue, confusion, headache, sleeping problems
CV: Orthostatic hypotension, dizziness, chest pain, weakness, edema
EENT: Nasal congestion, ptosis, blurred vision
GI: Nausea, vomiting, *diarrhea, constipation, dry mouth,* weight gain, *anorexia,* abdominal pain
GU: Ejaculation failure, impotence, nocturia, edema, *retention,* increased BUN, *frequency*
INTEG: Dermatitis, loss of scalp hair
MS: Aches, leg cramps
RESP: Dyspnea, cough, shortness of breath

Contraindications: Hypersensitivity, pheochromocytoma, recent MI, CHF, cardiac failure, sinus bradycardia

Precautions: Pregnancy **C**, lactation, peptic ulcer, asthma

---

Pharmacokinetics	
Absorption	Incompletely absorbed (up to 50%)
Distribution	Widely distributed, does not cross blood-brain barrier
Metabolism	Liver—partially
Excretion	Kidneys, breast milk (minimal)
Half-life	5 days

Pharmacodynamics	
Onset	4 wk
Peak	4 wk
Duration	4 wk

Interactions
Individual drugs
Alcohol: ↑ hypotension
Ephedrine: Blocks antihypertensive effect
Levodopa: ↑ hypotension
Metharaminol: ↑ pressor, mydriatic effects
Norepinephrine: ↑ pressor, mydriatic effects
Phenylephrine: ↑ pressor, mydriatic effects
Drug classifications
Amphetamines: ↑ pressor, mydriatic effects
Antidepressants, tricyclics: ↑ hypotension
Antihypertensives: ↑ hypotension
Contraceptives, oral: Blocks antihypertensive effect, ↑ hypertension
MAOIs: ↑ hypertension
Nitrates: ↑ hypotension
Phenothiazines: Blocks antihypertensive effect, ↑ hypertension
Lab test interferences
↑ BUN
↓ Blood glucose, ↓ VMA excretion, ↓ urinary norepinephrine

NURSING CONSIDERATIONS
Assessment
• Monitor blood studies: neutrophils, decreased platelets
• Monitor B/P, orthostatic hypotension, syncope
• Monitor renal studies: protein, BUN, creatinine; watch for increased levels that may indicate nephrotic syndrome; polyuria, oliguria, urinary frequency
• Obtain baselines of renal, liver function tests before therapy begins
• Obtain potassium levels, although hyperkalemia rarely occurs
• Check for edema in feet, legs daily; monitor I&O; check for decreasing output
• Assess for allergic reaction: rash, fever, pruritus, urticaria; drug should be discontinued if antihistamines fail to help
• Assess for symptoms of CHF: edema, dyspnea, wet rales, B/P, weight gain

Nursing diagnoses
☑ Cardiac output, decreased (uses)
☑ Injury, risk for (adverse reactions)
☑ Knowledge deficit (teaching)

Implementation
• Usually given as adjunct with other cardiovascular drugs (diuretics) to decrease edema
• Store in air-tight container at 86° F (30° C) or less

Patient/family education
• Instruct patient not to discontinue drug abruptly because withdrawal symptoms may occur: anxiety, increased B/P, headache, insomnia, increased pulse, tremors, nausea, sweating
• Teach patient to comply with dosage schedule even if feeling

G

better; drug controls symptoms, does not cure

• Caution patient to rise slowly to sitting or standing position to minimize orthostatic hypotension, especially in the **G** elderly

• Instruct patient to notify prescriber of sore throat, fever, swelling of hands or feet, irregular heartbeat, chest pain

• Caution patient that drug may cause dizziness, fainting, light-headedness may occur during first few days of therapy; that drug may cause dry mouth—use hard candy, saliva product, or frequent rinsing of mouth; that compliance is necessary—not to skip or stop drug unless directed by physician; that drug may cause skin rash or impaired perspiration

• Teach patient to avoid hazardous activities—drug may cause drowsiness, dizziness

Evaluation
Positive therapeutic outcome

• Decreased B/P in hypertension

Treatment of overdose: Administer vasopressors; discontinue drug

---

guanfacine (℞)
(gwahn'fa-seen)
Tenex
Func. class.: Antihypertensive
Chem. class.: Central α_2-adrenergic agonist

Pregnancy category B

Action: Stimulates central α_2-adrenergic receptors in the CNS resulting in decreased sympathetic outflow from brain

with decreased peripheral resistance

→**Therapeutic Outcome:** Decreased B/P in hypertension

Uses: Hypertension in individual using a thaizide diuretic

Dosage and routes
Adult: PO 1 mg/day hs; may increase dose in 2-3 wk to 2-3 mg/day

Available forms: Tab 1 mg

Adverse effects
CNS: Somnolence, dizziness, headache, fatigue
CV: Bradycardia, chest pain
EENT: Taste change, tinnitus, vision change, rhinitis, nasal congestion
GI: Dry mouth, constipation, cramps, nausea, diarrhea
GU: Impotence, urinary incontinence
INTEG: Dermatitis, pruritus, purpura
MS: Leg cramps
RESP: Dyspnea

Contraindications: Hypersensitivity

Precautions: Pregnancy **B,**
P lactation, children <12 yr, severe coronary insufficiency, recent MI, renal or hepatic **G** disease, CVA, elderly

Pharmacokinetics	
Absorption	Well absorbed (80%)
Distribution	Widely distributed
Metabolism	Liver (50%)
Excretion	Kidneys—unchanged (50%)
Half-life	17 hr

Pharmacodynamics	
Onset	Unknown
Peak	1-4 hr
Duration	Unknown

Interactions
Individual drugs
Alcohol: ↑ hypotension, ↑ sedation
Drug classifications
Analgesics, narcotic: ↑ sedation

Antidepressants, tricyclic: ↓ effectiveness of guanabenz

Antihypertensives: ↑ hypotension

β-Adrenergic blockers: ↑ bradycardia, CHF

MAOIs: ↓ effectiveness of guanabenz

Nitrates: ↑ nitrates

Sedatives/hypnotics: ↑ sedation

NURSING CONSIDERATIONS
Assessment
• Monitor blood studies: neutrophils, decreased platelets
• Monitor renal studies: protein, BUN, creatinine; watch for increased levels that may indicate nephrotic syndrome; polyuria, oliguria, frequency
• Obtain baselines in renal, liver function tests before therapy begins; potassium levels, although hyperkalemia rarely occurs
• Monitor B/P, pulse if the drug is being used for hypertension; notify prescriber of changes
• Assess for edema in feet, legs daily; monitor I&O; check weight for decreasing output
• Assess for allergic reaction: rash, fever, pruritus, urticaria; drug should be discontinued if antihistamines fail to help
• Assess for symptoms of CHF: edema, dyspnea, wet rales, BP, weight gain

Nursing diagnoses
☑ Cardiac output, decreased (uses)
☑ Injury, risk for (adverse reactions)
☑ Knowledge deficit (teaching)
☑ Noncompliance (teaching)

Implementation
• Give hs
• Store in air-tight container at room temp

Patient/family education
• Instruct patient not to discontinue drug abruptly, or withdrawal symptoms may occur: anxiety, increased B/P, headache, insomnia, increased pulse, tremors, nausea, sweating
• Caution patient not to use OTC (cough, cold, or allergy) products unless directed by prescriber
• Teach patient to comply with dosage schedule even if feeling better; drug controls symptoms, does not cure
• Caution patient (especially the elderly) to change position slowly, to rise slowly to sitting or standing position to minimize orthostatic hypotension
• Instruct patient to notify prescriber of sore throat, fever, swelling of hands or feet, irregular heartbeat, chest pain, increased weight
• Inform patient that drug may cause dizziness, fainting; light-headedness may occur during 1st few days of therapy; drug may cause dry mouth—use hard candy or saliva product, or rinse mouth frequently
• Teach patient that compliance is necessary; not to skip or stop drug unless directed by prescriber
• Caution patient that drug may cause skin rash

- Teach patient to avoid hazardous activities—drug may cause drowsiness; dizziness

Evaluation
Positive therapeutic outcome
- Decreased B/P

---

haloperidol (℞)
(hal-oh-pehr'ih-dol)
Apo-Haloperidol ✦, Haldol, Novo-Peridol ✦, Peridol ✦
haloperidol decanoate (℞)
Haldol Decanoate, Haldol LA ✦
haloperidol lactate (℞)
Haldol, Haloperidol Injection, Haloperidol Intensol
Func. class.: Antipsychotic/neuroleptic
Chem. class.: Butyrophenone

Pregnancy category C

Action: Depresses cerebral cortex, hypothalamus, limbic system, which control activity and aggression; blocks neurotransmission produced by dopamine at synapse; exhibits strong α-adrenergic, anticholinergic blocking action; mechanism for antipsychotic effects unclear

⊃Therapeutic Outcome: Decreased signs and symptoms of psychosis

Uses: Psychotic disorders, control of tics, vocal utterances in Gilles de la Tourette syndrome, short-term treatment **P** of hyperactive children showing excessive motor activity, prolonged parenteral therapy in chronic schizophrenia, control of severe nausea and vomiting in chemotherapy, organic mental syndrome with psychotic features, hiccups (short-term)

Dosage and routes
Psychosis
Adult: PO 0.5-5 mg bid or tid initially depending on severity of condition; increase to desired dosage, max 100 mg/day; IM 2-5 mg q1-8h

G *Geriatric:* 0.25-0.5 mg qd-bid, titrate q3-4 days by 0.25-0.5 mg/dose

P *Child 3-12 yr:* PO/IM 0.05-0.15 mg/kg/day

Chronic schizophrenia
Adult: IM 10-15 times the PO dosage q4 wk (decanoate)

P *Child 3-12 yr:* PO/IM 0.05-0.15 mg/kg/day

Tics/vocal utterances
Adult: PO 0.5-5 mg bid or tid, increased until desired response occurs

P *Child 3-12 yr:* PO 0.05-0.075 mg/kg/day

Hyperactive children
P *Child 3-12 yr:* PO 0.05-0.075 mg/kg/day

Available forms: Tabs 0.5, 1, 2, 5, 10, 20 mg; lactate: conc 2 mg/ml; inj 5 mg/ml, 50 mg base/ml, 100 mg base/ml

Adverse effects
CNS: Extrapyramidal symptoms: pseudoparkinsonism, akathisia, dystonia, tardive dyskinesia, drowsiness, headache, **seizures, neuroleptic malignant syndrome,** confusion
CV: Orthostatic hypotension, hypertension, **cardiac arrest,** ECG changes, **tachycardia**
EENT: Blurred vision, glaucoma, dry eyes

GI: Dry mouth, nausea, vomiting, anorexia, constipation, diarrhea, jaundice, weight gain, **ileus, hepatitis**

GU: Urinary retention, urinary frequency, enuresis, impotence, amenorrhea, gynecomastia

INTEG: Rash, photosensitivity, dermatitis

RESP: **Laryngospasm,** dyspnea, **respiratory depression**

Contraindications: Hypersensitivity, blood dyscrasias, coma, child <3 yr, brain damage, bone marrow depression, alcohol and barbiturate withdrawal states, Parkinson's disease, angina, epilepsy, urinary retention, narrow-angle glaucoma

Precautions: Pregnancy **C,** lactation, seizure disorders, hypertension, hepatic disease, cardiac disease, elderly

Do Not Confuse:
haloperidol/Halotestin, Haldol/Stadol

Pharmacokinetics

Absorption	Well absorbed (PO, IM); decanoate (IM) absorbed slowly
Distribution	High concentrations in liver, crosses placenta
Metabolism	Liver, extensively
Excretion	Kidneys, breast milk
Half-life	21-24 hr

Pharmacodynamics

	PO	IM	IM (decanoate)
Onset	Erratic	½ hr	3-9 days
Peak	2-6 hr	30-45 min	4-11 days
Duration	8-12 hr	4-8 hr	3 wk

Interactions
Individual drugs
Alcohol: ↑ effects of both drugs, oversedation
Aluminum hydroxide: ↓ absorption
Bromocriptine: ↓ antiparkinson activity
Disopyramide: ↑ anticholinergic effects
Epinephrine: ↑ toxicity
Guanethidine: ↓ antihypertensive response
Levodopa: ↓ antiparkinsonian activity
Lithium: ↓ haloperidol levels, ↑ extrapyramidal symptoms, masking of lithium toxicity
Magnesium hydroxide: ↓ absorption
Norepinephrine: ↓ vasoresponse, ↑ toxicity
Phenobarbital: ↓ effectiveness, ↑ metabolism
Drug classifications
Antacids: ↓ absorption
Anticholinergics: ↑ anticholinergic effects
Antidepressants: ↑ CNS depression
Antidiarrheals, adsorbent: ↓ absorption
Antihistamines: ↑ CNS depression
Antihypertensives: ↑ hypotension
Antithyroid agents: ↑ agranulocytosis
Barbiturate anesthetics: ↑ CNS depression
β-Adrenergic blockers: ↑ effects of both drugs
General anesthetics: ↑ CNS depression
MAOIs: ↑ CNS depression
Opiates: ↑ CNS depression
Sedative/hypnotics: ↑ CNS depression
Herb/drug
Kava: ↑ action

Lab test interferences

↑ Liver function tests, ↑ cardiac enzymes, ↑ cholesterol, ↑ blood glucose, ↑ prolactin, ↑ bilirubin, ↑ PBI, ↑ cholinesterase

↓ Hormones (blood and urine)

False positive: Pregnancy tests, PKU, urine bilirubin

False negative: Urinary steroids, 17-OHCS

NURSING CONSIDERATIONS
Assessment

• Assess mental status: orientation, mood, behavior, presence and type of hallucinations before initial administration and monthly; this drug should significantly reduce psychotic behavior

• Check for swallowing of PO medication; check for hoarding or giving of medication to other patients

• Monitor I&O ratio; palpate bladder if low urinary output

🅖 occurs, especially in elderly; urinalysis is recommended before, during prolonged therapy

• Monitor bilirubin, CBC, liver function studies monthly

• Assess affect, orientation, LOC, reflexes, gait, coordination, sleep pattern disturbances

• Monitor B/P with patient sitting, standing, and lying; take pulse and respirations q4h during initial treatment; establish baseline before starting treatment; report drops of 30 mm Hg; obtain baseline ECG, Q wave and T wave changes

• Check for dizziness, faintness, palpitations, tachycardia on rising; severe orthostatic hypotension is common

• Identify for neuroleptic malignant syndrome: hyperpyrexia, muscle rigidity, increased CPK, altered mental status; drug should be discontinued immediately

• Assess for extrapyramidal symptoms including akathisia (inability to sit still, no pattern to movements), tardive dyskinesia (bizarre movements of the jaw, mouth, tongue, extremities), pseudoparkinsonism (ragged tremors, pill rolling, shuffling gate); an antiparkinsonian drug should be prescribed

• Assess for constipation and urinary retention daily; if these occur, increase bulk, water in diet

Nursing diagnoses

☑ Thought processes, altered (uses)

☑ Coping, ineffective individual (uses)

☑ Knowledge deficit (teaching)

☑ Noncompliance (teaching)

Implementation
PO route

• Give drug in liquid form mixed in glass of juice or caffeine-free cola if hoarding is suspected; do not mix in caffeine drinks, tannics, pectins

🅖 • Give decreased dosage in elderly because of slower metabolism

• Give PO with full glass of water, milk; or give with food to decrease GI upset

• Store in tight, light-resistant container, oral sol in amber bottle

IM route

• Inject in deep muscle mass, do not give SC; use 21 G 2-inch needle; do not administer sol with a precipitate; give <3 ml per inj site; give slowly, may be painful

---

☑ Herb/drug   🅢 Do Not Crush   ◆ Alert   ◆🍸 Key Drug   🅖 Geriatric   🅟 Pediatric

Syringe compatibilities:
Hydromorphone, sufentanil

Y-site compatibilities:
Amifostine, amsacrine, aztreonam, cimetidine, cisatracurium, cladribine, dobutamine, dopamine, doxorubicin liposome, famotidine, filgrastim, fludarabine, granisetron, lidocaine, lorazepam, melphalan, midazolam, nitroglycerin, norepinephrine, ondansetron, paclitaxel, phenylephrine, propofol, remifentanil, sufentanil, tacrolimus, teniposide, theophylline, thiotepa, vinorelbine

Y-site incompatibilities:
Fluconazole, foscarnet, heparin, sargramostim

Patient/family education
• Teach patient to use good oral hygiene; use frequent rinsing of mouth, sugarless gum for dry mouth
• Advise patient to avoid hazardous activities until drug response is determined; dizziness, blurred vision are common
• Inform patient that orthostatic hypotension occurs often and to rise from sitting or lying position gradually; to remain lying down after IM inj for at least 30 min; tell patient to avoid hot tubs, hot showers, tub baths, since hypotension may occur; tell patient that in hot weather heat stroke may occur; take extra precautions to stay cool
• Instruct patient to avoid abrupt withdrawal of this drug, or extrapyramidal symptoms may result; drug should be withdrawn slowly
• Caution patient to avoid OTC preparations (cough, hay fever, cold) unless approved by prescriber, since serious drug interactions may occur; avoid use with alcohol, CNS depressants since increased drowsiness may occur
• Advise patient to use a sunscreen and sunglasses to prevent burns
• Teach patient about extrapyramidal symptoms and necessity of meticulous oral hygiene, since oral candidiasis may occur
• Instruct patient to take antacids 2 hr before or after this drug
• Tell patient to report sore throat, malaise, fever, bleeding, mouth sores; if these occur, CBC should be completed and drug discontinued

Evaluation
Positive therapeutic outcome
• Decrease in emotional excitement, hallucinations, delusions, paranoia, reorganization of patterns of thought, speech; improvement in specific behaviors
• Reorganization of patterns of thought, speech

Treatment of overdose:
Lavage if orally ingested; provide airway; *do not induce vomiting*

H

heparin ⊶ (℞)
(hep'a-rin)

Calcilean ✦, Calciparine, Hepalean ✦, Heparin Sodium and 0.45% Sodium Chloride, Heparin Sodium and 0.9% Sodium Chloride, Heparin Leo ✦, Heparin Lock Flush, Heparin Sodium, Hep-Lock, Hep-Lock U/P, Liquaemin Sodium

Func. class.: Anticoagulant

Pregnancy category   C

Action: Prevents conversion of fibrinogen to fibrin and prothrombin to thrombin by enhancing inhibitory effects of antithrombin III

Therapeutic Outcome: Prevention of thrombi

Uses: Deep vein thrombosis and pulmonary emboli (treatment and prevention), MI, open heart surgery, disseminated intravascular clotting syndrome, atrial fibrillation with embolization, as an anticoagulant in transfusion and dialysis procedures

Dosage and routes
Deep vein thrombosis/MI
Adult: IV push 5000-7000 U q4h then titrated to PTT or ACT level; **IV** bol 5000-7500 U, then **IV** inf; **IV** inf after bolus dose, then 1000 U/hr titrated to PTT or ACT level

P *Child:* IV inf 50 U/kg, maintenance 100 U/kg q4h or 20,000 U/m^2 qd

Anticoagulation
Adult: SC 5000 UIV then 10,000-20,000 U, then 8,000-10,000 U q8hr or 15,000-20,000 U q12hr

Pulmonary embolism
Adult: IV push 7500-10,000 q4h then titrated to PTT or ACT level; **IV** bol 7500-10,000, then **IV** inf; **IV** inf after bol dose, then 1000 U/hr titrated to PTT or ACT level

P *Child:* IV inf 50 U/kg; maintenance 100 U/kg q4h or 20,000 U/m^2 qd

Open heart surgery
Adult: IV inf 150-300 U/kg, prophylaxis for DVT/PE; SC 5,000 U q8-12h

Heparin flush
P *Adult/child:* IV 10-100 U

Available forms: Sodium: carpuject 5000 U/ml; disposable inj 1000, 2500, 5000, 7500, 10,000, 15,000, 20,000, 40,000 U/ml; unit dose 1000, 5000, 10,000, 20,000, 40,000 U/ml; vials 1000, 2000, 2500, 5000, 7500, 10,000, 20,000, 40,000 U/ml; flush, disposable syringes 10, 100 U/ml; vials 10, 100 U/ml; ampules 12,500 U/0.5 ml; 20,000 U/0.8 ml

Adverse effects
CNS: Fever, chills
GI: Diarrhea, nausea, vomiting, anorexia, stomatitis, abdominal cramps, **hepatitis**
GU: **Hematuria**
HEMA: **Hemorrhage, thrombocytopenia**
INTEG: Rash, dermatitis, urticaria, alopecia, pruritus
SYST: **Anaphylaxis**

Contraindications: Hypersensitivity, hemophilia, leukemia with bleeding, peptic ulcer disease, thrombocytopenic purpura, hepatic disease (severe), renal disease (severe), blood dyscrasias, severe hyper-

---

tension, subacute bacterial endocarditis, acute nephritis

Precautions: Alcoholism, **G** elderly, pregnancy **C**

Pharmacokinetics

Absorption	Well absorbed (SC)
Distribution	Unknown
Metabolism	Unknown
Excretion	Lymph, spleen
Half-life	1½ hr

Pharmacodynamics

	SC	IV
Onset	½-1 hr	5 min
Peak	2 hr	10 min
Duration	8-12 hr	2-6 hr

Lab test interferences
False ↑ T$_3$ uptake, ↑ serum thyroxine, ↑ BSP
↓ Uric acid
False negative: ^{125}I fibrinogen uptake

NURSING CONSIDERATIONS
Assessment
• Assess for blood studies (Hct, occult blood in stools) q3 mo if patient is on long-term therapy
• Monitor PPT, which should be 1½-2 times control, PTT; often done qd, APTT, ACT
• Monitor platelet count q2-3 days; thrombocytopenia may occur on 4th day of treatment and resolve, or continue to 8th day of treatment
❶• Assess for bleeding gums, petechiae, ecchymosis, black tarry stools, hematuria, epistaxis, decrease in Hct, B/P; may indicate bleeding and possible hemorrhage; notify prescriber immediately
• Monitor for hypersensitivity: fever, skin rash, urticaria; notify prescriber immediately

Nursing diagnoses
☑ Injury, risk for (uses, adverse reactions)
☑ Tissue perfusion, altered (uses)
☑ Knowledge deficit (teaching)

Implementation
Ⅳ IV route
• Give directly; **IV** loading dose over 1 min
• Give **IV** diluted in 0.9% NaCl, dextrose, Ringer's sol and by intermittent or cont inf; inf may run from 4-24 hr; use inf pump

Syringe compatibilities:
Aminophylline, amphotericin B, ampicillin, atropine, azlocillin, bleomycin, cefamandole, cefazolin, cefoperazone, cefotaxime, cefoxitin, chloramphenicol, cimetidine, cisplatin, clindamycin, cyclophosphamide, diazoxide, digoxin, dimenhydrinate, dobutamine, dopamine, epinephrine, fentanyl, fluorouracil, furosemide, leucovorin, lidocaine, lincomycin, methotrexate, metoclopramide, mezlocillin, mitomycin, moxalactam, nafcillin, naloxone, neostigmine, nitroglycerin, norepinephrine, pancuronium, penicillin G, phenobarbital, piperacillin, sodium nitroprusside, succinylcholine, trimethoprimsulfamethoxazole, verapamil, vincristine

Y-site compatibilities:
Acyclovir, aldesleukin, allopurinol, amifostine, aminophylline, ampicillin, ampicillin/sulbactam, atracurium, atropine, aztreonam, betamethasone, bleomycin, calcium gluconate, cefazolin, cefotetan, ceftazidime, ceftriaxone, cephalothin, cephapirin, chlordiazepoxide, chlorpromazine, cimetidine, cisplatin, cladri-

H

bine, clindamycin, conjugated estrogens, cyanocobalamin, cyclophosphamide, cytarabine, dexamethasone, digoxin, diphenhydramine, dopamine, doxorubicin liposome, edrophonium, enalaprilat, epinephrine, erythromycin, esmolol, ethacrynate, famotidine, fentanyl, fluconazole, fludarabine, fluorouracil, foscarnet, furosemide, gallium, granisetron, hydralazine, hydrocortisone, hydromorphone, regular insulin, isoproterenol, kanamycin, leucovorin, lidocaine, lorazepam, magnesium sulfate, melphalan, menadiol sodium, meperidine, meropenem, methicillin, methotrexate, methoxamine, methyldopa, methylergonovine, metoclopramide, metronidazole, midazolam, milrinone, minocycline, mitomycin, morphine, nafcillin, neostigmine, nitroglycerin, nitroprusside, norepinephrine, ondansetron, oxacillin, oxytocin, paclitaxel, pancuronium, penicillin G potassium, pentazocine, phytonadione, piperacillin, piperacillin/tazobactam, propofol, potassium chloride, prednisolone, procainamide, prochlorperazine, propofol, propranolol, pyridostigmine, ranitidine, remifentanil, sargramostim, scopolamine, sodium bicarbonate, streptokinase, succinylcholine, tacrolimus, teniposide, theophylline, thiopental, thiotepa, ticarcillin, ticarcillin/clavulanate, trimethobenzamide, vecuronium, vinblastine, vincristine, vinorelbine, warfarin, zidovudine

Y-site incompatibilities:
Alteplase, ciprofloxacin, dacarbazine, diazepam, dobutamine, doxorubicin, ergotamine, gentamicin, haloperidol, idarubicin, methotrimeprazine, phenytoin, promethazine, tobramycin, triflupromazine

Additive compatibilities:
Aminophylline, amphotericin, ascorbic acid, bleomycin, calcium gluconate, cefepime, cephapirin, chloramphenicol, clindamycin, colistimethate, dimenhydrinate, doxacillin, dopamine, enalaprilat, erythromycin, esmolol, floxacillin, fluconazole, flumazenil, furosemide, hydrocortisone, isoproterenol, lidocaine, lincomycin, magnesium sulfate, meropenem, methyldopa, methylprednisolone, metronidazole/sodium bicarbonate, nafcillin, norepinephrine, octreotide, penicillin G, potassium chloride, prednisolone, promazine, ranitidine, sodium bicarbonate, verapamil, vitamin B complex, vitamin B complex with C

Additive incompatibilities:
Amikacin, erythromycin lactobionate, gentamicin, kanamycin, meperidine, methadone, morphine, polymyxin B, streptomycin

Heparin lock route
• Inject 10-100 U/0.5-1 ml after each inf or q8-12h

SC route
• Give SC with at least 25 G ⅜-in needle; do not massage area or aspirate fluid when giving SC inj; give in abdomen between pelvic bones, rotate sites; do not pull back on plunger, leave in for 10 sec; apply gentle pressure for 1 min
• Give at same time each day to maintain steady blood levels
• Changing needles is not recommended

☑ Herb/drug 🚫 Do Not Crush ◆ Alert ⛐ Key Drug 🄶 Geriatric 🄿 Pediatric

Patient/family education

• Advise patient to avoid OTC preparations that may cause serious drug interactions unless directed by prescriber; may contain aspirin or other anticoagulants

• Tell patient that drug may be held during active bleeding (menstruation), depending on condition

• Caution patient to use soft-bristle toothbrush to avoid bleeding gums; avoid contact sports; use electric razor; avoid IM inj

• Instruct patient to carry a Medic Alert ID or other identification identifying drug taken and condition treated

• Advise patient to report any signs of bleeding: gums, under skin, urine, stools; or unusual bruising

Evaluation

Positive therapeutic outcome

• Decrease of deep vein thrombosis

• PTT of 1.5-2.5 times control

• Free-flowing **IV**

Treatment of overdose:

Withdraw drug, give protamine sulfate

---

hepatitis B immune globulin (R)

(hep-a-tite′iss)

H-BIG, Hep-B-Gammagee, Hyper Hep

Func. class.: Immune globulin

Pregnancy category   C

Action: Provides passive immunity to hepatitis B

➡ **Therapeutic Outcome:** Passive immunity to hepatitis B

Uses: Prevention of hepatitis B virus in exposed patients, including passive immunity in neonates born to HBsAg-positive mother

Dosage and routes

P *Adult and child:* IM 0.06 ml/kg within 1 wk of exposure, repeat after 4 wks, if patient refuses hepatitis B vaccine

P *Neonate:* IM 0.5 ml within 12 hr of birth

Available forms: 1, 4, 5 ml vials; 0.5 ml single dose syringe

Adverse effects

CNS: Headache, dizziness, fever, faintness, weakness
INTEG: Soreness at inj site, urticaria, erythema, swelling, pruritus
MS: Joint pain
SYST: **Anaphylaxis, angioedema**

Contraindications: Hypersensitivity to immune globulins, coagulation disorders

Precautions: Pregnancy **C**, elderly, lactation, children, active infection, IgA deficiency

Pharmacokinetics	
Absorption	Slowly absorbed
Distribution	Unknown
Metabolism	Unknown
Excretion	Unknown
Half-life	3 wk

Pharmacodynamics	
Onset	1-7 days
Peak	3-10 days
Duration	2-6 mo

Interactions
Drug classifications
Live vaccines: ↓ or ↑ immune response

NURSING CONSIDERATIONS
Assessment
• Assess for history of allergies, skin conditions (eczema, psoriasis, dermatitis), reactions to vaccinations
• Assess for skin reactions: rash, induration, urticaria
• Assess for sneezing, pruritus, angioedema, dysphagia, vomiting, abdominal pain
🔶• Assess for anaphylaxis: inability to breathe, bronchospasm, hypotension, wheezing, diaphoresis, fever, flushing; epinephrine and emergency equipment should be available

Nursing diagnoses
☑Infection, risk for (uses)
☑Knowledge deficit (teaching)

Implementation
• Give after rotating vial; do not shake
• Give in deltoid (adult) or anterolateral thigh for better protection; give 2-ml dose in two different sites; do not give **IV**
• Refrigerate unused portion; sol should be clear, light amber, and thick

Patient/family education
• Teach patient purpose of medication and expected results
• Give patient a list of adverse reactions that need to be reported immediately: wheezing, vomiting, sneezing, abdominal pain, sweating, tightness in chest
• Advise patient that pain, rash, swelling at inj site can be expected
• Give patient written record of immunization

Evaluation
Positive therapeutic outcome
• Prevention of hepatitis B

---

hetastarch (℞)
(het′a-starch)
Hespan
Func. class.: Plasma expander
Chem. class.: Synthetic polymer
Pregnancy category C

Action: Similar to human albumin, which expands plasma volume by colloidal osmotic pressure

➡**Therapeutic Outcome:** Increased plasma volume

Uses: Plasma volume expander for sepsis, trauma, burns, leukopheresis

Dosage and routes
Adult: **IV** inf 500-1000 ml (30-60 g); total dose not to exceed 1500 ml/day, not to exceed 20 ml/kg/hr (hemorrhagic shock)

Leukapheresis
Adult: **IV** inf 250-700 ml infused at 1:8 ratio with whole blood; may be repeated twice weekly up to 10 treatments

Available forms: 6% hetastarch/0.9% NaCl (6 g/ 100 ml)

Adverse effects
CNS: Headache
GI: Nausea, vomiting
HEMA: Decreased hematocrit, platelet function, increased bleeding/coagulation times, increased erythrosedimentation rate
INTEG: Rash, urticaria, pruritus, angioedema, chills, fever, flushing, peripheral edema
RESP: Wheezing, dyspnea, **bronchospasm, pulmonary edema**
SYST: **Anaphylaxis**

☑ Herb/drug   🚫 Do Not Crush   🔶 Alert   ⟳π Key Drug   🄶 Geriatric   🄿 Pediatric

Contraindications: Hypersensitivity, severe bleeding disorders, renal failure, CHF (severe)

Precautions: Pregnancy **C**, liver disease, pulmonary edema

Pharmacokinetics

Absorption	Completely absorbed
Distribution	Unknown
Metabolism	Degraded
Excretion	Kidneys, unchanged
Half-life	17 days (90%); 48 days (10%)

Pharmacodynamics

Onset	Immediate
Peak	Infusion's end
Duration	Over 24 hr

Interactions: None
Lab test interferences
False: ↑ Bilirubin

NURSING CONSIDERATIONS
Assessment
• Monitor VS q5 min for 30 min; CVP during inf (5-10 cm H_2O normal range); PCWP; urine output q1h: watch for increase which is common; if output does not increase, inf should be decreased or discontinued
• Monitor CBC with differential, Hgb, Hct, pro-time, PTT, platelet count, clotting time during treatment; treatment may increase clotting time, PTT, pro-time, sedimentary rates, Hct may drop due to increase volume and hemodilution; do not allow Hct to be <30% by volume
• Monitor I&O ratio and sp gr, urine osmolarity; if sp gr is very low, renal clearance is low; drug should be discontinued
• Assess for allergy: rash, urticaria, pruritus, wheezing, dyspnea, bronchospasm; drug should be discontinued immediately
◆• Assess for circulatory overload: increased pulse, respirations, SOB, wheezing, chest tightness, chest pain, increased CVP, jugular vein distention
• Assess for dehydration after inf; decreased output, increased temp, poor skin turgor, increased sp gr, dry skin

Nursing diagnoses
☑ Fluid volume deficit (uses)
☑ Tissue perfusion, altered (uses)
☑ Fluid volume excess (adverse reactions)
☑ Knowledge deficit (teaching)

Implementation
• Give by **IV** cont inf, undiluted, run at 20 ml/kg/hr; reduced rate in septic shock, burns; rate is calculated by blood volume and response of patient
• Give up to 20 ml kg (1.2 g/kg)/hr
• Store at room temp; discard unused portions; do not freeze; do not use if turbid or deep brown or precipitate forms

Y-site compatibilities: Cimetidine, diltiazem, doxycycline, enalaprilat

Y-site incompatibilities: Amikacin, cefamandole, cefoperazone, cefotaxime, cefoxitin, gentamicin, theophylline, tobramycin

Additive compatibilities: Cloxacillin, fosphenytoin

Patient/family education
• Teach patient the reason for administration and expected results
• Advise patient to notify prescriber if flulike symptoms or allergic symptoms occur

Evaluation
Positive therapeutic outcome
• Increased plasma volume as evidenced by higher B/P, blood volume, output

---

hydralazine (R)
(hye-dral′a-zeen)
Alazine, Apresoline, Dralzine, Novo-Hylazin ♣, hydralazine HCl, Rolzine, Supres ♣
Func. class.: Antihypertensive, direct-acting peripheral vasodilator
Chem. class.: Phthalazine
Pregnancy category C

Action: Vasodilates arterioles in smooth muscle by direct relaxation; reduces B/P with reflex increases in cardiac function

➡ **Therapeutic Outcome:** Decreased B/P in hypertension, decreased afterload in CHF

Uses: Essential hypertension; *parenteral:* severe essential hypertension, CHF

Dosage and routes
Adult: PO 10 mg qid 2-4 days, then 25 mg for rest of 1st wk, then 50 mg qid individualized to desired response, not to exceed 300 mg qd; **IV**/IM bol 20-40 mg q4-6h; administer PO as soon as possible; IM 20-40 mg q4-6h

🄿 *Child:* PO 0.75-3 mg/kg/day in 4 divided doses; max 7.5 mg/kg/24 hr; **IV** bol 0.10.2 mg/kg q4-6h; IM 0.1-0.2 mg/kg q4-6h

Available forms: Inj 20 mg/ml; tabs 10, 25, 50, 100 mg

Adverse effects
CNS: Headache, tremors, dizziness, anxiety, peripheral neuritis, depression
CV: Palpitations, reflex tachycardia, angina, **shock,** edema, rebound hypertension
GI: Nausea, vomiting, anorexia, diarrhea, constipation
GU: Impotence, urinary retention, Na⁺, H_2O retention
HEMA: **Leukopenia, agranulocytosis,** anemia, **thrombocytopenia**
INTEG: Rash, pruritus
MISC: Nasal congestion, muscle cramps, *lupuslike symptoms*

Contraindications: Hypersensitivity to hydralazines, coronary artery disease, mitral valvular rheumatic heart disease, rheumatic heart disease

Precautions: Pregnancy **C**, CVA, advanced renal disease, 🄖 elderly

🄽 **Do Not Confuse:**
Apresoline/allopurinol

Pharmacokinetics
Absorption	Rapidly absorbed (PO); well absorbed (IM); completely absorbed (**IV**)
Distribution	Widely distributed; crosses placenta
Metabolism	GI mucosa, liver extensively
Excretion	Kidneys
Half-life	2-8 hr

Pharmacodynamics
	PO	IM	IV
Onset	½ hr	10-30 min	5-20 min
Peak	1 hr	1 hr	10-80 min
Duration	2-4 hr	4-6 hr	4-6 hr

🄩 Herb/drug � Do Not Crush ◆ Alert ☰ Key Drug 🄖 Geriatric 🄿 Pediatric

Interactions
Individual drugs
Alcohol: ↑ hypotension
Drug classifications
Antihypertensives: ↑ hypotension
β-Adrenergic blockers: ↑ bradycardia, CHF
MAOIs: ↑ hypotension
Nitrates: ↑ action of nitrates
NSAIDs: ↓ antihypertensive effect

NURSING CONSIDERATIONS
Assessment
• Assess B/P q5 min for 2 hr, then q1h for 2 hr, then q4h; pulse, jugular venous distention q4h
• Monitor electrolytes, blood studies: potassium, sodium, chloride, carbon dioxide, CBC, serum glucose; LE prep, ANA titer before starting treatment
• Monitor weight daily, I&O; edema in feet, legs daily; check skin turgor, dryness of mucous membranes for hydration status
• Assess for rales, dyspnea, orthopnea; peripheral edema, fatigue, weight gain, jugular vein distention (CHF)
• For fever, joint pain, rash, sore throat (Lupus-like symptoms), notify prescriber

Nursing diagnoses
☑ Cardiac output, decreased (adverse reactions)
☑ Injury, risk for physical (side effects)
☑ Knowledge deficit (teaching)

Implementation
PO route
• Give with meals to enhance absorption
• Store protected from light and heat

IV IV route
• Give by **IV** undiluted through Y-tube or 3-way stopcock ≤10 mg/min
• Administer with patient in recumbent position; keep in that position for 1 hr after administration

Y-site compatibilities:
Heparin, hydrocortisone, potassium chloride, verapamil, vit B/C

Y-site incompatibilities:
Aminophylline, ampicillin, diazoxide, furosemide, paclitaxel

Additive incompatibilities:
Aminophylline, ampicillin, chlorothiazide, edetate calcium disodium, ethacrynate, hydrocortisone, melphalan, mephentermine, methohexital, nitroglycerin, phenobarbital, verapamil, vinorelbine

Additive compatibilities:
Dobutamine

Patient/family education
• Teach patient to take with food to increase bioavailability (PO)
• Teach patient to avoid OTC preparations unless directed by prescriber
• Advise patient to notify prescriber if chest pain, severe fatigue, fever, muscle or joint pain occur
• Advise patient to rise slowly to prevent orthostatic hypertension
• Advise patient to notify prescriber if pregnancy is suspected

Evaluation
Positive therapeutic outcome
• Decreased B/P in hypertension

H

Treatment of overdose: Administer vasopressors, volume expanders for shock; if PO, lavage or give activated charcoal, digitalization

---

hydrochlorothiazide
⚷ (R)
(hye-droe-klor-oh-thye′a-zide)
Diaqua, Diachlor H ✦, Esidrix, Hydro-Chlor, hydrochlorothiazide, HydroDiuril, Hydromal, Hydro-T, Hydrozide ✦, Microzide, Neo-Codema ✦, Novohydrazide ✦, Oretic, Thiuretic, Urozide ✦
Func. class: Diuretic, antihypertensive
Chem. class: Thiazide, sulfonamide derivative

Pregnancy category   B

Action: Acts on the distal tubule in the kidney, increasing excretion of sodium, water, chloride, magnesium, potassium, and bicarbonate

➡ **Therapeutic Outcome:** Decreased B/P, decreased edema in lung tissues peripherally

Uses: Edema in CHF, nephrotic syndrome; may be used alone or as adjunct with antihypertensives

Dosage and routes
Adult: PO 25-200 mg/day

🇬 *Elderly:* PO 12.5 mg/day, initially

🅿 *Child >6 mo:* PO 2 mg/kg/day

🅿 *Child <6 mo:* PO up to 4 mg/kg/day in divided doses

Available forms: Tabs 25, 50, 100 mg; sol 50 mg/5 ml, 100 mg/ml

Adverse effects
CNS: Drowsiness, paresthesia, anxiety, depression, headache, *dizziness, fatigue, weakness*
CV: Irregular pulse, orthostatic hypotension, palpitations, volume depletion, allergic myocarditis
EENT: Blurred vision
ELECT: Hypokalemia, hypercalcemia, hyponatremia, hypochloremia, hypomagnesemia
GI: Nausea, vomiting, anorexia, constipation, diarrhea, cramps, pancreatitis, GI irritation, **hepatitis**
GU: Frequency, polyuria, **uremia,** glucosuria
HEMA: **Aplastic anemia, hemolytic anemia, leukopenia, agranulocytosis, thrombocytopenia, neutropenia**
INTEG: Rash, urticaria, purpura, photosensitivity, fever, alopecia, erythema multiform
META: Hyperglycemia, hyperuricemia, increased creatinine, BUN

Contraindications: Hypersensitivity to thiazides or sulfonamides, anuria, renal decompensation, lactation

Precautions: Hypokalemia, renal disease, hepatic disease, gout, COPD, lupus erythematosus, diabetes mellitus, 🇬 elderly, hyperlipidemia, CrCl <25 ml/min, pregnancy **B**

Pharmacokinetics

	PO
Absorption	Variable
Distribution	Extracellular spaces; crosses placenta
Metabolism	Excreted unchanged in urine
Excretion	Breast milk
Half-life	6-15 hr

Pharmacodynamics

Onset	2 hr
Peak	4 hr
Duration	6-12 hr

Interactions
Individual drugs
Cholestyramine: ↓ absorption of hydrochlorothiazide
Colestipol: ↓ absorption of hydrochlorothiazide
Diazoxide: ↑ hyperglycemia, hyperuricemia, hypotension
Digitalis: ↑ toxicity
Lithium: ↑ toxicity
Mezlocillin: ↑ hypokalemia
Piperacillin: ↑ hypokalemia
Ticarcillin: ↑ hypokalemia
Drug classifications
Anticoagulants: ↓ effects of anticoagulants
Antidiabetics: ↓ effect of antidiabetic agent
Antihypertensives: ↑ antihypertensive effect
Diuretics, loop: ↑ effects of diuretic
Glucocorticoids: ↑ hypokalemia
NSAIDs: ↑ risk of renal failure
Sulfonylureas: ↓ effect of sulfonylurea
Food/drug
↑ absorption
Lab test interferences
↑ BSP retention, ↑ calcium, ↑ amylase, ↑ parathyroid test
↓ PBI, ↓ PSP

NURSING CONSIDERATIONS
Assessment
• Monitor glucose in urine if patient is diabetic
• Assess improvement in CVP q8h
• Check for rashes, temp elevation qd
• Assess for confusion, especially in elderly; take safety precautions if needed
• Monitor manifestations of hypokalemia: acidic urine, reduced urine, osmolality, nocturia; hypotension, broad T wave, U wave, ectopy, tachycardia, weak pulse; muscle weakness, altered LOC, drowsiness, apathy, lethargy, confusion, depression; anorexia, nausea, cramps, constipation, distention, paralytic ileus; hypoventilation, respiratory muscle weakness
• Monitor for manifestations of hypomagnesemia: agitation, muscle twitching, paresthesias, hyperactive reflexes, positive Babinski reflex, dysphagia, nystagmus seizures, tetany; nausea, vomiting, diarrhea, anorexia, abdominal distention; ectopy, tachycardia, broad, flat, or inverted T waves, depressed ST segment, prolonged QT, decreased cardiac output, hypotension
• Monitor for manifestations of hyponatremia: increased B/P, cold, clammy skin, hypovolemia or hypervolemia; anorexia, nausea, vomiting, diarrhea, abdominal cramps; lethargy, increased ICP, confusion, headache, seizures, coma, fatigue, tremors, hyperreflexia
• Monitor for manifestations of hyperchloremia: weakness, lethargy, coma, deep rapid breathing

• Assess fluid volume status: I&O ratios, record, count, or weigh diapers as appropriate, weight, distended red veins, crackles in lungs, color, quality and sp gr of urine, skin turgor, adequacy of pulses, moist mucous membranes, bilateral lung sounds, peripheral pitting edema; assess for dehydration symptoms of decreasing output, thirst, hypotension; dry mouth and mucous membranes should be reported

• Monitor electrolytes: potassium, sodium, calcium, magnesium; also include BUN, blood pH, ABGs, uric acid, CBC, blood sugar, renal function

• Assess B/P before and during therapy with patient lying, standing and sitting as appropriate; orthostatic hypotension can occur rapidly

Nursing diagnoses

☑ Altered urinary elimination (side effect)
☑ Fluid volume deficit (side effects)
☑ Fluid volume excess (uses)
☑ Knowledge deficit (teaching)

Implementation

• Give in AM to avoid interference with sleep

• Provide potassium replacement if potassium level is ≤3.0; give whole tab or use oral sol lightly; drug may be crushed if patient is unable to swallow

• Administer with food; if nausea occurs, absorption may be increased

Patient/family education

• Teach patient to take the medication early in the day to prevent nocturia

• Instruct the patient to take with food or milk if GI symptoms of nausea and anorexia occur

• Teach patient to maintain a weekly record of weight and notify prescriber of weight loss >5 lb

• Caution the patient that this drug causes a loss of potassium and that food rich in potassium should be added to the diet; refer to a dietician for assistance in planning

• Caution the patient not to exercise in hot weather or stand for prolonged periods since orthostatic hypotension will be enhanced

• Teach patient not to use alcohol or any OTC medications without prescriber's approval; serious drug reactions may occur

• Emphasize the need to contact prescriber immediately if muscle cramps, weakness, nausea, dizziness or numbness occurs

• Teach patient to take own B/P and pulse and record findings

• Caution the patient that orthostatic hypotension may occur; patient should rise slowly from sitting or reclining positions and lie down if dizziness occurs

• Teach patient to continue taking medication even if feeling better; this drug controls symptoms but does not cure the condition

• Advise the patient with hypertension to continue other medical treatment (exercise, weight loss, relaxation techniques, cessation of smoking)

Evaluation
Positive therapeutic outcome
- Decreased edema
- Decreased B/P
- Increased diuresis

Treatment of overdose:
Lavage if taken orally, monitor electrolytes, administer dextrose in saline, monitor hydration, CV, renal status

---

hydrocodone (℞)
(hye-droe-koe'done)
Hycodan ♣, Robidone ♣, Tussigon
Func. class.: Narcotic analgesic
Chem. class.: Opiate analgesic, antitussive

Pregnancy category   C
Controlled substance schedule   III

Action: Acts directly on cough center in medulla to suppress cough; binds to opiate receptors in the CNS to reduce pain

Therapeutic Outcome: Pain relief, decreased cough, decreased diarrhea

Uses: Hyperactive and nonproductive cough, mild pain

Dosages and routes
Adult: PO 5 mg q4h prn
Child: PO 2-12 mg 1.25-5 mg q4h prn or 0.2 mg/kg q3-4h

Available forms: Syrup 5 mg/5 ml; tabs 5 mg

Adverse effects
CNS: Drowsiness, dizziness, lightheadedness, confusion, headache, sedation, euphoria, dysphoria, weakness, hallucinations, disorientation, mood changes, dependence, **convulsions**
CV: Palpitations, tachycardia, bradycardia, change in B/P, **circulatory depression,** syncope
EENT: Tinnitus, blurred vision, miosis, diplopia
GI: Nausea, vomiting, anorexia, constipation, cramps, dry mouth
GU: Increased urinary output, dysuria, urinary retention
INTEG: Rash, urticaria, flushing, pruritus
RESP: **Respiratory depression**

Contraindications: Hypersensitivity, addiction (narcotic)

Precautions: Addictive personality, pregnancy **C**, lactation, increased intracranial pressure, MI (acute), severe heart disease, respiratory depression, hepatic disease, renal disease, child <18 yr

Do Not Confuse:
hydrocodone/hydrocortisone, Hycodan/Vicodin

Pharmacokinetics	
Absorption	Well absorbed
Distribution	Unknown; crosses placenta
Metabolism	Liver, extensively
Excretion	Kidneys
Half-life	3½-4½ hr

Pharmacodynamics		
	PO (analgesic)	PO (antitussive)
Onset	10-20 min	Unknown
Peak	30-60 min	Unknown
Duration	4-6 hr	4-6 hr

Interactions
Individual drugs
Alcohol: ↑ respiratory depression, hypotension, sedation
Cimetidine: ↑ recovery

H

Erythromycin: ↑ recovery
Nalbuphine: ↓ analgesia
Pentazocine: ↓ analgesia
Drug classifications
Antihistamines: ↑ respiratory depression, hypotension
CNS depressants: ↑ respiratory depression, hypotension
MAOIs: Do not use for 2 wk before taking hydrocodone
Phenothiazines: ↑ respiratory depression, hypotension
Sedative/hypnotics: ↑ respiratory depression, hypotension
Lab test interferences
↑ Amylase, ↑ lipase

NURSING CONSIDERATIONS
Assessment
• Assess pain: intensity, type, location, duration, precipitating factor
• Monitor VS after parenteral route; note muscle rigidity, drug history, liver, kidney function tests, cough and respiratory dysfunction: respiratory depression, character, rate, rhythm; notify prescriber if respirations are <10/min
• Monitor CNS changes: dizziness, drowsiness, hallucinations, euphoria, LOC, pupil reaction
• Monitor allergic reactions: rash, urticaria

Nursing diagnoses
☑Pain (uses)
☑Sensory-perceptual alteration: visual, auditory (adverse reactions)
☑Breathing pattern, ineffective (adverse reactions)
☑Knowledge deficit (teaching)

Implementation
• Give with antiemetic if nausea, vomiting occur
• Give when pain is beginning to return; determine dosage interval by patient response; continuous dosing of medication is more effective given prn
• Medication should be slowly withdrawn after long-term use to prevent withdrawal symptoms
• Store in light-resistant container at room temp
• May be given with food or milk to lessen GI upset
◙• Do not crush, chew caps

Patient/family education
• Instruct patient to report any symptoms of CNS changes, allergic reactions; to avoid CNS depressants: alcohol, sedative/hypnotics for at least 24 hr after taking this drug
• Teach patient that dizziness, drowsiness, and confusion are common and to avoid getting up without assistance
• Discuss in detail all aspects of the drug

Evaluation
Positive therapeutic outcome
• Decreased pain
• Decreased cough

Treatment of overdose:
Naloxone HCl (Narcan) 0.2-0.8 **IV**, O₂, **IV** fluids, vasopressors

---

hydrocortisone (Ŗ)
(hy-droh-kor'tih-sone)
Cortef, Cortenema,
Hydrocortone
**hydrocortisone
acetate** (Ŗ)
Cortifoam, Hydrocortone
Acetate
**hydrocortisone
cypionate** (Ŗ)
Cortef
**hydrocortisone
sodium phosphate** (Ŗ)
Hydrocortone Phosphate
**hydrocortisone
sodium succinate** (Ŗ)
A-hydroCort, Solu-Cortef
Func. class.: Short-acting
glucocorticoid
Chem. class.: Natural
nonfluorinated, group IV
potency (valerate), group
VI potency (acetate and
plain)
Pregnancy category   C

Action: Decreases inflammation by suppressing migration
of polymorphonuclear leukocytes and fibroblasts and re-
versing increased capillary
permeability and lysosomal
stabilization (systemic); antipruritic, antiinflammatory
(top)

Therapeutic Outcome: Decreased inflammation

Uses: Severe inflammation,
septic shock, adrenal insufficiency, ulcerative colitis, collagen disorders (systemic), psoriasis, eczema, contact
dermatitis, pruritus (top)

Dosage and routes
*Adrenal insufficiency/
inflammation*
Adult: PO 5-30 mg bid-qid;
IM/**IV** 100-250 mg (succinate), then 50-100 mg IM as
needed; IM/**IV** 15-240 mg
q12h (phosphate)

Shock
Adult: 500 mg-2 g q2-6h
(succinate)
P *Child:* IM/**IV** 0.186-1 mg/kg
bid-tid (succinate)

Colitis
Adult: Enema 100 mg nightly
for 21 days

Top
P *Adult and child >2 yr:* Apply
to affected area qd-qid

Available forms: Oint 0.5%,
1%, 2.5%; cream 0.25%, 0.5%,
1%, 2.5%; lotion 0.25%, 0.5%,
1%, 2%, 2.5%; gel 1%; sol 1%;
aerosol/pump spray 0.5%;
acetate: oint 0.5%, 1%, 2.5%;
cream 0.5%; lotion 0.05%;
aerosol 1%; *valerate:* oint 0.2%;
cream 0.2% (many others)

Adverse effects
CNS: Depression, flushing,
sweating, headache, mood
changes
CV: Hypertension, **circulatory
collapse, thrombophlebitis,
embolism,** tachycardia, edema
EENT: Fungal infections,
increased intraocular pressure,
blurred vision
GI: Diarrhea, nausea, abdominal distention, **GI hemorrhage,** increased appetite,
pancreatitis
HEMA: **Thrombocytopenia**
INTEG: Acne, poor wound
healing, ecchymosis, petechiae
(top) burning, dryness, itching, irritation, acne, folliculitis,
hypertrichosis, perioral dermatitis, hypopigmentation, atro-

H

phy, striae, miliaria, allergic contact dermatitis, secondary infection
MS: Fractures, osteoporosis, weakness

Contraindications: Psychosis, hypersensitivity, idiopathic thrombocytopenia, acute glomerulonephritis, amebiasis, fungal infections, nonasthmatic [P] bronchial disease, child <2 yr, AIDS, TB, fungal infections (top)

Precautions: Pregnancy **C**, diabetes mellitus, glaucoma, osteoporosis, seizure disorders, ulcerative colitis, CHF, myasthenia gravis, renal disease, esophagitis, peptic ulcer, lactation, (top) viral infections, bacterial infections

[N] **Do Not Confuse:**
hydrocortisone/hydrocodone

Pharmacokinetics

Absorption	Well absorbed (PO); systemic (top)
Distribution	Crosses placenta
Metabolism	Liver, extensively
Excretion	Kidney
Half-life	3-5 hr, adrenal suppression 3-4 days

Pharmacodynamics

	PO	IM	IV	TOP
Onset	1-2 hr	20 min	Rapid	Min to hr
Peak	1 hr	4-8 hr	Unkn	Hr to days
Duration	1½ days	1½ days	1½ days	Hr to days

Interactions
Individual drugs
Amphotericin B: ↑ hypokalemia
Cholestyramine: ↓ action of hydrocortisone
Colestipol: ↓ action of hydrocortisone

Ephedrine: ↓ action of hydrocortisone
Insulin: ↑ need for insulin
Mezlocillin: ↑ hypokalemia
Phenytoin: ↓ action, ↑ metabolism
Rifampin: ↓ action, ↑ metabolism
Theophylline: ↓ action of hydrocortisone
Ticarcillin: ↑ hypokalemia
Drug classifications
Anticoagulants: ↓ action of anticoagulant
Barbiturates: ↓ action, ↑ metabolism
Diuretics: ↑ hypokalemia
Hypoglycemic agents: ↑ need for hypoglycemic agents
NSAIDs: ↑ risk of GI bleeding
[☑] *Herb/drug*
Aloe: ↑ hypokalemia
Buckthorn: ↑ hypokalemia
Cascara sagrada: ↑ hypokalemia
Senna: ↑ hypokalemia
Lab test interferences
↑ Cholesterol, ↑ sodium, ↑ blood glucose, ↑ uric acid, ↑ calcium, ↑ urine glucose
↓ Calcium, ↓ potassium, ↓ T_4, ↓ T_3, ↓ thyroid ^{131}I uptake test, ↓ urine 17-OHCS, ↓ 17KS, ↓ PBI
False negative: Skin allergy tests

NURSING CONSIDERATIONS
Assessment
• Monitor potassium, blood sugar, urine glucose while patient on long-term therapy; hypokalemia and hyperglycemia may occur
• Monitor I&O ratio; be alert for decreasing urinary output and increasing edema; weigh daily; notify prescriber of weekly gain >5 lb or edema, hypertension, cardiac symptoms

---

• Monitor plasma cortisol levels during long-term therapy (normal level is 138-635 nmol/L when drawn at 8 AM); check adrenal function periodically for HPA axis suppression

• Assess for infection: increased temp, WBC even after withdrawal of medication; drug masks infection symptoms; if fever develops, drug should be discontinued

• Check for potassium depletion: paresthesias, fatigue, nausea, vomiting, depression, polyuria, dysrhythmias, weakness

• Assess mental status: affect, mood, behavioral changes, aggression

• Check nasal passages during long-term treatment for changes in mucus (nasal)

• Assess for systemic absorption: increased temp, inflammation, irritation (top)

Nursing diagnoses

☑ Infection, risk for (adverse reactions)

☑ Knowledge deficit (teaching)

☑ Noncompliance (teaching) (top/nasal preparation)

Implementation

PO route

• Give with food or milk to decrease GI symptoms

▣ IV route

• Give only sodium phosphate product **IV**; reconstitute with sol provided; give 100 mg over >1 min

• May be given by intermittent inf in compatible sol

• Give titrated dose; use lowest effective dosage

Sodium phosphate preparations

Syringe compatibilities:

Fluconazole, fludarabine, metoclopramide

Additive compatibilities:

Amikacin, amphotericin B, bleomycin, cephapirin, metaraminol, sodium bicarbonate, verapamil

Y-site compatibilities:

Allopurinol, amifostine, aztreonam, cefepime, cladribine, famotidine, filgrastim, fluconazole, fludarabine, granisetron, melphalan, ondansetron, paclitaxel, piperacillin/tazobactam, teniposide, thiotepa, vinorelbine

Sodium succinate preparations

Syringe compatibilities:

Metoclopramide, thiopental

Y-site compatibilities:

Acyclovir, allopurinol, amifostine, aminophylline, ampicillin, amphotericin B cholesteryl, amrinone, amsacrine, atracurium, atropine, aztreonam, betamethasone, calcium gluconate, cefepime, cefmetazole, cephalothin, cephapirin, chlordiazepoxide, chlorpromazine, cisatracurium, cladribine, cyanocobalamin, cytarabine, dexamethasone, digoxin, diphenhydramine, dopamine, doxorubicin liposome, droperidol, edrophonium, enalaprilat, epinephrine, esmolol, conjugated estrogens, ethacrynate, famotidine, fentanyl, fentanyl/droperidol, filgrastim, fludarabine, fluorouracil, foscarnet, furosemide, gallium, granisetron, heparin, hydralazine, regular insulin, isoproterenol, kanamycin, lidocaine, lorazepam, magnesium sulfate, melphalan, menadiol, meperidine, methicillin, methoxamine, methylergonovine, minocycline, morphine, neostigmine, norepinephrine, ondansetron, oxacillin, oxytocin, paclitaxel, pancuronium, penicillin G potassium, pentazocine, phytonadione, piperacillin/tazobactam, prednisolone, procainamide, prochlorperazine, propofol, propranolol, pyridostigmine, remifentanil, scopolamine, sodium bicarbonate, succinylcholine, tacrolimus, teniposide, theophylline, thiotepa, trimethaphan, trimethobenzamide, vecuronium, vinorelbine

Y-site incompatibilities:
Diazepam, ergotamine tartrate, idarubicin, phenytoin, sargramostim

Additive compatibilities:
Amikacin, aminophylline, amphotericin B, calcium chloride, calcium gluconate, cephalothin, cephapirin, chloramphenicol, clindamycin, cloxacillin, corticotropin, daunorubicin, diphenhydramine, dopamine, erythromycin, floxacillin, lidocaine, magnesium sulfate, mephentermine, metronidazole/sodium bicarbonate, mitomycin, mitoxantrone, netilmicin, netilmicin/potassium chloride, norepinephrine, penicillin G potassium/sodium, piperacillin, polymyxin B, potassium chloride, sodium bicarbonate, theophylline, thiopental, vancomycin, verapamil, vit B/C

Additive incompatibilities:
Bleomycin, doxorubicin
Rec route
• Use applicator provided
• Clean applicator after each use
Top route
• Apply only to affected areas; do not get in eyes
• Cleanse and dry area before applying medication, then

cover with occlusive dressing (only if prescribed); seal to normal skin; change q12h; syst absorption may occur; use only on dermatoses; do not use on weeping, denuded, or infected area
• Use for a few days after area has cleared
• Store at room temp
Nasal route
• Patient should clear nasal passages before administration; use decongestant if needed; shake inhaler, invert, tilt head backward, insert nozzle into nostril, away from septum; hold other nostril closed and depress activator, inhale through nose, exhale through mouth

Patient/family education
• Teach patient all aspects of drug usage, including cushingoid symptoms
• Advise patient that ID as steroid user should be carried; not to discontinue abruptly; adrenal crisis can result
• Instruct patient to notify prescriber if therapeutic response decreases; dosage adjustment may be needed
• Instruct patient to notify prescriber of signs of infection
• Caution patient to avoid OTC products unless directed by perscriber: salicylates, alcohol in cough products, cold preparations
• Teach patient symptoms of adrenal insufficiency: nausea, anorexia, fatigue, dizziness, dyspnea, weakness, joint pain, and when to notify prescriber
• Advise patient that long-term therapy may be needed to clear infection (1-2 mo depending on type of infection)

☑ Herb/drug ⑤ Do Not Crush ◆ Alert ⛬ Key Drug ⑥ Geriatric ⑨ Pediatric

Nasal route
• Instruct patient to clear nasal passages if sneezing attack occurs, then repeat dose; to continue using product even if mild nasal bleeding occurs; bleeding is usually transient
• Teach method of instillation after providing written instruction from manufacturer on instillation

Evaluation
Positive therapeutic outcome
• Decrease in runny nose (nasal)
• Ease of respirations, decreased inflammation
• Absence of severe itching, patches on skin, flaking (top)

---

hydromorphone (℞)
(hye-droe-mor'fone)
Dihydromorphinone, Dilaudid, Dilaudid-HP, Dilaudid Cough Syrup (combination with guaifenesin/alcohol)
Func. class.: Antitussive, narcotic; opioid analgesic agonist
Chem. class.: Phenanthrene derivative, guaifenesin

Pregnancy category   **C**
Controlled substance schedule   **II**

Action: Depresses pain impulse transmission at the spinal cord level by interacting with opioid receptors; increases respiratory tract fluid by decreasing surface tension and adhesiveness, which increases removal of mucus; analgesic, antitussive

➡ Therapeutic Outcome: Decreased cough, decreased pain

Uses: As an antitussive to suppress cough; moderate to severe pain

Dosage and routes
Antitussive
Adult: PO 1 mg q3-4h prn
P *Child 6-12 yr:* PO 0.5 mg q3-4h prn
Analgesic
Adult: PO 2 mg q3-6h prn; may increase to 4 mg q4-6h; SC/IM 1-2 mg q3-6h prn; may increase to 3-4 mg q4-6h; **IV** 0.5-1 mg q3h prn; rec 3 mg q4-8h prn

Available forms: Inj 1, 2, 3, 4, 10 mg/ml; tabs 1, 2, 3, 4, 8 mg; oral sol 5 mg/5 ml; syrup 1 mg/5 ml

Adverse effects
CNS: Dizziness, drowsiness, *sedation, confusion,* headache, euphoria, dreaming, hallucinations
CV: Hypotension, bradycardia
EENT: Miosis, diplopia, blurred vision
GI: Nausea, constipation, vomiting, anorexia
GU: Retention
INTEG: Urticaria, rash, sweating, flushing
RESP: **Respiratory depression**

Contraindications: Hypersensitivity, increased intracranial pressure, status asthmaticus

Precautions: Hypothyroidism, Addison's disease, CNS depression, brain tumor, asthma, hepatic disease, renal disease, COPD, psychosis, alcoholism, convulsive disorders, pregnancy **C**

⚠ Do Not Confuse:
Dilaudid/Demerol,
hydromorphone/meperidine,
hydromorphone/morphine

Pharmacokinetics

Absorption	Well absorbed (PO), complete (**IV**)
Distribution	Unknown; crosses placenta
Metabolism	Liver, extensively
Excretion	Kidneys
Half-life	2-3 hr

Pharmacodynamics

	PO/IM/SC	IV	REC
Onset	15-30 min	10-15 min	15-30 min
Peak	30-60 min	15-30 min	30-90 min
Duration	4-5 hr	2-3 hr	4-5 hr

Interactions
Individual drugs
Alcohol: ↑ respiratory depression, hypotension, sedation
Nalbuphine: ↓ analgesia
Pentazocine: ↓ analgesia
Drug classifications
Antidepressants: ↑ respiratory depression, hypotension
Antihistamines: ↑ respiratory depression, hypotension
CNS depressants: ↑ respiratory depression, hypotension
MAOIs: Serious reactions; dosage should be reduced
Phenothiazines: ↑ respiratory depression, hypotension
Sedative/hypnotics: ↑ respiratory depression, hypotension
☑ Herb/drug
Kava: ↑ action
Lab test interferences
↑ Amylase, ↑ lipase

NURSING CONSIDERATIONS
Assessment
• Monitor VS after parenteral route; note muscle rigidity, drug history, liver, kidney function tests, respiratory dysfunction: respiratory depression, character, rate, rhythm; notify prescriber if respirations are <10/min
• Monitor CNS changes: dizziness, drowsiness, hallucinations, euphoria, LOC, pupil reaction
• Monitor allergic reactions: rash, urticaria

Nursing diagnoses
☑ Pain (uses)
☑ Sensory-perceptual alteration: visual, auditory (adverse reactions)
☑ Breathing pattern, ineffective (adverse reactions)
☑ Knowledge deficit (teaching)

Implementation
• Give with antiemetic if nausea, vomiting occur
• Give when pain is beginning to return; determine dosage interval by patient response; continuous dosing of medication is more effective given prn; explain analgesic effect
• Withdraw medication slowly after long-term use to prevent withdrawal symptoms
• Store in light-resistant container at room temp
PO route
• May be given with food or milk to lessen GI upset
IM/SC route
• Do not give if sol is cloudy or a precipitate has formed; rotate inj sites
☒ IV route
• Give by direct **IV** after diluting with 5 ml or more sterile water or 0.9% NaCl for inj
• Give slowly at 2 mg over 3-5 min or less

Syringe compatibilities:
Atropine, bupivacaine, ceftazidime, chlorpromazine, cimetidine, dimenhydrinate, diphen-

hydramine, fentanyl, glycopyrrolate, haloperidol, hydroxyzine, lorazepam, midazolam, pentazocaine, pentobarbital, prochlorperazine, promethazine, ranitidine, scopolamine, tetracaine, thiethylperazine, trimethobenzamide

Y-site compatibilities:
Acyclovir, allopurinol, amifostine, amikacin, amsacrine, aztreonam, cefamandole, cefepime, cefmetazole, cefoperazone, cefotaxime, cefoxitin, ceftazidime, ceftizoxime, cefuroxime, cephalothin, cephapirin, chloramphenicol, cisplatin, cladribine, clindamycin, cyclophosphamide, cytarabine, diltiazem, dobutamine, dopamine, doxorubicin, doxycycline, epinephrine, erythromycin lactobionate, famotidine, fentanyl, filgrastim, fludarabine, foscarnet, furosemide, gentamicin, granisetron, heparin, kanamycin, labetalol, lorazepam, magnesium sulfate, melphalan, methotrexate, metronidazole, mezlocillin, midazolam, milrinone, morphine, moxalactam, nafcillin, nicardipine, nitroglycerin, norepinephrine, ondansetron, oxacillin, paclitaxel, penicillin G potassium, piperacillin, piperacillin/tazobactam, propofol, ranitidine, teniposide, thiotepa, ticarcillin, tobramycin, trimethoprim/sulfamethoxazole, vancomycin, vecuronium, vinorelbine

Y-site incompatibilities:
Ampicillin, diazepam, minocycline, phenobarbital, phenytoin, sargramostim

Additive compatibilities:
Bupivacaine, fluorouracil, midazolam, ondansetron, promethazine, verapamil

Additive incompatibilities:
Sodium bicarbonate, thiopental

Solution compatibilities:
D_5W, D_5/0.45% NaCl, D_5/0.9% NaCl, D_5/LR, D_5/Ringer's sol, 0.45% NaCl, 0.9% NaCl, Ringer's and lactated Ringer's sol

Patient/family education
• Instruct patient to report any symptoms of CNS changes, allergic reactions; to avoid CNS depressants: alcohol, sedative/hypnotics for at least 24 hr after taking this drug
• Advise patient that dizziness, drowsiness, and confusion are common and to avoid getting up without assistance
• Discuss in detail all aspects of the drug

Evaluation
Positive therapeutic outcome
• Decreased pain
• Decreased cough

Treatment of overdose:
Naloxone HCl (Narcan) 0.2-0.8 IV, O_2, **IV** fluids, vasopressors

---

hydroxyurea (℞)
(hye-drox-ee-yoo-ree'ah)
Droxia, Hydrea
Func. class.: Antineoplastic, antimetabolite
Chem. class.: Synthetic urea analog
Pregnancy category   D

Action: Acts by inhibiting DNA synthesis without interfering with RNA or protein synthesis; incorporates thymidine into DNA, causing direct damage to DNA strands; S phase specific of cell cycle

▶**Therapeutic Outcome:** Prevention of rapidly growing malignant cells

Uses: Melanoma, chronic myelocytic leukemia, recurrent or metastatic ovarian cancer, squamous cell carcinoma of the head and neck, sickle cell anemia, psoriasis

Dosage and routes
Solid tumors
Adult: PO 80 mg/kg as a single dose q 3 days or 20-30 mg/kg as a single dose qd

In combination with radiation
Adult: PO 80 mg/kg as a single dose q 3 days; should be started 7 days before irradiation

Resistant chronic myelocytic leukemia
Adult: PO 20-30 mg/kg/day as a single daily dose

Renal dose
CrCl 10-50 ml/min dose 50%; CrCl <10 ml/min dose 20%

Available forms: Cap 200, 300, 400, 500 mg

Adverse effects
CNS: Headache, confusion, hallucinations, dizziness, **convulsions**
CV: Angina, ischemia
GI: Nausea, vomiting, anorexia, diarrhea, stomatitis, constipation
GU: Increased BUN, uric acid, creatinine, temporary renal function impairment
HEMA: **Leukopenia, anemia, thrombocytopenia**
INTEG: *Rash,* urticaria, pruritus, dry skin

Contraindications: Hypersensitivity, leukopenia (<2500/mm^3), thrombocytopenia (<100,000/mm^3), anemia (severe), pregnancy **D**

Precautions: Renal disease (severe)

Pharmacokinetics	
Absorption	Well absorbed
Distribution	Crosses blood-brain barrier
Metabolism	Liver (50%)
Excretion	Kidneys, unchanged (50%)
Half-life	4 hr

Pharmacodynamics	
Onset	Unknown
Peak	2 hr
Duration	Unknown

Interactions
Individual drugs
Cyclophosphamide: ↑ cardiotoxicity, CHF
Radiation: ↑ toxicity, bone marrow suppression
Drug classifications
Antineoplastics: ↑ toxicity, bone marrow suppression
Lab test interferences
↑ Renal function studies

NURSING CONSIDERATIONS
Assessment
• Assess buccal cavity q8h for dryness, sores or ulceration, white patches, oral pain, bleeding, dysphagia; obtain prescription for viscous lidocaine (Xylocaine)
• Assess symptoms indicating severe allergic reaction: rash, pruritus, urticaria, purpuric skin lesions, itching, flushing
• Monitor CBC, differential, platelet count weekly; withhold drug if WBC count is <4000/mm^3 or platelet count is <100,000/mm^3; notify prescriber of results if WBC <20,000/mm^3, platelets <150,000/mm^3

• Assess for increased uric acid levels, swelling, joint pain primarily in extremities; patient should be well hydrated to prevent urate deposits

• Monitor renal function studies: BUN, creatinine, serum uric acid, urine CrCl before and during therapy; I&O ratio; report fall in urine output to <30 ml/hr

• Monitor temp q4h (may indicate beginning of infection)

• Monitor liver function tests before and during therapy (bilirubin, AST, ALT, LDH) as needed or monthly

• Assess for bleeding: hematuria, stool guaiac, bruising or petechiae, mucosa or orifices q8h; check for inflammation of mucosa, breaks in skin

Nursing diagnoses

☑ Injury, risk for (adverse reactions)

☑ Body image disturbance (adverse reactions)

☑ Infection, risk for (adverse reactions)

☑ Knowledge deficit (teaching)

Implementation

• Avoid contact with skin, very irritating; wash completely to remove

• Give fluids **IV** or PO before chemotherapy to hydrate patient

• Give antiemetic 30-60 min before giving drug and prn to prevent vomiting; antibiotics for prophylaxis of infection

• Provide liq diet: carbonated beverages; gelatin may be added if patient is not nauseated or vomiting

• Provide rinsing of mouth tid-qid with water, club soda; brushing of teeth bid-qid with soft brush or cotton-tipped applicators for stomatitis; use unwaxed dental floss

• For difficulty swallowing, cap contents may be mixed with water

🚫 • Do not crush or chew caps

Patient/family education

• Advise patient that contraceptive measures are recommended during therapy

• Teach patient to avoid use of products containing aspirin or ibuprofen, razors, commercial mouthwash, since bleeding may occur; instruct patient to report symptoms of bleeding (hematuria, tarry stools)

• Instruct patient to report signs of anemia (fatigue, headache, irritability, faintness, shortness of breath)

• Advise patient to report any changes in breathing or coughing even several mo after treatment; to avoid crowds and persons with respiratory tract or other infections

• Caution patient not to have any vaccinations without the advice of the prescriber, serious reactions can occur

Evaluation

Positive therapeutic outcome

• Prevention of rapid division of malignant cells

H

hydroxyzine (℞)
(hye-drox'i-zeen)
Apo-hydroxyzine ✿, Atarax,
Atarax 100, hydroxyzine HCl,
hydroxyzine pamoate,
Multipax ✿,
Novohydroxyzine ✿,
Vistaril, Vistazine 50
Func. class.: Antianxiety/
sedative/hypnotic/
antihistamine
Chem. class.: Piperazine
derivative

Pregnancy category C

Action: Depresses subcortical
levels of CNS, including limbic
system, reticular formation;
anticholinergic, antiemetic,
antihistaminic responses

Therapeutic Outcome: Absence of allergy symptoms,
rhinitis, pruritus, absence of
nausea/vomiting, sedation,
absence of anxiety

Uses: Anxiety preoperatively,
postoperatively to prevent
nausea, vomiting; to potentiate
narcotic analgesics; sedation;
pruritus; prevention of alcohol,
drug withdrawal

Dosage and routes
Adult: PO 25-100 mg tid-qid

G *Elderly:* PO 10 mg tid-qid
(pruritus)

P *Child >6 yr:* PO 50-100 mg/
day in divided doses

P *Child <6 yr:* PO 50 mg/day in
divided doses

*Preoperatively/
postoperatively*
Adult: IM 25-100 mg q4-6h

P *Child:* IM 0.5-1.1 mg/kg
q4-6h

Available forms: Tabs 10, 25,
50, 100 mg; caps 25, 50, 100
mg; syrup 10 mg/5 ml; oral
susp 25 mg/5 ml; inj 25, 50
mg/ml

Adverse effects
CNS: Dizziness, drowsiness,
confusion, headache, tremors,
fatigue, depression, **convulsions**
CV: Hypotension
GI: Dry mouth

Contraindications: Hypersensitivity to this drug or
cetirizine, early pregnancy,
lactation

G **Precautions:** Elderly, debilitated
patients, hepatic disease, renal
disease, pregnancy **C**

Do Not Confuse:
Vistaril/Versed

Pharmacokinetics	
Absorption	Well absorbed
Distribution	Not known
Metabolism	Liver, completely
Excretion	Feces, urine, bile
Half-life	3 hr

Pharmacodynamics	
	PO/IM
Onset	15-30 min
Peak	2-4 hr
Duration	4-6 hr

Interactions
Individual drugs
Alcohol: ↑ CNS depression
Atropine: ↑ anticholinergic
reactions
Disopyramide: ↑ anticholiner-
gic reactions
Haloperidol: ↑ anticholinergic
reactions
Quinidine: ↑ anticholinergic
reactions
Drug classifications
Antidepressants: ↑ anticholin-
ergic reactions
Antihistamines: ↑ anticholin-
ergic reactions

CNS depressants: ↑ CNS depression
Opiates: ↑ CNS depression
Phenothiazines: ↑ anticholinergic reactions
Sedative/hypnotics: ↑ CNS depression

☑ **Herb/drug**
Henbane: ↑ anticholinergic effect
Kava: ↑ action
Lab test interferences
False: ↑ 17-OHCS

NURSING CONSIDERATIONS
Assessment
• Assess respiratory status: rate, rhythm, increase in bronchial secretions, wheezing, chest tightness; provide fluids to 2 L/day to decrease secretion thickness
• Monitor I&O ratio: be alert for urinary retention, frequency, dysuria, especially in the elderly; drug should be discontinued if these occur
• Observe for drowsiness, dizziness
• Assess cough characteristics including type, frequency, thickness of secretions; evaluate response to this medication if using for cough

Nursing diagnoses
☑ Injury, risk for (side effects)
☑ Anxiety (uses)
☑ Knowledge deficit (teaching)

Implementation
PO route
• Give with meals if GI symptoms occur; absorption may be slightly decreased; cap may be opened and drug mixed with food/fluids for patients with swallowing difficulties
IM route
• Give IM inj in large muscle mass; aspirate to prevent **IV** administration; use Z-track

method; severe necrosis can result with improper technique; never give **IV**/SC

Syringe compatibilities:
Atropine, atropine/meperidine, benzquinamide, bupivacaine, butorphanol, chlorpromazine, cimetidine, codeine, diphenhydramine, doxapram, droperidol, fentanyl, fluphenazine, glycopyrrolate, hydromorphone, lidocaine, meperidine, meperidine/atropine, methotrimeprazine, metoclopramide, midazolam, morphine, nalbuphine, oxymorphone, pentazocine, perphenazine, procaine, prochlorperazine, promazine, promethazine, remifentanil, scopolamine, sufentanil, thiothixene

Syringe incompatibilities:
Aminophylline, chloramphenicol, dimenhydrinate, heparin, penicillin G potassium, pentobarbital, phenobarbital, phenytoin

Y-site compatibilities:
Aztreonam, ciprofloxacin, cladribine, famotidine, filgrastim, foscarnet, granisetron, melphalan, ondansetron, propofol, sufentanil, teniposide, thiotepa, vinorelbine

Y-site incompatibilities:
Paclitaxel

Additive compatibilities:
Cisplatin, cyclophosphamide, cytarabine, dimenhydrinate, etoposide, lidocaine, mesna, methotrexate, nafcillin

Patient/family education
• Caution patient to avoid hazardous activities and activities requiring alertness, since dizziness may occur; instruct patient to request assistance with ambulation

---

- Advise patient to avoid alcohol, other CNS depressants including cough, cold preparations; CNS depression may occur
- Teach all aspects of drug use; to notify prescriber if confusion, sedation, hypotension occur; to avoid driving and other hazardous activity if drowsiness occurs; to avoid alcohol and other CNS depressants that may potentiate effect
- Instruct patient to take 1 hr pc or 2 hr ac to facilitate absorption
- May crush if patient unable to swallow whole
- Caution patient not to exceed recommended dosage; dysrhythmias may occur
- Tell patient hard candy, gum, frequent rinsing of mouth may be used for dryness

Evaluation
Positive therapeutic outcome
- Absence of nausea, vomiting
- Decreased anxiety

Treatment of overdose:
Lavage if orally ingested, VS, supportive care, **IV** norepinephrine for hypotension

---

ibuprofen ⚷ (OTC)
(eye-byoo-proe′fen)
Aches-N-Pain, Actiprofen ✽,
Advil, Amersol ✽, Apo-
Ibuprofen ✽, Children's
Advil, Excedrin IB, Genpril,
Haltran, Ibuprin, ibuprofen,
Ibuprohm, I-Tab, Medipren,
Menadol, Midol-200, Motrin,
Motrin IB, Motrin Junior
Strength, Novoprosen ✽,
Nuprin, Pamprin-IB, Rufen,
Saleto-200, Saleto-400,
Saleto-600, Saleto-800,
Trendar
Func. class.: Nonsteroidal
antiinflammatory; nonnarcotic analgesic
Chem. class.: Propionic
acid derivative
Pregnancy category   **B**

Action: Inhibits prostaglandin synthesis by decreasing enzyme needed for biosynthesis; analgesic, antiinflammatory, antipyretic

Therapeutic Outcome: Decreased pain, inflammation, fever

Uses: Rheumatoid arthritis, osteoarthritis, primary dysmenorrhea, gout, dental pain, musculoskeletal disorders, fever

Dosage and routes
Analgesia
Adult: PO 200-400 mg q4-6h, not to exceed 3.2 g/day
P *Child:* PO 4-10 mg/kg/dose q6-8h
Antipyretic
P *Child 6 mo-12yr:* PO 5 mg/kg (temp <102.5° F), 10 mg/kg (temp >102.5° F), may repeat q4-6h; max 40 mg/kg/day

---

Antiinflammatory
Adult: PO 300-800 mg tid-qid; max 3.2 g/day

P *Child:* PO 30-40 mg/kg/day in 3-4 divided doses; max 50 mg/kg/day

Available forms: Tabs 100, 200, 300, 400, 600, 800 mg; oral susp 100 mg/5 ml, tab, chew 50, 100 mg

Adverse effects
CNS: Headache, dizziness, drowsiness, fatigue, tremors, confusion, insomnia, anxiety, depression
CV: Tachycardia, peripheral edema, palpitations, dysrhythmias
EENT: Tinnitus, hearing loss, blurred vision
GI: Nausea, anorexia, vomiting, diarrhea, jaundice, **cholestatic hepatitis,** constipation, flatulence, cramps, dry mouth, peptic ulcer
GU: **Nephrotoxicity;** dysuria, hematuria, oliguria, azotemia
HEMA: **Blood dyscrasias,** increased bleeding time
INTEG: Purpura, rash, pruritus, sweating

Contraindications: Hypersensitivity, asthma, severe renal disease, severe hepatic disease

Precautions: Pregnancy **B** 1st and 2nd trimesters, lactation,
P children, bleeding disorders, GI disorders, cardiac disorders, hypersensitivity to other antiin-
G flammatory agents, elderly, CHF, CrCl <25 ml/min

N **Do Not Confuse:**
Nuprin/Lupron

Pharmacokinetics

Absorption	Well absorbed
Distribution	Not known; crosses placenta
Metabolism	Liver, extensively
Excretion	Kidneys, unchanged (10%)
Half-life	3½ hr

Pharmacodynamics

Onset	½ hr
Peak	1-2 hr
Duration	4-6 hr

Interactions
Individual drugs
Acetaminophen (long-term use): ↑ renal reactions
Alcohol: ↑ adverse reactions
Aspirin: ↓ effectiveness, ↑ adverse reactions
Cyclosporine: ↑ toxicity
Digoxin: ↑ toxicity, levels
Furosemide: ↓ effect of furosemide
Insulin: ↓ insulin effect
Lithium: ↑ toxicity
Methotrexate: ↑ toxicity
Phenytoin: ↑ toxicity
Probenecid: ↑ toxicity
Radiation: ↑ risk of hematologic toxicity
Sulfonylurea: ↑ toxicity
Drug classifications
Anticoagulants: ↑ risk of bleeding
Antihypertensives: ↓ effect of antihypertensives
Antineoplastics: ↑ risk of hematologic toxicity
β-Adrenergic blockers: ↑ antihypertension
Cephalosporins: ↑ risk of bleeding
Diuretics: ↓ effectiveness of diuretics
Glucocorticoids: ↑ adverse reactions
Hypoglycemics: ↓ hypoglycemic effect
NSAIDs: ↑ adverse reactions

Potassium supplements:
↑ adverse reactions
Sulfonamides: ↑ toxicity
Lab test interferences
↑ Bleeding time

NURSING CONSIDERATIONS
Assessment
• Assess pain: location, duration, type, intensity before dose and 1 hr after
• Assess musculoskeletal status: ROM before dose and 1 hr after
• Monitor liver function studies: AST, ALT, bilirubin, creatinine if patient is on long-term therapy
• Monitor renal function studies: BUN, urine creatinine if patient is on long-term therapy
• Assess cardiac status: edema (peripheral), tachycardia, palpitations; monitor B/P, pulse for character, quality, rhythm
• Monitor blood studies: CBC, Hct, Hgb, pro-time if patient is on long-term therapy
• Check I&O ratio; decreasing output may indicate renal failure if patient is on long-term therapy
• Assess hepatotoxicity: dark urine, clay-colored stools, jaundice of skin and sclera, itching, abdominal pain, fever, diarrhea if patient is on long-term therapy
• Assess for history of peptic ulcer disorder; asthma, aspirin, hypersensitivity, check closely for hypersensitivity reactions
• Assess for allergic reactions: rash, urticaria; if these occur, drug may have to be discontinued
• Assess for ototoxicity: tinnitus, ringing, roaring in ears; audiometric testing needed before, after long-term therapy
• Assess for visual changes: blurring, halos; may indicate corneal, retinal damage
• Identify prior drug history; there are many drug interactions
• Identify fever: length of time in evidence and related symptoms

Nursing diagnoses
☑ Pain (uses)
☑ Mobility, impaired (uses)
☑ Injury, risk for (side effects)
☑ Knowledge deficit (teaching)

Implementation
• Administer to patient crushed or whole; 800-mg tab may be dissolved in water
• Give with food or milk to decrease gastric symptoms; give 30 min pc or 2 hr ac; absorption may be slowed

Patient/family education
• Teach patient to report any symptoms of hepatotoxicity, renal toxicity, visual changes, ototoxicity, allergic reactions, bleeding if patient is on long-term therapy
• Caution patient not to exceed recommended dosage; acute poisoning may result
• Advise patient to read label on other OTC drugs
• Inform patient that the therapeutic response takes 1 mo (arthritis)
• Caution patient to avoid alcohol ingestion, salicylates, NSAIDs; GI bleeding may occur
• Advise patient with allergies that allergic reactions may develop
• Advise patient to use sunscreen to prevent photosensitivity

☑ Herb/drug 🚫 Do Not Crush ◆ Alert 🔑 Key Drug G Geriatric P Pediatric

Evaluation
Positive therapeutic outcome
- Decreased pain
- Decreased inflammation
- Decreased fever
- Increased mobility

ibutilide (℞)
(eye-byoo'te-lide)
Corvert
Func. class.: Antidysrhythmic (Class III)
Pregnancy category   C

Action: Prolongs duration of action potential and effective refractory period; noncompetitive α- and β-adrenergic inhibition

➡ **Therapeutic Outcome:** Decreased amount and severity of atrial fibrillation/flutter

Uses: Atrial fibrillation/flutter

Dosage and routes
Adult: **IV** inf (≥60 kg) 1 vial (1 mg) given over 10 min; **IV** inf (<60 kg) 0.1 mg/kg (0.01 mg/kg) given over 10 min

Available forms: Inj 0.1 mg/ml

Adverse effects
CNS: Headache
CV: Hypotension, bradycardia, **sinus arrest, CHF, dysrhythmias,** hypertension, extrasystoles, ventricular tachycardia, bundle branch block, AV block
GI: Nausea

Contraindications: Hypersensitivity

Precautions: SN dysfunction, 2nd- or 3rd-degree AV block, electrolyte imbalances, pregnancy **C**, bradycardia, lactation, children <18 yr, renal/hepatic, disease, elderly

Pharmacokinetics

Absorption	Slow, variable
Distribution	Body tissues; crosses placenta
Metabolism	Liver
Excretion	Kidney
Half-life	15-100 days

Pharmacodynamics

Onset	1-3 wk
Peak	2-10 hr
Duration	Up to months

Interactions
Individual drugs
Digoxin: ↑ blood levels, ↑ toxicity
Disopyramide: ↑ levels, ↑ toxicity
Flecainide: ↑ levels, ↑ toxicity
Phenytoin: ↑ blood levels
Procainamide: ↑ levels, ↑ toxicity
Quinidine: ↑ levels, ↑ toxicity
Drug classifications
Antidepressants, tricyclic/ tetracyclic: prodysrhythmia
H₁-Receptor antagonists: ↑ prodysrhythmia
Phenothiazines: ↑ prodysrhythmia
Herb/drug
Aloe: ↑ action
Buckthorn: ↑ action
Cascara sagrada: ↑ action
Senna: ↑ action

NURSING CONSIDERATIONS
Assessment
- Monitor I&O ratio; monitor electrolytes: potassium, sodium, chloride
- Monitor liver function studies: AST, ALT, bilirubin, alkaline phosphatase
- Monitor ECG continuously to determine drug effectiveness; measure PR, QRS, QT intervals; check for PVCs, other dysrhythmias; monitor B/P continuously for

hypotension, hypertension; check for rebound hypertension after 1-2 hr; discontinue drug when atrial fibrillation/flutter ceases
• Monitor for dehydration or hypovolemia
• Assess for CNS symptoms: confusion, psychosis, numbness, depression, involuntary movements; if these occur drug should be discontinued
• Monitor cardiac rate, respiration; rate, rhythm, character, chest pain, ventricular tachycardia, supraventricular tachycardia or fibrillation

Nursing diagnoses
☑ Cardiac output, decreased (uses)
☑ Gas exchange, impaired (adverse reactions)
☑ Knowledge deficit (teaching)

Implementation
Ⓘ **IV route**
• Give reduced dosage slowly with ECG monitoring only
• Give undiluted or diluted in 50 ml 0.9% NaCl or D₅W (0.017 mg/ml), give over 10 min
• Solution is stable for 48 hr refrigerated or 24 hr at room temperature
• Do not admix with other solution, drugs

Patient/family education
• Instruct patient to report side effects immediately to prescriber

Evaluation
Positive therapeutic outcome
• Decrease in atrial fibrillation/flutter

---

idarubicin (℞)
(eye-da-roo'bi-sin)
Idamycin
Func. class.: Antineoplastic, antibiotic
Chem. class.: Anthracycline glycoside
Pregnancy category   D

Action: Inhibits DNS synthesis derived from daunorubicin by binding to DNA, which causes strand splitting; cell cycle specific (S phase); a vesicant

➡**Therapeutic Outcome:** Prevention of rapidly growing malignant cells

Uses: Used in combination with other antineoplastics for acute myelocytic leukemia in adults

Dosage and routes
Adult: **IV** 12 mg/m²/day × 3 days in combination with cytosine or 25 mg/m² **IV** bolus followed by 200 mg/m²/day × 5 days by cont inf

Available forms: Inj 5, 10 mg vials

Adverse effects
CNS: Fever, chills, headache
CV: **Dysrhythmias, CHF, pericarditis, myocarditis,** peripheral edema
GI: Nausea, vomiting, abdominal pain, mucositis, diarrhea, **hepatotoxicity**
HEMA: **Thrombocytopenia, leukopenia, anemia**
INTEG: Rash, extravasation, dermatitis, reversible alopecia, urticaria, thrombophlebitis at inj site

Contraindications: Hypersensitivity, pregnancy **D**

Precautions: Renal and hepatic disease, gout, bone marrow depression, children

Do Not Confuse:
Idamycin/Adriamycin,
idarubicin/doxorubicin

Pharmacokinetics

Absorption	Complete bioavailability
Distribution	Rapidly distributed; high tissue binding
Metabolism	Liver, extensively
Excretion	Bile
Half-life	22 hr

Pharmacodynamics
Unknown

Interactions
Individual drugs
Radiation: ↑ toxicity, bone marrow suppression
Drug classifications
Antineoplastics: ↑ toxicity, bone marrow suppression
Live virus vaccines: ↓ antibody response
Lab test interferences
↑ Uric acid

NURSING CONSIDERATIONS
Assessment
• Assess symptoms indicating severe allergic reaction: rash, pruritus, urticaria, purpuric skin lesions, itching, flushing; drug should be discontinued
• Assess for tachypnea, ECG changes, dyspnea, edema, fatigue
• Assess for cardiac toxicity: CHF, dysrhythmias, cardiomyopathy; cardiac studies should be done prior to and periodically during treatment; ECG, chest x-ray
• Monitor CBC, differential, platelet count weekly; withhold drug if WBC count is <4000/mm^3 or platelet count is <100,000/mm^3; notify pre-

scriber of results if WBC <20,000/mm^3, platelets <150,000/mm^3
• Monitor temp q4h (may indicate beginning of infection)
• Monitor liver function tests before and during therapy (bilirubin, AST, ALT, LDH) as needed or monthly; note jaundice of skin and sclera, dark urine, clay-colored stools, itchy skin, abdominal pain, fever, diarrhea; hepatoxicity can be severe
• Assess for bleeding: hematuria, stool guaiac, bruising or petechiae, mucosa or orifices q8h; assess for inflammation of mucosa, breaks in skin
• Identify effects of alopecia on body image; discuss feelings about body changes

Nursing diagnoses
✓ Injury, risk for (adverse reactions)
✓ Cardiac output, decreased (adverse reactions)
✓ Body image disturbance (adverse reactions)
✓ Infection, risk for (adverse reactions)
✓ Knowledge deficit (teaching)

Implementation
• Avoid contact with skin; very irritating; wash completely to remove
• Give fluids **IV** or PO before chemotherapy to hydrate patient
• Administer antiemetic 30-60 min before giving drug and prn to prevent vomiting; administer antibiotics for prophylaxis of infection
• Give a liq diet: carbonated beverages; gelatin may be added if patient is not nauseated or vomiting
• Provide rinsing of mouth tid-qid with water, club soda;

brushing of teeth bid-qid with soft brush or cotton-tipped applicators for stomatitis; use unwaxed dental floss
• Drug should be prepared by experienced personnel using proper precautions (biologic cabinet, wearing gown, gloves, mask)
• Give after reconstituting 5-mg vial with 5 ml 0.9% NaCl (1 mg/1 ml); give over 10-15 min through Y-tube or 3-way stopcock of inf of D_5 or normal saline; discard unused portion
• Inject hydrocortisone for extravasation; apply ice compress after stopping inf
• Store at room temp for 3 days after reconstituting or 7 days refrigerated

Y-site compatibilities:
Amifostine, amikacin, aztreonam, cimetidine, cladribine, cyclophosphamide, cytarabine, diphenhydramine, droperidol, erythromycin, filgrastim, granisetron, imipenem/cilastatin, magnesium sulfate, mannitol, melphalan, metoclopramide, potassium chloride, ranitidine, sargramostim, thiotepa, vinorelbine

Y-site incompatibilities:
Acyclovir, ampicillin/sulbactam, cefazolin, ceftazidine, clindamycin, dexamethasone, etoposide, furosemide, gentamicin, hydrocortisone, lorazepam, meperidine, methotrexate, mezlocillin, sargramostim, sodium bicarbonate, vancomycin, vincristine

Solution compatibilities:
$D_{3.3}$/0.3% NaCl, D_5/0.9% NaCl, D_5W, Ringer's, 0.9% NaCl, LR

Patient/family education
• Teach patient to avoid use of products containing aspirin or ibuprofen, razors, commercial mouthwash, since bleeding may occur; to report symptoms of bleeding (hematuria, tarry stools)
• Instruct patient to report signs of anemia (fatigue, headache, irritability, faintness, shortness of breath)
• Advise patient that hair may be lost during treatment; a wig or hair piece may make patient feel better; new hair may be different in color, texture
• Tell patient not to have any vaccinations without the advice of the prescriber; serious reactions can occur
• Advise patient that contraception is needed during treatment and for several mo after the completion of therapy

Evaluation
Positive therapeutic outcome
• Prevention of rapid division of malignant cells

ifosfamide (℞)
(i-foss'fa-mide)
Ifex
Func. class.: Antineoplastic alkylating agent
Chem. class.: Nitrogen mustard
Pregnancy category   D

Action: Alkylates DNA, RNA; inhibits enzymes that allow synthesis of amino acids in proteins; also responsible for cross-linking DNA strands; activity is not cell cycle stage specific

---

☑ Herb/drug   ⬡ Do Not Crush   ◆ Alert   ☛ Key Drug   ⒢ Geriatric   ⒫ Pediatric

Therapeutic Outcome: Prevention of rapidly growing malignant cells

Uses: Testicular cancer

Dosage and routes
Adult: **IV** 1.2 g/m^2/day × 5 days; repeat course q3 wk; give with mesna

Available forms: Inj 1, 3 g

Adverse effects
CNS: Facial paresthesia, fever, malaise, somnolence, confusion, depression, hallucinations, dizziness, disorientation, **seizures, coma**
GI: Nausea, vomiting, anorexia, **hepatotoxicity,** stomatitis, constipation
GU: **Hematuria, nephrotoxicity, hemorrhagic cystitis,** dysuria, urinary frequency
HEMA: **Thrombocytopenia, leukopenia, anemia**
INTEG: Dermatitis, alopecia, pain at inj site

Contraindications: Hypersensitivity, bone marrow suppression, pregnancy **D**

Precautions: Renal disease, lactation, children

Pharmacokinetics

Absorption	Complete bioavailability
Distribution	Saturation at high dosages
Metabolism	Liver
Excretion	Breast milk
Half-life	15 hr

Pharmacodynamics
Unknown

Interactions
Individual drugs
Allopurinol: ↑ toxicity
Radiation: ↑ toxicity, bone marrow suppression
Drug classifications
Antineoplastics: ↑ toxicity, bone marrow suppression

Barbiturates: ↑ toxicity
Live virus vaccines: ↓ antibody response

NURSING CONSIDERATIONS
Assessment
• Monitor CBC, differential, platelet count weekly; withhold drug if WBC is <2000 or platelet count is <50,000; notify prescriber of results if WBC <10,000/mm^3, platelets <100,000/mm^3
• Monitor renal function studies: BUN, serum uric acid, urine CrCl before, during therapy; I&O ratio; report fall in urine output of 30 ml/hr
• Monitor for cold, fever, sore throat (may indicate beginning infection); identify edema in feet and joints, stomach pain, shaking; prescriber should be notified
• Assess for bleeding: hematuria, guaiac, bruising or petechiae, mucosa or orifices q8h; no rec temp
• Monitor liver function studies prior to and during therapy (ALT, AST, LDH); jaundice of skin, sclera, dark urine, clay-colored stools, itching, abdominal pain, fever, diarrhea

Nursing diagnoses
✓ Injury, risk for (adverse reactions)
✓ Body image disturbance (adverse reactions)
✓ Infection, risk for (adverse reactions)
✓ Knowledge deficit (teaching)

Implementation
• Give fluids **IV** or PO before chemotherapy to hydrate patient
• Give antiemetic 30-60 min before giving drug and prn to prevent vomiting

- Provide liq diet: carbonated beverages; gelatin may be added if patient is not nauseated or vomiting
- Give **IV** after diluting 1 g/20 ml sterile or bacteriostatic water for inj with parabens or benzyl only; shake
- Give by intermittent inf after further diluting with D$_5$W, LR, 0.9% NaCl, sterile water for inj (1 g/20 ml = 50 mg/ml); (1 g/50 ml = 20 mg/ml; 1 g/200 ml = 5 mg/ml); give over ≥30 min; may also give as a continuous infusion over 72 hr
- Store powder at room temp; always give with mesna, increase fluids to 3L/day to prevent ifosfamide-induced hemorrhagic cystitis

Syringe compatibilities:
Mesna

Y-site compatibilities:
Allopurinol, amifostine, aztreonam, filgrastim, fludarabine, gallium, granisetron, melphalan, ondansetron, paclitaxel, piperacillin/tazobactam, propofol, sargramostim, teniposide, thiotepa, vinorelbine

Additive compatibilities:
Carboplatin, cisplatin, etoposide, fluorouracil, mesna

Patient/family education
- Teach patient to avoid use of products containing aspirin or NSAIDs, razors, commercial mouthwash, since bleeding may occur; to report symptoms of bleeding (hematuria, tarry stools)
- Instruct patient to report signs of anemia (fatigue, headache, irritability, faintness, shortness of breath)
- Advise patient to report any changes in breathing or coughing even several mo after

treatment; to avoid crowds and persons with respiratory tract or other infections
- Teach patient that hair loss is common; discuss the use of wigs or hair pieces
- Caution patient not to have any vaccinations without the advice of the prescriber; serious reactions can occur
- Advise patient contraception is needed during treatment and for several mo after the completion of therapy

Evaluation
Positive therapeutic outcome
- Prevention of rapid division of malignant cells
- Absence of swelling at night
- Increased appetite, increased weight

imipenem/cilastatin (℞)
(i-me-pen'em sye-la-stat'in)
Primaxin IM, Primaxin IV
Func. class.: Antiinfective; miscellaneous penicillin
Pregnancy category   C

Action: Interferes with cell wall replication of susceptible organisms; osmotically unstable cell wall swells and bursts from osmotic pressure; addition of cilastatin prevents renal inactivation that occurs with high urinary concentrations of imipenem

Therapeutic Outcome: Bactericidal action against the following: *Streptococcus pneumoniae,* group A β-hemolytic streptococci, *Staphylococcus aureus,* enterococcus; gram-negative organisms: *Klebsiella, Proteus, Escherichia coli, Acinetobacter, Serratia, Pseudomonas*

---

aeruginosa; Salmonella, Shigella

Uses: Serious infections caused by gram-positive or gram-negative organisms

Dosage and routes
Adult: **IV** 250-500 mg q6h; severe infections may require 1 g q6h; may give IM q12h (total daily IM dose >1500 mg not recommended); mild to moderate infections

P *Child:* **IV** 60-100 mg/kg/day max 4 g/day

Renal dose
Renal adjustment is needed at CrCl <70 ml/min

Available forms: **IV** inj 250, 500; IM inj 500, 750 mg

Adverse effects
CNS: Fever, somnolence, *seizures,* confusion, dizziness, weakness
CV: Hypotension, palpitations
GI: Diarrhea, nausea, vomiting, **pseudomembranous colitis, hepatitis,** glossitis
HEMA: **Eosinophilia, neutropenia,** decreased HGb, Hct
INTEG: Rash, urticaria, pruritus, pain at inj site, phlebitis, erythema at inj site
RESP: Chest discomfort, dyspnea, hyperventilation
SYST: **Anaphylaxis**

Contraindications: Hypersensitivity, IM hypersensitivity to local anesthetics of the amide type

Precautions: Pregnancy **C**, **G** lactation, elderly, hypersensitivity to penicillins, seizure disor- **P** ders, renal disease, children

N **Do Not Confuse:**
imipenem/Omnipen, Primaxin/Premarin

Pharmacokinetics
Absorption	Complete bioavailability (**IV**)
Distribution	Widely distributed; crosses placenta
Metabolism	Liver
Excretion	Kidneys, unchanged (70%-80%); breast milk
Half-life	1 hr; increased in renal disease

Pharmacodynamics
	IV	IM
Onset	Rapid	Unknown
Peak	½-1 hr	Unknown

Interactions
Individual drugs
Ganciclovir: ↑ risk of seizures
Probenecid: ↓ renal excretion, ↑ blood level
Drug classifications
β-Lactam antibiotics: ↑ toxicity
Cephalosporins: ↓ action
Penicillins: ↓ action
Lab test interferences
False: ↑ Creatinine (serum urine), ↑ urinary 17-KS
False positive: Urinary protein, direct Coombs' test, urine glucose
Interference: Cross-matching

NURSING CONSIDERATIONS
Assessment
• Assess patient for previous sensitivity reaction
• Assess patient for signs and symptoms of infection, including characteristics of wounds, sputum, urine, stool, WBC >10,000, fever; obtain baseline information before and during treatment
• Complete C&S tests before beginning drug therapy to identify if correct treatment has been initiated
• Assess for allergic reactions: rash, urticaria, pruritus, chills,

wheezing, laryngeal edema, fever, joint pain; angioedema may occur a few days after therapy begins; epinephrine, resuscitation equipment should be available for anaphylactic reaction

• Identify urine output; if decreasing, notify prescriber (may indicate nephrotoxicity); also check for increased BUN, creatinine

• Monitor blood studies: AST, ALT, CBC, Hct, bilirubin, LDH, alkaline phosphatase, Coombs' test monthly if patient is on long-term therapy

• Monitor electrolytes: potassium, sodium, chloride monthly if patient is on long-term therapy

• Assess bowel pattern qd; if severe diarrhea occurs, drug should be discontinued; may indicate pseudomembranous colitis

• Monitor for bleeding: ecchymosis, bleeding gums, hematuria, stool guaiac daily if on long-term therapy

• Assess for overgrowth of infection: perineal itching, fever, malaise, redness, pain, swelling, drainage, rash, diarrhea, change in cough, sputum

Nursing diagnoses
☑ Infection, risk for (uses)
☑ Diarrhea (adverse reactions)
☑ Injury, risk for (adverse reactions)
☑ Knowledge deficit (teaching)
☑ Noncompliance (teaching)

Implementation
IM route
• Reconstitute 500 mg/2 ml or 750 mg/3 ml lidocaine without epinephrine; shake well, withdraw and administer entire vial; give deep in large muscle mass, massage

IV route
• Reconstitute each 250 or 500 mg/10 ml of compatible diluent; shake well; transfer the resulting susp to not less than 100 ml of compatible diluent; add 10 ml to each previously reconstituted vial and shake to ensure all medication is used; transfer the remaining contents of the vial to the inf container; do not administer susp by direct inj; reconstitute 120-ml inf bottles/100 ml of a compatible diluent; shake until clear; may use 0.9% NaCl, D_5W, $D_{10}W$, D_5/0.2% sodium bicarbonate, D_5/0.9% NaCl, D_5/0.45% NaCl, D_5/0.225% NaCl, mannitol 2.5%, 5%, or 10%

• Give by intermittent inf: each 250- or 500-mg dose over 20-30 min, and each 1-g dose over 40-60 min; administer over 15-20 min for pediatric patients; do not administer direct **IV**; do not admix with other antibiotics

Y-site compatibilities:
Acyclovir, amifostine, aztreonam, cefepime, diltiazem, famotidine, fludarabine, foscarnet, granisetron, idarubicin, regular insulin, melphalan, methotrexate, ondansetron, propofol, tacrolimus, teniposide, thiotepa, vinorelbine, zidovudine

Y-site incompatibilities:
Fluconazole, meperidine, sargramostim

Additive incompatibilities:
Fluconazole, meperidine, sargramostim

Patient/family education
• Teach patient to report sore throat, bruising, bleeding,

---

joint pain; may indicate blood dyscrasias (rare)

• Advise patient to contact prescriber if vaginal itching, loose, foul-smelling stools, furry tongue occur; may indicate superinfection

• Advise patient to notify prescriber of diarrhea with blood or pus, which may indicate pseudomembranous colitis

Evaluation

Positive therapeutic outcome

• Absence of signs/symptoms of infection (WBC <10,000, temp WNL, absence of red, draining wounds)

• Reported improvement in symptoms of infection

Treatment of anaphylaxis: Epinephrine, antihistamines, resuscitate if needed

---

imipramine ⚖ (℞)

(im-ip'ra-meen)
Apo-Imipramine ✦, Imipramine HCl, Impril ✦, Janimine, Novo-Pramine ✦, SK-Pramine, Tipramine, Tofranil, Tofranil PM

Func. class.: Antidepressant, tricyclic
Chem. class.: Dibenzazepine, tertiary amine

Pregnancy category C

Action: Blocks reuptake of norepinephrine and serotonin into nerve endings, increasing action of norepinephrine and serotonin in nerve cells; has anticholinergic effects

➧Therapeutic Outcome: Decreased symptoms of depression after 2-3 wk; decreased bedwetting in children

Uses: Depression, enuresis in children

Investigational uses: Chronic pain, migraine headaches, cluster headaches as adjunct, incontinence

Dosage and routes

Adult: PO/IM 75-100 mg/day in divided doses; may increase by 25-50 mg up to 200 mg, not to exceed 300 mg/day; may give daily dose hs

Elderly: PO 25 mg hs, may increase to 100 mg/day in divided doses

Child: PO 25-75 mg/day

Enuresis

Child: PO 10 mg at hs, max 50 mg

Available forms: Tabs 10, 25, 50 mg; inj 25 mg/2 ml; caps 75, 100, 125, 150 mg

Adverse effects

CV: Orthostatic hypotension, ECG changes, tachycardia, hypertension, palpitations
CNS: Dizziness, drowsiness, confusion, headache, anxiety, tremors, stimulation, weakness, insomnia, nightmares, extrapyramidal symptoms (elderly), increased psychiatric symptoms, paresthesia
EENT: Blurred vision, tinnitus, mydriasis
GI: Diarrhea, dry mouth, nausea, vomiting, **paralytic ileus,** increased appetite, cramps, epigastric distress, jaundice, **hepatitis,** stomatitis
GU: Retention, **acute renal failure**
HEMA: **Agranulocytosis, thrombocytopenia, eosinophilia, leukopenia**
INTEG: Rash, urticaria, sweating, pruritus, photosensitivity

✦ Canada Only   Adverse effects: *italic* = common; **bold** = life-threatening

Contraindications: Hypersensitivity to tricyclic antidepressants, recovery phase of MI, convulsive disorders, prostatic hypertrophy

Precautions: Suicidal patients, severe depression, increased intraocular pressure, narrow-angle glaucoma, urinary retention, cardiac disease, hepatic disease, hyperthyroidism, electroshock therapy, elective **G** surgery, elderly, pregnancy **C**

Pharmacokinetics

Absorption	Well absorbed
Distribution	Widely distributed; crosses placenta
Metabolism	Liver, extensively
Excretion	Kidneys, breast milk
Half-life	6-20 hr

Pharmacodynamics

	PO	IM
Onset	1 hr	1 hr
Peak	Unknown	Unknown
Duration	Unknown	Unknown

Interactions
Individual drugs
Alcohol: ↑ CNS depression
Cimetidine: ↑ levels, toxicity
Clonidine: Severe hypotension; avoid use
Disulfiram: Organic brain syndrome
Fluoxetine: ↑ levels, toxicity
Guanethidine: ↓ effects
Drug classifications
Analgesics: ↑ CNS depression
Anticholinergics: ↑ side effects
Antihistamines: ↑ CNS depression
Antihypertensives: May block antihypertensive effect
Barbiturates: ↑ effects
Benzodiazepines: ↑ effects
CNS depressants: ↑ effects
MAOIs: Hypertensive crisis, convulsions

Oral contraceptives: ↑ effects, toxicity
Phenothiazines: ↑ toxicity
Sedative/hypnotics: ↑ CNS depression
Sympathomimetics, indirect acting: ↓ effects
☑ Herb/drug
Belladonna: ↑ anticholinergic effect
Henbane: ↑ anticholinergic effect
Kava: ↑ imipramine action
Scopolia: ↑ imipramine action
Smoking
↑ metabolism, ↓ effects
Lab test interferences
↑ Serum bilirubin, ↑ blood glucose, ↑ alkaline phosphatase
↓ VMA, ↓ 5-HIAA, ↓ blood glucose
False: ↑ Urinary catecholamines

NURSING CONSIDERATIONS
Assessment
• Monitor B/P (with patient lying, standing), pulse q4h; if systolic B/P drops 20 mm Hg, hold drug, notify prescriber; take vital signs q4h in patients with cardiovascular disease
• Monitor blood studies: CBC, leukocytes, differential, cardiac enzymes if patient is receiving long-term therapy
• Monitor hepatic studies: AST, ALT, bilirubin
• Check weight weekly; appetite may increase with drug
• Assess ECG for flattening of T wave, bundle branch block, AV block, dysrhythmias in cardiac patients
• Assess for extrapyramidal
G symptoms primarily in elderly: rigidity, dystonia, akathisia
• Assess mental status: mood, sensorium, affect, suicidal tendencies; increase in psychi-

---

☑ Herb/drug   🚫 Do Not Crush   ◆ Alert   🔑 Key Drug   **G** Geriatric   **P** Pediatric

atric symptoms: depression, panic
• Monitor urinary retention, constipation; constipation is ⓟ more likely to occur in children ⓖ or elderly
◆• Assess for withdrawal symptoms: headache, nausea, vomiting, muscle pain, weakness; do not usually occur unless drug was discontinued abruptly
• Identify alcohol consumption; if alcohol is consumed, hold dose until AM

Nursing diagnoses
☑ Coping, ineffective individual (uses)
☑ Injury, risk for physical (side effects)
☑ Knowledge deficit (teaching)
☑ Noncompliance (teaching)

Implementation
PO route
• Give with food or milk
⊘• Do not crush, chew caps
• Store at room temp; do not freeze
IM route
• Put ampule under warm running water for 1 min to dissolve crystals; sol may be yellow or red

Syringe compatibilities:
Doxapram

Y-site compatibilities:
Cladribine

Patient/family education
• Teach patient that therapeutic effects may take 2-3 wk
• Teach patient to use caution in driving and other activities requiring alertness because of drowsiness, dizziness, blurred vision; to avoid rising quickly from sitting position, especially ⓖ elderly
• Teach patient to avoid alcohol ingestion, other CNS depressants
• Teach patient not to discontinue medication quickly after long-term use: may cause nausea, headache, malaise
• Teach patient to wear sunscreen or large hat, since photosensitivity occurs
• Teach patient to increase fluids, bulk in diet if constipation, urinary retention occur, ⓖ especially elderly
• Teach patient to take gum, hard sugarless candy, or frequent sips of water for dry mouth

Evaluation
Positive therapeutic outcome
• Decreased depression
• Absence of suicidal thoughts
ⓟ• Decreased enuresis in children
• Decreased pain

Treatment of overdose:
ECG monitoring, induce emesis, lavage, activated charcoal, administer anticonvulsant

---

immune globulin (℞)
gamma globulin, Gamimune N, Gammagard S/D, Gammar-P I.V., Iveegam, polygam, polygam S/D, Sandoglobulin, Venoglobulin-I, immune serum globulin
Func. class.: Immune serum
Chem. class.: IgG
Pregnancy category **C**

Action: Provides passive immunity to hepatitis A, measles, varicella, rubella, immune globulin deficiency; contains γ-globulin antibodies (IgG)

➔**Therapeutic Outcome:** Absence of infection

Uses: Immunodeficiency syndrome, B-cell chronic lymphocytic leukemia, Kawasaki syndrome, bone marrow transplantation, pediatric HIV infection, agammaglobulinemia, hepatitis A, B exposure, measles exposure, measles vaccine complications, purpura, rubella exposure, chickenpox exposure

Dosage and routes
Adult: IM 30-50 ml q mo; **IV** 100 mg/kg q mo, 0.01-0.02 ml/kg/min over 30 min (Gamimune); **IV** 200 mg/kg qmo, 0.05-1 ml/min over 15-30 min, then increase to 1.5-2.5 ml/min (Sandoglobulin)

P *Child:* IM 20-40 ml q mo

Hepatitis A exposure
P *Adult and child:* IM 0.02-0.04 ml/kg or 0.1 mg/kg if treatment is delayed

Hepatitis B exposure
P *Adult and child:* IM 0.06 ml/kg within 1 wk, q mo

Measles (postexposure)
P *Child:* IM 0.25 ml/kg within 6 days

Immunoglobulin deficiency
P *Adult and child:* IM 1.3 ml/kg, then 0.66 ml/kg after 2-4 wk and q2-4 wk thereafter

Idiopathic thrombocytopenic purpura
P *Adult and child:* **IV** 0.4 g/kg/day × 5 days or 1g/kg/day × 1-2 days

Kawasaki syndrome
P *Child:* PO 2g/kg as a single dose

Available forms: IM inj 2, 10 ml/vial; **IV** inj 5% sol, 0.5, 1, 2.5, 3, 6, 10 g vials

Adverse effects
CNS: Headache, fatigue, malaise
GI: Abdominal pain
INTEG: Pain at inj site, rash, pruritus, chills, chest pain
MS: Arthralgia
SYST: Lymphadenopathy, **anaphylaxis**

Contraindications: Hypersensitivity

Precautions: Pregnancy **C**

Pharmacokinetics	
Absorption	Well absorbed (IM); completely absorbed (**IV**)
Distribution	Rapidly
Metabolism	Liver, catabolism
Excretion	Kidneys
Half-life	3-4 wk

Pharmacodynamics		
	IM	IV
Onset	Unknown	Rapid
Peak	Unknown	Unknown
Duration	Unknown	Unknown

Interactions
Live virus vaccines: Do not give within 3 mo

NURSING CONSIDERATIONS
Assessment
• Assess for exposure date: this drug should be given within 6 days of measles, 1 wk of hepatitis B, 14 days of hepatitis A; if the date of exposure is outside these limits, immune globulin will not be effective
• Monitor blood studies in leukemia, idiopathic thrombocytopenic purpura: WBCs (leukemia), platelets
• Identify the number of inj of this drug the patient has

received; multiple inj may lead to sensitization (diaphoresis, fever, chills, malaise)
• Assess for anaphylaxis in patient receiving **IV** immune globulin: diaphoresis, flushing, nausea, vomiting, wheezing, difficulty breathing, hypotension, chest tightness, fever, weakness, sneezing, abdominal pain; VS should be monitored during inf and 1 hr after beginning inf; emergency equipment should be available with epinephrine and antihistamines to treat anaphylaxis

Nursing diagnoses
☑ Infection, risk for (uses)
☑ Knowledge deficit (teaching)

Implementation

IM route
• Give IM (IGIM) in deltoid or anterolateral thigh in adults or anterolateral thigh in young children; if large amounts are given, several inj may be needed
• Do not give the IM preparation **IV**, SC, or intradermally
• Sol should be transparent and clear or slightly colored

IV route
• Warm to room temp before administration (diluent, powder for inj)
• A transfer device is provided by manufacturer; this drug should not be agitated or shaken
• Do not give the **IV** preparation SC, IM, or intradermally
• Check for adverse reaction during inf; stop inf if adverse reactions are present

Y-site compatibilities: Fluconazole, sargramostim

Gamimune N: Dilute **IV** with D$_5$; give 0.01 ml/kg/min; may increase to 0.02-0.04 ml/kg/min if no adverse reactions are present; may increase to 0.08 ml/kg/hr; sol should be refrigerated; do not freeze

Gammagard: Reconstitute with sterile water for inj (50 mg protein/ml); give within 2 hr of reconstitution; give 0.5 ml/kg/hr; may increase to 4 ml/kg/hr if no adverse reactions occur; use inf set provided

Gammar-IV: Give 0.01 ml/kg/min (50 mg/ml sol) over 15-30 min; may increase to 0.02 ml/kg/min; if adverse reactions are not present, may increase to 0.03-0.06 ml/kg/min; do not freeze; store at room temp

Iveegam (5%): Give 1-2 ml/min; refrigerate, do not freeze

Sandoglobulin: IV diluted with provided diluent; give 0.5-1 ml/min over 15-30 min; may increase to 1.5-2.5 ml/min; other inf may be given 2-2.5 ml/min; store at room temp

Venoglobulin-I: Give 50 mg/ml sol 0.01-0.02 ml/kg/min over 30 min if no adverse reactions; increase 0.04 ml/kg/min; store at room temp

Patient/family education
• Advise patient that passive immunity is temporary; explain reason for and expected results of this drug
• Advise patient that pain and tenderness may occur at inj site

Evaluation

Positive therapeutic outcome
• Prevention of infection
• Increased platelets

Adverse effects: *italic* = common; **bold** = life-threatening

Treatment of anaphylaxis:
Epinephrine, diphenhydramine, O_2, vasopressors, corticosteroids

---

inamrinone
See amrinone

---

indapamide (℞)
(in-dap'a-mide)
indapamide, Lozide ✦,
Lozol
Func. class.: Diuretic,
thiazide-like, antihypertensive
Chem. class.: Thiazide-like
sulfonamide derivative

Pregnancy category   B

Action: Acts on the distal
tubule and thick ascending
loop of Henle in the kidney,
increasing excretion of sodium,
water, chloride, magnesium,
potassium, and bicarbonate

⮞**Therapeutic Outcome:** Decreased B/P, decreased edema
in lung tissues, peripherally

Uses: May be used alone or as
adjunct with antihypertensives
(mild to moderate)

Dosage and routes
Edema
Adult: PO 2.5 mg qd in AM;
may be increased to 5 mg qd if
needed

Antihypertensive
Adult: PO 1.25-5 mg qd; may
increase to 5 mg/day over 8
wks

Available forms: Tabs 1.25,
2.5 mg

Adverse effects
CNS: Depression, *headache,
dizziness, fatigue, weakness,
nervousness, agitation*

CV: Orthostatic hypotension,
palpitations, volume depletion,
PVCs
EENT: Blurred vision, nasal
congestion, increased intraocular pressure
ELECT: Hypokalemia, hypercalcemia, hyponatremia, hypochloremia, hypomagnesemia
GI: Nausea, vomiting, anorexia, constipation, diarrhea,
cramps, GI irritation, abdominal pain
GU: Frequency, polyuria, nocturia
INTEG: Rash, *pruritus,*
META: Hyperglycemia, *hyperuricemia,* increased creatinine,
BUN
MS: Cramps

Contraindications: Hypersensitivity to thiazides or sulfonamides, anuria, lactation, hepatic coma

Precautions: Hypokalemia,
renal disease, hepatic disease,
ⓖ gout, diabetes mellitus, elderly,
ascites, dehydration, pregnancy **B**, lactation, CrCl <25
ml/min (not effective)

Pharmacokinetics

Absorption	Well absorbed
Distribution	Widely distributed
Metabolism	Liver; 7%
Excretion	Unchanged (urine)
Half-life	14-18 hr

Pharmacodynamics

Onset	1-2 hr
Peak	2 hr
Duration	Up to 36 hr

Interactions
Individual drugs
Alcohol: ↑ hypotension
Amphotericin B: ↓ effects
Lithium: ↑ toxicity
Mezlocillin: ↑ hypokalemia
Piperacillin: ↑ hypokalemia
Ticarcillin: ↑ hypokalemia

Drug classifications
Anticoagulants: ↓ effects
Antigout agents: ↓ effects
Antihypertensives: ↑ antihypertensive effect
Cardiac glycosides: ↑ hypokalemia, ↑ toxicity
Glucocorticoids: ↑ hypokalemia

☑ *Herb/drug*
Aloe: ↑ hypokalemia
Buckthorn: ↑ hypokalemia
Licorice: ↑ hypokalemia
Senna: ↑ hypokalemia

Lab test interferences
↑ Calcium, ↑ parathyroid test

NURSING CONSIDERATIONS
Assessment
• Check for rashes, temp elevation qd
• Monitor patients that receive cardiac glycosides for increased hypokalemia, toxicity
• Monitor manifestations of hypokalemia: acidic or reduced urine, osmolality, nocturia; hypotension, broad T wave, U wave, ectopy, tachycardia, weak pulse; muscle weakness, altered LOC, drowsiness, apathy, lethargy, confusion, depression; anorexia, nausea, cramps, constipation, distention, paralytic ileus; hypoventilation, respiratory muscle weakness
• Monitor for manifestations of hypomagnesemia: agitation, muscle twitching, paresthesias, hyperactive reflexes, positive Babinski reflex, dysphagia, nystagmus, seizures, tetany; nausea, vomiting, diarrhea, anorexia, abdominal distention; ectopy, tachycardia, broad, flat or inverted T waves, depressed ST segment, prolonged QT, decreased cardiac output, hypotension
• Monitor for manifestations of hyponatremia: increased B/P, cold, clammy skin, hypovolemia or hypervolemia; anorexia, nausea, vomiting, diarrhea, abdominal cramps; lethargy, increased ICP, confusion, headache, seizures, coma, fatigue, tremors, hyperreflexia
• Monitor for manifestations of hyperchloremia: weakness, lethargy, coma, deep rapid breathing
• Assess fluid volume status: I&O ratios and record, weight, distended red veins, crackles in lung, color, quality and sp gr of urine, skin turgor, adequacy of pulses, moist mucous membranes, bilateral lung sounds, peripheral pitting edema; dehydration symptoms of decreasing output, thirst, hypotension, dry mouth and mucous membranes should be reported
• Monitor electrolytes: potassium, sodium, calcium, magnesium; also include BUN, blood pH, ABGs, uric acid, CBC, blood sugar
• Assess B/P before and during therapy with patient lying, standing, and sitting as appropriate; orthostatic hypotension can occur rapidly

Nursing diagnoses
☑ Altered urinary elimination (side effect)
☑ Fluid volume deficit (side effects)
☑ Fluid volume excess (uses)
☑ Knowledge deficit (teaching)

Implementation
• Give in AM to avoid interference with sleep
• Provide potassium replacement if potassium level is <3.0; give whole
• Give with food; if nausea occurs, absorption may be increased

---

♣ Canada Only   Adverse effects: *italic* = common; **bold** = life-threatening

Patient/family education
• Teach patient to take the medication early in the day to prevent nocturia
• Instruct the patient to take with food or milk if GI symptoms of nausea and anorexia occur
• Teach patient to maintain weekly record of weight and notify prescriber of weight loss >5 lb
• Caution the patient that this drug causes a loss of potassium, so food rich in potassium should be added to the diet; refer to a dietician for assistance in planning
• Caution the patient not to exercise in hot weather or stand for prolonged periods, since orthostatic hypotension will be enhanced
• Teach patient not to use alcohol or any OTC medications without prescriber's approval; serious drug reactions may occur
• Emphasize the need to contact prescriber immediately if muscle cramps, weakness, nausea, dizziness, or numbness occurs
• Teach patient to take own B/P and pulse and record findings
• Caution the patient that orthostatic hypotension may occur and to rise slowly from sitting or reclining positions and lie down if dizziness occurs
• Teach patient to continue taking medication even if feeling better; this drug controls symptoms but does not cure the condition
• Advise the patient with hypertension to continue other medical treatment (exercise, weight loss, relaxation techniques, cessation of smoking)

Evaluation
Positive therapeutic outcome
• Decreased edema
• Decreased B/P
• Increased diuresis

Treatment of overdose:
Lavage, monitor electrolytes, administer **IV** fluids, monitor hydration, CV, renal status

---

indinavir (℞)
(en-den'a-veer)
Crixivan
Func. class.: Antiviral
Chem. class.: Synthetic peptide-like substrate analog

Pregnancy category   C

Action: Inhibits human immunodeficiency virus (HIV) protease, this prevents maturation of the infectious virus

➡**Therapeutic Outcome:**
Decreased signs/symptoms of HIV infection

Uses: HIV alone or in combination

Dosage and routes
Reduce dose in mild/moderate hepatic impairment and ketoconazole co-administration
Adult: PO 800 mg q8hr; if given with ddI, given 1 hr apart on empty stomach

Available forms: Caps 200, 400 mg

Adverse effects
CNS: Headache, insomnia, dizziness, somnolence
GI: Diarrhea, abdominal pain, nausea, vomiting, anorexia, dry mouth
INTEG: Rash
MS: Pain
OTHER: Asthenia

Contraindications: Hypersensitivity

Precautions: Liver disease, **P** pregnancy C, lactation, children, renal disease

Pharmacokinetics

Absorption	Unknown
Distribution	Unknown
Metabolism	Unknown
Excretion	Unknown
Half-life	Unknown

Pharmacodynamics

Unknown

Interactions
Individual drugs
Clarithromycin: ↑ levels of both drugs
Isoniazid: ↑ level of isoniazid
Ketoconazole: ↑ levels of both drugs
Midazolam: ↑ life-threatening dysrhythmias
Triazolam: ↑ life-threatening dysrhythmias
Drug classifications
Ergots: ↑ life-threatening dysrhythmias
Rifamycins: ↑ life-threatening dysrhythmias

Food/drug
High fat, high protein: ↓ absorption
Grapefruit: ↓ absorption

NURSING CONSIDERATIONS
Assessment
• Monitor signs of infection, anemia
• Monitor liver studies: ALT, AST
• Determine the presence of other sexually transmitted diseases
• Assess bowel pattern before, during treatment; if severe abdominal pain with bleeding occurs, drug should be discontinued; monitor hydration

• Assess skin eruptions; rash, urticaria, itching
• Assess allergies before treatment, reaction of each medication; place allergies on chart

Nursing diagnoses
☑ Infection, risk for (uses)
☑ Knowledge deficit (teaching)

Implementation
• Give with water, 1 hr ac or 2 hr pc

Patient/family education
• Advise to take as prescribed; if dose is missed, take as soon as remembered up to 1 hr before next dose; do not double dose
⊘ • Do not crush, chew caps
• Advise that drug must be taken in equal intervals around the clock to maintain blood levels for duration of therapy

Evaluation
Positive therapeutic outcome
• Decreased signs/symptoms of infection

---

indomethacin (℞)
(in-doe-meth'a-sin)
Apo-Indomethacin ✦,
Indameth ✦, Indocid ✦,
Indocin PDA ✦,
Novomethacin ✦,
indomethacin, Indocin,
Indocin SR, Indocin IV
Func. class.: NSAID
Chem. class.: Propionic acid derivative
Pregnancy category **B**

Action: Inhibits prostaglandin synthesis by decreasing enzyme needed for biosynthesis; analgesic, antiinflammatory, antipyretic

➔**Therapeutic Outcome:** Decreased pain, inflammation; or

---

closure of patent ductus
P arteriosus (premature infants)

Uses: Rheumatoid arthritis,
ankylosing rheumatoid spondylitis, acute gouty arthritis,
closure of patent ductus arteri-
P osus in premature infants

Dosage and routes
Arthritis/antiinflammatory
Adult: PO/rec 25-50 mg
bid-tid; may increase by 25
mg/day q wk, not to exceed
200 mg/day; sus rel 75 mg qd;
may increase to 75 mg bid

Acute arthritis
Adult: PO/rec 50 mg tid; use
only for acute attack, then
reduce dosage

Patent ductus arteriosus
Longer or repeated treatment
courses may be necessary for
P very premature infants

P *Infant <2 days:* **IV** 0.2 mg/
kg, then 0.1 mg/kg q12-24h

P *Infant 2-7 days:* **IV** 0.2 mg/
kg, then 0.2 mg × 2 doses after
12, 24 hr

P *Infant >7 days:* **IV** 0.2 mg/
kg, then 0.25 mg/kg × 2 doses
after 12, 24 hr

Available forms: Caps 25, 50
mg; sus rel cap 75 mg; oral
susp 25 mg/5 ml; rec supp 50
mg; inj 1 mg vials

Adverse effects
CNS: Dizziness, drowsiness,
fatigue, tremors, confusion,
insomnia, anxiety, depression,
headache
CV: Tachycardia, peripheral
edema, palpitations, dysrhythmias, hypertension
EENT: Tinnitus, hearing loss,
blurred vision
GI: Nausea, anorexia, *vomiting,* diarrhea, jaundice, **cholestatic hepatitis,** *constipation,*
flatulence, cramps, dry mouth,

peptic ulcer, **ulceration, perforation, GI bleeding**
GU: **Nephrotoxicity (dysuria,
hematuria, oliguria, azotemia)**
HEMA: **Blood dyscrasias,**
prolonged bleeding
INTEG: Purpura, rash, pruritus, sweating

Contraindications: Hypersensitivity, asthma, severe renal
disease, severe hepatic disease,
ulcer disease

Precautions: Lactation,
P children, bleeding disorders,
GI disorders, cardiac disorders,
hypersensitivity to other antiinflammatory agents, pregnancy
B (1st and 2nd trimesters),
depression

Pharmacokinetics	
Absorption	Well absorbed (PO); erratic (rec); complete (**IV**)
Distribution	Crosses blood-brain barrier; placenta, 99% plasma protein binding
Metabolism	Liver, extensively
Excretion	Breast milk
Half-life	2.6-11 hr

Pharmacodynamics			
	IV	PO	PO– EXT REL
Onset	2 day	1-2 hr	½ hr
Peak	Un-known	3 hr	Un-known
Dura-tion	Un-known	4-6 hr	4-6 hr

Interactions
Individual drugs
**Acetaminophen (long-term
use):** ↑ renal reactions
Alcohol: ↑ adverse reactions
Aspirin: ↓ effectiveness, ↑ ad-
verse reactions of indometha-
cin
Cyclosporine: ↑ nephrotoxi-
city
Digoxin: ↑ toxicity, levels

Insulin: ↓ insulin effect
Lithium: ↑ toxicity, levels
Methotrexate: ↑ toxicity
Phenytoin: ↑ toxicity
Probenecid: ↑ toxicity
Radiation: ↑ risk of hematologic toxicity
Triamterene: ↑ toxicity
Zidovudine: ↑ toxicity, levels

Drug classifications

Aminoglycosides: ↑ toxicity
Anticoagulants: ↑ risk of bleeding
Antihypertensives: ↓ effect of antihypertensives
Antineoplastics: ↑ risk of hematologic toxicity
β-Adrenergic blockers: ↑ antihypertension
Cephalosporins: ↑ risk of bleeding
Diuretics: ↓ effectiveness of diuretics
Glucocorticoids: ↑ adverse reactions
Hypoglycemics: ↓ hypoglycemic effect
NSAIDs: ↑ adverse reactions
Potassium supplements: ↑ adverse reactions
Sulfonamides: ↑ toxicity
Sulfonylureas: ↑ toxicity

NURSING CONSIDERATIONS
Assessment
* Assess for joint pain (duration, intensity, ROM), baseline and during treatment
* Assess for confusion, mood changes, hallucinations, especially in elderly
* Assess renal, liver, blood studies: BUN, creatinine, AST, ALT, Hgb before treatment and periodically thereafter; if renal function is ↓, do not give subsequent doses

Nursing diagnoses
☑ Pain (uses)
☑ Chronic pain (uses)
☑ Impaired mobility (uses)
☑ Knowledge deficit (teaching)

Implementation
PO route
🚫 • Administer to patient whole; do not crush, chew, or break sus rel cap
* Give with food or milk to decrease gastric symptoms, and prevent ulceration

Ⅳ IV route
* Give after diluting 1 mg/ml or more normal saline or sterile water for inj without preservative; give over ½ hr to avoid dramatic shift in cerebral blood flow; avoid extravasation

Y-site compatibilities:
Furosemide, insulin (regular), potassium chloride, sodium bicarbonate, sodium nitroprusside

Rec route
* Have patient retain rec supp for 1 hr after insertion

Patient/family education
* Advise patient to report change in vision, blurring, rash, tinnitus, black stools
* Tell patient not to use for any other condition than prescribed
* Advise patient to avoid use with OTC medications for pain unless approved by prescriber
* Advise patient to avoid hazardous activities, since dizziness or drowsiness can occur
* Instruct patient to use sunscreen to prevent photosensitivity

Evaluation
Positive therapeutic outcome
* Decreased stiffness
* Increased joint mobility
* Decreased pain

---

infliximab (℞)
(in-fliks'ih-mab)
Remicade
Func. class.: Monoclonal antibody
Pregnancy category   C

Action: Monoclonal antibody that neutralizes the activity of tumor necrosis factor alpha (TNFα) that has been found in Crohn's disease; decreased infiltration of inflammatory cells

➡ **Therapeutic Outcome:** Decreased cramping and blood in stools

Uses: Crohn's disease; fistulizing, moderate-severe

Dosage and routes
Crohn's disease (moderate-severe)
Adult: IV inf 5 mg/kg

Crohn's disease (fistulizing)
Adult: IV inf 5 mg/kg initially, then repeat dose 2 wk, 6 wk after 1st dose

Available forms: Powder for inj 100 mg

Adverse effects
CNS: Headache, dizziness, depression, vertigo, fatigue, anxiety, fever
CV: Chest pain, hypertension and hypotension, tachycardia
GU: Dysuria, frequency
HEMA: **Anemia**
INTEG: Rash, dermatitis, urticaria, dry skin, sweating, flushing, hematoma, pruritus
MS: Myalgia, back pain, arthralgia
RESP: URI, pharyngitis, bronchitis, cough, dyspnea, sinusitis
SYST: **Anaphylaxis**

Contraindications: Hypersensitivity to murines

P **Precautions:** Pregnancy **C,**
G lactation, children, elderly

Pharmacokinetics	
Absorption	Unknown
Distribution	Vascular compartment
Metabolism	Unknown
Excretion	Unknown
Half-life	9½ days

Pharmacodynamics	
Onset	Unknown
Peak	Unknown
Duration	Unknown

Interactions: Unknown

NURSING CONSIDERATIONS
Assessment
• Assess GI symptoms: nausea, vomiting, abdominal pain
• Take periodic blood counts: CBC
• Assess CV status: B/P, pulse, chest pain
• Assess for allergic reaction: rash, dermatitis, urticaria, fever, chills, dyspnea, hypotention; discontinue if severe, administer epinephrine corticosteroids
Nursing diagnoses
☑ Injury, risk for (uses)
☑ Diarrhea (uses)
☑ Knowledge deficit (teaching)
Implementation
IV inf route
• Administer immediately after reconstitution; reconstitute with 10 ml of sterile water for inj, further dilute total dose/ 250 ml 0.9% NaCl inj to a total conc of between 0.4 and 4 mg/ml; use 21G or smaller needle for reconstitution, direct sterile water at glass wall of vial, gently swirl
• Give over ≥2 hr, use polyethylene-lined infusion with in-line, sterile, low-protein-bind filter

• Provide refrigerated storage, do not freeze

Patient/family education
• Teach patient not to breast-feed while taking this drug
• Advise patient to notify prescriber of GI symptoms, hypersensitivity reactions

Evaluation
Positive therapeutic outcome
• Absence of blood in stool
• Reported improvement in comfort
• Weight gain

INSULINS

insulin, isophane suspension (NPH) ⊘π (℞)
Humulin N, Iletin NPH, Iletin II NPH ✿, Novolin ge NPH ✿, Novolin N, Novolin N PenFill, Novolin N Prefilled, NPH Iletin I, NPH Iletin II, NPH-N

insulin, isophane suspension and regular insulin (℞)
Humulin 70/30, Humalin 30/70 ✿, Novolin 70/30, Novolin 70/30 PenFill, Novolin 7/30 Prefilled, Novolin ge 30/70 ✿

insulin, regular ⊘π (℞)
Humulin R, Iletin I, Iletin II ✿, Novolin ge Toronto ✿, Novolin R, Novolin R PenFill, Novolin R Prefilled, Novolin R Velosulin, Regular Illetin I, Regular Illetin II, regular purified pork insulin, Velosulin Human BR

insulin lispro
Humalog

insulin, zinc suspension (lente) (℞)
Humulin L, Iletin ✿, Iletin II ✿, Lente Iletin I, Lente Iletin II, Lente L, Novolin ge Lente ✿, Novolin L

insulin, zinc suspension extended (ultralente) (℞)
Humulin U ✿, Humulin U Ultralente, Novolin ge Ultralente

isophane insulin suspension and insulin injection (℞)
Humalin 50/50, Novolin ge 50/50 ✿,

Func. class.: Pancreatic hormone
Chem. class.: Exogenous unmodified insulin
Pregnancy category   B

✿ Canada Only   Adverse effects: *italic* = common; **bold** = life-threatening

Action: Decreases blood sugar; by transport of insulin into cells and the conversion of glucose to glycogen indirectly increases blood pyruvate and lactate, decreases phosphate and potassium; insulin may be beef, pork, human (processed by recombinant DNA technologies)

⟞**Therapeutic Outcome:** Decreased blood glucose levels in diabetes mellitus

Uses: Adult-onset diabetes, juvenile diabetes, ketoacidosis types I and II, type II (non–insulin-dependent) diabetes mellitus, type I (insulin-dependent) diabetes mellitus

Dosage and routes
Insulin lispro
Adult: SC Give 15 min AC

Human reg
Adults: SC Give ½-1 AC

Insulin, isophane suspension
Adult: SC dosage individualized by blood, urine glucose; usual dose 7-26 U; may increase by 2-10 U/day if needed

Regular insulin
Ketoacidosis
Adult: IV 5-10 U, then 5-10 U/hr until desired response, then switch to SC dose; IV/inf 2-12 U (50 U/500 ml of normal saline)

P *Child:* IV 0.1 U/kg
Replacement
P *Adult and child:* SC 0.5-1 U/kg/day qid given 30 min pc

Adolescents: SC 0.8-1.2 mg/kg/day; this dosage is used during rapid growth

Available forms: NPH inj 100 U/ml; regular **IV**/IM/SC inj 100 U/ml; insulin analog inj 100 U/ml; insulin zinc susp, ext (ultralente) 100 U/ml; isophane insulin/insulin inj 100 U/ml; zinc susp 100 U/ml; insulin lispro 100 U/ml, 1.5 ml cartridges

Adverse effects
EENT: Blurred vision, dry mouth
INTEG: Flushing, rash, urticaria, warmth, *lipodystrophy,* lipohypertrophy, swelling, redness
META: *Hypoglycemia,* rebound hyperglycemia (Somogyi effect 12-72 hr or longer)
SYST: **Anaphylaxis**

Contraindications: Hypersensitivity to protamine

Precautions: Pregnancy **B**

☒ **Do Not Confuse:**
Novolin 70/30 Penfill, Novolin 70/30 Prefilled

Pharmacokinetics	
Absorption	Rapidly absorbed (SC)
Distribution	Widely distributed
Metabolism	Liver, muscle, kidney
Excretion	Kidneys
Half-life	Regular 3-5 min; NPH 10 min

Pharmacodynamics

	NPH	MIXTARD	INSULIN, REGULAR		INSULIN, REGULAR CONC	ZINC SUSP	ZINC SUSP CONC	ZINC SUSP PROMPT	LISPRO
			SC	IV				SC	
Onset	1-2 hr	½ hr	½-1 hr	10-30 min	½-1 hr	1-2½ hr	4-8 hr	1-1½ hr	rapid
Peak	4-12 hr	4-8 hr	2-4 hr	30-60 min	2-5 hr	7-15 hr	10-30 hr	5-10 hr	½-1 hr
Duration	18-24 hr	12-24 hr	5-7 hr	½-1 hr	5-7 hr	12-24 hr	7-36 hr	12-16 hr	3-4 hr

Interactions
Individual drugs
Alcohol: ↑ hypoglycemia
Diltiazem: ↑ insulin need
Dobutamine: ↑ insulin need
Fenfluramine: ↓ insulin need
Guanethidine: ↓ insulin need
Phenylbutazone: ↓ insulin need
Rifampin: ↑ insulin need
Sulfinpyrazone: ↓ insulin need
Tetracycline: ↓ insulin need
Drug classifications
Anabolic steroids: ↓ insulin need
β-Adrenergic blockers: Signs/symptoms of hypoglycemia may be masked
Estrogens: ↑ insulin need
Glucocorticoid steroids: ↑ insulin need
MAOIs: ↓ insulin need
Oral anticoagulants: ↓ insulin need
Oral hypoglycemics: ↑ hypoglycemia
Thiazide diuretics: ↑ insulin need
Thyroid hormones: ↑ insulin need
Herb/drug
Broom: ↓ hypoglycemic effect
Buchu: ↓ hypoglycemic effect
Chromium: ↑ or ↓ hypoglycemic effect
Dandelion: ↓ hypoglycemic effect
Fenugreek: ↑ or ↓ hypoglycemic effect

Ginseng: ↑ or ↓ hypoglycemic effect
Juniper: ↓ hypoglycemic effect
Karela: ↑ glucose tolerance
Smoking
↑ insulin need
Lab test interferences
↑ VMA
↓ Potassium, ↓ magnesium, ↓ inorganic phosphate
Interference: Liver function studies, thyroid function studies

NURSING CONSIDERATIONS
Assessment
• Monitor fasting blood glucose, 2 hr PP (80-150 mg/dl, normal fasting level; 70-130 mg/dl, normal 2-hr level); also glycosylated Hgb may be drawn to identify treatment effectiveness
• Monitor urine ketones during illness; insulin requirements may increase during stress, illness, surgery
• Assess for hypoglycemic reaction that can occur during peak time (sweating, weakness, dizziness, chills, confusion, headache, nausea, rapid weak pulse, fatigue, tachycardia, memory lapses, slurred speech, staggering gait, anxiety, tremors, hunger)
• Assess for hyperglycemia: acetone breath, polyuria, fa-

tigue, polydipsia, flushed, dry skin, lethargy

Nursing diagnoses
☑ Injury, risk for (adverse reactions)
☑ Knowledge deficit (teaching)
☑ Noncompliance (teaching)

Implementation
SC route
• Give after warming to room temp by rotating in palms to prevent injecting cold insulin; use only insulin syringes with markings or syringe matching U/ml; rotate inj sites within one area: abdomen, upper back, thighs, upper arm, buttocks; keep record of sites
• Give increased dosages if tolerance occurs; give human insulin to those allergic to beef or pork
• Give lispro 15 min ac
• Store at room temp for <1 mo; keep away from heat and sunlight; refrigerate all other supply; do not use if discolored; do not freeze

Ⅳ IV route, regular only
• Do not use if cloudy, thick, or discolored
• Give **IV** direct, undiluted via vein, Y-site, 3-way stopcock; give at 50 U/min or less
• Give by cont inf after diluting with **IV** sol and run at prescribed rate; use **IV** inf pump for correct dosing; give reduced dose at serum glucose level of 250 mg/100 ml

Syringe compatibilities:
Metoclopramide

Y-site compatibilities:
Amiodarone, ampicillin, ampicillin/sulbactam, aztreonam, cefazolin, cefotetan, dobutamine, esmolol, famotidine, gentamicin, heparin, heparin/hydrocortisone,

imipenen/cilastatin, indomethacin sodium trihydrate, magnesium sulfate, meperidine, meropenem, midazolam, morphine, nitroglycerin, nitroprusside, oxytocin, pentobarbital, potassium chloride, propofol, ritodrine, sodium bicarbonate, tacrolimus, terbutaline, ticarcillin, ticarcillin/clavulanate, tobramycin, vancomycin, vit B/C

Y-site incompatibilities:
Nafcillin

Additive compatibilities:
Bretylium, cimetidine, lidocaine, meropenem, ranitidine, verapamil

Additive incompatibilities:
Aminophylline, amobarbital, chlorothiazide, cytarabine, dobutamine, pentobarbital, phenobarbital, phenytoin, secobarbital, sodium bicarbonate, thiopental

Patient/family education
• Advise patient that blurred vision occurs; not to change corrective lenses until vision is stabilized after 1-2 mo of therapy
• Advise patient to keep insulin and equipment available at all times
• Advise patient to carry Medic Alert ID as diabetic
• Teach patient dosage, route, mixing instructions, disease process; tell patient to continue to use the same brand of insulin and to rotate inj sites
• Instruct patient to carry candy or lump of sugar to treat hypoglycemia; have glucagon emergency kit available; teach how to use these
• Teach patient symptoms of ketoacidosis: nausea, thirst, polyuria, dry mouth, decreased

B/P, dry, flushed skin, acetone breath, drowsiness, Kussmaul respirations; to have insulin available at all times
• Advise patient that a plan is necessary for diet, exercise; all food on diet should be eaten, exercise routine should not vary
• Teach patient to avoid OTC drugs and alcohol unless approved by a prescriber
• Instruct patient to notify prescriber if pregnancy is planned
• Caution patient that treatment is lifelong; insulin does not cure condition

Evaluation
Positive therapeutic outcome
• Decrease in polyuria, polydipsia, polyphagia; clear sensorium, absence of dizziness, stable gait
• Blood glucose level under control

Treatment of overdose: Glucose 25 g **IV**, via dextrose 50% sol, 50 ml or 1 mg glucagon

---

interferon alfa-2a/ interferon alfa-2b (℞)
(in-ter-feer′on)
Roferon-A/Intron-A
Func. class.: Miscellaneous antineoplastic
Chem. class.: Protein product

Pregnancy category   C

Action: Antiviral action inhibits viral replication by reprogramming virus; antitumor action suppresses cell proliferation; immunomodulating action phagocytizes target cells; may also inhibit virus replication

⮕ **Therapeutic Outcome:** Prevention of rapid growth of malignant cells; treatment of hepatitis non-A, non-B (liver function improvement)

Uses: Hairy cell leukemia in persons >18 yr, condylomata acuminata (alfa 2b), malignant melanoma, AIDS-related Kaposi's sarcoma, chronic hepatitis non-A, non-B (alfa 2b), chronic hepatitis B, C (alfa 2b)

Investigational uses: Bladder tumors, carcinoid tumors, non-Hodgkin's lymphoma, essential thrombocytopenia, cytomegaloviruses, herpes simplex

Dosage and routes
Hairy cell leukemia (2a)
Adult: SC/IM 3 million IU/day × 16-24 wk, then 3 million IU 3 times a wk maintenance

Hairy cell leukemia (2b)
2 million IU/m^2 3 times a wk; if severe adverse reactions occur, dose should be skipped or reduced by one half

Kaposi's sarcoma (2a)
Adult: SC/IM 36 million IU/day × 10-12 wk or 3 million IU/day × 3 days, then 9 million IU/day × 3 days, then 18 million IU/day × 3 days, then 36 million IU/day for the rest of the course; if severe reaction occurs reduce dose by one half

Condylomata acuminata (2b)
1 million IU/lesion 3 times a wk × 3 wk

Chronic hepatitis B (2b)
Adult: SC/IM 30-35 million IU/wk or 5 million IU/day or 10 million IU/3×/wk × 16 wk

---

Chronic hepatitis C
Adult: SC/IM 36 million IU
3 times a wk

Available forms: Alfa-2a inj
3, 6, 36 million IU/ml; alfa-2b
inj 3, 5, 10, 18, 25 million
U/vial, powder for inj 5, 10,
18, 25, 50, million U/vial

Adverse effects
*CNS: Dizziness, confusion,
numbness, paresthesias,* hallucinations, **convulsions, coma,**
amnesia, anxiety, mood
changes
CV: Edema, hypotension, hypertension, chest pain, palpitations, dysrhythmias, **CHF, MI,
CVA**
GI: Weight loss, taste changes
GU: Impotence
INTEG: Rash, dry skin, itching, alopecia, flushing, photosensitivity
*MISC: Flulike syndrome: fever,
fatigue, myalgias, headache,
chills*

Contraindications: Hypersensitivity

Precautions: Severe hypotension, dysrhythmia, tachycardia,
P pregnancy **C,** lactation, children, severe renal or hepatic
disease, convulsion disorder

N **Do Not Confuse:**
Roferon-A/Imferon

Pharmacokinetics

Absorption	80%-90% (SC/IM)
Distribution	Unknown
Metabolism	Renal tubular (degraded)
Excretion	Kidneys
Half-life	3.7-8.5 hr (2a); 2-7 hr (2b)

Pharmacodynamics

Onset	Unknown
Peak	3-8 hr
Duration	Unknown

Interactions
Individual drugs
Aminophylline: ↑ toxicity,
blood levels
Radiation: ↑ toxicity, bone
marrow suppression
Zidovudine: ↑ neutropenia
Drug classifications
Antineoplastics: ↑ toxicity,
bone marrow suppression
Lab test interferences
Interference: AST, ALT,
LDH, alkaline phosphatase,
WBC, platelets, granulocytes,
creatinine

NURSING CONSIDERATIONS
Assessment
• Assess cardiac status: lung
sounds; ECG before and during treatment, especially in
those with cardiac disease
• Assess bone marrow depression: bruising, bleeding,
blood in stools, urine, sputum,
emesis
• Assess mental status: depression, suicidal thoughts, hallucinations, amnesia
• Assess for symptoms of
infection; may be masked by
drug fever; fever, chills, headache, sore throat may occur 6
hr after dose; give acetaminophen for symptoms
• In AIDS patients with Kaposi's sarcoma, assess characteristics of lesions during
therapy; symptoms should
decrease
• Assess for bleeding: hematuria, stool guaiac, bruising or
petechiae, mucosa or orifices
q8h; check for inflammation of
mucosa, breaks in skin; avoid
IM injection, rectal temp, or
any other procedures that
break the skin
• Assess for CNS reaction:
LOC, mental status, dizziness,
confusion, poor coordination,

difficulty speaking, behavior changes; notify prescriber (alfa-2b)

Nursing diagnoses

☑ Injury, risk for (adverse reactions)

☑ Body image disturbance (adverse reactions)

☑ Infection, risk for (adverse reactions)

☑ Knowledge deficit (teaching)

Implementation

• Sol should be prepared by qualified personnel only under controlled conditions in biologic cabinet using gown, gloves, and mask

• Use Luer-Lok tubing to prevent leakage; do not let sol come in contact with skin; if contact occurs, wash well with soap and water

• Give at hs to minimize side effects

• Give acetaminophen as ordered to alleviate fever and headache

• Give by IM/SC after reconstituting 3-5 million IU/1 ml, 10 million IU/2 ml, 25 million IU/5 ml, of diluent provided; mix gently

Alfa-2a

• SC/IM after reconstituting 18 million U/3 ml of diluent provided (6 million U/ml)

• 36 million U/ml is used for Kaposi's sarcoma only

• Store reconstituted sol for 1 mo in refrigerator

Intralesional route (2b)

• Give by intralesional route after reconstituting 10 million IU/1 ml bacteriostatic water for inj; no more than 5 lesions can safely be treated at a time; using a 25 G needle inject 0.1 ml into base at center

Patient/family education

• Caution patient to avoid hazardous tasks, since confusion, dizziness may occur; fatigue is common; activity may have to be altered; to take hs to minimize flu-like symptoms; to take acetaminophen for fever; avoid prolonged sunlight

• Advise patient that brands of this drug should not be changed; each form is different, with different dosages

• Caution patient not to become pregnant while taking drug; possible mutagenic effects; impotence may occur during treatment but is temporary

• Advise patient to report signs of infection: sore throat, fever, diarrhea, vomiting

• Advise patient that emotional lability is common; notify prescriber if severe or incapacitating

Evaluation

Positive therapeutic outcome

• Leukocytes, Hgb, platelets, WNL

• Decreased amount of lesions in AIDS patients with Kaposi's sarcoma

• Decreased amount of genital warts

interferon alfa-n 1 lymphoblastoid
See Appendix A, Selected New Drugs

**interferon
alfacon-1 (R)**
(in-ter-feer'on al'fa-kon)
Infergen
Func. class.: Recombinant
type I interferon
Pregnancy category C

Action: Induces biologic responses and has antiviral, antiproliferative, and immunomodulatory effects

➡ **Therapeutic Outcome:** Decreased signs/symptoms of
hepatitis C

Uses: Chronic hepatitis C
infections

Investigational uses: Hairy
cell leukemia when used with
G-CSF

Dosage and routes
Adult: SC 9 micrograms as a
single inj 3×/wk × 24 wk

Available forms: Inj 9, 15 mg

Adverse effects
CNS: Headache, fatigue, fever,
rigors, insomnia, dizziness
CV: Hypertension, palpitation
EENT: Tinnitus, earache,
conjunctivitis, eye pain
GI: Abdominal pain, nausea,
diarrhea, anorexia, dyspepsia,
vomiting, constipation, flatulence, hemorrhoids, decreased
salivation
GU: Dysmenorrhea, vaginitis,
menstrual disorders
HEMA: **Granulocytopenia,
thrombocytopenia, leukopenia,** echymosis
INTEG: Alopecia, pruritus,
rash, erythema, dry skin
MS: Back, limb, neck, skeletal
pain
PSYCH: Nervousness, depression, anxiety, lability, abnormal
thinking

RESP: Pharyngitis, upper
respiratory infection, cough
sinusitis, rhinitis, respiratory
tract congestion, epistaxis,
dyspnea, bronchitis

Contraindications: Hypersensitivity to alpha interferons, or
products from *E. coli*

Precautions: Thyroid disorders, myelosuppression, hepatic, cardiac disease, lactation,
P pregnancy **C,** children <18 yrs

Pharmacokinetics	
Absorption	Unknown
Distribution	Unknown
Metabolism	Unknown
Excretion	Unknown
Half-life	Unknown

Pharmacodynamics	
Onset	Unknown
Peak	24-36 hr
Duration	Unknown

Interactions: None known

**NURSING CONSIDERATIONS
Assessment**
• Assess platelet counts, heme
concentration, ANC, serum
creatinine concentration, albumin, bilirubin, TSH, T4
• Assess for myelosuppression,
low dose is neutrophil count is
<500 × 10 6/1 or if platelets
are <50 × 10 9/L
• Assess for hypersensitivity;
discontinue immediately if
hypersensitivity occurs

Nursing diagnoses
✓ Infection, risk for (uses)
✓ Knowledge deficit (teaching)

Patient/family education
• Provide patient or family
member with written, detailed
instructions about the drug
• Caution patient to use contraception during treatment

Evaluation
Positive therapeutic outcome
• Decreased hepatitis C signs/symptoms

---

interferon β-1a (℞)
(in-ter-feer′on)
Avonex
interferon β-1b (℞)
Betaseron
Func. class.: Multiple sclerosis agent, immune modifier
Chem. class.: Escherichia coli derivative
Pregnancy category   C

Action: Antiviral, immunoregulatory; action not clearly understood; biologic response-modifying properties mediated through specific receptors on cells, inducing expression of interferon-induced gene products

➡**Therapeutic Outcome:** Correcting symptoms of multiple sclerosis

Uses: Ambulatory patients with relapsing or remitting multiple sclerosis

Investigational uses: May be useful in treatment of AIDS, AIDS-related Kaposi's sarcoma, malignant melanoma, metastatic renal cell carcinoma, cutaneous T cell lymphoma, acute non-A, non-B hepatitis

Dosage and routes
Interferon-β-1a
Adult: IM 30 µg qwk

Interferon-β-1b
Relapsing/remitting multiple sclerosis
Adult: SC 0.25 mg (8 IU) qod

Available forms: beta-1a 33 µg (6.6 million IU/vial; beta-1b powder for inj lyophilized 0.3 mg (9.6 mIU)

Adverse effects
CNS: Headache, fever, pain, chills, mental changes, hypertonia, **suicide attempts,** gait disturbances, depression
CV: Migraine, palpitations, hypertension, tachycardia, peripheral vascular disorders
EENT: Conjunctivitis, blurred vision, laryngitis
GI: Diarrhea, constipation, vomiting, abdominal pain
GU: Dysmenorrhea, irregular menses, metrorrhagia, cystitis, breast pain, spontaneous abortion
HEMA: **Decreased lymphocytes, WBC;** *lymphadenopathy*
INTEG: Sweating, inj site reaction, necrosis
MS: Myalgia, **myasthenia,** back pain
RESP: Sinusitis, dyspnea

Contraindications: Hypersensitivity to natural or recombinant interferon-β or human albumin

Precautions: Pregnancy **C,** lactation, child <18 yr, chronic progressive MS, depression, mental disorders

Pharmacokinetics	
Absorption	50% is absorbed
Distribution	Unknown
Metabolism	Unknown
Excretion	Unknown
Half-life	8 min-4½ hr

Pharmacodynamics	
Onset	Rapid
Peak	Up to 8 hr
Duration	Unknown

Interactions: None

NURSING CONSIDERATIONS
Assessment
• Monitor blood, renal, hepatic studies: CBC, differential, platelet counts, BUN, creatinine, ALT, urinalysis; if neutrophil count is <750/mm³, or if AST, ALT, is 10 times greater than upper normal limit, or if bilirubin is 5 times greater than upper normal limit; when neutrophil count exceeds 750/mm³ and liver function or renal studies return to normal, treatment may resume at 50% original dosage
• Assess for CNS symptoms: headache, fatigue, depression; if depression occurs and is severe, drug should be discontinued
• Assess for multiple sclerosis symptoms
• Assess mental status: depression, depersonalization, suicidal thoughts, insomnia
• Monitor GI status: diarrhea or constipation, vomiting, abdominal pain
• Monitor cardiac status: increased B/P, tachycardia

Nursing diagnoses
☑ Physical mobility, impaired (uses)
☑ Knowledge deficit (teaching)

Implementation
• Reconstitute 0.3 mg (9.6 million IU)/1.2 ml of supplied diluent (0.2 mg or 8 million IU concentration); rotate vial gently, do not shake; withdraw 1 ml using a syringe with 27 G needle; administer SC into hip, thigh, arm; discard unused portion

Interferon β-1a
• Reconstitute with 1.1 ml diluent, swirl, give within 6 hr

Interferon β-1b
• Reconstitute by injecting diluent provided (1.2 ml) into vial, swirl (8 mIU/ml), use 27-G needle for inj
• Give acetaminophen for fever, headache; use SC route only; do not give IM or **IV**
• Store reconstituted sol in refrigerator; do not freeze; do not use sol that contains precipitate or is discolored

Patient/family education
• Provide patient or family member with written, detailed instructions about the drug; provide initial and return demonstrations on inj procedure; give information on use and disposal of drug
• Inform patient that blurred vision, sweating may occur
• Advise women patients that irregular menses, dysmenorrhea, or metrorrhagia as well as breast pain may occur; use contraception during treatment; drug may cause spontaneous abortion
• Teach patient to use sunscreen to prevent photosensitivity
• Instruct patient to notify prescriber if pregnancy is suspected
• Teach patient inj technique and care of equipment
• Instruct patient to notify prescriber of increased temp, chills, muscle soreness, fatigue

Evaluation
Positive therapeutic outcome
• Decreased symptoms of multiple sclerosis

**interferon
gamma-1b** (℞)
(in-ter-feer′on)
Actimmune
Func. class.: Biologic
response modifier
Chem. class.: Lymphokine,
interleukin type
Pregnancy category   **C**

Action: Species-specific protein synthesized in response to
viruses; potent phagocyte-
activating effects; capable of
mediating the killing of *Staphylococcus aureus, Toxoplasma
gondii, Leishmania donovani,
Listeria monocytogenes,
Mycobacterium avium-
intracellulare;* enhances
oxidative metabolism of
macrophages; enhances
antibody-dependent cellular
cytotoxicity

⮞ **Therapeutic Outcome:** Decreased signs/symptoms of
infection (serious) in chronic
granulomatous disease

Uses: Serious infections associated with chronic granulomatous disease

Dosage and routes
Adult: SC 50 µg/m² (1.5
million U/m²) for patients
with a surface area of >0.5 m²;
1.5 µg/kg/dose for patient
with a surface area of <0.5/m²;
give on Monday, Wednesday,
Friday for 3 times a wk dosing

Available forms: Inj 100 µg
(3 million U)/single-dose vial

Adverse effects
CNS: Headache, fatigue,
depression, fever, chills
GI: Nausea, anorexia, abdominal pain, weight loss, diarrhea,
vomiting

INTEG: Rash, pain at inj site
MS: Myalgia, arthralgia

Contraindications: Hypersensitivity to interferon gamma, *E.
coli*–derived products

Precautions: Pregnancy **C,**
cardiac disease, seizure disorders, CNS disorders, myelosuppression, lactation, children

Pharmacokinetics

Absorption	Slowly absorbed; 89%
Distribution	Unknown
Metabolism	Unknown
Excretion	Unknown
Half-life	5.9 hr

Pharmacodynamics

Onset	Unknown
Peak	7 hr
Duration	Unknown

Interactions
Individual drugs
Radiation: ↑ toxicity, bone
marrow suppression
Drug classifications
Antineoplastics: ↑ toxicity,
bone marrow suppression

NURSING CONSIDERATIONS
Assessment
• Monitor blood, renal, hepatic studies: CBC with differential, platelet count, BUN,
creatinine, ALT, urinalysis
before and q3 mo during
treatment
• Assess for infection: headache, fever, chills, fatigue; these
are common adverse reactions
• Monitor CNS symptoms:
headache, fatigue, depression

Nursing diagnoses
☑ Infection, risk for (uses)
☑ Knowledge deficit (teaching)

Implementation
• Give at hs to minimize adverse reactions; administer

---

acetaminophen for fever, headache; use 50% of the dosage prescribed if severe reactions occur or discontinue treatment until reactions subside
• Give in right or left deltoid and anterior thigh; warm to room temp before use; do not leave at room temp over 12 hr (unopened vial); does not contain preservatives
• Store in refrigerator upon receipt; do not freeze; do not shake

Patient/family education
• Provide patient or family member with written, detailed instructions about the drug; provide initial and return demonstrations on inj procedure; give information on use and disposal of drug
• Caution patient to use contraception during treatment

Evaluation
Positive therapeutic outcome
• Decreased serious infections
• Improvement in existing infections and inflammatory conditions

---

ipecac syrup (OTC)
(ip'e-kak)
Func. class.: Emetic
Chem. class.: Cephaelis ipecacuanha derivative
Pregnancy category   C

Action: Acts on chemoreceptor trigger zone to induce vomiting; irritates gastric mucosa

➡ **Therapeutic Outcome:** Emesis

Uses: In poisoning from noncaustic substances to induce vomiting

Dosage and routes
Adult: PO 15-30 ml, then 200-300 ml water; may repeat ×1, if vomiting does not occur within 20 min

P *Child >1 yr:* PO 15 ml, then 200-300 ml water; may repeat in 30 min

P *Child 6-12 mo:* PO 5-10 ml, then 100-200 ml water; may repeat dose if needed

Available forms: Liq

Adverse effects
CNS: Depression, convulsions, coma
CV: Circulatory failure, atrial fibrillation, fatal myocarditis, dysrhythmias
GI: Nausea, vomiting, bloody diarrhea

Contraindications: Hypersensitivity, unconscious/semiconscious, depressed gag reflex, poisoning with petroleum products or caustic substances, convulsions, shock, alcohol intolerance

Precautions: Lactation, pregnancy C, child <6 mo
P

Pharmacokinetics	
Absorption	Not absorbed
Distribution	Unknown
Metabolism	Unknown
Excretion	Unknown
Half-life	Unknown

Pharmacodynamics	
Onset	15-30 min
Peak	Unknown
Duration	½ hr

Interactions
Individual drugs
Activated charcoal: ↓ effect; do not use together
Drug classifications
Antiemetics: ↓ effect, do not use together

☑ Herb/drug 🚫 Do Not Crush ◆ Alert ↻ Key Drug **G** Geriatric **P** Pediatric

Food/drug
Milk: ↓ effect
Carbonated drinks: ↑ abdominal distention

NURSING CONSIDERATIONS
Assessment
• Assess type of poisoning; do not administer if petroleum products or caustic substances have been ingested: kerosene, gasoline, lye, Drano
• Assess respiratory status before, during, after administration of emetic; check rate, rhythm, character; respiratory depression can occur rapidly
G with elderly or debilitated patients
• Monitor LOC; do not give to patients who are semiconscious or unconscious or if gag reflex is not present

Nursing diagnoses
✓ Injury, risk for (uses)
✓ Poisoning (uses)
✓ Knowledge deficit (teaching)

Implementation
PO route
◆• Give **ipecac** *syrup,* **not ipecac fluid,** which is 14 times stronger or death may occur
• Give activated charcoal after the patient has finished vomiting; may begin lavage after 10-15 min after 2 doses of ipecac syrup without results
• Give with the patient upright; give water immediately after the ipecac syrup (200-300 ml for adults; 100-
P 200 ml child <1 yr; 200-300 ml for a child >1 yr)

Patient family education
• Give patient phone number for poison control
• Give patient written guidelines on poisoning and when to induce vomiting; suggest patient keep ipecac syrup in

P house if young children are present
Evaluation
Positive therapeutic outcome
• Vomiting within 30 min

---

ipratropium (℞)
(i-pra-troe′pee-um)
Atrovent
Func. class.: Anticholinergic, bronchodilator
Chem. class.: Synthetic quaternary ammonium compound
Pregnancy category **B**

Action: Inhibits interaction of acetylcholine at receptor sites on the bronchial smooth muscle, resulting in decreased cyclic guanosine monophosphate (cGMP) and bronchodilatation

⇒**Therapeutic Outcome:** Bronchodilatation

Uses: Bronchodilatation during bronchospasm for patients with COPD; rhinorrhea in
P children 6-11 yr (nasal spray)

Dosage and routes
Adult: 2 inh qid, not to exceed 12 inh/24 hr; sol 500 μg (1 unit dose) given 3-4 ×1 day

P *Child 6-11 yr:* Nasal, 1 spray in each nostril

Available forms: Aerosol 18 μg/actuation; nasal spray 0.03%, 0.06%; sol for INH 0.02%

Adverse effects
CNS: Anxiety, dizziness, headache, nervousness
CV: Palpitations
EENT: Dry mouth, blurred vision
GI: Nausea, vomiting, cramps

INTEG: Rash
RESP: Cough, worsening of symptoms, **bronchospasm**

Contraindications: Hypersensitivity to this drug, atropine, soya lecithin

Precautions: Pregnancy **B**,
P lactation, children <12 yr, narrow-angle glaucoma, prostatic hypertrophy, bladder neck obstruction

⚠ Do Not Confuse:
Atrovent/Alupent

Pharmacokinetics	
Absorption	Minimal
Distribution	Does not cross blood-brain barrier
Metabolism	Liver, minimal
Excretion	Unknown
Half-life	2 hr

Pharmacodynamics	
Onset	5-15 min
Peak	1-1½ hr
Duration	3-6 hr

Interactions
Drug classifications
Bronchodilators, aerosol:
↑ action of bronchodilator

NURSING CONSIDERATIONS
Assessment
• Monitor respiratory function: vital capacity, FEV, ABGs, lung sounds, heart rate, rhythm (baseline and during treatment); if severe bronchospasm is present, a more rapid medication is needed
• Monitor for evidence of allergic reactions, paradoxic bronchospasm; withhold dose and notify prescriber; identify if patient is allergic to belladonna products or atropine; allergy to this drug may occur

Nursing diagnoses
☑ Airway clearance, ineffective (uses)
☑ Gas exchange, impaired (uses)
☑ Knowledge deficit (teaching)

Implementation
• Give after shaking container; have patient exhale, place mouthpiece in mouth, inhale slowly, hold breath, remove, exhale slowly; allow at least 1 min between inhalations
Nebulizer route
• Use solution in nebulizer with a mouthpiece rather than a face mask
Nasal route
• Prime pump, initially requires 7 actuations of the pump, priming again is not necessary if used regularly
• Store in light-resistant container; do not expose to temp over 86° F (30° C)

Patient/family education
• Advise patient not to use OTC medications unless approved by prescriber; extra stimulation may occur; to use this medication before other medications and allow at least 5 min between each to prevent overstimulation
• Teach patient that compliance is necessary with number of inhalations/24 hr, or overdose may occur
• Instruct patient to use spacer
G device if elderly
• Teach patient the proper use of the inhaler; review package insert with patient; to avoid getting aerosol in eyes; blurring may result; to wash inhaler in warm water qd and dry; to avoid smoking, smoke-filled rooms, persons with respiratory tract infections
• Teach patient if paradoxic bronchospasm occurs to stop

drug immediately and notify prescriber; to limit caffeine products such as chocolate, coffee, tea, and colas
• Instruct patient on administration of dose, not to use more than prescribed; serious side effects may occur; if dose is missed, take when remembered; space other doses on new time schedule; do not double doses

Evaluation
Positive therapeutic outcome
• Absence of dyspnea, wheezing after 1 hr
• Improved airway exchange
• Improved ABGs

---

irbesartan (Rx)
(er-be-sar′tan)
Avapro
Func. class.: Antihypertensive
Chem. class.: Angiotensin II receptor (Type AT$_1$)

Pregnancy category C (1st trimester); **D** (2nd/3rd trimesters)

Action: Blocks the vasoconstrictor and aldosterone-secreting effects of angiotensin II; selectively blocks the binding of angiotensin II to the AT$_1$ receptor found in tissues

➡ **Therapeutic Outcome:** Decreased B/P

Uses: Hypertension, alone or in combination

Investigational uses: Heart failure, hypertensive patients with diabetic nephropathy caused by type II diabetes

Dosage and routes
Adult: PO 150 mg qd; may be increased to 300 mg qd

Available forms: Tabs 75, 150, 300 mg

Adverse effects
CNS: Dizziness, anxiety, headache, fatigue
GI: Diarrhea, dyspepsia
RESP: cough, upper respiratory infection

Contraindications: Hypersensitivity, pregnancy **D** (2nd, 3rd trimesters)

Precautions: Hypersensitivity to ACE inhibitors; pregnancy **C** (1st trimester), ℙlactation, children, ℊelderly, renal disease

Pharmacokinetics	
Absorption	Well
Distribution	Bound to plasma proteins (90%)
Metabolism	Liver (minimal)
Excretion	Feces, urine
Half-life	11-15 hr

Pharmacodynamics
Unknown

Interactions: None significant

NURSING CONSIDERATIONS
Assessment
• Assess B/P, pulse q4h; note rate, rhythm, quality
• Monitor electrolytes: potassium, sodium, chloride
• Obtain baselines in renal liver function tests before therapy begins
• Monitor for edema in feet, legs daily
• Assess for skin turgor, dryness of mucous membranes for hydration status

Nursing diagnoses
✓Fluid volume deficit (side effects)
✓Noncompliance (teaching)
✓Knowledge deficit (teaching)

Implementation
• Administer without regard to meals
• Give **IV** 0.9% NaCl and place supine for severe hypotension

Patient/family education
• Advise patient to comply with dosage schedule, even if feeling better
• Inform patient that drug may cause dizziness, fainting; lightheadedness may occur
• Caution patient to rise slowly to sitting or standing position to minimize orthostatic hypotension
• Advise patient to notify prescriber if pregnancy is suspected

Evaluation
Positive therapeutic outcome
• Decreased B/P

---

irinotecan (℞)
(ear-een-oh-tee'kan)
Camptosar
Func. class.: Antineoplastic hormone
Chem. class.: Topoisomerase inhibitor

Pregnancy category D

Action: Cytotoxic by producing damage to double-strand DNA during DNA synthesis

▶Therapeutic Outcome: Prevention in growth of tumor size

Uses: Metastatic carcinoma of the colon or rectum

Dosage and routes
Adult: **IV** 125 mg/m² given over 1½ hr qwk × 4 wk, then 2 wk rest period, may be repeated; 4 wk or 2 wk off, dosage adjustments may be made to 150 mg/m² (high) or 50 mg/m² (low); adjustments should be made in increments of 25-50 mg/m² depending on patient's tolerance

Available forms: Inj 20 mg/ml

Adverse effects
CNS: Fever, headache, chills, dizziness
CV: Vasodilation
GI: Diarrhea, nausea, vomiting, anorexia, constipation, cramps, flatus, stomatitis, dyspepsia
HEMA: **Leukopenia,** anemia, **neutropenia**
INTEG: Irritation at site, rash, sweating
RESP: Dyspnea, increased cough, rhinitis
MISC: Edema, asthenia, weight loss

Contraindications: Hypersensitivity, pregnancy **D**

P Precautions: Lactation, children, **G** elderly, myelosuppression, irradiation

Pharmacokinetics	
Absorption	Complete
Distribution	Widely, 30%-68% bond to plasma proteins
Metabolism	Unknown
Excretion	Urine/bile
Half-life	Unknown

Pharmacodynamics
Unknown

Interactions
Individual drugs
Dexamethensone: ↑ lymphocytopenia
Prochlorperazine: ↑ akathisia
Radiation: ↑ myelosuppression

Drug classifications
Antineoplastics: ↑ myelosuppression, diarrhea
Diuretics: ↑ dehydration

NURSING CONSIDERATIONS
Assessment
- Assess for CNS symptoms: fever, headache, chills, dizziness
- Assess CBC, differential, platelet count weekly; withhold drug if WBC is <2000/mm³, or platelet count <100,000/mm³, Hgb ≤ g/dl, neutrophil ≤1000/mm³; notify prescriber of these results, drug should be discontinued and colony-stimulating factor given
- Assess buccal cavity q8h for dryness, sores or ulceration, white patches, oral pain, bleeding, dysphagia
- Assess GI symptoms: frequency of stools; cramping
- Assess signs of dehydration: rapid respirations, poor skin turgor, decreased urine output; dry skin, restlessness, weakness
- Assess for bone marrow depression: bruising, bleeding, blood in stools, urine, sputum, emesis

Nursing diagnoses
☑Infection, risk for (adverse reactions)
☑Knowledge deficit (teaching)

Implementation
- Give antiemetics and dexamethasone 10 mg at least ½ hr before antineoplastics
- Give after preparing in biologic cabinet using gloves, mask, gown

Ⅳ IV route
- Give by intermittent inf after diluting with 0.9% NaCl or D₅W (0.12-1.1 mg/ml); give over 1½ hr

- Do not admix with other solutions or medications
- Provide increased fluid intake to 2-3 L/day to prevent dehydration, unless contraindicated
- Change **IV** site q48h
- Provide rinsing of mouth tid-qid with water, club soda; brushing of teeth bid-tid with soft brush or cotton-tipped applicator for stomatitis; use unwaxed dental floss
- Provide nutritious diet with iron, vitamin supplement, low fiber, few dairy products

Patient/family education
- Advise to avoid foods with citric acid or hot or rough texture if stomatitis is present; to drink adequate fluids
- Advise to report stomatitis; any bleeding, white spots, ulcerations in mouth; tell patient to examine mouth qd, report symptoms
- Advise to report signs of anemia: fatigue, headache, faintness, shortness of breath, irritability
- Advise to use contraception during therapy
- Advise patient to avoid vaccinations while taking this drug
- Instruct patient to report diarrhea that occurs 24 hr after administration; severe dehydration can occur rapidly
- Teach patient to avoid salicylates, NSAIDs, alcohol; bleeding may occur
- Teach patient about alopecia; advise that when hair grows back, it will be of different texture, thickness

Evaluation
Positive therapeutic outcome
- Decrease in tumor size, decrease in spread of cancer

Treatment of overdose:
Induce vomiting, provide
supportive care

iron dextran (℞)
DexFerrum, Imferon ✦,
InFed
Func. class.: Hematinic
Chem. class.: Ferric hy-
droxide complex with
dextran
Pregnancy category   C

Action: Iron is carried by
transferrin to the bone marrow,
where it is incorporated into
hemoglobin

➤**Therapeutic Outcome:** Prevention and resolution of
iron-deficiency anemia

Uses: Iron-deficiency anemia
in patients who cannot take
oral preparations

Dosage and routes
P *Adult and child:* IM 0.5 ml as
a test dose by Z-track, then no
more than the following per
day:

Adult <50 kg: IM 100 mg

Adult >50 kg: IM 250 mg

P *Infant <5 kg:* IM 25 mg

P *Child 5-9 kg:* IM 50 mg

Adult: IV 0.5 ml (25 mg) test
dose, then 100 mg qd after 2-3
days; IV 250/1000 ml of
NaCl; give 25 mg test dose,
wait 5 min, then inf over 6-12
hr or follow equation:

$$0.3 \times weight \ (lb) \times$$
$$\frac{100\text{-Hgb (g/dl)} \times 100}{14.8}$$

Patients <30 lb (66 kg) should
be given 80% of above formula
dose

Available forms: Inj IM/**IV**
50 mg/ml; inj IM only 50
mg/ml

Adverse effects
CNS: Headache, paresthesia,
dizziness, shivering, weakness,
seizures
CV: Chest pain, **shock,** hypotension, tachycardia
GI: Nausea, vomiting, metallic
taste, abdominal pain
HEMA: Leukocytosis
INTEG: Rash, pruritus, urticaria, fever, sweating, chills,
brown skin discoloration, pain
at inj site, necrosis, sterile
abscesses, phlebitis
MISC: Anaphylaxis
RESP: Dyspnea

Contraindications: Hypersensitivity, all anemias excluding
iron-deficiency anemia, hepatic
disease

Precautions: Acute renal
P disease, children, asthma,
lactation, rheumatoid arthritis
P (**IV**), infants <4 mo, pregnancy C

✂ **Do Not Confuse:**
Imferon/Imuran, Imferon/
Roferon-A

Pharmacokinetics	
Absorption	Well absorbed; lym- phatics over wk or mo
Distribution	Crosses placenta
Metabolism	Slow; blood loss, desquamation
Excretion	Breast milk, feces, urine, bile
Half-life	6 hr

Pharmacodynamics
Unknown

Interactions
Individual drugs
Chloramphenicol: ↓ reticulo-
cyte response

☑ Herb/drug ⓢ Do Not Crush ◆ Alert ⊶ Key Drug �G Geriatric P Pediatric

Oral iron: Do not use together

Penicillamine: ↓ absorption of penicillamine

Vitamin E: ↓ reticulocyte response

Lab test interferences
False ↑ Serum bilirubin
False ↓ Serum calcium
False positive: ^{99m}Tc diphosphate bone scan, iron test (large doses >2 ml)

NURSING CONSIDERATIONS
Assessment
• Monitor blood studies: Hct, Hgb, reticulocytes, transferrin, plasma iron concentrations, ferritin, total iron-binding bilirubin before treatment, at least monthly
• Assess for allergic reaction and **anaphylaxis;** rash, pruritus, fever, chills, wheezing, notify prescriber immediately, keep emergency equipment available
• Assess cardiac status: anginal pain, hypotension, tachycardia
• Assess for nutrition: amount of iron in diet (meat, dark green leafy vegetables, dried fruits, eggs); cause of iron loss or anemia, including salicylates, sulfonamides
• Monitor pulse, B/P during **IV** administration
• Assess for toxicity: nausea, vomiting, diarrhea, fever, abdominal pain (early symptoms); cyanotic lips, nailbeds, seizures, CV collapse (late symptoms)

Nursing diagnoses
☑ Fatigue (uses)
☑ Activity intolerance (uses)
☑ Knowledge deficit (teaching)

Implementation
IM route
• D/C oral iron before parenteral; give only after test dose of 25 mg by preferred route; wait at least 1 hr before giving remaining portion
• Give IM deep in large muscle mass; use Z-track method and 19-20 G 2-, 3-inch needle; ensure needle is long enough to place drug deep in muscle; change needles after withdrawing medication and injecting to prevent skin and tissue staining

IV route
• Give **IV** after flushing tubing with 10 ml of 0.9% NaCl; give undiluted; give 1 ml (50 mg) or less over 1 min or more; flush line after use with 10 ml of 0.9% NaCl; patient should remain recumbent for 30-60 min to prevent orthostatic hypotension
• **IV** inj requires single-dose vial without preservative; verify on label **IV** use is approved
• Give by cont inf after diluting in 50-250 normal saline for inf; administer over 4-5 hr
• Give only with epinephrine available in case of anaphylactic reaction during dose
• Store at room temp in cool environment

Additive compatibilities:
Netilmicin

Patient/family education
• Caution patient that iron poisoning may occur if increased beyond recommended level; to not take oral iron preparation unless approved by prescriber
• Advise patient that delayed reaction may occur 1-2 days after administration and last 3-4 days (**IV**) or 3-7 days (IM); report fever, chills, malaise,

muscle, joint aches, nausea, vomiting, backache

Evaluation
Positive therapeutic outcome
• Increased serum iron levels, Hct, Hgb

Treatment of overdose:
• Discontinue drug, treat allergic reaction, give diphenhydramine or epinephrine as needed for anaphylaxis; give iron-chelating drug in acute poisoning

---

isoniazid ⚷ (Ⓡ)
(eye-soe-nye´a-zid)
INH, isoniazid, Isotamine ✦, Laniazid, Laniazid C.T., Nydrazid, PMS-Isoniazid ✦, Tubizid
Func. class.: Antitubercular
Chem. class.: Isonicotinic acid hydrazide
Pregnancy category **C**

Action: Inhibits RNA synthesis, decreases tubercle bacilli replication

➢ Therapeutic Outcome: Resolution of TB infection

Uses: Pulmonary TB as an adjunct; other infections caused by mycobacteria

Dosage and routes
Treatment
Adult: PO/IM 5 mg/kg qd as single dose for 9-24 mo, not to exceed 300 mg/day

P *Child and infant:* PO/IM 10-20 mg/kg qd as single dose for 18-24 mo, not to exceed 300 mg/day

Prevention
Adult: PO 300 mg qd as single dose × 12 mo

P *Child and infant:* PO/IM 10 mg/kg qd as single dose for 12 mo, not to exceed 300 mg/day

Available forms: Tabs 100, 300 mg; inj 100 mg/ml; powder 50 mg/5 ml; syrup 50 mg/5 ml

Adverse effects
Hypersensitivity: fever, skin eruptions, lymphadenopathy, vasculitis
CNS: Peripheral neuropathy, dizziness, memory impairment, **toxic encephalopathy, convulsions,** psychosis
EENT: Blurred vision, optic neuritis, visual disturbance
GI: Nausea, vomiting, epigastric distress, jaundice, **fatal hepatitis**
HEMA: **Agranulocytosis, hemolytic anemia, aplastic anemia, thrombocytopenia, eosinophilia, methemoglobinemia**
MISC: Dyspnea, vitamin B_6 deficiency, pellagra, hyperglycemia, metabolic acidosis, gynecomastia, rheumatic syndrome, SLE-like syndrome

Contraindications: Hypersensitivity, acute liver disease

Precautions: Pregnancy **C**, renal disease, diabetic retinopathy, cataracts, ocular defects, **P** hepatic disease, child <13 yr

Pharmacokinetics	
Absorption	Well
Distribution	Widely
Metabolism	Liver
Excretion	Kidneys
Half-life	1-4 hr

Pharmacodynamics		
	PO	IM
Onset	Rapid	Rapid
Peak	1-2 hr	45-60 min
Duration	6-8 hr	6-8 hr

Interactions
Individual drugs
Alcohol: ↑ toxicity
BCG vaccine: ↓ effectiveness of BCG vaccine
Carbamazepine: ↑ toxicity
Cycloserine: ↑ toxicity
Ethionamide: ↑ toxicity
Ketoconazole: ↓ effectiveness of BCG vaccine
Phenytoin: ↓ metabolism of phenytoin
Rifampin: ↑ toxicity
Warfarin: ↑ toxicity
Drug classifications
Antacids, aluminum: ↓ absorption
Benzodiazepines: ↑ toxicity
Food/drug
Tyramine foods: ↑ toxicity

NURSING CONSIDERATIONS
Assessment
• Obtain C&S tests, including sputum tests, before treatment; monitor every mo to detect resistance
• Monitor liver studies weekly: ALT, AST, bilirubin; renal studies during treatment and monthly before: BUN, creatinine, output, sp gr, urinalysis, uric acid
• Assess mental status often: affect, mood, behavioral changes; psychosis may occur with hallucinations, confusion
• Assess hepatic status: decreased appetite, jaundice, dark urine, fatigue
• Assess for visual disturbance that may indicate optic neuritis: blurred vision, change in color perception; may lead to blindness

Nursing diagnoses
☑ Infection, risk for (uses)
☑ Diarrhea (adverse reactions)
☑ Injury, risk for (adverse reactions)
☑ Knowledge deficit (teaching)
☑ Noncompliance (teaching)

Implementation
• Give antiemetic for vomiting
PO route
• Give with meals to decrease GI symptoms; it is better to take on empty stomach for better absorption, 1 hr ac or 2 hr pc
IM route
• Give deep in large muscle mass, massage; rotate inj sites

Patient/family education
• Instruct patient that compliance with dosage schedule for duration is necessary; not to skip or double doses; that scheduled appointments must be kept or relapse may occur
• Caution patient to avoid alcohol while taking drug or hepatoxicity may result; to avoid ingestion of aged cheeses, fish or hypertensive crisis may result; give patient written directions on which foods to avoid while taking this medication
• Tell patient to report peripheral neuritis: weakness, tingling/numbness of hands/feet, fatigue, hepatoxicity: loss of appetite, nausea, vomiting, jaundice of skin or eyes

Evaluation
Positive therapeutic outcome
• Decreased symptoms of TB
• Culture negative for TB

Treatment of overdose: Pyridoxine

isoproterenol (℞)
(eye-soe-proe-ter'e-nole)
Aerolone, Dispos-a-Med,
Isoproterenol HCl, Isuprel,
Isuprel Glossets, Isuprel
Mistometer, Medihaler-Iso,
Vapo-Iso
Func. class.: β-Adrenergic-
agonist, antidysrhythmic,
inotropic
Chem. class.: Catechol-
amine

Pregnancy category **C**

Action: Has β_1- and β_2-
adrenergic action; relaxes
bronchial smooth muscle and
dilates the trachea and main
bronchi by increasing levels of
cAMP, which relaxes smooth
muscles; causes increased contractility and heart rate by
acting on β-receptors in heart

Therapeutic Outcome: Bronchodilatation, increased heart
rate and cardiac output from
action on β-receptors in the
heart

Uses: Bronchospasm, asthma,
heart block, ventricular dysrhythmias, shock

Dosage and routes
Asthma, bronchospasm
Adult: SL tab 10-20 mg q6-
8h; inh 1 puff; may repeat in
2-5 min; maintenance 1-2
puffs 4-6 times/day; **IV** 1020
mg during anesthesia

P **Child:** SL tab 5-10 mg q6-8h;
inh 1 puff; may repeat in 2-5
min; maintenance 1-2 puffs
4-6 times/day

*Heart block/ventricular
dysrhythmias*
Adult: **IV** 0.02-0.06 mg, then
0.01-0.2 mg or 5 µg/ min
HCl; 0.2 mg, then 0.02-1 mg
as needed

Shock
Adult: **IV** inf 0.5-5 µg/min (1
mg/500 ml D₅W) titrate to
B/P, CVP, hourly urine output

Available forms: Sol for
nebulization 1:400 (0.25%),
1:200 (0.5%), 1:100 (1%);
aerosol 0.25%, 0.2%; powder
for inh 0.1 mg/cartridge; inj
1:5000 (0.2 mg/ml) **IV**; glossets (SL) 10, 15 mg

Adverse effects
CNS: *Tremors, anxiety,* insomnia, headache, dizziness, stimulation
CV: Palpitations, tachycardia,
hypertension, **cardiac arrest**
GI: Nausea, vomiting
META: Hyperglycemia
RESP: Bronchial irritation,
edema, dryness of oropharynx,
bronchospasms (overuse)

Contraindications: Hypersensitivity to sympathomimetics,
narrow-angle glaucoma

Precautions: Pregnancy **C**,
cardiac disorders, hyperthyroidism, diabetes mellitus,
G prostatic hypertrophy, elderly

Pharmacokinetics	
Absorption	Erratic (SL, rec), rapid (inh, **IV**)
Distribution	Unknown
Metabolism	Lungs, liver, GI tract
Excretion	Kidneys, unchanged (50%)
Half-life	Unknown

Pharmacodynamics				
	SL	INH	IV	REC
Onset	1-2 hr	Rapid	Rapid	2-4 hr
Peak	Un-known	Un-known	Un-known	Un-known
Dura-tion	2 hr	1 hr	10 min	3-4 hr

Interactions
Drug classifications
β-Adrenergic blockers: Block therapeutic effect

Bronchodilators, aerosol: ↑ action of bronchodilator

MAOIs: ↑ chance of hypertensive crisis

Sympathomimetics: ↑ adrenergic side effects

NURSING CONSIDERATIONS
Assessment
• Assess respiratory function: vital capacity, FEV, ABGs, lung sounds, heart rate, rhythm (baseline and during therapy)
• Monitor for evidence of allergic reactions, paradoxic bronchospasm; withhold dose; notify prescriber

Nursing diagnoses
✓ Airway clearance, ineffective (uses)
✓ Impaired gas exchange (uses)
✓ Knowledge deficit (teaching)

Implementation
SL route
• Give ≤q3-4hr or no more than tid

Inh route
• Give after diluting dose in sterile water or 0.9% NaCl, 0.45% NaCl; give over 15-20 min
• Store in light-resistant container; do not expose to temp over 86° F (30° C)

IV route
• Give by direct IV after diluting 0.2 mg or 1 ml (1:5000 sol)/10 ml 0.9% NaCl for inj or D₅W (1:50,000 sol); give 1:50,000 sol over 1 min
• Give by cont inf by diluting 2 mg or 10 ml (1:5000 sol)/500 ml 0.9% NaCl, D₅W, D₁₀W, 0.45% NaCl, Ringer's, LR (1:250,000 sol); give at a rate of 1 ml/min by inf pump;

ratio is adjusted according to patient response

Syringe compatibilities:
Ranitidine

Y-site compatibilities:
Amiodarone, amrinone, atracurium, bretylium, cisatracurium, famotidine, heparin, hydrocortisone, pancuronium, potassium chloride, propofol, remifentanil, tacrolimus, vecuronium, vit B/C

Additive compatibilities:
Atracurium, calcium chloride, calcium gluceptate, cephalothin, cimetidine, dobutamine, floxacillin, heparin, magnesium sulfate, multivitamins, netilmicin, potassium chloride, ranitidine, succinylchloride, verapamil, vit B/C

Patient/family education
• Caution patient not to use OTC medications before consulting prescriber; extra stimulation may occur
• Instruct patient to use this medication before other medications and allow at least 5 min between each; to prevent overstimulation by limiting caffeine products such as chocolate, coffee, tea, and colas
• Teach patient use of inhaler; review package insert with patient; advise patient to avoid getting aerosol in eyes, as blurring may result; instruct patient to wash inhaler in warm water qd and dry; to rinse mouth after using; to avoid smoking, smoke-filled rooms, persons with respiratory tract infections
• Teach patient to use spacer device if elderly
• Instruct patient if paradoxic bronchospasm occurs to stop drug immediately and notify

prescriber; to limit caffeine products such as chocolate, coffee, tea, and colas
• Instruct patient on administration of dose; not to use more than prescribed; serious side effects may occur; if taking PO regularly and dose is missed, take when remembered; space other doses on new time schedule; do not double doses

Evaluation
Positive therapeutic outcome
• Absence of dyspnea, wheezing
• Improved airway exchange
• Improved ABGs

Treatment of overdose: Administer a β_2-adrenergic blocker

---

isosorbide dinitrate (℞)
(eye-soe-sor'bide)
Apo-ISDN ✦, Cedocard-SR ✦, Coronex ✦, Dilatrate-SR, ISDN, Iso-Bid, Isonate, Isorbid, Isordil, Isordil Tembids, Isordil Titradose, Isosorbide Dinitrate, Isotrate Timecelles, Novasorbide, Sorbitrate, Sorbitrate SA
isosorbide mononitrate (℞)
Imdur, ISMO, Monoket
Func. class.: Antianginal, vasodilator
Chem. class.: Nitrate
Pregnancy category C

Action: Decreases preload, afterload, thus decreasing LVEDP, systemic vascular resistance, and reducing cardiac O_2 demand

◢**Therapeutic Outcome:** Relief and prevention of angina pectoris

Uses: Chronic stable angina pectoris, prophylaxis of angina pain

Dosage and routes
Adult: PO 5-40 mg qid; SL tab 2.5-10 mg; may repeat q2-3h; chew tab 5-10 mg prn or q2-3h as prophylaxis; sus rel cap 40-80 mg q8-12h

Available forms: Sus rel caps 40 mg; ext rel tabs 40, 60 mg; tabs 5, 10, 20, 30, 40 mg; chew tabs 5, 10 mg; SL tabs 2.5, 5, 10 mg

Adverse effects
CNS: Vascular headache, flushing, dizziness, weakness, faintness
CV: Postural hypotension, tachycardia, **collapse,** syncope
GI: Nausea, vomiting
INTEG: Pallor, sweating, rash
MISC: Twitching, hemolytic anemia, **methemoglobinemia**

Contraindications: Hypersensitivity to this drug or nitrates, severe anemia, increased intracranial pressure, cerebral hemorrhage, acute MI

Precautions: Postural hypotension, pregnancy **C**, lactation, children

Pharmacokinetics	
Absorption	Well
Distribution	Unknown
Metabolism	Liver
Excretion	Urine, metabolites
Half-life	Dinitrate 1 hr, mononitrate 5 hr

Pharmacodynamics

	SUS REL	SL	PO
Onset	20-45 min	2-5 min	15-30 min
Peak	Un-known	Un-known	Un-known
Duration	8-12 hr	1-4 hr	4-6 hr

Interactions
Individual drugs
Alcohol: ↑ hypotension
Drug classifications
Antihypertensives: ↑ hypotension
β-Adrenergic blockers: ↑ hypotension
Calcium channel blockers: ↑ hypotension
Phenothiazines: ↑ hypotension

NURSING CONSIDERATIONS
Assessment
• Monitor for orthostatic B/P, pulse at baseline and during treatment
• Assess for pain: duration, time started, activity being performed, character, intensity
Nursing diagnoses
☑ Cardiac output, decreased (uses)
☑ Tissue perfusion, decreased (uses)
☑ Knowledge deficit (teaching)
Implementation
SL route
• Hold SL tab under tongue until dissolved (a few min); do not take anything PO when SL tab is in place
PO route
• Give 1 hr ac or 2 hr pc with 8 oz of water
🚫• Sus rel tab should not be chewed, broken, or crushed; chew tab should be chewed thoroughly

Patient/family education
• Instruct patient to swallow sus rel tab whole, do not chew; SL tab should be dissolved under tongue, do not swallow; chew tab should be chewed thoroughly; do not skip or double doses; if dose is missed take when remembered if 2 hr before next dose (dinitrate), 6 hr before next dose (sus rel), or 8 hr before next dose (mononitrate)
• Caution patient to avoid alcohol and OTC medications unless approved by prescriber
• Inform patient that drug may be taken before stressful activity: exercise, sexual activity
• Advise patient that SL tab may sting mucous membranes
• Caution patient to avoid driving and hazardous activities if dizziness occurs
• Advise patient to comply with complete medical regimen
• Caution patient to make position changes slowly to prevent orthostatic hypotension

Evaluation
Positive therapeutic outcome
• Decrease in, prevention of anginal pain

---

isradipine (℞)
(is-ra'di-peen)
DynaCirc, DynaCirc CR
Func. class.: Calcium channel blocker, antihypertensive
Chem. class.: Dihydropyridine
Pregnancy category C

Action: Inhibits calcium ion influx across cell membrane during cardiac depolarization;

---

produces relaxation of coronary vascular smooth muscle and peripheral vascular smooth muscle; dilates coronary vascular arteries; increases myocardial oxygen delivery in patients with vasospastic angina

⮕ **Therapeutic Outcome:** Decreased B/P

Uses: Hypertension, pectoris, vasospastic angina

Dosage and routes
Adult: PO 2.5 mg bid; increase at 3-4 wk intervals up to 10 mg bid or 5 mg qd cont rel, may be increased q2-4wk, max 20 mg/day

Available forms: Caps 2.5, 5 mg; cont rel tabs 5, 10 mg

Adverse effects
CNS: Headache, fatigue, dizziness, fainting, sleep disturbances
CV: Peripheral edema, tachycardia, hypotension, chest pain, **CHF, dysrhythmias**
GI: Nausea, vomiting, diarrhea, gastric upset, constipation, hepatitis
GU: Nocturia, polyuria, **acute renal failure**
HEMA: **Thrombocytopenia, leukopenia, anemia**
INTEG: Rash, pruritus, urticaria, photosensitivity, hair loss, **Stevens-Johnson syndrome**
MISC: Flushing

Contraindications: Sick sinus syndrome, 2nd- or 3rd-degree heart block, hypotension less than 90 mm Hg systolic, hypersensitivity

Precautions: CHF, hypotension, hepatic disease, pregnancy **C**, lactation, children, renal disease, elderly

Pharmacokinetics	
Absorption	Well absorbed
Distribution	High plasma protein binding (95%)
Metabolism	Liver, extensively and rapidly
Excretion	Kidney
Half-life	8 hr

Pharmacodynamics	
Onset	1-2 hr
Peak	2-3 hr
Duration	12 hr

Interactions
Individual drugs
Alcohol: ↑ hypotension
Fentanyl: ↑ hypotension
Drug classifications
Antihypertensives: ↑ hypotension
Nitrates: ↑ hypotension
NSAIDs: ↓ antihypertensive effect

NURSING CONSIDERATIONS
Assessment
• Assess fluid volume status: I&O ratio and record, weight, distended red veins, crackles in lung, color, quality and sp gr of urine, skin turgor, adequacy of pulses, moist mucous membranes, bilateral lung sounds, peripheral pitting edema; dehydration symptoms of decreasing output, thirst, hypotension, dry mouth and mucous membranes should be reported
• Monitor ALT, AST, bilirubin; if these are elevated, hepatotoxicity is suspected
• Assess renal, hepatic, electrolytes prior to and during treatment
• Monitor cardiac status: B/P, pulse, respiration, ECG; assess anginal pain, precipitating, ameliorating factors

---

Nursing diagnoses

☑ Cardiac output, decreased (uses)

☑ Knowledge deficit (teaching)

Implementation

• Give once a day, with food for GI symptoms

🚫• Do not crush, chew caps, cont rel tabs

Patient/family education

• Instruct patient to avoid hazardous activities until stabilized on drug and dizziness is no longer a problem

• Instruct patient to limit caffeine consumption; to avoid alcohol and OTC drugs unless directed by prescriber

• Advise patient to comply in all areas of medical regimen: diet, exercise, stress reduction, drug therapy; to notify prescriber of irregular heart beat, shortness of breath, swelling of feet and hands, pronounced dizziness, constipation, nausea, hypotension

• Teach patient to use as directed even if feeling better

• Teach patient to take with a full glass of water

Evaluation

Positive therapeutic outcome

• Decreased B/P

Treatment of overdose:
Defibrillation, atropine for AV block, vasopressor for hypotension

---

itraconazole (℞)

(it-tra-kon′a-zol)

Sporanox

Func. class.: Antifungal (systemic)

Chem. class.: Triazole derivative

Pregnancy category **C**

Action: Increases cell membrane permeability in susceptible organisms by binding sterols in fungal cell membrane; decreases potassium, sodium, and nutrients in cell

➡**Therapeutic Outcome:** Fungistatic against *Histoplasma capsulatum, Blastomyces dermatitis, Cryptococcus neoformans, Aspergillus fumigatus, Candida*

Uses: Systemic candidiasis, chronic mucocandidiasis, oral thrush, candiduria, coccidioidomycosis, histoplasmosis, chromomycosis, paracoccidioidomycosis, blastomycosis (pulmonary and extrapulmonary)

Investigational uses: Dermatophytoses, pityriasis versicolor, sebopsoriasis, vaginal candidias, cryptococcal, subcutaneous mycoses, dimorphic infections, Leishmaniasis, fungal keratitis, alternariosis, zygomyeosis

Dosage and routes
Adult: PO 200 mg qd with food; may increase to 400 mg qd if needed; life-threatening infections may require a loading dose of 200 mg tid × 3 days; **IV** 200 mg bid ×4 doses, then 200mg qd; give each dose over 1 hr

---

P *Child:* PO 3-5 mg/kg/day

Available forms: Cap 100 mg; oral sol 10 mg/ml; inj 10 mg/ml

Adverse effects

CNS: Headache, dizziness, insomnia, somnolence, depression

GI: Nausea, vomiting, anorexia, diarrhea, cramps, abdominal pain, flatulence, **GI bleeding, hepatotoxicity**

GU: Gynecomastia, impotence, decreased libido

INTEG: Pruritus, fever, rash

MISC: Edema, fatigue, malaise, hypertension, hypokalemia, tinnitus

Contraindications: Hypersensitivity, lactation, fungal meningitis, coadministration with terfenadine

Precautions: Hepatic disease, achlorhydria or hypochlorhydria (drug-induced), children, pregnancy **C**

Pharmacokinetics	
Absorption	Variable
Distribution	Tissue, plasma, CSF
Metabolism	Liver, extensively
Excretion	Feces, breast milk
Half-life	20-21 hr

Pharmacodynamics	
Onset	Unknown
Peak	4 hr
Duration	Unknown

Interactions

Individual drugs

Buspirone: ↑ buspirone levels

Carbamazepine: ↑ metabolism, ↓ effect of itraconazole

Cyclosporine: ↑ effects of cyclosporine

Didanosine: ↓ antifungal action

Digoxin: ↑ effects of digoxin

Isoniazid: ↑ metabolism, ↓ effect of itraconazole

Midazolam: ↑ sedation

Omeprazole: ↓ action of itraconazole

Phenobarbital: ↑ metabolism, ↓ effect of itraconazole

Phenytoin: ↑ metabolism, ↓ effect of itraconazole

Rifampin: ↑ metabolism, ↓ effect of itraconazole

Sucralfate: ↓ action of itraconazole

Tacrolimus: ↑ tacrolimus effect

Terfenadine: ↑ dysrhythmias

Triazolam: ↑ sedation

Warfarin: ↑ effects of warfarin

Drug classifications

Antacids: ↓ action of itraconazole

Calcium channel blockers: ↑ edema

Cardiac glycosides: ↑ effects of cardiac glycosides

H₂-receptor antagonists: ↓ action of itraconazole

Oral hypoglycemics: ↑ effects of oral hypoglycemics

Food/drug

↑ absorption

NURSING CONSIDERATIONS

Assessment

◆• Monitor for hepatotoxicity: increasing AST, ALT, alkaline phosphatase, bilirubin

• Monitor for allergic reaction: dermatitis, rash; drug should be discontinued, antihistamines (mild reaction) or epinephrine (severe reaction) administered; check inj site for thrombophlebitis

• Monitor for hypokalemia: anorexia, drowsiness, weakness, decreased reflexes, dizziness, increased urinary output, increased thirst, paresthesias; if these occur, drug should be decreased or discontinued and potassium administered

Nursing diagnoses

☑ Infection, risk for (uses)
☑ Injury, risk for physical (adverse reaction)
☑ Knowledge deficit (teaching)

Implementation

• Oral sol: patient should swish in mouth vigorously
• Give with food or milk to prevent nausea and vomiting
🚫 • Do not crush, chew caps
• Store in tight container at room temp
• Oral sol and caps are not interchangeable on a mg/mg basis

IV IV route

• **IV** after adding full contents 25 ml to 50 ml NaCl, mix gently, use flow control device, give over 1 hr; use separate line, flush after use

Patient/family education

• Advise patient that long-term therapy may be needed to clear infection (1 wk-6 mo depending on type of infection)
• Teach patient side effects and when to notify prescriber
• Instruct patient to avoid hazardous activities if dizziness occurs
• Instruct patient to take 2 hr administration of other drugs that increase gastric pH (antacids, H_2-blockers, omeprazole, sucralfate, anticholinergics)
• Teach patient importance of compliance with drug regimen
• Instruct patient to notify prescriber of GI symptoms, signs of liver dysfunction (fatigue, nausea, anorexia, vomiting, dark urine, pale stools)
🚫 • Tell patient not to break, crush, or chew caps

Evaluation

Positive therapeutic outcome

• Decreased fever, malaise, rash
• Negative C&S for infectious organism

---

kanamycin (℞)
(kan-a-mye'sin)
kanamycin sulfate, Kantrex
Func. class.: Antiinfective
Chem. class.: Aminoglycoside

Pregnancy category   C

Action: Interferes with protein synthesis in bacterial cell by binding to the 30S ribosomal subunit, causing inaccurate peptide sequence to form in protein chain, resulting in bacterial death

Therapeutic Outcome: Bactericidal effects for *Escherichia coli, Acinetobacter, Proteus, Serratia, Pseudomonas aeruginosa*

Uses: Severe systemic infections of CNS, respiratory tract, GI tract, urinary tract, bone, skin, soft tissues; also used as adjunct in hepatic coma, peritonitis, preoperatively to sterilize bowel; decreases ammonia-producing bacteria in bowel and intraperitoneally after fecal spill during surgery

Dosage and routes
Severe systemic infections
P *Adult and child:* **IV** inf 15 mg/kg/day in divided doses q8-12h; diluted 500 mg/200 ml of NS or D_5W given over 30-60 min, not to exceed 1.5 g/day; IM 15 mg/kg/day in divided doses q8-12h, not to exceed 1.5 g/day; irrigation not to exceed 1.5 g/day

K

Hepatic coma
Adult: PO 8-12 g/day in divided doses
Preoperative bowel sterilization
Adult: PO 1 g qh × 4 doses, then q6h × 36-72 hr

Available forms: Inj 75, 500 mg/2 ml, 1 g/3 ml; cap 500 mg

Adverse effects
CNS: Confusion, depression, numbness, tremors, **convulsions**, muscle twitching, **neurotoxicity**
CV: Hypotension
EENT: Ototoxicity, deafness, visual disturbances, dizziness, vertigo, tinnitus
GI: Nausea, vomiting, anorexia, increased ALT, AST, bilirubin, hepatomegaly, **hepatic necrosis,** splenomegaly
GU: **Oliguria, hematuria, renal damage, azotemia, renal failure, nephrotoxicity**
HEMA: **Agranulocytosis, thrombocytopenia, leukopenia, eosinophilia, anemia**
INTEG: Rash, burning, urticaria, dermatitis, alopecia
RESP: Respiratory depression

Contraindications: Bowel obstruction, severe renal disease, hypersensitivity

P **Precautions:** Neonates, myasthenia gravis, hearing deficits, mild renal disease, lactation, Parkinson's disease, pregnancy C

Do Not Confuse:
kanamycin/Garamycin

Pharmacokinetics

Absorption	Well absorbed IM; not absorbed PO
Distribution	Widely distributed in extracellular fluids; crosses placenta
Metabolism	Liver, minimally
Excretion	Kidneys, mostly unchanged (79%)
Half-life	2-3 hr; increased in renal disease

Pharmacodynamics

	IM	IV
Onset	Rapid	Rapid
Peak	1-2 hr	1-2 hr

Interactions
Individual drugs
Amphotericin B: ↑ ototoxicity, neurotoxicity, nephrotoxicity
Cisplatin: ↑ ototoxicity, neurotoxicity, nephrotoxicity
Ethacrynic acid: ↑ ototoxicity, neurotoxicity, nephrotoxicity
Furosemide: ↑ ototoxicity, neurotoxicity, nephrotoxicity
Mannitol: ↑ ototoxicity, neurotoxicity, nephrotoxicity
Methoxyflurane: ↑ ototoxicity, neurotoxicity, nephrotoxicity
Polymyxin: ↑ ototoxicity, neurotoxicity, nephrotoxicity
Succinylcholine: ↑ neuromuscular blockade, respiratory depression
Vancomycin: ↑ ototoxicity, neurotoxicity, nephrotoxicity
Drug classifications
Aminoglycosides: ↑ ototoxicity, nephrotoxicity, neurotoxicity
Anesthetics: ↑ neuromuscular blockade, respiratory depression
Nondepolarizing neuromuscular blockers: ↑ neuromuscular blockade, respiratory depression
Penicillins: ↑ ototoxicity, neurotoxicity, nephrotoxicity

NURSING CONSIDERATIONS
Assessment
- Assess patient for previous sensitivity reaction
- Assess patient for signs and symptoms of infection including characteristics of wounds, sputum, urine, stool, WBC >10,000, fever; obtain baseline information and during treatment
- Obtain C&S tests before beginning drug therapy to identify if correct treatment has been initiated
- Assess for allergic reactions: rash, urticaria, pruritus, chills, fever, joint pain; angioedema may occur a few days after therapy begins
- Identify urine output; if decreasing, notify prescriber (may indicate nephrotoxicity); also check for increased BUN, creatinine, urine CrCl <80 ml/min
- Monitor blood studies: AST, ALT, CBC, Hct, bilirubin, LDH, alkaline phosphatase, Coombs' test monthly if patient is on long-term therapy
- Monitor electrolytes: potassium, sodium, chloride, calcium, magnesium monthly if patient is on long-term therapy
- Assess bowel pattern qd; if severe diarrhea occurs, drug should be discontinued; may indicate pseudomembranous colitis
- Monitor for bleeding: ecchymosis, bleeding gums, hematuria, stool guaiac daily if on long-term therapy
- Assess for overgrowth of infection: perineal itching, fever, malaise, redness, pain, swelling, drainage, rash, diarrhea, change in cough, sputum
- Obtain weight before treatment; calculation of dosage is usually based on ideal body weight, but may be calculated on actual body weight
- Monitor I&O ratio; perform urinalysis daily for proteinuria, cells, casts; report sudden change in urine output
- Monitor VS during inf; watch for hypotension, change in pulse
- Assess **IV** site for thrombophlebitis including pain, redness, swelling q30 min; change site if needed; apply warm compresses to discontinued site
- Obtain serum peak, drawn at 30-60 min after **IV** inf or 60 min after IM inj; draw trough level just before next dose; blood level should be 2-4 times bacteriostatic level
- Assess hearing by audiometric testing, ringing, roaring in ears, vertigo before, during, after treatment
- Assess for dehydration: high sp gr, decrease in skin turgor, dry mucous membranes, dark urine
- Assess vestibular dysfunction: nausea, vomiting, dizziness, headache; drug should be discontinued if severe

Nursing diagnoses
☑ Infection, risk for (uses)
☑ Diarrhea (adverse reactions)
☑ Injury, risk for (adverse reactions)
☑ Knowledge deficit (teaching)

Implementation
PO route
- Give in even doses around the clock; if GI upset occurs, give with food; drug must be given for 10-14 days to ensure organism death and prevent superinfection; store in tight container

K

✤ Canada Only   Adverse effects: *italic* = common; **bold** = life-threatening

IM route
- Inject deep in large muscle mass

IV **IV route**
- Dilute 500 mg/100-200 ml; or 1 g/200-400 ml D_5W, $D_{10}W$, $D_5/0.9\%$ NaCl, 0.9% NaCl, LR
- Do not admix; give aminoglycosides and penicillin at least 1 hr apart
- Give by intermittent inf over 30-60 min; flush with 0.9% NaCl or D_5W after inf is complete

Syringe compatibilities:
Penicillin G sodium

Syringe incompatibilities:
Ampicillin, carbanicillin, heparin

Y-site compatibilities:
Cyclophosphamide, furosemide, heparin with hydrocortisone, hydromorphone, magnesium sulfate, meperidine, morphine, perphenazine, potassium chloride

Additive compatibilities:
Ascorbic acid, cefoxitin, chloramphenicol, clindamycin, dopamine, furosemide, penicillin G potassium, penicillin G sodium, polymyxin B, sodium bicarbonate, tetracycline, vit B/C; admixing is not recommended

Additive incompatibilities:
Amphotericin B, cephalothin, cephapirin, chlorpheniramine, heparin, methohexital

Patient/family education
- Teach patient to report sore throat, bruising, bleeding, joint pain, may indicate blood dyscrasias (rare)
- Advise patient to contact prescriber if vaginal itching, loose, foul-smelling stools, furry tongue occur; may indicate superinfection

Evaluation
Positive therapeutic outcome
- Absence of signs/symptoms of infection (WBC <10,000, temp WNL, absence of red, draining wounds)
- Reported improvement in symptoms of infection

Treatment of overdose:
Withdraw drug, hemodialysis, monitor serum levels of drug

---

kaolin/pectin (OTC)
(kay'-oh-lin pek'tin)
Donnagel-MB ♣, **Kaodene, Kao-Spen, Kapectolin**
Func. class.: Antidiarrheal
Chem. class.: Hydrous magnesium aluminum silicate
Pregnancy category   C

Action: Decreases gastric motility, water content of stool; adsorbent, demulcent

➡ **Therapeutic Outcome:** Absence of diarrhea

Uses: Diarrhea (cause undetermined)

Dosage and routes
Adult: PO 60-120 ml (45-90 ml conc) after each loose bowel movement

P *Child >12 yrs:* PO 60 ml after each loose bowel movement

P *Child 6-12 yrs:* PO 30-60 ml (15 ml conc) after each loose bowel movement

P *Child 3-6 yrs:* PO 15-30 ml (7.5 ml conc) after each loose bowel movement

Available forms: Susp kaolin 0.87 g/5 ml, pectin 43 mg/5

---

ml; kaolin 0.98 g/5 ml, pectin 21.7 mg/5 ml

Adverse effects
GI: Constipation (chronic use)

Contraindications: Child <3 yr, severe abdominal pain

Precautions: Pregnancy **C**

Pharmacokinetics	
Absorption	Not absorbed
Distribution	Unknown
Metabolism	Unknown
Excretion	Unknown
Half-life	Unknown

Pharmacodynamics	
Onset	½ hr
Peak	Unknown
Duration	6 hr

Interactions
All drugs: ↓ action of all other drugs

NURSING CONSIDERATIONS
Assessment
• Assess bowel pattern before, during treatment; for rebound constipation after termination of medication; check bowel sounds
• Assess for dehydration in children
• Check response after 48 hr; if no response, drug should be discontinued and other treatment initiated

Nursing diagnoses
☑ Diarrhea (uses)
☑ Constipation (adverse reactions)
☑ Knowledge deficit (teaching)
☑ Noncompliance (teaching)

Implementation
• Shake susp before use
• Administer for 48 hr only

Patient/family education
• Advise patient not to exceed recommended dosage; to take

all other medications ≥2 hr apart

Evaluation
Positive therapeutic outcome
• Decreased diarrhea

---

ketoconazole (℞)
(kee-toe-koe′na-zole)
Nizoral
Func. class.: Antifungal
Chem. class.: Imidazole derivative
Pregnancy category   C

Action: Alters cell membrane and inhibits several fungal enzymes; prevents production of adrenal sterols; prevents fungal metabolism

Therapeutic Outcome: Fungistatic/fungicidal against susceptible organisms: *Blastomycoses, Candida, Coccidioides, Cryptococcus, Histoplasma;* top route: *tinea cruris, tinea corporis, tinea versicolor, pityrosporum ovale*

Uses: Systemic candidiasis, chronic mucocandidiasis, oral thrush, candiduria, coccidioidomycosis, histoplasmosis, chromomycosis, paracoccidioidomycosis, blastomycosis

Investigational uses: Cushing's syndrome, advanced prostatic cancer

Dosage and routes
Adult: PO 200-400 mg once daily for 1-2 wk (candidiasis), 6 wk (other infections)

Children >2 yr: 3.3-6.6 mg/kg/day as single daily dose; <2 yr daily dose not established

Adult and child >2 yr: Top 2% cream applied qd or bid

K

Adult: Massage shampoo into scalp 1 min, reapply × 3 min, rinse; continue treatment twice/wk × 1 mo, no more than once q3 days

Available forms: Tab 200 mg; oral susp ♣ 100 mg/5 ml; cream 2%, shampoo 2%

Adverse effects

CNS: Headache, dizziness, somnolence

GI: Nausea, vomiting, anorexia, diarrhea, abdominal pain, **hepatotoxicity**

GU: Gynecomastia, impotence

HEMA: **Thrombocytopenia, leukopenia, hemolytic anemia**

INTEG: Pruritus, fever, chills, photophobia, rash, dermatitis, purpura, urticaria

SYST: **Anaphylaxis**

Contraindications: Hypersensitivity, lactation, fungal meningitis; coadministration with terfenadine

Precautions: Renal disease, hepatic disease, achlorhydria (drug induced), pregnancy **C**, children <2 yr, other hepatotoxic agents including terfenadine

Pharmacokinetics	
Absorption	pH dependent; ↓ pH ↑ absorption
Distribution	Widely distributed; crosses placenta
Metabolism	Liver, partially
Excretion	Feces, bile, breast milk
Half-life	Biphasic: 2 hr, 8 hr

Pharmacodynamics	
Onset	Unknown
Peak	1-3 hr
Duration	Unknown

Interactions

Individual drugs

Alcohol: ↑ hepatotoxicity

Carbamazepine: ↑ metabolism, ↓ effects of itraconazole

Cimetidine: ↓ absorption

Cyclosporine: ↑ effects of cyclosporine

Digoxin: ↑ effects of digoxin

Famotidine: ↓ absorption

Isoniazid: ↑ metabolism, ↓ effect of itraconazole

Nizatidine: ↓ absorption

Omeprazole: ↓ absorption

Paclitaxel: ↓ metabolism

Phenobarbital: ↑ metabolism, ↓ effect of itraconazole

Phenytoin: ↑ metabolism, ↓ effect of itraconazole

Ranitidine: ↓ absorption

Rifampin: ↑ metabolism, ↓ effect of itraconazole

Theophylline: ↓ effectiveness

Warfarin: ↑ effects of warfarin

Drug classifications

Anticholinergics: ↓ ketoconazole action

Cardiac glycosides: ↑ effects of cardiac glycosides

Oral anticoagulants: ↑ effects of oral anticoagulants

Oral hypoglycemics: ↑ effects of oral hypoglycemics

Food/drug

↑ absorption

☑ *Herb/drug*

Yew: ↓ ketoconazole action

NURSING CONSIDERATIONS

Assessment

• Assess for signs and symptoms of infection: drainage, sore throat, urinary pain, hematuria, fever

• Obtain cultures for C&S before beginning treatment; therapy may be started after culture is taken

---

☑ Herb/drug ⬡ Do Not Crush ◆ Alert ⬤☞ Key Drug ⑤ Geriatric ⓟ Pediatric

◆• Monitor for hepatotoxicity: increased AST, ALT, alkaline phosphatase, bilirubin; drug is discontinued if hepatotoxicity occurs

Nursing diagnoses
☑ Infection, risk for (uses)
☑ Injury, risk for (adverse reactions)
☑ Knowledge deficit (teaching)

Implementation
PO route
• Give in the presence of acid products only; do not use alkaline products, proton pump inhibitors, H_2 antagonists, or antacids within 2 hr of drug; may give coffee, tea, acidic fruit juices, cola; give with food to decrease GI symptoms; dissolve tab/4 ml of aqueous sol 0.2 N HCl, use straw to avoid contact with, rinse with water afterward and swallow
• Give with hydrochloric acid if achlorhydria is present
• Store in tight container at room temp

Top route
• Use enough medication to cover fungally infected area and surrounding area; rub in; do not use occlusive dressing; do not get in eyes

Shampoo
• Hair should be wet; apply shampoo, lather, rub gently into scalp and hair for 1 min; rinse; reapply × 3 min; continue treatment 2 times/wk for 1 mo, no more than once q3 days

Patient/family education
• Advise patient that long-term therapy may be needed to clear infection (1 wk-6 mo depending on infection)

• Advise patient to avoid hazardous activities if dizziness occurs
• Instruct patient to take 2 hr before administration of other drugs that increase gastric pH (antacids, H_2-blockers, omeprazole, sucralfate, anticholinergics)
• Stress the importance of compliance with drug regimen
• Advise patient to notify prescriber of GI symptoms, signs of liver dysfunction (fatigue, nausea, anorexia, vomiting, dark urine, pale stools)
• Teach patient proper hygiene: hand washing, nail care, use of concomitant top agents if prescribed
• Caution patient to avoid alcohol, since nausea, vomiting, hypertension may occur
• Advise patient to use sunscreen or avoid direct sunlight to prevent photosensitivity
• Advise patient to notify prescriber of sore throat, fever, skin rash, which may indicate superinfection
• Advise patient to use sunglasses to prevent photophobia

Evaluation
Positive therapeutic outcome
• Decreased oral candidiasis, fever, malaise, rash
• Negative C&S for infectious organism
• Absence of dandruff, scaling

K

---

ketoprofen (OTC, ℞)
(ke-to-proe′fen)
Actron, Apo-Keto ✦, Apo-
Keto-E ✦, Ketoprofen,
Orudis, Orudis-E ✦, Orudis-
KT, Orudis-SR ✦, Oruvail,
Rhodis ✦
Func. class.: NSAID;
nonopioid analgesic
Chem. class.: Propionic
acid derivative

Pregnancy category   B

Action: Inhibits prostaglandin
synthesis by decreasing enzyme
needed for biosynthesis; analgesic, antiinflammatory

Therapeutic Outcome: Decreased pain, inflammation

Uses: Mild to moderate pain,
osteoarthritis, rheumatoid
arthritis, dysmenorrhea

Dosage and routes
Antiinflammatory
Adult: PO 150-300 mg in
divided doses tid-qid, not to
exceed 300 mg/day or ext rel
150-200 mg qd

Analgesic
Adult: PO 25-50 mg q6-8h

Available forms: Caps 12.5,
25, 50, 75 mg; ext rel cap 100,
150, 200 mg

Adverse effects
CNS: Dizziness, drowsiness,
fatigue, tremors, confusion,
insomnia, anxiety, depression,
headache
CV: Tachycardia, peripheral
edema, palpitations, dysrhythmias, hypertension
EENT: Tinnitus, hearing loss,
blurred vision
*GI: Nausea, anorexia, vomit-
ing, diarrhea,* jaundice, **cholestatic hepatitis,** constipation,
flatulence, cramps, dry mouth,
peptic ulcer
GU: **Nephrotoxicity: dysuria,
hematuria, oliguria, azotemia**
HEMA: **Blood dyscrasias**
INTEG: Purpura, rash, pruritus, sweating

Contraindications: Hypersensitivity, asthma, severe renal
disease, severe hepatic disease,
ulcer disease

Precautions: Pregnancy **B** (1st
trimester), lactation, children,
bleeding disorders, GI disorders, cardiac disorders, hypersensitivity to other antiinflammatory agents, elderly

Do Not Confuse:
Oruvail/Clinoril, Oruvail/
Elavil

Pharmacokinetics

Absorption	Well absorbed
Distribution	Not known
Metabolism	Liver
Excretion	Kidneys
Half-life	2-4 hr

Pharmacodynamics

Onset	Unknown
Peak	2 hr
Duration	Unknown

Interactions
Individual drugs
**Acetaminophen (long-term
use):** ↑ renal reactions
Alcohol: ↑ adverse reactions
Aspirin: ↓ effectiveness, ↑ ad-
verse reactions
Coumadin: ↑ anticoagulant
effects
Cyclosporine: ↑ toxicity
Digoxin: ↑ toxicity, levels
Insulin: ↓ insulin effect
Lithium: ↑ toxicity
Methotrexate: ↑ toxicity
Phenytoin: ↑ toxicity
Probenecid: ↑ toxicity

Radiation: ↑ risk of hematologic toxicity

Sulfonylurea: ↑ toxicity

Drug classifications

Anticoagulants: ↑ risk of bleeding

Antihypertensives: ↓ effect of antihypertensives

Antineoplastics: ↑ risk of hematologic toxicity

β-Adrenergic blockers: ↑ antihypertension

Cephalosporins: ↑ risk of bleeding

Diuretics: ↓ effectiveness of diuretics

Glucocorticoids: ↑ adverse reactions

Hypoglycemics: ↓ hypoglycemic effect

NSAIDs: ↑ adverse reactions

Potassium supplements: ↑ adverse reactions

Sulfonamides: ↑ toxicity

Lab test interferences

↑ Bleeding time, ↑ liver function studies, ↑ serum uric acid, ↑ amylase, ↑ CO_2, ↑ urinary protein

↓ Serum potassium, ↓ PBI, ↓ cholesterol

Interference: Urine catecholamines, pregnancy test, urine glucose tests (Clinistix, Tes-Tape)

NURSING CONSIDERATIONS
Assessment

• Assess for pain: type, location, intensity; ROM before and 1-2hr after treatment

• Monitor liver function, renal function, studies: AST, ALT, bilirubin, creatinine, BUN, urine creatinine, CBC Hct, Hgb, pro-time if patient is on long-term therapy

• Check I&O ratio; decreasing output may indicate renal failure (long-term therapy)

• Assess hepatotoxicity: dark urine, clay-colored stools, jaundice of skin and sclera, itching, abdominal pain, fever, diarrhea if patient is on long-term therapy

• Assess for allergic reactions: rash, urticaria; if these occur, drug may have to be discontinued

• Assess for ototoxicity: tinnitus, ringing, roaring in ears; audiometric testing needed before, after long-term therapy

• Assess for visual changes: blurring, halos; may indicate corneal, retinal damage

• Assess for GI bleeding: blood in sputum, emesis, stools

• Check edema in feet, ankles, legs

• Identify prior drug history; there are many drug interactions

• Monitor pain: location, duration, type, intensity, before dose and 1 hr after; ROM before dose and after

Nursing diagnoses

☑ Pain (uses)

☑ Mobility, impaired physical (uses)

☑ Injury, risk for (adverse reactions)

☑ Knowledge deficit (teaching)

Implementation

⊘ • Administer to patient whole; do not crush, break, chew, or open cap

• Give with food or milk to decrease gastric symptoms; give 30 min ac or 2 hr pc; absorption may be slowed

Patient/family education

• Teach patient to report any symptoms of hepatotoxicity, renal toxicity, visual changes, ototoxicity, allergic reactions, bleeding (long-term therapy)

• Advise patient to take with 8 oz of water and sit upright for

K

30 min after dose to prevent ulceration

• Caution patient not to exceed recommended dosage; acute poisoning may result; to take as prescribed; do not double dose

• Advise patient to read label on other OTC drugs; many contain other antiinflammatories

• Advise patient to use sunscreen to prevent photosensitivity

• Inform patient that the therapeutic response takes 2 wk (arthritis)

• Teach patient to report tinnitus, confusion, diarrhea, sweating, hyperventilation, blurred vision, fever, joint aches

• Caution patient to avoid alcohol ingestion; GI bleeding may occur

Evaluation
Positive therapeutic outcome
• Decreased pain
• Decreased inflammation
• Increased mobility
• Decreased fever

---

ketorolac (R)
(kee'toe-role-ak)
Acular, Toradol
Func. class.: NSAID, nonopioid analgesic
Chem. class.: Pyrrolopyrrole

Pregnancy category   C

Action: Inhibits prostaglandin synthesis by decreasing an enzyme needed for biosynthesis; analgesic, needed for biosynthesis; analgesic, antiinflammatory, antipyretic effects

⇨**Therapeutic Outcome:** Decreased pain, inflammation, ocular itching

Uses: Mild to moderate pain (short term); decreased ocular itching in seasonal allergic conjunctivitis

Dosage and routes
Adult (multiple dosing): **IV** bol/IM 30 mg q6h; max 120 mg/day, with transition of 20 mg PO (1st dose) then 10 mg q4-6h; *≥65 yr, renal impairment or weight <50 kg:* 15 mg q6hr, max 60 mg

Adult (single dose): **IV** bol/IM 30 mg **IV** or 60 mg IM, then 20 mg transition dose, not to exceed 40 mg/day; then 10 mg q4-6hr; *≥65 yr, renal impairment or weight <50 kg:* IM 30 mg **IV** 15 mg

Ophth
Adult: 1 gtt (0.25 mg) qid × 7 days

P *Child:* **IV** 1 mg/kg then 0.5 mg/kg q6h

Available forms: Inj 15, 30 mg/ml (prefilled syringes); ophth 0.5% sol; tab 10 mg

Adverse effects
CV: Hypertension, flushing, syncope, pallor, edema, vasodilation
CNS: Dizziness, *drowsiness,* tremors
EENT: Tinnitus, hearing loss, blurred vision
GI: Nausea, anorexia, vomiting, diarrhea, constipation, flatulence, cramps, dry mouth, peptic ulcer, **GI bleeding, perforation,** taste change
GU: **Nephrotoxicity: dysuria, hematuria, oliguria, azotemia**
HEMA: **Blood dyscrasias,** prolonged bleeding

☑ Herb/drug 🚫 Do Not Crush ◆ Alert ☞ Key Drug G Geriatric P Pediatric

INTEG: Purpura, rash, pruritus, sweating

Contraindications: Hypersensitivity, asthma, severe renal disease, severe hepatic disease, peptic ulcer disease

Precautions: Pregnancy **C**, 🅿 lactation, children, bleeding disorders, GI disorders, cardiac disorders, hypersensitivity to other antiinflammatory agents, 🅶 elderly, CrCl <25 ml/min

🔃 **Do Not Confuse:**
Toradol/Tegretol, Toradol/Inderal, Toradol/Torecan, Toradol/tramadol

Pharmacokinetics	
Absorption	Rapidly, completely absorbed
Distribution	Bound to plasma proteins (99%)
Metabolism	Liver (<50%)
Excretion	Kidney, metabolites (92%); breast milk (6%); feces
Half-life	6 hr (IM); increased in renal disease

Pharmacodynamics		
	IM	OPHTH/PO
Onset	Up to 10 min	Unknown
Peak	50 min IM; 2-3 hr PO	Unknown
Duration	4-6 hr PO	Unknown

Interactions
Individual drugs
Heparin: ↑ bleeding
Lithium: ↑ toxicity
Methotrexate: ↑ effects
Phenytoin: ↑ effects
Sulfinpyrazone: ↓ effects
Drug classifications
ACE inhibitors: ↑ renal impairment
Anticoagulants: ↑ effects
Diuretics: ↓ antihypertensive effect
NSAIDs: ↑ gastric ulcers

Salicylates: ↓ blood sugar levels
Sulfonamides: ↓ effects
Lab test interferences
↑ Coagulation studies, ↑ liver function studies, ↑ serum uric acid, ↑ amylase, ↑ CO_2, ↑ urinary protein
↓ Serum potassium, ↓ PBI, ↓ cholesterol
Interference: Urine catecholamines, pregnancy test, urine glucose tests (Clinistix, Tes-Tape)

NURSING CONSIDERATIONS
Assessment
◆•　Monitor blood counts during therapy; watch for decreasing platelets; if low, therapy may need to be discontinued and restarted after hematologic recovery; assess for blood dyscrasia (thrombocytopenia): bruising, fatigue, bleeding, poor healing
• Monitor for aspirin sensitivity, asthma; these patients may be more likely to develop hypersensitivity to NSAIDs
• Assess patient's eyes: redness swelling, tearing, itching
• Monitor for pain: type, location, intensity, ROM before and 1 hr after treatment
• Assess for GI bleeding: blood in sputum, emesis, stools

Nursing diagnoses
☑ Pain (uses)
☑ Mobility, impaired physical (uses)
☑ Injury, risk for (adverse reactions)
☑ Knowledge deficit (teaching)

Implementation
PO route
• Administer to patient crushed or whole
• Give with food or milk to decrease gastric symptoms;

give 30 min ac or 2 hr pc; absorption may be slowed

IV **IM/IV route**
• **IV**-Give undiluted ≥15 sec
• Give IM/**IV** for 5 days or less, continue with PO

Y-site compatibilities:
Cisatracurium, remifentanil, sufentanil

Syringe incompatibilities:
Morphine, meperidine, promethazine, hydroxyzine

Solution compatibilities:
D_5W, 0.9% NaCl, LR

Patient/family education
• Teach patient that drug must be continued for prescribed time to be effective; to avoid aspirin, alcoholic beverages, other NSAIDs, acetaminophen
• Caution patient to report bleeding, bruising, fatigue, malaise, since blood dyscrasias do occur
• Instruct patient to use caution when driving; drowsiness, dizziness may occur
• Teach patient to take with a full glass of water to enhance absorption; do not crush, break, or chew
• Caution patient that this drug may cause eye redness, burning if soft contact lenses are worn

Evaluation
Positive therapeutic outcome
• Decreased pain
• Decreased inflammatory response
• Increased mobility
• Decreased ocular itching

labetalol (℞)
(la-bet'a-lole)
Normodyne, Trandate
Func. class.: Antihypertensive
Chem. class.: α- and β-blocker
Pregnancy category **C**

Action: Competitively blocks stimulation of β-adrenergic receptor within vascular smooth muscle; produces chronotropic, inotropic activity (decreases rate of SA node discharge, increases recovery time), slows conduction of AV node, decreases heart rate, which decreases O_2 consumption in myocardium; also has α-adrenergic blocking activity

⇒**Therapeutic Outcome:** Decreased B/P

Uses: Mild to moderate hypertension; treatment of severe hypertension (**IV**)

Investigational uses: Angina pectoris (PO), hypotension during surgery (**IV**)

Dosage and routes
Hypertension
Adult: PO 100 mg bid; may be given with a diuretic; may increase to 200 mg bid after 2 days; may continue to increase q1-3 days; max 400 mg bid

Hypertensive crisis
Adult: **IV** inf 200 mg/160 ml D_5W, run at 2 ml/min; stop inf after desired response obtained; repeat q6-8h as needed; **IV** bol 20 mg over 2 min; may repeat 40-80 mg q10 min, not to exceed 300 mg

Available forms: Tabs 100, 200, 300 mg; inj 5 mg/ml in 20 ml ampules

---

☑ Herb/drug 🚫 Do Not Crush ◆ Alert ☞ Key Drug **G** Geriatric **P** Pediatric

Adverse effects

CNS: Dizziness, mental changes, drowsiness, fatigue, headache, catatonia, depression, anxiety, nightmares, paresthesias, lethargy

CV: Orthostatic hypotension, **bradycardia, CHF,** chest pain, **ventricular dysrhythmias,** AV block

EENT: Tinnitus, visual changes, sore throat, double vision, dry burning eyes

GI: Nausea, vomiting, diarrhea

GU: Impotence, dysuria, ejaculatory failure

HEMA: **Agranulocytosis, thrombocytopenia, purpura** (rare)

INTEG: Rash, alopecia, urticaria, pruritus, fever

RESP: **Bronchospasm,** dyspnea, wheezing

Contraindications: Hypersensitivity to β-blockers, cardiogenic shock, heart block (2nd or 3rd degree), sinus bradycardia, CHF, bronchial asthma

Precautions: Major surgery, pregnancy **C,** lactation, diabetes mellitus, renal disease, thyroid disease, COPD, well-compensated heart failure, CAD, nonallergic broncho-🇬spasm, elderly, hepatic disease

Pharmacokinetics

Absorption	Bioavailability 25% (PO); complete (**IV**)
Distribution	Crosses placenta, CNS
Metabolism	Liver, extensively
Excretion	Breast milk, kidneys, bile
Half-life	6-8 hr

Pharmacodynamics

	PO	IV
Onset	1-2 hr	5 min
Peak	2-4 hr	15 min
Duration	8-12 hr	2-4 hr

Interactions

Individual drugs

Alcohol: ↑ hypotension (large amounts)

Cimetidine: ↑ effect of labetolol

Epinephrine: α-Adrenergic stimulation

Glutethimide: ↓ effect of labetolol

Hydralazine: ↑ hypotension, bradycardia

Indomethacin: ↓ antihypertensive effect

Insulin: ↑ hypoglycemia

Methyldopa: ↑ hypotension, bradycardia

Prazosin: ↑ hypotension, bradycardia

Reserpine: ↑ hypotension, bradycardia

Thyroid: ↓ effect of labetolol

Verapamil: ↑ myocardial depression

Drug classifications

Antidiabetics: ↑ hypoglycemia

Antihypertensives: ↑ hypertension

β₂-Agonists: ↓ bronchodilatation

Cardiac glycosides: ↑ bradycardia

Hydantoins: ↑ myocardial depression

MAOIs: Do not use within 2 wk

Nitrates: ↑ hypotension

NSAIDs: ↓ antihypertensive effect

Theophyllines: ↓ bronchodilatation

Lab test interferences

False: ↑ Urinary catecholamines

NURSING CONSIDERATIONS
Assessment

• Monitor B/P at beginning of treatment, periodically thereafter; pulse q4h; note rate, rhythm, quality: apical/

---

radial pulse before administration; notify prescriber of any significant changes (pulse <50 bpm)
• Check for baselines in renal, liver function tests before therapy begins
• Assess for edema in feet, legs daily, monitor I&O, daily weight; check for jugular vein distention, rales bilaterally, dyspnea (CHF)
• Monitor skin turgor, dryness of mucous membranes for hydration status, especially G elderly

Nursing diagnoses
☑ Cardiac output, decreased (uses)
☑ Injury, potential for physical (side effects)
☑ Knowledge deficit (teaching)
☑ Noncompliance (teaching)

Implementation
PO route
• Given ac, hs, tab may be crushed or swallowed whole; give with food to prevent GI upset; reduce dosage in renal dysfunction
• Store protected from light, moisture; place in cool environment
IV IV route
• Give **IV** undiluted 20 mg/2 min; may increase q10 min 40-80 mg until desired effect
• Give **IV** cont inf by diluting in LR, D_5W, D_5 in 0.2%, 0.9%, 0.33% NaCl or Ringer's inj; inf is titrated to patient response; 200 mg of drug/160 ml sol (1 mg/ml); 300 mg of drug/240 ml sol (1 mg/ml); 200 mg of drug/250 ml sol (2 mg/3ml); use inf pump
• Keep patient recumbent during and for 3 hr after inf

Y-site compatibilities:
Amikacin, aminophylline, amiodarone, ampicillin, butorphanol, calcium gluconate, cefazolin, ceftazidime, ceftizoxime, chloramphenicol, cimetidine, clindamycin, diltiazem, dobutamine, dopamine, enalaprilat, epinephrine, erythromycin, esmolol, famotidine, fentanyl, gentamicin, hydromorphone, lidocaine, lorazepam, magnesium sulfate, meperidine, metronidazole, midazolam, milrinone, morphine, nicardipine, nitroglycerin, nitroprusside, norepinephrine, oxacillin, penicillin G potassium, piperacillin, potassium chloride, potassium phosphate, propofol, ranitidine, sodium acetate, tobramycin, trimethoprim-sulfamethoxazole, vancomycin, vecuronium

Y-site incompatibilities:
Cefoperazone, nafcillin

Solution compatibilities:
D_5R, D_5LR, $D_{2\frac{1}{2}}$/0.45% NaCl, D_5/0.2% NaCl, D_5/0.33% NaCl, D_5/0.9% NaCl, D_5W, Ringer's, LR

Solution incompatibilities:
Sodium bicarbonate 5%

Patient/family education
• Teach patient not to discontinue drug abruptly, or precipitate angina might occur; taper over 2 wk
• Teach patient not to use OTC products containing α-adrenergic stimulants (such as nasal decongestants, cold preparations); to avoid alcohol, smoking and to limit sodium intake as prescribed
• Teach patient how to take pulse and B/P at home; advise when to notify prescriber

---

☑ Herb/drug Ⓢ Do Not Crush ◆ Alert ✦☛ Key Drug G Geriatric P Pediatric

• Instruct patient to comply with weight control, dietary adjustments, modified exercise program

• Advise patient to carry/wear Medic Alert ID to identify drug being taken, allergies; teach patient drug controls symptoms but does not cure

• Caution patient to avoid hazardous activities if dizziness, drowsiness are present

• Teach patient to report symptoms of CHF: difficult breathing, especially on exertion or when lying down, night cough, swelling of extremities, bradycardia, dizziness, confusion, depression, fever

• Teach patient to take drug as prescribed, not to double or skip doses; take any missed doses as soon as remembered if at least 4 hr until next dose

Evaluation
Positive therapeutic outcome
• Decreased B/P in hypertension (after 1-2 wk)
• Absence of dysrhythmias

Treatment of overdose: Lavage, **IV** atropine for bradycardia, **IV** theophylline for bronchospasm, digitalis, O_2, diuretic for cardiac failure, hemodialysis, **IV** glucose for hyperglycemia, **IV** diazepam (or phenytoin) for seizures

---

lactulose (℞)
(lak′tyoo-lose)
Cephulac, Cholac, Chronulac, Constilac, Constulose, Duphalac Emulose, Enulose, Lactulax ✦
Func. class.: Laxative (hyperosmotic/ammonia detoxicant)
Chem. class.: Lactose synthetic derivative
Pregnancy category   B

Action: Increases osmotic pressure; draws fluid into colon; prevents absorption of ammonia in colon; increases water in stool

➡ Therapeutic Outcome: Decreased constipation, decreased blood ammonia level

Uses: Chronic constipation, portal-systemic encephalopathy in patients with hepatic disease

Dosage and routes
Constipation
Adult: PO 15-60 ml qd

ⓟ Child: PO 7.5 ml qd

Encephalopathy
Adult: PO 20-30 g tid or qid until stools are soft; retention enema 30-45 ml in 100 ml of fluid

ⓟ Infant: 2.5-10 ml/day in divided doses

ⓟ Child: 40-90 ml/day in divided doses given 2-4×/day

Available forms: Oral sol, rec sol 3.33 g/5 ml; syrup 10 g/15 ml

Adverse effects
GI: Nausea, vomiting, anorexia, abdominal cramps, diarrhea, flatulence, *distention, belching*

Contraindications: Hypersensitivity, low-galactose diet

Precautions: Pregnancy **B**, lactation, diabetes mellitus, elderly and debilitated patient

Pharmacokinetics

Absorption	Poorly absorbed
Distribution	Not known
Metabolism	Colonic bacteria to acids
Excretion	Kidneys, unchanged
Half-life	Unknown

Pharmacodynamics
Unknown

Interactions
Individual drugs
Neomycin: ↓ effectiveness (portal-systemic encephalopathy)
Drug classifications
Laxatives: Do not use together (portal-systemic encephalopathy)

NURSING CONSIDERATIONS
Assessment
• Monitor glucose levels in diabetic (increases)
• Monitor blood, urine, electrolytes if used often by patient; may cause diarrhea, hypokalemia, hypernatremia; check I&O ratio to identify fluid loss
• Assess cramping, rec bleeding, nausea, vomiting; if these symptoms occur, drug should be discontinued; identify cause of constipation; identify whether fluids, bulk, or exercise is missing from lifestyle
• Monitor blood ammonia level (30-70 mg/100 ml); monitor for clearing of confusion, lethargy, restlessness, irritability (hepatic encephalopathy); may decrease ammonia level by 50%

Nursing diagnoses
☑ Constipation (uses)
☑ Diarrhea (adverse reactions)
☑ Knowledge deficit (teaching)
☑ Noncompliance (teaching)

Implementation
PO route
• Give with full glass fruit juice, water, milk to increase palatability of oral form; give increased fluids of 2 L/day; do not give with other laxatives; if diarrhea occurs, reduce dosage
Rec route
• Administer retention enema by diluting 300 ml lactulose/700 ml of water or 0.9% NaCl; administer by rec balloon catheter; retain for 30-60 min; repeat if evacuated too quickly

Patient/family education
• Discuss with the patient that adequate fluid consumption is necessary
• Teach patient that normal bowel movements do not always occur daily
• Teach patient not to use in presence of abdominal pain, nausea, vomiting; tell patient to notify prescriber if constipation unrelieved or if symptoms of electrolyte imbalance occur: muscle cramps, pain, weakness, dizziness, excessive thirst
• Teach patient not to use laxatives for long-term therapy; bowel tone will be lost
• Do not give at hs as a laxative; may interfere with sleep
• Notify prescriber if diarrhea occurs; may indicate overdosage

Evaluation
Positive therapeutic outcome
• Decreased constipation
• Decreased blood ammonia level
• Clearing of mental state

lamivudine (3TC) (R)
(lam-i'vue-dine)
Epivir, Epivir-HBV, 3TC
Func. class.: Antiviral
Chem. class.: Nucleoside reverse transcriptase inhibitor

Pregnancy category C

Action: Inhibits replication of HIV virus by incorporating into cellular DNA by viral reverse transcriptase, thereby terminating the cellular DNA chain

➡Therapeutic Outcome: Improved symptoms of HIV infection

Uses: HIV infection in combination with zidovudine (Epivir); chronic hepatitis B (Epivir-HBV)

Dosage and routes
Adult/adolescents (12-16 yr): PO 150 mg bid with zidovudine; <50 kg: PO 2 mg/kg bid with zidovudine

P *Child 3 mo-12 yr:* PO 4 mg/kg bid; may give 150 mg bid with zidovudine

Renal dose
Dosage reduction needed in renal disease (CrCl <50 ml/min)

Available forms: Tabs 150 mg; oral sol 5, 10 mg/ml; tabs 100 mg (Epivir-HBV)

Adverse effects
CNS: Fever, headache, malaise, dizziness, insomnia, depression, fatigue, chills
EENT: Taste change, hearing loss, photophobia
GI: Nausea, vomiting, diarrhea, anorexia, cramps,
P dyspepsia, **pancreatitis** (pediatrics)

HEMA: **Neutropenia,** anemia, **thrombocytopenia**
INTEG: Rash
MS: Myalgia, arthralgia, pain
RESP: Cough

Contraindications: Hypersensitivity

Precautions: Granulocyte count <1000/mm³ or Hgb <9.5 g/dl, pregnancy **C,** lacta-
P tion, children, renal disease, severe hepatic function, pancreatitis

Pharmacokinetics
Absorption	Rapidly absorbed
Distribution	Extravascular space
Metabolism	Unknown
Excretion	Unchanged in urine
Half-life	Unknown

Pharmacodynamics
Unknown

Interactions
Individual drugs
Trimethoprim-sulfamethoxazole: ↑ level of lamivudine
Zidovudine: ↑ level of zidovudine when given with lamivudine

NURSING CONSIDERATIONS
Assessment
• Monitor blood counts q2wk; watch for neutropenia, thrombocytopenia, Hgb, CD4, viral load, lipase, triglycerides periodically during treatment; if low, therapy may have to be discontinued and restarted after hematologic recovery; blood transfusions may be required
• Monitor liver studies: AST, ALT, bilirubin; amylase
P • Monitor children for pancreatitis

Nursing diagnoses

☑ Infection, risk for (uses)
☑ Injury, risk for (adverse reactions)
☑ Knowledge deficit (teaching)

Implementation

• Administer PO bid
• Give with other antiretrovirals only
• Store in cool environment; protect from light

Patient/family education

• Teach patient that GI complaints and insomnia resolve after 3-4 wk of treatment
• Tell patient that drug is not a cure for AIDS but will control symptoms
• Inform patient to notify prescriber of sore throat, swollen lymph nodes, malaise, fever; other infections may occur
• Teach patient that patient is still infective, may pass AIDS virus to others
• Encourage patient that follow-up visits must be continued since serious toxicity may occur; blood counts must be done q2wk
• Teach patient that drug must be taken tid, even if feeling better
• Tell patient that other drugs may be necessary to prevent other infections
• Teach patient that drug may cause fainting or dizziness

Evaluation

Positive therapeutic outcome

• Absence of infection, symptoms of HIV infection

---

lamotrigine (℞)

(lam-o-trye′geen)

Lamictal, Lamictal chewable

Func. class.: Anticonvulsant

Chem. class.: Phenyltriazine

Pregnancy category   C

Action: Unknown; may inhibit voltage-sensitive sodium channels

Therapeutic Outcome: Decrease in intensity and amount of seizures

Uses: Adjunct in the treatment of partial seizures; children with Lennox-Gastaut syndrome

Investigational uses: Refractory bipolar disorder, generalized tonic-clonic, absence, atypical absence and myoclonic seizures

Dosage and routes

Monotherapy

Adult: PO 50 mg/day for weeks 1 and 2, then increase to 100 mg divided bid for weeks 3 and 4; maintenance 300-500 mg/day

Child: 2 mg/kg/day in 2 divided doses × 2 wk, then 10 mg/kg/day, max 15 mg/kg/day or 400 mg/day

Multiple therapy

Adult: PO 25 mg every other day, weeks 1 through 4, then 150 mg/day in divided doses

Child: 0.1-0.2 mg/kg/day initially, then increase q2wk as needed to 2 mg/kg/day or 150 mg/day

Available forms: Tabs 25, 100, 150, 200 mg; chew tabs 5, 25 mg

---

☑ Herb/drug   Ⓢ Do Not Crush   ◆ Alert   ⚷ Key Drug   Ⓖ Geriatric   Ⓟ Pediatric

Adverse effects

CNS: Fever, insomnia, tremor, depression, anxiety, *dizziness,* ataxia, *headache*

EENT: Nystagmus, **diplopia,** *blurred vision*

GI: Nausea, vomiting, anorexia, abdominal pain

GU: Dysmenorrhea

INTEG: **Rash (potentially life-threatening),** alopecia, photosensitivity

RESP: Rhinitis, pharyngitis, cough

SYST: **Stevens-Johnson syndrome**

Contraindications: Hypersensitivity

Precautions: Pregnancy C, ☒ lactation, children <16 yr, renal, hepatic disease

☒ **Do Not Confuse:**
Lamictal/Lomotil, Lamictal/Lamisil

Pharmacokinetics

Absorption	Well absorbed
Distribution	Unknown
Metabolism	Unknown
Excretion	Unknown
Half-life	Varies, depending on dose

Pharmacodynamics
Unknown

Interactions
Individual drugs

Carbamazepine: ↑ metabolic clearance of lamotrigine

Phenobarbital: ↑ metabolic clearance of lamotrigine

Phenytoin: ↑ metabolic clearance of lamotrigine

Primidone: ↑ metabolic clearance of lamotrigine

Valproic acid: ↓ metabolic clearance of lamotrigine

NURSING CONSIDERATIONS
Assessment
◆● Assess for rash (Stevens-Johnson syndrome or toxic ☒ epidermal necrolysis) in pediatric patients, drug should be discontinued at first sign of rash
• Assess for seizure activity: duration, type, intensity, halo before seizure
• Assess for hypersensitive reactions

Nursing diagnoses
☑ Injury, risk for (uses)
☑ Knowledge deficit (teaching)

Implementation
• May be given with food or fluids
• Dispersible tabs should be swallowed whole, chewed, dispersed in water or diluted fruit juice; if chewed, a small amount of water should be taken

Patient/family education
• Teach patient to take PO doses divided with or after meals to decrease adverse effects
• Caution patient not to discontinue drug abruptly; seizures may occur
• Caution patient to avoid hazardous activities until stabilized on drug
• Advise patient to notify prescriber of skin rash or increased seizure activity
• Instruct patient to report to prescriber if pregnant or if patient intends to become pregnant
• Teach patient to use sunscreen and protective clothing, photosensitivity occurs
• Advise patient to carry Medic Alert ID stating drug use

L

Evaluation
Positive therapeutic outcome
• Decrease in severity of seizures

---

lansoprazole (℞)
(lan-soe′prah-zole)
Prevacid
Func. class.: Anti-ulcer–proton pump inhibitor
Chem. class.: Benzimidazole

Pregnancy category   B

Action: Suppresses gastric secretion by inhibiting hydrogen/potassium ATPase enzyme system in gastric parietal cell; characterized as gastric acid pump inhibitor since it blocks final step of acid production

Therapeutic Outcome: Reduction in gastric pain, swelling, fullness

Uses: Gastroesophageal reflux disease (GERD), severe erosive esophagitis, poorly responsive systemic GERD, pathologic hypersecretory conditions (Zollinger-Ellison syndrome, systemic mastocytosis, multiple endocrine adenomas); possibly effective for treatment of duodenal, gastric ulcers, maintenance of healed duodenal ulcers

Dosage and routes
NG tube
Adult: Use intact granules mixed in 40 ml of apple juice injected through NG tube, then flush with apple juice

Duodenal ulcer
Adult: PO 15 mg qd ac for 4 wk, then 15 mg qd to maintain healing of ulcers, associated with *Helicobacter pylori*—30 mg lansoprazole, 500 mg clarithromycin, 1 g amoxicillin bid × 14 days or 30 mg lansoprazole, 1 gm amoxicillin tid × 14 days

Erosive esophagitis
Adult: PO 30 mg qd ac for up to 8 wk, may use another 8 wk course if needed

Pathological hypersecretory conditions
Adult: PO 60 mg qd, may give up to 90 mg bid

Available forms: Caps, delayed rel 15, 30 mg

Adverse effects
CNS: Headache, dizziness, confusion, agitation, amnesia, depression
CV: Chest pain, angina, tachycardia, bradycardia, palpitations, **CVA,** hypertension/hypotension, **MI,** shock, vasodilation
EENT: Tinnitus, taste perversion, deafness, eye pain, otitis media
GI: Diarrhea, abdominal pain, vomiting, nausea, constipation, flatulence, acid regurgitation, anorexia, irritable colon
GU: Hematuria, glycosuria, impotence, kidney calculus, breast enlargement
HEMA: **Hemolysis,** anemia
INTEG: Rash, urticaria, pruritus, alopecia
META: Weight gain/loss, gout
RESP: Upper respiratory infections, cough, epistaxis, asthma, bronchitis, dyspnea

Contraindications: Hypersensitivity

Precautions: Pregnancy **B,** lactation, children

Pharmacokinetics

Absorption	Rapid after granules leave stomach
Distribution	Protein binding 97%
Metabolism	Liver extensively
Excretion	Urine, feces; clearance decreased in 🅖 elderly, renal, hepatic disease
Half-life	Plasma 1.5 hr

Pharmacodynamics

Unknown

Interactions
Individual drugs
Ampicillin: ↓ absorption of ampicillin
Digoxin: ↓ absorption of digoxin
Iron: ↓ absorption of iron
Ketoconazole: ↓ absorption of ketoconazole
Sucralfate: Delayed absorption of lansoprazole
Theophylline: ↓ clearance of theophylline

NURSING CONSIDERATIONS
Assessment
• Assess GI system; bowel sounds q8h, abdomen for pain, swelling, anorexia
• Monitor hepatic enzymes: AST, ALT, alk phosphatase during treatment

Nursing diagnoses
☑ Pain (uses)
☑ Knowledge deficit (teaching)

Implementation
• Administer before eating; swallow capsule whole
🚫• Do not open, chew, crush

Patient/family education
• Instruct patient to report severe diarrhea; drug may have to be discontinued
• Inform diabetic patient that hypoglycemia may occur

• Encourage patient to avoid hazardous activities; dizziness may occur
• Tell patient to avoid alcohol, salicylates, ibuprofen; may cause GI irritation

Evaluation
Positive therapeutic outcome
• Absence of gastric pain, swelling, fullness

---

leflunomide (℞)
(leh-floo'noh-mide)
Arava
Chem. class.: Pyrimidine synthesis inhibitor
Pregnancy category   X

Action: Inhibits an enzyme involved in pyrimidine synthesis and has antiproliferative effect

⮞ **Therapeutic Outcome:** Decreased pain, joint swelling, increased mobility

Uses: Rheumatoid arthritis

Dosage and routes
Adult: **PO** loading dose 100 mg/day × 3 days maintenance 20 mg/day, may be decreased to 10 mg/day if not well tolerated

Available forms: Tabs 10, 20, 100 mg

Adverse effects
CNS: Dizziness, insomnia, depression, paresthesia, anxiety, migraine, neuralgia
CV: Palpitations, hypertension, chest pain, angina pectoris, migraine, peripheral edema
EENT: Pharyngitis, oral candidiasis, stomatitis, dry mouth, blurred vision
HEMA: Anemia, ecchymosis, hyperlipidemia

L

GI: *Nausea, anorexia, vomiting, constipation, flatulence, diarrhea, LFTs*
INTEG: *Rash, pruritus,* alopecia, acne, hematoma, herpes infections
RESP: *Pharyngitis, rhinitis,* bronchitis, cough, respiratory infection, pneumonia, sinusitis

Contraindications: Hypersensitivity, pregnancy **X,** lactation

Precautions: Hepatic, renal disorders

Pharmacokinetics	
Absorption	Unknown
Distribution	Unknown
Metabolism	Liver
Excretion	Kidneys
Half-life	Unknown

Pharmacodynamics	
Onset	Unknown
Peak	Unknown
Duration	Unknown

Interactions
Individual drugs
Activated charcoal: ↓ effect of leflunomide
Cholestyramine: ↓ effect of leflunomide
Methotrexate: ↑ side effects
Drug classifications
NSAIDs: ↑ NSAID effect
Hepatotoxic agents: ↑ side effects of leflunomide

NURSING CONSIDERATIONS
Assessment
• Monitor liver function studies: if ALT elevations are > twofold ULN, reduce dose to 10 mg/day
Nursing diagnoses
☑ Mobility, impaired (uses)
☑ Pain (uses)
☑ Knowledge deficit (teaching)

Implementation
PO route
• Give PO with food for GI upset

Patient/family education
• Teach patient that drug must be continued for prescribed time to be effective
• Instruct patient to take with food, milk, or antacids to avoid GI upset
• Advise patient to use caution when driving; drowsiness, dizziness may occur
• Advise patient to take with a full glass of water to enhance absorption
• Advise patient to avoid pregnancy while taking this drug

Evaluation
Positive therapeutic outcome
• Increased joint mobility without pain
• Decreased joint swelling

lepirudin (℞)
(lep-ih-roo′din)
Refludan
Func. class.: Anticoagulant
Chem. class.: Hirudin
Pregnancy category   B

Action Direct inhibitor of thrombin that is highly specific

➨**Therapeutic Outcome:** Absence of thrombocytopenia, stroke, MI, or other thromboembolic conditions

Uses: Heparin-induced thrombocytopenia and other thromboembolic conditions

Dosage and routes
Adult: **IV** 0.4 mg/kg (≤110 kg) over 15-20 sec; then 0.15 mg/kg (≤110 kg/hr) as a cont inf for 2-10 days or longer

---

☑ Herb/drug   🚫 Do Not Crush   ◆ Alert   ⟐ Key Drug   **G** Geriatric   **P** Pediatric

Available forms: Powder for inj 50 mg

Adverse effects

CNS: Fever

CV: Heart failure, pericardial effusion, ventricular fibrillation

GI: GI bleeding, abnormal LFTs

GU: Hematuria, abnormal kidney function

HEMA: Hemorrhage, thrombocytopenia

INTEG: Allergic skin reactions

RESP: Pneumonia

SYST: Multiorgan failure, sepsis

Contraindications: Hypersensitivity to hirudins

Precautions: Intracranial bleeding, renal function impairment, lactation, children, hepatic disease, pregnancy **B**

Pharmacokinetics	
Absorption	Unknown
Distribution	Unknown
Metabolism	Possibly by the release of amino acids during catabolism
Excretion	50% unchanged in urine
Half-life	Unknown

Pharmacodynamics	
Onset	Unknown
Peak	Unknown
Duration	Unknown

Interactions

Drug classifications

Coumadin derivatives: ↑ risk of bleeding

Thrombolytics: ↑ action of lepirudin

NURSING CONSIDERATIONS

Assessment

• Obtain baseline in APTT before treatment; do not start treatment if APTT ratio is ≥2.5, then APTT 4 hr after initiation of treatment and at least qd thereafter; if APTT is above target, stop infusion for 2 hr, then restart at 50%, take APTT in 4 hr; if below target, increase inf rate by 20%, take APTT in 4 hr, do not exceed inf rate of 0.21 mg/kg/hr without checking for coagulation abnormalities

• Monitor APTT, which should be 1.5-2.5 × control

◆• Assess bleeding gums, petechiae, ecchymosis, black tarry stools, hematuria/epistaxis, B/P, vaginal bleeding, puncture sites; indicate bleeding and possible hemorrhage

• Assess fever, skin rash, urticaria

Nursing diagnoses

☑ Tissue perfusion, altered (uses)

☑ Injury, risk for (side effects)

☑ Knowledge deficits (teaching)

Implementation

• Administer after reconstitution and further dilution under sterile conditions; use water for inj or 0.9% NaCl; for further dilution 0.9% NaCl or D_5; for rapid and complete reconstitution, inject 1 ml of diluent into vial and shake gently, use immediately, warm to room temp before use

• Avoid all IM injections that may cause bleeding

IV route

• Administer **IV** bol: Use sol with conc. of 5 mg/ml, reconstitute 5 mg (1 vial)/1 ml of water for inj or 0.9% NaCl, use body wt for correct calculation as to weight

• Administer **IV** inf: Use sol with a conc. of 0.2 or 0.4 mg/ml; reconstitute 100 mg (2 vials) with 1 ml each (2 ml) water for inj or 0.9% NaCl,

L

transfer to inf. bag with either 500 or 250 ml of 0.9% NaCl or D$_5$

Patient/family education
• Teach patient to use soft-bristle toothbrush to avoid bleeding gums, avoid contact sports, use electric razor, avoid IM injection
• Teach patient to report any signs of bleeding: gums, under skin, urine, stools

Evaluation
Positive therapeutic outcome
• Absence of thrombocytopenia without significant bleeding

---

letrozole (℞)
(let'tro-zohl)
Femara
Func. class.: Antineoplastic, nonsteroidal aromatase inhibitor

Pregnancy category D

Action: Binds to the heme group of aromatase; inhibits conversion of androgens to estrogens to reduce plasma estrogen levels; 30% of breast cancers decrease in size when deprived of estrogen

➔ **Therapeutic Outcome:** Decreased spread of malignancy

Uses: Metastatic breast cancer in postmenopausal women

Dosage and routes
Adult: PO 2.5 mg qd

Available forms: Tab 2.5 mg

Adverse effects
CNS: Somnolence, dizziness, depression, anxiety, *headache, lethargy*
CV: Hypertension
GI: Nausea, vomiting, an-

orexia, **hepatotoxicity,** constipation, heartburn, diarrhea
INTEG: Rash, pruritus, alopecia, sweating, hot flashes
RESP: Dyspnea, cough

Contraindications: Hypersensitivity, pregnancy **D**

Precautions: Hepatic disease, respiratory disease

Pharmacokinetics	
Absorption	Well absorbed
Distribution	Widely
Metabolism	Liver
Excretion	Kidneys
Half-life	Unknown

Pharmacodynamics
Unknown

NURSING CONSIDERATIONS
Assessment
• Monitor renal function studies: BUN, serum uric acid, urine CrCl, electrolytes before, during therapy; I&O ratio; report fall in urine output of 30 ml/hr
• Monitor temperature q4h; may indicate beginning infection
• Monitor liver function tests before, during therapy (bilirubin, AST, ALT, LDH) as needed or monthly; RBC, Hct, Hgb, since these may be decreased; lymphocyte count, thyroid function tests
• Monitor inflammation of mucosa, breaks in skin, yellowing of skin and sclera, dark urine, clay-colored stools, itchy skin, abdominal pain, fever, diarrhea

Nursing diagnoses
☑ Injury, risk for (adverse reactions)
☑ Body image disturbance (adverse reactions)

☑ Infection, risk for (adverse reactions)

☑ Knowledge deficit (teaching)

Implementation
- Give with food or fluids for GI upset
- Give in equal intervals q6h

Patient/family education
- Instruct patient to report side effects
- Advise patient to avoid use of alcohol, which potentiates this drug

Evaluation

Positive therapeutic outcome
- Prevention of rapid division of malignant cells, postmenopausal cancer, prostate cancer

Treatment of overdose: Induce vomiting, provide supportive care

---

leucovorin (R)

(loo-koe-vor'in)

Citrovorum Factor, 5-Formyl Tetrahydrofolate, Folinic Acid, leucovorin calcium, Wellcovorin

Func. class.: Vitamin/folic acid antagonist antidote

Chem. class.: Tetrahydrofolic acid derivative

Pregnancy category   C

Action: Needed for normal growth patterns; prevents toxicity during antineoplastic therapy by protecting normal cells

➡**Therapeutic Outcome:** Reversal of severe toxic effects of folic acid antagonists

Uses: Megaloblastic or macrocytic anemia caused by folic acid deficiency, overdose of folic acid antagonist, methotrexate toxicity, toxicity caused by pyrimethamine or trimethoprim, pneumocystosis, toxoplasmosis

Dosage and routes

Megaloblastic anemia caused by enzyme deficiency

P *Adult and child:* PO/IM/**IV** up to 1 mg/day

Megaloblastic anemia caused by deficiency of folate

P *Adult and child:* IM 1 mg or less qd until adequate response

Methotrexate toxicity

P *Adult and child:* PO/IM/**IV** given 6-36 hr after dose of methotrexate 10 mg/m^2, then 10 mg/m^2 q6h × 72 hr

Pyrimethamine toxicity

P *Adult and child:* PO/IM 5 mg qd

Trimethoprim toxicity

P *Adult and child:* PO/IM 400 μg qd

Available forms: Tabs 5, 10, 15, 25 mg; inj 3, 5 mg/ml; powder for inj 10 mg/ml

Adverse effects

INTEG: Rash, pruritus, erythema, thrombocytosis, urticaria

RESP: Wheezing

Contraindications: Hypersensitivity, anemias other than megaloblastic not associated with vitamin B$_{12}$ deficiency

Precautions: Pregnancy **C**

🚫 **Do Not Confuse:**
leucovorin/Leukeran, leucovorin/Leukine

L

Pharmacokinetics

Absorption	Rapidly absorbed (PO); completely absorbed (**IV**)
Distribution	Widely distributed
Metabolism	Liver
Excretion	Kidney
Half-life	3½ hr

Pharmacodynamics

	PO/IM/IV
Onset	Up to 5 min
Peak	Unknown
Duration	4-6 hr

Interactions
Individual drugs
Chloramphenicol: ↓ folate levels
Phenobarbital: ↑ metabolism of phenobarbital, ↓ effect
Drug classifications
Hydantoins: ↑ metabolism of hydantoins, ↓ effect

NURSING CONSIDERATIONS
Assessment
• Obtain CrCl before leucovorin rescue and qd to detect nephrotoxicity
• Monitor I&O; watch for nausea and vomiting; if vomiting occurs IM or **IV** route may be necessary
• Assess diet for inclusion of bran, yeast, dried beans, nuts, fruits, fresh vegetables, asparagus, which have high folic acid levels
• Assess drugs currently taken: alcohol, hydantoins, trimethoprim may cause increased folic acid use by body
• Assess for allergic reactions: rash, dyspnea, wheezing

Nursing diagnoses
☑ Injury, risk for (uses)
☑ Nutrition, altered: less than body requirements (uses)
☑ Knowledge deficit (teaching)

Implementation
PO route
• Use PO route only if patient is not vomiting
IM route
• Give within 1 hr of folic acid antagonist, no reconstitution needed
• Give increased fluid intake if used to treat folic acid inhibitor overdose
• Provide protection from light and heat when storing ampules

Ⅳ IV route
• Reconstitute 50 mg/5 ml bacteriostatic water or sterile water for inj (10 mg/ml) or 100 mg/10 ml; use immediately if sterile water for inj is used to reconstitute
• Give by direct **IV** over 160 mg/min or less (16 ml of 10 mg/ml sol/min)
• Give by intermittent inf after diluting in 100-500 ml of 0.9% NaCl, D_5W, $D_{10}W$, LR, Ringer's

Syringe compatibilities:
Bleomycin, cisplatin, cyclophosphamide, doxorubicin, fluorouracil, furosemide, heparin, methotrexate, metoclopramide, mitomycin, vinblastine, vincristine

Y-site compatibilities:
Amifostine, aztreonam, bleomycin, cefepime, cisplatin, cladribine, cyclophosphamide, doxorubicin, filgrastim, fluconazole, fluorouracil, furosemide, granisetron, heparin, methotrexate, metoclopramide, mitomycin, piperacillin/tazobactam, tacrolimus, teniposide, thiotepa, vinblastine, vincristine

Additive compatibilities:
Cisplatin, cisplatin/floxuridine, floxuridine

Patient/family education
• Advise patient to take drug exactly as prescribed; to notify prescriber of side effects immediately
• Advise patient to report signs of hyposensitivity reaction immediately
• Instruct patient about leucovorin rescue; have patient drink 3 L of fluid each day of rescue
• Advise patient with folic acid deficiency to eat folic acid–rich foods: bran, yeast, dried beans, nuts, fruits, fresh green leafy vegetables, asparagus

Evaluation
Positive therapeutic outcome
• Increased weight
• Improved orientation, well-being
• Absence of fatigue

---

leuprolide (R)
(loo-proe'lide)
Leupron Depo Ped, Lupron Depot, Lupron, Lupron Depot-3 month,
Func. class.: Antineoplastic hormone
Chem. class.: Gonadotropin-releasing hormone

Pregnancy category   X (depot)

Action: Causes initial increase in circulating levels of LH, FSH; continuous administration results in decreased LH, FSH; in men testosterone is reduced to castration levels; in premenopausal women estrogen is reduced to menopausal levels

➡**Therapeutic Outcome:** Prevention of rapidly growing malignant cells in prostate

cancer, decreased pain in endometriosis, resolution of central precocious puberty (CPP)

Uses: Metastatic prostate cancer, management of endometriosis (depot), central precocious puberty

Dosage and routes
Prostate cancer
Adult: SC 1 mg/day; IM 7.5 mg/dose qmo
Endometriosis
Adult: IM 3.5 mg once a month or 11.25 mg q3mo
Central precocious puberty
P **Child:** SC 50 µg/kg/day; increase as needed by 10 µg/kg/day
P **Child:** >37.5 kg: IM 15 mg q4wk
25-37.5 kg: IM 11.25 mg q4wk
≤25 kg: 7.5 mg q4wk

Available forms: Inj (depot) 3.75 mg, 7.5 mg single-dose, multiple-dose vials (5 mg/ml); single-use kit 11.25 mg vial; pediatric depot 7.5, 11.25, 15 mg; 3 mo depot 22.5 mg single use

Adverse effects
CV: **MI, pulmonary emboli, dysrhythmias**
GI: Anorexia, diarrhea, **GI bleeding**
GU: Edema, hot flashes, impotence, decreased libido, amenorrhea, vaginal dryness, gynecomastia

Contraindications: Hypersensitivity to GnRH or analogs, thromboembolic disorders, pregnancy **X**, lactation, undiagnosed vaginal bleeding

Precautions: Edema, hepatic disease, CVA, MI, seizures, hypertension, diabetes mellitus

---

✦ Canada Only   Adverse effects: *italic* = common; **bold** = life-threatening

⊠ Do Not Confuse:
Lupron/Nuprin, Lupron/
Lopurin

Pharmacokinetics	
Absorption	Rapidly absorbed (SC); slowly absorbed (IM depot)
Distribution	Unknown
Metabolism	Unknown
Excretion	Unknown
Half-life	3-4 hr

Pharmacodynamics
Unknown

Interactions
Individual drugs
Megestrol: ↑ antineoplastic
action
Flutamide: ↑ antineoplastic
action

NURSING CONSIDERATIONS
Assessment
• Assess for symptoms of
endometriosis/fibroids including lower abdominal pain if
drug is given for the diagnosis
of endometriosis
• If giving this drug for CPP,
the diagnosis should have been
confirmed by development of
secondary sex characteristics in
P child <9 yr; also included to
confirm the diagnosis of CPP is
estradiol/testosterone, GnRH
test, tomography of head,
adrenal steroid, chorionic
gonadotropin, wrist x-ray,
height, weight; patients diagnosed with CPP display the
signs of testicular growth,
facial, body hair (males), breast
development, menses (females)
• Monitor liver function tests
before, during therapy (bilirubin, AST, ALT, LDH) as
needed or monthly; PSA in
prostate cancer
• Monitor pituitary gonado-

tropic and gonadal function
during therapy and 4-8 wk
after therapy is decreased;
check LH, FSH, acid phos-
phate at beginning of treatment
• Monitor worsening of signs
and symptoms (normal during
beginning therapy): fatigue,
increased pulse, pallor, lethargy, edema in feet, joints,
stomach pain, shaking
• Monitor renal status: I&O
ratio, check for bladder distention daily during beginning
therapy (renal obstruction)

Nursing diagnoses
✓ Sexual dysfunction (adverse
reactions)
✓ Injury, risk for (adverse reac-
tions)
✓ Knowledge deficit (teaching)

Implementation
• Use syringe and drug pack-
aged together; give deep in
large muscle mass; rotate sites
• Use depot only IM; never
give SC
• Reconstitute vial (single
dose)/1 ml of diluent; shake
(appearance should be white);
withdraw and use immediately
• Unused vials may be stored
at room temp

Patient/family education
• Advise patient to notify
prescriber if menstruation
continues; menstruation
should stop; to use a nonhormonal method of contraception during therapy
• Instruct patient to report any
complaints, side effects to
nurse or prescriber; hot flashes
are common
• Teach patient how to prepare, administer; to rotate sites
for SC inj; to keep accurate
records of dosing (prostate
cancer)

• Instruct patient that tumor flare may occur: increase in size of tumor, increased bone pain; tell patient that bone pain disappears after 1 wk; may take analgesics for pain; premenopausal women must use mechanical birth control; ovulation may be induced

Evaluation
Positive therapeutic outcome
• Decreased size, spread of malignancy
• Decreased pain in endometriosis
• Decreased signs of CPP

---

levalbuterol
See Appendix A, Selected New Drugs

---

levamisole (R)
(lee-vam′i-sol)
Ergamisol
Func. class.: Antineoplastic, immunomodulator
Pregnancy category   C

Action: May increase the action of macrophages, monocytes, and T cells, which restore immune function; complete action is unknown; cholinergic properties

Therapeutic Outcome: Prevention of rapid growth of malignant cells when used with fluorouracil

Uses: Treatment of Dukes' stage C colon cancer when given with fluorouracil after surgical resection

Investigational uses: Malignant melanoma (advanced)

Dosage and routes
Adult: PO 50 mg q8h × 3 days; begin treatment at least 1 wk but no more than 4 wk after resection; give with fluorouracil 450 mg/m^2/day

Available forms: Tab 50 mg (base)

Adverse effects
CNS: Dizziness, headache, paresthesia, somnolence, depression, anxiety, *fatigue,* fever, mental changes, ataxia, insomnia
CV: Chest pain, edema
EENT: Blurred vision, conjunctivitis
GI: Nausea, vomiting, anorexia, diarrhea, stomatitis, constipation, flatulence, dyspepsia, abdominal pain
HEMA: **Granulocytopenia, leukopenia, thrombocytopenia**
INTEG: Rash, pruritus, *alopecia, dermatitis,* urticaria
META: Hyperbilirubinemia
MISC: Rigors, infection, altered sense of smell, arthralgia, myalgia

Contraindications: Hypersensitivity

Precautions: Pregnancy **C**, lactation, children, blood dyscrasias

Pharmacokinetics

Absorption	Rapidly absorbed
Distribution	Unknown
Metabolism	Liver, extensively
Excretion	Unknown
Half-life	3-4 hr

Pharmacodynamics

Onset	Unknown
Peak	1½-2 hr
Duration	Unknown

L

Interactions
Individual drugs
Alcohol: ↑ disulfiram reaction
Phenytoin: ↑ plasma levels, toxicity
Radiation: ↑ bone marrow depression
Warfarin: ↑ warfarin effect
Drug classifications
Antineoplastics: ↑ bone marrow depression

NURSING CONSIDERATIONS
Assessment
◆• Monitor CBC, differential, platelet count weekly; withhold drug if WBC is <4000 or platelet count is <100,000; notify prescriber of results; drug should be discontinued and restarted after recovery
• Monitor renal function studies: BUN, serum uric acid, urine CrCl before, during therapy; I&O ratio; report fall in urine output of 30 ml/hr; check for decreased hyperuricemia
• Monitor for cold, fever, sore throat (may indicate beginning infection)
• Assess for bleeding: hematuria, guaiac, bruising or petechiae, mucosa or orifices q8h; no rec temp
• Identify inflammation of mucosa, breaks in skin; use viscous lidocaine (Xylocaine) for oral pain

Nursing diagnoses
☑ Injury, risk for (adverse reactions)
☑ Body image disturbance (adverse reactions)
☑ Infection, risk for (adverse reactions)
☑ Knowledge deficit (teaching)

Implementation
• Give 7-20 days after surgery; start fluorouracil with 2nd course of levamisole; begin no sooner than 21 days and no later than 35 days after surgery; if levamisole therapy begins 21-30 days after resection, fluorouracil should be given with 1st course; apply pressure to venipuncture sites for 10 min, especially if platelets are low

Patient/family education
• Advise patient to call prescriber if sore throat, swollen lymph nodes, malaise, fever occur, since other infections may develop
• Advise patient that contraceptive measures are recommended during therapy and 4 mo after; teratogenic effects are possible
• Caution patient to avoid ingestion of alcohol, since disulfiram reaction may occur with flushing, severe nausea, vomiting, pounding headache; death can result; advise patient that tyramine-containing foods and cold, hay fever, weight-reducing products may cause hypertensive crisis
• Caution patient to avoid use of products containing aspirin or ibuprofen, razors, commercial mouthwash, since bleeding may occur; to report symptoms of bleeding (hematuria, tarry stools)
• Advise patient to report signs of anemia (fatigue, headache, irritability, faintness, shortness of breath) and CNS reactions including confusion, psychosis, nightmares, seizures, severe headaches
• Inform patient that hair may be lost during treatment; a wig or hair piece may make patient feel better; new hair may be different in color, texture

---

☑ Herb/drug   ⓢ Do Not Crush   ◆ Alert   ⚛ Key Drug   🅖 Geriatric   🅟 Pediatric

• Teach patient the reason for medication use and expected results

Evaluation
Positive therapeutic outcome
• Decreased spread of malignant cells when used with fluorouracil

---

levetiracetam
See Appendix A, Selected New Drugs

---

levobupivacaine
See Appendix A, Selected New Drugs

---

levodopa ⚕ (℞)
(lee'voe-doe-pa)
Dopar, Larodopa, L-Dopa
Func. class.: Antiparkinsonian agent
Chem. class.: Catecholamine, dopamine agonist
Pregnancy category C

Action: Decarboxylation to dopamine, which increases dopamine levels in brain

⮕ **Therapeutic Outcome:** Decreased symptoms of Parkinson's disease (involuntary movements)

Uses: Parkinsonism

Dosage and routes
Adult: PO 0.5-1 g qd divided bid-qid with meals; may increase by up to 0.75 g q3-7 days, not to exceed 8 g/day unless closely supervised

Available forms: Caps 100, 250, 500 mg; tabs 100, 250, 500 mg

Adverse effects
CNS: Involuntary choreiform movements, hand tremors, fatigue, headache, anxiety, twitching, numbness, weakness, confusion, agitation, insomnia, nightmares, psychosis, hallucinations, hypomania, severe depression, dizziness
CV: Orthostatic hypotension, tachycardia, hypertension, palpitations
EENT: Blurred vision, diplopia, dilated pupils
GI: Nausea, vomiting, anorexia, abdominal distress, dry mouth, flatulence, dysphagia, bitter taste, diarrhea, constipation
HEMA: Hemolytic anemia, leukopenia, agranulocytosis
INTEG: Rash, sweating, alopecia
MISC: Urinary retention, incontinence, weight change, dark urine

Contraindications: Hypersensitivity, narrow-angle glaucoma, undiagnosed skin lesions

Precautions: Renal disease, cardiac disease, hepatic disease, respiratory disease, MI with dysrhythmias, convulsions, peptic ulcer, pregnancy **C,** asthma, endocrine disease, affective disorders, psychosis, lactation, children <12 yr peptic ulcer

▣ **Do Not Confuse:**
L-Dopa/methyldopa

Pharmacokinetics	
Absorption	Well absorbed
Distribution	Widely distributed
Metabolism	Liver, GI tract, extensively
Excretion	Kidneys to metabolites; breast milk
Half-life	1 hr

Pharmacodynamics	
Onset	10-15 min
Peak	1-3 hr
Duration	Up to 24 hr

Interactions
Individual drugs
Haloperidol: ↓ effects of levodopa
Methyldopa: ↑ CNS toxicity
Papaverine: ↓ effects of levodopa
Phenytoin: ↓ effects of levodopa
Pyridoxine: ↓ effects of levodopa
Reserpine: ↓ effects of levodopa
Selegiline: ↑ adverse reaction
Drug classifications
Anticholinergics: ↓ effects of levodopa
Antihypertensives: ↑ hypotension
Hydantoins: ↓ effects of levodopa
MAOIs: Hypertensive crisis
☑ Herb/drug
Kava: ↑ parkinson's symptoms
Food/drug
↑ pyridoxine will ↓ levodopa effect
↑ protein food will ↓ absorption
Lab test interferences
False positive: Urine ketones, urine glucose, Coombs' test, urine, norepinephrine
False negative: Urine glucose (glucose oxidase)
False: ↑ Uric acid, false ↑ urine protein
↓ VMA

NURSING CONSIDERATIONS
Assessment
• Monitor B/P, respiration during initial treatment; hypotension or hypertension should be reported
• Assess mental status: affect, mood, behavioral changes, depression; complete suicide assessment
• Monitor liver function enzymes: AST, ALT, alkaline phosphatase; also check LDH, bilirubin, CBC
• Assess for involuntary movements in parkinsonism: akinesia, tremors, staggering gait, muscle rigidity, drooling; these symptoms should improve with levodopa therapy
◆• Assess for levodopa toxicity: mental, personality changes, increased twitching, grimacing, tongue protrusion; these should be reported to prescriber

Nursing diagnoses
☑ Mobility, impaired (uses)
☑ Injury, risk for (uses)
☑ Knowledge deficit (teaching)
☑ Noncompliance (teaching)

Implementation
• Levodopa/carbidopa should not be started until this drug is withheld for 8 hr; toxicity may result if the two drugs are taken close together
• Give drug until NPO before surgery
• Adjust dosage to patient response
• Give with meals to decrease GI upset; limit protein taken with drug
• Give only after MAOIs have been discontinued for 2 wk

Patient/family education
• Advise patient that therapeutic effects may take several wk to a few mo
• Caution patient to change positions slowly to prevent orthostatic hypotension
• Instruct patient to report side effects: twitching, eye spasms; indicate overdose
• Instruct patient to use drug

exactly as prescribed; if drug is discontinued abruptly, parkinsonian crisis may occur
• Inform patient that urine, sweat may darken
• Advise patient to avoid vitamin B_6 preparations, vitamin-fortified foods containing B_6; these foods can reverse effects of levodopa; also OTC preparations should be avoided unless approved by prescriber

Evaluation
Positive therapeutic outcome
• Decreased akathisia, other involuntary movements
• Increased mood

---

levofloxacin (℞)
(lev-o-floks′a-sin)
Levaquin
Func. class.: Antiinfective
Chem. class.: Fluoroquinolone antibacterial
Pregnancy category **C**

Action: Interferes with conversion of intermediate DNA fragments into high-molecular-weight DNA in bacteria; DNA gyrase inhibitor

▶ **Therapeutic Outcome:** Bacterial action against the following: *Streptococcus pneumoniae, Haemophilus influenzae, H. parainfluenzae, Moraxella catarrhalis, Staphylococcus aureus, Klebsiella pneumonia, Mycoplasma pneumoniae*

Uses: Adult urinary tract infections (including complicated); lower respiratory, skin infection

Dosage and routes
Adult: **IV** inf 500 mg by slow inf over 1 hr q24hr × 7-14 days depending on infection; PO

500 mg q24h × 7 days depending on infection
Renal dose
CrCl 20-49 ml/min initial 500 mg, then 250 mg q24h; CrCl 10-19 ml/min 250 or 500 mg, depending on condition, then 250 mg q48h

Available forms: Single-use vials (500 mg), 25 mg/ml 20 ml vials, premixed flexible container; tabs 250, 500 mg

Adverse effects:
CNS: Headache, dizziness, *insomnia,* anxiety, **seizures,** encephalopathy, paresthesia
CV: Chest pain, palpitations, vasodilation
GI: Nausea, flatulence, *vomiting,* diarrhea, abdominal pain, **pseudomembranous colitis**
GU: Vaginitis, crystalluria
HEMA: Eosinophilia, **hemolytic anemia,** lymphophemia
INTEG: Rash, pruritus, urticaria, photosensitivity, **Stevens-Johnson syndrome**
RESP: Pneumonitis

Contraindications: Hypersensitivity to quinolones

Precautions: Pregnancy C, lactation, children, renal disease

Pharmacokinetics
Absorption	Unknown
Distribution	Unknown
Metabolism	Liver
Excretion	Kidneys unchanged
Half-life	6-8 hr

Pharmacodynamics
Onset	Immediate
Peak	Infusion's end

Interactions
Individual drugs
Caffeine: ↑ toxicity
Calcium: ↓ absorption of levofloxacin

L

P

Cimetidine: ↑ effect of levofloxacin

Cyclosporine: ↑ toxicity

Digoxin: ↑ toxicity

Iron: ↓ absorption of levofloxacin

Probenecid: ↑ effect of levofloxacin

Sucralfate: ↓ absorption of levofloxacin

Theophylline: ↓ theophylline clearance

Warfarin: ↑ toxicity, bleeding

Zinc: ↓ absorption of levofloxacin

Drug classifications

Antacids: ↓ absorption of levofloxacin

Antidiabetics: Altered blood glucose levels

NSAIDs: ↑ CNS stimulation, seizures

Lab test interferences

Interference: ↓ glucose, ↓ lymphocytes

NURSING CONSIDERATIONS
Assessment

• Assess patient for previous sensitivity reaction

• Assess patient for signs and symptoms of infection including characteristics of wounds, sputum, urine, stool, WBC >10,000, fever; obtain baseline information before and during treatment

• Obtain C&S before beginning drug therapy to identify if correct treatment has been initiated

• Assess for allergic reactions: rash, urticaria, pruritus, chills, fever, joint pain; may occur a few days after therapy begins; epinephrine and resuscitation equipment should be available for anaphylactic reaction

• Identify urine output; if decreasing, notify prescriber (may indicate nephrotoxicity); also check for increased BUN, creatinine

• Monitor blood studies: AST, ALT, CBC, Hct, bilirubin, LDH, alkaline phosphatase, Coombs' test monthly if patient is on long-term therapy

• Monitor electrolytes: potassium, sodium, chloride monthly if patient is on long-term therapy

• Assess bowel pattern qd; if severe diarrhea occurs, drug should be discontinued

• Monitor for bleeding: ecchymosis, bleeding gums, hematuria, stool guaiac daily if on long-term therapy

• Assess for overgrowth of infection: perineal itching, fever, malaise, redness, pain, swelling, drainage, rash, diarrhea, change in cough, sputum

Nursing diagnoses

☑ Infection, risk for (uses)
☑ Diarrhea (side effects)
☑ Injury, risk for (side effects)
☑ Knowledge deficit (teaching)
☑ Noncompliance (teaching)

Implementation

• Give PO 4 hr before or 2 hr after antacids, iron, calcium, zinc

• Check for irritation, extravasation, phlebitis daily

Patient/family education

• Teach patient to report sore throat, bruising, bleeding, joint pain; may indicate blood dyscrasias (rare)

• Advise patient to contact prescriber if vaginal itching, loose foul-smelling stools, furry tongue occur, may indicate superinfection; report itching, rash, pruritus, urticaria

• Instruct patient to take all medication prescribed for the length of time ordered; drug must be taken around the clock to maintain blood levels; do not give medication to others

• Advise patient to notify prescriber of diarrhea with blood or pus

• Instruct patient to take 4 hr before antacids, iron, calcium, zinc products

• Tell patient to complete full course of therapy

Evaluation
Positive therapeutic outcome
• Absence of signs/symptoms of infection (WBC <10,000, temp WNL)

• Reported improvement in symptoms of infection

levorphanol (℞)
(lee-vor' fan-ole)
Levo-Dromoran, Levorphan
Func. class.: Opioid analgesic agonist
Chem. class.: Opiate, synthetic morphine derivative

Pregnancy category B
Controlled substance schedule II

Action: Inhibits ascending pain pathways in limbic system, thalamus, midbrain, hypothalamus by binding to opiate receptor sites, altering pain perception and response

Therapeutic Outcome: Relief of pain

Uses: Moderate to severe pain

Dosage and routes
Adult: PO/SC/**IV** 2-3 mg q4-5h prn; PCA 0.1 mg/ml

Available forms: Inj 2 mg/ml; tab 2 mg

Adverse effects
CNS: Drowsiness, dizziness, confusion, headache, sedation, euphoria
CV: Palpitations, bradycardia, change in B/P
EENT: Tinnitus, blurred vision, miosis, diplopia
GI: Nausea, vomiting, anorexia, constipation, cramps
GU: Urinary retention, dysuria
INTEG: Rash, urticaria, diaphoresis, pruritus
RESP: **Respiratory depression**

Contraindications: Hypersensitivity, addiction (narcotic)

Precautions: Addictive personality, pregnancy **B,** lactation, increased intracranial pressure, MI (acute), severe heart disease, respiratory depression, hepatic disease, renal disease, child <18 yr

Pharmacokinetics
Absorption	Well absorbed (SC, PO); completely absorbed (**IV**)	
Distribution	Unknown	
Metabolism	Liver, extensively	
Excretion	Kidneys	
Half-life	12-16 hr	

Pharmacodynamics
	PO	SC	IV
Onset	½-1½ hr	Unknown	Unknown
Peak	½-1 hr	½-1 hr	20 min
Duration	6-8 hr	6-8 hr	6-8 hr

Interactions
Individual drugs
Alcohol: ↑ respiratory depression, hypotension, sedation
Nalbuphine: ↓ analgesia
Pentazocine: ↓ analgesia
Drug classifications
Antihistamines: ↑ respiratory depression, hypotension

Antidepressants: ↑ respiratory depression, hypotension
CNS depressants: ↑ respiratory depression, hypotension
MAOIs: ↑ respiratory depression, do not use together
Sedative/hypnotics: ↑ respiratory depression, hypotension
☑ Herb/drug
Kava: ↓ analgesia
Lab test interferences
↑ Amylase

NURSING CONSIDERATIONS
Assessment
• Monitor VS after parenteral route; note muscle rigidity, drug history, liver, kidney function tests, respiratory dysfunction: respiratory depression, character, rate, rhythm; notify prescriber if respirations are <10/min
• Monitor CNS changes: dizziness, drowsiness, hallucinations, euphoria, LOC, pupil reaction
• Monitor allergic reactions: rash, urticaria
Nursing diagnoses
☑ Pain (uses)
☑ Sensory-perceptual alteration: visual, auditory (adverse reactions)
☑ Breathing pattern, ineffective (adverse reactions)
☑ Injury, risk for (adverse reactions)
☑ Knowledge deficit (teaching)
Implementation
• Give with antiemetic if nausea, vomiting occur
• Administer when pain is beginning to return, determine dosage interval by patient response; continuous dosing of medication is more effective given prn; explain analgesic effect

• Medication should be slowly withdrawn after long-term use to prevent withdrawal symptoms
• Store in light-resistant container at room temp
PO route
• May be given with food or milk to lessen GI upset
ⅣV route
• Give **IV** directly; give through Y-tube or 3-way stopcock over 5 min; do not administer rapidly or circulatory collapse may occur
• Store in light-resistant area at room temp
Syringe compatibilities:
Glycopyrrolate, propofol
Additive incompatibilities:
Aminophylline, ammonium chloride, amobarbital, chlorothiazide, heparin, methicillin, pentobarbital, phenobarbital, phenytoin, secobarbital, sodium bicarbonate, sodium iodine, thiopental
Patient/family education
• Caution patients to avoid CNS depressants: alcohol, sedative/hypnotics for at least 24 hr after taking this drug
• Discuss with patient that dizziness, drowsiness, confusion are common; to avoid getting up without assistance
• Discuss in detail all aspects of the drug and what to expect after anesthesia
• Advise patient to make position changes carefully to lessen orthostatic hypotension
Evaluation
Positive therapeutic outcome
• Decreased pain
Treatment of overdose:
Narcan 0.2-0.8 mg **IV**, O_2, **IV** fluids, vasopressors

☑ Herb/drug   Ⓢ Do Not Crush   ◆ Alert   ☞ Key Drug   Ⓖ Geriatric   Ⓟ Pediatric

levothyroxine 🔑 (Rx)
(lee-voe-thye-rox'een)
Eltroxin ✦, Levo-T,
Levothroid, levothyroxine
sodium, Levoxine, Levoxyl,
PMS-Levothyroxine Sodium
✦, Synthroid, T_4
Func. class.: Thyroid
hormone
Chem. class.: Levoisomer
of thyroxine
Pregnancy category **A**

Action: Controls protein
synthesis; increases metabolic
rate, cardiac output, renal
blood flow, O_2 consumption,
body temp, blood volume,
growth, development at cellular level

Therapeutic Outcome: Correction of lack of thyroid hormone

Uses: Hypothyroidism, myxedema coma, thyroid hormone
replacement, cretinism, thyrotoxicosis, congenital hypothyroidism, some types of thyroid
cancer

Dosage and routes
Severe hypothyroidism
Adult: PO 12.5-50 µg qd,
increased by 0.05-0.1 mg q1-4
wk until desired response;
maintenance dosage 75-125 µg
qd, IM/**IV** 50-100 µg/day as
a single dose

P *Child >12 yr:* PO 2-3 µg/kg/
day given as a single dose AM

P *Child 6-12 yr:* PO 4-5 µg/
kg/day given as a single
dose AM

P *Child 1-5 yr:* PO 5-6 µg/kg/
day given as a single dose AM

P *Child 6-12 mo:* PO 6-8 µg/
kg/day give as a single dose AM

P *Child to 6 mo:* PO 8-10 µg/
kg/day given as a single
dose AM

Myxedema coma
Adult: **IV** 200-500 µg; may
increase by 100-300 µg after
24 hr; place on oral medication
as soon as possible; maintenance 50-100 µg/day

Available forms: Inj 50, 200,
500 µg/vial; tabs 0.025, 0.05,
0.075, 0.088, 0.1, 0.112,
0.125, 0.137, 0.15, 0.175,
0.2, 0.3 mg

Adverse effects
*CNS: Anxiety, insomnia, trem-
ors,* headache, **thyroid storm**
*CV: Tachycardia, palpitations,
angina, dysrhythmias,* hypertension, **cardiac arrest**
GI: Nausea, diarrhea, increased
or decreased appetite, cramps
MISC: Menstrual irregularities,
weight loss, sweating, heat
intolerance, fever

Contraindications: Adrenal
insufficiency, MI, thyrotoxicosis, hypersensitivity to beef,
alcohol intolerance (inj only)

G **Precautions:** Elderly, angina
pectoris, hypertension, ischemia, cardiac disease, pregnancy **A**, lactation

N **Do Not Confuse:**
Synthroid/Symmetrel

Pharmacokinetics	
Absorption	Erratic (PO); complete (**IV**)
Distribution	Widely distributed
Metabolism	Liver; enterohepatic recirculation
Excretion	Feces via bile; breast milk (small amounts)
Half-life	6-7 days

Pharmacodynamics		
	PO	IV
Onset	Unknown	6-8 hr
Peak	12-48 hr	12-48 hr
Duration	Unknown	Unknown

Interactions
Individual drugs
Cholestyramine: ↓ absorption of thyroid hormone
Colestipol: ↓ absorption of levothyroxine
Digitalis: ↓ effect of digitalis
Insulin: ↑ requirement for insulin
Phenytoin (IV): ↑ release of thyroid hormone
Drug classifications
Amphetamines: ↑ CNS, cardiac stimulation
β-Adrenergic blockers: ↓ effect of β-blockers
Decongestants: ↑ CNS, cardiac stimulation
Oral anticoagulants: ↑ requirements for anticoagulants
Vasopressors: ↑ CNS, cardiac stimulation
☑ Herb/drug
Bugleweed: Do not give together
Lab test interferences
↑ CPK, ↑ LDH, ↑ AST, ↑ PBI, ↑ blood glucose
↓ thyroid function tests

NURSING CONSIDERATIONS
Assessment
• Identify if the patient is taking anticoagulants, antidiabetic agents; document on chart
• Take B/P, pulse before each dose; monitor I&O ratio and weight every day in same clothing, using same scale, at same time of day
• Monitor height, weight, psychomotor development and growth rate if given to a **P** child
• Monitor T_3, T_4, FTIs, which are decreased; radioimmunoassay of TSH, which is increased; radio uptake, which is increased if patient is on too low a dosage of medication
• Monitor pro-time (may require decreased anticoagulant); check for bleeding, bruising
• Assess for increased nervousness, excitability, irritability, which may indicate too high a dosage of medication, usually after 1-3 wk of treatment
• Assess cardiac status: angina, palpitations, chest pain, change **G** in VS; the elderly patient may have undetected cardiac problems and baseline ECG should be completed before treatment

Nursing diagnoses
☑ Knowledge deficit (teaching)
☑ Noncompliance (teaching)

Implementation
PO route
• Give in AM if possible as a single dose to decrease sleeplessness; give at same time each day to maintain drug level
• Give crushed and mixed with water, non-soy formula, or **P** breast milk for infants/children
• Give only for hormone imbalances; not to be used for obesity, male infertility, menstrual conditions, lethargy; give lowest dosage that relieves symptoms; lower dosage for **G** the elderly and in cardiac diseases
• Store in tight, light-resistant container
• Remove medication 4 wk before RAIU test
IV IV route
• Give **IV** after diluting with provided diluent (0.9% NaCl),

---

0.5 mg/5 ml; shake well; give through Y-tube or 3-way stopcock; give 0.1 mg or less over 1 min; do not add to IV inf; 0.1 mg = 1 ml; discard any unused portion

Patient/family education
• Teach patient that drug is not a cure but controls symptoms and treatment is long term
• Instruct patient to report excitability, irritability, anxiety, sweating, heat intolerance, chest pain, palpitations, which indicate overdose
• Advise patient not to switch brands unless approved by prescriber; bioavailability may differ; do not take with food; absorption will be decreased
• Teach patient that drug may be discontinued after giving birth; thyroid panel will be evaluated after 1-2 mo
• Teach patient or parent that **P** hyperthyroid child will show almost immediate behavior/ personality change; that hair loss will occur in child but is temporary
• Caution patient that drug is not to be taken to reduce weight
• Caution patient to avoid OTC preparations with iodine; read labels; other medications should not be used unless approved by prescriber
• Teach patient to avoid iodine-rich food: iodized salt, soybeans, tofu, turnips, some seafood, some bread

Evaluation
Positive therapeutic outcome
• Absence of depression
• Weight loss, increased diuresis, pulse, appetite
• Absence of constipation, peripheral edema, cold intoler-ance, pale, cool dry skin, brittle nails, alopecia, coarse hair, menorrhagia, night blindness, paresthesias, syncope, stupor, coma, rosy cheeks
• Improved levels of T_3, T_4 by laboratory tests
P • Child: age-appropriate weight, height and psychomotor development

Treatment of overdose: Withhold dose for up to 1 wk: acute overdose: gastric lavage or induced emesis, activated charcoal; provide supportive treatment to control symptoms

---

lidocaine ⚷ (R)
(lye'doe-kane)
Anestacon, Baylocaine, L-Caine, Lidocaine HCl IV for Cardiac Arrhythmias, Lidopen Auto-Injector, Xylocaine HCl IM for Cardiac Arrhythmias, Xylocaine HCl IV for Cardiac Arrhythmias
Func. class.: Antidysrhythmic (Class IB); local anesthetic
Chem. class.: Aminoacyl amide

Pregnancy category B

Action: Increases electrical stimulation threshold of ventricle and His-Purkinje system, which stabilizes cardiac membrane and decreases automaticity; locally produces anesthesia by preventing initiation and conduction of nerve impulses

Therapeutic Outcome: Decreased ventricular dysrhythmia; produces anesthesia locally

Uses: Ventricular tachycardia, ventricular dysrhythmias during cardiac surgery, MI, digitalis toxicity, cardiac catheterization; anesthesia locally

Dosage and routes
Adult: **IV** bol 50-100 mg (1 mg/kg) over 2-3 min; repeat q3-5 min, not to exceed 300 mg in 1 hr; begin **IV** inf 20-50 μg/kg/min; **IM** 200-300 mg (4.3 mg/kg) in deltoid muscle, may repeat in 1-1½ hr if needed

G *Elderly with CHF, reduced liver function:* **IV** bol give ½ adult dose

P *Child:* **IV** bol 1 mg/kg, then **IV** inf 30 μg/kg/min

P *Adult and child:* Top apply as needed to affected areas

Available forms: **IV** inf 0.2% (2 mg/ml), 0.4% (4 mg/ml), 0.8% (8 mg/ml); **IV** admixture 4% (40 mg/ml), 10% (100 mg/ml), 20% (200 mg/ml); **IV** dir 1% (10 mg/ml), 2% (20 mg/ml); IM 300 mg/3 ml; ointment (top) 2.5, 5%; cream (top) 0.5%; spray 10%; jelly 2%; viscous sol 2%; local infiltrative inj 0.5, 1%

Adverse effects
CNS: Headache, dizziness, involuntary movement, confusion, tremor, *drowsiness,* euphoria, **convulsions**
CV: Hypotension, bradycardia, **heart block, cardiovascular collapse, arrest**
EENT: Tinnitus, blurred vision
GI: Nausea, vomiting, anorexia
INTEG: Rash, urticaria, edema, swelling, burning, stinging
MISC: Febrile response, phlebitis at inj site

Contraindications: Hypersensitivity to amides, severe heart block, supraventricular dysrhythmias, Adams-Stokes syndrome, Wolff-Parkinson-White syndrome

Precautions: Pregnancy **B,**
P lactation, children, renal disease, liver disease, CHF, respiratory depression, malignant hyperthermia

Pharmacokinetics

Absorption	Complete bioavailability (**IV**)
Distribution	Erythrocytes, cardiovascular endothelium
Metabolism	Liver
Excretion	Kidneys
Half-life	Biphasic 8 min, 1-2 hr

Pharmacodynamics

	IV	IM	TOP
Onset	2 min	5-15 min	Unknown
Peak	Unknown	½ hr	5 min
Duration	20 min	1½ hr	½-1 hr

Interactions
Individual drugs
Cimetidine: ↓ metabolism, ↑ toxicity
Phenytoin: ↑ toxicity
Procainamide: ↑ toxicity
Propranolol: ↑ toxicity
Quinidine: ↑ toxicity
Drug classifications
β-Adrenergic blockers: ↑ toxicity
☑ *Herb/drug*
Aloe: ↑ action of lidocaine
Buckthorn: ↑ action of lidocaine
Cascara sagrada: ↑ action of lidocaine
Senna: ↑ action of lidocaine
Lab test interferences
↑ Liver function tests

☑ Herb/drug **☒** Do Not Crush **◆** Alert **☞** Key Drug **G** Geriatric **P** Pediatric

NURSING CONSIDERATIONS
Assessment
- Assess for oxygenation or perfusion deficit: decreased B/P, chest pain, dizziness, loss of consciousness
- Assess respiratory status: auscultate lung fields for bibasilar crackles in patients with advanced CHF
- Assess for urinary retention: check for pain, abdominal absorption, palpate bladder; check males with benign prostatic hypertrophy; anticholinergic reaction may cause retention
- Monitor I&O ratio, electrolytes (potassium, sodium, chloride); watch for decreasing urinary output, possible retention
- Monitor liver function studies: AST, ALT, bilirubin, alkaline phosphatase
- Monitor ECG continuously to determine drug effectiveness, measure PR, QRS, QT intervals, check for PVCs, other dysrhythmias; monitor B/P continuously for hypotension, hypertension; check for rebound hypertension after 1-2 hr, prolonged PR/QT intervals, QRS complex; if QT or QRS increases by 50% or more, withhold next dose, notify prescriber
- Monitor for CNS symptoms: confusion, numbness, depression, involuntary movements; if these occur, drug should be discontinued
- Monitor blood levels (therapeutic level 1.5-5 μg/ml), notify prescriber of abnormal results

Nursing diagnoses
- ☑ Cardiac output, decreased (uses)
- ☑ Impaired gas exchange (adverse reactions)
- ☑ Knowledge deficit (teaching)

Implementation
IM route
- Administer in deltoid, aspirate to prevent **IV** administration
- Check site daily for extravasation

☑ IV route
- Give **IV** bolus undiluted (1%, 2% only); give 6 mg or less over 1 min; if using an **IV** line, use port near insertion site, flush with normal saline (50 ml)
- Store at room temp; sol should be clear
- Give by cont inf after adding 1 g/250-1000 ml D_5W; give 1-4 mg/min; use inf pump for correct dosage; pediatric inf is 120 mg of lidocaine/100 ml of D_5W; 1-2.5 ml/kg/hr = 20-50 μg/kg/min; use only 1%, 2% sol

Solution compatibilities:
D_5W, D_5/0.9% NaCl, D_5/0.45% NaCl, D_5/LR, 0.9% NaCl, 0.45% NaCl

Syringe compatibilities:
Cloxacillin, glycopyrrolate, heparin, hydroxyzine, methicillin, metoclopramide, milrinone, moxalactam, nalbuphine

Syringe incompatibilities:
Cefazolin

Y-site compatibilities:
Alteplase, amiodarone, amrinone, cefazolin, ciprofloxacin, diltiazem, dobutamine, dopamine, enalaprilat, etomidate, famotidine, haloperidol, heparin, heparin with hydrocortisone, labetalol, meperidine, morphine, nitroglycerin, nitroprusside, potassium chloride,

propofol, streptokinase, theophylline, vit B/C, warfarin

Additive compatibilities:
Alteplase, aminophylline, amiodarone, atracurium, bretylium, calcium chloride, calcium gluceptate, calcium gluconate, chloramphenicol, chlorothiazide, cimetidine, dexamethasone, digoxin, diphenhydramine, dobutamine, dopamine, ephedrine, erythromycin, floxacillin, flumazenil, furosemide, heparin, hydrocortisone, nafcillin, hydroxyzine, regular insulin, mephentermine, metaraminol, nafcillin, nitroglycerin, penicillin G potassium, pentobarbital, phenylephrine, potassium chloride, procainamide, prochlorperazine, promazine, ranitidine, sodium bicarbonate, sodium lactate, theophylline, verapamil, vit B/C

Additive incompatibilities:
Methohexital, phenytoin; do not admix with blood transfusions

Infiltration
Physician may order lidocaine with epinephrine to minimize systemic absorption and prolong local anesthesia

Patient/family education
• Teach patient or family reason for use of medication and expected results
• Instruct patient in at-home use of Lidopen Auto-Injector; patient should call prescriber before use if heart attack is imminent

Evaluation
Positive therapeutic outcome
• Decreased B/P, dysrhythmias
• Decreased heart rate
• Normal sinus rhythm

Treatment of overdose:
Oxygen, artificial ventilation, ECG, administer dopamine for circulatory depression, diazepam or thiopental for convulsions, decreased drug or discontinuation may be required

---

lindane (OTC)
(lin-dane)
Bio-Well, GBH ✤, G-Well, Kwell, Kwellada ✤, Kwildane, lindane, Scabene, Thionex
Func. class.: Scabicide/pediculicide
Chem. class.: Chlorinated hydrocarbon (synthetic)
Pregnancy category B

Action: Stimulates nervous system of arthropods, resulting in seizures, death of organism

➥**Therapeutic Outcome:** Resolution of infestation

Uses: Scabies, lice (head/pubic/body), nits

Dosage and routes
Lice
P *Adult and child:* Cream/lotion: wash area with soap and water 8-12 hr after application; may reapply in 1 wk if needed; shampoo using 30 ml: work into lather, rub for 5 min, rinse, dry with towel; use fine-toothed comb to remove nits

Scabies
P *Adult and child:* Top apply 1% cream/lotion to skin from neck to bottom of feet, toes; repeat in 1 wk if necessary

Available forms: Lotion, shampoo, cream (1%)

Adverse effects

CNS: Tremors, **convulsions,** stimulation, dizziness (chronic inhalation of vapors)
CV: Ventricular fibrillation (chronic inhalation of vapors)
GI: Nausea, vomiting, diarrhea, liver damage (inhalation of vapors)
HEMA: Aplastic anemia (chronic inhalation of vapors)
INTEG: Pruritus, rash, irritation, contact dermatitis

Contraindications: Hypersensitivity, premature neonate, patients with known seizure disorders, inflammation of skin, abrasions, or breaks in skin

Precautions: Pregnancy **B,** children <10 yr, infants, lactation; avoid contact with eyes

Pharmacokinetics

Absorption	20%
Distribution	Fat
Metabolism	Liver
Excretion	Kidneys
Half-life	18 hr

Pharmacodynamics

Onset	Rapid
Peak	Rapid
Duration	3 hr

Interactions
Oil-based hair dressing:
↑ absorption; wash, rinse, and dry hair before using lindane

NURSING CONSIDERATIONS
Assessment
• Assess head, hair for lice and nits before and after treatment; if scabies are present, check all skin surfaces
• Identify source of infection: school, family members, sexual contacts

Nursing diagnoses
☑ Skin integrity, impaired (uses)
☑ Knowledge deficit (teaching)

Implementation
• Apply to body areas, scalp only; do not apply to face, lips, mouth, eyes, any mucous membrane, anus, or meatus
• Give top corticosteroids as ordered to decrease contact dermatitis; provide antihistamines
• Apply menthol or phenol lotions to control itching
• Give top antibiotics for infection
• Provide isolation until areas on skin, scalp have cleared and treatment is completed
• Remove nits by using a fine-toothed comb rinsed in vinegar after treatment; use gloves

Patient/family education
• Advise patient to wash all inhabitants' clothing, using insecticide; preventive treatment may be required of all persons living in same house, using lotion or shampoo to decrease spread of infection; use rubber gloves when applying drug
• Instruct patient that itching may continue for 4-6 wk; that drug must be reapplied if accidently washed off, or treatment will be ineffective
• Advise patient not to apply to face; if accidental contact with eyes occurs, flush with water
• Advise patient that sexual contacts should be treated simultaneously

Evaluation
Positive therapeutic outcome
• Decreased crusts, nits, brownish trails on skin, itching papules in skinfolds

L

• Decreased itching after several wk

Treatment of ingestion:
Gastric lavage, saline laxatives, **IV** diazepam (Valium) for convulsions (if taken orally)

liothyronine (T₃) (℞)
(lye-oh-thye'roe-neen)
Cytomel, ʟ-Triiodothyronine, liothyronine sodium, Triostat, T₃
Func. class.: Thyroid hormone
Chem. class.: Synthetic T₃
Pregnancy category   A

Action: Controls protein synthesis; increases metabolic rates, cardiac output, renal blood flow, O₂ consumption, body temp, blood volume, growth, development at cellular level

Therapeutic Outcome: Correction of lack of thyroid hormone

Uses: Hypothyroidism, myxedema coma, thyroid hormone replacement, nontoxic goiter, T₃ suppression test, congenital hypothyroidism

Dosage and routes
Adult: PO 25 μg qd, increased by 12.5-25 μg q1-2 wk until desired response, maintenance dosage 25-75 μg qd

G *Elderly:* PO 5 μg/day, increase by 5 μg/day q1-2 wk

Congenital hypothyroidism
P *Child >3 yr:* PO 50-100 μg qd

P *Child <3 yr:* PO 5 μg qd, increased by 5 μg q3-4 days titrated to response

Myxedema, severe hypothyroidism
Adult: PO 5 μg qd; may increase by 5-10 μg q1-2 wk; maintenance dosage 50-100 μg qd

Myxedema coma/precoma
Adult: IV 25-50 μg initially; 5 **G** μg in elderly; 10-20 μg in cardiac disease; give doses q4-12h

Nontoxic goiter
Adult: PO 5 μg qd, increased by 12.5-25 μg q1-2 wk; maintenance dosage 75 μg qd

Suppression test (T₃)
Adult: PO 75-100 μg qd × 1 wk; ¹³¹I is given before and after 1st wk dose

Available forms: Tabs 5, 25, 50 μg; inj 10 μg/ml

Adverse effects
CNS: Insomnia, tremors, headache, **thyroid storm**
CV: Tachycardia, palpitations, angina, dysrhythmias, hypertension, cardiac arrest
GI: Nausea, diarrhea, increased or decreased appetite, cramps
MISC: Menstrual irregularities, weight loss, sweating, heat intolerance, fever

Contraindications: Adrenal insufficiency, MI, thyrotoxicosis

G **Precautions:** Elderly, angina pectoris, hypertension, ischemia, cardiac disease, pregnancy **A**, lactation

Pharmacokinetics	
Absorption	Well (PO); complete (IV)
Distribution	Widely distributed; does not cross placenta
Metabolism	Liver
Excretion	Feces via bile, breast milk
Half-life	6-7 days

Pharmacodynamics	
	PO/IV
Onset	Unknown
Peak	12-24 hr
Duration	72 hr

Interactions
Individual drugs
Cholestyramine: ↓ absorption of thyroid hormone
Colestipol: ↓ absorption of thyroid hormone
Digitalis: ↓ effect of digitalis
Insulin: ↑ requirement for insulin
Phenytoin (IV): ↑ release of thyroid hormone
Drug classifications
Amphetamines: ↑ CNS, cardiac stimulation
β-Adrenergic blockers: ↓ effect of β-blockers
Decongestants: ↑ CNS, cardiac stimulation
Oral anticoagulants: ↑ requirements for anticoagulants
Vasopressors: ↑ CNS, cardiac stimulation
⬚ Herb/drug
Bugleweed: Do not use together
Lab test interferences
↑ CPK, ↑ LDH, ↑ AST, ↑ PBI, ↑ blood glucose
↓ thyroid function tests

NURSING CONSIDERATIONS
Assessment
• Identify if the patient is taking anticoagulants, antidiabetic agents; document on patient record
• Take B/P, pulse before each dose; monitor I&O ratio and weight every day in same clothing, using same scale, at same time of day
• Monitor height, weight, psychomotor development, and growth rate if given to a child
• Monitor T$_3$, T$_4$, FTIs, which are decreased; radioimmunoassay of TSH, which is increased; RAIU, which is increased if patient is on too low a dosage of medication
• Monitor pro-time; may require decreased anticoagulant; check for bleeding, bruising
• Assess for increased nervousness, excitability, irritability, which may indicate too high a dosage, usually after 1-3 wk of treatment
• Assess cardiac status: angina, palpitations, chest pain, change in VS; elderly patients may have undetected cardiac problems, and baseline ECG should be completed before treatment

Nursing diagnoses
☑ Knowledge deficit (teaching)
☑ Noncompliance (teaching)

Implementation
PO route
• Give in AM if possible as a single dose to decrease sleeplessness; give at same time each day to maintain drug level
• Give only for hormone imbalances; not to be used for obesity, male infertility, menstrual conditions, lethargy; give lowest dosage that relieves symptoms; give lower dosage to the elderly and for cardiac diseases
• Store in air-tight, light-resistant container
IV route
• Administer **IV** for myxedema coma and precoma; do not give IM or SC; give q4-12h; use PO dose as soon as feasible

Patient/family education
• Teach patient that drug is not a cure but controls symp-

toms, and treatment is long term

• Instruct patient to report excitability, irritability, anxiety, sweating, heat intolerance, chest pain, palpitations, which indicate overdose

• Advise patient not to switch brands unless approved by prescriber; bioavailability may differ; do not take with food or absorption will be decreased

• Teach patient that drug may be discontinued after giving birth; thyroid panel will be evaluated after 1-2 mo

🄿 • Teach patient that hyperthyroid child will show almost immediate behavior/personality change; that hair loss will occur in child but is temporary

• Caution patient that drug is not to be taken to reduce weight

• Caution patient to avoid OTC preparations with iodine; read labels; other medications should not be used unless approved by prescriber

• Teach patient to avoid iodine-rich food: iodized salt, soybeans, tofu, turnips, some seafood, some bread

Evaluation
Positive therapeutic outcome
• Absence of depression
• Weight loss
• Increased diuresis, pulse, appetite
• Absence of constipation, peripheral edema, cold intolerance, pale, cool dry skin, brittle nails, alopecia, coarse hair, menorrhagia, night blindness, paresthesias, syncope, stupor, coma, rosy cheeks
• Improved levels of T_3, T_4 by laboratory tests

🄿 • Child: age-appropriate weight, height, and psychomotor development

Treatment of overdose:
Withhold dose for up to 1 wk; for acute overdose: gastric lavage or induce emesis, then activated charcoal; provide supportive treatment to control symptoms

liotrix (℞)
(lye′oh-trix)
Euthroid, T_3/T_4, Thyrolar
Func. class.: Thyroid hormone
Chem. class.: Levothyroxine/liothyronine (synthetic T_4, T_3)
Pregnancy category **A**

Action: Controls protein synthesis; increases metabolic rates, cardiac output, renal blood flow, O_2 consumption, body temp, blood volume, growth, development at cellular level

➡ **Therapeutic Outcome:** Correction of lack of thyroid hormone

Uses: Hypothyroidism, thyroid hormone replacement

Dosage and routes
🄿 *Adult and child:* PO 15-30 mg qd, increased by 15-30 mg q1-2 wk until desired response; may increase by 15-30 mg q2 wk in child

🄶 *Elderly:* PO 15 mg initially, increase q2-4 wk by 15 mg until desired response

Available forms: Euthroid ½, 1, 2, 3 gr; Thyrolar ¼, ½, 1, 2, 3, gr; ½ grain = 30 mg

---

☑ Herb/drug 🄢 Do Not Crush ◆ Alert ☯ Key Drug 🄶 Geriatric 🄿 Pediatric

Adverse effects
CNS: Insomnia, tremors, headache, thyroid storm
CV: Tachycardia, palpitations, angina, dysrhythmias, hypertension, cardiac arrest
GI: Nausea, diarrhea, increased or decreased appetite, cramps
MISC: Menstrual irregularities, weight loss, sweating, heat intolerance, fever

Contraindications: Adrenal insufficiency, MI, thyrotoxicosis

G Precautions: Elderly, angina pectoris, hypertension, ischemia, cardiac disease, pregnancy **A,** lactation

N Do Not Confuse:
Thyrolar/Thyrar

Pharmacokinetics

Absorption	50%-80% (T_4); 95% (T_3)
Distribution	Widely distributed; does not cross placenta
Metabolism	Liver, tissues
Excretion	Feces via bile; breast milk
Half-life	6-7 days (T_4); 2 days (T_3)

Pharmacodynamics

	PO (T_4)	PO (T_3)
Onset	Unknown	Unknown
Peak	Unknown	24-72 hr
Duration	Unknown	72 hr

Interactions
Individual drugs
Cholestyramine: ↓ absorption of thyroid hormone
Colestipol: ↓ absorption of liotrix
Digitalis: ↓ effect of digitalis
Insulin: ↑ requirement for insulin
Phenytoin (IV): ↑ release of thyroid hormone

Drug classifications
Amphetamines: ↑ CNS, cardiac stimulation
β-Adrenergic blockers: ↓ effect of β-blockers
Decongestants: ↑ CNS, cardiac stimulation
Oral anticoagulants: ↑ requirements for anticoagulants
Vasopressors: ↑ CNS, cardiac stimulation
☑ Herb/drug
Bugleweed: Do not use together
Lab test interferences
↑ CPK, ↑ LDH, ↑ AST, ↑ PBI, ↑ blood glucose
↓ thyroid function tests

NURSING CONSIDERATIONS
Assessment
• Identify if the patient is taking anticoagulants, antidiabetic agents; document on chart
• Take B/P, pulse before each dose; monitor I&O ratio and weight every day in same clothing, using same scale, at same time of day
• Monitor height, weight, psychomotor development, and growth rate if given to a
P child
• Monitor T_3, T_4, FTIs, which are decreased; radioimmunoassay of TSH, which is increased; RAIU, which is increased if patient is on too low a dosage of medication
• Monitor pro-time; may require decreased anticoagulant; check for bleeding, bruising
• Assess for increased nervousness, excitability, irritability, which may indicate too high a dosage of medication, usually after 1-3 wk of treatment

L

• Assess cardiac status: angina, palpitations, chest pain, change in VS; the elderly patient may have undetected cardiac problems, and baseline ECG should be completed before treatment

Nursing diagnoses
✓ Knowledge deficit (teaching)
✓ Noncompliance (teaching)

Implementation
• Give in AM if possible as a single dose to decrease sleeplessness; give at same time each day to maintain drug level
• Give only for hormone imbalances; not to be used for obesity, male infertility, menstrual conditions, lethargy; give lowest dosage that relieves symptoms; give lower dosage to the elderly and for cardiac diseases
• Store in airtight, light-resistant container
• Remove medication 4 wk before RAIU test

Patient/family education
• Teach patient that drug is not a cure but controls symptoms, and treatment is long term
• Instruct patient to report excitability, irritability, anxiety, sweating, heat intolerance, chest pain, palpitations, which indicate overdose
• Advise patient not to switch brands unless approved by prescriber; bioavailability may differ; do not take with food or absorption will be decreased
• Teach patient that drug may be discontinued after giving birth; thyroid panel will be evaluated after 1-2 mo
• Teach patient that hyperthyroid child will show almost immediate behavior/personality change; that hair loss will occur in child but is temporary
• Caution patient that drug is not to be taken to reduce weight
• Caution patient to avoid OTC preparations with iodine; read labels; other medications should not be used unless approved by prescriber
• Teach patient to avoid iodine-rich food: iodized salt, soybeans, tofu, turnips, some seafood, some bread

Evaluation
Positive therapeutic outcome
• Absence of depression
• Weight loss
• Increased diuresis, pulse, appetite
• Absence of constipation, peripheral edema, cold intolerance, pale, cool dry skin, brittle nails, alopecia, coarse hair, menorrhagia, night blindness, paresthesias, syncope, stupor, coma, rosy cheeks
• Improved levels of T_3, T_4 by laboratory tests
• Child: age-appropriate weight, height, and psychomotor development

Treatment of overdose:
Withhold dose for up to 1 wk; acute overdose: gastric lavage or induce emesis, then activated charcoal; provide supportive treatment to control symptoms

---

lisinopril (℞)
(lyse-in'oh-pril)
Prinivil, Zestril
Func. class.: Antihypertensive, angiotensin converting enzyme (ACE) inhibitor
Chem. class.: Enalaprilat lysine analog

Pregnancy category
C (1st trimester),
D (2nd/3rd trimesters)

Action: Selectively suppresses renin-angiotensin-aldosterone system; inhibits ACE; prevents conversion of angiotensin I to angiotensin II; results in dilatation of arterial, venous vessels

▶**Therapeutic Outcome:** Decreased B/P in hypertension, decreased preload, afterload in CHF

Uses: Mild to moderate hypertension, adjunctive therapy of systolic CHF

Dosage and routes
Hypertension
Adult: PO 10-40 mg qd; may increase to 80 mg qd if required

G *Elderly:* PO 2.5-5 mg/day, increase q7 days

CHF
Adult: PO 2.5-5 mg initially with diuretics/digitalis

Available forms: Tabs 5, 10, 20, 40 mg

Adverse effects
CNS: Vertigo, depression, stroke, insomnia, paresthesias, *headache,* fatigue, asthenia
EENT: Blurred vision, nasal congestion
GI: Nausea, vomiting, anorexia, constipation, flatulence, GI irritation

GU: **Proteinuria, renal insufficiency,** sexual dysfunction, impotence
HEMA: **Agranulocytopenia,** neutropenia
INTEG: Rash, pruritus
RESP: Dry cough, dyspnea
SYST: **Angioedema**

Contraindications: Hypersensitivity, pregnancy **D**, (2nd/3rd trimesters)

Precautions: Pregnancy **C**, (1st trimester), lactation, renal disease, hyperkalemia, renal artery stenosis

◨ **Do Not Confuse:**
Prinivil/Plendil, Prinivil/Proventil, Prinivil/Prilosec

Pharmacokinetics	
Absorption	Variable
Distribution	Unknown
Metabolism	Not metabolized
Excretion	Kidneys, unchanged
Half-life	12 hr

Pharmacodynamics	
Onset	1 hr
Peak	6-8 hr
Duration	24 hr

Interactions
Individual drugs
Alcohol: ↑ hypotension (large amounts)
Allopurinol: ↑ hypersensitivity
Digoxin: ↑ serum levels
Hydralazine: ↑ toxicity
Indomethacin: ↓ antihypertensive effect
Lithium: ↑ levels of lithium
Prazosin: ↑ toxicity
Drug classifications
Adrenergic blockers: ↑ hypotension
Antacids: ↓ absorption
Antihypertensives: ↑ hypotension
Diuretics: ↑ hypotension
Diuretics, potassium-sparing: ↑ toxicity

L

Ganglionic blockers: ↑ hypotension
Potassium supplements: ↑ toxicity
Sympathomimetics: ↑ toxicity
Food/drug
High-potassium diet (bananas, orange juice, avocados, broccoli, nuts, spinach) should be avoided; hyperkalemia may occur
Lab test interferences
False positive: Urine acetone

NURSING CONSIDERATIONS
Assessment
• Monitor B/P, check for orthostatic hypotension, syncope; if changes occur, dosage change may be required
• Monitor renal studies: protein, BUN, creatinine; watch for increased levels that may indicate nephrotic syndrome and renal failure; monitor renal symptoms: polyuria, oliguria, frequency, dysuria
• Establish baselines in renal, liver function tests before therapy begins
• Check potassium levels throughout treatment, although hyperkalemia rarely occurs
• Check for edema in feet, legs daily
• Assess for allergic reactions: rash, fever, pruritus, urticaria; drug should be discontinued if antihistamines fail to help

Nursing diagnoses
☑ Cardiac output, decreased (uses)
☑ Injury, risk for (side effects)
☑ Knowledge deficit (teaching)
☑ Noncompliance (teaching)

Implementation
• Store in tight container at 86° F (30° C) or less
• Severe hypotension may

occur after 1st dose of this medication; it may be prevented by reducing or discontinuing diuretic therapy 3 days before beginning lisinopril therapy

Patient/family education
• Caution patient not to discontinue drug abruptly; advise patient to inform all health care providers about taking this drug
• Teach patient not to use OTC products (cough, cold, allergy) unless directed by prescriber; serious side effects can occur
• Teach patient the importance of complying with dosage schedule, even if feeling better; to continue with medical regimen to decrease B/P: exercise, cessation of smoking, decreasing stress, diet modifications
• Teach patient to notify prescriber of mouth sores, sore throat, fever, swelling of hands or feet, irregular heartbeat, chest pain, coughing, shortness of breath
• Caution patient to report excessive perspiration, dehydration, vomiting, diarrhea; may lead to fall in B/P
• Emphasize the need to rise slowly to sitting or standing position to minimize orthostatic hypotension; not to exercise in hot weather or increased hypotension can occur
• Caution patient that drug may cause dizziness, fainting, light-headedness; may occur during 1st few days of therapy; to avoid activities that may be hazardous
• Teach patient how to take B/P, and normal readings for

---

age group; advise patient to take B/P regularly

• Instruct patient to avoid increasing K in the diet

Evaluation
Positive therapeutic outcome
• Decreased B/P in hypertension
• Decreased CHF symptoms

Treatment of overdose: 0.9% NaCl **IV** inf, hemodialysis

---

lithium (℞)
(li'thee-um)
Carbolith ✦, Cibalith-S, Duralith ✦, Eskalith, Eskalith CR, Lithane, lithium carbonate, Lithizine ✦, Lithonate, Lithotabs
Func. class.: Antimanic
Chem. class.: Alkali metal ion salt

Pregnancy category   D

Action: May alter sodium, potassium ion transport across cell membrane in nerve, muscle cells; may balance biogenic amines of norepinephrine, serotonin in CNS areas involved in emotional responses

➡ Therapeutic Outcome: Stable mood

Uses: Manic-depressive illness (manic phase), prevention of bipolar manic-depressive psychosis

Dosage and routes
Adult: PO 300-600 mg tid; maintenance 300 mg tid or qid; slow rel tab 300 mg bid; dosage should be individualized to maintain blood levels at 0.5-1.5 mEq/L

G Elderly: PO 300 mg bid, increase q7 days by 300 mg to desired dose

P Child: PO 15-20 mg (0.4-0.5 mEq)/kg/day in 2-3 divided doses, increase as needed, do not exceed adult doses

Renal dose
PO CrCl 10-50 ml/min 50-75% of dose; CrCl <10 ml/min 25%-50% of dose

Available forms: Caps 300, 600 mg; tab 300 mg; controlled rel tab 450 mg; syrup 300 mg/5 ml (8 mEq/5 ml); slow rel caps 300 mg ✦

Adverse effects
CNS: Headache, drowsiness, dizziness, tremors, twitching, ataxia, **seizure,** slurred speech, restlessness, *confusion,* stupor, memory loss, clonic movements, *fatigue*
CV: Hypotension, ECG changes, **dysrhythmias, circulatory collapse, edema**
EENT: Tinnitus, blurred vision, aphasia, dysarthria
ENDO: Hypothyroidism, goiter, hyperglycemia, hyperthyroidism
GI: Dry mouth, anorexia, nausea, vomiting, diarrhea, incontinence, abdominal pain, metallic taste
GU: **Polyuria, glycosuria, proteinuria, albuminuria,** urinary incontinence, polydipsia, edema, **renal toxicity**
HEMA: **Leukocytosis**
INTEG: Drying of hair, alopecia, rash, pruritus, hyperkeratosis, *acneiform rash, folliculitis*
MS: Muscle weakness, rigidity
SYST: Hyponatremia

Contraindications: Hepatic disease, renal disease, brain trauma, OBS, pregnancy **D,** lactation, schizophrenia, severe cardiac disease, severe renal disease, severe dehydration

L

G Precautions: Elderly, thyroid disease, seizure disorders, diabetes mellitus, syst infection, urinary retention, **P** children <12 yr

Pharmacokinetics

Absorption	Completely absorbed
Distribution	Reabsorbed by renal tubules (80%); crosses blood-brain barrier; crosses placenta
Metabolism	Unknown
Excretion	Urine, unchanged
Half-life	18-36 hr depending on age

Pharmacodynamics

Onset	Rapid
Peak	½-4 hr
Duration	Unknown

Interactions
Individual drugs
Acetazolamide: ↑ renal clearance
Aminophylline: ↑ renal clearance
Calcium iodide: ↑ hypothyroid effect
Carbamazepine: ↑ lithium toxicity
Fluoxetine: ↑ lithium toxicity
Haloperidol: ↑ neurotoxicity
Iodinated glycerol: ↑ hypothyroid effect
Indomethacin: ↑ toxicity
Losartan: ↑ toxicity
Mannitol: ↑ renal clearance
Methyldopa: ↑ lithium toxicity
Potassium: ↑ hypothyroid effect
Sodium bicarbonate: ↑ renal clearance
Thioridazine: Brain damage
Urea: ↑ toxicity
Drug classifications
NSAIDs: ↑ lithium toxicity
Phenothiazines: ↑ effect of phenothiazines

Theophyllines: ↓ effect of lithium
Thiazides: ↑ lithium toxicity
⊘ Herb/drug
Broom: ↑ lithium effect
Buchu: ↑ lithium effect
Dandelion: ↑ lithium effect
Juniper: ↑ lithium effect
Food/drug
Significant changes in sodium intake will alter lithium excretion

Lab test interferences
↑ Potassium excretion, ↑ urine glucose, ↑ blood glucose, ↑ protein, ↑ BUN
↓ VMA, ↓ T_3, ↓ T_4, ↓ PBI, ↓ ^{131}I

NURSING CONSIDERATIONS
Assessment
• Assess for minor lithium toxicity: vomiting, diarrhea, poor coordination, fine motor tremors, weakness, lassitude; major toxicity: coarse tremors, severe thirst, tinnitus, dilute urine
• Assess weight daily; check for edema in legs, ankles, wrists; report if present; check skin turgor at least daily
• Monitor sodium intake; decreased sodium intake with decreased fluid intake may lead to lithium retention; increased sodium and fluids may decrease lithium retention
• Monitor urine for albuminuria, glycosuria, uric acid during beginning treatment, q2 mo thereafter
• Assess neuro status: LOC, gait, motor reflexes, hand tremors
• Monitor serum lithium levels weekly initially, then q2 mo (therapeutic level: 0.5-1.5 mEq/L); toxicity and therapeutic levels are very close; toxicity may occur rapidly;

---

blood levels are drawn before the AM dose

Nursing diagnoses
- ☑ Ineffective individual coping (uses)
- ☑ Thought processes, altered (uses)
- ☑ Knowledge deficit (teaching)
- ☑ Noncompliance (teaching)

Implementation
- 🅖 Administer reduced dosage to elderly; give with meals to avoid GI upset
- Provide adequate fluids (2-3 L/day) to prevent dehydration during initial treatment, 1-2 L/day during maintenance

Patient/family education
- Provide patient with written information on symptoms of minor toxicity: vomiting, diarrhea, poor coordination, fine motor tremors, weakness, lassitude; major toxicity: coarse tremors, severe thirst, tinnitus, dilute urine
- Advise patient to monitor urine sp gr; emphasize need for follow-up care to determine lithium effects
- Advise patient that contraception is necessary, since lithium may harm fetus
- Caution patient not to operate machinery until lithium levels are stable and response determined; that beneficial effects may take 1-3 wk
- Provide to the patient a list of drugs that interact with lithium and discuss need for adequate, stable intake of salt and fluid
- 🚫 Advise patient not to crush, chew caps

Evaluation
Positive therapeutic outcome
- Decrease in excitement, poor

judgment, insomnia (manic phase)
- Decreased mood swings and lability

Treatment of overdose: Induce emesis or lavage, maintain airway, respiratory function; dialysis for severe intoxication

---

lomefloxacin (℞)
(lome-flocks'a-sin)
Maxaquin
Func. class.: Antiinfective
Chem. class.: Fluoroquinolone

Pregnancy category C

Action: Interferes with conversion of intermediate DNA fragments into high-molecular-weight DNA in bacteria; DNA gyrase inhibitor

Therapeutic Outcome: Bactericidal for gram-negative organisms *Aeromonas, Citrobacter, Enterobacter, Escherichia coli, Haemophilus influenzae, Klebsiella, Legionella, Moraxella catarrhalis, Morganella morganii, Proteus vulgaris, P. mirabilis, Providencia alcalifaciens, P. rettgeri, Pseudomonas aeruginosa, Serratia;* gram-positive organisms *Staphylococcus aureus, S. epidermidis, S. saprophyticus* (methicillin-resistant strains also)

Uses: Treatment of lower respiratory tract infections (pneumonia, bronchitis), genitourinary tract infections (prostatitis, UTIs), preoperatively to reduce urinary tract infections in transurethral surgical procedures

---

Dosage and routes
Adult: PO 400 mg/day × 7-14 days depending on type of infection

In renal impairment
Adult: PO 200 mg/day

Surgical prophylaxis of UTI
Adult: PO 400 mg 2-6 hr before surgery

Available forms: Tab 400 mg

Adverse effects
CNS: Dizziness, headache, somnolence, depression, insomnia, nervousness, confusion, agitation
EENT: Visual disturbances
GI: Diarrhea, *nausea,* vomiting, anorexia, flatulence, heartburn, dry mouth, increased AST, ALT, constipation, abdominal pain, oral thrush, glossitis, stomatitis
INTEG: Rash, pruritus, urticaria, *photosensitivity*

Contraindications: Hypersensitivity to quinolones

P G **Precautions:** Pregnancy C, lactation, children, elderly, renal disease, seizure disorders, excessive exposure to sunlight

Pharmacokinetics
Absorption	Well absorbed
Distribution	Widely distributed
Metabolism	Unknown
Excretion	Kidney, unchanged
Half-life	6-8 hr; increased in renal disease

Pharmacodynamics
Onset	Unknown
Peak	1-2 hr

Interactions
Individual drugs
Caffeine: ↑ levels
Calcium: ↓ effects of lomefloxacin
Cimetidine: ↑ lomefloxacin levels, toxicity
Cyclosporine: ↑ levels of cyclosporine, toxicity
Nitrofurantoin: ↓ lomefloxacin levels
NSAIDs: ↑ CNS stimulation, seizures
Probenicid: ↑ lomefloxacin levels, toxicity
Sucralfate: ↓ lomefloxacin levels
Theophylline: ↑ levels
Warfarin: ↑ levels of warfarin, toxicity

Drug classifications
Antacids: ↓ levels of lomefloxacin
Iron sulfate: ↓ levels of lomefloxacin
Zinc sulfate: ↓ levels of lomefloxacin

NURSING CONSIDERATIONS
Assessment
• Assess patient for previous sensitivity reaction
• Assess patient for signs and symptoms of infection: characteristics of wounds, sputum, urine, stool, WBC >10,000, fever; obtain baseline information before and during treatment
• Obtain C&S before beginning drug therapy to identify if correct treatment has been initiated
• Assess for allergic reactions: rash, urticaria, pruritus
• Monitor blood studies: AST, ALT, CBC, Hct, bilirubin, LDH, alkaline phosphatase, Coombs' test monthly if patient is on long-term therapy
• Assess bowel pattern qd; if severe diarrhea occurs, drug should be discontinued
• Assess for overgrowth of infection: perineal itching, fever, malaise, redness, pain,

---

☑ Herb/drug   Ⓢ Do Not Crush   ◆ Alert   ☛ Key Drug   Ⓖ Geriatric   Ⓟ Pediatric

swelling, drainage, rash, diarrhea, change in cough, sputum
• Assess for CNS symptoms: insomnia, vertigo, headaches, agitation, confusion

Nursing diagnoses
☑ Infection, risk for (uses)
☑ Diarrhea (adverse reactions)
☑ Injury, risk for (adverse reactions)
☑ Knowledge deficit (teaching)
☑ Noncompliance (teaching)

Implementation
• Give with food for GI symptoms; give with 8 oz of water
• Give 2 hr before or 2 hr after iron, calcium, zinc, magnesium products or antacids, which decrease absorption

Patient/family education
• Instruct patient to take all medication prescribed for the length of time ordered; drug must be taken around the clock to maintain blood levels; do not give medication to others
• Teach patient to use sunscreen when outdoors to decrease phototoxicity
• Advise patient to increase fluids to 2 L/day to prevent crystalluria
• Caution patient to avoid driving and other hazardous activities until response is known; dizziness, confusion, drowsiness may occur

Evaluation
Positive therapeutic outcome
• Negative C&S, absence of signs/symptoms of infection (WBC <10,000, temp WNL)
• Reported improvement in symptoms of infection

lomustine (℞)
(loe-mus′teen)
CCNU, CeeNU
Func. class.: Antineoplastic alkylating agent
Chem. class.: Nitrosourea
Pregnancy category **D**

Action: Changes essential cellular ions to covalent bonding with resultant alkylation; this interferes with normal biologic function of DNA; activity is not phase specific; action is due to myelosuppression

▶**Therapeutic Outcome:** Prevention of rapid growth of malignant cells in chronic myelocytic leukemia

Uses: Hodgkin's disease, lymphomas, multiple myeloma

Investigational uses: Brain, breast, renal, GI tract, bronchogenic carcinoma; melanomas

Dosage and routes
Adult: PO 100, 130 mg/m² as a single dose q6 wk; titrate dosage to WBC level; do not give repeat dose unless WBCs are >4000/mm³, platelet count >100,000/mm³

Available forms: Caps 10, 40, 100 mg

Adverse effects
GI: Nausea, vomiting, anorexia, stomatitis, **hepatotoxicity**
GU: Azotemia, renal failure
HEMA: **Thrombocytopenia, leukopenia, myelosuppression, anemia**
INTEG: Burning at inj site
RESP: **Fibrosis, pulmonary infiltrate**

L

Contraindications: Radiation, chemotherapy, lactation, pregnancy **D** (3rd trimester), "blastic" phase of chronic myelocytic leukemia, hypersensitivity

Precautions: Childbearing age men and women, leukopenia, thrombocytopenia, anemia, hepatotoxicity, renal toxicity

---

Pharmacokinetics

Absorption	Rapidly absorbed
Distribution	Widely
Metabolism	Liver
Excretion	Kidneys, breast milk
Half-life	16-48 hr

Pharmacodynamics
Unknown

Interactions
Individual drugs
Radiation: ↑ toxicity, bone marrow suppression
Drug classifications
Antineoplastics: ↑ toxicity, bone marrow suppression
Lab test interferences
False positive: Cytology tests for breast, bladder, cervix, lung

NURSING CONSIDERATIONS
Assessment
◆• Monitor CBC, differential, platelet count weekly; withhold drug if WBC is <4000 or platelet count is <100,000; notify prescriber of results if WBC <20,000 /mm^3, platelets <150,000/mm^3
• Monitor pulmonary function tests, chest x-ray films before, during therapy; chest film should be obtained q2 wk during treatment; assess for dyspnea, rales, unproductive cough, chest pain, tachypnea
• Monitor renal function studies: BUN, serum uric acid, urine CrCl before, during

therapy; I&O ratio; report fall in urine output of 30 ml/hr; check for decreased hyperuricemia
• Monitor for cold, fever, sore throat (may indicate beginning infection); identify edema in feet, joint and stomach pain, shaking; prescriber should be notified
• Assess for bleeding: hematuria, guaiac, bruising or petechiae, mucosa or orifices q8h, no rec temp

Nursing diagnoses
☑ Injury, risk for (adverse reactions)
☑ Body image disturbance (adverse reactions)
☑ Infection, risk for (adverse reactions)
☑ Knowledge deficit (teaching)

Implementation
• Give drug after evening meal, before hs; administer antiemetic 30-60 min before giving drug to prevent vomiting
• Antiinfectives for prophylaxis of infection may be prescribed since infection potential is high
• Store in tight container

Patient/family education
• Teach patient to avoid use of products containing aspirin or ibuprofen, razors, commercial mouthwash, since bleeding may occur; to report symptoms of bleeding (hematuria, tarry stools)
• Advise patient to report signs of anemia (fatigue, headache, irritability, faintness, shortness of breath)
• Caution patient to report any changes in breathing or coughing even several mo after treatment; to avoid crowds and persons with respiratory tract or other infections

---

• Caution patient not to have any vaccinations without the advice of prescriber; serious reactions can occur

• Tell patient contraception is needed during treatment and for several mo after the completion of therapy

Evaluation
Positive therapeutic outcome
• Decreased tumor sizes
• Decreased spread of malignancy

Ioperamide (OTC, ℞)
(loe-per'a-mide)
Ioperamide solution, Imodium, Imodium A-D, Imodium A-D Caplet, Loperamide, A-D Kaopectate II Caplets, Maalox Antidiarrheal Caplets, Pepto Diarrhea Control
Func. class.: Antidiarrheal
Chem. class.: Piperidine derivative

Pregnancy category   B

Action: Direct action on intestinal muscles to decrease GI peristalsis; reduces volume, increases bulk; electrolytes are not lost

▶**Therapeutic Outcome:** Absence of diarrhea

Uses: Diarrhea (cause undetermined), chronic diarrhea, ileostomy discharge

Dosage and routes
Adult: PO 4 mg, then 2 mg after each loose stool, not to exceed 16 mg/day

🅿 *Child 2-5 yr:* PO 1 mg on day 1, then 0.1 mg/kg after each loose stool

🅿 *Child 5-8 yr:* PO 2 mg bid on day 1, then 0.1 mg/kg after each loose stool

🅿 *Child 8-12 yr:* PO 2 mg tid on day 1, then 0.1 mg/kg after each loose stool

Available forms: Cap 2 mg; liq 1 mg/5 ml; tab 2 mg

Adverse effects
CNS: Dizziness, drowsiness, fatigue, fever
GI: Nausea, dry mouth, vomiting, constipation, abdominal pain, anorexia, **toxic megacolon**
INTEG: Rash

Contraindications: Hypersensitivity, severe ulcerative colitis, pseudomembranous colitis, acute diarrhea associated with *E. coli*

Precautions: Pregnancy **B,**
🅿 lactation, children <2 yr, liver disease, dehydration, bacterial disease

L

Pharmacokinetics	
Absorption	Poor
Distribution	Unknown
Metabolism	Liver
Excretion	Feces, unchanged; small amount in urine
Half-life	7-14 hr

Pharmacodynamics	
Onset	½-1 hr
Peak	Unknown
Duration	4-5 hr

Interaction
Solutions: Do not mix with other oral sol

NURSING CONSIDERATIONS
Assessment
• Monitor electrolytes (potassium, sodium, chloride) if patient is on long-term

---

therapy; check fluid status, skin turgor

• Assess bowel pattern before, during treatment; check for rebound constipation after termination of medication; check bowel sounds

• Check response after 48 hr; if no response, drug should be discontinued and other treatment initiated

• Assess for abdominal distention, toxic megacolon, which may occur in ulcerative colitis

Nursing diagnoses
☑ Diarrhea (uses)
☑ Constipation (adverse reactions)
☑ Knowledge deficit (teaching)
☑ Noncompliance (teaching)

Implementation
🚫 • Do not chew, crush caps
• Store in airtight containers

Patient/family education
• Caution patient to avoid alcohol and OTC products unless directed by prescriber; may cause increased CNS depression

• Advise patient not to exceed recommended dosage; drug may be habit forming

• Advise patient that drug may cause drowsiness and to avoid hazardous activities until response to drug is determined

• Teach patient that dry mouth can be decreased by frequent sips of water, hard candy, sugarless gum

Evaluation
Positive therapeutic outcome
• Decreased diarrhea

---

loratadine (℞)
(lor-a'ti-deen)
Claritin
Func. class.: Antihistamine (2nd-generation)
Chem. class.: Selective histamine (H_1) receptor antagonist
Pregnancy category B

Action: Binds to peripheral histamine receptors, which provides antihistamine action without sedation

➡**Therapeutic Outcome:** Decreased nasal stuffiness, itching, swollen eyes

Uses: Seasonal rhinitis

Dosage and routes
P *Adult and child ≥12 yr:* PO 10 mg qd, tabs rapid-disintegrating 10 mg; syrup 1 mg/ml

P *Child 6-12 yr:* PO 10 mg (10 ml) qd

Available forms: Tab 10 mg; tabs rapid-disintegrating 10 mg; syrup 5 mg/5 ml

Adverse effects
CNS: Sedation (more common with increased dosages), headache

Contraindications: Hypersensitivity, acute asthma attacks, lower respiratory tract disease

Precautions: Pregnancy **B**, increased intraocular pressure, bronchial asthma

Pharmacokinetics
Absorption	Well absorbed
Distribution	Unknown
Metabolism	Liver, extensively, to active metabolites
Excretion	Kidneys
Half-life	8½-28 hr

☑ Herb/drug 🚫 Do Not Crush ◆ Alert ⊶ Key Drug G Geriatric P Pediatric

Pharmacodynamics	
Onset	Unknown
Peak	1½ hr
Duration	Unknown

Interactions
Individual drugs
Alcohol: ↑ CNS depression
Cimetidine: ↑ loratadine levels
Drug classifications
Antibiotics, macrolide: ↑ CV effects
Antifungals, azole: ↑ CV effects
CNS depressants: ↑ CNS depression
MAOIs: ↑ anticholinergic sedative effects
Opiates: ↑ CNS depression
Sedative/hypnotics: ↑ CNS depression
Food/drug
↑ absorption
⊘ Herb/drug
Henbane: ↑ anticholinergic effect
Lab test interferences
False negative: Skin allergy tests (discontinue antihistamine 3 days before testing)

NURSING CONSIDERATIONS
Assessment
• Assess respiratory status: rate, rhythm, increase in bronchial secretions, wheezing, chest tightness; provide fluids to 2 L/day to decrease secretion thickness
Nursing diagnoses
☑ Airway clearance, ineffective (uses)
☑ Knowledge deficit (teaching)
☑ Noncompliance (teaching, overuse)
Implementation
• Give on an empty stomach, 1 hr ac or 2 hr pc to facilitate absorption
• Place rapidly disintegrating tabs on tongue, then swallow after disintegrated with or without water
• Store in tight, light-resistant container

Patient/family education
• Teach all aspects of drug uses; to notify prescriber if confusion, sedation, hypotension occur; to avoid driving and other hazardous activity if drowsiness occurs; to avoid alcohol and other CNS depressants that may potentiate effect
• Teach patient to take 1 hr ac or 2 hr pc to facilitate absorption
• Caution patient not to exceed recommended dosage; dysrhythmias may occur
• Teach patient hard candy, gum, frequent rinsing of mouth may be used for dryness

Evaluation
Positive therapeutic outcome
• Absence of running or congested nose

lorazepam (℞)
(lor-az'e-pam)
Alzapam, Apo-Lorazepam ✦, Ativan, Loraz, lorazepam, Novolorazem ✦
Func. class.: Sedative/hypnotic, antianxiety agent
Chem. class.: Benzodiazepine
Pregnancy category D
Controlled substance schedule IV

Action: Potentiates the actions of GABA, an inhibitory neurotransmitter, especially in the limbic system and reticular

---

✦ Canada Only   Adverse effects: *italic* = common; **bold** = life-threatening

formation, which depresses the CNS

➡ Therapeutic Outcome: Decreased anxiety, relaxation

Uses: Anxiety, irritability in psychiatric or organic disorders, preoperatively, insomnia

Investigational uses: Antiemetic prior to chemotherapy, status epilepticus

Dosage and routes
Anxiety
Adult: PO 2-6 mg/day in divided doses, not to exceed 10 mg/day

G Elderly: PO 0.5-1 mg/day in divided doses; or 0.5-1 mg hs

P Child: PO 0.05 mg/kg/dose, q4-8hr

Insomnia
Adult: PO 2-4 mg hs; only minimally effective after 2 wk continuous therapy

G Elderly: PO 1-2 mg initially

Preoperatively
Adult: IM 50 µg/kg 2 hr before surgery; **IV** 44 µg/kg 15-20 min before surgery

P Child: 0.05 mg/kg

Status epilepticus
P Neonate: 0.05 mg/kg

P Child: 0.1 mg/kg up to 4 mg/dose

Available forms: Tabs 0.5, 1, 2 mg; inj 2, 4 mg/ml; conc sol 2 mg/ml

Adverse effects
CNS: Dizziness, drowsiness, confusion, headache, anxiety, tremors, stimulation, fatigue, depression, insomnia, hallucinations, weakness, unsteadiness
CV: Orthostatic hypotension, **ECG changes, tachycardia,** hypotension

EENT: Blurred vision, tinnitus, mydriasis
GI: Constipation, dry mouth, nausea, vomiting, anorexia, diarrhea
INTEG: Rash, dermatitis, itching

Contraindications: Hypersensitivity to benzodiazepines, narrow-angle glaucoma, psy-
P chosis, pregnancy **D,** child <12 yr, history of drug abuse, COPD

G Precautions: Elderly, debilitated patients, hepatic disease, renal disease

N Do Not Confuse:
lorazepam/alprazolam

Pharmacokinetics

Absorption	Well absorbed (PO); completely absorbed (IM)
Distribution	Widely distributed; crosses placenta, blood-brain barrier
Metabolism	Liver, extensively
Excretion	Kidneys, breast milk
Half-life	14 hr

Pharmacodynamics

	PO	IM	IV
Onset	½ hr	15-30 min	5-15 min
Peak	1-3 hr	1-1½ hr	Unknown
Duration	3-6 hr	3-6 hr	3-6 hr

Interactions
Individual drugs
Alcohol: ↑ CNS depression
Cimetidine: ↑ action
Disulfiram: ↑ action
Fluoxetine: ↑ action
Levodopa: ↓ action of levodopa
Drug classifications
Antidepressants: ↑ CNS depression

☑ Herb/drug ◐ Do Not Crush ◆ Alert ✜ Key Drug **G** Geriatric **P** Pediatric

Antihistamines: ↑ CNS depression
Opiates: ↑ CNS depression
Smoking
↑ metabolism, ↓ effect
Herb/drug
Kava: ↑ action
Lab test interferences
↑ AST, ↑ ALT, ↑ serum bilirubin
False: ↑ 17-OHCS
↓ RAIU

NURSING CONSIDERATIONS
Assessment

• Assess degree of anxiety; what precipitates anxiety and whether drug controls symptoms; other signs of anxiety: dilated pupils, inability to sleep, restlessness, inability to focus
• Assess for alcohol withdrawal symptoms, including hallucinations (visual, auditory), delirium, irritability, agitation, fine to coarse tremors
• Monitor B/P (with patient lying/standing), pulse, check respiratory rate; if systolic B/P drops 20 mm Hg, hold drug, notify prescriber; respirations q5-15 min if given **IV**
• Monitor CBC during long-term therapy; blood dyscrasias have occurred (rarely)
• Monitor for seizure control; type, duration, and intensity of convulsions; what precipitates seizures
• Monitor hepatic studies: AST, ALT, bilirubin, creatinine, LDH, alkaline phosphatase
• Assess mental status: mood, sensorium, affect, sleeping pattern, drowsiness, dizziness, suicidal tendencies, and ability of drug to control these symptoms; check for tolerance, withdrawal symptoms: headache, nausea, vomiting, muscle pain, weakness after long-term use

Nursing diagnoses
☑ Sleep pattern disturbance (uses)
☑ Coping, ineffective individual (uses)
☑ Knowledge deficit (teaching)
☑ Noncompliance (teaching)

Implementation
PO route

• Give with food or milk for GI symptoms; crush tab if patient is unable to swallow medication whole; provide sugarless gum, hard candy, frequent sips of water for dry mouth
• Use by SL route for rapid response (investigational use)
IM route
• Give deep in muscle mass; if using for preoperative sedation, give 2 hr or more before surgical procedure
IV route
• Dilute with sterile water for inj, 0.9% NaCl, or D_5W just before using; give by Y-site or 3-way stopcock at 2 mg/min
• Do not use sol that is discolored or contains a precipitate

Syringe compatibilities:
Cimetidine, hydromorphone
Y-site incompatibilities:
Idarubicin, ondansetron, sargramostim
Y-site compatibilities:
Acyclovir, albumin, allopurinol, amifostine, amikacin, amoxicillin, amoxicillin/clavulanate, amsacrine, atracurium, bumetanide, cefepime, cefmetazole, cefotaxime, ciprofloxacin, cisatracurium, cisplatin, cladribine, clonidine, cyclophosphamide, cytarabine, dexamethasone, diltiazem, dobutamine, dopamine, doxo-

L

rubicin, epinephrine, erythromycin, etomidate, famotidine, fentanyl, filgrastim, fluconazole, fludarabine, furosemide, gentamicin, granisetron, haloperidol, heparin, hydrocortisone, hydromorphone, ketanserin, labetalol, melphalan, methotrexate, metronidazole, midazolam, milrinone, morphine, nicardipine, nitroglycerin, norepinephrine, paclitaxel, pancuronium, piperacillin, piperacillin/tazobactam, potassium chloride, propofol, ranitidine, tacrolimus, teniposide, thiotepa, trimethoprim-sulfamethoxazole, vancomycin, vecuronium, vinorelbine, zidovudine

Patient/family education

• Advise patient that drug may be taken with food; that drug is not to be used for everyday stress or used longer than 4 mo unless directed by a prescriber; to take no more than prescribed amount; may be habit forming

• Caution patient to avoid OTC preparations unless approved by prescriber; to avoid alcohol, other psychotropic medications unless prescribed by physician; not to discontinue medication abruptly after long-term use

• Inform patient to avoid driving and activities that require alertness; drowsiness may occur; to rise slowly or fainting **G** may occur, especially in elderly

• Inform patient that drowsiness may worsen at beginning of treatment

Evaluation

Positive therapeutic outcome

• Decreased anxiety, restlessness, insomnia

Treatment of overdose:

Lavage, VS, supportive care

---

losartan (℞)
(low-sar'tan)
Cozaar
Func. class.: Antihypertensive
Chem. class.: Angiotensin II receptor (Type AT_1)
Pregnancy category C (1st trimester); D (2nd/3rd trimesters)

Action: Blocks the vasoconstrictor and aldosterone-secreting effects of angiotensin II; selectively blocks the binding of angiotensin II to the AT_1 receptor found in tissues

Therapeutic Outcome: Decreased B/P

Uses: Hypertension, alone or in combination

Dosage and routes

Adult: PO 50 mg qd alone or 25 mg qd when used in combination

Hepatic dose
25 mg qd

Available forms: Tabs 25, 50 mg

Adverse effects

CNS: Dizziness, insomnia, anxiety, confusion, abnormal dreams, migraine, tremor, vertigo

CV: Angina pectoris, 2nd-degree AV block, **cerebrovascular accident,** hypotension, **myocardial infarction, dysrhythmias**

EENT: Blurred vision, burning eyes, conjunctivitis, task perversion

GI: Diarrhea, dyspepsia, anorexia, constipation, dry mouth, flatulence, gastritis, vomiting

---

GU: Impotence, nocturia, urinary frequency, urinary tract infection
HEMA: Anemia
INTEG: Alopecia, dermatitis, dry skin, flushing, photosensitivity, rash, pruritus, sweating
META: Gout
MS: Cramps, myalgia, pain, stiffness
RESP: Cough, upper respiratory infection, congestion, dyspnea, bronchitis

Contraindications: Hypersensitivity, pregnancy **D** (2nd, 3rd trimesters)

Precautions: Hypersensitivity to ACE inhibitors; pregnancy **P** **C** (1st trimester); lactation, **G** children, elderly

N **Do Not Confuse:**
Cozaar/Zocor

Pharmacokinetics	
Absorption	Well
Distribution	Bound to plasma proteins
Metabolism	Extensive
Excretion	Feces, urine
Half-life	Biphasic, 2 hr, 6-9 hr

Pharmacodynamics
Unknown

Interactions
Individual drugs
Lithium: ↑ toxicity

NURSING CONSIDERATIONS
Assessment
• Assess B/P, pulse q4h; note rate, rhythm, quality
• Monitor electrolytes: potassium, sodium, chloride
• Obtain baselines in renal, liver function tests before therapy begins
• Monitor for edema in feet, legs daily

• Assess for skin turgor, dryness of mucous membranes for hydration status

Nursing diagnoses
✓ Fluid volume deficit (side effects)
✓ Noncompliance (teaching)
✓ Knowledge deficit (teaching)

Implementation
• Administer without regard to meals

Patient/family education
• Teach patient to avoid sunlight or wear sunscreen if in sunlight; photosensitivity may occur
• Advise patient to comply with dosage schedule, even if feeling better
• Teach patient to notify prescriber of mouth sores, fever, swelling of hands or feet, irregular heartbeat, chest pain
• Advise patient excessive perspiration, dehydration, vomiting, diarrhea may lead to fall in blood pressure—consult prescriber if these occur
• Inform patient that drug may cause dizziness, fainting; light-headedness may occur
• Caution patient to rise slowly to sitting or standing position to minimize orthostatic hypotension

Evaluation
Positive therapeutic outcome
• Decreased B/P

L

lovastatin ⚷ (R)
(loe'va-sta-tin)
Mevacor
Func. class.: Antilipemic
Chem. class.: Aspergillus terreus strain derivative
Pregnancy category   X

Action: By inhibiting HMG-CoA reductase, inhibits biosynthesis of VLDL and LDL, which are responsible for cholesterol development

➥**Therapeutic Outcome:** Decreased cholesterol levels and LDLs, increased HDLs

Uses: As an adjunct in primary hypercholesterolemia (types IIa, IIb), mixed hyperlipidemia, other osclerosis

Dosage and routes
(Patient should first be placed on a cholesterol-lowering diet)
Adult: PO 20 mg qd with evening meal; may increase to 20-80 mg/day in single or divided doses; not to exceed 80 mg/day; dosage adjustments should be made monthly; reduce dose in renal disease

Available forms: Tabs 10, 20, 40 mg

Adverse effects
CNS: Dizziness, headache, tremor
EENT: Blurred vision, dysgeusia, lens opacities
GI: Nausea, constipation, diarrhea, dyspepsia, flatus, abdominal pain, heartburn, **liver dysfunction**
HEMA: **Thrombocytopenia, hemolytic anemia, leukopenia**
INTEG: Rash, pruritus, photosensitivity

MS: Muscle cramps, myalgia, **myositis, rhabdomyolysis**
Contraindications: Hypersensitivity, pregnancy **X**, lactation, active liver disease

Precautions: Past liver disease, alcoholism, severe acute infections, trauma, hypotension, uncontrolled seizure disorders, severe metabolic disorders, electrolyte imbalances, visual condition, children **P**

Pharmacokinetics

Absorption	Poorly absorbed, erratic
Distribution	Crosses placenta, blood-brain barrier
Metabolism	Liver, extensively
Excretion	Feces, kidneys
Half-life	3-4 hr

Pharmacodynamics

Onset	Unknown
Peak	2-4 hr
Duration	Unknown

Interactions
Individual drugs
Cholestyramine: ↓ action of lovastatin
Cyclosporine: ↑ risk of myopathy
Erythromycin: ↑ risk of myopathy
Gemfibrozil: ↑ risk of myopathy
Niacin: ↑ risk of myopathy
Propranolol: ↓ antihyperlipidemic effect
Warfarin: ↑ bleeding
Food/drug
↑ levels of lovastatin with food
Lab test interferences
↑ CPK, ↑ liver function tests

NURSING CONSIDERATIONS
Assessment
• Assess nutrition: fat, protein, carbohydrates; nutritional

☒ Herb/drug 🚫 Do Not Crush ◆ Alert ⚷ Key Drug G Geriatric P Pediatric

analysis should be completed by dietician before treatment
• Monitor bowel pattern daily; diarrhea may be a problem
• Monitor triglycerides, fasting cholesterol LDL, HDL at baseline and throughout treatment; LDL and VLDL should be watched closely; if increased, drug should be discontinued

Nursing diagnoses
☑ Diarrhea (adverse reactions)
☑ Knowledge deficit (teaching)
☑ Noncompliance (teaching)

Implementation
• Give with evening meal; if dosage is increased, take with breakfast and evening meal
• Store in cool environment in airtight, light-resistant container

Patient/family education
• Inform patient that compliance is needed for positive results to occur; not to double doses
• Inform patient that blood work and eye exam will be necessary during treatment
• Teach patient that risk factors should be decreased: high-fat diet, smoking, alcohol consumption, absence of exercise
• Advise patient to report if pregnancy is suspected
• Advise patient to notify prescriber if the GI symptoms of diarrhea, abdominal or epigastric pain, nausea, vomiting occur; or if chills, fever, sore throat, blurred vision, dizziness, headache, muscle pain, weakness occur

Evaluation
Positive therapeutic outcome
• Decreased cholesterol levels, serum triglyceride
• Improved ratio of HDLs

loxapine (℞)
(lox′a-peen)
Loxapac ✦, loxapine succinate, Loxitane IM, Loxitane, Loxitane-C
Func. class.: Antipsychotic/neuroleptic
Chem. class.: Dibenzoxazepine
Pregnancy category C

Action: Depresses cerebral cortex, hypothalamus, limbic system, which control activity and aggression; blocks neurotransmission produced by dopamine at synapse; exhibits strong α-adrenergic, anticholinergic blocking action; mechanism for antipsychotic effects is unclear

➡**Therapeutic Outcome:** Decreased psychotic behavior

Uses: Psychotic disorders, nonpsychotic symptoms associated with dementia

Investigational uses: Depression, anxiety

Dosage and routes
Adult: PO 10 mg bid-qid initially; may be rapidly increased depending on severity of condition; maintenance 60-100 mg/day; IM 12.5-50 mg q4-6h or more until desired response, then start PO form

🅖*Elderly:* PO 5-10 mg qd bid, increase q4-7 days by 5-10 mg, max 125 mg

Available forms: Caps 5, 10, 25, 50 mg; conc 25 mg/ml; inj 50 mg/ml

Adverse effects
CNS: Extrapyramidal symptoms: pseudoparkinsonism, akathisia, dystonia, tardive

L

---

dyskinesia, drowsiness, headache, **seizures,** confusion, **neuroleptic malignant syndrome**
CV: Orthostatic hypotension, **cardiac arrest,** ECG changes, tachycardia
EENT: Blurred vision, glaucoma
GI: Dry mouth, nausea, vomiting, anorexia, constipation, diarrhea, jaundice, weight gain
GU: Urinary retention, urinary frequency, enuresis, impotence, amenorrhea, gynecomastia
HEMA: **Anemia, leukopenia, leukocytosis, agranulocytosis**
INTEG: Rash, photosensitivity, dermatitis
RESP: **Laryngospasm,** dyspnea, **respiratory depression**

Contraindications: Hypersensitivity, blood dyscrasias, coma, brain damage, bone marrow depression, alcohol and barbiturate withdrawal states

Precautions: Pregnancy **C,** lactation, seizure disorders, hepatic disease, cardiac disease, prostatic hypertrophy, **P** cardiac conditions, child <16 yr, glaucoma, GI obstruction, **G** elderly

Pharmacokinetics

Absorption	Well absorbed (PO)
Distribution	Unknown
Metabolism	Liver, extensively
Excretion	Kidneys
Half-life	Biphasic 5 hr, 19 hr

Pharmacodynamics

	PO	IM
Onset	½ hr	15-30 min
Peak	2-4 hr	15-20 min
Duration	12 hr	12 hr

Interactions
Individual drugs
Alcohol: ↑ effects of both drugs, oversedation
Aluminum hydroxide: ↓ absorption
Epinephrine: ↑ toxicity
Guanadrel: ↓ antihypertensive response
Guanethidine: ↓ antihypertensive response
Magnesium hydroxide: ↓ absorption
Drug classifications
Anticholinergics: ↑ anticholinergic effects
Antidepressants: ↑ CNS depression
Antihistamines: ↑ CNS depression
Barbiturate anesthetics: ↑ CNS depression
MAOIs: ↑ CNS depression
Opiates: ↑ CNS depression
Sedatives/hypnotics: ↑ CNS depression
☑ *Herb/drug*
Kava: ↑ action

NURSING CONSIDERATIONS
Assessment
• Assess mental status: orientation, mood, behavior, presence and type of hallucinations before initial administration and monthly; this drug should significantly reduce psychotic behavior
• Check for swallowing of PO medication; check for hoarding or giving of medication to other patients
• Monitor I&O ratio; palpate bladder if low urinary output **G** occurs, especially in elderly; urinalysis recommended before, during prolonged therapy
• Monitor bilirubin, CBC, liver function studies monthly
• Assess affect, orientation, LOC, reflexes, gait, coor-

---

dination, sleep pattern disturbances
• Monitor B/P with patient sitting, standing, and lying; take pulse and respirations q4h during initial treatment; establish baseline before starting treatment; report drops of 30 mm Hg
• Check for dizziness, faintness, palpitations, tachycardia on rising; severe orthostatic hypotension is common
◆• Identify for neuroleptic malignant syndrome: hyperpyrexia, muscle rigidity, increased CPK, altered mental status; drug should be discontinued
• Assess for EPS including akathisia (inability to sit still, no pattern to movements), tardive dyskinesia (bizarre movements of the jaw, mouth, tongue, extremities), pseudoparkinsonism (ragged tremors, pill rolling, shuffling gait); an antiparkinsonian drug should be prescribed
• Assess for constipation, urinary retention daily; if these occur, increase bulk, water in diet

Nursing diagnoses
☑ Thought processes, altered (uses)
☑ Coping, ineffective individual (uses)
☑ Knowledge deficit (teaching)
☑ Noncompliance (teaching)

Implementation
PO route
• Administer drug in liq form mixed in glass of juice or cola if hoarding is suspected; do not mix in caffeine drinks, tannics, pectins
• Administer lowered dose in 🅖 elderly, since metabolism is slowed

• Administer with full glass of water or milk; or give with food to decrease GI upset
• Store in airtight, light-resistant container, oral sol in amber bottle
IM route
• Inject deep in muscle mass; do not give SC; do not administer sol with a precipitate; amber-colored sol can be used

Patient/family education
• Teach patient to use good oral hygiene; suggest frequent rinsing of mouth, sugarless gum for dry mouth
• Caution patient to avoid hazardous activities until drug response is determined; dizziness, blurred vision may occur
• Inform patient that orthostatic hypotension occurs often and to rise from sitting or lying position gradually; to remain lying down after IM inj for at least 30 min; caution patient to avoid hot tubs, hot showers, tub baths, since hypotension may occur; tell patient that in hot weather heat stroke may occur; take extra precautions to stay cool
• Advise patient to avoid abrupt withdrawal of this drug, or EPS may result; drug should be withdrawn slowly
• Advise patient to avoid use with alcohol, CNS depressants; increased drowsiness may occur
• Advise patient to use a sunscreen and sunglasses to prevent burns
• Teach patient about EPS and necessity of meticulous oral hygiene, since oral candidiasis may occur
• Suggest patient take antacids 2 hr before or after taking this drug

L

✦ Canada Only   Adverse effects: *italic* = common; **bold** = life-threatening

• Instruct patient to report sore throat, malaise, fever, bleeding, mouth sores; if these occur, CBC should be drawn and drug discontinued

Evaluation
Positive therapeutic outcome
• Decrease in emotional excitement, hallucinations, delusions, paranoia
• Reorganization of patterns of thought, speech

Treatment of overdose:
Lavage if orally ingested; barbiturates; provide airway, **IV** fluids; do not use epinephrine, which may increase hypotension

---

magaldrate (OTC)
(mag′al-drate)
Antiflux ❦, Losopan ❦, Lowsium, Riopan, Riopan Extra Strength ❦
Func. class.: Antacid
Chem. class.: Aluminum/ magnesium hydroxide
Pregnancy category   C

Action: Neutralizes gastric acidity; drug is dissolved in gastric contents; this drug is a combination of aluminum and magnesium

➡ **Therapeutic Outcome:** Decreased pain of ulcers

Uses: Antacid, peptic ulcer disease (adjunct), indigestion/heartburn, duodenal and gastric ulcers, reflex esophagitis, hyperacidity

Dosage and routes
Adult: Susp 5-10 ml (400-800 mg) with water between meals, hs, not to exceed 100 ml/day
Available forms: Susp 540 mg/5 ml; liquid 540 mg/5 ml

Adverse effects
GI: Constipation, diarrhea
META: Hypermagnesemia, hypophosphatemia

Contraindications: Hypersensitivity to this drug or aluminum products

G Precautions: Elderly, fluid restriction, decreased GI motility, GI obstruction, dehydration, renal disease, sodium-restricted diets, pregnancy **C**

Pharmacokinetics	
Absorption	Not absorbed
Distribution	Not distributed
Metabolism	Not metabolized
Excretion	Kidneys
Half-life	Unknown

Pharmacodynamics	
Onset	Unknown
Peak	½ hr
Duration	1 hr

Interactions
Individual drugs
Chlordiazepoxide: ↓ absorption of chlordiazapoxide
Cimetidine: ↓ absorption of cimetidine
Ketoconazole: ↓ effect of ketoconazole
Phenytoin: ↓ absorption of phenytoin
Tetracycline: ↓ effect of tetracycline
Drug classifications
Anticholinergics: ↓ absorption of anticholinergics
Corticosteroids: ↓ absorption of corticosteroids
Iron salts: ↓ absorption of iron salts
Phenothiazines: ↓ absorption of phenothiazines
Salicylates: ↓ absorption of salicylates

NURSING CONSIDERATIONS
Assessment
• Assess GI status: location of pain, intensity, characteristics, what aggravates, ameliorates pain; heartburn/indigestion; hematemesis
• Monitor serum magnesium levels with impaired renal function
• Assess for constipation: increase bulk in diet if needed or obtain order for stool softener

Nursing diagnoses
☑ Pain (uses)
☑ Knowledge deficit (teaching)

Implementation
• Give laxatives or stool softeners if constipation occurs
• Give susp after shaking; give between meals and hs
• Give when stomach is empty pc and hs

Patient/family education
• Advise patient to separate ingestion of enteric-coated drugs and antacid by 2 hr
• Advise patient to use 2 wk or less; drug should not be used for long periods
• Teach patient to notify prescriber immediately if coffeeground emesis, emesis with frank blood, or black tarry stools occur

Evaluation
Positive therapeutic outcome
• Absence of abdominal pain
• Decreased acidity

---

magnesium salts (OTC)
(mag-neez′ee-um)
magnesium chloride (OTC)
Chloromag, Slo-Mag
magnesium citrate (OTC)
Citrate of Magnesia, Citroma, Citromag ✦, Evac-Q-Mag
magnesium hydroxide (OTC)
Phillips Magnesium Tablets, Phillips Milk of Magnesia, MOM
magnesium oxide (OTC)
Mag-Ox 400, Maox, Uro-Mag
magnesium sulfate (OTC)
Epsom Salt
Func. class.: Laxative, saline; antacid
Pregnancy category A

Action: Increases osmotic pressure, draws fluid into colon, neutralizes HCl

➡ **Therapeutic Outcome:** Magnesium levels within normal limits, absence of constipation

Uses: Constipation, bowel preparation before surgery or exam, electrolyte, anticonvulsant

Dosage and routes
Laxative
Adult: PO 30-60 ml hs (Milk of Magnesia), 300 mg
P *Adult and child >6 yr:* PO 15 g in 8 oz H_2O (magnesium sulfate); PO 10-20 ml (Concentrated Milk of Magnesia); PO 5-10 oz hs (magnesium citrate)
P *Child 2-6 yr:* 5-15 ml (Milk of Magnesia)

M

Prevention of magnesium deficiency

P *Adult and child ≥10 yr:* PO male: 270-400 mg/day; female: 280-300 mg/day; lactation: 335-350 mg/day; pregnancy 320 mg/day

P *Child 8-10 yr:* PO 170 mg/day

P *Child 4-7 yr:* PO 120 mg/day

P *Infant to 4 yr:* 40-80 mg/day

Deficiency
Adult: PO 200-400 mg in divided doses tid-qid; IM 1 g q6h × 4 doses; **IV** 5 g (severe)

P *Child 6-12 yr:* 3-6 mg/kg/day in divided doses tid-qid

Pre-eclampsia/eclampsia magnesium sulfate
Adult: IM/**IV** 4-5 g **IV** inf; with 5 g IM in each gluteus, then 5 g q4h or 4 g **IV** inf then 1-2 g/hr cont inf

Available forms: *Chloride:* sus-rel-tab 535 mg (64 mg Mg); enteric tabs 833 mg (100 mg Mg); inj 200 mg/ml
Citrate: 240, 296, 300 ml/bottle (77 mEq Mg/100 ml)
Hydroxide: 400 mg/5 ml (164 mg Mg/5 ml); conc liquid 800 mg/5 ml (328 mg Mg/5 ml); chew tab 300 mg (130 Mg), 600 mg (260 Mg)
Oxide: tabs 400 mg (241.3 mg Mg); caps 140 mg (84.5 mg Mg)
Sulfate: pwdr for oral; bulk packages; Epsom salts, bulk packages; inj 10, 12.5, 25, 50%

Adverse effects
CNS: Muscle weakness, flushing, sweating, confusion, sedation, depressed reflexes, **flaccidity, paralysis, hypothermia**
CV: Hypotension, heart block, **circulatory collapse**

GI: *Nausea, vomiting, anorexia, cramps*
META: Electrolyte, fluid imbalances

Contraindications: Hypersensitivity, renal diseases, abdominal pain, nausea/vomiting, obstruction, acute surgical abdomen, rectal bleeding

Precautions: Pregnancy **A**

Pharmacokinetics	
PO	Onset 3-6 hr
IM	Onset 1 hr, duration 4 hr
IV	Duration ½ hr

Interactions
Drug classifications
Antiinfectives, other: ↓ absorption
Neuromuscular blockers: ↑ effect
Tetracyclines: ↓ absorption

NURSING CONSIDERATIONS
Assessment
• Assess I&O ratio; check for decrease in urinary output
• Assess cause of constipation; lack of fluids, bulk, exercise
• Assess cramping, rectal bleeding, nausea, vomiting; drug should be discontinued
◆• Assess Mg toxicity: thirst, confusion, decrease in reflexes
• Assess visual changes: blurring, halos, corneal and retinal damage
• Assess edema in feet, ankles, legs
• Assess prior drug history; there are many drug interactions

Implementation
PO route
• Administer with 8 oz H_2O
• Administer to patient

---

crushed or whole; chewable tablets may be chewed
• Administer with food or milk to decrease gastric symptoms; give 30 min before or 2 hr after antacids

IV IV route
• Administer only when calcium gluconate available for magnesium toxicity
• Administer **IV** undiluted 1.5 ml of 10% sol over 1 min; may dilute to 20% sol, infuse over 3 hr
• Administer **IV** at less than 150 mg/min; circulatory collapse may occur

Y-site compatibilities: Acyclovir, aldesleukin, amifostine, amikacin, ampicillin, aztreonam, cefamandole, cefazolin, cefmetazole, cefoperazone, cefotaxime, cefoxitin, cephalothin, cephapirin, chloramphenicol, cisatracurium, clindamycin, dobutamine, doxycycline, doxorubicin liposome, enalaprilat, erythromycin, esmolol, famotidine, fludarabine, gallium, gentamicin, granisetron, heparin, hydrocortisone, hydromorphone, idarubicin, insulin, kanamycin, labetalol, meperidine, metronidazole, minocycline, morphine, moxalactam, nafcillin, ondansetron, oxacillin, paclitaxel, penicillin G potassium, piperacillin, piperacillin/tazobactam, potassium chloride, propofol, remifentanil, sargramostim, thiotepa, ticarcillin, tobramycin, trimethoprim/sulfamethoxazole, vancomycin, vit B complex/C

Additive compatibilities: Calcium gluconate, cephalothin, chloramphenicol, cisplatin, heparin, hydrocortisone, isoproterenol, meropenem, methyldopa, norepinephrine, penicillin G potassium, potassium phosphate, verapamil

Patient/family education
• Inform patient to report any symptoms of hepatotoxicity, renal toxicity, visual changes, ototoxicity, allergic reactions, bleeding (long-term therapy)
• Inform patient not to exceed recommended dosage; acute poisoning may result
• Inform patient to read label on other OTC drugs; many contain aspirin
• Inform patient that therapeutic response takes 2 wk (arthritis)
• Inform patient to avoid alcohol ingestion; GI bleeding may occur
• Inform patient that if anticoagulants are given with this drug, both should be discontinued 2 wk before surgery

Evaluation
Positive therapeutic outcomes
• Decreased pain, fever

Treatment of overdose: Lavage, activated charcoal, monitor electrolytes, VS

M

mannitol (℞)
(man′i-tole)
mannitol, Osmitrol, Resectisol
Func. class.: Osmotic diuretic
Chem. class.: Hexahydric alcohol

Pregnancy category C

Action: Increases osmolarity of glomerular filtrate, which raises osmotic pressure of fluid in renal tubules; there is a decrease in reabsorption of water, electrolytes; increases in urinary output, sodium, chloride, potassium, calcium, phosphorus, uric acid, urea, magnesium

Uses: Edema; promote systemic diuresis in cerebral edema, decrease intraocular pressure, improve renal function in acute renal failure, chemical poisoning

Dosage and routes
Oliguria, prevention
Adult: **IV** 50-100 g of a 5%-25% sol

Oliguria, treatment
Adult: **IV** 300-400 mg/kg of a 20%-25% sol up to 100 g of a 15%-20% sol over 30-60 min
P *Child:* **IV** 0.25-2 g/kg as a 15%-20% sol, run over 2-6 hr

Intraocular pressure/ intracranial pressure
Adult: **IV** 1.5-2 g/kg of a 15%-25% sol over 30-60 min
P *Child:* **IV** 1-2 g/kg (30-60 g/m^2) as a 15%-20% sol run over 30-60 min

Renal failure
Adult: **IV** 50-200 g/24 hr, adjusting to maintain output of 30-50 mg/hr

Diuresis in drug intoxication
P *Adult and child >12 yr:* 5%-10% sol continuously up to 200 g **IV,** while maintaining 100-500 ml urine output/hr

Available forms: Inj 5%, 10%, 15%, 20%, 25%; irrigation 5%

Adverse effects
CNS: Dizziness, headache, *convulsions,* **rebound increased intracranial pressure,** confusion
CV: Edema, hypotension, hypertension, **tachycardia, CHF,** thrombophlebitis
EENT: Loss of hearing, blurred vision, nasal congestion, decreased intraocular pressure
ELECT: Fluid, electrolyte imbalances, **acidosis,** electrolyte loss, dehydration
GI: Nausea, vomiting, dry mouth, diarrhea
GU: Marked diuresis, urinary retention, thirst
RESP: Pulmonary congestion

Contraindications: Active intracranial bleeding, hypersensitivity, anuria, severe pulmonary congestion, edema, severe dehydration, progressive heart, renal failure

Precautions: Dehydration, pregnancy **C,** severe renal disease, CHF, lactation

Pharmacokinetics	
Absorption	Complete
Distribution	Extracellular spaces
Metabolism	Minimal
Excretion	Renal
Half-life	100 min

Pharmacodynamics	
Onset	½-1 hr
Peak	1 hr
Duration	6-8 hr

Interactions
Individual drugs
EDTA: ↑ effects
Lithium: ↓ action, ↑ excretion
Food/drug
Potassium foods: ↑ hyperkalemia
Lab test interferences
Interference: Inorganic phosphorus, ethylene glycol

NURSING CONSIDERATIONS
Assessment
• Assess neurologic status: LOC, intracranial pressure

---

reading, pupil size and reaction when drug is given for increased intracranial pressure
• Assess for visual changes or eye discomfort or pain before and during treatment; (increases intraocular pressure); neuro checks, intracranial pressure during treatment (increased intracranial pressure)
• Assess patient for tinnitus, hearing loss, ear pain; periodic testing of hearing is needed when high doses of this drug are given by **IV** route
• Monitor manifestations of hypokalemia: acidic urine, reduced urine osmolality, nocturia, polyuria, polydipsia; hypotension, broad T wave, U wave, ectopy, tachycardia, weak pulse; muscle weakness, altered LOC, drowsiness, apathy, lethargy, confusion, depression; anorexia, nausea, cramps, constipation, distention, paralytic ileus; hypoventilation, respiratory muscle weakness
• Monitor for manifestations of hyponatremia: increased B/P, cold, clammy skin, hypovolemia or hypervolemia; anorexia, nausea, vomiting, diarrhea, abdominal cramps; lethargy, increased intracranial pressure, confusion, headache, seizures, coma, fatigue, tremors, hyperreflexia
• Assess fluid volume status: check I&O ratios and record hourly urine values, CVP, breath sounds, weight, distended red veins, crackles in lung, color, quality and sp gr of urine, skin turgor, adequacy of pulses, moist mucous membranes, bilateral lung sounds, peripheral pitting edema

• Assess for dehydration; symptoms of decreasing output, thirst, hypotension, dry mouth and mucous membranes should be reported
• Monitor electrolytes: potassium, sodium, calcium, magnesium; also include BUN, ABGs, CVP, PAP, CBC; regularly monitor serum and urine levels of sodium and potassium
• Assess B/P before and during therapy with patient lying, standing, and sitting as appropriate; orthostatic hypotension can occur rapidly
• Monitor for rebound intracranial pressure: headache, confusion

Nursing diagnoses
☑ Urinary elimination, altered (adverse reactions)
☑ Fluid volume deficit (adverse reactions)
☑ Fluid volume excess (uses)
☑ Knowledge deficit (teaching)

M

Implementation
• Administer potassium replacement if potassium level is less than 3 mg/ml
• Use an in-line filter for 15%, 20%, 25% give with inf pump; check **IV** patency at inf site before and during administration; do not use sol that is yellow or has a precipitate or crystals; to redissolve, run bottle in hot water and shake vigorously; cool to body temp before giving
• Run at 30-50 ml/hr in oliguria
• Run over 30-60 min in increased intracranial pressure
• Run over 30 min for intraocular pressure; 60-90 min after surgery

Irrigation
- Use 100 ml of 25%/900 ml of sterile water for inj (2.5% sol)

Y-site compatibilities:
Allopurinol, amifostine, aztreonam, cladribine, fludarabine, fluorouracil, gallium, idarubicin, melphalan, ondansetron, paclitaxel, piperacillin, propofol, sargramostim, teniposide, thiotepa, vinorelbine

Y-site incompatibilities:
Amsacrine, bleomycin, doxorubicin, fluconazole, gentamicin, quinidine, vinblastine, vincristine

Additive compatibilities:
Amikacin, bretylium, cefamandole, cefoxitin, cimetidine, cisplatin, dopamine, fosphenytoin, furosemide, gentamicin, metoclopramide, netilmicin, nizatidine, ofloxacin, ondansetron, sodium bicarbonate, tobramycin, verapamil

Additive incompatibilities:
Blood, blood products, imipenem/cilastatin, potassium chloride, sodium chloride

Patient/family education
- Teach patient reason for and method of treatment

Evaluation
Positive therapeutic outcome
- Decreased intracranial pressure
- Decreased intraocular pressure
- Prevention of hypokalemia (diuretic use)
- Decreased edema
- Decreased ICP
- Increased diuresis of >30 ml/hr
- Increased excretion of toxic substances

Treatment of overdose:
Discontinue inf, correct fluid, electrolyte imbalances, hemodialysis, monitor hydration, CV, renal function

---

mebendazole (R)
(me-ben′da-zole)
Vermox
Func. class.: Anthelmintic
Chem. class.: Carbamate
Pregnancy category   C

Action: Inhibits glucose uptake, degeneration of cytoplasmic microtubules in the cell; interferes with absorption, secretory function

Therapeutic Outcome: Parasite, cyst, egg death

Uses: Infestation with pinworms, roundworms, hookworms, whipworms, threadworms, pork tapeworms, dwarf tapeworms, beef tapeworms; hydatid cyst

Dosage and routes
P *Adult and child >2 yr:* PO 100 mg as a single dose or bid × 3 days, depending on type of infestation; course may be repeated in 3 wk if needed

Available forms: Chew tab 100 mg

Adverse effects
CNS: Dizziness, fever, headache
GI: Transient diarrhea, abdominal pain, nausea, vomiting

Contraindication: Hypersensitivity

P **Precautions:** Child <2 yr, lactation, pregnancy **C** (1st trimester)

Pharmacokinetics

Absorption	Minimal
Distribution	Highly bound to plasma proteins
Metabolism	Liver
Excretion	Feces in metabolites (>95%); urine, unchanged
Half-life	2½-9 hr; increased in hepatic disease

Pharmacodynamics

Onset	Unknown
Peak	½-7 hr
Duration	Unknown

Interactions
Individual drugs
Carbamazepine: ↓ effect of mebendazole
Drug classifications
Hydantoins: ↓ effect of hydantoins
Food/drug
High-fat foods: ↑ absorption

NURSING CONSIDERATIONS
Assessment
• Assess stools during entire treatment; specimens must be sent to lab while still warm, also 1-3 wk after treatment is completed; monitor for diarrhea during expulsion of worms; avoid self-contamination with patient's feces

• Assess for allergic reaction: rash (rare)

• Identify infestation in other family members, since transmission from person to person is common

• If pinworms are suspected, place a piece of cellophane tape over the anal area at night for 1 wk after treatment at night to identify ova; negative perianal swabs taken every AM for 3 days confirm that the patient is no longer infested

• Monitor blood studies: AST, ALT, alkaline phosphatase, BUN, CBC during treatment

Nursing diagnoses
✓ Infection, risk for (uses)
✓ Knowledge deficit (teaching)

Implementation
• Tabs may be chewed if patient is unable to swallow whole

• Give PO after meals to avoid GI symptoms, since absorption is not decreased by food

• Give second course after 3 wk if needed; usually recommended (pinworms)

• Store in airtight container

Patient/family education
• Teach patient proper hygiene after BM, including handwashing technique; tell patient to avoid putting fingers in mouth; clean fingernails

• Advise patient that infested person should sleep alone; do not shake bed linen; wash bed linen daily in hot water; change and wash undergarments daily; that all members of the family should be treated (pinworms)

• Advise patient to clean toilet daily with disinfectant (green soap sol)

• Inform patient that compliance is needed with dosage schedule, duration of treatment

• Tell patient to wear shoes, wash all fruits and vegetables well before eating, use commercial fruit and vegetable cleaner solution

Evaluation
Positive therapeutic outcome
• Expulsion of worms
• Three negative stool cultures after completion of treatment

M

mechlorethamine (℞)
(me-klor-eth'a-meen)
Mustargen, Nitrogen
Mustard
Func. class.: Antineoplastic
alkylating agent
Chem. class.: Nitrogen
mustard

Pregnancy category **D**

Action: Alkylates DNA, RNA;
inhibits enzymes that allow
synthesis of amino acids in
proteins; activity is not cell
cycle phase specific; a vesicant

→**Therapeutic Outcome:** Prevention of rapidly growing
malignant cells

Uses: Hodgkin's disease,
lymphomas, leukemias,
lymphosarcoma; ovarian,
breast, lung carcinoma; neoplastic effusions

Dosage and routes
Adult: **IV** 0.4 mg/kg as 1 dose
or 2-4 divided doses over 2-4
days; second course after 3 wk
depending on blood cell count

Neoplastic effusions
Adult: Intracavity 10-20 mg
(may be 200-400 µg/kg)

Available forms: Inj 10 mg/
vial

Adverse effects
*CNS: Headache, dizziness,
drowsiness, paresthesia,* peripheral neuropathy, **coma**
EENT: Tinnitus, hearing loss
GI: Nausea, vomiting, diarrhea, stomatitis, weight loss,
colitis, **hepatotoxicity**
HEMA: **Thrombocytopenia,
leukopenia, agranulocytosis,**
anemia
INTEG: Alopecia, pruritus,
herpes zoster, extravasation

Contraindications: Lactation,
pregnancy **D**, myelosuppression, acute herpes zoster

Precautions: Radiation therapy, chronic lymphocytic leukopenia

Pharmacokinetics

Absorption	Complete (**IV**)
Distribution	Unknown
Metabolism	Tissues/fluids
Excretion	Kidneys
Half-life	Unknown

Pharmacodynamics

	IV
Onset	1 day
Peak	1-2 wk
Duration	1-3 wk

Interactions
Individual drugs
Radiation: ↑ toxicity, bone
marrow suppression
Drug classifications
Antineoplastics: ↑ toxicity,
bone marrow suppression
**Bone marrow–suppressing
drugs:** ↑ bone marrow suppression
Live vaccines: ↑ adverse reactions, ↓ antibody reaction
Lab test interferences
↑ Uric acid

NURSING CONSIDERATIONS
Assessment
• Monitor CBC, differential,
platelet count weekly; withhold
drug if WBC is <1000/mm³
or platelet count is <75,000/
mm³; notify prescriber of
results if WBC <20,000/mm³,
platelets <150,000/mm³
• Monitor pulmonary function
tests, chest x-ray films before,
during therapy; chest film
should be obtained q2 wk
during treatment; assess for
dyspnea, rales, unproductive
cough, chest pain, tachypnea

☑ Herb/drug ⬚ Do Not Crush ◆ Alert ⟳ Key Drug **G** Geriatric **P** Pediatric

• Assess for increased uric acid levels, swelling, joint pain primarily in extremities; patient should be well hydrated to prevent urate deposits
• Monitor renal function studies: BUN, serum uric acid, urine CrCl before, during therapy; I&O ratio; report fall in urine output of 30 ml/hr; for decreased hyperuricemia
• Monitor for cold, fever, sore throat (may indicate beginning infection); identify edema in feet, joint and stomach pain, shaking; prescriber should be notified
• Assess for bleeding: hematuria, guaiac, bruising or petechiae, mucosa or orifices q8h; no rec temp

Nursing diagnoses
☑ Injury, risk for (adverse reactions)
☑ Body image disturbance (adverse reactions)
☑ Infection, risk for (adverse reactions)
☑ Knowledge deficit (teaching)

Implementation
• Give fluids **IV** or PO before chemotherapy to hydrate patient
• Give antacid before oral agent; give drug after evening meal, before hs; administer antiemetic 30-60 min before giving drug and prn to prevent vomiting; give antibiotics for prophylaxis of infection
• Give top or syst analgesics for pain
• Give in AM so drug can be eliminated before hs
• Use a liq diet: carbonated beverages; gelatin may be added if patient is not nauseated or vomiting

IV IV route
• Give **IV** after diluting 10 mg/10 ml sterile water or 0.9% NaCl; leave needle in vial, shake, withdraw dose, give through Y-tube or 3-way stopcock or directly over 3-5 min into running **IV** of 0.9% NaCl

Y-site compatibilities:
Amifostine, aztreonam, filgrastim, fludarabine, granisetron, melphalan, ondansetron, sargramostim, teniposide, vinorelbine

Additive incompatibilities:
Methohexital

Solution incompatibilities:
D_5W, 0.9% NaCl (**IV** only)
Intracavity route
• Further dilute in 100 ml 0.9% NaCl; administration is completed by prescriber
• Watch for infiltration; if infiltration occurs, infiltrate area with isotonic sodium thiosulfate or 1% lidocaine; apply ice for 6-12 hr

Patient/family education
• Teach patient to avoid use of products containing aspirin or ibuprofen, razors, commercial mouthwash, since bleeding may occur; to report symptoms of bleeding (hematuria, tarry stools)
• Teach patient to report signs of anemia (fatigue, headache, irritability, faintness, shortness of breath)
• Advise patient to report any changes in breathing or coughing even several mo after treatment; to avoid crowds and persons with respiratory tract or other infections
• Tell patient hair loss is common; discuss the use of wigs or hair pieces

M

- Caution patient not to have any vaccinations without the advice of the presciber, serious reactions can occur
- Advise patient contraception is needed during treatment and for several mo after the completion of therapy
- Have patient rinse mouth tid-qid with water, club soda; brush teeth bid-qid with soft brush or cotton-tipped applicators for stomatitis; use unwaxed dental floss

Evaluation
Positive therapeutic outcome
- Decreased size of tumor
- Decreased spread of malignancy
- Improved blood values
- Absence of sweating at night
- Increased appetite, increased weight

---

medroxyprogesterone
(℞)
(me-drox-ee-proe-jess'te-rone)
Amen, Curretab, Cycrin, Depo-Provera, medroxyprogesterone acetate, Provera
Func. class.: Hormone—progestogen; contraceptive; antineoplastic
Chem. class.: Progesterone derivative

Pregnancy category   X

Action: Inhibits secretion of pituitary gonadotropins, which prevents follicular maturation and ovulation; stimulates growth of mammary tissue; antineoplastic action against endometrial cancer

▶**Therapeutic Outcome:** Decreased abnormal uterine bleeding, absence of amenorrhea

Uses: Uterine bleeding (abnormal), secondary amenorrhea, endometrial cancer, renal cancer, contraceptive, prevention of endometrial changes associated with estrogen replacement therapy (ERT)

Investigational uses: Pickwickian syndrome, sleep apnea, hypersomnolence

Dosage and routes
Secondary amenorrhea
Adult: PO 5-10 mg qd × 5-10 days

Endometrial/renal cancer
Adult: IM 400-1000 mg/wk

Uterine bleeding
Adult: PO 5-10 mg qd × 5-10 days starting on 16th day of menstrual cycle

Contraceptive
Adult: Inj q3 mo

With ERT
Adult: PO monophasic 2.5 mg qd; biphasic 5 mg days 15-28 of cycle

Available forms: Tabs 2.5, 5, 10, 100 ✦ mg; inj susp 50, 100, 150, 400 mg/ml; contraceptive injectable

Adverse effects
CNS: Dizziness, headache, migraines, depression, fatigue
CV: Hypotension, thrombophlebitis, edema, **thromboembolism, stroke, pulmonary embolism, myocardial infarction**
EENT: Diplopia
GI: *Nausea,* vomiting, anorexia, cramps, increased weight, **cholestatic jaundice**
GU: Amenorrhea, cervical erosion, breakthrough bleed-

---

ing, dysmenorrhea, vaginal candidiasis, breast changes, *gynecomastia, testicular atrophy, impotence,* endometriosis, **spontaneous abortion**
INTEG: Rash, urticaria, acne, hirsutism, alopecia, oily skin, seborrhea, purpura, melasma, photosensitivity
META: Hyperglycemia

Contraindications: Breast cancer, hypersensitivity, thromboembolic disorders, reproductive cancer, genital bleeding (abnormal, undiagnosed), pregnancy **X**

Precautions: Lactation, hypertension, asthma, blood dyscrasias, gallbladder disease, CHF, diabetes mellitus, bone disease, depression, migraine headache, convulsive disorders, hepatic disease, renal disease, family history of cancer of breast or reproductive tract

🔌 **Do Not Confuse:**
Amen/Ambien, medroxyprogesterone/ methylprednisolone, Provera/ Premarin

Pharmacokinetics

Absorption	Unknown
Distribution	Unknown
Metabolism	Unknown
Excretion	Unknown
Half-life	Unknown

Pharmacodynamics

	PO	IM
Onset	Unknown	Unknown
Peak	Unknown	Unknown
Duration	2-4 hr	Unknown

Interactions
Individual drugs
Aminoglutethimide: ↓ contraceptive effect
Bromocriptine: ↓ effectiveness

Lab test interferences
↑ Alkaline phosphatase, ↑ pregnanediol, ↑ amino acids ↓ GTT, ↓ HDL

NURSING CONSIDERATIONS
Assessment
• Monitor B/P at beginning of treatment and periodically; check weight daily; notify prescriber of weekly weight gain >5 lb
• Monitor I&O ratio: be alert for decreasing urinary output, increasing edema, hypertension
• Assess liver function studies: ALT, AST, bilirubin, periodically during long-term therapy
• Assess for edema, hypertension, cardiac symptoms, jaundice
• Assess mental status: affect, mood, behavioral changes, depression

Nursing diagnoses
☑ Sexual dysfunction (uses)
☑ Tissue perfusion, altered (adverse reactions)
☑ Injury, risk for (adverse reactions)
☑ Knowledge deficit (teaching)

M

Implementation
PO route
• Give with food or milk to decrease GI symptoms
IM route
• Store in dark area
• Give titrated dosage; use lowest effective dosage; give oil sol deep in large muscle mass (IM); rotate sites; use after warming to dissolve crystals

Patient/family education
• Advise patient to avoid sunlight or use sunscreen; photosensitivity and melasma (brown patches on the face) can occur
• Teach patient about cushingoid symptoms

• Teach patient to report breast lumps, vaginal bleeding, edema, jaundice, dark urine, clay-colored stools, dyspnea, headache, blurred vision, abdominal pain, numbness or stiffness in legs, chest pain; male to report impotence or gynecomastia
• Teach patient to report suspected pregnancy immediately

Evaluation
Positive therapeutic outcome
• Decreased abnormal uterine bleeding
• Absence of amenorrhea
• Prevented pregnancy
• Arrested spread of malignant cells

---

megestrol (℞)
(me-jess′trole)
Megace, megestrol acetate
Func. class.: Antineoplastic
Chem. class.: Hormone, progestin

Pregnancy category D (tabs), X (susp)

Action: Affects endometrium by antiluteinizing effect; this is thought to bring about cell death

➤Therapeutic Outcome: Prevention of rapidly growing malignant cells; weight gain, increased appetite in AIDS

Uses: Breast, endometrial, renal cell cancer; increase weight, decrease cachexia and anorexia associated with AIDS

Dosage and routes
Endometrial/ovarian carcinoma
Adult: PO 40-320 mg/day in divided doses

Breast carcinoma
Adult: PO 40 mg qid

Anorexia (AIDS)
Adult: PO 800 mg qd (oral susp)

Available forms: Tabs 20, 40 mg; oral susp 200 mg/5 ml

Adverse effects
CNS: Mood swings
CV: **Thrombophlebitis, thrombembolism**
GI: Nausea, vomiting, diarrhea, abdominal cramps, weight gain
GU: Gynecomastia, fluid retention, **hypercalcemia,** vaginal bleeding, discharge, impotence, decreased libido
INTEG: Alopecia, rash, pruritus, purpura, itching

Contraindications: Hypersensitivity, pregnancy **X** (susp), **D** (tabs)

▧ Do Not Confuse:
Megace/Reglan

Pharmacokinetics	
Absorption	Well absorbed
Distribution	Unknown
Metabolism	Liver, completely
Excretion	Unknown
Half-life	1 hr

Pharmacodynamics	
Onset	Several wk-mo
Peak	Unknown
Duration	1-3 days

Interactions: None
Lab test interferences
↑ Alkaline phosphatase, ↑ urinary pregnanediol, ↑ plasma amino acids
False positive: Urine glucose
↓ HDL, ↓ glucose tolerance test

NURSING CONSIDERATIONS
Assessment
- Monitor effects of alopecia on body image; discuss feelings about body changes
- In AIDS patients monitor calorie counts, weight, appetite
- Assess for thrombophlebitis: pain, redness, swelling in legs; notify prescriber if these occur

Nursing diagnoses
☑ Knowledge deficit (teaching)

Implementation
- Administer with meals for GI symptoms
- Oral susp is usually used for AIDS patients

Patient/family education
- Teach patient to report any complaints or side effects to prescriber
- Advise patient that contraceptive measures must be used during and several mo after treatment; drug is teratogenic
- Explore with patient the need for wig or hair piece for hair loss
- Caution patient to report vaginal bleeding to prescriber
- Review with patient the need to comply with dosage schedule, not to miss or double doses; missed doses may be taken up to 1 hr before next dose

Evaluation
Positive therapeutic outcome
- Decreased spread of malignant cells
- Weight gain, increased appetite in AIDS patients

melphalan (℞)
(mel'fa-lan)
Alkeran, Alkeran IV, ʟ-Pam, ʟ-Sarcolysin
Func. class.: Antineoplastic, alkylating agent
Chem. class.: Nitrogen mustard
Pregnancy category **D**

Action: Alkylates DNA, RNA; inhibits enzymes that allow synthesis of amino acids in proteins; activity is not cell cycle phase specific

Therapeutic Outcome: Prevention of rapidly growing malignant cells

Uses: Multiple myeloma, malignant melanoma, advanced ovarian cancer

Investigational uses: Breast, testicular, prostate carcinoma; osteogenic sarcoma, chronic myelogenous leukemia

Dosage and routes
Multiple myeloma
Adult: PO 6 mg qd × 2-3 wk; stop drug for 4 wk or until WBC level begins to rise; do not administer if WBC <3000/mm³ or platelets <100,000/mm³; may be given 0.15 mg/kg/day × 7 days; wait until platelets and WBCs rise, then 0.05 mg/kg/day

Ovarian carcinoma
Adult: **IV** inf 16 mg/m²; reduce in renal insufficiency; give over 15-20 min; give at 2-wk intervals × 4 doses, then at 4-wk intervals

Available forms: Tabs 2 mg; inj 50 mg

Adverse effects
GI: Nausea, vomiting, stomatitis, diarrhea

M

GU: Amenorrhea, hyperuricemia, gonadal suppression
HEMA: **Thrombocytopenia, neutropenia, leukopenia,** anemia
INTEG: Rash, urticaria, alopecia, pruritus
RESP: **Fibrosis, dysplasia**
SYST: **Anaphylaxis,** allergic reaction

Contraindications: Lactation, pregnancy **D**, hypersensitivity to this drug or other nitrogen mustards

Precautions: Radiation therapy, bone marrow depression, infection, renal disease, **P** children

Pharmacokinetics	
Absorption	Variable; incompletely absorbed
Distribution	Rapidly distributed
Metabolism	Bloodstream
Excretion	Kidneys, unchanged (10%)
Half-life	1½ hr

Pharmacodynamics
Unknown

Interactions
Individual drugs
Radiation: ↑ toxicity, bone marrow suppression
Drug classifications
Antineoplastics: ↑ toxicity, bone marrow suppression
Bone marrow–suppressing drugs: ↑ bone marrow suppression
Live vaccines: ↑ adverse reactions, ↓ antibody reaction

Lab test interferences
Increase: Uric acid

NURSING CONSIDERATIONS
Assessment
• Monitor CBC, differential, platelet count weekly; withhold drug if WBC is <3000/mm³ or platelet count is <100,000/mm³; notify prescriber of results if WBC <20,000/mm³, platelets <100,000/mm³
• Monitor pulmonary function tests, chest x-ray films before, during therapy; chest film should be obtained q2 wk during treatment; check for dyspnea, rales, unproductive cough, chest pain, tachypnea
• Assess for increased uric acid levels, swelling, joint pain primarily in extremities; patient should be well hydrated to prevent urate deposits
• Monitor renal function studies: BUN, serum uric acid, urine CrCl before, during therapy; check I&O ratio; report fall in urine output of 30 ml/hr; check for decreased hyperuricemia; monitor AST, ALT
• Monitor for cold, fever, sore throat (may indicate beginning infection); identify edema in feet, joint and stomach pain, shaking; prescriber should be notified
• Assess for bleeding: hematuria, guaiac, bruising or petechiae, mucosa or orifices q8h; no rec temp

Nursing diagnoses
☑ Injury, risk for (adverse reactions)
☑ Body image disturbance (adverse reactions)
☑ Infection, risk for (adverse reactions)
☑ Knowledge deficit (teaching)

Implementation
• Give fluids **IV** or PO before chemotherapy to hydrate patient
• Give antacid before oral agent; give drug after evening meal, before hs; provide anti-

emetic 30-60 min before giving drug and prn to prevent vomiting; give antibiotics for prophylaxis of infection

• Give in AM so drug can be eliminated before hs

• Use a liq diet: carbonated beverages; gelatin may be added if patient is not nauseated or vomiting

PO route

• Give 1 hr ac or 2 hr pc to prevent nausea/vomiting

IV **IV route**

• Give as intermittent inf: reconstitute with provided diluent (10 ml) to 5 mg/ml; shake until clear; further dilute with 0.9% NaCl to <0.45 mg/ml; give over 15 min

Y-site compatibilities:

Acyclovir, amikacin, aminophylline, ampicillin, aztreonam, bleomycin, bumetanide, buprenorphine, butorphanol, calcium gluconate, carboplatin, carmustine, cefazolin, cefepime, cefoperazone, cefotaxime, cefotetan, ceftazidime, ceftizoxime, ceftriaxone, cefuroxime, cimetidine, cisplatin, clindamycin, cyclophosphamide, cytarabine, dacarbazine, dactinomycin, daunorubicin, dexamethasone, diphenhydramine, doxorubicin, doxycycline, droperidol, enalaprilat, etoposide, famotidine, floxuridine, fluconazole, fludarabine, fluorouracil, furosemide, gallium, ganciclovir, gentamicin, granisetron, haloperidol, heparin, hydrocortisone sodium phosphate, hydromorphone, hydroxyzine, idarubicin, ifosfamide, imipenem-cilastatin, lorazepam, mannitol, mechlorethamine, meperidine, mesna, methylprednisolone, metoclopramide, methotrexate, metro-nidazole, miconazole, minocycline, mitomycin, mitoxantrone, morphine, nalbuphine, netilmicin, ondansetron, pentostatin, piperacillin, plicamycin, potassium chloride, prochlorperazine, promethazine, ranitidine, sodium bicarbonate, streptozocin, teniposide, thiotepa, ticarcillin, ticarcillin/clavulanate, tobramycin, trimethoprim-sulfamethoxazole, vancomycin, vinblastine, vincristine, vinorelbine, zidovudine

Patient/family education

• Teach patient to avoid use of products containing aspirin or ibuprofen, razors, commercial mouthwash, since bleeding may occur; to report symptoms of bleeding (hematuria, tarry stools)

• Instruct patient to report signs of anemia (fatigue, headache, irritability, faintness, shortness of breath)

• Instruct patient to report any changes in breathing or coughing even several mo after treatment; to avoid crowds and persons with respiratory tract or other infections

• Tell patient hair loss is common; discuss the use of wigs or hair pieces

• Caution patient not to have any vaccinations without the advice of the prescriber; serious reactions can occur

• Advise patient that contraception is needed during treatment and for several mo after the completion of therapy

• Teach patient to rinse mouth tid-qid with water, club soda; brush teeth bid-qid with soft brush or cotton-tipped applicators for stomatitis; use unwaxed dental floss

M

Evaluation
Positive therapeutic outcome
• Decreased size of tumor
• Decreased spread of malignancy

---

menotropins (℞)
(men-oh-troe′pinz)
HMG, Pergonal, Repronex
Func. class.: Gonadotropin
Chem. class.: Exogenous gonadotropin
Pregnancy category **X**

Action: In women, increases follicular growth, maturation; in men, when given with HCG, stimulates spermatogenesis; contains FSH and LH

▸**Therapeutic Outcome:** Pregnancy, ovulation

Uses: Infertility, anovulation in women; stimulates spermatogenesis in men; usually used with HCG

Dosage and routes
Infertility
Adult (men): IM 1 ampule 3 times a wk with HCG 2000 U 2 times a wk × 4 mo

Anovulation
Adult (women): IM 75 IU of FSH, LH qd × 9-12 days, then 10,000 U HCG 1 day after these drugs; repeat × 2 menstrual cycles, then increase to 150 IU of FSH, LH qd × 9-12 days, then 10,000 U HCG 1 day after these drugs × 2 menstrual cycles

Available forms: Powder for inj 17 IU/ampule

Adverse effects
CNS: Fever
CV: **Hypovolemia,** thrombophlebitis, **pulmonary embolism, thromboembolism**

GI: Nausea, vomiting, diarrhea, anorexia, abdominal distention/pain
GU: **Ovarian enlargement,** multiple births, ovarian hyperstimulation, sudden ovarian enlargement, ascites with or without pain, pleural effusion, gynecomastia in men
HEMA: **Hemoperitoneum, arterial thromboembolism**
RESP: **ARDs, pulmonary embolism, pulmonary infarction**
OTHER: **Anaphylaxis**

Contraindications: Primary ovarian failure, abnormal bleeding, thyroid/adrenal dysfunction, organic intracranial lesion, ovarian cysts, primary testicular failure, pregnancy **X**

Pharmacokinetics	
Absorption	Well absorbed
Distribution	Unknown
Metabolism	Unknown
Excretion	Kidneys, unchanged (8%)
Half-life	70 hr (FSH); 4 hr (LH)

Pharmacodynamics	
Unknown	

Interactions: None

NURSING CONSIDERATIONS
Assessment
• Monitor weight qd; notify prescriber if weight gain increases rapidly
• Monitor estrogen excretion level; if >100 µg/24 hr, drug is withheld; hyperstimulation syndrome may occur
• Monitor I&O ratio; be alert for decreasing urinary output
• Assess for ovarian enlargement, abdominal distention/pain; report symptoms immediately

---

Nursing diagnoses
☑ Sexual dysfunction (uses)
☑ Knowledge deficit (teaching)

Implementation
• Give after reconstituting with 1-2 ml sterile saline inj; use immediately

Patient/family education
• Advise patient that multiple births are possible; if pregnancy occurs, it is usually 4-6 wk after start of treatment
• Instruct patient to keep daily appointment for 2 wk during treatment

Evaluation
Positive therapeutic outcome
• Pregnancy

---

meperidine ⚭ (℞)
(me-per′i-deen)
Demerol, meperidine HCl, Pethandol, Pethidine
Func. class.: Opiate analgesic
Chem. class.: Phenylpiperidine derivative

Pregnancy category B
Controlled substance schedule II

Action: Depresses pain impulse transmission at the spinal cord level by interacting with opioid receptors; produces CNS depression

⇒ Therapeutic Outcome: Relief of pain

Uses: Moderate to severe pain, preoperatively, during labor

Dosage and routes
Pain
Adult: PO/SC/IM 50-150 mg q3-4h prn; dosage should be decreased if given **IV**

P *Child:* PO/SC/IM 1 mg/kg q4-6h prn, not to exceed 100 mg q4h

Preoperatively
Adult: IM/SC 50-100 mg q30-90 min before surgery; dosage should be reduced if given **IV**

P *Child:* IM/SC 1-2.2 mg/kg 30-90 min before surgery

Renal dose
CrCl 10-50 ml/min 75% of dose; CrCl <10 ml/min 50% of dose

Labor analgesia
Adult: SC/IM 50-100 mg given when contractions are regulary spaced, repeat q1-3h prn

Available forms: Inj 10, 50, 75, 100 mg/ml; tabs 50, 100 mg; syr 50 mg/5 ml

Adverse effects
CNS: Drowsiness, dizziness, confusion, headache, sedation, euphoria, **increased intracranial pressure, seizures**
CV: Palpitations, bradycardia, change in B/P, tachycardia (**IV**)
EENT: Tinnitus, blurred vision, miosis, diplopia, depressed corneal reflex
GI: Nausea, vomiting, anorexia, constipation, cramps
GU: Urinary retention, dysuria
INTEG: Rash, urticaria, bruising, flushing, diaphoresis, pruritus
RESP: Respiratory depression

Contraindications: Hypersensitivity, addiction (opiate)

Precautions: Addictive personality, pregnancy **B**, lactation, increased intracranial pressure, MI (acute), severe heart disease, respiratory

M

Adverse effects: *italic* = common; **bold** = life-threatening

depression, hepatic disease,
P renal disease, child <18 yr,
G elderly

N Do Not Confuse:
Demerol/Dilaudid,
meperidine/hydromorphone

Pharmacokinetics	
Absorption	Well absorbed (IM, SC); 50% (PO)
Distribution	Widely distributed; crosses placenta
Metabolism	Liver, extensively
Excretion	Kidneys; breast milk
Half-life	3-4 hr

Pharmacodynamics			
	PO	IM/SC	IV
Onset	15 min	10 min	Rapid
Peak	½-1 hr	½-1 hr	5-7 min
Duration	2-4 hr	2-4 hr	2-4 hr

Interactions
Individual drugs
Alcohol: ↑ respiratory depression, hypotension, sedation
Cimetidine: ↑ recovery
Erythromycin: ↑ recovery
Nalbuphine: ↓ analgesia
Pentazocine: ↓ analgesia
Procarbazine: Fatal reaction, do not use together
Drug classifications
Antihistamines: ↑ respiratory depression, hypotension
Barbiturates: ↑ respiratory depression
CNS depressants: ↑ respiratory depression, hypotension
MAOIs: Do not use for 2 wk before taking meperidine
Phenothiazines: ↑ respiratory depression, hypotension
Sedative/hypnotics: ↑ respiratory depression, hypotension
Lab test interferences
↑ Amylase

NURSING CONSIDERATIONS
Assessment
• Assess pain: location, duration, intensity before and 1 hr after administration
• Assess renal function prior to initiating therapy; poor renal function can lead to accumulation of toxic metabolite and seizures
• Monitor VS after parenteral route; note muscle rigidity, drug history, liver, kidney function tests, respiratory dysfunction: respiratory depression, character, rate, rhythm; notify prescriber if respirations are <10/min
• Monitor CNS changes: dizziness, drowsiness, hallucinations, euphoria, LOC, pupil reaction; these are due to metabolite produced
• Monitor allergic reactions: rash, urticaria

Nursing diagnoses
☑ Pain (uses)
☑ Sensory perceptual alteration: visual, auditory (adverse reactions)
☑ Breathing pattern, ineffective (adverse reactions)
☑ Injury, risk for (adverse reactions)
☑ Knowledge deficit (teaching)

Implementation
• Give with antiemetic if nausea, vomiting occur
• Administer when pain is beginning to return; determine dosage interval by patient response; continuous dosing of medication is more effective given prn
• Medication should be slowly withdrawn after long-term use to prevent withdrawal symptoms
• Store in light-resistant container at room temp

☑ Herb/drug   ◎ Do Not Crush   ◆ Alert   ⚷ Key Drug   **G** Geriatric   **P** Pediatric

PO route
• May be given with food or milk to lessen GI upset
• Syrup should be mixed with 4 oz of water

IM/SC route
• Do not give if cloudy or a precipitate has formed
• Patient should remain recumbent for 1 hr after administration

IV IV route
• Give by direct **IV** after diluting to 10 mg/ml with sterile water, 0.9% NaCl for inj; give slowly at 25 mg/1 min; rapid administration may cause respiratory depression, hypotension, circulatory collapse
• Give cont inf after diluting to 1 mg/ml with D_5W, $D_{10}W$, dextrose/saline combinations, dextrose/Ringer's, inj combinations, 0.45% NaCl, 0.9% NaCl, Ringer's, LR; give by inf pump; titrate according to response

Syringe compatibilities:
Atropine, benzquinamide, butorphanol, chlorpromazine, cimetidine, dimenhydrinate, diphenhydramine, droperidol, fentanyl, glycopyrrolate, hydroxyzine, ketamine, metoclopramide, midazolam, pentazocine, perphenazine, prochlorperazine, promazine, promethazine, ranitidine, scopolamine

Syringe incompatibilities:
Heparin, morphine, pentobarbital

Additive compatibilities:
Cefazolin, dobutamine, ondansetron, scopolamine, succinylcholine, triflupromazine, verapamil

Y-site compatibilities:
Amifostine, amikacin, ampicillin, atenolol, aztreonam, bumetanide, cefamandole, cefazolin, cefmetazole, cefotaxime, cefotetan, cefoxitin, ceftazidime, ceftizoxime, ceftriaxone, cefuroxime, cephalothin, cephapirin, chloramphenicol, cladribine, clindamycin, dexamethasone, diltiazem, diphenhydramine, dobutamine, dopamine, doxycycline, droperidol, erythromycin lactobionate, famotidine, filgrastim, fluconazole, fludarabine, gallium, gentamicin, granisetron, heparin, hydrocortisone, regular insulin, kanamycin, labetalol, lidocaine, magnesium sulfate, melphalan, methyldopate, methylprednisolone, metoclopramide, metoprolol, metronidazole, moxalactam, ondansetron, oxacillin, oxytocin, paclitaxel, penicillin G potassium, piperacillin, potassium chloride, propofol, propranolol, ranitidine, sargramostim, teniposide, thiotepa, ticarcillin, ticarcillin/clavulanate, tobramycin, trimethoprim/sulfamethoxazole, vancomycin, verapamil, vinorelbine

Y-site incompatibilities:
Cefoperazone, idarubicin, imipenem/cilastatin, mezlocillin, minocycline

Patient/family education
• Advise patients to avoid CNS depressants (alcohol, sedative/hypnotics) for at least 24 hr after taking this drug
• Discuss with patient that dizziness, drowsiness, and confusion are common; to avoid getting up without assistance
• Discuss in detail with the patient all aspects of the drug, including its purpose and what to expect

M

- Caution patient to make position changes carefully to lessen orthostatic hypotension

Evaluation
Positive therapeutic outcome
- Decreased pain

Treatment of overdose: Narcan 0.2-0.8 mg **IV**, O₂, **IV** fluids, vasopressors

---

meprobamate (℞)
(me-proe-ba′mate)
Apo-Meprobamate ✤, Equanil, Meditran ✤, meprobamate, Meprospan, Miltown, Miltown 400, Miltown 600, Neuramate, Neo-Tran ✤, Novomepro ✤, Sedabamate, Trancot
Func. class.: Sedative/hypnotic; antianxiety
Chem. class.: Propanediol carbamate derivative

Pregnancy category   D
Controlled substance schedule   IV

Action: Produces widespread depression of the CNS

➡**Therapeutic Outcome:** Decreased anxiety, sedation

Uses: Anxiety, sedation

Dosage and routes
Adult: PO 1.2-1.6 g/day in 2-3 divided doses, not to exceed 2.4 g/day or 800-1600 mg/day in 2 divided doses (sus rel); max 2.4 g/day

G *Elderly:* PO 200 mg bid-tid, adjust to lowest possible dose

P *Child 6-12 yr:* PO 100-200 mg bid-tid or 200 mg (sus rel) bid

Available forms: Tabs 200, 400, 600 mg; sus rel caps 200, 400 mg

Adverse effects
CNS: Dizziness, drowsiness, headache, **convulsions,** ataxia
CV: Hypotension, tachycardia, palpitations, **hyperthermia**
EENT: Blurred vision, tinnitus, mydriasis, slurred speech
GI: Nausea, vomiting, anorexia, diarrhea, stomatitis
HEMA: **Thrombocytopenia, leukopenia, eosinophilia**
INTEG: Urticaria, pruritus, maculopapular rash

Contraindications: Hypersensitivity, renal failure, porphyria, pregnancy **D**, history of drug abuse or dependence

Precautions: Suicidal patients, severe depression, renal disease, hepatic disease, elderly

Pharmacokinetics	
Absorption	Well absorbed
Distribution	Widely distributed; crosses placenta
Metabolism	Liver
Excretion	Kidneys, feces, breast milk
Half-life	6-16 hr

Pharmacodynamics		
	PO	PO–SUS REL
Onset	1 hr	Unknown
Peak	1-3 hr	Unknown
Duration	6-12 hr	Up to 12 hr

Interactions
Individual drugs
Alcohol: ↑ CNS depression
Fluoxetine: ↑ action
Propoxyphene: ↑ action
Drug classifications
Antidepressants: ↑ CNS depression
Antihistamines: ↑ CNS depression

⊘ Herb/drug   Ⓢ Do Not Crush   ✦ Alert   ⟜ Key Drug   **G** Geriatric   **P** Pediatric

Opiates: ↑ CNS depression
Sedative/hypnotics: ↑ CNS depression
Lab test interferences
False: ↑ 17-OHCS
False positive: Phentolamine test

NURSING CONSIDERATIONS
Assessment
• Assess patient's sleep pattern and note physical (sleep apnea, obstructed airway, pain/discomfort, urinary frequency) and psychologic (fear, anxiety) circumstances that interrupt sleep
• Assess patient's bedtime routine, presleep cues, props
• Assess potential for abuse; this drug may lend to physical and psychologic dependency; amount of drug should be limited
• Monitor blood studies: Hct, Hgb, RBCs, serum folate (if on long-term therapy), protime in patients receiving anticoagulants, since action of anticoagulant may be increased
• Monitor mental status: mood, sensorium, affect, memory (long, short)
• Monitor physical dependency: more frequent requests for medication, shakes, anxiety, pinpoint pupils
• Monitor respiratory dysfunction: respiratory depression, character, rate, rhythm; hold drug if respirations are <10/min or if pupils are dilated (rare)
• Assess for blood dyscrasias: fever, sore throat, bruising, rash, jaundice, epistaxis (rare)
• Assess previous history of substance abuse, cardiac disease, or gastritis

Nursing diagnoses
☑ Anxiety (uses)
☑ Knowledge deficit (teaching)
☑ Noncompliance (teaching)

Implementation
• Give with food to minimize GI symptoms
⊘• Do not break, crush, or chew sus rel cap
• Store in tight container in cool environment

Patient/family education
• Advise patient to avoid driving and other activities requiring alertness; to avoid alcohol and CNS depressants; serious CNS depression may result, as well as tachycardia, flushing, headache, hypotension
• Caution patient not to discontinue medication quickly after long-term use; drug should be tapered over 1-2 wk; effects may take 2 nights for benefits to be noticed; withdrawal symptoms include tremors, anxiety, hallucinations, delirium
• Teach patient alternate measures to improve sleep (reading, exercise several hr before hs, warm bath, warm milk, TV, self-hypnosis, deep breathing)
• Instruct patient that hangover is common in elderly but less common than with barbiturates
• Teach patient symptoms of withdrawal: nausea, vomiting, anxiety, hallucinations, insomnia, tachycardia, fever, cramps, tremors, seizures
• Teach patient to watch for blood dyscrasias: fever, sore throat, bruising, rash, jaundice (rare)
• Teach patient to watch for allergic reaction (rash); discontinue drug if rash occurs

M

Evaluation
Positive therapeutic outcome
• Decreased anxiety, restlessness, insomnia
Treatment of overdose:
Lavage, VS, supportive care

---

mercaptopurine (℞)
(mer-kap-toe-pyoor'een)
6-MP, Purinethol
Func. class.: Antineoplastic, antimetabolite
Chem. class.: Purine analog
Pregnancy category **D**

Action: Inhibits purine metabolism at multiple sites, which inhibits DNA and RNA synthesis S phase of cell cycle

⊳**Therapeutic Outcome:** Prevention of rapidly growing malignant cells

Uses: Chronic myelocytic leukemia, acute lymphoblastic **P** leukemia in children, acute myelogenous leukemia

Investigational uses: Polycythemia vera, psoriatic arthritis, colitis, lymphoma

Dosage and routes
Adult: PO 2.5 mg/kg/day, not to exceed 5 mg/kg/day; maintenance 1.5-2.5 mg/kg/day
P *Child:* 75 mg/m^2/day (2.5 mg/kg/day)

Available forms: Tab 50 mg
Adverse effects
CNS: Fever, headache, weakness
GI: Nausea, vomiting, anorexia, diarrhea, stomatitis, **hepatotoxicity** (with high doses), jaundice, gastritis
GU: **Renal failure,** hyperuricemia, **oliguria,** crystalluria, **hematuria**
HEMA: **Thrombocytopenia, leukopenia, myelosuppression, anemia**
INTEG: Rash, dry skin, urticaria

Contraindications: Patients with prior drug resistance, leukopenia (<2500/mm^3), thrombocytopenia (<100,000/mm^3), anemia, pregnancy **D**
Precautions: Renal disease

Pharmacokinetics	
Absorption	Variable
Distribution	Widely-body water
Metabolism	Liver-extensively
Excretion	Kidneys unchanged (small amounts)
Half-life	Unknown

Pharmacodynamics
Unknown

Interactions
Individual drugs
Allopurinol: ↑ toxicity
Cyclophosphamide: ↑ cardiotoxicity, CHF
Radiation: ↑ toxicity, bone marrow suppression
Warfarin: ↑ or ↓ effect of warfarin
Drug classifications
Antineoplastics: ↑ toxicity, bone marrow suppression
Hepatotoxic agents: ↑ hepatotoxicity
Live virus vaccines: ↓ antibodies
Nondepolarizing muscle relaxants: Reversal of neuromuscular blockade

NURSING CONSIDERATIONS
Assessment
• Assess buccal cavity q8h for dryness, sores or ulceration, white patches, oral pain, bleeding, dysphagia; obtain prescrip-

tion for viscous lidocaine (Xylocaine)

⚕ Assess symptoms indicating severe allergic reaction: rash, pruritus, urticaria, purpuric skin lesions, itching, flushing

• Monitor CBC, differential, platelet count weekly; withhold drug if WBC count is <4000/mm^3 or platelet count is <100,000/mm^3; notify prescriber of results if WBC <20,000/mm^3, platelets <150,000/mm^3

• Assess for increased uric acid levels, swelling, joint pain primarily in extremities; patient should be well hydrated to prevent urate deposits

• Monitor renal function studies: BUN, creatinine, serum uric acid, urine CrCl before and during therapy; check I&O ratio; report fall in urine output to <30 ml/hr

• Monitor temp q4h (may indicate beginning of infection)

• Monitor liver function tests before and during therapy (bilirubin, AST, ALT, LDH) as needed or monthly; check for yellowing of skin or sclera, dark urine, clay-colored stools, itchy skin, abdominal pain, fever, diarrhea

• Assess for bleeding: hematuria, stool guaiac, bruising or petechiae; mucosa or orifices q8h; check for inflammation of mucosa, breaks in skin

Nursing diagnoses

☑Injury, risk for (adverse reactions)
☑Body image disturbance (adverse reactions)
☑Infection, risk for (adverse reactions)
☑Knowledge deficit (teaching)

Implementation

• Give fluids IV or PO before chemotherapy to hydrate patient

• Give antiemetic 30-60 min before giving drug and prn to prevent vomiting; give antibiotics for prophylaxis of infection

• Give in AM so drug can be eliminated before hs

• Provide liq diet: carbonated beverages; gelatin may be added if patient is not nauseated or vomiting

• Encourage patient to rinse mouth tid-qid with water, club soda; brush teeth bid-qid with soft brush or cotton-tipped applicators for stomatitis; use unwaxed dental floss

• Tab may be crushed and added to fluids or food to facilitate swallowing

Patient/family education

• Advise patient that contraceptive measures are recommended during therapy; serious teratogenic effects may occur, to avoid breastfeeding

• Teach patient to avoid use of products containing aspirin or NSAIDs, razors, commercial mouthwash, since bleeding may occur; to report symptoms of bleeding (hematuria, tarry stools)

• Instruct patient to report signs of anemia (fatigue, headache, irritability, faintness, shortness of breath)

• Instruct patient to report any changes in breathing or coughing even several mo after treatment; to avoid crowds and persons with respiratory tract or other infections

• Caution patient not to have any vaccinations without the

M

---

advice of the prescriber; serious reactions can occur

Evaluation
Positive therapeutic outcome
• Prevention of rapid division of malignant cells

---

meropenem (Rx)
(mer-oh-pen'em)
Merrem **IV**
Func. class.: Antiinfective-misc.

Pregnancy category **B**

Action: Interferes with cell wall replication of susceptible organisms; osmotically unstable cell wall swells and bursts from osmotic pressure

➡Therapeutic Outcome: Bactericidal action against the following: *Streptococcus pneumoniae*, group A β-hemolytic streptococci, *viridans* group streptococci, enterococcus; gram-negative organisms: *Klebsiella, Proteus, Escherichia coli, Pseudomonas aeruginosa, Bacteroides fragilis, B. thetaiotamicron*, bacterial **P** meningitis (>3 mo old)

Uses: Serious infections caused by gram-positive or gram-negative organisms (appendicitis, peritonitis)

Dosage and routes
Adult: IV 1 g q8h, given over 15-30 min or as an **IV** bolus 5-20 ml given over 3-5 min

Renal dose
CrCl 26-50 ml/min 1 g q12h; CrCl 10-25 ml/min 500 mg q12h; CrCl <10 ml/min 500 mg q24h

P *Child ≥ 3 mo:* IV 20-40 mg/kg q8h (max 2 g q8h meningitis)

P *Child >50 kg:* **IV** 1 g q8h (intraabdominal infection) or 2 g q8h (meningitis) given over 15-30 min or as an **IV** bolus 5-20 ml over 3-5 min

Available forms: Inj 500 mg

Adverse effects
CNS: Fever, somnolence, *seizures,* dizziness, weakness, *headache*
CV: Hypotension, palpitations
GI: Diarrhea, nausea, vomiting, **pseudomembranous colitis, hepatitis,** glossitis
HEMA: **Eosinophilia, neutropenia,** decreased Hgb, Hct
INTEG: Rash, urticaria, *pruritus,* pain at inj site, phlebitis, erythema at inj site
RESP: Chest discomfort, dyspnea, hyperventilation
SYST: **Anaphylaxis**

Contraindications: Hypersensitivity to meropenem or imipenem

Precautions: Pregnancy **B,**
G lactation, elderly, renal disease

Pharmacokinetics	
Absorption	Complete bioavailability
Distribution	Widely distributed
Metabolism	Liver
Excretion	Kidneys
Half-life	1 hr; increased in renal disease

Pharmacodynamics	
Onset	Rapid
Peak	Dose dependent

Interactions
Individual drugs
Probenecid: ↓ renal excretion, ↑ blood level
Lab test interferences
False: ↑ Creatinine (serum urine), false ↑ urinary 17-KS

False positive: Urinary protein, direct Coombs' test, urine glucose
Interference: Cross-matching

NURSING CONSIDERATIONS
Assessment
• Assess patient for previous sensitivity reaction to carbapenem antiinfectives, penicillins
• Assess patient for signs and symptoms of infection, including characteristics of wounds, sputum, urine, stool, WBC >10,000, fever; obtain baseline information before and during treatment
• Complete C&S tests before beginning drug therapy to identify if correct treatment has been initiated
• Assess for allergic reactions: rash, urticaria, pruritus, chills, fever, joint pain; angioedema may occur a few days after therapy begins; epinephrine, resuscitation equipment should be available for anaphylactic reaction
• Identify urine output; if decreasing, notify prescriber (may indicate nephrotoxicity); also check for increased BUN, creatinine
• Monitor blood studies: AST, ALT, CBC, Hct, bilirubin, LDH, alkaline phosphatase, Coombs' test monthly if patient is on long-term therapy
• Monitor electrolytes: potassium, sodium, chloride monthly if patient is on long-term therapy
• Assess bowel pattern qd; if severe diarrhea occurs, drug should be discontinued; may indicate pseudomembranous colitis
• Monitor for bleeding: ecchymosis, bleeding gums, hematuria, stool guaiac daily if on long-term therapy
• Assess for overgrowth of infection: perineal itching, fever, malaise, redness, pain, swelling, drainage, rash, diarrhea, change in cough, sputum

Nursing diagnoses
☑ Infection, risk for (uses)
☑ Diarrhea (adverse reactions)
☑ Injury, risk for (adverse reactions)
☑ Knowledge deficit (teaching)
☑ Noncompliance (teaching)

Implementation
IV route
• Reconstitute with 0.9% NaCl, D_5W, LR, dilute in 5-20 ml of compatible sol; give by direct **IV** over 3-5 mins
• Give by intermittent inf, dilute in 5-20 ml of compatible sol, give over 15-30 min

Patient/family education
• Teach patient to report sore throat, bruising, bleeding, joint pain; may indicate blood dyscrasias (rare)
• Advise patient to contact prescriber if vaginal itching, loose foul-smelling stools, furry tongue occur; may indicate superinfection
• Advise patient to notify prescriber of diarrhea with blood or pus, may indicate pseudomembranous colitis

Additive compatibilities:
Aminophylline, atropine, cimetidine, dexamethasone, dobutamine, dopamine, enalaprilat, fluconazole, furosemide, gentamicin, heparin, insulin (regular), magnesium sulfate, metoclopramide, morphine, norepinephrine, phenobarbital, ranitidine, vancomycin

M

Y-*site compatibilities:* Aminophylline, atenolol, atropine, cimetidine, dexamethasone, digoxin, diphenhydramine, enalaprilat, fluconazole, furosemide, gentamicin, heparin, insulin (regular), metoclopramide, morphine, norepinephrine, phenobarbital, vancomycin

Evaluation
Positive therapeutic outcome
• Absence of signs/symptoms of infection (WBC <10,000, temp WNL, absence of red draining wounds)
• Reported improvement in symptoms of infection

Treatment of anaphylaxis: Epinephrine, antihistamines, resuscitate if needed

---

mesalamine (℞)
(mez-al′a-meen)
Asacol, Pentasa, Rowasa, Salofulk ✦
Func class.: GI antiinflammatory
Chem class.: 5-Aminosalicylic acid
Pregnancy category   B

Action: May diminish inflammation by blocking cyclooxygenase, inhibiting prostaglandin production in colon, local action only

➡**Therapeutic Outcome:** Decreased cramping, pain in GI conditions

Uses: Mild to moderate active distal ulcerative colitis, proctosigmoiditis, proctitis

Dosage and routes
Adult: Rec 60 ml (4 g) hs, retained for 8 hr × 3-6 wk; PO 800 mg tid for 6 wk; supp 500 mg bid for 3-6 wk

Available forms: Rec susp 4 g/60 ml; supp 500 mg; delayed rel tab 400 mg; cap con rel 250 mg (Pentasa)

Adverse effects
CNS: Headache, fever, dizziness, insomnia, asthenia, weakness, fatigue
CV: Pericarditis, myocarditis
EENT: Sore throat, cough, pharyngitis, rhinitis
GI: Cramps, gas, nausea, diarrhea, rec pain, constipation
INTEG: Rash, itching, acne
SYST: Flu, malaise, back pain, peripheral edema, leg and joint pain, arthralgia, dysmenorrhea

Contraindications: Hypersensitivity to this drug or salicylates

Precautions: Renal disease,
Ppregnancy **B**, lactation, children, sulfite sensitivity

N Do Not Confuse:
Asacol/Ansaid

Pharmacokinetics	
Absorption	20%-30% (PO), 10%-25% (rec)
Distribution	Unknown
Metabolism	Unknown
Excretion	Feces
Half-life	1 hr; metabolite 5-10 hr

Pharmacodynamics
Unknown

Interactions: None

NURSING CONSIDERATIONS
Assessment
• Assess for GI symptoms: cramping, gas, nausea, diarrhea, rec pain, abdominal pain; if severe, the drug should be discontinued
• Assess renal function prior to treatment

Nursing diagnoses
- ✓ Pain (uses)
- ✓ Diarrhea (uses)
- ✓ Knowledge deficit (teaching)

Implementation
PO route
- 🚫• Do not crush, chew tabs
- • May give orally

Rec route (susp)
- • Give hs, retained until AM
- • Store at room temp
- • Usual course of therapy is 3-6 wk
- • Give after shaking bottle well

Patient/family education
- • Advise patient to notify prescriber if abdominal pain, cramping, diarrhea with blood, headache, fever, rash, chest pain occur; drug should be discontinued
- • Teach correct administration for PO, or enema

Evaluation
Positive therapeutic outcome
- • Absence of pain, bleeding from GI tract

---

mesoridazine (℞)
(mez-oh-rid'a-zeen)
Serentil
Func. class.: Antipsychotic/neuroleptic
Chem. class.: Phenothiazine, piperidine
Pregnancy category C

Action: Depresses cerebral cortex, hypothalamus, limbic system, which control activity, aggression; blocks neurotransmission produced by dopamine at synapse; exhibits strong α-adrenergic, anticholinergic blocking action; mechanism for antipsychotic effects is unclear

➡Therapeutic Outcome: Decreased signs and symptoms of psychosis, reorganization of thought patterns

Uses: Psychotic disorders, schizophrenia, anxiety, alcoholism, behavioral problems in mental deficiency, chronic brain syndrome

Dosage and routes
Schizophrenia
Adult: PO 50 mg tid; optimum dosage 100-400 mg/day; IM 25 mg; may repeat in 30-60 min; dosage range 25-200 mg/day

Behavior problems
Adult: PO 25 mg tid; optimum dosage 75-300 mg/day

🅖*Elderly:* PO 10 mg qd bid, increase q3-7 days by 10-25 mg to desired dose

Alcoholism
Adult: PO 25 mg bid; optimum dosage 50-200 mg/day

Schizoaffective disorders
Adult: PO 10 mg tid; optimum dosage 30-150 mg/day

Available forms: Tabs 10, 25, 50, 100 mg; conc 25 mg/ml; inj 25 mg/ml

Adverse effects
CNS: Extrapyramidal symptoms: pseudoparkinsonism, akathisia, dystonia, tardive dyskinesia, drowsiness, headache, **neuroleptic malignant syndrome**
CV: Orthostatic hypotension, hypertension, **cardiac arrest,** ECG changes, tachycardia
EENT: Blurred vision, glaucoma
GI: Dry mouth, nausea, vomiting, anorexia, constipation, diarrhea, jaundice, weight gain
GU: Urinary retention, urinary

M

---

frequency, enuresis, impotence, amenorrhea, gynecomastia
HEMA: **Anemia, leukopenia, leukocytosis, agranulocytosis**
INTEG: *Rash,* photosensitivity, dermatitis
RESP: **Laryngospasm,** dyspnea, **respiratory depression**

Contraindications: Hypersensitivity, circulatory collapse, liver damage, cerebral arteriosclerosis, coronary disease, severe hypertension/hypotension, blood dyscrasias, coma, brain damage, bone marrow depression, narrow-angle glaucoma

Precautions: Pregnancy **C,** lactation, seizure disorders, hypertension, hepatic disease, cardiac disease, prostatic hypertrophy, intestinal obstruction, respiratory conditions

◪ Do Not Confuse:
Serentil/Sinequan

Pharmacokinetics

Absorption	Well absorbed (PO, IM)
Distribution	Widely distributed; crosses placenta, blood-brain barrier
Metabolism	Liver, extensively
Excretion	Kidneys, breast milk
Half-life	Unknown

Pharmacodynamics

	PO	IM
Onset	Erratic	15-30 min
Peak	2 hr	30 min
Duration	4-6 hr	6-8 hr

Interactions
Individual drugs
Alcohol: ↑ effects of both drugs, oversedation
Aluminum hydroxide: ↓ absorption
Bromocriptine: ↓ antiparkinsonian activity

Disopyramide: ↑ anticholinergic effects
Guanethidine: ↓ antihypertensive response
Levodopa: ↓ antiparkinsonian activity
Magnesium hydroxide: ↓ absorption
Norepinephrine: ↓ vasoresponse, ↑ toxicity
Phenobarbital: ↓ effectiveness, ↑ metabolism
Drug classifications
Antacids: ↓ absorption
Anticholinergics: ↑ anticholinergic effects
Antidepressants: ↑ CNS depression
Antidiarrheals, adsorbent: ↓ absorption
Antihistamines: ↑ CNS depression
Antihypertensives: ↑ hypotension
Barbiturate anesthetics: ↑ CNS depression
General anesthetics: ↑ CNS depression
MAOIs: ↑ CNS depression
Opiates: ↑ CNS depression
Sedative/hypnotics: ↑ CNS depression
◪ Herb/drug
Henbane: ↑ anticholinergic effect
Lab test interferences
↑ Liver function tests, ↑ cardiac enzymes, ↑ cholesterol, ↑ blood glucose, ↑ prolactin, ↑ bilirubin, ↑ PBI, ↑ cholinesterase ^{131}I, ↑ alkaline phosphatase, ↑ leukocytes, ↑ granulocytes, ↑ platelets
↓ Hormones (blood and urine)
False positive: Pregnancy tests, PKU
False negative: Urinary steroids, 17-OHCS

NURSING CONSIDERATIONS
Assessment
- Assess mental status: orientation, mood, behavior, presence and type of hallucinations before initial administration and monthly; this drug should significantly reduce psychotic behavior
- Check for swallowing of PO medication; check for hoarding or giving of medication to other patients
- Monitor I&O ratio; palpate bladder if low urinary output **G** occurs, especially in elderly; urinalysis recommended before, during prolonged therapy
- Monitor bilirubin, CBC, liver function studies monthly
- Assess affect, orientation, LOC, reflexes, gait, coordination, sleep pattern disturbances
- Monitor B/P with patient sitting, standing, and lying; take pulse and respirations q4h during initial treatment; establish baseline before starting treatment; report drops of 30 mm Hg; obtain baseline ECG, Q wave and T wave changes
- Check for dizziness, faintness, palpitations, tachycardia on rising; severe orthostatic hypotension is common
- Identify for neuroleptic malignant syndrome: hyperpyrexia, muscle rigidity, increased CPK, altered mental status; drug should be discontinued
- Assess for EPS including akathisia (inability to sit still, no pattern to movements), tardive dyskinesia (bizarre movements of the jaw, mouth, tongue, extremities), pseudoparkinsonism (ragged tremors, pill rolling, shuffling gait); an antiparkinsonism drug should be prescribed
- Assess for constipation, urinary retention daily; if these occur, increase bulk, water in diet

Nursing diagnoses
☑ Thought processes, altered (uses)
☑ Coping, ineffective individual (uses)
☑ Knowledge deficit (teaching)
☑ Noncompliance (teaching)

Implementation
PO route
- Administer drug in liq form mixed in glass of juice or cola if hoarding is suspected; do not mix in caffeine drinks or with tannics, pectins
- Administer lowest possible **G** dose to elderly to minimize side effects, since metabolism is slowed
- Reduce dose in patients treated for behavior problems
- Administer PO with full glass of water, milk; or give with food to decrease GI upset
- Store in airtight, light-resistant container, oral sol in bottle
IM route
- Inject deeply in large muscle mass; do not give SC; do not administer sol with a precipitate

Patient/family education
- Teach patient to use good oral hygiene; frequent rinsing of mouth, sugarless gum for dry mouth
- Tell patient to avoid hazardous activities until drug response is determined; dizziness, blurred vision may occur
- Inform patient that orthostatic hypotension occurs often and to rise from sitting or lying position gradually; to remain lying down after IM inj for at

M

---

least 30 min; tell patient to avoid hot tubs, hot showers, tub baths, since hypotension may occur; tell patient that in hot weather heat stroke may occur; take extra precautions to stay cool

• Caution patient to avoid abrupt withdrawal of this drug, or EPS may result; drug should be withdrawn slowly

• Teach patient to avoid OTC preparations (cough, hay fever, cold) unless approved by prescriber, since serious drug interactions may occur; avoid use with alcohol, CNS depressants; increased drowsiness may occur

• Caution patient to use a sunscreen and sunglasses in case of photosensitivity

• Teach patient about EPS and necessity of meticulous oral hygiene, since oral candidiasis may occur

• Advise patient to take antacids 2 hr before or after taking this drug

• Instruct patient to report sore throat, malaise, fever, bleeding, mouth sores; if these occur, CBC should be drawn and drug discontinued

• Teach patient that urine may turn pink or red

Evaluation
Positive therapeutic outcome
• Decrease in emotional excitement, hallucinations, delusions, paranoia
• Reorganization of patterns of thought, speech

Treatment of overdose:
Lavage if orally ingested; provide airway; *do not induce vomiting or use epinephrine*

---

metaproterenol (Ŗ)
(met-a-proe-ter'e-nole)
Alupent, Arm-A-Med, metaproterenol sulfate, Metaprel
Func. class.: Selective β₂-agonist, bronchodilator
Pregnancy category C

Action: Relaxes bronchial smooth muscle by direct action on β_2-adrenergic receptors, with increased levels of cAMP and increased bronchodilatation, diuresis, and cardiac and CNS stimulation

Therapeutic Outcome: Bronchodilatation with ease of breathing

Uses: Bronchial asthma, bronchospasm

Dosage and routes
P *Adult and child >12 yr:* Inh 2-3 puffs; may repeat q3-4h, not to exceed 12 puffs/day

Asthma/bronchospasm
Adult: PO 20 mg q6-8h

G *Elderly:* PO 10 mg tid-qid, initially

P *Child >9 yr or >27 kg:* PO 20 mg q6-8h or 0.4-0.9 mg/kg tid

P *Child 6-9 yr or <27 kg:* PO 10 mg q6-8h or 0.4-0.9 mg/kg tid

P *Child 2-6 yr:* PO 1.3-2.6 mg/kg divided q6-8h

Available forms: Tabs 10, 20 mg; aerosol 0.65 mg/dose; syr 10 mg/5 ml; sol for inh 0.4%, 0.6%, 5%

Adverse effects
CNS: Tremors, anxiety, insomnia, headache, dizziness, stimulation

---

☑ Herb/drug ⊗ Do Not Crush ◆ Alert ⟳ Key Drug **G** Geriatric **P** Pediatric

CV: Palpitations, tachycardia, hypertension, **dysrhythmias, cardiac arrest**
GI: Nausea, vomiting
RESP: **Paradoxical broncho-spasm**

Contraindications: Hypersensitivity to sympathomimetics, narrow-angle glaucoma

Precautions: Pregnancy **C**, cardiac disorders, hyperthyroidism, diabetes mellitus, prostatic hypertrophy

◼ Do Not Confuse:
Alupent/Atrovent

Pharmacokinetics	
Absorption	Well absorbed (PO)
Distribution	Unknown
Metabolism	Liver, tissues
Excretion	Unknown
Half-life	2-4 hr

Pharmacodynamics		
	PO	INH
Onset	15 min	5 min
Peak	1 hr	1 hr
Duration	4 hr	4 hr

Interactions
Drug classifications
β-Adrenergic blockers: Block therapeutic effect
Bronchodilators, aerosol: ↑ action of bronchodilator
MAOIs: ↑ chance of hypertensive crisis
Sympathomimetics: ↑ adrenergic side effects
☑ *Herb/drug*
Ephedra: ↑ effect

NURSING CONSIDERATIONS
Assessment
• Monitor respiratory function: vital capacity, FEV, ABGs, lung sounds, heart rate, rhythm (baseline)
• Determine that patient has not received theophylline

therapy before giving dose; identify client's ability to self-medicate
• Monitor for evidence of allergic reactions; paradoxic bronchospasm; withhold dose; notify prescriber

Nursing diagnoses
☑ Airway clearance, ineffective (uses)
☑ Impaired gas exchange (uses)
☑ Knowledge deficit (teaching)

Implementation
Aerosol route
• Give after shaking, exhale, place mouthpiece in mouth, inhale slowly, hold breath, remove, exhale slowly; allow at least 1 min between inh
• Store in light-resistant container, do not expose to temp over 86° F (30° C)
• Provide spacer device for **◼**elderly

PO route
• Give PO with meals to decrease gastric irritation; syrup **◼** to children (no alcohol, sugar)

Patient/family education
• Advise patient not to use OTC medications; excess stimulation may occur; to use this medication before other medications and allow at least 5 min between each to prevent overstimulation
• Teach patient use of inhaler; review package insert with patient; teach patient to avoid getting aerosol in eyes, since blurring may result; to wash inhaler in warm water qd and dry; to avoid smoking, smoke-filled rooms, persons with respiratory tract infections
• Advise patient that paradoxic bronchospasm may occur and to stop drug immediately and notify prescriber; to limit caf-

M

feine products such as chocolate, coffee, tea, and colas
- Instruct patient on administration of dose; not to use more than prescribed; serious side effects may occur

Evaluation
Positive therapeutic outcome
- Absence of dyspnea, wheezing after 1 hr
- Improved airway exchange
- Improved ABGs

Treatment of overdose: Administer a β_1-adrenergic blocker

---

metformin (R)
(met-for′min)
glucophage
Func. class.: Antidiabetic, oral
Chem. class.: Biguanide
Pregnancy category   B

Action: Inhibits hepatic glucose production and increases sensitivity of peripheral tissue to insulin

Therapeutic Outcome: Blood glucose at normal levels

Uses: Stable adult-onset diabetes mellitus (NIDDM)

Dosage and routes
Adult: PO 500 mg bid initially, then increase to desired response 1-3 g; dosage adjustment q2-3wk or 850 mg qd with morning meal with dosage increased every other week, max 2550 mg/day

Available forms: Tabs 500, 850 mg

Adverse effects:
CNS: Headache, weakness, dizziness, drowsiness, tinnitus, fatigue, vertigo, *agitation*

ENDO: **Lactic acidosis**
GI: Nausea, vomiting, diarrhea, heartburn, anorexia, metallic taste
HEMA: **Thrombocytopenia,** decreased vit B_{12} concentration
INTEG: Rash

Contraindications: Hypersensitivity, hepatic, renal disease, alcoholism, cardiopulmonary disease, history of lactic acidosis

Precautions: Pregnancy **B,** elderly, thyroid disease, previous hypersensitivity to phenformin or buformin, CHF, renal disease

Pharmacokinetics	
Absorption	Unknown
Distribution	Unknown
Metabolism	Unknown
Excretion	Kidneys, unchanged (35-50%)
Half-life	1½-5, Terminal 9-17 hr

Pharmacodynamics	
Onset	Unknown
Peak	1-3 hr
Duration	Unknown

Interactions
Individual drugs
Acetazolamide: ↑ blood glucose levels
Cimetidine: ↑ hypoglycemia
Ethanol: ↑ risk of lactic acidosis
Drug classifications
Glucocorticoids: ↑ risk of lactic acidosis

NURSING CONSIDERATIONS
Assessment
- Assess for hypoglycemic reactions (sweating, weakness, dizziness, anxiety, tremors, hunger), hyperglycemic reactions soon after meals
- Monitor CBC (baseline, q3mo) during treatment; check

---

liver function tests periodically AST, LDH, renal studies: BUN, creatinine during treatment
• Monitor for lactic acidosis: malaise, myalgia, abdominal distress; risk increases with age, poor renal function

Nursing diagnoses
☑ Knowledge deficit (teaching)

Implementation
• Conversion from other oral hypoglycemic agents; change may be made without gradual dosage change; monitor serum or urine glucose and ketones tid during conversion
• Give twice a day with meals to decrease GI upset and provide best absorption
• Give tabs crushed and mixed with meal or fluids for patients with difficulty swallowing
• Store in tight container in cool environment

Patient/family education
• Teach patient to use capillary blood glucose test or Chemstrip tid
• Teach patient symptoms of hypo/hyperglycemia, what to do about each
• Advise patient that drug must be continued on daily basis; explain consequence of discontinuing drug abruptly
• Advise patient to take drug in morning to prevent hypoglycemic reactions at night
• Advise patient to avoid OTC medications unless approved by the prescriber
• Teach patient that diabetes is a lifelong illness; that this drug is not a cure; only controls symptoms
• Teach patient that all food included in diet plan must be eaten to prevent hypoglycemia

• Teach patient to carry Medic Alert ID and glucagon emergency kit for emergencies

Evaluation
• Therapeutic response: decrease in polyuria, polydipsia, polyphagia; clear sensorium; absence of dizziness; stable gait, blood glucose at normal level

Treatment of overdose: Glucose 25 g **IV** via dextrose 50% sol, 50 ml or 1 mg glucagon

methadone (℞)
(meth'a-done)
Dolophine, methadone HCl, Methadose
Func. class.: Opiate analgesic
Chem. class.: Synthetic diphenylheptane derivative
Pregnancy category   B
Controlled substance schedule   II

Action: Depresses pain impulse transmission at the spinal cord level by interacting with opioid receptors; produces CNS depression

▶**Therapeutic Outcome:** Relief of pain; successful opiate withdrawal

Uses: Severe pain, opiate withdrawal

Dosage and routes
Pain
Adult: PO/SC/IM 2.5-10 mg q4-12h prn

Narcotic withdrawal
Adult: PO 15-40 mg/day individualized initially, then 20-120 mg/day titrated to patient response

P *Child:* 0.05-0.1 mg/kg/dose q6-12h

Renal dose
CrCl 10-50 ml/min dose q8h; CrCl <10 ml/min dose q8-12h

Available forms: Inj 10 mg/ml; tabs 5, 10 mg; oral sol 5, 10 mg/5 ml; dispersible tab 40 mg; oral cap 10 mg/ml

Adverse effects
CNS: Drowsiness, dizziness, confusion, headache, sedation, euphoria
CV: Palpitations, bradycardia, change in B/P
EENT: Tinnitus, blurred vision, miosis, diplopia
GI: Nausea, vomiting, anorexia, constipation, cramps, biliary tract spasm
GU: Increased urinary output, dysuria, urinary retention
INTEG: Rash, urticaria, bruising, flushing, diaphoresis, pruritus
RESP: Respiratory depression

Contraindications: Hypersensitivity to this drug, or hypersensitivity to chlorobutanol (inj route), addiction (opiate)

Precautions: Addictive personality, pregnancy **B**, lactation, increased intracranial pressure, MI (acute), severe heart disease, respiratory de-**P**pression, hepatic disease, renal **G**disease, child <18 yr, elderly

N **Do Not Confuse:**
methadone/methylphenidate

Pharmacokinetics	
Absorption	Well absorbed (PO, SC, IM)
Distribution	Widely distributed; crosses placenta
Metabolism	Liver, extensively
Excretion	Kidneys, breast milk
Half-life	15-30 hr; extended interval with continued dosing

Pharmacodynamics		
	PO	IM/SC
Onset	½-1hr	20 min
Peak	1½-2 hr	1½-2 hr
Duration	4-12 hr	4-6 hr

Interactions
Individual drugs
Alcohol: ↑ respiratory depression, hypotension, sedation
Cimetidine: ↑ recovery
Erythromycin: ↑ recovery
Nalbuphine: ↓ analgesia
Pentazocine: ↓ analgesia
Drug classifications
Antihistamines: ↑ respiratory depression, hypotension
CNS depressants: ↑ respiratory depression, hypotension
MAOIs: Do not use for 2 wk before taking methadone
Phenothiazines: ↑ respiratory depression, hypotension
Sedative/hypnotics: ↑ respiratory depression, hypotension
Lab test interferences
↑ Amylase, ↑ lipase

NURSING CONSIDERATIONS
Assessment
• Assess for pain: type, location, intensity, grimacing before and 1½-2 hr after administration; use pain scoring
• Monitor VS after parenteral route; note muscle rigidity, drug history, liver, kidney function tests, respiratory dysfunction: respiratory depression, character, rate, rhythm; notify prescriber if respirations are <10/min
• Monitor CNS changes: dizziness, drowsiness, hallucinations, euphoria, LOC, pupil reaction
• Monitor allergic reactions: rash, urticaria

☑Herb/drug ⊘Do Not Crush ◆Alert ☞Key Drug **G**Geriatric **P**Pediatric

Nursing diagnoses
- ✓ Pain (uses)
- ✓ Sensory-perceptual alteration: visual, auditory (adverse reactions)
- ✓ Breathing pattern, ineffective (adverse reactions)
- ✓ Knowledge deficit (teaching)

Implementation
- Medication should be slowly withdrawn after long-term use to prevent withdrawal symptoms

PO route
- May be given with food or milk to lessen GI upset
- Store in light-resistant container at room temp

IM/SC route
- Do not give if cloudy or a precipitate has formed
- Give deeply in large muscle mass; rotate inj sites

Patient/family education
- Instruct patient to report any symptoms of CNS changes, allergic reactions; to avoid CNS depressants: alcohol, sedative/hypnotics for at least 24 hr after taking this drug
- Discuss with patient that dizziness, drowsiness, and confusion are common; to avoid getting up without assistance
- Discuss in detail with patient all aspects of the drug
- Caution patient to make position changes slowly to prevent orthostatic hypotension

Evaluation
Positive therapeutic outcome
- Decreased pain
- Successful narcotic withdrawal

Treatment of overdose: Naloxone (Narcan) 0.2-0.8 mg **IV**, O_2, **IV** fluids, vasopressors

methimazole (℞)
(meth-im′a-zole)
Tapazole
Func. class.: Thyroid hormone antagonist (antithyroid)
Chem. class.: Thioamide
Pregnancy category D

Action: Inhibits synthesis of thyroid hormones by decreasing iodine use in the manufacture of thyroglobin and iodothyronine; does not affect already formed hormones

Therapeutic Outcome: Decreased T_4 levels, hyperthyroid symptoms

Uses: Hyperthyroidism, preparation for thyroidectomy, thyrotoxic crisis, thyroid storm

Dosage and routes
Hyperthyroidism
Adult: PO 5-20 mg tid depending on severity of condition; continue until euthyroid; maintenance dosage 5-10 mg qd-tid; max dosage 150 mg qd

Child: PO 0.4 mg/kg/day in divided doses q8h; continue until euthyroid; maintenance dosage 0.2 mg/kg/day in divided doses q8h

Preparation for thyroidectomy
Adult and child: PO same as above; iodine may be added for 10 days before surgery

Thyrotoxic crisis
Adult and child: PO same as hyperthyroidism with iodine and propranolol

Available forms: Tabs 5, 10 mg

M

Adverse effects
CNS: Drowsiness, headache, vertigo, fever, paresthesias, neuritis
ENDO: Enlarged thyroid
GI: Nausea, diarrhea, vomiting, jaundice, **hepatitis,** loss of taste
GU: Nephritis
HEMA: **Agranulocytosis, leukopenia, thrombocytopenia, hypothrombinemia, lymphadenopathy,** bleeding, vasculitis
INTEG: Rash, urticaria, pruritus, alopecia, hyperpigmentation, lupuslike syndrome
MS: Myalgia, arthralgia, nocturnal muscle cramps

Contraindications: Hypersensitivity, pregnancy **D,** lactation

Precautions: Infection, bone marrow depression, hepatic disease, patient >40 yr

Pharmacokinetics

Absorption	Rapidly absorbed
Distribution	Crosses placenta
Metabolism	Liver, extensively
Excretion	Kidneys, unchanged; breast milk
Half-life	1-2 hr

Pharmacodynamics

Onset	½ hr
Peak	Unknown
Duration	2-4 hr

Interactions
Individual drugs
Amiodarone: ↓ effectiveness
Digitalis: Altered response
Lithium: ↑ antithyroid effect
Potassium iodide: ↑ antithyroid effect, ↓ effectiveness
Radiation: ↑ bone marrow depression
Warfarin: Altered response

Drug classifications
Antineoplastics: ↑ bone marrow depression
Phenothiazines: ↑ granulocytosis
Lab test interferences
↑ Pro-time, ↑ AST, ↑ ALT, ↑ alkaline phosphatase

NURSING CONSIDERATIONS
Assessment
• Monitor pulse, B/P, temp; check I&O ratio; check for edema (puffy hands, feet, periorbits); indicates hypothyroidism
• Check weight qd; same clothing, scale, time of day
• Monitor T_3, T_4, which are increased; serum TSH, which is decreased; free thyroxine index, which is increased if dosage is too low; discontinue drug 3-4 wk before RAIU
• Monitor blood work: CBC for blood dyscrasias (leukopenia, thrombocytopenia, agranulocytosis); liver function tests
◆• Assess for overdose (peripheral edema, heat intolerance, diaphoresis, palpitations, dysrhythmias, severe tachycardia, increased temp, delirium, CNS irritability); drug should be discontinued
• Assess for hypersensitivity (rash, enlarged cervical lymph nodes); drug may have to be discontinued
• Assess for hypoprothrombinemia (bleeding, petechiae, ecchymosis)
• Monitor clinical response: after 3 wk should include increased weight, pulse, decreased T_4
• Assess for bone marrow depression: sore throat, fever, fatigue

Nursing diagnoses
☑ Knowledge deficit (teaching)
☑ Noncompliance (teaching)

Implementation
• Give with meals to decrease GI upset; give at same time each day to maintain drug level
• Give lowest dosage that relieves symptoms
• Store in light-resistant container
• Increase fluids to 3-4 L/day, unless contraindicated

Patient/family education
• Advise patient to abstain from breastfeeding after delivery; drug appears in breast milk
• Instruct patient to take pulse daily; to keep graph of weight, pulse, mood
• Advise patient to report redness, swelling, sore throat, mouth lesions, which indicate blood dyscrasias
• Caution patient to avoid OTC products that contain iodine; that seafood and other iodine-containing products may be restricted by prescriber
• Caution patient not to discontinue this medication abruptly; thyroid crisis may occur; stress patient compliance
• Advise patient that response may take several mo if thyroid is large
• Teach patient symptoms/signs of overdose: periorbital edema, cold intolerance, mental depression; notify prescriber at once
• Teach patient symptoms of inadequate dosage: tachycardia, diarrhea, fever, irritability; prescriber should be notified to adjust
• Teach patient to take medication exactly as prescribed, not to skip or double doses; missed doses should be taken when remembered up to 1 hr before next dose
• Instruct patient to carry identification (Medic Alert) describing medication taken and condition being treated

Evaluation
Positive therapeutic outcome
• Decreased weight gain
• Decreased pulse
• Decreased T_4
• Decreased B/P

---

methocarbamol (℞)
(meth-oh-kar′ba-mole)
Carbacot, methocarbamol, Robaxin
Func. class.: Skeletal muscle relaxant, central acting
Chem. class.: Carbamate derivative

Pregnancy category   C

Action: Depresses multisynaptic pathways in the spinal cord, causing skeletal muscle relaxation

Therapeutic Outcome: Decreased pain, spasm

Uses: Adjunct for relief of spasm and pain in musculoskeletal conditions, tetanus management

Dosage and routes
Pain of muscle spasm
Adult: PO 1.5 g × 2-3 days, then 1 g qid; IM 500 mg in each gluteal region; may repeat q8h; **IV** bol 1-3 g/day at 3 ml/min; **IV** inf 1 g/250 ml D_5W or NS, not to exceed 3 g/day
Elderly: PO 500 mg qid, titrate to needed dose

Tetanus
Adult: **IV** inf 1-3 g/L of sol q6h; **IV** bol 1-2 g injected into running **IV**

P *Child:* **IV** 15 mg/kg q6h

Available forms: Tabs 500, 750 mg; inj 100 mg/ml

Adverse effects

CNS: Dizziness, weakness, drowsiness, headache, tremor, depression, insomnia, **seizures**
CV: Postural hypotension, bradycardia
EENT: Diplopia, temporary loss of vision, blurred vision, nystagmus
GI: Nausea, vomiting, hiccups, anorexia, metallic taste
GU: Brown, black, green urine
HEMA: Hemolysis, increased hemoglobin (**IV** only)
INTEG: Rash, pruritus, fever, facial flushing, urticaria
MISC: **Anaphylaxis**

Contraindications: Hypersensitivity, child <12 yr, intermittent porphyria

Precautions: Renal disease, hepatic disease, addictive personalities, pregnancy **C,** myasthenia gravis, epilepsy

Pharmacokinetics	
Absorption	Rapidly absorbed (PO)
Distribution	Widely distributed; crosses placenta
Metabolism	Liver, partially
Excretion	Kidney, unchanged
Half-life	1-2 hr

Pharmacodynamics			
	PO	IM	IV
Onset	½ hr	Rapid	Rapid
Peak	1-2 hr	Unknown	Inf end
Duration	>8 hr	Unknown	Unknown

Interactions
Individual drugs
Alcohol: CNS depression
Drug classifications
Antidepressants, tricyclic: ↑ CNS depression
Barbiturates: ↑ CNS depression
Narcotics: ↑ CNS depression
Sedative/hypnotics: ↑ CNS depression
Lab test interferences
False: ↑ VMA, false ↑ urinary 5 HIAA

NURSING CONSIDERATIONS
Assessment
• Assess for pain and spasm: location, duration, intensity, range of motion
• Monitor during and after inj: CNS effects, rash, conjunctivitis, and nasal congestion may occur
• Monitor ECG in epileptic patients; poor seizure control has occurred in patients taking this drug
• Assess allergic reactions: rash, fever, respiratory distress; check for severe weakness, numbness in extremities
• Assess for tolerance: increased need for medication, more frequent requests for medication, increased pain
• Assess for CNS depression: dizziness, drowsiness, psychiatric symptoms

Nursing diagnoses
☑ Physical mobility, impaired (uses)
☑ Injury, risk for (adverse reactions)
☑ Knowledge deficit (teaching)
Implementation
PO route
• Give with meals if GI symptoms occur

• Store in tight container at room temp

IV **IV route**
• Give **IV** undiluted over 1 min or more; give 300 mg or less/1 min or longer; may be diluted in 250 ml or less D$_5$ or isotonic NaCl sol
• Give by slow **IV** to prevent phlebitis; keep recumbent for 15 min to prevent orthostatic hypotension; check for extravasation

IM route
• Give deep in large muscle mass; rotate sites

Patient/family education
• Advise patient not to discontinue medication quickly; insomnia, nausea, headache, spasticity, tachycardia will occur; drug should be tapered off over 1-2 wk
• Inform patient that urine may turn green, black, or brown
• Caution patient not to take with alcohol, other CNS depressants; increased CNS depression can occur
• Advise patient to avoid altering activities while taking this drug
• Caution patient to avoid hazardous activities if drowsiness, dizziness occur; driving should be avoided until drug response is known
• Advise patient to avoid using OTC medications that are CNS depressants (cough preparations, antihistamines) unless directed by prescriber; CNS depression can occur

Evaluation
Positive therapeutic outcome
• Decreased pain, spasticity

Treatment of overdose:
Induce emesis in conscious patient; lavage, dialysis; have epinephrine, antihistamines, and corticosteroids available

methotrexate ☠ (℞)
(meth-oh-trex′ate)
Amethopterin, Folex PFS, methotrexate, methotrexate LPF, Rheumatrex Dose Pack
Func. class.: Antineoplastic, antimetabolite
Chem. class.: Folic acid antagonist
Pregnancy category   X

Action: Inhibits an enzyme that reduces folic acid, which is needed for nucleic acid synthesis in all cells; S phase of cell cycle specific; immunosuppressive

Therapeutic Outcome: Prevention of rapidly growing malignant cells; immunosuppression

Uses: Acute lymphocytic leukemia, in combination for breast, lung, head, neck carcinoma, lymphosarcoma, gestational choriocarcinoma, hydatidiform mole, psoriasis, rheumatoid arthritis, mycosis fungoides

Dosage and routes
Leukemia
Adult and child: PO 3.3 mg/m^2/day given with prednisone IT 12 mg/m^2; maintenance 30 mg/m^2/day 2 times a wk; **IV** 2.5 mg/kg q2 wk

Choriocarcinoma
Adult and child: PO 15-30 mg/ m^2 qd × 5 days, then off 1 wk; may repeat

Breast cancer
Adult: **IV** 40 mg/m^2 on day 1 and 8 with other antineoplastics

M

Arthritis
Adult: PO 7.5 mg/wk

Osteosarcoma
🅿 *Adult and child:* **IV** 12 g/m² given over 4 hr, then leucovorin rescue is given

Mycosis fungoides
Adult: PO 2.5-10 mg/day until cleared (may be many mo); IM 50 mg q wk or 25 mg 2 times a wk

Psoriasis
Adult: PO/IM/**IV** 10 mg q wk; may increase to 25 mg q wk

Available forms: Tab 2.5 mg; inj 25 mg/ml; powder for inj 20, 25, 50, 100, 250 mg/g; sodium inj 2.5, 25 mg/ml

Adverse effects
CNS: Dizziness, **convulsions,** headache, confusion, hemiparesis, malaise, fatigue, chills, fever
GI: Nausea, vomiting, anorexia, diarrhea, stomatitis, **hepatotoxicity,** cramps, ulcer, gastritis, **GI hemorrhage,** abdominal pain, hematemesis
GU: Urinary retention, **renal failure,** menstrual irregularities, defective spermatogenesis, **hematuria, azotemia, uric acid nephropathy**
HEMA: Leukopenia, **thrombocytopenia, myelosuppression, anemia**
INTEG: Rash, alopecia, dry skin, urticaria, photosensitivity, folliculitis, vasculitis, petechiae, ecchymosis, acne, alopecia

Contraindications: Hypersensitivity, leukopenia (<2500/mm³), thrombocytopenia (<100,000/mm³), anemia, psoriatic patients with severe renal/hepatic disease, pregnancy **X,** alcoholism, HIV

Precautions: Renal disease, lactation

🔳 **Do Not Confuse:**
methotrexate/metolazone

Pharmacokinetics	
Absorption	Well absorbed (GI)
Distribution	Widely distributed; crosses placenta
Metabolism	Not metabolized
Excretion	Kidneys, unchanged; breast milk (minimal)
Half-life	2-4 hr; increased in renal disease

Pharmacodynamics			
	PO	IM/IV	IT
Onset	Unknown	Unknown	Unknown
Peak	1-4 hr	½-2 hr	Unknown
Duration	Unknown	Unknown	Unknown

Interactions
Individual drugs
Acyclovir: ↑ neurologic reactions (IT route)
Allopurinol: ↑ toxicity
Asparaginase: ↓ effects of methotrexate
Chloramphenicol: ↑ toxicity
Cyclophosphamide: ↑ cardiotoxicity, CHF
Phenylbutazone: ↑ toxicity
Phenytoin: ↑ toxicity
Probenecid: ↑ toxicity
Radiation: ↑ toxicity, bone marrow suppression
Warfarin: ↑ or ↓ effect of warfarin
Drug classifications
Antineoplastics: ↑ toxicity, bone marrow suppression
Hepatotoxic agents: ↑ hepatotoxicity
Live virus vaccines: ↓ antibodies
Nephrotoxic drugs: ↑ toxicity
Nondepolarizing muscle relaxants: Reversal of neuromuscular blockade

---

☑ Herb/drug 🚫 Do Not Crush ◆ Alert ☛ Key Drug 🅖 Geriatric 🅿 Pediatric

NSAIDs: ↑ toxicity
Penicillins: ↑ toxicity
Salicylates: ↑ toxicity
Sulfonylureas: ↑ toxicity
Tetracylines: ↑ toxicity

NURSING CONSIDERATIONS
Assessment
• Assess buccal cavity q8h for dryness, sores or ulceration, white patches, oral pain, bleeding, dysphagia; obtain prescription for viscous lidocaine (Xylocaine)
• Assess symptoms indicating severe allergic reaction: rash, pruritus, urticaria, purpuric skin lesions, itching, flushing
• Assess tachypnea, ECG changes, dyspnea, edema, fatigue; identify dyspnea, rales, unproductive cough, chest pain, tachypnea
• Monitor CBC, differential, platelet count weekly; withhold drug if WBC count is <4000/mm³ or platelet count is <100,000/mm³; notify prescriber of results if WBC <20,000/mm³, platelets <150,000/mm³
• Assess for increased uric acid levels, swelling, joint pain primarily in extremities; patient should be well hydrated to prevent urate deposits
• Monitor renal function studies: BUN, creatinine, serum uric acid, urine CrCl before and during therapy; check I&O ratio; report fall in urine output to <30 ml/hr
• Monitor temp q4h (may indicate beginning of infection)
• Monitor liver function tests before and during therapy (bilirubin, AST, ALT, LDH) as needed or monthly; check for jaundice skin and sclera, dark urine, clay-colored stools, itchy skin, abdominal pain, fever, diarrhea (hepatotoxicity)
• Assess for bleeding: hematuria, stool guaiac, bruising or petechiae, mucosa or orifices q8h; check for inflammation of mucosa, breaks in skin
• Identify effects of alopecia on body image; discuss feelings about body changes
• Identify edema in feet, joint and stomach pain, shaking; prescriber should be notified

Nursing diagnoses
☑ Injury, risk for (adverse reactions)
☑ Body image disturbance (adverse reactions)
☑ Infection, risk for (adverse reactions)
☑ Knowledge deficit (teaching)

Implementation
• Avoid contact with skin, since drug is very irritating; wash completely to remove
◆• Administer leucovorin calcium within 12 hr of giving this drug to prevent tissue damage; check agency policy
• Give fluids **IV** or PO before chemotherapy to hydrate patient
• Give antacid before oral agent; give drug after evening meal, before hs; give antiemetic 30-60 min before giving drug and prn to prevent vomiting; administer antibiotics for prophylaxis of infection
• Give in AM so drug can be eliminated before hs
• Provide liq diet: carbonated beverages; gelatin may be added if patient is not nauseated or vomiting
• Encourage patient to rinse mouth tid-qid with water, club soda; brush teeth bid-qid with soft brush or cotton-tipped

M

applicators for stomatitis; use unwaxed dental floss

PO route
• Give 1 hr ac or 2 hr pc to prevent vomiting

IM route
• Give deeply in large muscle mass

IV IV route
• Give **IV** after diluting 5 mg/2 ml of sterile water for inj; give through Y-tube or 3-way stopcock at 10 mg or less/min
• Give **IV** inf after diluting in 0.9% NaCl, D_5W, D_5/0.9% NaCl and give as prescribed

Syringe compatibilities:
Bleomycin, cisplatin, cyclophosphamide, doxapram, doxorubicin, fluorouracil, furosemide, heparin, leucovorin, mitomycin, vinblastine, vincristine

Syringe incompatibilities:
Droperidol, ranitidine

Y-site compatibilities:
Allopurinol, amifostine, asparaginase, aztreonam, bleomycin, cefepime, ceftriaxone, cimetidine, cisplatin, cyclophosphamide, cytarabine, daunorubicin, dexchlorpheniramine, diphenhydramine, doxorubicin, etoposide, famotidine, filgrastim, fludarabine, fluorouracil, furosemide, gallium, ganciclovir, granisetron, heparin, hydromorphone, imipenem-cilastatin, leucovorin, lorazepam, melphalan, mesna, methylprednisolone, metoclopramide, mitomycin, morphine, ondansetron, oxacillin, paclitaxel, piperacillin/tazobactam, prochlorperazine, ranitidine, sargramostim, teniposide, thiotepa, vinblastine, vincristine, vinorelbine

Y-site incompatibilities:
Droperidol, idarubicin

Additive compatibilities:
Cephalothin, cyclophosphamide, cytarabine, fluorouracil, hydroxyzine, mercaptopurine, ondansetron, sodium bicarbonate, vincristine

Additive incompatibilities:
Bleomycin, prednisolone

Solution compatibilities:
Amino acids, 4.25%/D_{25}, D_5W, sodium bicarbonate 0.05 mol/L, sodium chloride 0.9%

Patient/family education
• Advise patient that contraceptive measures are recommended during therapy; drug is teratogenic; contraception should be used for 3 mo (male) and 4-6 wk (female)
• Teach patient to avoid use of products containing aspirin or NSAIDs, razors, commercial mouthwash, since bleeding may occur; to report symptoms of bleeding (hematuria, tarry stools)
• Caution patient to report signs of anemia (fatigue, headache, irritability, faintness, shortness of breath)
• Advise patient to report any changes in breathing or coughing even several mo after treatment; to avoid crowds and persons with respiratory tract or other infections
• Teach patient that hair may be lost during treatment; a wig or hair piece may make patient feel better; new hair may be different in color, texture
• Caution patient not to have any vaccinations without the advice of the prescriber; serious reactions can occur

Evaluation
Positive therapeutic outcome
• Prevention of rapid division of malignant cells

methyldopa/ methyldopate (℞)
(meth-ill-doe′pa)
Aldomet, Apo-methyldopa ✤, Dopamet ✤, methyldopa/methyldopate HCl, Novamedopa, Nu-Medopa ✤
Func. class.: Antihypertensive
Chem. class.: Centrally acting α-adrenergic inhibitor
Pregnancy category C

Action: Stimulates central α_2-adrenergic receptors in the CNS, resulting in decreased sympathetic outflow from the brain with decreased peripheral resistance

Therapeutic Outcome: Decreased B/P in hypertension

Uses: Hypertension

Dosage and routes
Adult: PO 250-500 mg bid or tid, then adjusted q2 days prn, 0.5-2 g qd in 2-4 divided doses (maintenance), not to exceed 3 g/day; IV 250-500 mg in 100 ml D_5W q6h, run over 30-60 min, not to exceed 1 g q6h
Elderly: PO 125 mg bid tid, increase q2 days as needed, max 3 g/day
Child: PO 10 mg/kg/day in 2-4 divided doses, not to exceed 65 mg/kg or 3 g/day, whichever is less; IV 20-40 mg/kg/day in 4 divided doses, not to exceed 65 mg/kg or 3 g, whichever is less

Available forms: Methyldopa tabs 125, 250, 500 mg; oral susp 50 mg/ml; methyldopate inj 50 mg/ml (250 mg/5 ml)

Adverse effects
CNS: Drowsiness, weakness, dizziness, sedation, headache, depression, psychosis, paresthesias, parkinsonism, Bell's palsy, nightmares
CV: Bradycardia, **myocarditis,** orthostatic hypotension, angina, edema, weight gain, CHF
EENT: Nasal congestion, eczema
ENDO: Breast enlargement, gynecomastia, lactation, amenorrhea
GI: Nausea, vomiting, diarrhea, constipation, **hepatic dysfunction,** sore or "black" tongue, **pancreatitis**
GU: Impotence, failure to ejaculate
HEMA: Leukopenia, **thrombocytopenia, hemolytic anemia, granulocytopenia,** positive Coombs' test
INTEG: Lupuslike syndrome, rash, toxic epidural necrolysis

Contraindications: Active hepatic disease, hypersensitivity, blood dyscrasias

Precautions: Pregnancy **C,** liver disease, eclampsia, severe cardiac disease

Do Not Confuse:
methyldopa/L-Dopa (levodopa)

Pharmacokinetics	
Absorption	50% (PO)
Distribution	Crosses placenta, blood-brain barrier
Metabolism	Liver, moderately
Excretion	Kidneys, unchanged (partially)
Half-life	1½ hr

Pharmacodynamics		
	PO	**IV**
Onset	Unknown	Unknown
Peak	2-4 hr	2 hr
Duration	12-24 hr	10-16 hr

Interactions
Individual drugs
Alcohol: ↑ hypotension
Haloperidol: ↑ psychosis
Levodopa: ↑ hypotension, toxicity
Lithium: ↑ lithium toxicity
Tolbutamide: ↑ hypoglycemia
Drug classifications
Amphetamines: ↓ antihypertensive effect
Antidepressants, tricyclic: ↓ effects of methyldopa
Antihypertensives: ↑ hypotension
β-Adrenergic blockers: ↑ B/P
Barbiturates: ↓ effects of methyldopa
MAOIs: ↑ pressor effect
Nitrates: ↑ hypotension
NSAIDs: ↓ antihypertensive effect
Phenothiazines: ↓ antihypertensive effect
Lab test interferences
Interference: Urinary uric acid, serum creatinine, AST
False: ↑ Urinary catecholamines

NURSING CONSIDERATIONS
Assessment
• Monitor blood studies: neutrophils, decreased platelets
• Monitor renal studies: protein, BUN, creatinine; watch for increased levels that may indicate nephrotic syndrome: polyuria, oliguria, frequency
• Obtain baselines in renal, liver function tests before therapy begins; check potassium levels, although hyperkalemia rarely occurs
• Monitor B/P, pulse if the drug is being used for hypertension; notify prescriber of changes
• Monitor edema in feet, legs daily; monitor I&O; check weight for decreasing output
• Assess for allergic reaction: rash, fever, pruritus, urticaria; drug should be discontinued if antihistamines fail to help
• Monitor CNS symptoms, **G** especially in the elderly

Nursing diagnoses
☑ Cardiac output, decreased (uses)
☑ Injury, risk for (side effects)
☑ Knowledge deficit (teaching)
☑ Noncompliance (teaching)

Implementation
PO route
• Give ac
• Shake susp before using
• Store in tight container at room temp
IV IV route
• Give by intermittent inf after diluting in 100 ml 0.9% NaCl, D$_5$W, D$_5$/0.9% NaCl, 5% sodium bicarbonate, Ringer's sol; administer over 30-60 min

Y-site compatibilities:
Esmolol, heparin, meperidine, morphine, theophylline

Additive compatibilities:
Aminophylline, ascorbic acid, chloramphenicol, diphenhydramine, heparin, magnesium sulfate, multivitamins, netilmicin, potassium chloride, promazine, sodium bicarbonate, succinylcholine, verapamil, vit B/C

☑ Herb/drug   Ⓢ Do Not Crush   ◆ Alert   ⚷ Key Drug   **G** Geriatric   **P** Pediatric

Acetaminophen/Codeine

Tylenol with Codeine
300/15mg: McNeil

Tylenol with Codeine
300/30mg: McNeil

Tylenol with Codeine
300/60mg: McNeil

**Acetaminophen/
Hydrocodone**

Lorcet Plus
650/7.5mg: Forest

Lorcet
650/10mg: Forest

Vicodin
500/5mg: Knoll

Vicodin ES
750/7.5mg: Knoll

Anexsia
650/7.5mg: Monarch

Lortab
500/5mg: Whitby

Lortab
500/7.5mg: Whitby

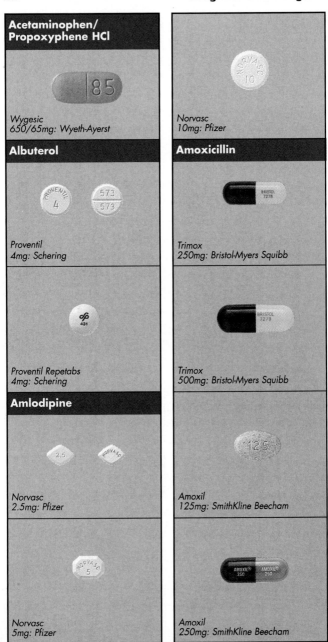

Acetaminophen/ Propoxyphene HCl

Wygesic
650/65mg: Wyeth-Ayerst

Albuterol

Proventil
4mg: Schering

Proventil Repetabs
4mg: Schering

Amlodipine

Norvasc
2.5mg: Pfizer

Norvasc
5mg: Pfizer

Norvasc
10mg: Pfizer

Amoxicillin

Trimox
250mg: Bristol-Myers Squibb

Trimox
500mg: Bristol-Myers Squibb

Amoxil
125mg: SmithKline Beecham

Amoxil
250mg: SmithKline Beecham

Amoxil
250mg: SmithKline Beecham

Amoxil
500mg: SmithKline Beecham

Amoxicillin/Clavulanate

Augmentin
125/31.25mg: SmithKline Beecham

Augmentin
250/62.5mg: SmithKline Beecham

Augmentin
250/125mg: SmithKline Beecham

Augmentin
500/125mg: SmithKline Beecham

Augmentin
875/125mg: SmithKline Beecham

Azithromycin

Zithromax
250mg: Pfizer

Zithromax
250mg: Pfizer

Cephalexin

Keflex
250mg: Dista

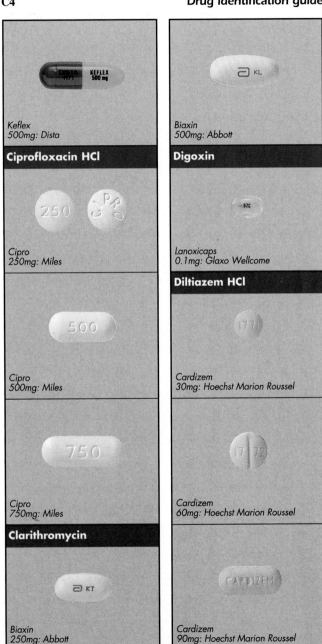

Keflex
500mg: Dista

Ciprofloxacin HCl

Cipro
250mg: Miles

Cipro
500mg: Miles

Cipro
750mg: Miles

Clarithromycin

Biaxin
250mg: Abbott

Biaxin
500mg: Abbott

Digoxin

Lanoxicaps
0.1mg: Glaxo Wellcome

Diltiazem HCl

Cardizem
30mg: Hoechst Marion Roussel

Cardizem
60mg: Hoechst Marion Roussel

Cardizem
90mg: Hoechst Marion Roussel

Drug identification guide

Cardizem CD
120mg: Hoechst Marion Roussel

Cardizem CD
180mg: Hoechst Marion Roussel

Cardizem CD
240mg: Hoechst Marion Roussel

Dilacor XR
180mg: Rhone-Poulenc Rorer

Dilacor XR
240mg: Rhone-Poulenc Rorer

Enalapril

Vasotec
2.5mg: Merck

Vasotec
5mg: Merck

Vasotec
10mg: Merck

Vasotec
20mg: Merck

Estrogens, Conjugated

Premarin
0.3mg: Wyeth-Ayerst

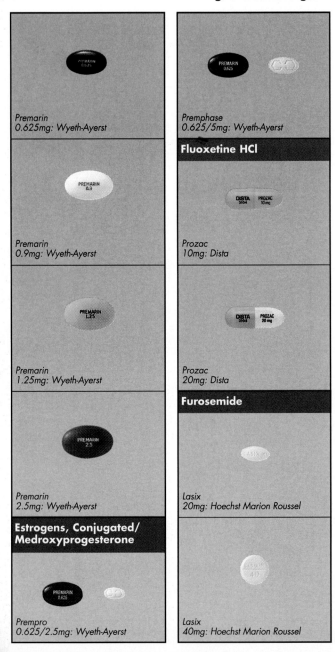

Premarin
0.625mg: Wyeth-Ayerst

Premphase
0.625/5mg: Wyeth-Ayerst

Fluoxetine HCl

Premarin
0.9mg: Wyeth-Ayerst

Prozac
10mg: Dista

Premarin
1.25mg: Wyeth-Ayerst

Prozac
20mg: Dista

Furosemide

Premarin
2.5mg: Wyeth-Ayerst

Lasix
20mg: Hoechst Marion Roussel

**Estrogens, Conjugated/
Medroxyprogesterone**

Prempro
0.625/2.5mg: Wyeth-Ayerst

Lasix
40mg: Hoechst Marion Roussel

Lasix
80mg: Hoechst Marion Roussel

Generic
20mg: Rugby

Generic
40mg: Rugby

Generic
80mg: Rugby

Levothyroxine

Levothroid
0.025mg: Forest

Levothroid
0.05mg: Forest

Levothroid
0.075mg: Forest

Levothroid
0.088mg: Forest

Levothroid
0.1mg: Forest

Levothroid
0.112mg: Forest

Levothroid
0.125mg: Forest

Synthroid
0.025mg: Knoll

Levothroid
0.137mg: Forest

Synthroid
0.05mg: Knoll

Levothroid
0.150mg: Forest

Synthroid
0.075mg: Knoll

Levothroid
0.2mg: Forest

Synthroid
0.1mg: Knoll

Levothroid
0.3mg: Forest

Synthroid
0.112mg: Knoll

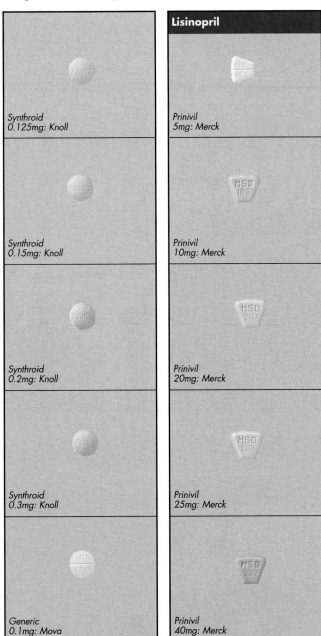

Synthroid *0.125mg: Knoll*	**Lisinopril** *Prinivil* *5mg: Merck*
Synthroid *0.15mg: Knoll*	*Prinivil* *10mg: Merck*
Synthroid *0.2mg: Knoll*	*Prinivil* *20mg: Merck*
Synthroid *0.3mg: Knoll*	*Prinivil* *25mg: Merck*
Generic *0.1mg: Mova*	*Prinivil* *40mg: Merck*

Drug identification guide

Zestril
5mg: Stuart

Zestril
10mg: Stuart

Zestril
20mg: Stuart

Zestril
40mg: Stuart

Zestril
2.5mg: Zeneca

Loratadine

Claritin
10mg: Schering

Metformin HCl

Glucophage
500mg: Lipha

Glucophage
850mg: Lipha

Nifedipine

Adalat CC
30mg: Miles

Adalat CC
60mg: Miles

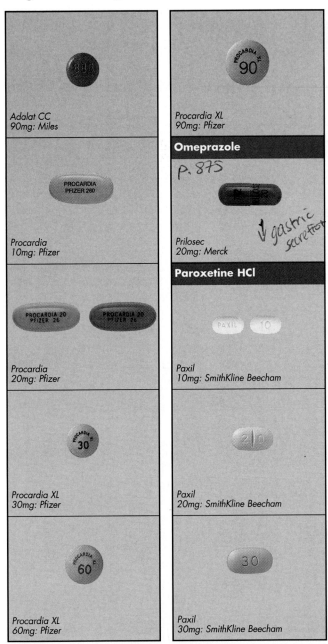

Adalat CC
90mg: Miles

Procardia
10mg: Pfizer

Procardia
20mg: Pfizer

Procardia XL
30mg: Pfizer

Procardia XL
60mg: Pfizer

Procardia XL
90mg: Pfizer

Omeprazole

P. 875

↓ gastric secretion

Prilosec
20mg: Merck

Paroxetine HCl

Paxil
10mg: SmithKline Beecham

Paxil
20mg: SmithKline Beecham

Paxil
30mg: SmithKline Beecham

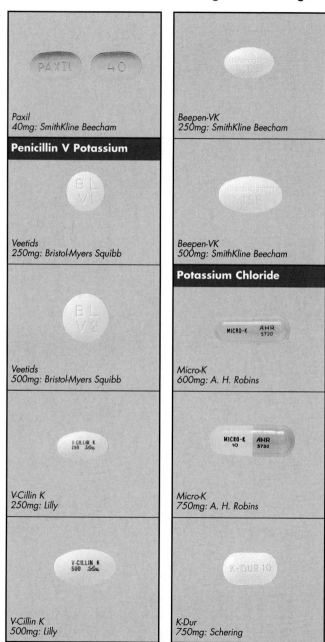

Paxil
40mg: SmithKline Beecham

Penicillin V Potassium

Veetids
250mg: Bristol-Myers Squibb

Veetids
500mg: Bristol-Myers Squibb

V-Cillin K
250mg: Lilly

V-Cillin K
500mg: Lilly

Beepen-VK
250mg: SmithKline Beecham

Beepen-VK
500mg: SmithKline Beecham

Potassium Chloride

Micro-K
600mg: A. H. Robins

Micro-K
750mg: A. H. Robins

K-Dur
750mg: Schering

Drug identification guide

C13

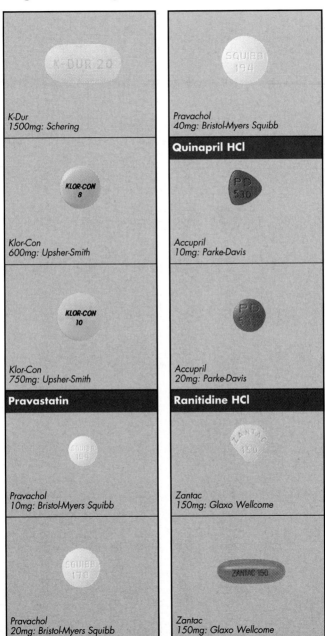

K-Dur
1500mg: Schering

Klor-Con
600mg: Upsher-Smith

Klor-Con
750mg: Upsher-Smith

Pravastatin

Pravachol
10mg: Bristol-Myers Squibb

Pravachol
20mg: Bristol-Myers Squibb

Pravachol
40mg: Bristol-Myers Squibb

Quinapril HCl

Accupril
10mg: Parke-Davis

Accupril
20mg: Parke-Davis

Ranitidine HCl

Zantac
150mg: Glaxo Wellcome

Zantac
150mg: Glaxo Wellcome

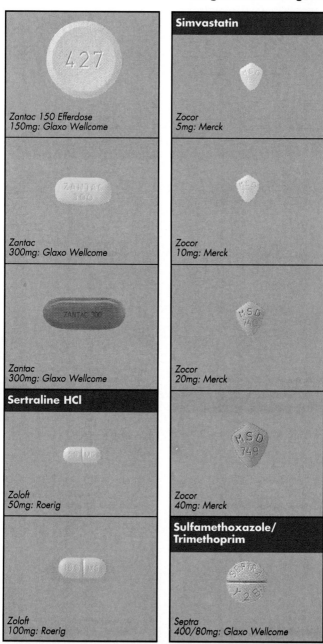

Zantac 150 Efferdose
150mg: Glaxo Wellcome

Zantac
300mg: Glaxo Wellcome

Zantac
300mg: Glaxo Wellcome

Sertraline HCl

Zoloft
50mg: Roerig

Zoloft
100mg: Roerig

Simvastatin

Zocor
5mg: Merck

Zocor
10mg: Merck

Zocor
20mg: Merck

Zocor
40mg: Merck

**Sulfamethoxazole/
Trimethoprim**

Septra
400/80mg: Glaxo Wellcome

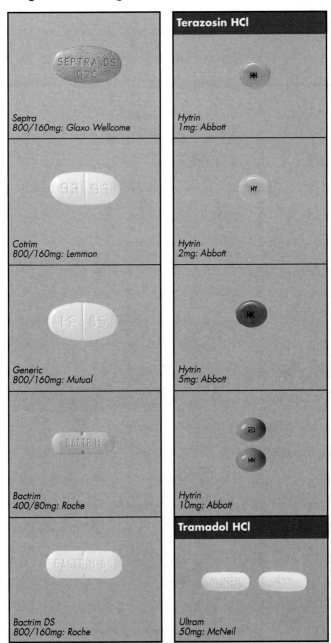

Septra
800/160mg: Glaxo Wellcome

Cotrim
800/160mg: Lemmon

Generic
800/160mg: Mutual

Bactrim
400/80mg: Roche

Bactrim DS
800/160mg: Roche

Terazosin HCl

Hytrin
1mg: Abbott

Hytrin
2mg: Abbott

Hytrin
5mg: Abbott

Hytrin
10mg: Abbott

Tramadol HCl

Ultram
50mg: McNeil

Warfarin Sodium

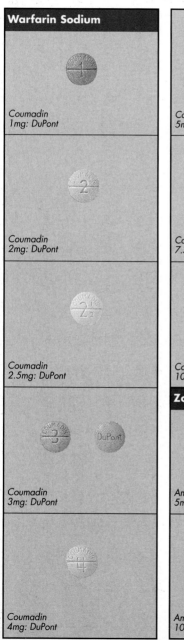

Coumadin
1mg: DuPont

Coumadin
2mg: DuPont

Coumadin
2.5mg: DuPont

Coumadin
3mg: DuPont

Coumadin
4mg: DuPont

Coumadin
5mg: DuPont

Coumadin
7.5mg: DuPont

Coumadin
10mg: DuPont

Zolpidem

Ambien
5mg: Searle

Ambien
10mg: Searle

Standard Precautions

In 1996, the Centers for Disease Control and Prevention published a set of recommendations to protect health care workers, patients, and others from the spread of infection. These recommendations are called *Standard Precautions*. The precautions are used in the care of all patients regardless of their diagnosis or disease. The precautions will not work if they are not used correctly. It is the health care worker's responsibility to select the correct personal protective equipment for the procedure being performed. The principles of standard precautions are also applied when handling or cleaning equipment or supplies that are potentially contaminated.

1. Wear gloves any time that you may contact blood, any moist body fluid (except sweat), secretions, excretions, nonintact skin, or mucous membranes.

2. Remove your gloves, wash your hands, and reapply clean gloves if your gloves become soiled with infective material.

3. Even if you are wearing gloves, remove them, wash your hands, and apply clean gloves *immediately before* contact with mucous membranes or nonintact skin.

4. Wear a protective cover gown of waterproof material if your clothing is likely to have substantial contact with infective material or if splashing of body fluids is likely.

5. Wear a face shield or goggles to protect your eyes if splashing of secretions is likely.

6. Any time a face shield or goggles is worn, wear a surgical mask to protect the mucous membranes of your nose and mouth. A surgical mask may be worn in certain sterile procedures without protective eyewear. However, protective eyewear is *never* worn without a surgical mask.

7. Handle needles, razors, broken glass, and other sharp objects with care. Needles should never be recapped. All sharps should be disposed of in a puncture-resistant sharps container.

8. Wash your hands before and after each patient contact.

9. Wash your hands before you apply and after you remove gloves. Do not assume that handwashing is unnecessary because gloves were worn. Do not wash your hands with gloves on them.

10. Gloves are used for the care of one patient only, then discarded.

---

*Except where indicated otherwise, all color plates are from Potter PA and Perry AG: *Fundamentals of Nursing: Concepts, Process, and Practice*, ed. 4; St. Louis, 1997, Mosby.

11. Follow your facility policy for disposal of gloves and other contaminated items. These items are generally not disposed of in open trash containers. Facilities have designated disposal sites for these biohazardous waste materials.

12. Use resuscitation barrier devices as an alternative to mouth-to-mouth resuscitation.

13. Linen should be handled in a manner that prevents contamination of the outside of the container. Linen from isolation rooms was previously doubled bagged. Double bagging is no longer recommended, since all linen is handled as potentially infectious. Double bag linen only if the outside of the bag becomes contaminated during the bagging process.

Plate 1 Preparing an injection from a vial. **A,** Remove needle cap from syringe. Pull back on the plunger to draw amount of air into syringe equivalent to volume of medication to be aspirated from vial. **B,** Insert tip of needle, with bevel pointing up, through center of rubber seal. Apply pressure on tip of needle during insertion.   *Continued*

Plate 1, cont'd C, Allow air pressure to fill syringe gradually with medication. Pull back slightly on plunger if necessary.

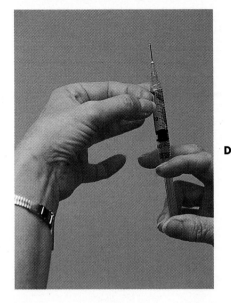

D

Plate 1, cont'd D, Remove remaining air from syringe by holding it and needle upright. Tap barrel to dislodge air bubbles. Draw back slightly on plunger and then push plunger upward to eject air. Do not eject fluid.

Plate 2 Administering an injection. Cleanse site with antiseptic swab. Apply swab at center of site and rotate outward in circular direction for about 5 cm (2 in).

A

Plate 3 A, For a subcutaneous injection, hold the syringe between the thumb and forefinger of the dominant hand as a dart, with the palm down. *Continued*

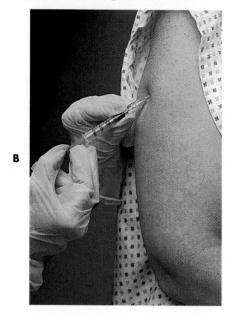

B

Plate 3, cont'd B, After injecting the needle at a 45- to 90-degree angle, grasp lower end of syringe barrel with nondominant hand to end of plunger. Avoid moving syringe while slowly pulling back on plunger to aspirate drug. If blood appears in syringe, remove needle, discard medication and syringe, and repeat procedure. *Exception:* do not aspirate when giving heparin.

Plate 4 For an intradermal injection, note formation of small bleb approximately 6 mm (½ in) in diameter at injection site.

Plate 5 A, Site of IM injection into the left dorsogluteal muscle. Imaginary diagonal line extending from the posterior iliac spine to the greater trochanter is the landmark for selecting the dorsogluteal injection site. **B,** Giving IM injection in left dorsogluteal site (client is prone).

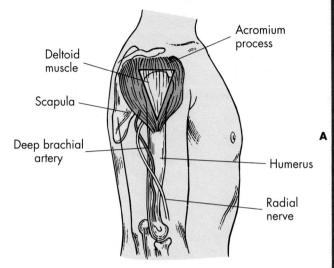

Plate 6 A, Landmarks for IM injection into the deltoid muscle.   *Continued*

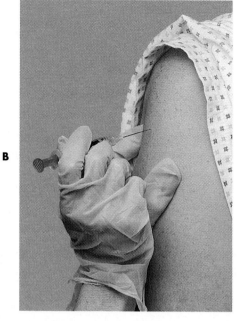

Plate 6, cont'd B, Giving IM injection in deltoid muscle.

Plate 7 A, Landmarks for IM injection in vastus lateralis.
B, Giving IM injection in vastus lateralis site.

A

B

Plate 8 A, Anatomical view of ventrogluteal site. **B,** Giving IM injection into ventrogluteal muscle to avoid major nerves and blood vessels.

Air lock

Medication

A

During Injection

Injection tract seals
as skill is released

Skin

Subcutaneous
tissue

B

Air lock

Muscle

Medication

After Release

Plate 9 Z-track method of injection. **A,** Pulling on overlying skin during IM injection moves tissues to prevent later tracking. **B,** The Z-track left after injection prevents the deposit of medication through sensitive tissue.

Plate 10 Administering IM injection by the air-lock technique prevents tracing of medication through SQ tissue.

Plate 11 Sites recommended for SQ injections. (From Potter PA and Perry AG: *Basic Nursing: A Critical Thinking Approach, ed 4.* St. Louis, 1999, Mosby.)

Plate 12 Comparison of angles of insertion for IM (90 degrees), SQ (45 degrees), and ID (15 degrees) injections. (From Potter PA and Perry AG: *Basic Nursing: A Critical Thinking Approach, ed 4.* St. Louis, 1999, Mosby.)

Plate 13 Administering medication by IV bolus (push).
A, Needle system: insert small-gauge needle of syringe containing prepared drug through center of injection port.
B, Needleless system: Remove cap of needleless injection port. Connect tip of syringe directly.

Continued

Plate 13, cont'd C, Occlude IV line by pinching tubing just above injection port. Pull back gently on syringe's plunger to aspirate blood return. **D,** After noting blood return, continue to occlude tubing and inject medication slowly over several minutes (read directions on drug package). Use watch to time administration.   *Continued*

E

Plate 13, cont'd E, IV lock: Insert needle of syringe containing prepared drug through center of diaphragm.

Plate 14 Administering IV medication by piggyback, volume administration sets or miniinfusors (syringe pump). Use needle-lock device to secure needle of secondary piggyback line through injection port of main line.

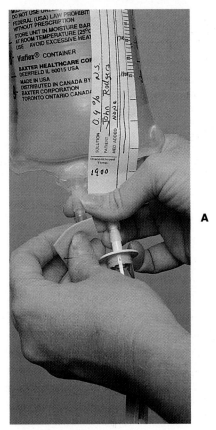

Plate 15 Adding medications to IV fluid containers. **A,** Wipe off port or injection site with alcohol or antiseptic swab.

Continued

Plate 15, cont'd B, Remove needle cap from syringe and insert needle of syringe through center of injection port or site, and inject medication.

Additive incompatibilities:
Amphotericin B, barbiturates, methohexital, sulfonamides

Solution compatibilities:
D_5W, $D_5/0.9\%$ NaCl, Ringer's, sodium bicarbonate 5%, 0.9% NaCl, amino acids 4.25%/D_{25}, Dextran$_6$/0.9% NaCl, Normosol R, Normosol M/D_5W

Patient/family education
• Instruct patient not to discontinue drug abruptly, or withdrawal symptoms may occur: anxiety, increased B/P, headache, insomnia, increased pulse, tremors, nausea, sweating
• Caution patient not to use OTC (cough, cold, or allergy) products unless directed by prescriber
• Teach patient to comply with dosage schedule even if feeling better; drug controls symptoms, does not cure
• Caution patient to change position slowly, to rise slowly to sitting or standing position to minimize orthostatic hypo-**G** tension, especially elderly
• Teach patient about excessive perspiration, dehydration, vomiting, diarrhea, may lead to fall in B/P; consult prescriber if these occur
• Advise patient that drug may cause dizziness, fainting; lightheadedness may occur during 1st few days of therapy; that drug may cause dry mouth; use hard candy, saliva product, or frequent rinsing of mouth
• Caution patient that compliance is necessary; not to skip or stop drug unless directed by prescriber
• Teach patient that drug may cause skin rash

• Teach patient to avoid hazardous activities, since drug may cause drowsiness, dizziness
• Teach patient to take ac

Evaluation
Positive therapeutic outcome
• Decreased B/P

Treatment of overdose:
Gastric evacuation, sympathomimetics, may be indicated if severe; hemodialysis

---

methylergonovine (℞)
(meth-ill-er-goe-noe′veen)
Methergine,
methylergonovine
Func. class.: Oxytocic
Chem. class.: Ergot alkaloid
Pregnancy category   C

Action: Stimulates uterine and vascular smooth muscle, causing contractions, decreased bleeding

▶**Therapeutic Outcome:** Absence of hemorrhage

Uses: Treatment of hemorrhage postpartum or after abortion

Dosage and routes
Adult: IM 0.2 mg q2-5h, not to exceed 5 doses; **IV** 0.2 mg given over 1 min; PO 0.2 mg given over 1 min; PO 0.2-0.4 mg q6-12h × 2-7 days after initial IM or **IV** dose

Available forms: Inj 0.2 mg/ml; tab 0.2 mg

Adverse effects
CNS: Headache, dizziness
CV: Chest pain, palpitations, hypertension, *hypotension,* **dysrhythmias**
EENT: Tinnitus

M

GI: Nausea, vomiting
GU: Cramping
INTEG: Sweating, rash, allergic reactions
RESP: Dyspnea

Contraindications: Hypersensitivity to ergot preparations, indication of labor, before delivery of placenta, hypertension, pelvic inflammatory disease, respiratory disease, cardiac disease, peripheral vascular disease

Precautions: Pregnancy **C**, severe hepatic disease, severe renal disease, jaundice, diabetes mellitus, convulsive disorders

Pharmacokinetics

Absorption	Well absorbed (PO, IM)
Distribution	Unknown
Metabolism	Liver, possibly
Excretion	Unknown
Half-life	½-2 hr

Pharmacodynamics

	PO	IM	IV
Onset	5-15 min	5 min	Immediate
Peak	Unknown	Unknown	Unknown
Duration	3 hr	3 hr	Unknown

Interactions
Individual drugs
Cyclopropane anesthesia:
↑ hypotension
Drug classifications
Vasopressors: ↑ hypertension
Smoking
↑ vasoconstriction

NURSING CONSIDERATIONS
Assessment
• Monitor B/P, pulse; watch for change that may indicate hemorrhage; check respiratory rate, rhythm, depth; notify prescriber of abnormalities
• Assess fundal tone, nonphasic contractions; check for relaxation or severe cramping
• Assess for ergotism or overdose: nausea, vomiting, weakness, muscular pain, insensitivity to cold, paresthesia of extremities; drug should be decreased or inf discontinued
• Before administering ergonovine, check calcium levels; if hypocalcemia is present, correction should be made to increase effectiveness of this drug
• Monitor prolactin levels and for decreased breast milk production

Nursing diagnoses
☑ Tissue perfusion, decreased (uses)
☑ Injury, risk for (adverse reactions)
☑ Knowledge deficit (teaching)

Implementation
PO route
• PO is the preferred route
IM route
• Give deeply in large muscle mass
IV IV route
• Give by this route for severe, life-threatening hemorrhage
• Give directly undiluted or diluted with 5 ml 0.9% NaCl given through Y-site or 3-way stopcock; give 0.2 mg/min; use clear, colorless sol
• Store up to 2 mo if unused

Y-site compatibilities:
Heparin, hydrocortisone sodium succinate, potassium chloride, vit B/C

Patient/family education
• Advise patient to stop smoking, since increased vasoconstriction will result
• Inform patient that abdominal cramps are a side effect of this medication

---

- Instruct patient to notify prescriber if chest pain, nausea, vomiting, headache, muscle pain, weakness or cold, numb extremities occur

Evaluation
Positive therapeutic outcome
- Prevention of hemorrhage

---

methylphenidate ⚷☞
(**R**)
(meth-ill-fen′i-date)
Methidate, Ritalin, Ritalin SR
Func. class.: Cerebral stimulant
Chem. class.: Piperidine derivative

Pregnancy category C
Controlled substance schedule II

Action: Increases release of norepinephrine and dopamine in cerebral cortex to reticular activating system; exact action not known

➔**Therapeutic Outcome:** Increased alertness, decreased fatigue, ability to stay awake (narcolepsy), increased attention span, decreased hyperactivity (ADHD)

Uses: Attention deficit disorder with hyperactivity, narcolepsy

Investigational uses: Depression in the elderly, cancer, stroke

Dosage and routes
ADHD
Adult: PO 5-20 bid-tid

P *Child >6 yr:* PO 5 mg before breakfast and lunch, increasing by 5-10 mg/wk, not to exceed 60 mg/day; sus rel 20 mg qd-tid

Narcolepsy
Adult: PO 10 mg bid-tid, 30-45 min ac; may increase up to 40-60 mg/day

Depression
G *Elderly:* PO 2.5 mg q AM, increase q 3rd day by 2.5 mg to desired dose, max 20 mg/day

Available forms: Tabs 5, 10, 20 mg; sus rel tab 20 mg

Adverse effects
CNS: Hyperactivity, insomnia, restlessness, talkativeness, dizziness, headache, akathisia, dyskinesia, masking or worsening of Gilles de la Tourette's syndrome
CV: Palpitations, tachycardia, B/P changes, angina, **dysrhythmias, thrombocytopenic purpura**
ENDO: Growth retardation
GI: Nausea, anorexia, dry mouth, weight loss, abdominal pain
GU: **Uremia**
HEMA: **Leukopenia,** anemia
INTEG: **Exfoliative dermatitis,** urticaria, rash, erythema multiforme
MISC: Fever, arthralgia, scalp hair loss

Contraindications: Hypersensitivity, anxiety, history of Gilles de la Tourette's
P syndrome; children <6 yr, glaucoma

Precautions: Hypertension, depression, pregnancy **C,** seizures, lactation, drug abuse

N **Do Not Confuse:**
methylphenidate/methadone

M

Pharmacokinetics

Absorption	Well absorbed (PO); delayed (sus rel)
Distribution	Widely distributed; crosses placenta
Metabolism	Liver
Excretion	Kidneys
Half-life	1-3 hr

Pharmacodynamics

	PO	PO–SUS REL
Onset	½-1 hr	2 hr
Peak	1-3 hr	4 hr
Duration	4-6 hr	6-8 hr

Interactions
Drug classifications
Anticonvulsants: ↓ effects
Antidepressants, tricyclics: ↓ effects
MAOIs: Hypertensive crisis
Oral anticoagulants: ↓ effects
Sympathomimetics: ↑ effects
Vasopressors: Hypertensive crisis
Food/drug
Caffeine: ↑ stimulation

NURSING CONSIDERATIONS
Assessment
• Monitor VS, B/P, since this drug may reverse antihypertensives; check patients with cardiac disease more often for increased B/P
• Perform CBC, urinalysis; for diabetic patients monitor blood sugar, urine sugar; insulin changes may be required, since eating will decrease
• Monitor height and weight q3 mo since growth rate in children may be decreased; appetite is suppressed, weight loss is common during the first few mo of treatment
• Monitor mental status: mood sensorium, affect, stimulation, insomnia; aggressiveness may occur; depression with crying spells may occur after drug has worn off
• Assess for tolerance; should not be used for extended time except in ADHD; dosage should be discontinued gradually to prevent withdrawal symptoms
• Assess for narcoleptic symptoms before medication and after; ability to stay awake should increase significantly
• In children or adults with ADHD, monitor for improved organizational skills, attention span, attending to tasks, impulse control, socialization, and ability to get along better with others
• Assess for withdrawal symptoms: headache, nausea, vomiting, muscle pain, weakness; drug tolerance will develop after long-term use; dosage should not be increased if tolerance develops
• Assess appetite, sleep, speech patterns

Nursing diagnoses
☑ Thought processes, altered (uses, adverse reactions)
☑ Coping, ineffective individual (uses)
☑ Knowledge deficit (teaching)
☑ Family coping, impaired (uses)

Implementation
• Give at least 6 hr before hs to avoid sleeplessness; titrate to patient's response; lowest dosage should be used to control symptoms
🚫• Do not chew, crush time-rel tabs
• Give gum, hard candy, frequent sips of water for dry mouth at beginning of treatment; these symptoms tend to lessen with time

Patient/family education
• Teach patient to decrease caffeine consumption (coffee, tea, cola, chocolate), which may increase irritability and stimulation; to avoid OTC preparations unless approved by prescriber; to avoid alcohol ingestion; these may cause serious drug interactions
• Advise patient to taper off drug over several wk, or depression, increased sleeping, lethargy may occur
• Caution patient to avoid hazardous activities until stabilized on medication
• Instruct patient not to double doses if medication is missed; prescriber may suggest drug holidays (ADHD) during the school year to assess progress and determine continued drug necessity
• Instruct patient/family to notify presciber if significant side effects occur: tremors, insomnia, palpitations, restlessness; drug changes may be needed
• Inform patient that if dry mouth occurs to use frequent sips of water, sugarless gum, hard candy during beginning therapy; dry mouth lessens with continued treatment
• Encourage patient to get needed rest; patients will feel more tired at end of day; to take last dose at least 6 hr before hs to avoid insomnia

Evaluation
Positive therapeutic outcome
• Decreased activity in ADHD
• Improved attention span in ADHD
• Absence of sleeping during day in narcolepsy

Treatment of overdose: Administer fluids, hemodialysis, peritoneal dialysis, antihypertensives for increased B/P

---

methylprednisolone/ methylprednisolone acetate/ methylprednisolone sodium succinate (℞)
(meth-ill-pred-niss'oh-lone)
Medrol/Depo-Medrol, Duralone, Medralone, Rep-Pred/A-Methapred, Solu-Medrol
Func. class.: Corticosteroid
Chem. class.: Glucocorticoid, immediate acting

Pregnancy category   C

Action: Decreases inflammation by suppression of migration of polymorphonuclear leukocytes, fibroblasts; reverses increased capillary permeability and lysosomal stabilization; antipruritic, antiinflammatory (top)

▷**Therapeutic Outcome:** Decreased inflammation

Uses: Severe inflammation, shock, adrenal insufficiency, collagen disorders, psoriasis, eczema, contact dermatitis, pruritus (top)

Dosage and routes
Adrenal insufficiency/ inflammation
Adult: PO 2-60 mg in 4 divided doses; IM 40-80 mg (acetate); IM/**IV** 10-250 mg (succinate); intraarticular 4-30 mg (acetate)

P *Child:* **IV** 117 μg-1.66 mg/kg in 3-4 divided doses (succinate)

M

Shock
Adult: IV 100-250 mg q2-6h (succinate)

Pruritus
P Adult and child: TOP apply to affected area qd-qid

Available forms: Tabs 2, 4, 6, 8, 16, 24, 32 mg; inj 20, 40, 80 mg/ml acetate; inj 40, 125, 500, 1000 mg/vial succinate, 1%; dosepack 4 mg tabs

Adverse effects
CNS: Depression, flushing, sweating, headache, mood changes
CV: Hypertension, **circulatory collapse, thrombophlebitis, embolism,** tachycardia
EENT: Fungal infections, increased intraocular pressure, blurred vision, cataracts
GI: Diarrhea, nausea, abdominal distention, **GI hemorrhage,** increased appetite, **pancreatitis**
HEMA: **Thrombocytopenia**
INTEG: Burning, dryness, itching, irritation, acne, folliculitis, hypertrichosis, perioral dermatitis, hypopigmentation, atrophy, striae, miliaria, allergic contact dermatitis, secondary infection, poor wound healing, ecchymosis, petechiae
MS: Fractures, osteoporosis, weakness

Contraindications: Hypersensitivity to corticosteroids, fungal infections, psychosis, idiopathic thrombocytopenia, acute glomerulonephritis, amebiasis, nonasthmatic bronchial disease, child <2 yr, AIDS, TB

Precautions: Pregnancy **C**, lactation, viral or bacterial infections, diabetes mellitus, glaucoma, osteoporosis

⊠ Do Not Confuse:
methylprednisolone/prednisone, methylprednisolone/medroxyprogesterone

Pharmacokinetics	
Absorption	Well absorbed (PO); systemic (top)
Distribution	Crosses placenta
Metabolism	Liver, extensively
Excretion	Kidney
Half-life	3-5 hr; adrenal suppression 3-4 days

Pharmacodynamics				
	PO	IM	IV	TOP
Onset	Unknown	Unknown	Rapid	Min to hr
Peak	2 hr	4-8 days	Unknown	Hr to days
Duration	1½ days	1-4 wk	Unknown	Hr to days

Interactions
Individual drugs
Amphotericin B: ↑ hypokalemia
Insulin: ↑ need for insulin
Mezlocillin: ↑ hypokalemia
Phenytoin: ↓ action, ↑ metabolism
Rifampin: ↓ action, ↑ metabolism
Ticarcillin: ↑ hypokalemia
Drug classifications
Barbiturates: ↓ action, ↑ metabolism
Diuretics: ↑ hypokalemia
Hypoglycemic agents: ↑ need for hypoglycemic agents
⊘ Herb/drug
Aloe: ↑ hypokalemia
Buckthorn: ↑ hypokalemia
Cascara sagrada: ↑ hypokalemia
Rhubarb root: ↑ hypokalemia
Senna: ↑ hypokalemia
Lab test interferences
↑ Cholesterol, ↑ sodium, ↑ blood glucose, ↑ uric acid, ↑ calcium, ↑ urine glucose
↓ calcium, ↓ potassium, ↓ T_4,

⊘ Herb/drug   ⊗ Do Not Crush   ◆ Alert   ⚫⊓ Key Drug   **G** Geriatric   **P** Pediatric

↓ T_3, ↓ thyroid RAIU test, ↓ urine 17-OHCS, ↓ 17-KS, ↓ PBI

False negative: Skin allergy tests

NURSING CONSIDERATIONS
Assessment
• Monitor potassium, blood sugar, urine glucose while patient is on long-term therapy; hypokalemia and hyperglycemia
• Monitor weight daily; notify prescriber of weekly gain >5 lb
• Monitor B/P q4h, pulse; notify prescriber if chest pain occurs
• Monitor I&O ratio; be alert for decreasing urinary output and increasing edema
• Monitor plasma cortisol levels during long-term therapy (normal level 138-635 nmol/L when drawn at 8 AM)
• Monitor adrenal function periodically for HPA axis suppression
• Assess for infection: increased temp, WBC even after withdrawal of medication; drug masks infection symptoms
• Assess for potassium depletion: paresthesias, fatigue, nausea, vomiting, depression, polyuria, dysrhythmias, weakness
• Assess for edema, hypertension, cardiac symptoms
• Assess mental status: affect, mood, behavioral changes, aggression
• Check temp; if fever develops, drug should be discontinued
• Assess for syst absorption: increased temp, inflammation, irritation (top)

Nursing diagnoses
☑ Infection, risk for (adverse reactions)
☑ Knowledge deficit (teaching)
☑ Noncompliance (teaching)

Implementation
☒ **IV route**
• Give **IV**, use only sodium phosphate product; give >1 min; may be given by **IV** inf in compatible sol
• Give after shaking susp (parenteral)
• Give titrated dosage; use lowest effective dosage

Syringe compatibilities: Granisetron, metoclopramide

Y-site compatibilities: Acyclovir, amifostine, amrinone, aztreonam, cefepime, cisplatin, cladribine, cyclophosphamide, cytarabine, dopamine, doxorubicin, enalaprilat, famotidine, fludarabine, granisetron, heparin, melphalan, meperidine, methotrexate, metronidazole, midazolam, morphine, piperacillin/tazobactam, sodium bicarbonate, tacrolimus, teniposide, theophylline, thiotepa, vitamin B with C

Y-site incompatibilities: Ondansetron, paclitaxel, sargramostim, vinorelbine

Additive compatibilities: Chloramphenicol, cimetidine, clindamycin, dopamine, granisetron, heparin, norepinephrine, penicillin G potassium, ranitidine, theophylline, verapamil

IM route
• Give IM inj deep in large muscle mass; rotate sites; avoid deltoid; use 21 G needle
• Give in one dose in AM to prevent adrenal suppression; avoid SC administration; may damage tissue

PO route
• Give with food or milk to decrease GI symptoms

M

Inh route

• Give inh with water to decrease possibility of fungal infections

• Give titrated dosage; use lowest effective dosage

• Clean aerosol top daily with warm water; dry thoroughly

• Store in cool environment; do not puncture or incinerate container

Top route

• Cleanse area before applying drug

• Apply only to affected areas; do not get in eyes

• Apply medication, then cover with occlusive dressing (only if prescribed); seal to normal skin; change q12h; syst absorption may occur

• Apply only to dermatoses; do not use on weeping, denuded, or infected area

• Apply treatment for a few days after area has cleared

• Store at room temp

Patient/family education

• Teach patient that ID as steroid user should be carried

• Advise patient to notify prescriber if therapeutic response decreases; dosage adjustment may be needed

• Caution patient not to discontinue abruptly; adrenal crisis can result

• Caution patient to avoid OTC products: salicylates, alcohol in cough products, cold preparations unless directed by prescriber

• Teach patient all aspects of drug usage including cushingoid symptoms

• Teach patient symptoms of adrenal insufficiency: nausea, anorexia, fatigue, dizziness, dyspnea, weakness, joint pain

• Inform patient that long-term therapy may be needed to clear infection (1-2 mo depending on type of infection)

Nasal route

• Advise patient to clear nasal passages if sneezing attack occurs; repeat dose

• Advise patient to continue using product even if mild nasal bleeding occurs; is usually transient

• Teach patient method of instillation after providing written instructions from manufacturer

Top route

• Advise patient to avoid sunlight on affected area; burns may occur

Evaluation

Positive therapeutic outcome

• Ease of respirations, decreased inflammation

• Absence of severe itching, patches on skin, flaking (top)

---

methysergide (℞)

(meth-i-ser′jide)

Sansert

Func. class.: Adrenergic blocker, serotonin antagonist

Chem. class.: Ergot derivative

Pregnancy category C

Action: Competitively blocks serotonin hydroxytryptamine receptors in CNS and periphery; potent vasoconstrictor

➡**Therapeutic Outcome:** Absence of migraines and other vascular headaches

Uses: Prophylaxis for migraine and other vascular headaches; if no improvement is noted in 3

---

wk, drug is unlikely to be beneficial

Dosage and routes
Adult: PO 2 mg bid with meals

Available forms: Tab 2 mg

Adverse effects
CNS: Tremors, anxiety, insomnia, headache, dizziness, euphoria, confusion, depersonalization, hallucinations, paresthesias, drowsiness
CV: **Retroperitoneal fibrosis,** valvular thickening, palpitations, tachycardia, postural hypertension, angina, thrombophlebitis, ECG changes, **cardiac fibrosis**
GI: Nausea, vomiting, weight gain
HEMA: **Blood dyscrasias**
INTEG: Flushing, rash, alopecia
MS: Arthralgia, myalgia

Contraindications: Hypersensitivity to ergot, tartrazine, peripheral vascular occlusion, CAD, hepatic disease, renal disease, peptic ulcer, hypertension, connective tissue disease, fibrotic pulmonary disease

Precautions: Pregnancy **C,** lactation, children

Pharmacokinetics
Absorption	Rapidly absorbed
Distribution	Widely distributed
Metabolism	Liver
Excretion	Kidneys, breast milk
Half-life	10 hr

Pharmacodynamics
Unknown

Interactions
Drug classifications
β-Adrenergic blockers: ↑ vasoconstriction
Opiates: ↓ effect of narcotics

Smoking
↑ vasoconstriction

NURSING CONSIDERATIONS
Assessment
• Monitor stress level, activity, reaction, coping mechanisms of patient
• Assess neurologic status: LOC, blurring vision, nausea, vomiting, tingling in extremities preceding headache
• Assess for ingestion of tyramine-containing foods (pickled products, beer, wine, aged cheese), food additives, preservatives, colorings, artificial sweeteners, chocolate, caffeine, which may precipitate these types of headaches

Nursing diagnoses
☑ Pain, chronic (uses)
☑ Injury, risk for (adverse reactions)
☑ Knowledge deficit (teaching)

Implementation
• Provide quiet, calm environment with decreased stimulation; no noise, bright lights, or excessive talking
• Give with or pc to avoid GI symptoms
• Store in dark area

Patient/family education
• Caution patient to avoid OTC medications and alcohol; serious drug interactions may occur
• Caution patient to maintain dosage at approved level; not to increase even if drug does not relieve headache
• Advise patient that an increase in headaches may occur when this drug is discontinued after long-term use
• Caution patient to keep drug out of the reach of children; death may occur

M

- Caution patient to use drug for less than 6 mo continuously; a 3-4 wk drug-free period must follow each 6 mo period

Evaluation
Positive therapeutic outcome
- Decrease in frequency, severity of headache

---

metoclopramide (℞)
(met-oh-kloe-pra′mide)
Apo-Metoclop ✦, Clopra, Emex ✦, Maxeran ✦, Maxolon, metoclopramide, Octamide, Octamide PFS, Reclomide, Reglan
Func. class.: Cholinergic, antiemetic
Chem. class.: Central dopamine receptor antagonist

Pregnancy category   B

Action: Enhances response to acetylcholine of tissue in upper GI tract, which causes contraction of gastric muscle, relaxes pyloric, duodenal segments, increases peristalsis without stimulating secretions, blocks dopamine in chemoreceptor trigger zone of CNS

Therapeutic Outcome: Decreased symptoms of delayed gastric emptying, decreased nausea, vomiting

Uses: Prevention of nausea, vomiting induced by chemotherapy, radiation; delayed gastric emptying, gastroesophageal reflux

Investigational uses: Hiccups, migraines

Dosage and routes
Nausea/vomiting
Adult: **IV** 2 mg/kg q2h × 5 doses 30 min before administration of chemotherapy
P *Child:* **IV** 0.1-0.2 mg/kg/dose
Delayed gastric emptying
Adult: PO 10 mg 30 min ac, hs × 2-8 wk
G *Elderly:* PO 5 mg ½hr ac hs, increase to 10 mg if needed
Gastroesophageal reflux
Adult: PO 10-15 mg qid 30 min ac
P *Child:* 0.4-0.8 mg/kg/day divided in 4 doses
Renal dose: CrCl <40 ml/min 50% of dose

Available forms: Tabs 5, 10 mg; syr 5 mg/5 ml; inj 5 mg/ml

Adverse effects
CNS: Sedation, fatigue, restlessness, headache, sleeplessness, dystonia, dizziness, drowsiness
CV: Hypotension, **supraventricular tachycardia**
GI: Dry mouth, constipation, nausea, anorexia, vomiting, diarrhea
GU: Decreased libido, prolactin secretion, amenorrhea, galactorrhea
HEMA: **Neutropenia, leukopenia**
INTEG: Urticaria, rash

Contraindications: Hypersensitivity to this drug or procaine or procainamide, seizure disorder, pheochromocytoma, breast cancer (prolactin dependent), GI obstruction

Precautions: Pregnancy **B**, lactation, GI hemorrhage, CHF, Parkinson's disease

---

Do Not Confuse:
metoclopramide/metolazone,
Reglan/Megace

Pharmacokinetics

Absorption	Well absorbed (PO)
Distribution	Widely distributed; crosses blood-brain barrier, placenta
Metabolism	Liver, minimally
Excretion	Kidneys, breast milk
Half-life	4 hr

Pharmacodynamics

	PO	IM	IV
Onset	½-1 hr	10-15 min	1-3 min
Peak	Unknown	Unknown	Unknown
Duration	1-2 hr	1-2 hr	1-2 hr

Interactions
Individual drugs
Alcohol: ↓ action of metoclopramide
Cyclosporine: ↑ risk of toxicity
Digoxin: ↓ action
Haloperidol: ↑ extrapyramidal reaction
Drug classifications
Anticholinergics: ↓ action of metoclopramide
Antidepressants: ↑ CNS depression
Antihistamines: ↑ CNS depression
CNS depressants: ↑ sedation
MAOIs: Avoid use
Opiates: ↑ sedation
Phenothiazines: ↑ extrapyramidal reaction
Sedative/hypnotics: ↑ CNS depression
Lab test interferences
↑ Prolactin, ↑ aldosterone, ↑ thyrotropin

NURSING CONSIDERATIONS
Assessment
• Assess GI complaints: nausea, vomiting, anorexia, constipation, abdominal distention before and after administration
• Assess for EPS and tardive dyskinesia, more likely to occur in elderly patient: rigidity, grimacing, shuffling gait, tremors, rhythmic involuntary movements of tongue, mouth, jaw, feet, hands; these side effects should be reported to prescriber immediately; some effects may be irreversible
• Assess mental status: depression, anxiety, irritability during treatment

Nursing diagnoses
☑ Injury, risk for (adverse reactions)
☑ Knowledge deficit (teaching)

Implementation
IV route
• Give IV undiluted if dose is <10 mg; give over 2 min
• Dilute 10 mg or more in 50 ml or more D_5W, NaCl, Ringer's, LR and given over 15 min or more
• Discard open ampules

Syringe compatibilities:
Aminophylline, ascorbic acid, atropine, benztropine, bleomycin, butorphanol, chlorpromazine, cisplatin, cyclophosphamide, cytarabine, dexamethasone, dimenhydrinate, diphenhydramine, doxorubicin, droperidol, fentanyl, fluorouracil, heparin, hydrocortisone, hydroxyzine, regular insulin, leucovorin, lidocaine, magnesium sulfate, meperidine, methotrimeprazine, methylprednisolone, midazolam, mitomycin, morphine, pentazocine, perphenazine, prochlorperazine, promazine,

promethazine, ranitidine, scopolamine, sufentanil, vinblastine, vincristine, vit B/C
Syringe incompatibilities:
Ampicillin, calcium gluconate, cephalothin, chloramphenicol, furosemide, penicillin G potassium, sodium bicarbonate
Y-site compatibilities:
Acyclovir, aldesleukin, amifostine, aztreonam, bleomycin, ciprofloxacin, cisplatin, cladribine, cyclophosphamide, cytarabine, diltiazem, doxorubicin, droperidol, famotidine, filgrastim, fluconazole, fludarabine, fluorouracil, foscarnet, gallium, granisetron, heparin, idarubicin, leucovorin, melphalan, meperidine, meropenem, methotrexate, mitomycin, morphine, ondansetron, paclitaxel, piperacillin/tazobactam, propofol, sargramostim, sufentanil, tacrolimus, teniposide, thiotepa, vinblastine, vincristine, vinorelbine, zidovudine
Y-site incompatibilities:
Furosemide
Additive compatibilities:
Clindamycin, meropenem, morphine, multivitamins, potassium acetate/chloride/phosphate, verapamil
Additive incompatibilities:
Cisplatin, erythromycin, tetracycline
PO route
• Give 30-60 min ac for better absorption and at hs
• Use gum, hard candy, frequent rinsing of mouth for dryness of oral cavity
Patient/family education
• Instruct patient to avoid driving, other hazardous activities until stabilized on this medication

• Advise patient to avoid alcohol and other CNS depressants that enhance sedating properties of this drug
• Advise patient to notify prescriber if involuntary movements occur
Evaluation
Positive therapeutic outcome
• Absence of nausea, vomiting, anorexia, fullness

---

metolazone (R_x)
(me-tole′a-zone)
MyKrox, Zaroxolyn
Func. class.: Diuretic, antihypertensive
Chem. class.: Thiazide-like quinazoline derivative
Pregnancy category **B**

Action: Acts on the distal tubule and cortical thick ascending limb of the loop of Henle in the kidney, increasing excretion of sodium, water, chloride, magnesium, potassium, and bicarbonate

➡**Therapeutic Outcome:** Decreased B/P, decreased edema in lung tissue and peripherally

Uses: Edema in CHF, nephrotic syndrome; may be used alone or as adjunct with antihypertensives for mild to moderate hypertension

Dosage and routes
Edema
Adult: PO 5-20 mg/day
Hypertension
Adult: PO 2.5-5 mg/day (Zaroxolyn)
P *Child:* PO 0.2-0.4 mg/kg/day divided q12-24h
Adult: PO 0.5 mg (MyKrox) qd in AM: may increase to 1 mg

Available forms: MyKrox tab 0.5; Zaroxolyn 2.5, 5, 10 mg

Adverse effects

CNS: Drowsiness, paresthesia, anxiety, depression, headache, *dizziness, fatigue, weakness*

CV: Irregular pulse, orthostatic hypotension, palpitations, volume depletion, chest pain

EENT: Blurred vision

ELECT: Hypokalemia, hypercalcemia, hyponatremia, hypochloremia, hypomagnesemia, hypophosphatemia

GI: Nausea, vomiting, anorexia, constipation, diarrhea, cramps, **pancreatitis,** GI irritation, **hepatitis**

GU: Frequency, polyuria, **uremia,** glucosuria

HEMA: **Aplastic anemia, hemolytic anemia, leukopenia, agranulocytosis, neutropenia**

INTEG: Rash, urticaria, purpura, photosensitivity, fever

META: Hyperglycemia, hypomagnesemia, increased creatinine, BUN

Contraindications: Hypersensitivity to thiazides or sulfonamides, anuria, renal decompensation

Precautions: Hypokalemia, renal disease, hepatic disease, gout, COPD, lupus erythematosus, diabetes mellitus, elderly, pregnancy **B,** lactation

Do Not Confuse:

metolazone/methotrexate, metolazone/metoclopramide

Pharmacokinetics

Absorption	GI tract (10%-20%)
Distribution	Crosses placenta
Metabolism	Urine, unchanged
Excretion	Breast milk
Half-life	8 hr (extended); 14 hr (prompt)

Pharmacodynamics

Onset	1 hr
Peak	2 hr
Duration	12-24 hr

Interactions

Individual drugs

Amphotericin B: ↑ hypokalemia

Cholestyramine: ↓ absorption of metolazone

Colestipol: ↓ absorption of metolazone

Diazoxide: ↓ hyperglycemia, hyperuricemia, hypotension

Digoxin: ↑ toxicity

Indomethacin: ↓ hypotensive response

Lithium: ↑ toxicity

Mezlocillin: ↑ hypokalemia

Piperacillin: ↑ hypokalemia

Ticarcillin: ↑ hypokalemia

Drug classifications

Antidiabetics: ↓ effect of antidiabetic agent

Antihypertensives: ↑ antihypertensive effect

Cardiac glycosides: ↑ hypokalemia

Glucocorticoids: ↑ hypokalemia

Nitrates: ↑ hypotension

Nondepolarizing skeletal muscle relaxants: ↑ toxicity

Sulfonylureas: ↓ effect of sulfonylurea

Food/drug

↑ absorption

Lab test interferences

Interference: Urine steroid tests

↑ BSP retention, ↑ calcium, ↑ amylase, ↑ parathyroid test ↓ PBI, ↓ PSP

NURSING CONSIDERATIONS

Assessment

• Monitor blood glucose if patient is diabetic

• Check for rashes, temp elevation qd

M

- Monitor patients that receive cardiac glycosides for increased hypokalemia
- Monitor manifestations of hypokalemia; acidic urine, reduced urine, osmolality, nocturia; hypotension, broad T wave, U wave, ectopy, tachycardia, weak pulse; muscle weakness, altered LOC, drowsiness, apathy, lethargy, confusion, depression; anorexia, nausea, cramps, constipation, distention, paralytic ileus; hypoventilation, respiratory muscle weakness
- Monitor for manifestations of hypomagnesemia: agitation, muscle twitching, paresthesias, hyperactive reflexes, positive Babinski reflex, dysphagia, nystagmus seizures, tetany; nausea, vomiting, diarrhea, anorexia, abdominal distention; ectopy, tachycardia, broad, flat, or inverted T waves, depressed ST segment, prolonged QT, decreased cardiac output, hypotension
- Monitor for manifestations of hyponatremia; increased B/P, cold, clammy skin, hypovolemia or hypervolemia; anorexia, nausea, vomiting, diarrhea, abdominal cramps; lethargy, increased ICP, confusion, headache, seizures, coma, fatigue, tremors, hyperreflexia
- Monitor for manifestations of hyperchloremia: weakness, lethargy, coma, deep rapid breathing
- Assess and record fluid volume status: I&O ratios; monitor weight, distended red veins, crackles in lung, color, quality and sp gr of urine, skin turgor, adequacy of pulses, moist mucous membranes, bilateral lung sounds, peripheral pitting edema; dehydration symptoms of decreasing output, thirst, hypotension, dry mouth and mucous membranes should be reported
- Monitor electrolytes: potassium, sodium, calcium, magnesium; also include BUN, blood pH, ABGs, uric acid, CBC, blood sugar
- Assess B/P before and during therapy with patient lying, standing, and sitting as appropriate; orthostatic hypotension can occur rapidly

Nursing diagnoses
✓ Altered urinary elimination (adverse reactions)
✓ Fluid volume deficit (adverse reactions)
✓ Fluid volume excess (uses)
✓ Knowledge deficit (teaching)

Implementation
- Give in AM to avoid interference with sleep
- Provide potassium replacement if potassium level is 3.0; drug may be crushed if patient is unable to swallow
- Give with food; if nausea occurs, absorption may be increased; extended release product is Zaroxolyn; prompt action product is MyKrox; the two formulations are not equivalent

Patient/family education
- Teach patient to take the medication early in the day to prevent nocturia
- Instruct patient to take with food or milk if GI symptoms of nausea and anorexia occur
- Teach patient to maintain a weekly record of weight and notify prescriber of weight loss >5 lb
- Caution patient that this drug causes a loss of potassium, so food rich in potassium should be added to the diet;

refer to a dietician for assistance in planning

• Caution the patient not to exercise in hot weather or stand for prolonged periods, since orthostatic hypotension will be enhanced

• Teach patient not to use alcohol or any OTC medications without prescriber's approval; serious drug reactions may occur

• Emphasize the need to contact prescriber immediately if muscle cramps, weakness, nausea, dizziness, or numbness occurs

• Teach patient to take own B/P and pulse and record

• Advise patient to use sunscreen to prevent burns

• Caution the patient that orthostatic hypotension may occur and to rise slowly from sitting or reclining positions, lie down if dizziness occurs

• Teach patient to continue taking medication even if feeling better; this drug controls symptoms but does not cure the condition

• Advise patient with hypertension to continue other medical treatment (exercise, weight loss, relaxation techniques, cessation of smoking)

Evaluation
Positive therapeutic outcome
• Decreased edema
• Decreased B/P

Treatment of overdose:
Lavage if taken orally, monitor electrolytes; administer dextrose in saline; monitor hydration, CV, renal status

metoprolol (℞)
(met-oh-proe'lole)
Apo-Metoprolol ✥,
Betaloc ✥, Betaloc
Durules ✥, Lopressor,
Lopressor SR ✥,
Novometoprol ✥, Toprol XL
Func. class.: Antihypertensive, antianginal
Chem. class.: β_1-Adrenergic blocker
Pregnancy category **C**

Action: Competitively blocks stimulation of β_1-adrenergic receptor within vascular smooth muscle; produces chronotropic, inotropic activity (decreases rate of SA node discharge, increases recovery time), slows conduction of AV node, decreases heart rate, which decreases O_2 consumption in myocardium; also decreases renin-aldosterone-angiotensin system at high doses

➡**Therapeutic Outcome:** Decreased B/P, heart rate, AV conduction

Uses: Mild to moderate hypertension, acute MI to reduce cardiovascular mortality, angina pectoris

Investigational uses: Dysrhythmias, hypertrophic cardiomyopathy, mitral valve prolapse, pheochromocytoma, tremors, prevention of vascular headaches, aggression

Dosage and routes
Hypertension
Adult: PO 50 mg bid, or 100 mg qd; may give 200-450 mg in divided doses; ext rel tabs give qd

G *Elderly:* PO 25 mg/day initially, increase weekly as needed

M

MI
Adult: Early treatment, **IV** bol 5 mg q2 min × 3 doses, then 50 mg PO 15 min after last dose and q6h × 48 hr; late treatment, PO maintenance 100 mg bid for 3 mo

Available forms: Tabs 50, 100 mg; inj 1 mg/ml; ext rel tabs 50, 100, 200 mg

Adverse effects
CNS: Insomnia, *dizziness,* mental changes, hallucinations, **depression,** anxiety, headaches, nightmares, confusion, fatigue
CV: **CHF,** *palpitations,* dysrhythmias, **cardiac arrest, AV block,** hypotension, **bradycardia**
EENT: Sore throat, dry burning eyes
GI: Nausea, vomiting, colitis, cramps, *diarrhea,* constipation, flatulence, dry mouth, *hiccups*
GU: Impotence
HEMA: **Agranulocytosis, eosinophilia, thrombocytopenic purpura**
INTEG: Rash, purpura, alopecia, dry skin, urticaria, pruritus
RESP: **Bronchospasm,** dyspnea, wheezing

Contraindications: Hypersensitivity to β-blockers, cardiogenic shock, heart block (2nd-3rd-degree), sinus bradycardia, CHF, bronchial asthma

Precautions: Major surgery, pregnancy **C,** lactation, diabetes mellitus, renal disease, thyroid disease, COPD, heart failure, CAD, nonallergic bronchospasm, hepatic disease

◼ **Do Not Confuse:**
metoprolol/misoprostol

Pharmacokinetics

Absorption	Well absorbed (PO); completely absorbed (**IV**)
Distribution	Crosses blood-brain barrier, placenta
Metabolism	Liver, extensively
Excretion	Kidneys, breast milk
Half-life	3-4 hr

Pharmacodynamics

	PO	IV
Onset	15 min	Immediate
Peak	2-4 hr	20 min
Duration	6-19 hr	5-8 hr

Interactions
Individual drugs
Alcohol: ↑ hypotension (large amounts)
Dobutamine: ↓ effect of dobutamine
Dopamine: ↓ dopamine
Epinephrine: α-Adrenergic stimulation
Hydralazine: ↑ hypotension, bradycardia
Indomethacin: ↓ antihypertensive effect
Insulin: ↑ hypoglycemia
Methyldopa: ↑ hypotension, bradycardia
Prazosin: ↑ hypotension, bradycardia
Reserpine: ↑ hypotension, bradycardia
Thyroid: ↓ effectiveness
Verapamil: ↑ myocardial depression
Drug classifications
Amphetamines: ↑ hypertension, bradycardia
Antidiabetics: ↑ hypoglycemia
Antihypertensive: ↑ hypotension
β₂-Agonists: ↓ bronchodilatation
Cardiac glycosides: ↑ bradycardia
MAOIs: Do not use together
Nitrates: ↑ hypotension

◩ Herb/drug ◎ Do Not Crush ◆ Alert ⌖ Key Drug 🄶 Geriatric 🄿 Pediatric

Sulfonylureas: ↓ hypoglycemic effect
Theophyllines: ↓ bronchodilatation

Lab test interferences
False: ↑ Urinary catecholamines

NURSING CONSIDERATIONS
Assessment
• Monitor B/P during beginning treatment, periodically thereafter; pulse q4h; note rate, rhythm, quality; check apical/radial pulse before administration; notify prescriber of any significant changes (pulse <50 bpm)
• Check for baselines in renal, liver function tests before therapy begins and periodically thereafter
• Assess for edema in feet, legs daily; monitor I&O, daily weight; check for jugular vein distention, rales bilaterally, dyspnea (CHF)
• Monitor skin turgor, dryness of mucous membranes for hydration status, especially
🅖 elderly

Nursing diagnoses
☑Cardiac output, decreased (uses)
☑Injury, risk for (adverse reactions)
☑Knowledge deficit (teaching)
☑Noncompliance (teaching)

Implementation
PO route
• Given ac, hs; tab may be crushed or swallowed whole; give with food to prevent GI upset; reduced dosage in renal dysfunction
• Do not crush or chew ext rel tab
• Store protected from light, moisture; place in cool environment

🅜**IV route**
• Give by direct **IV** 5 mg/2 min or more; keep patient recumbent for 3 hr

Y-site compatibilities:
Alteplase, meperidine, morphine

Patient/family education
• Teach patient not to discontinue drug abruptly; taper over 2 wk; may cause precipitate angina if stopped abruptly
• Teach patient not to use OTC products containing α-adrenergic stimulants (such as nasal decongestants, cold preparations); to avoid alcohol, smoking and to limit sodium intake as prescribed
• Teach patient how to take pulse and B/P at home; advise when to notify prescriber
• Instruct patient to comply with weight control, dietary adjustments, modified exercise program
• Tell patient to carry/wear Medic Alert ID to identify drug being taken, allergies; tell patient drug controls symptoms but does not cure
• Caution patient to avoid hazardous activities if dizziness, drowsiness is present, to avoid driving until drug response is known
• Teach patient to report symptoms of CHF; difficult breathing, especially on exertion or when lying down, night cough, swelling of extremities or bradycardia, dizziness, confusion, depression, fever
• Teach patient to take drug as prescribed, not to double doses or skip doses; take any missed doses as soon as remembered if at least 4 hr until next dose

Evaluation

Positive therapeutic outcome
• Decreased B/P in hypertension (after 1-2 wk)
• Absence of dysrhythmias

Treatment of overdose:
Lavage, **IV** atropine for bradycardia, **IV** theophylline for bronchospasm, digitalis, O_2, diuretic for cardiac failure, hemodialysis, **IV** glucose for hyperglycemia, **IV** diazepam (or phenytoin) for seizures

---

metronidazole (℞)
(me-troe-ni'da-zole)
Apo-Metronidazole ✦,
Flagyl, Flagyl IV, Flagyl IV
RTU, Metro IV,
Metronidazole,
Metronidazole Redi-
Infusion, Metryl, Neo-
Metric ✦, Novonidazole ✦,
PMS-Metronidazole ✦,
Protostat, Satric,
Trikacide ✦
Func. class.: Trichomonacide, amebicide, antiinfective
Chem. class.: Nitroimidazole derivative
Pregnancy category   C

Action: Direct-acting amebicide/trichomonacide; binds, degrades DNA in organism

Therapeutic Outcome:
Trichomonacidal, amebicidal, bactericidal for the following susceptible organisms: *Bacteroides, Clostridium, Trichomonas vaginalis, Giardia lamblia, Entamoeba histolytica*

Uses: Intestinal amebiasis, amebic abscess, trichomoniasis, refractory trichomoniasis, bacterial anaerobic infections, giardiasis; septicemia, endocarditis, bone, joint, and lower respiratory tract infections

Dosage and routes
Trichomoniasis
Adult: PO 250 mg tid × 7 days or 2 g in single dose; do not repeat treatment for 4-6 wk

P *Child:* PO 15 mg/kg/day in divided doses × 7-10 days

Refractory trichomoniasis
Adult: PO 250 mg bid × 10 days

Amebic abscess
Adult: PO 500-750 mg tid × 5-10 days

P *Child:* PO 35-50 mg/kg/day in 3 divided doses × 10 days

Intestinal amebiasis
Adult: PO 750 mg tid × 5-10 days

P *Child:* PO 35-50 mg/kg/day in 3 divided doses × 10 days; then oral iodoquinol

Anaerobic bacterial infections
Adult: **IV** inf 15 mg/kg/over 1 hr, then 7.5 mg/kg **IV** or PO q6h, not to exceed 4 g/day; first maintenance dose should be administered 6 hr following loading dose

Giardiasis
Adult: PO 250 mg tid × 5 days

P *Child:* PO 5 mg/kg tid × 5 days

Antibiotic-associated pseudomembranous colitis
Adult: PO 250-500 mg 3-4 ×/day × 10-14 days

P *Child:* PO 20 mg/kg/day (max 2 g) divided q6h

Available forms: Tabs 250, 500 mg; film-coated tabs 250, 1500 mg; inj 5 mg/vial; HCl inj 500 mg

Adverse effects

CNS: Headache, dizziness, confusion, irritability, restlessness, ataxia, depression, fatigue, drowsiness, insomnia, paresthesia, peripheral neuropathy, **convulsions,** incoordination, depression

CV: Flat T waves

EENT: Blurred vision, sore throat, retinal edema, dry mouth, metallic taste, furry tongue, glossitis, stomatitis

GI: Nausea, vomiting, diarrhea, epigastric distress, *anorexia,* constipation, *abdominal cramps,* metallic taste, **pseudomembranous colitis**

GU: Darkened urine, vaginal dryness, polyuria, **albuminuria,** dysuria, cystitis, decreased libido, **nephrotoxicity,** incontinence, dyspareunia

HEMA: **Leukopenia, bone marrow depression, aplasia**

INTEG: Rash, pruritus, urticaria, flushing

SYST: Superinfection

Contraindications: Hypersensitivity to this drug, renal disease, hepatic disease, contracted visual or color fields, blood dyscrasias, lactation, CNS disorders

Precautions: Candidal infections, pregnancy **C** (2nd, 3rd trimesters)

Pharmacokinetics

Absorption	80% (PO)
Distribution	Widely distributed, crosses placenta
Metabolism	Liver
Excretion	Urine, unchanged; feces
Half-life	6-11 hr

Pharmacodynamics

	PO	IV
Onset	Rapid	Immediate
Peak	1-2 hr	Infusion's end

Interactions
Individual drugs
Alcohol: ↑ disulfiram-like reaction
Azathioprine: ↑ leukopenia
Cimetidine: ↓ action of metronidazole
Disulfiram: ↑ risk of psychosis
Fluorouracil: ↑ leukopenia
Phenobarbital: ↓ effect of metronidazole
Phenytoin: ↓ action of metronidazole
Drug classifications
Anticoagulants, oral: ↑ risk of bleeding
Lab test interferences
↓ AST, ↓ ALT

NURSING CONSIDERATIONS
Assessment
• Assess patient for signs and symptoms of infection including characteristics of wounds, WBC >10,000, vaginal secretions, fever; obtain baseline information and during treatment
• Obtain C&S before beginning drug therapy to identify if correct treatment has been initiated
• Assess for allergic reactions: rash, urticaria, pruritus
• Identify urine output; if decreasing, notify prescriber (may indicate nephrotoxicity);

M

also check for increased BUN, creatinine
• Assess bowel pattern qd; if severe diarrhea occurs, drug should be discontinued
• Assess for overgrowth of infection: perineal itching, fever, malaise, redness, pain, swelling, drainage, rash, diarrhea, change in cough, sputum

Nursing diagnoses

✓ Infection, risk for (uses)
✓ Diarrhea (adverse reactions)
✓ Injury, risk for (adverse reactions)
✓ Knowledge deficit (teaching)
✓ Noncompliance (teaching)

Implementation

IV IV route
• Give intermittent **IV** prediluted; for Flagyl **IV** dilute with 4.4 ml sterile water or 0.9% NaCl; must be diluted further with 8 mg/ml or more 0.9% NaCl, D_5W, or LR; must neutralize with 5 mEq $NaHCO_3$/500 mg; CO_2 gas will be generated and may require venting; run over 1 hr; primary **IV** must be discontinued; may be given as cont inf; do not use aluminum products; **IV** may require venting

Y-site compatibilities:
Acyclovir, allopurinol, amifostine, amiodarone, cefepime, cyclophosphamide, diltiazem, dopamine, enalaprilat, esmolol, fluconazole, foscarnet, granisetron, heparin, hydromorphone, labetalol, lorazepam, magnesium sulfate, melphalan, meperidine, methylprednisolone, midazolam, morphine, perphenazine, piperacillin/tazobactam, sargramostim, tacrolimus, teniposide, theophylline, thiotepa, vinorelbine

Additive compatibilities:
Amikacin, aminophylline, cefazolin, cefotaxime, cefotiam, ceftazidime, ceftizoxime, ceftriaxone, cefuroxime, chloramphenicol, ciprofloxacin, clindamycin, disopyramide, floxacillin, fluconazole, gentamicin, heparin, moxalactam, multielectrolyte concentrate, multivitamins, netilmicin, penicillin G potassium, tobramycin

Top route
• A thin coating should be applied to affected area after cleaning with soap and water and patting dry

PO route
• Give with or pc to avoid GI symptoms, metallic taste; crush tab if needed
• Store in light-resistant container; do not refrigerate

Patient/family education

• Teach patient to report sore throat, bruising, bleeding, joint pain; may indicate blood dyscrasias (rare)
• Advise patient to contact prescriber if vaginal itching, loose, foul-smelling stools, furry tongue occur; may indicate superinfection
• Advise patient to notify physician of numbness or tingling of extremities
• Teach trichomoniasis patient that both partners need to be treated; condoms should be used during intercourse to prevent reinfection
• Advise patient of disulfiram-like reaction to alcohol ingestion; alcohol should not be used when taking this anti-infective
• Inform patient drug has a metallic taste and urine may turn dark

---

- Advise patient to contact prescriber if pregnancy is suspected

Evaluation

Positive therapeutic outcome
- Decreased symptoms of infection

---

mexiletine (R)
(mex-il'e-teen)
Mexitil
Func. class.: Antidysrhythmic (Class IB)
Chem. class.: Lidocaine analog
Pregnancy category   C

Action: Increases electrical stimulation threshold of ventricle and His-Purkinje system, which stabilizes cardiac membrane and decreases automaticity

➤**Therapeutic Outcome:** Decreased ventricular dysrhythmia

Uses: Ventricular tachycardia, ventricular dysrhythmias during cardiac surgery, MI

Dosage and routes
Adult: PO 400 mg (loading dose), then 200 mg q8h, then 200-400 mg q8h

Available forms: Caps 150, 200, 250 mg

Adverse effects
CNS: Headache, dizziness, confusion, **convulsions,** tremors, psychosis, nervousness, paresthesias, weakness, fatigue, coordination difficulties, change in sleep habits
CV: Hypotension, bradycardia, angina, PVCs, **heart block, cardiovascular collapse, arrest,** sinus node slowing, **left ventricular failure,** syncope, **cardiogenic shock**
EENT: Blurred vision, hearing loss, tinnitus
GI: Nausea, vomiting, anorexia, diarrhea, abdominal pain, **hepatitis,** dry mouth, peptic ulcer, altered taste, GI bleeding
GU: Urinary hesitancy, decreased libido
HEMA: **Thrombocytopenia, leukopenia, agranulocytosis, hypoplastic anemia,** SLE syndrome
INTEG: Rash, alopecia, dry skin
MISC: Edema, arthralgia, fever
RESP: Dyspnea, **fibrosis, embolism,** pneumonia

Contraindications: Hypersensitivity to amides, cardiogenic shock, blood dyscrasias, severe heart block

Precautions: Pregnancy **C,** lactation, children, renal disease, liver disease, CHF, respiratory depression, myasthenia gravis

Pharmacokinetics	
Absorption	Well absorbed
Distribution	Body tissues
Metabolism	Liver, extensively
Excretion	Kidneys, unchanged (10%)
Half-life	12 hr

Pharmacodynamics	
Onset	½-2 hr
Peak	2-3 hr
Duration	8-12 hr

Interactions
Individual drugs
Cimetidine: ↑ toxicity
Digoxin: ↑ blood levels, toxicity
Disopyramide: ↑ levels, toxicity

M

Flecainide: ↑ levels, toxicity
Lidocaine: Bradycardia, cardiac arrest
Metoclopramide: ↑ effects of mexiletine
Phenobarbital: ↓ effectiveness
Phenytoin: ↑ effectiveness
Procainamide: ↑ levels, toxicity
Quinidine: ↑ levels, toxicity
Rifampin: ↓ effectiveness
Warfarin: ↑ level, bleeding
Drug classifications
Analgesics, opioid: ↓ absorption
Antacids: ↓ absorption
Theophyllines: ↑ theophylline levels
Smoking
↓ effectiveness
☑ *Herb/drug*
Aloe: ↑ hypokalemia, ↑ antidysrhythmic action
Buckthorn: ↑ hypokalemia, ↑ antidysrhythmic action
Cascara sagrada: ↑ hypokalemia, ↑ antidysrhythmic action
Rhubarb: ↑ hypokalemia, ↑ antidysrhythmic action
Senna: ↑ hypokalemia, ↑ antidysrhythmic action
Lab test interferences
↑ CPK

NURSING CONSIDERATIONS
Assessment
• Assess for oxygenation or perfusion deficit: decreased B/P, chest pain, dizziness, loss of consciousness
• Assess respiratory status: auscultate lung fields for bibasilar crackles in patients with advanced CHF
• Assess for urinary retention: check for pain, abdominal absorption, palpate bladder; check males with benign prostatic hypertrophy; anticholinergic reaction may cause retention

• Monitor I&O ratio; electrolytes potassium, sodium, chloride; watch for decreasing urinary output, possible retention
• Monitor liver function studies: AST, ALT, bilirubin, alkaline phosphatase
• Monitor ECG periodically to determine drug effectiveness; measure PR, QRS, QT intervals; check for PVCs, other dysrhythmias; assess B/P for hypotension, hypertension, for rebound hypertension after 1-2 hr; for prolonged PR/QT intervals, QRS complex, if QT or QRS increase by 50% or more, withhold next dose, notify prescriber
• Monitor for dehydration and hypovolemia
• Monitor blood levels (therapeutic level 0.5-2 μg/ml), notify prescriber of abnormal results
• Assess pulmonary toxicity: dyspnea, fatigue, cough, fever, chest pain; drug should be discontinued
• Assess cardiac rate, respiration: rate, rhythm, character, chest pain, ventricular tachycardia, supraventricular tachycardia, fibrillation

Nursing diagnoses
☑ Cardiac output, decreased (uses)
☑ Impaired gas exchange (adverse reactions)
☑ Knowledge deficit (teaching)

Implementation
• Give with meals for GI upset

Patient/family education
• Teach patient to report side effects immediately to prescriber; to take exactly as prescribed; if dose is missed, take when remembered if within 3-4 hr of next dose; do not double doses

---

• Caution patient to avoid temp extremes; impairment of heat-regulating mechanism can occur
• Encourage patient to complete follow-up appointment with health care provider, including pulmonary function studies, chest x-ray
• Instruct patient that dry mouth may be relieved by frequent sips of water, hard candy, sugarless gum
• Caution patient to make position changes from lying to standing slowly to prevent orthostatic hypotension

Evaluation
Positive therapeutic outcome
• Decreased B/P, dysrhythmias
• Decreased heart rate
• Normal sinus rhythm

Treatment of overdose:
O_2, artificial ventilation, ECG, administer dopamine for circulatory depression, administer diazepam or thiopental for convulsions, isoproterenol

---

mezlocillin (R̤)
(mez-loe-sill'in)
Mezlin
Func. class.: Antiinfective, broad-spectrum
Chem. class.: Extended-spectrum penicillin
Pregnancy category **B**

Action: Interferes with cell wall replication of susceptible organisms; osmotically unstable cell wall swells, bursts from osmotic pressure

Uses: Infection due to penicillinase-producing staphylococci, streptococci; respiratory tract, skin, skin structure, urinary tract, bone, joint infections; sinusitis, endocarditis, septicemia, meningitis; may be combined with an aminoglycoside for *Pseudomonas* infection

⇒**Therapeutic Outcome:** Bactericidal effects on the following: gram-positive cocci *Staphylococcus aureus, Streptococcus viridans, S. faecalis, S. pneumoniae,* gram-negative coccus *Neisseria gonorrhoeae,* gram-positive bacilli *Clostridium perfringens, C. tetani,* gram-negative bacilli *Bacteroides, Escherichia coli, Haemophilus influenzae, Klebsiella, Proteus mirabilis, Peptococcus, Peptostreptococcus, Morganella morganii, Enterobacter, Serratia, Pseudomonas, Proteus vulgaris, P. rettgeri, Shigella, Citrobacter, Veillonella*

Dosage and routes
Adult: IM/**IV** 3-4 g q4-6h or **IV** 500 mg q8h; may give up to 24 g/day for severe infections
🅟 *Child:* IM/**IV** 50 mg/kg q4-6h
🅟 *Infants >8 days:* >2000 g, 75 mg/kg q6h; <2000 g, 75 mg/kg q8h
🅟 *Infants <8 days:* 75 mg/kg q12h
Renal dose
Dose reduction indicated if CrCl <30 ml/min
Hepatic dose
Give 50% of dose
Available forms: Powder for inj 1, 2, 3, 4 g; **IV** inf 2, 3, 4 g
Adverse effects
CNS: Lethargy, hallucinations, anxiety, depression, twitching, **coma, convulsions**

M

GI: *Nausea, vomiting, diarrhea,* increased AST, ALT, abdominal pain, glossitis, colitis, abnormal taste
GU: Oliguria, proteinuria, hematuria vaginitis, moniliasis, **glomerulonephritis,** increased BUN, creatinine
HEMA: Anemia, increased bleeding time, **bone marrow depression, granulocytopenia**
META: Hyperkalemia, hypokalemia, alkalosis, hypernatremia

Contraindications: Hypersensitivity to penicillins

Precautions: Pregnancy **B,** hypersensitivity to cephalosporins, neonates, renal disease

Pharmacokinetics

Absorption	Well absorbed
Distribution	Widely distributed; crosses placenta
Metabolism	Liver, small amounts
Excretion	Kidneys, unchanged (40%-70%); breast milk, bile (15%-30%)
Half-life	50-55 min; increased in renal disease

Pharmacodynamics

	IM	IV
Onset	Rapid	Rapid
Peak	5 min	Inf end

Interactions
Individual drugs
Aspirin: ↑ mezlocillin levels, ↓ renal excretion
Chloramphenicol: ↑ half-life of chloramphenicol, ↓ effectiveness of mezlocillin
Cholestyramine: ↓ effectiveness of mezlocillin
Colestipol: ↓ effectiveness of mezlocillin
Digoxin: ↑ hypokalemia
Heparin: ↑ effect
Lithium: ↓ excretion, ↑ toxicity

Probenecid: ↑ mezlocillin levels, ↓ renal excretion
Vecuronium: ↑ effect
Drug classifications
Aminoglycosides: ↓ effectiveness of aminoglycosides if mixed together
Diuretics: ↑ hypokalemia
Erythromycins: ↓ antimicrobial effectiveness
Oral anticoagulants: ↑ anticoagulant effects
Oral contraceptives: ↓ contraceptive effectiveness
Tetracyclines: ↓ antimicrobial effectiveness
Food
Food, carbonated drinks, citrus fruit juices: ↓ absorption
Herb/drug
Khat: ↓ absorption
Lab test interferences
False positive: Urine glucose, urine protein

NURSING CONSIDERATIONS
Assessment
• Assess patient for previous sensitivity reaction to penicillins or other cephalosporins; cross-sensitivity between penicillins and cephalosporins is common
• Assess patient for signs and symptoms of infection including characteristics of wounds, sputum, urine, stool, WBC >10,000, fever; obtain baseline information and during treatment
• Obtain C&S before beginning drug therapy to identify if correct treatment has been initiated
• Assess for allergic reactions: rash, urticaria, pruritus, chills, fever, joint pain; angioedema may occur a few days after therapy begins; epinephrine, resuscitation equipment should

be available for anaphylactic reaction
• Identify urine output; if decreasing, notify prescriber (may indicate nephrotoxicity); also check for increased BUN, creatinine
• Monitor blood studies: AST, ALT, CBC, Hct, bilirubin, LDH, alkaline phosphatase, Coombs' test monthly if patient is on long-term therapy
• Monitor electrolytes: potassium, sodium, chloride monthly if patient is on long-term therapy
• Assess bowel pattern qd; if severe diarrhea occurs, drug should be discontinued; may indicate pseudomembranous colitis
• Monitor for bleeding: ecchymosis, bleeding gums, hematuria, stool guaiac daily if on long-term therapy
• Assess for overgrowth of infection: perineal itching, fever, malaise, redness, pain, swelling, drainage, rash, diarrhea, change in cough, sputum

Nursing diagnoses
☑ Infection, risk for (uses)
☑ Diarrhea (adverse reactions)
☑ Injury, risk for (adverse reactions)
☑ Knowledge deficit (teaching)
☑ Noncompliance (teaching)

Implementation
IV **IV route**
• Dilute 1g or less/10 ml of sterile water, for inj; D₅, 0.9% NaCl, for inj; shake, dilute further with D₅W or 0.45 NaCl, give over 3-5 min

Syringe compatibilities:
Heparin

Y-site compatibilities:
Amifostine, aztreonam, cyclophosphamide, famotidine, fludarabine, granisetron, hydromorphone, morphine, perphenazine, sargramostim, tacrolimus, teniposide, thiotepa

Patient/family education
• Teach patient to report sore throat, bruising, bleeding, joint pain; may indicate blood dyscrasias (rare)
• Advise patient to contact prescriber if vaginal itching, loose, foul-smelling stools, furry tongue occur; may indicate superinfection
• Advise patient to notify prescriber of diarrhea with blood or pus, which may indicate pseudomembranous colitis

Evaluation
Positive therapeutic outcome
• Absence of signs/symptoms of infection (WBC <10,000, temp WNL, absence of red, draining wounds)
• Reported improvement in symptoms of infection

Treatment of anaphylaxis:
Withdraw drug, maintain airway, administer epinephrine, aminophylline, O₂, **IV** corticosteroids

mibefradil (℞)
(mi-be-fray'dill)
Posicor
Func. class.: Calcium channel blocker; antihypertensive; antianginal
Chem. class.: Benzimidazoyle-substituted tetraline derivative

Pregnancy category   C

Action: Inhibits calcium ion influx across cell membrane during cardiac depolarization; produces relaxation of coronary vascular smooth muscle; peripheral vascular smooth muscle; dilates coronary vascular arteries; increases myocardial oxygen delivery in patients with vasospastic angina; only calcium channel blocker that blocks both T-type and L-type

→ **Therapeutic Outcome:** Decreased angina pectoris

Uses: Chronic stable angina pectoris

Dosage and routes
Adult: PO 50-100 mg qd

Available forms: Tabs 50, 100 mg

Adverse effects
CNS: Headache, dizziness
CV: Bradycardia, hypotension, palpitation, AV block, Wenckebach episodes
GI: Gastric upset, heartburn
HEMA: **Intravascular hemolysis**

Contraindications: Sick sinus syndrome, 2nd- or 3rd-degree heart block, hypotension less than 90 mm Hg systolic, cardiogenic shock, severe CHF

Precautions: CHF, hypotension, hepatic injury, pregnancy **P** C, lactation, children, renal disease, concomitant β-blocker **G** therapy, elderly

Pharmacokinetics	
Absorption	Unknown
Distribution	Unknown
Metabolism	Liver
Excretion	Kidneys
Half-life	27 hr

Pharmacodynamics	
Onset	Unknown
Peak	2 hr
Duration	24 hr

Interactions
Drug classifications
β-Adrenergic blockers: ↑ depressant effects on myocardial contractility

NURSING CONSIDERATIONS
Assessment
• Assess fluid volume status: I&O ratio and record; weight; distended red veins; crackles in lung; color; quality, and sp gr of urine; skin turgor; adequacy of pulses; moist mucous membranes; bilateral lung sounds; peripheral pitting edema—dehydration symptoms of decreasing output, thirst, hypotension, dry mouth, and mucous membranes should be reported
• Monitor if platelets are <150,000/mm³—if so, drug is usually discontinued and another drug started
• Assess for extravasation: change site q48h
• Monitor cardiac status: B/P, pulse, respiration, ECG

Nursing diagnoses
☑ Cardiac output, decreased (uses)
☑ Knowledge deficit (teaching)

Implementation
• Give once a day, with food for GI symptoms

Patient/family education
• Caution patient to avoid hazardous activities until stabilized on drug, dizziness is no longer a problem
• Instruct patient to limit caffeine consumption; to avoid alcohol and OTC drugs unless directed by prescriber
• Advise patient to comply with medical regimen: diet, exercise, stress reduction, drug therapy; to notify prescriber of irregular heart beat, shortness of breath, swelling of feet and

---

☑ Herb/drug   🚫 Do Not Crush   ◆ Alert   ☛ Key Drug   **G** Geriatric   **P** Pediatric

hands, pronounced dizziness, constipation, nausea, hypotension
• Teach patient to use as directed even if feeling better; may be taken with other cardiovascular drugs (nitrates, β-blockers)

Evaluation
Positive therapeutic outcome
• Decreased anginal pain

Treatment of overdose:
Defibrillation, atropine for AV block, vasopressor for hypotension

miconazole ♥π (OTC)
(mi-kon'a-zole)
Monistat, Monistat I.V.; topical: Micatin, Micatin Liquid, miconazole Nitrate, Monistat-Derm, Monistat 3, Monistat 7, Monistat Dual-Pak
Func. class.: Antifungal
Chem. class.: Imidazole

Pregnancy category   C

Action: Alters cell membranes, inhibits fungal enzymes, inhibits sterols so intracellular contents are lost, prevents biosynthesis of phospholipids/triglycerides

Therapeutic Outcome:
Fungistatic/fungicidal against: *Aspergillus, Coccidioides, Cryptococcus, Candida, Dermatophytes, Histoplasma*

Uses: Coccidioidomycosis, candidiasis, cryptococcosis, paracoccidioidomycosis, chronic mucocutaneous candidiasis, fungal meningitis; **IV** used for severe infections only; (top) tinea pedis, tinea cruris, tinea corporis, tinea versicolor, vaginal or vulva candidal infections

Dosage and routes
Adult: **IV** inf 200-3600 mg/day; may be divided in 3 inf at 200-1200 mg/inf; may have to repeat course; IT 20 mg given simultaneously with **IV** for fungal meningitis q1-2d

🄿 *Child:* **IV** 20-40 mg/kg/day, not to exceed 15 mg/kg/day

🄿 *Adult and child:* Top apply to affected area bid × 2-4 wk

Adult: Intravag give 1 applicator or suppository × 7 days hs

Available forms: Inj 10 mg/ml; aerosol 2%; cream 2%; lotion 2%; powder 2%; spray 2%; vag cream 2%; vag supp 100, 200 mg

Adverse effects
CNS: Drowsiness, headache, lethargy
CV: Tachycardia, **dysrhythmias** (rapid **IV**)
GI: Nausea, vomiting, anorexia, diarrhea, cramps
GU: Vulvovaginal burning, itching, hyponatremia, pelvic cramps (topical forms)
HEMA: **Decreased Hct, thrombocytopenia, hyperlipidemia**
INTEG: Pruritus, rash, fever, flushing, hives
SYST: **Anaphylaxis**

Contraindications: Hypersensitivity

Precautions: Renal disease, hepatic disease, pregnancy **C**

Pharmacokinetics	
Absorption	Poorly absorbed (PO)
Distribution	Widely distributed (**IV**); bound to serum proteins (90%)
Metabolism	Liver, extensively
Excretion	Unknown
Half-life	Triphasic: 0.4, 2.1, 24 hr

Pharmacodynamics			
	IV	TOP	VAG
Onset	Rapid	Unknown	Unknown
Peak	Infusion's end	Unknown	Unknown

Interactions
Individual drugs
Amphotericin B: ↓ effect of miconazole and amphotericin B
Coumadin: ↑ anticoagulant effect
Isoniazid: ↓ effect of miconazole
Phenytoin: ↑ effect
Rifampin: ↓ effect of miconazole
Warfarin: ↑ effect
Drug classifications
Sulfonylureas: ↑ effect
Lab test interferences
False positive: Urine glucose, urine protein

NURSING CONSIDERATIONS
Assessment
• Assess for signs and symptoms of infection: drainage, sore throat, urinary pain, hematuria, fever
• Obtain cultures for C&S before beginning treatment; therapy may be started after culture is taken; monitor signs of infection before and throughout treatment
• Monitor bowel pattern before and during treatment; diarrhea may occur
• Monitor cardiac system: B/P, pulse; watch for increasing pulse, cardiac dysrhythmias; drug should be discontinued
• Monitor blood studies: WBC, RBC, Hgb, Hct, bleeding time; patients taking anticoagulants may need a decreased dosage; monitor liver and renal studies periodically for patients on long-term therapy
• Monitor I&O ratio; watch for decreasing urinary output, change in sp gr; discontinue drug to prevent renal damage; patients with renal disease may require lowered dose
• Monitor **IV** for thrombophlebitis; site should be changed q48-72h
• Monitor for allergies before initiation of treatment and reaction to each medication; highlight allergies on chart; check for allergic reaction: burning, stinging, swelling, redness (top); observe for skin eruptions after administration of drug to 1 wk after discontinuing drug

Nursing diagnoses
☑ Skin integrity, impaired (uses)
☑ Infection, risk (uses)
☑ Injury, risk for (adverse reactions)
☑ Knowledge deficit (teaching)

Implementation
• Have adrenalin, suction, tracheostomy set, endotracheal intubation equipment available
IV **IV route**
• Give 200 mg initially to prevent severe hypersensitive reaction
• Give **IV** after diluting ≤1 g/10 ml sterile water, D_5W, or 0.45% NaCl over 3-5 min
• Give by intermittent **IV** after diluting in 200 ml or more, D_5W or 0.9% NaCl; give over 30-60 min
• Store at room temp; reconstituted sol is stable for 24 hr refrigerated

Y-site incompatibilities:
Fludarabine

☑ Herb/drug ⓢ Do Not Crush ◆ Alert ⊶ Key Drug ⓖ Geriatric ⓟ Pediatric

Y-site compatibilities:
Allopurinol, filgrastim, foscarnet, granisetron, melphalan, ondansetron, propofol, sargramostim, teniposide, thiotepa, vinorelbine

Top route
• Apply after cleansing area with soap and water before each application; use enough medication to cover lesions completely; dry well
• Store at room temp in dry place

Vag route
• Administer 1 applicatorful every night high into the vagina
• Store at room temp in dry place

Patient/family education
• Inform patient that culture may be taken after completed course of medication
• Advise patient to notify nurse of diarrhea, symptoms of candidal vaginitis

Top route
• Teach patient to use medical asepsis (hand washing) before, after each application; to apply with glove to prevent further infection; to avoid contact with eyes; not to use occlusive dressings
• Caution patient to avoid use of OTC creams, ointments, lotions unless directed by prescriber
• Instruct patient to notify prescriber if no improvement in condition in 4 wk or if symptoms return in 2 mo; pregnancy or a serious medical condition may be the cause
• Teach patient to use for full prescribed treatment time, or reinfection may occur

Vag route
• Instruct patient in asepsis (hand washing) before, after each application
• Teach patient to apply with applicator only; to avoid use of any other vag product unless directed by prescriber; sanitary napkin may prevent soiling of undergarments; to abstain from sexual intercourse until treatment is completed; reinfection and irritation may occur
• Instruct patient to notify prescriber if symptoms persist

Evaluation
Positive therapeutic outcome
• Decreasing oral candidiasis, fever, malaise, rash
• Negative C&S for infectious organism
• Decrease in size, number of lesions
• Decrease in itching or white discharge (vaginal)

Treatment of overdose:
Withdraw drug; maintain airway; administer epinephrine, aminophylline, O_2, **IV** corticosteroids for anaphylaxis

M

---

midazolam (℞)
(mid′ay-zoe-lam)
Versed
Func. class.: Sedative/hypnotic
Chem. class.: Benzodiazepine, short-acting

Pregnancy category   D
Controlled substance schedule   IV

Action: Depresses subcortical levels in CNS; may act on limbic system, reticular formation; may potentiate

GABA by binding to specific benzodiazepine receptors

➡ **Therapeutic Outcome:** Sedation for anesthesia induction and procedures

Uses: Preoperative sedation, general anesthesia induction, sedation for diagnostic endoscopic procedures, intubation

Investigational uses: Epileptic seizures, refractory status epilepticus

Dosage and routes
Preoperative sedation
Adult: IM 0.07-0.08 mg/kg 30-60 min before general anesthesia

P *Child:* IM 0.1-0.15 mg/kg, may give up to 0.5 mg/kg if needed

Induction of general anesthesia
P *Adult and child 12-16 yr:* Unpremedicated patients, **IV** 0.3-0.35 mg/kg over 30 sec, wait 2 min, follow with 25% of initial dose if needed; premedicated patients, 0.15-0.35 mg/kg over 20-30 sec, allow 2 min for effect

P *Child 6-12 yr:* **IV** 0.025-0.05 mg/kg, total dose up to 0.4 mg/kg if needed

P *Child 6 mo-5 yr:* **IV** 0.05-0.1 mg/kg, total dose up to 0.6 mg/kg may be needed

P *Child <6 mo:* Titrate with small increments

Available forms: Inj 1, 5 mg/ml; syrup 2 mg/ml

Adverse effects
CNS: Retrograde amnesia, euphoria, confusion, headache, anxiety, insomnia, slurred speech, paresthesia, tremors, weakness, chills
CV: Hypotension, PVCs, tachycardia, bigeminy, nodal rhythm
EENT: Blurred vision, nystagmus, diplopia, blocked ears, loss of balance
GI: Nausea, vomiting, increased salivation, hiccups
INTEG: Urticaria, pain, swelling at inj site, rash, pruritus
RESP: Coughing, **apnea, bronchospasm, laryngospasm,** dyspnea

Contraindications: Pregnancy **D,** hypersensitivity to benzodiazepines, shock, coma, alcohol intoxication, acute narrow-angle glaucoma

Precautions: COPD, CHF, chronic renal failure, chills, G debilitated, elderly, children, P lactation

🔲 **Do Not Confuse:** Versed/Vepesid, Versed/Vistaril

Pharmacokinetics

Absorption	Well absorbed
Distribution	Crosses placenta, blood-brain barrier
Metabolism	Liver
Excretion	Kidneys, breast milk
Half-life	1-12 hr

Pharmacodynamics

	IM	IV
Onset	15 min	3-5 min
Peak	½-1 hr	Unknown
Duration	2-6 hr	2-6 hr

Interactions
Individual drugs
Alcohol: ↑ CNS depression
Cimetidine: ↑ levels of midazolam
Fluvoxamine: ↑ respiratory depression
Indinavir: ↑ respiratory depression
Ritonavir: ↑ respiratory depression

Verapamil: ↑ respiratory depression

Drug classifications

Antifungals, azole: ↑ levels of midalozam

Antihistamines: ↑ CNS depression

Antihypertensives: ↑ hypotension

Nitrates: ↑ hypotension

Opiates: ↑ CNS depression

Sedative/hypnotics: ↑ CNS depression

Theophyllines: ↓ effect of midazolam

NURSING CONSIDERATIONS
Assessment
• Monitor B/P, pulse, respiration during **IV**; O_2 and emergency equipment should be nearby
• Monitor inj site for redness, pain, swelling
• Assess degree of amnesia in ⒼＬ elderly; may be increased
• Assess anterograde amnesia
• Assess vital signs for recovery period in obese patient, since half-life may be extended
• Assess for apnea, respiratory depression, which may be ⒼＬ increased in the elderly

Nursing diagnoses
☑ Knowledge deficit (teaching)

Implementation
Ⓘ**IV route**
• Give **IV** undiluted or after diluting with D_5W or 0.9% NaCl to a conc of 0.25 mg/ml; give over 2 min (conscious sedation) or over 30 sec (anesthesia induction)
• Ensure immediate availability of resuscitation equipment, O_2 to support airway; do not give by rapid bol

Syringe compatibilities:
Atracurium, atropine, benzquinamide, buprenorphine, butorphanol, chlorpromazine, cimetadine, diphenhydramine, droperidol, fentanyl, glycopyrrolate, hydromorphine, hydroxyzine, meperidine, metoclopramide, morphine, nalbuphine, promazine, promethazine, scopolamine, sufentanil, thiethylperazine, trimethobenzamide

Syringe incompatibilities:
Dimenhydrinate, pentobarbital, perphenazine, prochlorperazine, ranitidine

Y-site compatibilities:
Amikacin, amiodarone, atracurium, calcium gluconate, cefazolin, cefmetazole, cefotaxime, cimetidine, ciprofloxacin, clindamycin, digoxin, diltiazem, dopamine, epinephrine, erythromycin, esmolol, etomidate, famotidine, fentanyl, fluconazole, gentamicin, haloperidol, heparin, hydromorphone, insulin (regular), labetalol, lorazepam, methylprednisolone, metronidazole, milrinone, morphine, nicardipine, nitroglycerin, norepinephrine, pancuronium, piperacillin, potassium chloride, ranitidine, sodium nitroprusside, sufentanil, theophylline, tobramycin, vancomycin, vecuronium

Y-site incompatibilities:
Foscarnet
IM route
• Give IM deep in large muscle mass
• Store at room temp

Patient/family education
• Inform patient that amnesia occurs; events may not be remembered
• Caution patient to avoid CNS depressants including

Ⓜ

alcohol for 24 hr after taking this drug

Evaluation
Positive therapeutic outcome
• Induction of sedation, amnesia

Treatment of overdose: O_2, vasopressors, physostigmine, resuscitation; flumazenil will reverse effects

---

midodrine (℞)
(mye′doh-dreen)
ProAmatine
Func. class.: Prodrug
Pregnancy category **C**

Action: Activates α-adrenergic receptors of arteriolar venous vasculature

➡ **Therapeutic Outcome:** Decreased feeling of faintness upon rising, absence of significant change in B/P

Uses: Orthostatic hypotension

Dosage and routes
Adult: PO 10 mg

Renal dose
Adult: PO 2.5 mg tid

Available forms: Tabs 2.5, 5 mg

Adverse effects
CNS: Drowsiness, restlessness, headache, paresthesia, pain, chills
CV: Supine hypertension
EENT: Dry mouth, blurred vision
GI: Nausea, anorexia
GU: Urinary urgency
INTEG: Pruritus, piloerection, rash

Contraindications: Hypersensitivity, severe organic heart disease, acute renal disease, urinary retention, pheochromocytoma, thyrotoxicosis, persistent/excessive supine hypertension

P **Precautions:** Children, urinary retention, lactation, prostatic hypertrophy, pregnancy **C**

Pharmacokinetics	
Absorption	Unknown
Distribution	Unknown
Metabolism	Unknown
Excretion	Unknown
Half-life	3-4 hr

Pharmacodynamics	
Onset	Unknown
Peak	1-2 hr
Duration	Unknown

Interactions
Drug classifications
α-Agonists: ↑ pressor effects
β-Adrenergic blockers: ↑ bradycardia
Cardiac glycosides: ↑ bradycardia
Psychopharmacologics: ↑ bradycardia
Steroids: ↑ intraocular pressure

NURSING CONSIDERATIONS
Assessment
• Monitor VS, B/P (standing, supine)
• Observe for drowsiness, dizziness, LOC

Implementation
• Tablets may be swallowed whole, chewed, or allowed to dissolve
• Administer upon arising, at midday, and in late afternoon (no later than 6 PM)
• Avoid administering if patient is to be supine during day

Nursing diagnoses
✓ Knowledge deficit (teaching)

Patient/family education
• Advise to avoid hazardous activities; activities requiring alertness; dizziness may occur; instruct patient to request assistance with ambulation
• Advise to avoid alcohol, other depressants

Evaluation
Positive therapeutic outcome
• Decreased orthostatic hypotension

---

miglitol (℞)
(mig′le-tol)
Glyset
Func. class.: Oral hypoglycemic
Chem. class.: α-glucosidase inhibitor
Pregnancy categeory **B**

Action: Delays the digestion of ingested carbohydrates, results in a smaller rise in blood glucose after meals; does not increase insulin production

Therapeutic Outcome: Decreased blood glucose levels in diabetes mellitus

Uses: Stable adult-onset diabetes mellitus (type II) NIDDM

Dosage and routes
Initial dose
Adult: PO 25 mg tid with first bite of meal

Maintenance dose
Adult: PO may be increased to 50 mg tid; may increase to 100 mg tid if needed only in patients >60 kg; dosage adjustment at 4-8 wk intervals

Available forms: Tabs 25, 50, 100 mg

Adverse effects
GI: Abdominal pain, diarrhea, flatulence, **hepatotoxicity**

HEMA: Low iron
INTEG: Rash

Contraindications: Hypersensitivity, diabetic ketoacidosis, cirrhosis, inflammatory bowel disease, colonic ulceration, partial intestinal obstruction, chronic intestinal disease

Precautions: Pregnancy **B,** renal disease, lactation, children, hepatic disease

Pharmacokinetics	
Absorption	Unknown
Distribution	Unknown
Metabolism	Not metabolized
Excretion	Kidneys, unchanged drug
Half-life	2 hr

Pharmacodynamics
Unknown

Interactions
Individual drugs
Digoxin: ↓ levels of digoxin
Insulin: ↑ hypoglycemia
Propranolol: ↓ levels of propranolol
Ranitidine: ↓ levels of ranitidine
Drug classifications
Adsorbents, intestinal: ↓ miglitol levels; do not use together
Enzymes, digestive: ↓ miglitol levels; do not use together
Sulfonylureas: ↑ hypoglycemia
Herb/drug
Broom: ↓ hypoglycemia
Buchu: ↓ hypoglycemia
Chromium: ↑ or ↓ hypoglycemic effect
Dandelion: ↓ hypoglycemia
Fenugreek: ↑ or ↓ hypoglycemic effect
Ginseng: ↑ or ↓ hypoglycemic effect
Juniper: ↓ hypoglycemia

M

Karela: improved glucose tolerance

NURSING CONSIDERATIONS
Assessment
• Assess for hypoglycemia, hyperglycemia; even though this drug does not cause hypoglycemia, if on a sulfonylurea or insulin, hypoglycemia may be additive
• Monitor blood glucose levels, glycosylated hemoglobin, LFTs

Nursing diagnoses
✓ Nutrition altered, more than body requirements (uses)
✓ Nutrition altered, less than body requirements (adverse reactions)
✓ Knowledge deficit (teaching)
✓ Noncompliance (teaching)

Implementation
• Give tid with first bite of each meal
• Provide storage in tight container in cool environment

Patient/family education
• Teach patient the symptoms of hypoglycemia, hyperglycemia and what to do about each
• Instruct that medication must be taken as prescribed; explain consequences of discontinuing the medication abruptly; that during periods of stress, infection, surgery, insulin may be required
• Tell patient to avoid OTC medications unless approved by prescriber
• Teach patient that diabetes is a life-long illness; drug will not cure condition
• Instruct patient to carry/wear Medic Alert ID as diabetic
• Teach patient that diet and exercise regimen must be followed

Evaluation
Positive therapeutic outcome
• Decreased signs, symptoms of diabetes mellitus (polyuria, polydipsia, polyphagia, clear sensorium, absence of dizziness, stable gait)

milrinone (R)
(mill-re′none)
Primacor
Func. class.: Inotropic/vasodilator agent with phosphodiesterase activity
Chem. class.: Bipyridine derivative

Pregnancy category   C

Action: Positive inotropic agent with vasodilator properties; reduces preload and afterload by direct relaxation of vascular smooth muscle; increases myocardial contractility

Therapeutic Outcome: Increased inotropic effect resulting in increased cardiac output

Uses: Short-term management of CHF that has not responded to other medication; can be used with digitalis products

Dosage and routes
Adult: **IV** bol 50 µg/kg given over 10 min; start inf of 0.375-0.75 µg/kg/min; reduce dosage in renal impairment

Available forms: Inj 1 mg/ml

Adverse effects
CV: Dysrhythmias, hypotension, chest pain
GI: Nausea, vomiting, anorexia, abdominal pain, **hepatotoxicity,** jaundice
HEMA: **Thrombocytopenia**
MISC: Headache, hypokalemia, tremor

Contraindications: Hypersensitivity to this drug, severe aortic disease, severe pulmonic valvular disease, acute MI

Precautions: Lactation, pregnancy **C**, children, renal disease, hepatic disease, atrial flutter/fibrillation, elderly

Pharmacokinetics

Absorption	Completely absorbed
Distribution	Unknown
Metabolism	Liver (50%)
Excretion	Kidney, unchanged and metabolites (60%-90%)
Half-life	3½-6 hr; increased in CHF

Pharmacodynamics

Onset	2-5 min
Peak	10 min
Duration	Variable

Interactions: None

NURSING CONSIDERATIONS
Assessment
• Monitor manifestations of hypokalemia: acidic urine, reduced urine, osmolality, nocturia; hypotension, broad T wave, U wave, ectopy, tachycardia, weak pulse; muscle weakness, altered LOC, drowsiness, apathy, lethargy, confusion, depression; anorexia, nausea, cramps, constipation, distention, paralytic ileus; hypoventilation, respiratory muscle weakness
• Assess fluid volume status: complete I&O ratio and record; note weight, distended red veins, crackles in lung, color, quality and sp gr of urine, skin turgor, adequacy of pulses, moist mucous membranes, bilateral lung sounds, peripheral pitting edema; dehydration symptoms of decreasing output, thirst, hypotension, dry mouth and mucous membranes should be reported
• Monitor electrolytes: potassium, sodium, calcium, magnesium; also include BUN, blood pH, ABGs
• Monitor B/P and pulse, PCWP, CVP, index, often during inf; if B/P drops 30 mm Hg, stop inf and call prescriber
• Monitor ALT, AST, bilirubin daily; if these are elevated, hepatoxicity is suspected
• Monitor platelets; if <150,000/mm³, drug is usually discontinued and another drug started
• Assess for extravasation: change site q48h

Nursing diagnoses
☑Cardiac output, decreased (uses)
☑Fluid volume excess (uses)
☑Knowledge deficit (teaching)

Implementation
• Do not mix directly with glucose sol; chemical reaction occurs over 24 hr; precipitate forms if milrinone and furosemide come in contact
• Administer by direct **IV** into inf through Y-connector or directly into tubing; may give undiluted over 2-3 min
• Give by cont inf diluted with 0.9% NaCl to conc of 1-3 mg/ml, run at prescribed rate; give by inf pump for doses other than bol
• Administer potassium supplements if ordered for potassium levels <3.0

Syringe compatibilities:
Atropine, calcium chloride, digoxin, epinephrine, lidocaine, morphine, propranolol, sodium bicarbonate, verapamil

M

Y-site compatibilities:
Digoxin, diltiazem, dobutamine, dopamine, epinephrine, fentanyl, heparin, hydromorphone, labetalol, lorazepam, midazolam, morphine, nicardipine, nitroglycerin, norepinephrine, propranolol, quinidine, ranitidine, thiopental, vecuronium

Additive compatibilities:
Quinidine

Patient/family education
• Teach patient reason for medication and expected results
• Instruct patient to make position changes slowly; orthostatic hypotension may occur
• Teach patient signs and symptoms of hypersensitivity reactions and hypokalemia

Evaluation
Positive therapeutic outcome
• Increased cardiac output
• Decreased PCWP, adequate CVP
• Decreased dyspnea, fatigue, edema, ECG

Treatment of overdose:
Discontinue drug, support circulation

minocycline (℞)
(min-oh-sye'kleen)
Minocin, Minocin IV
Func. class.: Antiinfective
Chem. class.: Tetracycline
Pregnancy category   D

Action: Inhibits protein synthesis and phosphorylation in microorganisms by binding to 30S ribosomal subunits and reversibly binding to 50S ribosomal subunits; bacteriostatic

Therapeutic Outcome: Bactericidal action against susceptible organisms, including *Neisseria meningitidis, N. gonorrhoeae, Treponema pallidum, Chlamydia trachomatis, Ureaplasma urealyticum, Mycoplasma pneumoniae, Nocardia, Rickettsia*

Uses: Syphilis, chlamydial infection, gonorrhea, lymphogranuloma venereum, rickettsial infections, inflammatory acne, meningitis carriers

Dosage and routes
Adult: PO/**IV** 200 mg, then 100 mg q12h or 50 mg q6h, not to exceed 400 mg/24h **IV**
P *Child >8 yr:* PO/**IV** 4 mg/kg then 4 mg/kg/day PO in divided doses q12h

Gonorrhea
Adult: PO 200 mg, then 100 mg q12h × 4 days

Chlamydia trachomatis infection
Adult: PO 100 mg bid × 7 days

Syphilis
Adult: PO 200 mg, then 100 mg q12h × 10-15 days

Available forms: Tabs 50, 100 mg; caps 50, 100 mg; oral susp 50 mg/5 ml; powder for inj 100 mg/vial

Adverse effects
CNS: Dizziness, fever, lightheadedness, vertigo
CV: Pericarditis
EENT: Dysphagia, glossitis, decreased calcification, permanent discoloration of deciduous teeth, oral candidiasis
GI: Nausea, abdominal pain, *vomiting, diarrhea,* anorexia, enterocolitis, **hepatotoxicity,** flatulence, abdominal cramps, epigastric burning, stomatitis

GU: Increased BUN, polyuria, polydipsia, **renal failure, nephrotoxicity**
HEMA: Eosinophilia, neutropenia, thrombocytopenia, hemolytic anemia
INTEG: Rash, urticaria, photosensitivity, increased pigmentation, **exfoliative dermatitis,** pruritus, angioedema, bluegray color of skin and mucous membranes

Contraindications: Hypersensitivity to tetracyclines,
P children <8 yr, pregnancy **D**

Precautions: Hepatic disease, lactation

Pharmacokinetics

Absorption	Well absorbed (PO)
Distribution	Widely distributed (70%-75% protein bound); some distribution in CSF, crosses placenta
Metabolism	Liver, some
Excretion	Kidneys, unchanged (20%), bile, feces
Half-life	11-17 hr

Pharmacodynamics

	PO	IV
Onset	Rapid	Rapid
Peak	2-3 hr	Infusion's end

Interactions
Individual drugs
Calcium: Forms chelates, ↓ absorption
Carbamazepine: ↓ effect
Iron: Forms chelates, ↓ absorption
Magnesium: Forms chelates, ↓ absorption
Phenytoin: ↓ effect
Warfarin: ↑ effect
Drug classifications
Antidiarrheals, adsorbent: ↓ absorption
Barbiturates: ↓ effect

Contraceptives, oral: ↓ effect of oral contraception
Penicillins: ↓ effect
Lab test interferences
False negative: Urine glucose with Clinistix, Tes-Tape

NURSING CONSIDERATIONS
Assessment
• Assess patient for previous sensitivity reaction
• Assess patient for signs and symptoms of infection including characteristics of wounds, sputum, urine, stool, WBC >10,000, fever; obtain baseline information, before and during treatment
• Obtain C&S before beginning drug therapy to identify if correct treatment has been initiated
• Assess for allergic reactions: rash, urticaria, pruritus
• Monitor blood studies: AST, ALT, CBC, Hct, bilirubin, alkaline phosphatase, amylase monthly if patient is on long-term therapy
• Assess bowel pattern qd; if severe diarrhea occurs, drug should be discontinued
• Monitor for bleeding: ecchymosis, bleeding gums, hematuria, stool guaiac daily if on long-term therapy; blood dyscrasias may occur
• Assess for overgrowth of infection: perineal itching, fever, malaise, redness, pain, swelling, drainage, rash, diarrhea, change in cough, sputum; black, furry tongue

Nursing diagnoses
☑ Infection, risk for (uses)
☑ Diarrhea (adverse reactions)
☑ Knowledge deficit (teaching)
☑ Noncompliance (teaching)

M

Implementation
PO route
• Give around the clock to maintain proper blood levels; give with food to increase absorption of drug; do not give within 3 hr of other agents; drug interactions may occur
• Give with 8 oz of water 1 hr before hs to prevent ulceration
• Shake liquid preparation well before giving; use calibrated device for proper dosing
• Do not give with iron, calcium, magnesium products or antacids, which decrease absorption and form insoluble chelate

IV route
• Check for irritation, extravasation, phlebitis daily; change site q72hr
• For intermittent inf, dilute each 100 mg/10 ml 0.9% NaCl, sterile water for inj; further dilute in 500-1000 ml 0.9% NaCl, D_5W, Ringer's, LR, D_5/LR; give over 6 hr

Y-site compatibilities: Cyclophosphamide, fludarabine, granisetron, heparin, hydrocortisone, magnesium sulfate, melphalan, perphenazine, potassium chloride, sargramostim, sodium succinate, vinorelbine, vit B/C

Y-site incompatibilities: Aztreonam, filgrastim, hydromorphone, meperidine, morphine, teniposide

Patient/family education
• Teach patient to use sunscreen when outdoors to decrease photosensitivity reaction
• Teach patient to report sore throat, bruising, bleeding, joint pain; may indicate blood dyscrasias (rare)
• Advise patient to contact prescriber if vaginal itching, loose, foul-smelling stools, furry tongue occur; may indicate superinfection; report itching, rash, pruritus, urticaria
• Instruct patient to take all medication prescribed for the length of time ordered; drug must be taken around the clock to maintain blood levels; do not give medication to others; take with a full glass of water; may take with food
• Advise patient to use a form of contraception other than hormonal

Evaluation
Positive therapeutic outcome
• Absence of signs/symptoms of infection (WBC <10,000, temp WNL, absence of red, draining wounds)
• Reported improvement in symptoms of infection

---

minoxidil (℞, OTC)
(mi-nox'i-dill)
Loniten, Minodyl, minoxidil, Rogaine
Func. class.: Antihypertensive, hair growth stimulant
Chem. class.: Vasodilator, peripheral

Pregnancy category C

Action: Directly relaxes arteriolar smooth muscle, causing vasodilatation; increased cutaneous blood flow; stimulation of hair follicles

▶ **Therapeutic Outcome:** Decreased B/P in hypertension; hair growth

Uses: Severe hypertension unresponsive to other therapy (use with diuretic); topically to treat alopecia

---

Herb/drug Do Not Crush Alert Key Drug G Geriatric P Pediatric

Dosage and routes
Severe hypertension
Adult: PO 5 mg/day not to exceed 100 mg daily; usual range 10-40 mg/day in single doses

G *Elderly:* PO 2.5 mg qd, may be increased gradually

P *Child <12 yr:* Initial, 0.2 mg/kg/day; effective range, 0.25-1 mg/kg/day; max, 50 mg/day

Alopecia
Adult: Apply top, rub into scalp daily

Available forms: Tabs 2.5, 10 mg; top 20, 50 mg/ml

Adverse effects
CNS: Drowsiness, dizziness, sedation, headache, depression, fatigue
CV: Severe rebound hypertension, tachycardia, angina, increased T wave, **CHF, pulmonary edema, pericardial effusion,** edema, sodium retention, water retention
GI: Nausea, vomiting
GU: Gynecomastia, breast tenderness
HEMA: Hct, Hgb, erythrocyte count may decrease initially
INTEG: Pruritus, **Stevens-Johnson syndrome,** rash, hirsutism

Contraindications: Acute MI, dissecting aortic aneurysm, hypersensitivity, pheochromocytoma

Precautions: Pregnancy **C**
P (PO), lactation, children, renal disease, CAD, CHF

N Do Not Confuse:
Loniten/Lotensin, minoxidil/Monopril

Pharmacokinetics
Absorption	Well absorbed (PO); minimally absorbed (top)
Distribution	Widely distributed
Metabolism	Liver
Excretion	Kidneys, breast milk
Half-life	4.2 hr

Pharmacodynamics
	PO	TOP
Onset	½ hr	4 mo
Peak	2-3 hr	Unknown
Duration	75 hr	4 mo

Interactions
Individual drugs
Alcohol: ↑ hypotension
Drug classifications
Antihypertensives: ↑ hypotension
Glucocorticoids (top route): ↑ absorption
Nitrates: ↑ nitrates
NSAIDs: ↓ antihypertensive effect
Retinoids (top route): ↑ absorption

M

NURSING CONSIDERATIONS
Assessment
• Monitor B/P, pulse, jugular venous distention periodically throughout treatment
• Monitor electrolytes, blood studies: potassium, sodium, chloride, carbon dioxide, CBC, serum glucose
• Monitor weight daily, I&O; assess edema in feet, legs daily; check skin turgor, dryness of mucous membranes for hydration status
• Assess for rales, dyspnea, orthopnea, peripheral edema, fatigue, weight gain, jugular vein distention (CHF)
• Assess for signs of hyperglycemia: acetone breath, increased urinary output, severe thirst, lethargy, dizziness

Nursing diagnoses
- ☑ Cardiac output, decreased (adverse reactions)
- ☑ Injury, risk for (side effects)
- ☑ Knowledge deficit (teaching)

Implementation
PO route
- Give with meals to decrease GI symptoms
- Give with β-blockers and/or diuretic for hypertension
- Store protected from light and heat

Top route
- Administer 1 ml dose no matter how much balding has occurred; increasing dose does not speed hair growth
- Treatment must continue long term or new hair will be lost again

Patient/family education
Top route
- Teach patient that new hair will be soft and hardly visible
- Caution patient not to use on other parts of the body; drug is to be used on the scalp only
- Instruct patient that hair should be clean before applying medication; do not get on clothing
- Caution patient not to get medication near mucous membranes (mouth, nose, eyes) and to contact prescriber if burning, stinging, or rash occurs

Evaluation
Positive therapeutic outcome
- Decreased B/P in hypertension
- Hair growth (top)

---

mirtazapine (℞)
(mer-ta′za-peen)
Remeron
Func. class.: Antidepressant
Chem. class.: Tetracyclic
Pregnancy category   C

Action: Blocks reuptake of norepinephrine, serotonin into nerve endings, increasing action of norepinephrine, serotonin in nerve cells; has anticholinergic action

Therapeutic Outcome: Decreased symptoms of depression after 2-3 wk

Uses: Depression, dysthymic disorder, bipolar disorder: depression, agitated depression

Dosage and routes
Adult: PO 15 mg/day at hs, maintenance to continue for 6 mo

G *Elderly:* PO 7.5 mg qhs, increase by 7.5 mg q1-2 wk to desired dose, max 45 mg/day

Available forms: Tabs 15, 30 mg

Adverse effects
CNS: Dizziness, drowsiness, confusion, headache, anxiety, tremors, stimulation, weakness, insomnia, nightmares, EPS
G (elderly), increased psychiatric symptoms, *seizures*
CV: Orthostatic hypotension, ECG changes, tachycardia, hypertension, palpitations
EENT: Blurred vision, tinnitus, mydriasis
GI: Diarrhea, dry mouth, nausea, vomiting, **paralytic ileus,** increased appetite; cramps, epigastric distress, jaundice, *hepatitis,* stomatitis
GU: Retention, **acute renal failure**

☑ Herb/drug 🚫 Do Not Crush ◆ Alert ☛ Key Drug **G** Geriatric **P** Pediatric

HEMA: **Agranulocytosis, thrombocytopenia, eosinophilia, leukopenia**
INTEG: Rash, urticaria, sweating, pruritus, photosensitivity

Contraindications: Hypersensitivity to tricyclic antidepressants, recovery phase of MI, convulsive disorders, prostatic hypertrophy

Precautions: Suicidal patients, severe depression, increased intraocular pressure, narrow-angle glaucoma, urinary retention, cardiac disease, hepatic disease, hypothyroidism, hyperthyroidism, electroshock therapy, elective surgery, **G** elderly, pregnancy **C**

Pharmacokinetics

Absorption	Slow, complete
Distribution	Widely distributed; crosses placenta
Metabolism	Liver, extensively
Excretion	Feces; breast milk
Half-life	20-40 hr

Pharmacodynamics

Onset	Unknown
Peak	2 hr
Duration	Unknown

Interactions
Individual drugs
Alcohol: ↑ CNS depression
Cimetidine: ↑ levels, ↑ toxicity
Clonidine: Severe hypotension; avoid use
Disulfiram: Organic brain syndrome
Fluoxetine: ↑ levels, toxicity
Guanethidine: ↓ effects
Drug classifications
Analgesics: ↑ CNS depression
Anticholinergics: ↑ side effects
Antihistamines: ↑ CNS depression

Antihypertensives: May block antihypertensive effect
Barbiturates: ↑ effects
CNS depressants: ↑ effects
MAOIs: Hypertensive crisis, convulsions
Oral contraceptives: ↑ effects, toxicity
Phenothiazines: ↑ toxicity
Sedative/hypnotics: ↑ CNS depression
Smoking
↑ metabolism, ↓ effects

Herb/drug
Belladonna: ↑ anticholinergic effect
Henbane: ↑ anticholinergic effect
Scopolia: ↑ antidepressant effect
Lab test interferences
↑ Serum bilirubin, ↑ blood gluclose, ↑ alkaline phosphatase
↓ VMA, ↓ 5-HIAA
False: ↑ Urinary catecholamines

M

NURSING CONSIDERATIONS
Assessment
• Monitor B/P (with patient lying, standing), pulse q4h during beginning treatment; if systolic B/P drops 20 mm Hg, hold drug, notify prescriber; take VS q4h in patients with cardiovascular disease
• Monitor blood studies: CBC, leukocytes, differential, cardiac enzymes if patient is receiving long-term therapy
• Monitor hepatic studies: AST, ALT, bilirubin
• Check weight weekly, drug may increase appetite
• Assess ECG for flattening of T wave, bundle branch block, AV block, dysrhythmias in cardiac patients

- Assess for EPS primarily in **G** elderly: rigidity, dystonia, akathisia
- Assess mental status: mood, sensorium, affect, suicidal tendencies; assess increase in psychiatric symptoms: depression, panic
- Monitor urinary retention, constipation; constipation is **P** more likely to occur in children **G** and elderly
- Assess for withdrawal symptoms: headache, nausea, vomiting, muscle pain, weakness; do not usually occur unless drug was discontinued abruptly
- Identify alcohol consumption; if alcohol is consumed, hold dose until AM

Nursing diagnoses
☑ Coping, ineffective individual (uses)
☑ Injury, risk for (side effects)
☑ Knowledge deficit (teaching)
☑ Noncompliance (teaching)

Implementation
- Give with food or milk for GI symptoms; crush if patient is unable to swallow medication whole
- Give dose hs if oversedation occurs during day; may take **G** entire dose hs; elderly may not tolerate once/day dosing
- Store at room temp; do not freeze

Patient/family education
- Inform patient that therapeutic effects may take 2-3 wk
- Advise patient to use caution in driving and other activities requiring alertness because of drowsiness, dizziness, blurred vision; to avoid rising quickly from sitting to standing, espe- **G** cially elderly
- Caution patient to avoid alcohol ingestion, other CNS depressants

- Caution patient not to discontinue medication quickly after long-term use: may cause nausea, headache, malaise
- Teach patient to wear sunscreen or large hat, since photosensitivity occurs
- Teach patient to increase fluids, bulk in diet if constipation, urinary retention occur, **G** especially elderly
- Teach patient to take gum, hard sugarless candy, or frequent sips of water for dry mouth

Evaluation
Positive therapeutic outcome
- Decrease in depression
- Absence of suicidal thoughts

Treatment of overdose:
ECG monitoring, induce emesis, lavage, activated charcoal, administer anticonvulsant

---

misoprostol (℞)
(mye-soe-prost'ole)
Cytotec
Func. class.: Gastric mucosa protectant; antiulcer
Chem. class.: Prostaglandin E_1 analog
Pregnancy category   X

Action: Inhibits gastric acid secretion; may protect gastric mucosa; can increase bicarbonate, mucus production

➡ **Therapeutic Outcome:** Prevention of gastric ulcers

Uses: Prevention of NSAID-induced gastric ulcers

Dosage and routes
Adult: PO 200 µg qid with food for duration of NSAID therapy; if 200 µg is not tolerated, 100 µg may be given

---

Available forms: Tabs 100, 200 μg

Adverse effects
GI: Diarrhea, nausea, vomiting, flatulence, constipation, dyspepsia, abdominal pain
GU: Spotting, cramps, hypermenorrhea, menstrual disorders

Contraindications: Hypersensitivity, pregnancy **X**

P Precautions: Lactation, children, elderly, renal disease

Do Not Confuse:
Cytotec/Cytoxan, misoprostol/metoprolol

Pharmacokinetics	
Absorption	Well absorbed
Distribution	Unknown
Metabolism	Liver
Excretion	Kidneys
Half-life	½-1 hr

Pharmacodynamics	
Onset	½ hr
Peak	Unknown
Duration	3 hr

Interactions
Drug classifications
Antacids, magnesium: ↑ diarrhea

NURSING CONSIDERATIONS
Assessment
• Assess patient for GI symptoms: hematemesis, occult or frank blood in stools, also severe abdominal pain, cramping, severe diarrhea
• Obtain a negative pregnancy test in women of childbearing age before starting medication; miscarriages are common

Nursing diagnoses
☑ Pain (uses)
☑ Knowledge deficit (teaching)

Implementation
• Give with meals for prolonged drug effect; avoid use of magnesium antacids

Patient/family education
• Advise patient to avoid black pepper, caffeine, alcohol, harsh spices, extremes in temp of food, which may aggravate condition
• Caution patient to avoid OTC preparations: aspirin, cough, cold preparations; condition may worsen
• Teach patient that drug must be continued for prescribed time to be effective and taken exactly as prescribed; doses are not to be doubled
• Instruct patient to report to prescriber diarrhea, black tarry stools, abdominal pain, cramping, menstrual disorders
• Caution patient to prevent pregnancy while taking this drug; spontaneous abortion may occur

Evaluation
Positive therapeutic outcome
• Prevention of ulcers

mitomycin (℞)
(mye-toe-mye′sin)
mitomycin, Mutamycin
Func. class.: Antineoplastic, antibiotic
Pregnancy category D

Action: Inhibits DNA synthesis, primarily; derived from *Streptomyces caespitosus;* appears to cause cross-linking of DNA, a vesicant

Therapeutic Outcome: Prevention of rapidly growing malignant cells

M

Uses: Pancreas, stomach, head and neck, breast cancer

Investigational uses: Palliative treatment of head, neck, colon, breast, biliary, cervical, lung malignancies

Dosage and routes
Adult: **IV** 20 mg/m²/day × 5 days, stop drug for 2 days, then repeat cycle; or 10-20 mg/m² as a single dose; repeat cycle in 6-8 wk; stop drug if platelets are <75,000/mm³ or WBC is <3000/mm³

Available forms: Inj 5, 20, 40 mg/vial

Adverse effects
CNS: Fever, headache, confusion, drowsiness, syncope, fatigue
EENT: Blurred vision, drowsiness, syncope
GI: Nausea, vomiting, anorexia, stomatitis, **hepatotoxicity,** diarrhea
GU: Urinary retention, **renal failure,** edema
HEMA: **Thrombocytopenia, leukopenia, anemia**
INTEG: Rash, alopecia, *extravasation*
RESP: **Fibrosis, pulmonary infiltrate,** dyspnea

Contraindications: Hypersensitivity, pregnancy **D** (1st trimester), as a single agent, thrombocytopenia, coagulation disorders

Precautions: Renal disease, bone marrow depression

Pharmacokinetics

Absorption	Complete bioavailability
Distribution	Widely distributed; concentrates in tumor
Metabolism	Liver, extensively
Excretion	Kidneys, unchanged
Half-life	1 hr

Pharmacodynamics
Unknown

Interactions
Individual drugs
Radiation: ↑ toxicity, bone marrow suppression
Drug classifications
Antineoplastics: ↑ toxicity, bone marrow suppression

NURSING CONSIDERATIONS
Assessment
• Assess buccal cavity q8h for dryness, sores or ulceration, white patches, oral pain, bleeding, dysphagia; obtain prescription for viscous lidocaine (Xylocaine)
• Assess symptoms indicating severe allergic reaction: rash, pruritus, urticaria, purpuric skin lesions, itching, flushing
• Monitor CBC, differential, platelet count weekly; withhold drug if WBC count is <4000/mm³ or platelet count is <100,000/mm³, notify prescriber of results if WBC <20,000/mm³, platelets <150,000/mm³
• Monitor renal function studies: BUN, creatinine, serum uric acid, urine CrCl before and during therapy; check I&O ratio; report fall in urine output to <30 ml/hr
• Monitor temp q4h (may indicate beginning of infection)
• Monitor liver function tests before and during therapy (bilirubin, AST, ALT, LDH) as needed or monthly; check for jaundiced skin and sclera, dark urine, clay-colored stools, itchy skin, abdominal pain, fever, diarrhea
• Assess for bleeding: hematuria, stool guaiac, bruising or

☑ Herb/drug   ⊘ Do Not Crush   ◆ Alert   ☠ Key Drug   **G** Geriatric   **P** Pediatric

petechiae, mucosa or orifices q8h; inflammation of mucosa, breaks in skin
• Identify effects of alopecia on body image; discuss feelings about body changes
• Identify edema in feet, joint pain, stomach pain, shaking; check for inflammation of mucosa, breaks in skin

Nursing diagnoses
☑ Injury, risk for (adverse reactions)
☑ Body image disturbance (adverse reactions)
☑ Infection, risk for (adverse reactions)
☑ Knowledge deficit (teaching)

Implementation
• Avoid contact with skin, since medication is very irritating; wash completely to remove
• Give fluids **IV** or PO before chemotherapy to hydrate patient
• Provide antacid before oral agent; give drug after evening meal, before hs; administer antiemetic 30-60 min before giving drug and prn to prevent vomiting; use antibiotics for prophylaxis of infection
• Give top or syst analgesics for pain
• Give in AM so drug can be eliminated before hs
• Provide a liq diet: carbonated beverages; gelatin may be added if patient is not nauseated or vomiting
• Encourage patient to rinse mouth tid-qid with water, club soda, brush teeth bid-qid with soft brush or cotton-tipped applicators for stomatitis, use unwaxed dental floss
• Drug should be prepared by experienced personnel using proper precautions in a bio-

logic cabinet using gown, gloves, mask
• Give by direct **IV** after diluting 5 mg/10 sterile water for inj; shake, allow to stand, give through Y-tube or 3 way stopcock; give over 5-10 min through running D₅W, 0.9% NaCl **IV**

• Apply ice compress for extravasation

Syringe compatibilities:
Bleomycin, cisplatin, cyclophosphamide, doxorubicin, droperidol, fluorouracil, furosemide, heparin, leucovorin, methotrexate, metoclopramide, vinblastine, vincristine

Y-site compatibilities:
Allopurinol, amifostine, bleomycin, cisplatin, cyclophosphamide, doxorubicin, droperidol, fluorouracil, furosemide, granisetron, heparin, leucovorin, melphalan, methotrexate, metoclopramide, ondansetron, teniposide, thiotepa, vinblastine, vincristine

Y-site incompatibilities:
Sargramostim, vinorelbine

Additive compatibilities:
Dexamethasone, hydrocortisone

Additive incompatibilities:
Bleomycin

Solution compatibilities:
LR, 0.3% NaCl, 0.5% NaCl

Patient/family education
• Teach patient to avoid use of products containing aspirin or ibuprofen, razors, commercial mouthwash, since bleeding may occur; to report symptoms of bleeding (hematuria, tarry stools)
• Caution patient to report signs of anemia (fatigue, head-

M

ache, irritability, faintness, shortness of breath)
• Advise patient to report any changes in breathing or coughing even several mo after treatment; to avoid crowds and persons with respiratory tract or other infections
• Inform patient that hair may be lost during treatment; a wig or hair piece may make patient feel better; new hair may be different in color, texture
• Advise patient not to have any vaccinations without the advice of the prescriber, serious reactions can occur
• Teach patient that contraception is needed during treatment and for several mo after completion of therapy

Evaluation
Positive therapeutic outcome
• Prevention of rapid division of malignant cells

mitoxantrone (℞)
(mye-toe-zan′trone)
Novantrone
Func. class.: Antineoplastic-antibiotic
Chem. class.: Synthetic anthraquinone
Pregnancy category   D

Action: DNA reactive agent; cytocidal effect on both proliferating and nonproliferating cells, suggesting lack of cell cycle phase specificity; a vesicant

➡ **Therapeutic Outcome:** Prevention of rapidly growing malignant cells

Uses: Acute nonlymphocytic leukemia (adult), relapsed leukemia, breast cancer

Investigational uses: Breast and liver malignancies, non-Hodgkin's lymphoma

Dosage and routes
Induction
Adult: **IV** inf 12 mg/m^2/day on days 1-3, and 100 mg/m^2 cytosine arabinoside × 7 days as a cont 24-hr inf; if complete remission occurs, 2nd inductor may be used

Consolidation
Adult: **IV** inf 12 mg/m^2/ day × 2 days, given with cytosine arabinoside 100 mg/m^2/ day × 5 days as cont inf usually 6 wk after induction

Available forms: Inj 2 mg/ml

Adverse effects
CNS: Headache, seizures
CV: **CHF, cardiomyopathy, dysrhythmias,** ECG changes
EENT: Conjunctivitis, blue-green sclera
GI: Nausea, vomiting, diarrhea, anorexia, mucositis, **hepatoxicity**
HEMA: **Thrombocytopenia, leukopenia, myelosuppression, anemia**
INTEG: Rash, necrosis at inj site, alopecia, dermatitis, thrombophlebitis at inj site
MISC: Fever, hypersensitivity, hyperuricemia
RESP: Cough, dyspnea

Contraindications: Hypersensitivity, pregnancy **D**

Precautions: Myelosuppression, lactation, cardiac disease, children, renal, hepatic disease, gout

---

☒ Herb/drug 🚫 Do Not Crush ◆ Alert ☛ Key Drug 🄶 Geriatric 🄿 Pediatric

Pharmacokinetics

Absorption	Completely absorbed
Distribution	Widely distributed
Metabolism	Liver
Excretion	Bile; kidneys, unchanged (<10%)
Half-life	24-72 hr

Pharmacodynamics

Unknown

Interactions
Individual drugs
Radiation: ↑ toxicity, bone marrow suppression
Drug classifications
Antineoplastics: ↑ toxicity, bone marrow suppression
Live virus vaccines: ↑ adverse reactions

NURSING CONSIDERATIONS
Assessment
• Monitor ECG; watch for ST-T wave changes, low QRS and T, possible dysrhythmias (sinus tachycardia, heart block, PVCs)

• Assess buccal cavity q8h for dryness, sores or ulceration, white patches, oral pain, bleeding, dysphagia; obtain prescription for viscous lidocaine (Xylocaine)

• Assess symptoms indicating severe allergic reaction: rash, pruritus, urticaria, purpuric skin lesions, itching, flushing

• Assess tachypnea, ECG changes, dyspnea, edema, fatigue

• Monitor CBC, differential, platelet count weekly; withhold drug if WBC count is <4000/mm^3 or platelet count is <100,000/mm^3, notify prescriber of results if WBC <20,000/mm^3, platelets <150,000/mm^3

• Assess for increased uric acid levels, swelling, joint pain primarily in extremities; patient should be well hydrated to prevent urate deposits

• Monitor renal function studies: BUN, creatinine, urine CrCl before and during therapy; determine I&O ratio

• Monitor temp q4h (may indicate beginning of infection)

• Monitor liver function tests before and during therapy (bilirubin, AST, ALT, LDH) as needed or monthly; check for jaundiced skin and sclera, dark urine, clay-colored stools, itchy skin, abdominal pain, fever, diarrhea

• Assess for bleeding: hematuria, stool guaiac, bruising or petechiae, mucosa or orifices q8h; check for inflammation of mucosa, breaks in skin

• Identify effects of alopecia on body image; discuss feelings about body changes

Nursing diagnoses
☑ Injury, risk for (adverse reactions)
☑ Body image disturbance (adverse reactions)
☑ Infection, risk for (adverse reactions)
☑ Knowledge deficit (teaching)

Implementation
• Avoid contact with skin, since medication is very irritating; wash completely to remove

• Give fluids **IV** or PO before chemotherapy to hydrate patient

• Give antacid before oral agent; give drug after evening meal, before hs; provide antiemetic 30-60 min before giving drug and prn to prevent vomiting; administer antibiotics for prophylaxis of infection

M

- Give top or syst analgesics for pain
- Liq diet: carbonated beverages; gelatin may be added if patient is not nauseated or vomiting
- Encourage patient to rinse mouth tid-qid with water, club soda, brush teeth bid-qid with soft brush or cotton-tipped applicators for stomatitis, use unwaxed dental floss
- Sol should be prepared by qualified personnel only under controlled conditions in a biologic cabinet using mask, gloves, gown
- Use Luer-Lok tubing to prevent leakage; do not let sol come in contact with skin; if contact occurs wash well with soap and water
- Give by direct **IV** after diluting with 50 ml or more normal saline or D_5W; give over 3-5 min, running **IV** of D_5W or 0.9% NaCl
- Intermittent inf may be diluted further in D_5W, 0.9% NaCl and run over 15-30 min; check for extravasation

Y-site compatibilities:
Allopurinol, amifostine, cladribine, filgrastim, fludarabine, granisetron, melphalan, ondansetron, sargramostim, teniposide, thiotepa, vinorelbine

Y-site incompatibilities:
Paclitaxel

Additive compatibilities:
Cyclophosphamide, cytarabine, fluorouracil, hydrocortisone, potassium chloride

Additive incompatibilities:
Heparin

Solution compatibilities:
D_5/0.9 NaCl, D_5W, 0.9% NaCl

Patient/family education
- Teach patient to avoid use of products containing aspirin or NSAIDs, razors, commercial mouthwash, since bleeding may occur; to report symptoms of bleeding (hematuria, tarry stools)
- Caution patient to report signs of anemia (fatigue, headache, irritability, faintness, shortness of breath)
- Inform patient that hair may be lost during treatment; a wig or hair piece may make patient feel better; new hair may be different in color, texture
- Caution patient not to have any vaccinations without the advice of the prescriber; serious reactions can occur
- Advise patient that contraception is needed during treatment and for several mo after completion of therapy

Evaluation
Positive therapeutic outcome
- Prevention of rapid division of malignant cells

mivacurium (R)
(mi-va-kure'ee-um)
Mivacron
Func. class.: Nondepolarizing neuromuscular blocker

Pregnancy category   C

Action: Inhibits transmission of nerve impulses by binding with cholinergic receptor sites, antagonizing action of acetylcholine; no analgesic response

➔**Therapeutic Outcome:** Paralysis of all skeletal muscles

Uses: Facilitation of endotracheal intubation; skeletal mus-

⊘ Herb/drug ⬡ Do Not Crush ◆ Alert ⊶ Key Drug �G Geriatric P Pediatric cle relaxation during mechanical ventilation, surgery, or general anesthesia; reduction of fractures/dislocations

Dosage and routes
Adult: IV 0.15 mg/kg; maintenance q15 min

P *Child 2-12:* IV 0.2 mg/kg for a 10-min block

Available forms: 5, 10 ml single-use vial (2 mg/ml); premixed inf in D_5W 50 ml flex container

Adverse effects
CV: Decreased B/P, bradycardia, tachycardia
EENT: Diplopia
INTEG: Rash, urticaria
MS: Weakness, prolonged skeletal muscle relaxation, **paralysis**
RESP: **Prolonged apnea, bronchospasm, wheezing, respiratory depression**

Contraindications: Hypersensitivity

Precautions: Pregnancy **C**, renal or hepatic disease, lactation, children <3 mo, fluid and electrolyte imbalances, neuromuscular disease, respiratory disease, obesity, elderly

N **Do Not Confuse:**
Mivacron/Mazicon

Pharmacokinetics
Absorption	Completely absorbed
Distribution	Extracellular spaces; crosses placenta
Metabolism	Plasma
Excretion	Kidneys
Half-life	2 hr

Pharmacodynamics
Onset	2-2½ min
Peak	2-3 min
Duration	20-30 min

Interactions
Individual drugs
Clindamycin: ↑ paralysis length and intensity
Colistin: ↑ paralysis length and intensity
Lidocaine: ↑ paralysis length and intensity
Lithium: ↑ paralysis length and intensity
Magnesium: ↑ paralysis length and intensity
Polymyxin B: ↑ paralysis length and intensity
Procainamide: ↑ paralysis length and intensity
Quinidine: ↑ paralysis length and intensity
Succinylcholine: ↑ paralysis length and intensity
Drug classifications
Aminoglycosides: ↑ paralysis length and intensity
β-Adrenergic blockers: ↑ paralysis length and intensity
Diuretics, potassium-losing: ↑ paralysis length and intensity
General anesthesia: ↑ paralysis length and intensity

NURSING CONSIDERATIONS
Assessment
• Monitor VS (B/P, pulse, respirations, airway) until fully recovered; rate, depth, pattern of respirations, strength of hand grip; patient should be intubated before use
• Monitor for electrolyte imbalances (potassium, magnesium) before drug is used; electrolyte imbalances may lead to increased action of this drug
• Monitor for recovery: decreased paralysis of face, diaphragm, leg, arm, rest of body; residual weakness and respiratory problems may occur during recovery period

M

• Assess for hypersensitive reactions: rash, fever, respiratory distress, pruritus; drug should be discontinued

Nursing diagnoses
☑ Breathing pattern, ineffective (uses)
☑ Communication, impaired verbal (adverse reactions)
☑ Fear (adverse reactions)
☑ Knowledge deficit (teaching)

Implementation
• Use peripheral nerve stimulator (anesthesiologist) to determine neuromuscular blockade; deep tendon reflexes should be monitored during extended periods
• Give direct **IV** undiluted over 5-15 min
• Give cont **IV** diluted to 0.5 mg ml in D₅W, 0.9% NaCl, D₅/0.9% NaCl, LR, D₅/LR and give as an inf at prescribed rate (only by qualified person, usually an anesthesiologist); do not administer IM
• Store in light-resistant container
• Give anticholinesterase to reverse neuromuscular blockade

Y-site compatibilities:
Etomidate, thiopental

Y-site incompatibilities:
Barbiturates

Patient/family education
• Provide reassurance if communication is difficult during recovery from neuromuscular blockade
• Provide explanation to patients regarding all procedures or treatments; patient will remain conscious if anesthesia is not given also

Evaluation
Positive therapeutic outcome
• Paralysis of jaw, eyelid, head, neck, rest of body as evaluated by peripheral nerve stimulator

Treatment of overdose:
Edrophonium or neostigmine, atropine; monitor VS; may require mechanical ventilation

modafinil
See Appendix A, Selected New Drugs

moexipril (℞)
(moe-ex'i-pril)
Univasc
Func. class.: Antihypertensive
Chem. class.: Angiotensin-converting enzyme inhibitor

Pregnancy category C (1st trimester) D (2nd/3rd trimesters)

Action: Selectively suppresses renin-angiotensin-aldosterone system; inhibits ACE; prevents conversion of angiotensin I to angiotensin II; results in dilation of arterial, venous vessels

Therapeutic Outcome: Decreased B/P in hypertension

Uses: Hypertension, alone or in combination with thiazide diuretics

Dosage and routes
Initial treatment
Adult: PO 7.5 mg 1 hr ac, may be increased or divided depending on B/P response

Maintenance
Adult: PO 7.5-30 mg qd in
1-2 divided doses 1 hr ac

Renal dose
CrCl <40 ml/min 3.75 mg/
day titrate to desired dose

Available forms: Tabs 7.5,
15 mg

Adverse effects
CNS: Fever, chills
CV: Hypotension, postural
hypotension
GI: Loss of taste
GU: Impotence, dysuria, noc-
turia, proteinura, nephrotic
syndrome, acute reversible
renal failure, polyuria, oliguria,
frequency
HEMA: Neutropenia
INTEG: Rash
META: Hypokalemia
RESP: Bronchospasm, dys-
pnea, dry cough
SYST: Angioedema

Contraindications: Hypersensitivity, children, lactation,
heart block, bilateral renal
stenosis, K-sparing diuretics,
pregnancy **D** (2nd/3rd trimesters)

Precautions: Dialysis patients,
hypovolemia, leukemia, scleroderma, lupus erythematosus,
blood dyscrasias, CHF, diabetes mellitus, renal disease,
thyroid disease, COPD,
asthma, pregnancy **C** (1st
trimester)

Pharmacokinetics	
Absorption	Unknown
Distribution	Unknown
Metabolism	Liver to metabolites
Excretion	Via kidneys, crosses placenta, excreted in breast milk
Half-life	Unknown

Pharmacodynamics	
Unknown	

Interactions
Drug classification
Adrenergic blockers: ↑ hypo-
tension
Antihypertensives: ↑ hypoten-
sion
Diuretics: ↑ hypotension
Diuretics, potassium-sparing:
Do not use together
Ganglionic blockers: ↑ hypo-
tension
Potassium supplements: Do
not use together
Sympathomimetics: Do not
use together
Lab test interferences
False positive: Urine acetone

NURSING CONSIDERATIONS
Assessment
• Monitor blood studies:
neutrophils, decreased platelets
• Monitor B/P
• Monitor renal studies: protein, BUN, creatinine; watch
for increased levels that may
indicate nephrotic syndrome
• Monitor baselines in renal,
liver function tests before
therapy begins
• Monitor K levels, although
hyperkalemia rarely occurs
• Assess edema in feet, legs
daily
• Assess allergic reaction:
rash, fever, pruritus, urticaria;
drug should be discontinued
if antihistamines fail to help
• Assess for symptoms of
CHF: edema, dyspnea, wet
rales, B/P
• Monitor for renal symptoms:
polyuria, oliguria, frequency
Implementation
• Give PO 1 hr ac
• Store in tight container at
86° F or less

M

Nursing diagnoses
☑ Knowledge deficit (teaching)

Patient/family education
• Teach patient to take 1 hr ac
• Instruct patient not to discontinue drug abruptly
• Tell patient not to use OTC (cough, cold, allergy) products unless directed by prescriber
• Teach patient to comply with dosage schedule, even if feeling better
• Encourage patient to rise slowly to sitting or standing position to minimize orthostatic hypotension
• Teach patient to notify prescriber of mouth sores, sore throat, fever, swelling of hands or feet, irregular heartbeat, chest pain, signs of angioedema
• Tell patient that excessive perspiration, dehydration, vomiting, diarrhea may lead to fall in B/P; consult prescriber if this occurs
• Teach patient that dizziness, fainting, lightheadedness may occur during first few days of therapy
• Tell patient that skin rash or impaired perspiration may occur
• Teach patient how to take B/P

Evaluation
Positive therapeutic outcome
• Decreased B/P in hypertension

Treatment of overdose: 0.9% NaCl **IV** inf, hemodialysis

---

montelukast (℞)
(mon-teh-loo'kast)
Singulair
Func. class.: Leukotriene receptor
Chem. class.: Cysteinyl

Pregnancy category   B

Action: Inhibits leukotriene (LTD$_4$) formation; leukotrienes exert their effects by increasing neutrophil, eosinophil migration; aggregation of neutrophils, monocytes; smooth muscle contraction, capillary permeability; these actions further lead to bronchoconstriction, inflammation, edema

▶**Therapeutic Outcome:** Ability to breathe with ease

Uses: Chronic asthma

Dosage and routes
Asthma
P *Adult and child ≥15 yr:* PO 10 mg qd PM

P *Child 6-14 yr:* PO 5 mg chew tab qd PM

Available forms: Tabs 10 mg; tabs, chew 5 mg

Adverse effects
CNS: Dizziness, fatigue, headache
GI: Abdominal pain, dyspepsia
INTEG: Rash
MS: Asthenia
RESP: Influenza, cough, nasal congestion

Contraindications: Hypersensitivity

Precautions: Acute attacks of asthma, alcohol consumption, P pregnancy **B,** lactation, child <6 yr, aspirin sensitivity

---

☑ Herb/drug   ⑤ Do Not Crush   ◆ Alert   Key Drug   Ⓖ Geriatric   Ⓟ Pediatric

Pharmacokinetics

Absorption	Rapidly
Distribution	Protein binding 99%
Metabolism	Liver
Excretion	Bile
Half-life	2.7-5.5 hr

Pharmacodynamics

Onset	Unknown
Peak	3-4 hr
Duration	Unknown

Interactions
Individual drugs
Phenobarbitol: ↑ montelukast levels
Rifampin: ↑ montelukast levels

NURSING CONSIDERATIONS
Assessment
◀•• Assess adult patients carefully for symptoms of Churg-Strauss syndrome (rare), including eosinophilia, vasculitic rash, worsening pulmonary symptoms, cardiac complications, and/or neuropathy
• Monitor CBC, blood chemistry during treatment
• Assess respiratory rate, rhythm, depth; auscultate lung fields bilaterally; notify prescriber of abnormalities
• Assess allergic reactions: rash, urticaria; drug should be discontinued

Nursing diagnoses
☑ Airway clearance, ineffective (uses)
☑ Activity intolerance (uses)
☑ Knowledge deficit (teaching)

Implementation
PO route
• Give PO in PM qd

Patient/family education
• Instruct patient to check OTC and current prescription medications for ephedrine, which will increase stimulation; to avoid alcohol
• Advise patient to avoid hazardous activities; dizziness may occur
• Teach patient that drug is not to be used for acute asthma attacks

Evaluation
Positive therapeutic outcome
• Increased ease of breathing
• Decreased bronchospasm

---

moricizine (℞)
(more-i′siz-een)
Ethmozine
Func. class.: Antidysrhythmic, group I
Chem. class.: Phenothiazine

Pregnancy category **B**

M

Action: Decreased rate of rise of action potential, prolonging refractory period and shortening the action potential duration; depression of inward influx if sodium mediates the effects; may slow atrial and AV nodal conduction

➡ **Therapeutic Outcome:** Resolution of life-threatening dysrhythmias

Uses: Life-threatening dysrhythmias

Dosage and routes
Adult: PO 10-15 mg/kg/day in 2-3 divided doses or 600-900 mg/day given in 2-3 divided doses

Available forms: Film-coated tabs 200, 250, 300 mg

Adverse effects
CNS: Dizziness, headache, fatigue, perioral numbness, euphoria, nervousness, sleep disorders, depression, tinnitus, fatigue
CV: Palpitations, chest pain, CHF, hypertension, syncope, **dysrhythmias**, bradycardia, **MI**, thrombophlebitis
GI: Nausea, abdominal pain, vomiting, diarrhea
GU: Sexual dysfunction, difficult urination, dysuria, incontinence
MISC: Sweating, musculoskeletal pain
RESP: Dyspnea, hyperventilation, **apnea**, asthma, pharyngitis, cough

Contraindications: 2nd- to 3rd-degree AV block, right bundle branch block, cardiogenic shock, hypersensitivity

Precautions: CHF, hypokalemia, hyperkalemia, sick sinus syndrome, pregnancy **B,** lactation, children, impaired hepatic and renal function, cardiac dysfunction

Pharmacokinetics

Absorption	Well absorbed
Distribution	Plasma protein binding (95%)
Metabolism	Liver, extensively
Excretion	Kidneys, breast milk
Half-life	1½-3½ hr

Pharmacodynamics

Onset	Unknown
Peak	½-2 hr
Duration	8-12 hr

Interactions
Individual drugs
Cimetidine: ↑ effect of moricizine
Theophylline: ↓ effect of theophylline

☑ Herb/drug
Aloe: ↑ hypokalemia, ↑ antidysrhythmic effect
Buckthorn: ↑ hypokalemia, ↑ antidysrhythmic effect
Cascara sagrada: ↑ hypokalemia, ↑ antidysrhythmic effect
Henbane: ↑ anticholinergic effect
Rhubarb: ↑ hypokalemia, ↑ antidysrhythmic effect
Senna: ↑ hypokalemia, ↑ antidysrhythmic effect

NURSING CONSIDERATIONS
Assessment
• Monitor ECG at baseline and periodically to determine drug effectiveness; measure PR, QRS, QT intervals, check for PVCs, other dysrhythmias; check B/P for hypotension, hypertension and for rebound hypertension after 1-2 hr; check for dehydration or hypovolemia
◆• Monitor I&O ratio and electrolytes: potassium, sodium, chloride; check weight daily and for signs of CHF or pulmonary toxicity: dyspnea, fatigue, cough, fever, chest pain; drug should be discontinued
• Monitor liver function studies: AST, ALT, bilirubin, alkaline phosphatase
• Monitor cardiac rate; monitor respiration rate, rhythm, character, and chest pain; watch for ventricular tachycardia, supraventricular tachycardia, or fibrillation

Nursing diagnoses
☑ Cardiac output, decreased (uses)
☑ Impaired gas exchange (adverse reactions)
☑ Knowledge deficit (teaching)

Implementation
- Give with meals for GI upset; may be given in 2 divided doses if adverse reactions are minimal
- Make dosage adjustment q 3 days or more

Patient/family education
- Instruct patient to report side effects immediately to prescriber
- Instruct patient to complete follow-up appointment with health care provider including pulmonary function studies, chest x-ray, ophth and otoscopic examinations
- Advise patient to carry identification (Medic Alert) indicating condition and treatment
- Caution patient to avoid driving and other hazardous activities until drug response is determined
- Instruct patient to take medication as prescribed, not to double doses; missed doses may be taken up to 6 hr after previous dose

Treatment of overdose:
O_2, artificial ventilation, ECG, administer dopamine for circulatory depression, administer diazepam or thiopental for convulsions, isoproterenol

---

morphine ⚷ (℞)
(mor′feen)
Astramorph PF, Duramorph, Epimorph ✦, Infumorph 200, Infumorph 500, Morphine H.P. ✦, morphine sulfate, Morphitec ✦, M.O.S. ✦, M.O.S.-S.R. ✦, MS Contin, MSIR, MSIR, OMS Concentrate, Oramorph SR, RMS, Roxanol, Roxanol 100, Roxanol Rescudose, Roxanol SR
Func. class.: Opioid analgesic
Pregnancy category B
Controlled substance schedule II

Action: Depresses pain impulse transmission at the spinal cord level by interacting with opioid receptors, produces CNS depression

▷**Therapeutic Outcome:** Decreased pain

M

Uses: Severe pain; often given after or during an MI

Dosage and routes
Adult: SC/IM 4-15 mg q4h prn; PO 10-30 mg q4h prn; ext rel q8-12h; rec 10-20 mg q4h prn; IV 4-10 mg diluted in 4-5 ml water for inj, over 5 min; epidural 2-10 mg/day

P *Child:* SC/IV 0.1-0.2 mg/kg, not to exceed 15 mg; IM/IV 50-100 µg/kg, max 10 mg/dose initially; PO 0.2-0.5 mg/kg q4-6h (reg rel), q12h (sus rel)

Available forms: Inj 2, 4, 5, 8, 10, 15 mg/ml; sol tabs 10, 15, 30 mg; oral sol 10, 20 mg/5 ml, 20 mg/10 ml, 20 mg/ml; oral tabs 15, 30 mg; rec supp 5, 10, 20, 30 mg; ext

---

rel tabs 15, 30, 60, 100, 200 mg; caps 15, 30 mg

Adverse effects

CNS: Drowsiness, dizziness, *confusion,* headache, *sedation,* euphoria, hallucinations, dysphoria

CV: Palpitations, bradycardia, *hypotension*

EENT: Tinnitus, blurred vision, miosis, diplopia

GI: Nausea, vomiting, anorexia, *constipation,* cramps, biliary tract pressure

GU: Urinary retention

INTEG: Rash, urticaria, bruising, flushing, diaphoresis, pruritus

RESP: **Respiratory depression**

Contraindications: Hypersensitivity, addiction (narcotic), hemorrhage, bronchial asthma, increased intracranial pressure

Precautions: Addictive personality, pregnancy **B,** lactation, acute MI, severe heart **G** disease, elderly, respiratory depression, hepatic disease, **P** renal disease, child <18 yr

Do Not Confuse:
morphine/hydromorphone, Roxanol/Roxicet

Interactions
Individual drugs
Alcohol: ↑ respiratory depression, hypotension, sedation
Nalbuphine: ↓ analgesia
Pentazocine: ↓ analgesia
Rifampin: ↓ analgesic action
Drug classifications
Antihistamines: ↑ respiratory depression, hypotension
CNS depressants: ↑ respiratory depression, hypotension
MAOIs: Reduce dosage; unpredictable reaction may occur
Sedative/hypnotics: ↑ respiratory depression, hypotension
Lab test interferences
↑ Amylase

NURSING CONSIDERATIONS
Assessment
• Assess pain: location, type, character, intensity; give dose before pain becomes extreme
• Monitor I&O ratio; check for decreasing output; may indicate urinary retention; check for constipation; increase fluids, bulk in diet if needed or stool softeners may be prescribed
• Monitor CNS changes: dizziness, drowsiness, hallucinations, euphoria, LOC, pupil reactions
• Monitor allergic reactions: rash, urticaria
• Assess respiratory dysfunction: depression, character, rate, rhythm; notify prescriber if respirations are <10/min

Pharmacokinetics	
Absorption	Variably absorbed (PO); well absorbed (IM, SC, rec); completely absorbed (**IV**)
Distribution	Widely distributed; crosses placenta
Metabolism	Liver, extensively
Excretion	Kidneys
Half-life	1½-2 hr

Pharmacodynamics							
	PO	PO–EXT REL	IM	SC	REC	IV	IT
Onset	Variable	Unknown	10-30 min	20 min	Unknown	Rapid	Rapid
Peak	1 hr	Unknown	½-1 hr	1-1½ hr	½-1 hr	20 min	Unknown
Duration	4-5 hr	8-12 hr	3-7 hr	4-5 hr	4-5 hr	4-5 hr	Ext

Nursing diagnoses
☑ Pain (uses)
☑ Sensory-perceptual alteration: visual, auditory (adverse reactions)
☑ Breathing pattern, ineffective (adverse reactions)
☑ Knowledge deficit (teaching)

Implementation
• Give with antiemetic if nausea, vomiting occur
• Administer when pain is beginning to return; determine dosage interval by patient response; continuous dosing of medication is more effective than giving prn
• Withdraw medication slowly after long-term use to prevent withdrawal symptoms
• Store in light-resistant container at room temp

PO route
• May be given with food or milk to lessen GI upset; may be crushed and mixed with food or fluids; ext rel tabs should be swallowed whole

IM/SC route
• Do not give if cloudy or a precipitate has formed

Ⅳ IV route
• Give direct **IV** by diluting with ≥5 ml of sterile water or 0.9% NaCl for inj; give 2.5-15 mg/4-5 min; rapid administration may lead to increased respiratory depression, death
• Give cont inf by adding to D_5W, $D_{10}W$, 0.9% NaCl, 0.45% NaCl, Ringer's, LR, any dextrose/saline sol, or any dextrose/Ringer's, 0.1-1 mg/ml
• Give by inf pump to deliver correct dosage; titrate to provide adequate pain relief without serious sedation, respiratory depression, hypotension
• May be given by patient-controlled analgesia (PCA) pump in terminal illnesses; patient is able to control amount of morphine
• Administer epidurally with caution in the elderly

Syringe compatibilities:
Atropine, benzquinamide, bupivacaine, butorphanol, cimetidine, dimenhydrinate, diphenhydramine, droperidol, fentanyl, glycopyrrolate, hydroxyzine, ketamine, metoclopramide, midazolam, milrinone, pentazocine, perphenazine, promazine, ranitidine, scopolamine

Syringe incompatibilities:
Meperidine, thiopental

Y-*site compatibilities:*
Allopurinol, amifostine, amikacin, aminophylline, amiodarone, ampicillin, ampicillin/sulbactam, amsacrine, atenolol, atracurium, aztreonam, bumetanide, calcium chloride, cefamandole, cefazolin, cefmetazole, cefoperazone, cefotaxime, cefotetan, cefoxitin, ceftazidime, ceftizoxime, ceftriaxone, cefuroxime, cephalothin, cephapirin, chloramphenicol, cisplatin, cladribine, clindamycin, cyclophosphamide, cytarabine, dexamethasone, digoxin, diltiazem, dobutamine, dopamine, doxycycline, enalaprilat, epinephrine, erythromycin, esmolol, etomidate, famotidine, fentanyl, filgrastim, fluconazole, fludarabine, foscarnet, gentamicin, granisetron, heparin, hydrocortisone, hydromorphone, IL-2, insulin (regular), kanamycin, labetalol, lidocaine, lorazepam, magnesium sulfate, melphalan, meropenem, methotrexate, methyldopate, methylprednisolone, metoclopramide, metoprolol,

M

metronidazole, mezlocillin, midazolam, milrinone, moxalactam, nafcillin, nicardipine, nitroglycerin, norepinephrine, ondansetron, oxacillin, oxytocin, paclitaxel, pancuronium, penicillin G potassium, piperacillin, piperacillin/tazobactam, potassium chloride, propofol, propranolol, ranitidine, sodium bicarbonate, sodium nitroprusside, teniposide, thiotepa, ticarcillin, ticarcillin/clavulanate, tobramycin, trimethoprim-sulfamethoxazole, vancomycin, vecuronium, vinorelbine, vit B/C, warfarin, zidovudine

Y-site incompatibilities:
Furosemide, minocycline, tetracycline

Additive compatibilities:
Alteplase, atracurium, baclofen, bupivacaine, dobutamine, fluconazole, furosemide, meropenem, metoclopramide, ondansetron, succinylcholine, verapamil

Additive incompatibilities:
Aminophylline

Patient/family education
• Advise patient to report any symptoms of CNS changes, allergic reactions
• Caution patients to avoid CNS depressants (alcohol, sedative/hypnotics) for at least 24 hr after taking this drug
• Discuss with patient that dizziness, drowsiness, and confusion are common; to avoid getting up without assistance
• Discuss in detail all aspects of the drug and expected response

Evaluation
Positive therapeutic outcome
• Decreased pain

Treatment of overdose:
Naloxone (Narcan) 0.2-0.8 **IV**, O_2, **IV** fluids, vasopressors

---

moxifloxacin
See Appendix A,
Selected New Drugs

---

multivitamins
(PO, OTC, **IV**, ℞)
Adavite, Dayalets, LKV Drops, Multi-75, Multi-Day, One-A-Day, Optilets, Poly-Vi-Sol, Quintabs, Rulets, Sesame Street Vitamins, Tab-A-Vite, Therabid, Theragran, Unicaps, Vita-Bob, Vita-Kid, many other brands; Berocca Parenteral, M.V.C. 9+3, M.V.I. Pediatric
Func. class.: Vitamins, multiple

Pregnancy category   A

Action: Needed for adequate metabolism

Therapeutic Outcome: Prevention and treatment of vitamin deficiencies

Uses: Prevention and treatment of vitamin deficiencies

Dosage and routes
Adult and child: PO depends on brand

Available forms: Many forms available

Adverse effects
Rare at recommended dosage

Precautions: Pregnancy **A**

Do Not Confuse:
Theragran/Phenergan

Pharmacokinetics	
Absorption	Well absorbed (PO)
Distribution	Widely distributed; crosses placenta
Metabolism	Widely metabolized
Excretion	Kidney, unchanged (water soluble)
Half-life	Unknown

Pharmacodynamics	
Unknown	

Interactions
Individual drugs
Levodopa: ↓ effect of levodopa (large amounts of B_6)

NURSING CONSIDERATIONS
Assessment
• Assess patient for vitamin deficiency; usually more than one vitamin is deficient

Nursing diagnoses
☑ Nutrition, less than body requirements (uses)
☑ Knowledge deficit (teaching)

Implementation
PO route
• Liq multivitamins can be diluted or dropped into patients' mouth using dropper provided with some brands
• Chew tab should be chewed and not swallowed whole

Ⓜ IV route
• Give by cont inf only after diluting 5-10 ml (multivitamins)/500-1000 ml of D_5W, $D_{10}W$, $D_{20}W$, LR, D_5/LR, $D_5/0.9\%$ NaCl, 0.9% NaCl, 3% NaCl
• Do not use sol with crystals, precipitate or color other than bright yellow

Y-site compatibilities:
Acyclovir, ampicillin, cefazolin, cephalothin, cephapirin, diltiazem, erythromycin, fludarabine, gentamicin, tacrolimus, tetracycline

Additive compatibilities:
Cefoxitin, isoproterenol, methyldopate, metoclopramide, metronidazole, netilmicin, norepinephrine, sodium bicarbonate, verapamil

Additive incompatibilities:
Penicillin G, erythromycin, tetracycline, kanamycin, streptomycin, doxycycline, lincomycin should not be admixed

Patient/family education
• Advise patient that adequate nutrition must be maintained to prevent further deficiencies; to comply with treatment regimen
• Advise patient to avoid treating flavored multivitamins as Ⓟ candy; child may overdose
• Caution patient to store Ⓟ vitamins out of children's reach

Evaluation
Positive therapeutic outcome
• Check each individual vitamin for guidelines
• Absence of vitamin deficiencies

Ⓜ

---

muromonab-CD3 (℞)
(mur-oe-mone'ab)
Orthoclone OKT3
Func. class.: Immunosuppressive
Chem. class.: Murine monoclonal antibody
Pregnancy category **C**

▷ **Action:** Reverses graft rejection by blocking T cell function

▷ **Therapeutic Outcome:** Prevention of graft rejection

Uses: Acute allograft rejection in renal, cardiac/hepatic transplant patients

---

Dosage and routes
Adult: **IV** bol 5 mg/day × 10-14 days; usually methylprednisolone sodium succinate, 1 mg/kg **IV**, is given before muromonab-CD3, 100 mg **IV** hydrocortisone sodium succinate is given 30 min after muromonab-CD3

P *Child:* **IV** 100 µg/kg/day × 10-14 day

Cardiac/hepatic allograft rejection, steroid resistant
Adult: **IV** bol 5 mg/day × 10-14 days; begin when it is known that rejection has not been reversed by steroids

Available forms: Inj 5 mg/5 ml

Adverse effects
CNS: Pyrexia, chills, tremors, **aseptic meningitis**
CV: Chest pain
GI: Vomiting, nausea, diarrhea
MISC: Infection, cytokine release syndrome
RESP: Dyspnea, wheezing, **pulmonary edema**

Contraindications: Hypersensitivity to murine origin, fluid overload

Precautions: Pregnancy **C,**
P child <2 yr, fever

Pharmacokinetics	
Absorption	Completely absorbed
Distribution	Unknown
Metabolism	Unknown
Excretion	Unknown
Half-life	Unknown

Pharmacodynamics
Unknown

Interactions
Individual drugs
Allopurinol: ↑ toxicity
Azathioprine: ↑ risk of infection

Cyclosporine: ↑ myelosuppression
Drug classifications
Antineoplastics: ↑ myelosuppression
Corticosteroids: ↑ risk of infection
Immunosuppressants: ↑ immunosuppressant
Live virus vaccines: ↓ antibody response

NURSING CONSIDERATIONS
Assessment
◆• Assess for cytosine release syndrome (CRS): nausea, vomiting, chills, fever, joint pain, weakness, dizziness, diarrhea, tremors, abdominal pain; occurs 30-60 min after first dose; methylprednisolone sodium succinate may be prescribed to lessen this reaction
• Assess for hypersensitivity reaction: dyspnea, bronchospasm, urticaria, tachycardia, hypotension, angioedema; discontinue drug; all emergency equipment must be nearby
• Assess for headache, photophobia, fever, rigidity; indicate aseptic meningitis has developed
• Assess for sore throat, fever, chills, rash, dysuria, which may indicate infection; therapy may be discontinued
• Assess for fluid overload: edema, pulmonary edema, increasing weight
• Monitor blood studies: CBC with differential, platelets, BUN, creatinine, alkaline phosphatase, bilirubin during treatment monthly
• Monitor AST, ALT, BUN, creatinine, alkaline phosphatase, bilirubin

---

• Obtain human-mouse antibody; if titer is over 1:1000, this drug should not be used
• Monitor T cell with CD_3, CD_4, CD_8 antigen qd; report should be CD_3 positive and T cells $<25/mm^3$

Nursing diagnoses
☑ Infection, risk for (uses)
☑ Knowledge deficit (teaching)

Implementation
• Give by direct **IV** undiluted; withdraw with a 0.2-0.22 low–protein binding µm filter; discard and use new needle for administration; give over 1 min
• Give for several days before transplant surgery

Patient/family education
• Instruct patient to report fever, chills, sore throat, fatigue, since serious infections may occur
• Advise patient to use contraceptive measures during treatment for 12 wk after ending therapy; drug is mutagenic
• Advise patient to avoid crowds and persons with known infections to reduce risk of infection
• Advise patient to report symptoms of cytokine release syndrome, aseptic meningitis
• Instruct patient to avoid vaccinations during treatment

Evaluation
Positive therapeutic outcome
• Absence of graft rejection

---

mycophenolate mofetil (R)
(mie-koe-feen'oh-late moe-feh-til)
CellCept
Func. class.: Immunosuppressant
Pregnancy category   C

Action: Inhibits inflammatory responses that are mediated by the immune system; prolongs survival of allogenic transplants

➤**Therapeutic Outcome:** Absence of graft rejection

Uses: Organ transplants to prevent rejection (renal); prophylaxis of rejection in allogenic cardiac transplants

Dosage and routes
Adult: PO; give initial dose 72 hr prior to transplantation; 1 gm bid given to renal transplant patients in combination with corticosteroids and cyclosporine

Available forms: Cap 250 mg; tab 500 mg; inj (powder) 500 mg

Adverse effects
CNS: Tremor, dizziness, insomnia, headache, fever
CV: Hypertension, chest pain
GI: Nausea, vomiting, stomatitis, *diarrhea, constipation*
GU: UTI, hematuria, **renal tubular necrosis**
HEMA: **Leukopenia, thrombocytopenia, anemia, pancytopenia**
INTEG: Rash
META: Peripheral edema, hypercholesteremia, hypophosphatemia, edema, hyperkalemia, hypokalemia, hyperglycemia
MS: Arthralgia, muscle wasting
RESP: Dyspnea, respiratory infection, increased cough,

M

---

pharyngitis, bronchitis, pneumonia
SYST: **Lymphoma, nonmelanoma skin carcinoma**

Contraindications: Hypersensitivity to this drug or mycophenolic acid

Precautions: Lymphomas, malignancies, neutropenia, renal disease, pregnancy **C**, lactation

Pharmacokinetics

Absorption	Rapidly and completely absorbed
Distribution	Unknown
Metabolism	To active metabolite (MPA)
Excretion	Urine, feces
Half-life	Unknown

Pharmacodynamics

Unknown

Interactions
Individual drugs
Acyclovir: ↑ concentration of both drugs
Azathioprine: Avoid use
Cholestyramine: ↓ levels of mycophenolate
Ganciclovir: ↑ concentration of both drugs
Phenytoin: ↓ protein binding of phenytoin
Probenecid: ↑ levels of mycophenolate
Theophylline: ↓ protein binding of theophylline
Drug classifications
Antacids: ↓ levels of mycophenolate
Salicylates: ↑ levels of mycophenolate

NURSING CONSIDERATIONS
Assessment
• Monitor blood studies: CBC during treatment monthly
• Monitor liver function

studies: alk phosphatase, AST, ALT, bilirubin
Nursing diagnoses
☑ Infection, risk for (uses)
☑ Knowledge deficit (teaching)

Implementation
• Give 72 hrs prior to transplantation; may be given in combination with corticosteroids and cyclosporine
PO route
• Give alone for better absorption
🚫• Do not crush, chew tabs, do not open caps
IV **IV route**
• Do not give by rapid or bolus inj: reconstitute and dilute to 6 mg/ml with D_5, give over ≥2 hr
• Do not admix with mycophenolate **IV** in infusion catheter or with other **IV** drug or infusion admixtures

Patient/family education
• Teach patient to report fever, rash, severe diarrhea, chills, sore throat, fatigue, since serious infections may occur
• Instruct patient to avoid crowds to reduce risk of infection
• Advise patient that repeated lab tests are necessary
• Advise to limit exposure to sunlight/UV light
• Instruct to use contraception before, during, and 6 wk after therapy

Evaluation
Positive therapeutic outcome
• Absence of graft rejection

nabumetone (℞)

(na-byoo′me-tone)

Relafen

Func. class.: Nonsteroidal antiinflammatory

Chem. class.: Acetic acid derivative

Pregnancy category   C

Action: Inhibits prostaglandin synthesis by decreasing an enzyme needed for biosynthesis; analgesic, antiinflammatory

➔Therapeutic Outcome: Decreased pain, swelling of joints

Uses: Osteoarthritis, rheumatoid arthritis, acute or chronic treatment

Dosage and routes

Adult: PO 1 g as a single dose; may increase to 1.5-2 g/day if needed; may give qd or bid (as a divided dose)

Available forms: Tabs 500, 750 mg

Adverse effects

CNS: Dizziness, headache, drowsiness, fatigue, tremors, confusion, insomnia, anxiety, depression, nervousness

CV: Tachycardia, peripheral edema, palpitations, **dysrhythmias, CHF**

EENT: Tinnitus, hearing loss, blurred vision

GI: Nausea, anorexia, vomiting, diarrhea, jaundice, cholestatic hepatitis, constipation, flatulence, cramps, dry mouth, peptic ulcer, gastritis, **ulceration, perforation**

GU: **Nephrotoxicity, dysuria, hematuria, oliguria, azotemia,** cystitis

HEMA: **Blood dyscrasias**

INTEG: Purpura, rash, pruritus, sweating, photosensitivity

RESP: Dyspnea, pharyngitis, **bronchospasm**

Contraindications: Hypersensitivity to this drug or aspirin, iodides, NSAIDs, asthma, severe renal disease

Precautions: Pregnancy **C** (1st/2nd trimesters), lactation, children, bleeding disorders, GI disorders, cardiac disorders, renal disorders hepatic dysfunction, elderly

Pharmacokinetics	
Absorption	Well absorbed
Distribution	Unknown
Metabolism	Liver, extensively, to inactive metabolite
Excretion	Unknown
Half-life	22-30 hr

Pharmacodynamics	
Onset	Unknown
Peak	2½-4 hr
Duration	Unknown

Interactions

Individual drugs

Acetaminophen (long-term use): ↑ renal reactions

Alcohol: ↑ adverse reactions

Aspirin: ↓ effectiveness, ↑ adverse reactions

Cefamandole: ↑ bleeding

Cefoperazone: ↑ bleeding

Cefotetan: ↑ bleeding

Digoxin: ↑ toxicity, levels

Insulin: ↓ insulin effect

Lithium: ↑ toxicity

Methotrexate: ↑ toxicity

Phenytoin: ↑ toxicity

Plicamycin: ↑ bleeding

Probenecid: ↑ toxicity

Radiation: ↑ risk of hematologic toxicity

Sulfonylurea: ↑ toxicity

Valproic acid: ↑ bleeding

Drug classifications

Anticoagulants: ↑ risk of bleeding

N

Antihypertensives: ↓ effect of antihypertensives
Antineoplastics: ↑ risk of hematologic toxicity
Cephalosporins: ↑ risk of bleeding
Diuretics: ↓ effectiveness of diuretics
Glucocorticoids: ↑ adverse reactions
Hypoglycemics, oral: ↓ hypoglycemic effect
NSAIDs: ↑ adverse reactions
Potassium supplements: ↑ adverse reactions
Salicylates: possible ↑ action or toxicity
Sulfonamides: ↑ toxicity
Thrombolytics: ↑ bleeding

NURSING CONSIDERATIONS
Assessment
• Assess for pain: frequency, characteristics, location, duration, intensity, relief of pain after med; and for inflammation of joints, ROM
• Monitor blood counts during therapy; watch for decreasing platelets; if low, therapy may need to be discontinued, restarted after hematologic recovery; check for blood dyscrasias (thrombocytopenia): brusing, fatigue, bleeding, poor healing; monitor liver function tests: AST, ALT, alkaline phosphatase, LDH, blood glucose, WBC, platelets, CrCl
• Assess for asthma, aspirin sensitivity, nasal polyps; increased hypersensitivity reactions

Nursing diagnoses
☑ Pain (uses)
☑ Mobility, impaired (uses)
☑ Injury, risk for (adverse reactions)
☑ Knowledge deficit (teaching)

Implementation
• Administer tab to patient crushed or whole
• Give with food or milk to decrease gastric symptoms

Patient/family education
• Tell patient that drug must be continued for prescribed time to be effective; to avoid aspirin, alcoholic beverages, ibuprofen, and OTC medications unless approved by prescriber
• Caution patient to report bleeding, bruising, fatigue, malaise, since blood dyscrasias do occur
• Instruct patient to use caution when driving; drowsiness, dizziness may occur
• Advise patient to use sunscreen, hat, and other protective clothing to prevent burning

Evaluation
Positive therapeutic outcome
• Decreased pain
• Decreased inflammation
• Increased mobility

---

nadolol (R)
(nay-doe'lole)
Corgard
Func. class.: Antihypertensive, antianginal
Chem. class.: β-Adrenergic receptor blocker
Pregnancy category   C

Action: Competitively blocks stimulation of β-adrenergic receptor within vascular smooth muscle; produces chronotropic, inotropic activity (decreases rate of SA node discharge, increases recovery time), slows conduction of AV node, decreases heart rate, which decreases O_2 consumption in myocardium; also decreases renin-aldosterone-angiotensin system at high doses, inhibits β_2-receptors in bronchial system

▶ **Therapeutic Outcome:** Decreased B/P, heart rate

Uses: Chronic stable angina pectoris, mild to moderate hypertension

Investigational uses: Tachydysrhythmias, aggression, anxiety, tremors, esophageal varices (rebleeding only), prophylaxis of migraine headaches

Dosage and routes
Adult: PO 40 mg qd; increase by 40-80 mg q3-7 days; maintenance 40-240 mg/day for angina, 40-320 mg/day for hypertension

G *Elderly:* PO 20 mg/day, may increase by 20 mg until desired dose

Renal dose
CrCl 31-50 ml/min give q24-36h; CrCl 10-30 ml/min give q24-48h

Available forms: Tabs 20, 40, 80, 120, 160 mg

Adverse effects
CNS: Depression, hallucinations, dizziness, fatigue, lethargy, paresthesia, headache
CV: Bradycardia, hypotension, **CHF,** palpitations, AV block, chest pain, peripheral ischemia, flushing, edema, vasodilatation, conduction disturbances
EENT: Sore throat
GI: Nausea, vomiting, diarrhea, colitis, constipation, cramps, dry mouth, flatulence, hepatomegaly, **pancreatitis,** taste distortion

HEMA: **Agranulocytosis, thrombocytopenia**
INTEG: Rash, pruritus, fever
RESP: Dyspnea, respiratory dysfunction, **bronchospasm,** cough, wheezing, nasal stuffiness, pharyngitis, **laryngospasm**

Contraindications: Hypersensitivity to this drug, cardiac failure, cardiogenic shock, 2nd- or 3rd-degree heart block, bronchospastic disease, sinus bradycardia, CHF, COPD

Precautions: Diabetes mellitus, pregnancy **C,** renal disease, lactation, hyperthyroidism, peripheral vascular disease, myasthenia gravis

◼ **Do Not Confuse:**
Corgard/Cognex

Pharmacokinetics	
Absorption	Variably absorbed
Distribution	Crosses placenta; minimal concentration in CNS
Excretion	Kidneys, unchanged
Half-life	10-24 hr; increased in renal disease

Pharmacodynamics	
Onset	Variable
Peak	3-4 hr
Duration	17-24 hr

Interactions
Individual drugs
Alcohol: ↑ hypotension (large amounts)
Epinephrine: α-Adrenergic stimulation
Hydralazine: ↑ hypotension, bradycardia
Insulin: ↑ hypoglycemia
Methyldopa: ↑ hypotension, bradycardia
Prazosin: ↑ hypotension, bradycardia

N

Reserpine: ↑ hypotension, bradycardia
Thyroid: ↓ effect of nadolol
Verapamil: ↑ myocardial depression

Drug classifications
Amphetamines: ↑ hypotension, bradycardia
Antihypertensives: ↑ hypertension
β₂-Agonists: ↓ bronchodilatation
Cardiac glycosides: ↑ bradycardia
MAOIs: ↑ bradycardia, do not use together
Nitrates: ↑ hypotension
NSAIDs: ↓ antihypertensive effect
Theophyllines: ↓ bronchodilatation

Lab test interferences
False ↑ Urinary catecholamines

NURSING CONSIDERATIONS
Assessment
• Monitor B/P at beginning of treatment, periodically thereafter; note rate, rhythm, quality of apical/radial pulse before administration; notify prescriber of any significant changes (pulse <55 bpm)
• Check for baselines in renal, liver function tests before therapy begins
• Assess for edema in feet, legs daily; monitor I&O, daily weight; check for jugular vein distention and rales bilaterally, dyspnea (CHF)
• Monitor skin turgor, dryness of mucous membranes for hydration status, especially **G** elderly

Nursing diagnoses
☑ Cardiac output, decreased (uses)
☑ Injury, potential for (adverse reactions)

☑ Knowledge deficit (teaching)
☑ Noncompliance (teaching)

Implementation
• Given ac, hs, tab may be crushed or swallowed whole; give with food to prevent GI upset; give reduced dosage in renal dysfunction
• Store protected from light, moisture; place in cool environment

Patient/family education
• Teach patient not to discontinue drug abruptly; taper over 2 wk; may cause precipitate angina if stopped abruptly
• Teach patient not to use OTC products containing α-adrenergic stimulants (such as nasal decongestants, cold preparations); to avoid alcohol, smoking and to limit sodium intake as prescribed
• Teach patient how to take pulse and B/P at home; advise when to notify prescriber
• Instruct patient to comply with weight control, dietary adjustments, modified exercise program
• Advise patient to carry/wear Medic Alert ID to identify drug being taken, allergies; teach patient drug controls symptoms but does not cure condition
• Caution patient to avoid hazardous activities if dizziness, drowsiness present; to rise slowly to prevent orthostatic hypotension
• Teach patient to report symptoms of CHF: difficult breathing, especially on exertion or when lying down, night cough, swelling of extremities or bradycardia, dizziness, confusion, depression, fever
• Teach patient to take drug as prescribed, not to double

doses, skip doses; take any missed doses as soon as remembered if at least 4 hr until next dose

Evaluation
Positive therapeutic outcome
• Decreased B/P in hypertension

---

nafcillin (R)
(naf-sill'in)
Nafcil, nafcillin sodium, Nallpen, Unipen
Func. class.: Antiinfective, broad-spectrum
Chem. class.: Penicillinase-resistant penicillin
Pregnancy category   B

Action: Interferes with cell wall replication of susceptible organisms; osmotically unstable cell wall swells, bursts from osmotic pressure

➔**Therapeutic Outcome:** Bactericidal effects for gram-positive cocci *Staphylococcus aureus, Streptococcus viridans, S. pneumoniae* and infections caused by penicillinase-producing *Staphylococcus*

Uses: Infections caused by penicillinase-producing staphylococci, streptococci; respiratory tract, skin, skin structure, urinary tract, bone, joint infections, sinusitis, endocarditis, septicemia, meningitis

Dosage and routes
Adult: PO 250-1000 mg q4-6h; IM 500 mg q4-6h; **IV** 500-1500 mg q4-6h

P *Child and infants, most infections:* PO 6.25-12.5 mg/kg q6h; pharyngitis PO 250 mg q8h; IM 25 mg/kg

q12h; **IV** most infections 10-20 mg/kg q4h or 20-40 mg/kg q8h, max 200 mg/kg/day

P *Neonates:* PO 10 mg/kg q6-8h; IM 10 mg/kg q12h; **IV:** most infections 10-20 mg/kg q4h or 20-40 mg/kg q8h, max 200 mg/kg/day

Meningitis
P *Neonates ≥2 kg:* 50 mg/kg q8h × 1 wk of life, then 50 mg/kg q6h

P *Neonates <2 kg:* 25-50 mg/kg q12h × 1 wk of life, then 50 mg/kg q8h

Available forms: Cap 250 mg; tab 500 mg; powder for oral susp 250 mg/5 ml; powder for inj 500 mg, 1, 2, 10 g; **IV** 1, 1.5, 2, 4 g

Adverse effects
CNS: Lethargy, hallucinations, anxiety, depression, muscle twitching, **coma, convulsions**
GI: Nausea, vomiting, diarrhea, increased AST, ALT, abdominal pain, glossitis, **pseudomembranous colitis**
GU: Oliguria, **proteinuria, hematuria, vaginitis, moniliasis, glomerulonephritis,** interstitial nephritis
HEMA: Anemia, increased bleeding time, **bone marrow depression, granulocytopenia**

Contraindications: Hypersensitivity to penicillins

Precautions: Pregnancy **B,** hypersensitivity to cephalosporins, neonates

N

Pharmacokinetics

Absorption	Well absorbed (IM); erratic (PO)
Distribution	Widely distributed; crosses placenta
Metabolism	Not metabolized
Excretion	Kidneys, unchanged; breast milk
Half-life	1 hr; increased in renal disease

Pharmacodynamics

	PO	IM	IV
Onset	½ hr	½ hr	Immediate
Peak	1-2 hr	1-2 hr	Inf end

Interactions
Individual drugs
Aspirin: ↑ nafcillin levels, ↓ renal excretion
Dilsulfiram: ↑ nafcillin concentrations
Probenecid: ↑ nafcillin levels, ↓ renal excretion
Drug classifications
Oral anticoagulants: ↑ anticoagulant effects
Oral contraceptives: ↓ contraceptive effectiveness
Food/drug
Food, carbonated drinks, citrus fruit juices: ↓ absorption
Herb/drug
Khat: ↓ absorption
Lab test interferences
False positive: Urine glucose, urine protein

NURSING CONSIDERATIONS
Assessment
• Assess patient for previous sensitivity reaction to penicillins or other cephalosporins; cross-sensitivity between penicillins and cephalosporins is common
• Assess patient for signs and symptoms of infection including characteristics of wounds, sputum, urine, stool, WBC >10,000, earache, fever; obtain baseline information and during treatment
• Obtain C&S before beginning drug therapy to identify if correct treatment has been initiated
• Assess for allergic reactions: rash, urticaria, pruritus, chills, fever, joint pain; angioedema may occur a few days after therapy begins; epinephrine, resuscitation equipment should be available for anaphylactic reaction
• Assess renal studies: urinalysis, protein, blood, BUN, creatinine
⬧• Identify urine output; if decreasing, notify prescriber (may indicate nephrotoxicity)
• Monitor blood studies: AST, ALT, CBC, Hct, bilirubin, LDH, alkaline phosphatase, Coombs' test monthly if patient is on long-term therapy
• Monitor electrolytes: potassium, sodium, chloride monthly if patient is on long-term therapy
• Assess bowel pattern qd; if severe diarrhea occurs, drug should be discontinued; may indicate pseudomembranous colitis
• Monitor for bleeding: ecchymosis, bleeding gums, hematuria, stool guaiac daily if on long-term therapy
• Assess for overgrowth of infection: perineal itching, fever, malaise, redness, pain, swelling, drainage, rash, diarrhea, change in cough, sputum
Nursing diagnoses
☑ Infection, risk for (uses)
☑ Diarrhea (adverse reactions)
☑ Injury, risk for (adverse reactions)
☑ Knowledge deficit (teaching)
☑ Noncompliance (teaching)

Implementation
PO route
- Give in even doses around the clock; if GI upset occurs, give with food; drug must be given for 10-14 days to ensure organism death and prevent superinfection; store in tight container.
- Do not crush, chew caps
- Shake susp; store in refrigerator for 2 wk, 1 wk at room temp

IM route
- Reconstitute 500 mg/1.7-1.8 ml; 1 g/3.4 ml; 2 g/6.6-6.8 ml with sterile water or bacteriostatic water for a conc of 250 mg/ml; store unused portion in refrigerator for up to 7 days
- Give deep in large muscle mass

IV route
- Reconstitute 500 mg/1.7 ml; 1 g/3.4 ml; 2 g/6.6-6.8 ml with sterile water or bacteriostatic water for a conc of 250 mg/ml; store unused portion in refrigerator for up to 7 days
- Give by direct **IV** by diluting reconstituted sol with 15-30 ml of sterile water or 0.9% NaCl; give over 5-10 min
- Give by intermittent inf by diluting to a conc of 2-40 mg/ml with 0.9% NaCl, D_5W, $D_{10}W$, D_5/0.9% NaCl, D_5/LR, LR, Ringer's; store in refrigerator for up to 96 hr or 24 hr room temp; run over 30-60 min

Syringe compatibilities:
Cimetidine, heparin

Y-site compatibilities:
Acyclovir, atropine, cyclophosphamide, diazepam, enalaprilat, esmolol, famotidine, fentanyl, fluconazole, foscarnet, hydromorphone, magnesium sulfate, morphine, perphenazine, propofol, theophylline, zidovudine

Y-site incompatibilities:
Droperidol, fentanyl/droperidol, labetalol, nalbuphine, pentazocine, regular insulin, verapamil

Additive compatibilities:
Chloramphenicol, chlorothiazide, dexamethasone, diphenhydramine, ephedrine, heparin, hydroxyzine, lidocaine, potassium chloride, prochlorperazine, sodium bicarbonate, sodium lactate

Additive incompatibilities:
Ascorbic acid, aztreonam, bleomycin, cytarabine, gentamicin, hydrocortisone sodium succinate, methylprednisolone sodium succinate, promazine

Patient/family education
- Teach patient to report sore throat, bruising, bleeding, joint pain; may indicate blood dyscrasias (rare)
- Advise patient to contact prescriber if vaginal itching, loose, foul-smelling stools, furry tongue occur; may indicate superinfection
- Instruct patient to take all medication prescribed for the length of time ordered
- Advise patient to notify prescriber of diarrhea with blood or pus, which may indicate pseudomembranous colitis

Evaluation
Positive therapeutic outcome
- Absence of signs/symptoms of infection (WBC <10,000, temp WNL, absence of red, draining wounds, earache)
- Reported improvement in symptoms of infection

Treatment of anaphylaxis:
Withdraw drug, maintain airway, administer epinephrine, aminophylline, O$_2$, **IV** corticosteroids

nalbuphine (Ŗ)
(nal'byoo-feen)
Nubain, nalbuphine HCl
Func. class.: Opioid analgesic
Chem. class.: Synthetic opioid agonist/antagonist
Pregnancy category   C

Action: Inhibits ascending pain pathways in limbic system, thalamus, midbrain, hypothalamus by binding to opiate receptor sites, thus altering pain perception and response

Therapeutic Outcome: Relief of pain

Uses: Moderate to severe pain, labor analgesia, balanced anesthesia (adjunct)

Dosage and routes
Analgesic
Adult: SC/IM/**IV** 10-20 mg q3-6h prn, not to exceed 160 mg/day

Balanced anesthesia supplement
Adult: **IV** 0.3-3 mg/kg given over 10-15 min; may give 0.25-0.5 mg/kg as needed (maintenance)

Available forms: Inj 10, 20 mg/ml

Adverse effects
CNS: Drowsiness, dizziness, confusion, headache, sedation, euphoria, dysphoria (high doses), hallucinations, dreaming, tolerance, physical and psychologic dependency
CV: Palpitations, bradycardia, change in B/P, orthostatic hypotension
EENT: Tinnitus, blurred vision, miosis (high doses), diplopia
GI: Nausea, vomiting, anorexia, constipation, cramps
GU: Increased urinary output, dysuria, urinary retention, urgency
INTEG: Rash, urticaria, bruising, flushing, *diaphoresis,* pruritus
RESP: **Respiratory depression**

Contraindications: Hypersensitivity, addiction (narcotic)

Precautions: Addictive personality, pregnancy **C**, lactation, increased intracranial pressure, MI (acute), severe heart disease, respiratory depression, hepatic disease, renal disease

Pharmacokinetics	
Absorption	Well absorbed (SC, IM); completely absorbed (**IV**)
Distribution	Crosses placenta
Metabolism	Liver, extensively
Excretion	Feces, kidneys, unchanged (small amounts); breast milk
Half-life	5 hr

Pharmacodynamics			
	IM	SC	IV
Onset	Up to 15 min	Up to 15 min	Rapid
Peak	1 hr	Unknown	½ hr
Duration	3-6 hr	3-6 hr	3-6 hr

Interactions
Individual drugs
Alcohol: ↑ respiratory depression, hypotension, sedation
Drug classifications
Antihistamines: ↑ respiratory depression, hypotension

CNS depressants: ↑ respiratory depression, hypotension
MAOIs: Use cautiously, results are unpredictable
Opiates: ↑ opioid withdrawals (dependency)
Phenothiazines: ↑ respiratory depression, hypotension
Sedative/hypnotics: ↑ respiratory depression, hypotension
Lab test interferences
↑ Amylase, ↑ lipase

NURSING CONSIDERATIONS
Assessment
• Assess pain characteristics (location, intensity, type) before medication administration and following treatment
• Monitor VS after parenteral route; note muscle rigidity, drug history, liver, kidney function tests; respiratory dysfunction: respiratory depression, character, rate, rhythm; notify prescriber if respirations are <10/min
• Monitor CNS changes: dizziness, drowsiness, hallucinations, euphoria, LOC, pupil reaction
• Monitor allergic reactions: rash, urticaria

Nursing diagnoses
✓Pain (uses)
✓Sensory-perceptual alteration: visual, auditory (adverse reactions)
✓Breathing pattern, ineffective (adverse reactions)
✓Knowledge deficit (teaching)

Implementation
• Give by inj (IM, **IV**), only with resuscitative equipment available; give slowly to prevent rigidity
• Store in light-resistant area at room temp

IM route
• Give deeply in large muscle mass; rotate inj sites
▮IV route
• Give direct **IV** undiluted 10 mg or less over 3-5 min or more

Syringe compatibilities:
Atropine, cimetidine, diphenhydramine, droperidol, glycopyrrolate, hydroxyzine, lidocaine, midazolam, prochlorperazine, promethazine, ranitidine, scopolamine, trimethobenzamide

Syringe incompatibilities:
Diazepam, pentobarbital

Y-site compatibilities:
Amifostine, aztreonam, cefmetazole, cladribine, filgrastim, fludarabine, granisetron, melphalan, paclitaxel, propofol, teniposide, thiotepa, vinorelbine

Y-site incompatibilities:
Nafcillin, sargramostim

Patient/family education
• Instruct patient to report any symptoms of CNS changes, allergic reactions
• Caution patients to avoid CNS depressants: alcohol, sedative/hypnotics for at least 24 hr after taking this drug
• Discuss with patient that dizziness, drowsiness, confusion are common; to avoid getting up without assistance
• Discuss in detail all aspects of the drug: reason for taking drug and expected results
• Instruct patient to change position slowly to prevent orthostatic hypotension
• Teach patient to turn, cough, deep breathe after surgery to prevent atelectasis

N

Evaluation
Positive therapeutic outcome
• Relief of pain

Treatment of overdose:
Naloxone (Narcan) 0.2-0.8 **IV**, O_2, **IV** fluids, vasopressors

---

naloxone (R)
(nal-oks'one)
naloxone HCl, Narcan
Func. class.: Opioid antagonist
Chem. class.: Thebaine derivative

Pregnancy category   **B**

Action: Competes with opioids at opioid receptor sites

➔**Therapeutic Outcome:** Absence of opioid overdose

Uses: Respiratory depression induced by narcotics, pentazocine, propoxyphene; refractory circulatory shock

Dosage and routes
Opioid-induced respiratory depression, CNS depression
Adult: **IV**/SC/IM 0.4-2 mg; repeat q2-3 min if needed
P *Child:* **IV**/SC/IM 0.5-2 μg/kg as small, frequent q/min bolus or as an inf titrated to response

Postoperative respiratory depression
Adult: **IV** 0.1-0.2 mg q2-3 min prn
P *Child:* **IV**/IM/SC 0.01 mg/kg q2-3 min prn

Asphyxia neonatorum
P *Neonates:* **IV** 0.01 mg/kg given into umbilical vein after delivery; may repeat in q2-3 min × 3 doses

Available forms: Inj 0.4, 1 **P** mg/ml; neonatal inj 0.02 mg/ml

Adverse effects
CNS: Drowsiness, nervousness
CV: **Ventricular tachycardia, fibrillation,** increased systolic B/P (high doses)
GI: Nausea, vomiting
RESP: Hyperpnea

Contraindications: Hypersensitivity, respiratory depression

Precautions: Pregnancy **B**, **P** children, cardiovascular disease, opioid dependency, lactation

Do Not Confuse:
Narcan/Norcuron

Pharmacokinetics	
Absorption	Well absorbed (SC, IM); completely absorbed (**IV**)
Distribution	Rapidly distributed; crosses placenta
Metabolism	Liver
Excretion	Kidneys
P Half-life	1 hr; up to 3 hr (neonates)

Pharmacodynamics		
	IV	IM/SC
Onset	1 min	2-5 min
Peak	Unknown	Unknown
Duration	45 min	45-60 min

Interactions
Drug classifications
Analgesics, opioids: ↑ withdrawal in those addicted to opioids
Lab test interferences
Interference: Urine VMA, 5-HIAA, urine glucose

NURSING CONSIDERATIONS
Assessment
• Assess for signs of opioid withdrawal in drug dependent individuals: cramping, hyper-

---

tension, anxiety, vomiting; may occur up to 2 hr after administration
• Monitor VS q3-5 min; ABGs including Po_2, Pco_2
• Assess cardiac status: tachycardia, hypertension; monitor ECG
• Assess for pain: duration, intensity, location before and after administration; may be used for respiratory depression
• Assess for respiratory dysfunction: respiratory depression, character, rate, rhythm; if respirations are <10/min, probably due to opioid overdose, administer naloxone; monitor LOC

Nursing diagnoses
☑ Breathing pattern, ineffective (uses)
☑ Coping, ineffective individual (uses)
☑ Pain (adverse reactions)
☑ Knowledge deficit (teaching)

Implementation
IV **IV route**
• Give by direct **IV** undiluted; give 0.4 mg or less over 15 sec or titrate inf to response
• Give cont **IV** further diluted with 0.9% NaCl and D_5 and give as an inf
• Give only with resuscitative equipment, O_2 nearby
• Use only sol prepared within 24 hr
• Store at room temp in darkness

Syringe compatibilities:
Benzquinamide, heparin
Y-site compatibilities:
Propofol
Additive compatibilities:
Verapamil

Patient/family education
• Explain reason for and expected results of medication when patient alert

Evaluation
Positive therapeutic outcome
• Reversal of respiratory depression
• LOC: alert

naproxen (R)
(na-prox′en)
Apo-Naproxen ✤, EC-Naprosyn, Naprelan, Napron X, Naprosyn, Naprosyn-E ✤, Naprosyn-SR ✤, Naxen ✤, Novo-Naprox ✤, Nu-Naprox ✤
naproxen sodium
Aleve, Anaprox, Anaprox DS, Apo-Napro-Na ✤, Apo-Napro-Na DS, Naprelan, Novo-Naprox Sodium ✤, Novo-Naprox Sodium DS ✤, Synflex ✤, Synflex DS ✤
Func. class.: Nonsteroidal antiinflammatory, non-opioid analgesic
Chem. class.: Propionic acid derivative
Pregnancy category   B

Action: Inhibits prostaglandin synthesis by decreasing enzyme needed for biosynthesis; analgesic, antiinflammatory
➡ **Therapeutic Outcome:** Decreased pain, inflammation
Uses: Mild to moderate pain, osteoarthritis, rheumatoid arthritis, gouty arthritis, juvenile arthritis, primary dysmenorrhea
Dosage and routes
Adult: PO 250-500 mg bid, not to exceed 1 g/day (base); 525 mg, then 275 mg q6-8h

prn, not to exceed 1475 mg (sodium)

P *Child:* PO 10 mg/kg in 2 divided doses

Available forms: Naproxen, tabs 250, 375, 500 mg; DR 375, 500 mg; oral susp 125 mg/5 ml; naproxen sodium, tabs 220, 275, 550 mg

Adverse effects

CNS: Dizziness, drowsiness, fatigue, tremors, confusion, insomnia, anxiety, depression

CV: Tachycardia, peripheral edema, palpitations, **dysrhythmias**

EENT: Tinnitus, hearing loss, blurred vision

GI: Nausea, anorexia, vomiting, diarrhea, jaundice, **cholestatic hepatitis,** constipation, flatulence, cramps, dry mouth, peptic ulcer, **GI ulceration, bleeding, perforation**

GU: **Nephrotoxicity: dysuria, hematuria, oliguria, azotemia**

HEMA: **Blood dyscrasias**

INTEG: Purpura, rash, pruritus, sweating

Contraindications: Hypersensitivity, asthma, severe renal disease, severe hepatic disease, ulcer disease

Precautions: Pregnancy **B** (1st trimester), lactation, **P** children <2 yr, bleeding disorders, GI disorders, cardiac disorders, hypersensitivity to other antiinflammatory agents, **G** elderly, CrCl <25 ml/min

Pharmacokinetics

Absorption	Completely absorbed
Distribution	Crosses placenta, 99% protein binding
Metabolism	Liver, extensively
Excretion	Breast milk
Half-life	10-20 hr

Pharmacodynamics

Onset	1 hr
Peak	2-4 hr
Duration	<7 hr

Interactions

Individual drugs

Acetaminophen (long-term use): ↑ renal reactions

Alcohol: ↑ adverse reactions

Aspirin: ↓ effectiveness, ↑ adverse reactions

Cefamandole: ↑ bleeding

Cefoperazone: ↑ bleeding

Cefotetan: ↑ bleeding

Digoxin: ↑ toxicity, levels

Insulin: ↓ insulin effect

Lithium: ↑ toxicity

Methotrexate: ↑ toxicity

Phenytoin: ↑ toxicity

Probenecid: ↑ toxicity

Radiation: ↑ risk of hematologic toxicity

Sulfonylurea: ↑ toxicity

Valproic acid: ↑ bleeding

Drug classifications

Anticoagulants: ↑ risk of bleeding

Antihypertensives: ↓ effect of antihypertensives

Antineoplastics: ↑ risk of hematologic toxicity

β-Adrenergic blockers: ↑ antihypertension

Cephalosporins: ↑ risk of bleeding

Diuretics: ↓ effectiveness of diuretics

Glucocorticoids: ↑ adverse reactions

Hypoglycemics, oral: ↓ hypoglycemic effect

NSAIDs: ↑ adverse reactions

Potassium supplements: ↑ adverse reactions

Sulfonamides: ↑ toxicity

Lab test interferences

↑ BUN, ↑ alkaline phosphatase

False: ↑ 5-HIAA, false ↑ 17KS

NURSING CONSIDERATIONS
Assessment

• Monitor liver function, renal function, other blood studies: AST, ALT, bilirubin, creatinine, BUN, CBC, Hct, Hgb, pro-time, LDH, blood glucose, WBC, platelets if patient is on long-term therapy
• Check I&O ratio; decreasing output may indicate renal failure (long-term therapy)
• Assess hepatotoxicity: dark urine, clay-colored stools, yellowing of the skin and sclera, itching, abdominal pain, fever, diarrhea if patient is on long-term therapy
• Assess for allergic reactions: rash, urticaria; if these occur, drug may have to be discontinued
• Assess for ototoxicity: tinnitus, ringing, roaring in ears; audiometric testing needed before, after long-term therapy
• Assess for visual changes: blurring, halos; may indicate corneal, retinal damage
• Check for edema in feet, ankles, legs
• Identify prior drug history; there are many drug interactions
• Monitor pain: location, frequency, duration, characteristics, type, intensity before dose and 1 hour after; assess ROM before dose and after
• Assess for asthma, aspirin hypersensitivity, or nasal polyps, increased risk of hypersensitivity

Nursing diagnoses

☑Pain (uses)
☑Mobility, impaired (uses)
☑Injury, risk for (adverse reactions)
☑Knowledge deficit (teaching)

Implementation

• Administer to patient crushed or whole
• Give with food or milk to decrease gastric symptoms; give ½ hr ac or 2 hr pc for better absorption

Patient/family education

• Teach patient to report any symptoms of hepatotoxicity, renal toxicity, visual changes, ototoxicity, allergic reactions, bleeding (long-term therapy)
• Advise patient to take with 8 oz of water and sit upright for 30 min after dose to prevent ulceration
• Caution patient not to exceed recommended dosage; acute poisoning may result; to take as prescribed, do not double dose
• Advise to use sunscreen to prevent photosensitivity reactions
• Teach patient to read label on other OTC drugs; many contain other antiinflammatories; caution patient to avoid alcohol ingestion; GI bleeding may occur
• Inform patient that the therapeutic response takes 2 wk (arthritis)
• Teach patient to report tinnitus, confusion, diarrhea, sweating, hyperventilation, blurred vision, fever, joint aches, black stools, flu-like symptoms

Evaluation
Positive therapeutic outcome

• Decreased pain
• Decreased inflammation
• Increased mobility

N

naratriptan (R)
(nair'ah-trip-tan)
Amerge
Func. class.: Migraine agent
Chem. class.: 5-HT$_1$-like receptor agonist
Pregnancy category C

Action: Binds selectively to the vascular 5-HT$_1$ receptor subtype, exerts antimigraine effect; causes vasoconstriction in cranial arteries

➔**Therapeutic Outcome:** Decreased intensity and incidence of migraines

Uses: Acute treatment of migraine with or without aura

Dosage and routes
Adult: PO 1 or 2.5 mg with fluids, if headache returns, repeat once after 4 hr, max 5 mg/24 hr

Hepatic/renal dose
Max 2.5 mg/24 hr

Available forms: Tab 1, 2.5 mg

Adverse effects
CV: Increased B/P, palpitations, **tachydysrhythmias, PR, QT$_C$, prolongation, ST/T wave changes, PVCs, atrial flutter, fibrillation, coronary vasospasm**
EENT: EENT infections, photophobia
GI: Nausea, vomiting
MISC: Temperature change sensations, tightness, pressure sensations
MS: Weakness, neck stiffness, myalgia
NEURO: Dizziness, sedation, fatigue

Contraindications: Angina pectoris, history of MI, docu-mented silent ischemia, ischemic heart disease, concurrent ergotamine-containing preparations, uncontrolled hypertension, hypersensitivity, severe renal disease (CrCl <15 ml/min); severe hepatic disease **P** (child-Pugh grade C)

Precautions: Postmenopausal women, men >40 yr, risk factors for CAD, hypercholesterolemia, obesity, diabetes, impaired hepatic or renal function, pregnancy **C,** lacta-**P** tion, children, elderly, periph-**G** eral vascular disease

Pharmacokinetics	
Absorption	Unknown
Distribution	28%-31% protein binding
Metabolism	Liver (metabolite)
Excretion	Urine/feces
Half-life	6 hr

Pharmacodynamics	
Onset	Unknown
Peak	2-3 hr
Duration	Unknown

Interactions
Drug classifications
5-HT Agonists: ↑ vasospastic effect
Ergot derivatives: ↑ vasospastics effects
Oral contraceptives: ↑ naratriptan levels
SSRIs: ↑ weakness, hyperreflexia, incoordination
Smoking: ↑ clearance of naratriptan

NURSING CONSIDERATIONS
Assessment
• Assess for stress level, activity, recreation, coping mechanisms
• Assess neurologic status: LOC blurred vision, nausea,

vomiting, tingling in extremities preceding headache

Nursing diagnoses
☑ Pain (uses)
☑ Knowledge deficit (teaching)
☑ Noncompliance (teaching)

Implementation
- Give with fluids
- Provide a quiet, calm environment with decreased stimulation for noise, bright light, excessive talking

Patient/family education
- Teach patient to report any side effect to prescriber
- Teach patient to use contraception while taking drug
- Advise patient not to use if another 5-HT agonist or an ergot preparation has been used in the past 24 hrs

Evaluation
Positive therapeutic outcome
- Absence of migraine headaches

---

nedocromil (℞)
(ned-o-kroe'mil)
Tilade
Func. class.: Antiasthmatic
Chem. class.: Mast cell stabilizer
Pregnancy category   B

Action: Stabilizes the membrane of the sensitized mast cell, preventing release of chemical mediators after an antigen-IgE interaction

▶ **Therapeutic Outcome:** Reduced symptoms of asthma

Uses: Allergic rhinitis, severe perennial bronchial asthma, exercise-induced bronchospasm (prevention), prevention of acute bronchospasm induced by environmental pollutants, mastocytosis

Dosage and routes
Bronchospasm
▣ *Adult and child >12 yr:* 2 inh 2-4 times a day at regular intervals to provide 14 g/day

Bronchial asthma
▣ *Adult and child >12 yr:* Same as above

Available forms: 1.75 mg nedocromil per activation in 16.2-g canisters providing at least 112 metered inh

Adverse effects
CNS: Headache, dizziness, neuritis, dysphonia
EENT: Throat irritation, cough, nasal congestion, burning eyes, rhinitis
GI: Nausea, vomiting, anorexia, dry mouth, bitter taste

Contraindications: Hypersensitivity to this drug or lactose, status asthmaticus

Precautions: Pregnancy **B**, ▣ lactation, children

N

Pharmacokinetics
Absorption	Poorly, 3%
Distribution	Unknown
Metabolism	Not usually metabolized
Excretion	Small amounts in bile, urine unchanged
Half-life	80 min

Pharmacodynamics
Onset	Unknown
Peak	15 min
Duration	4-6 hr

Interactions: None

NURSING CONSIDERATIONS
Assessment
- Assess pulmonary function testing baseline

• Assess respiratory status: respiratory rate, rhythm, characteristics, cough, wheezing, dyspnea

Nursing diagnoses

☑ Airway clearance, ineffective (uses)

☑ Knowledge deficit (teaching)

Implementation
• Give by inh only with spacer device if needed
• Encourage patient to gargle, sip water to decrease irritation in throat

Patient/family education
• Instruct patient to clear mucus before using
• Teach patient proper inh technique: exhale; using inhaler, inhale deeply with head tipped back to open airway; remove, hold breath, exhale
• Inform patient that therapeutic effect may take up to 4 wk
• Teach patient that drug is preventive only, not restorative

Evaluation
Positive therapeutic outcome
• Decrease in asthmatic symptoms

---

nefazodone (℞)

(nef-az′oe-done)

Serzone

Func. class.: Antidepressant-misc

Chem. class.: Phenylpiperazine

Pregnancy category C

Action: Selectively inhibits serotonin uptake by brain, potentiates behavioral changes, occupies central HT_2 receptors

▷**Therapeutic Outcome:** Decreased symptoms of depression after 2-3 wk

Uses: Major depression

Dosage and routes
Adult: PO 200 mg/day (100 mg bid); dosage may be increased to 300 mg/day (150 bid); max 600 mg/day

G *Elderly:* PO 100 mg/day (50 mg bid); increase to 100 mg bid after 2 wk to desired dose

Available forms: Tabs 100, 150, 200, 250 mg

Adverse effects
CNS: Dizziness, headache, insomnia
CV: Postural hypotension
EENT: Blurred vision
GI: Nausea, constipation, dry mouth
GU: Urinary frequency, retention, UTI
RESP: Pharyngitis, cough

Contraindications: Hypersensitivity to this drug or phenylpiperazines

Precautions: Pregnancy **C**,
P lactation, children, elderly,
G cardiovascular disease, seizure disorder

Pharmacokinetics	
Absorption	Well absorbed
Distribution	Widely distributed; crosses placenta
Metabolism	Liver, extensively, to metabolites
Excretion	Kidneys, breast milk
Half-life	2-4 hr

Pharmacodynamics	
Onset	Unknown
Peak	1-3 hr
Duration	Unknown

Interactions

Individual drugs

Alcohol: ↑ CNS depression
Alprazolam: ↑ toxicity
Midazolam: ↑ toxicity
Phenytoin: ↑ toxicity
Triazolam: ↑ toxicity

Drug classifications

Benzodiazepines: ↑ plasma concentrations
Barbiturates: ↑ effects
CNS depressants: ↑ effects
MAOIs: ↑ toxicity

NURSING CONSIDERATIONS
Assessment

* Monitor B/P (with patient lying, standing), pulse q4h; if systolic B/P drops 20 mm Hg hold drug, notify prescriber; take vital signs q4h in patients with cardiovascular disease
* Monitor blood studies: CBC, leukocytes, differential, cardiac enzymes if patient is receiving long-term therapy
* Monitor hepatic studies: AST, ALT, bilirubin
* Assess mental status: mood, sensorium, affect, suicidal tendencies; increase in psychiatric symptoms: depression, panic
* Monitor urinary retention, constipation is more likely to occur in the
G elderly
◑● Assess for withdrawal symptoms: headache, nausea, vomiting, muscle pain, weakness; do not usually occur unless drug was discontinued abruptly
* Identify alcohol consumption; if alcohol is consumed, hold dose until AM

Nursing diagnoses

☑ Coping, ineffective individual (uses)

☑ Knowledge deficit (teaching)
☑ Noncompliance (teaching)

Implementation

* Give with food or milk for GI symptoms
* Give crushed if patient is unable to swallow medication whole
* Store at room temp; do not freeze

Patient/family education

* Teach patient that therapeutic effects may take 3-4 wk
* Teach patient to use caution in driving and other activities requiring alertness because of drowsiness, dizziness; to avoid rising quickly from sitting to
G standing, especially elderly
* Teach patient to avoid alcohol ingestion, other CNS depressants, benzodiazepines
* Teach patient not to discontinue medication quickly after long-term use; may cause nausea, headache, malaise
* Teach patient to increase bulk in diet if constipation
G occurs, especially elderly
* Teach patient to take gum, hard sugarless candy, or frequent sips of water for dry mouth

Evaluation

Positive therapeutic outcome

* Decrease in depression
* Absence of suicidal thoughts

Treatment of overdose:

ECG monitoring, induce emesis, lavage, activated charcoal, administer anticonvulsant

N

nelfinavir (R)
(nell-fin'a-ver)
Viracept
Func. class.: Antiviral
Chem. class.: HIV protease inhibitor

Pregnancy category   B

Action: Inhibits human immunodeficiency virus (HIV) protease

➡ **Therapeutic Outcome:** Prevents maturation of the infectious virus

Uses: HIV alone or in combination

Dosage and routes
Adult: PO 750 mg tid

P *Child 2-13 yr:* PO 20-30 mg/kg tid

Available forms: Tabs 250 mg; oral powder 50 mg/g

Adverse effects
CNS: Headache, poor concentration, fatigue, anxiety, depression, **seizures**
CV: Bleeding
ENDO: Hypoglycemia, hyperlipidemia
GI: Diarrhea, nausea, anorexia, dyspepsia
HEMA: **Anemia, leukopenia, thrombocytopenia, Hgb abnormalities**
INTEG: Rash, dermatitis
OTHER: Asthenia

Contraindications: Hypersensitivity to protease inhibitors

Precautions: Liver disease, pregnancy **B**, lactation, hemophilia, PKU, renal disease

Pharmacokinetics

Absorption	Unknown
Distribution	98% protein binding
Metabolism	Liver, (minimal)
Excretion	Feces
Half-life	3½-5 hr

Pharmacodynamics

Onset	Unknown
Peak	2-4 hr
Duration	Unknown

Interactions
Individual drugs
Carbamazepine: ↓ nelfinavir levels
Dexamethasone: ↓ nelfinavir levels
Indinavir: ↑ nelfinavir effect
Lamivudine: ↓ effect of lamivudine
Midazolam: ↑ serious dysrhythmias
Nevirapine: ↓ nelfinavir effect
Phenobarbital: ↓ nelfinavir level
Phenytoin: ↓ nelfinavir level
Rifamycin: ↓ nelfinavir levels
Ritonavir: ↑ nelfinavir effect
Triazolam: ↑ serious dysrhythmias
Zidovudine: ↓ effect of zidovudine
Drug classifications
Ergots: ↑ serious dysrhythmias
Oral contraceptives: ↓ effect of contraceptive

NURSING CONSIDERATIONS
Assessment
• Assess signs of infection, anemia
• Monitor liver studies: ALT, AST
• Monitor C&S before drug therapy; drug may be taken as soon as culture is taken; repeat C&S after treatment; determine the presence of other sexually transmitted diseases

- Assess bowel pattern before, during treatment; if severe abdominal pain with bleeding occurs, drug should be discontinued; monitor hydration
- Assess skin eruptions, rash, urticaria, itching
- Assess allergies before treatment, reaction of each medication; place allergies on chart

Nursing diagnoses

✓ Infection, risk for (uses)

✓ Knowledge deficit (teaching)

Implementation

- Administer with food
- Oral powder can be mixed with fluids, do not mix with juice or acidic fluids, stable mixed for 6 hr

Patient/family education

- Advise patient to take with meal or snack; if dose is missed, take as soon as remembered up to 1 hr before next dose; do not double dose
- Advise to avoid taking with other medications, unless directed by prescriber
- Teach that drug does not cure, but manages symptoms
- Teach to use nonhormonal form of contraception while taking this drug

---

neomycin (℞)

(nee-oh-mye′sin)

Mycifradin, Myciguent

Func. class.: Antiinfective

Chem. class.: Aminoglycoside

Pregnancy category   C

Action: Interferes with protein synthesis in bacterial cell by binding to 30S ribosomal subunit causing inaccurate

peptide sequence to form in protein chain, resulting in bacterial death

▶**Therapeutic Outcome:** Bactericidal effects for *Pseudomonas aeruginosa, Escherichia coli, Enterobacter,* enteropathogenic *E. coli, Klebsiella pneumoniae, Proteus vulgaris*

Uses: Severe systemic infections of CNS, respiratory tract, GI tract, urinary tract, eye, bone, skin, soft tissues, also used for hepatic coma, preoperatively to sterilize bowel, infectious diarrhea; minor skin infections (top)

Dosage and routes

Hepatic coma

Adult: PO 4-12 g/day in divided doses times 5-6 days

P *Child:* PO 50-100 mg/kg/day in divided doses

Preoperative bowel sterilization

Adult: PO on 3rd day of a 3-day regimen; give 1 g early PM; repeat in 1 hr; repeat at hs (given with erythromycin); give saline cathartic before giving this drug

Skin infection

P *Adult and child:* Top 0.5% cream or ointment qd-tid

Available forms: Tab 500 mg; top 500 mg; oral sol 125 mg/5 ml

Adverse effects

CNS: Confusion, depression, numbness, tremors, **convulsions,** muscle twitching, **neurotoxicity,** dizziness, vertigo

CV: Hypotension, hypertension, palpitations

EENT: Ototoxicity, deafness, visual disturbances, tinnitus

GI: Nausea, vomiting, anorexia, increased ALT, AST,

---

bilirubin, hepatomegaly, **hepatic necrosis,** splenomegaly
GU: **Oliguria, hematuria, renal damage, azotemia, renal failure, nephrotoxicity**
HEMA: **Agranulocytosis, thrombocytopenia,** leukopenia, eosinophilia, anemia
INTEG: Rash, burning, urticaria, photosensitivity, dermatitis, alopecia

Contraindications: Bowel obstruction (oral use), severe renal disease, hypersensitivity, **P** infants, children

Precautions: Mild renal disease, pregnancy **C,** hearing deficits, lactation, myasthenia gravis, Parkinson's disease

Pharmacokinetics

Absorption	Well absorbed (IM); minimally absorbed (top)
Distribution	Unknown
Metabolism	Liver, minimal
Excretion	Feces, unchanged
Half-life	2-3 hr

Pharmacodynamics

	IM
Onset	Rapid
Peak	1-2 hr
Duration	6-8 hr

Interactions
Individual drugs
Amphotericin B: ↑ ototoxicity, neurotoxicity, nephrotoxicity
Cisplatin: ↑ ototoxicity, neurotoxicity, nephrotoxicity
Ethacrynic acid: ↑ ototoxicity, neurotoxicity, nephrotoxicity
Furosemide: ↑ ototoxicity, neurotoxicity, nephrotoxicity
Mannitol: ↑ ototoxicity, neurotoxicity, nephrotoxicity
Methoxyflurane: ↑ ototoxicity, neurotoxicity, nephrotoxicity

Polymyxin: ↑ ototoxicity, neurotoxicity, nephrotoxicity
Succinylcholine: ↑ neuromuscular blockade, respiratory depression
Vancomycin: ↑ ototoxicity, neurotoxicity, nephrotoxicity
Drug classifications
Aminoglycosides: ↑ ototoxicity, neurotoxicity, nephrotoxicity
Anesthetics, inhalation: ↑ neuromuscular blockade, respiratory depression
Nondepolarizing neuromuscular blockers: ↑ neuromuscular blockade, respiratory depression

NURSING CONSIDERATIONS
Assessment
- Assess patient for previous sensitivity reaction
- Assess patient for signs and symptoms of infection: characteristics of skin; obtain baseline information and during treatment
- Obtain C&S before beginning drug therapy to identify if correct treatment has been initiated
- Assess for allergic reactions: rash, urticaria, pruritus, chills, fever, joint pain

Nursing diagnoses
☑ Infection, risk for (uses)
☑ Knowledge deficit (teaching)
☑ Noncompliance (teaching)

Implementation
PO route
- Give as a preoperative medication before bowel surgery

Patient/family education
- Instruct patient to take all medication prescribed for the length of time ordered
- Advise patient to report headache, dizziness, symptoms of overgrowth of infection and

loss of hearing, ringing or roaring in ears

Evaluation
Positive therapeutic outcome
- Reported improvement in symptoms of infection (top)

Treatment of overdose: Withdraw drug; hemodialysis; monitor serum levels of drug

---

neostigmine (R)
(nee-oh-stig'meen)
neostigmine, Prostigmin
Func. class.: Cholinergic stimulant; anticholinesterase
Chem. class.: Quaternary compound
Pregnancy category   C

Action: Inhibits destruction of acetylcholine, which increases concentration at sites where acetylcholine is released; this facilitates transmission of impulses across the myoneural junction

➡️**Therapeutic Outcome:** Increased strength in myasthenia gravis, reversal of nondepolarizing muscular blockers

Uses: Myasthenia gravis, nondepolarizing neuromuscular blocker antagonist, bladder distention, postoperative ileus

Dosage and routes
Myasthenia gravis
Adult: PO 15-375 mg/day; IM/**IV** 0.5-2 mg q1-3h
🅟 *Child:* PO 2 mg/kg/day q3-4h

Nondepolarizing neuromuscular blocker antagonist
Adult: **IV** 0.5-2 mg slowly; may repeat if needed (give

0.6-1.2 mg atropine before this drug)
🅟 *Infant/child:* **IV** 0.025-0.1 mg/kg/dose

Abdominal distention/ postoperative ileus
Adult: IM/SC 0.25-1 mg (1:4000) q4-6h depending on condition × 2-3 days

Renal dose
CrCl 10-50 ml/min 50% of dose; CrCl <10 ml/min 25% of dose

Available forms: Tab 15 mg; inj 1:1000, 1:2000, 1:4000

Adverse effects
CNS: Dizziness, headache, sweating, weakness, **convulsions,** incoordination, **paralysis,** drowsiness, LOC
CV: Tachycardia, **dysrhythmias,** bradycardia, hypotension, AV block, ECG changes, **cardiac arrest,** syncope
EENT: Miosis, blurred vision, lacrimation, visual changes
GI: Nausea, diarrhea, vomiting, cramps, increased peristalsis, salivary and gastric secretions
GU: Frequency, incontinence, urgency
INTEG: Rash, urticaria, flushing
RESP: **Respiratory depression, bronchospasm, constriction, laryngospasm, respiratory arrest, dyspnea**

Contraindications: Obstruction of intestine, renal system, bromide sensitivity, peritonitis

Precautions: Bradycardia, hypotension, seizure disorders, bronchial asthma, coronary occlusion, hyperthyroidism, dysrhythmias, peptic ulcer, pregnancy **C,** megacolon,

N

poor GI motility, lactation,
P children

Pharmacokinetics

Absorption	Poorly absorbed (PO), completely absorbed (**IV**)
Distribution	Unknown
Metabolism	Liver
Excretion	Kidneys
Half-life	40-90 min

Pharmacodynamics

	PO	IM	IV
Onset	45-75 min	10-30 min	4-8 min
Peak	Unknown	30 min	30 min
Duration	2½-4 hr	2½-4 hr	2-4 hr

Interactions
Individual drugs
Atropine: ↓ action of atropine
Mecamylamine: ↓ action of neostigmine
Polymyxin: ↓ action of neostigmine
Procainamide: ↓ action of neostigmine
Quinidine: ↓ action of neostigmine
Drug classifications
Antidepressants: ↑ antagonism
Antihistamines: ↑ antagonism
Cholinesterase inhibitors: ↑ toxicity
Muscle relaxants, depolarizing: ↑ action of muscle relaxants
Phenothiazines: ↑ antagonism

NURSING CONSIDERATIONS
Assessment
• Monitor VS, respiration during rest
◆• Monitor for bradycardia, hypotension, bronchospasm, headache, dizziness, convulsions, respiratory depression;

drug should be discontinued if toxicity occurs
Nursing diagnoses
☑ Breathing pattern, ineffective (uses)
☑ Knowledge deficit (teaching)
Implementation
PO route
• Give only after all other cholinergics have been discontinued
• Increased dosage may be needed if tolerance develops
• Give larger doses after exercise or fatigue
• Administer on empty stomach for better absorption
• Store at room temp
IV IV route
• Give direct **IV** undiluted, through Y-tube or 3-way stopcock; give 0.5 mg or less over 1 min
• Give only with atropine sulfate available for cholinergic crisis

Syringe compatibilities:
Glycopyrrolate, heparin, pentobarbital, thiopental

Y-site compatibilities:
Heparin, hydrocortisone sodium succinate, potassium chloride, vit B/C

Additive compatibilities:
Netilmicin

Patient/family education
• Teach patient to wear Medic Alert ID specifying myasthenia gravis, drugs taken, prescriber's phone number

Evaluation
Positive therapeutic outcome
• Increased muscle strength, hand grasp
• Improved gait
• Absence of labored breathing (if severe)

Treatment of overdose:
Respiratory support, **IV** atropine 1-4 mg

nevirapine (℞)
(ne-veer′a-peen)
Viramune
Func. class.: Antiviral
Chem. class: Nonnucleoside reverse transcriptase inhibitor
(NNRTI)
Pregnancy category C

Action: Binds directly to reverse transcriptase and blocks
RNA, DNA causing a disruption of the enzyme's site

▷**Therapeutic Outcome:** Improvement of HIV-1 infection

Uses: HIV-1 in combination
with nucleoside analogs in
those experiencing deterioration

Dosage and routes
Adult: PO 200 mg qd × 2 wk,
then 200 mg bid in combination with nucleoside analogs

Available forms: Tabs 200
mg

Adverse effects
CNS: Paresthesia, headache,
fever, peripheral neuropathy
GI: Diarrhea, abdominal pain,
nausea, stomatitis, hepatitis
HEMA: Neutropenia, anemia, thrombocytopenia
INTEG: Rash
MS: Pain, myalgia

Contraindications: Hypersensitivity

Precautions: Liver disease,
P pregnancy **C,** lactation, children, renal disease

Pharmacokinetics
Absorption	Rapid
Distribution	60% bound to plasma proteins
Metabolism	Liver
Excretion	Unknown
Half-life	Unknown

Pharmacodynamics
Unknown

Interactions
Drug classifications
Oral contraceptives: ↓ action
Protease inhibitors: ↓ action
Rifamycins: ↓ nevirapine levels

NURSING CONSIDERATIONS
Assessment
• Assess signs of infection,
anemia
• Assess liver, renal, blood studies: ALT, AST; viral load, CD_4
• Assess C&S before drug
therapy; drug may be taken as
soon as culture is taken; repeat
C&S after treatment; determine the presence of other
sexually transmitted disease
• Assess bowel pattern before,
during treatment; if severe
abdominal pain with bleeding
occurs, drug should be discontinued; monitor hydration
• Assess skin eruptions; rash,
urticaria, itching
• Assess allergies before treatment, reaction to each medication; place allergies on chart

Nursing diagnoses
☑ Infection, risk for (uses)
☑ Diarrhea (side effects)
☑ Knowledge deficit (teaching)

Implementation
• Give without regard to meals

Patient/family education
• Instruct patient to report any
right quadrant pain, jaundice,
rash immediately

N

• Inform patient that drug may be taken with food, antacids, didanosine
• Advise patient to take as prescribed; if dose is missed, take as soon as remembered up to 1 hr before next dose; do not double dose
• Advise patient that drug must be taken in equal intervals around the clock to maintain blood levels for duration of therapy
• Advise patient that drug is not a cure, controls symptoms of HIV
• Instruct patient to avoid OTC agents unless approved by prescriber
• Advise patient to use a non-hormonal form of contraception during treatment

---

niacin (nicotinic acid)/ niacinamide (PO, OTC; IV/IM/SC, ℞)

(nye'a-sin) (nye-a-sin'a-mide)

Nia-Bid, Niac, Niacels, Niacin TD, SpaN Niacin, Niacin TR, Niacor, Niaspan, Nico-400, Nicobid, Nicolar, Nicotinex, nicotinic acid, Novaniacin ✦, Slo-Niacin, Tri-B₃ ✦, Vitamin B₃, Nicothamide

Func. class.: Vitamin B_3
Chem. class.: Water-soluble vitamin, lipid-lowering drug

Pregnancy category **C**

Action: Needed for conversion of fats, protein, carbohydrates by oxidation-reduction; acts directly on vascular smooth muscle, causing vasodilatation; high dosages decrease serum lipids

▸**Therapeutic Outcome:** Decreasing cholesterol and low-density lipoprotein levels, vitamin B_3 supplementation

Uses: Pellagra, hyperlipidemias, peripheral vascular disease

Dosage and routes
Niacin deficiency
Adult: PO up to 500 mg/day in divided doses; IM/SC 5-100 mg 5 or more times a day; **IV** 25-100 mg bid or tid

P *Child:* PO up to 300 mg/day in divided doses

Adjunct in hyperlipidemia
Adult: PO 500 mg qd in 3 divided doses pc; may be increased to 4 g/day

Pellagra
Adult: PO 300-500 mg, qd in divided doses

P *Child:* PO 100-300 mg qd in divided doses

Peripheral vascular disease
Adult: PO 250-800 mg qd in divided doses

Available forms: Niacin, tabs 25, 50, 100, 125, 500 mg; time rel caps 125, 250, 300, 400, 500 mg; time ext tabs 125, 250, 375, 500, 750, 1000 mg; elix 50 mg/5 ml; cap, ext rel 125, 250, 300, 400, 500 mg; nicotinamide, tabs 50, 100, 125, 250, 500 mg

Adverse effects
CNS: Paresthesias, headache, dizziness, anxiety
CV: Postural hypotension, vasovagal attacks, dysrhythmias, vasodilatation
EENT: Blurred vision, ptosis
GI: Nausea, vomiting, an-

orexia, flatulence, xerostomia, *jaundice,* diarrhea, peptic ulcer
GU: Hyperuricemia, **glycosuria, hypoalbuminemia**
INTEG: Flushing, dry skin, rash, pruritus
RESP: Wheezing

Contraindications: Hypersensitivity, peptic ulcer, hepatic disease, lactation, hemorrhage, severe hypotension

Precautions: Glaucoma, cardiovascular disease, CAD, diabetes mellitus, gout, schizophrenia, pregnancy **C**

Do Not Confuse:
Nicobid/Nitro-Bid

Pharmacokinetics

Absorption	Well absorbed (PO)
Distribution	Widely distributed
Metabolism	Converted to niacinamide
Excretion	Urine, unchanged (30%); breast milk
Half-life	45 min

Pharmacodynamics

	PO	IV
Onset	Unknown	Unknown
Peak	30-70 min	Unknown
Duration	Unknown	Unknown

Interactions
Individual drugs
Guanadrel: ↑ hypotension
Guanethidine: ↑ hypotension
Lovastatin: ↑ myopathy
Probenecid: ↑ uricosuric effects
Sulfinpyrazone: ↑ uricosuric effects
Lab test interferences
↑ Bilirubin, ↑ alkaline phosphatase, ↑ liver enzymes, ↑ LDH, ↑ uric acid
↓ Cholesterol
False: ↑ Urinary catecholamines
False positive: Urine glucose

NURSING CONSIDERATIONS
Assessment
• Assess for niacin deficiency (pellagra): nausea, vomiting, stomatitis, confusion, hallucinations before and throughout treatment
• Assess for symptoms of niacin deficiency: nausea, vomiting, anemia, poor memory, confusion, dermatitis
• Assess for lipid, triglyceride, cholesterol level, if using for hyperlipidemia
• Assess nutrition: fat, protein, carbohydrates, nutritional analysis should be completed by dietician
• Monitor liver function studies: AST, ALT, bilirubin, uric acid, alkaline phosphatase; blood glucose before and during treatment; liver dysfunction: clay-colored stools, itching, dark urine, jaundice
• Monitor niacin levels during administration of this drug
• Monitor cardiac status: rate, rhythm, quality; postural hypotension, dysrhythmias
• Monitor nutritional status: liver, yeast, legumes, organ meat, lean poultry; high-level niacin products should be included in the diet
• Assess for CNS symptoms: headache, paresthesias, blurred vision

Nursing diagnoses
✓ Nutrition, less than body requirements (uses)
✓ Knowledge deficit (teaching)
✓ Noncompliance (teaching)

Implementation
PO route
• Give with meals or milk for GI symptoms, and 325 mg aspirin ½ h before dose to decrease flushing

N

🚫 • Do not crush, break, or chew ext rel products

IV IV route

• Give by direct **IV** after diluting to 2 mg/ml at a rate of ≤2 mg/min

• Give by inf by adding 500 ml of 0.9% NaCl at a rate of ≤2 mg/min

Additive incompatibilities:
Acids (strong), alkalis, erythromycin, kanamycin, streptomycin

Additive compatibilities:
TPN sol

Patient/family education

• Advise patient that flushing and increase in feelings of warmth will occur several hr after taking drug (PO); after 2 wk of therapy these side effects diminish

• Instruct patient to remain recumbent if postural hypotension occurs; to rise slowly from sitting or recumbent

• Caution patient to abstain from alcohol if drug is prescribed for hyperlipidemia

• Caution patient to avoid sunlight if skin lesions are present

Evaluation

Positive therapeutic outcome

• Decreased lipid levels

• Warm extremities

• Absence of numbness in extremities

---

nicardipine (℞)
(nye-card′i-peen)
Cardene, Cardene IV, Cardene SR
Func. class.: Calcium channel blocker, antianginal, antihypertensive
Chem. class.: Dihydropyridine
Pregnancy category C

Action: Inhibits calcium ion influx across cell membrane during cardiac depolarization, produces relaxation of coronary vascular smooth muscle and peripheral vascular smooth muscle, dilates coronary arteries, increases myocardial oxygen delivery in patients with vasospastic angina

➡ **Therapeutic Outcome:** Decreased angina pectoris, decreased B/P in hypertension

Uses: Chronic stable angina pectoris, hypertension

Dosage and routes
Adult: PO 20 mg tid initially; may increase after 3 days (range 20-40 mg tid) or 30 mg bid sus rel, may increase to 60 mg bid

Available forms: Caps 20, 30 mg; sus rel caps 30, 45, 60 mg; inj 2.5 mg/ml

Adverse effects
CNS: Headache, fatigue, drowsiness, dizziness, anxiety, depression, weakness, insomnia, confusion, paresthesia, somnolence
CV: **Dysrhythmia,** edema, **CHF,** bradycardia, hypotension, palpitations, **MI, pulmonary edema**
GI: Nausea, vomiting, diarrhea, gastric upset, constipa-

---

tion, **hepatitis,** abdominal cramps
GU: Nocturia, polyuria, **acute renal failure**
INTEG: Rash, pruritus, urticaria, photosensitivity, hair loss
MISC: Blurred vision, flushing, nasal congestion, sweating, shortness of breath, gynecomastia, hyperglycemia, sexual difficulties, **Stevens-Johnson syndrome**

Contraindications: Sick sinus syndrome, 2nd- or 3rd-degree heart block, hypotension less than 90 mm Hg systolic, hypersensitivity

Precautions: CHF, hypotension, hepatic injury, pregnancy
P **C,** lactation, children, renal
G disease, elderly

Do Not Confuse:
Cardene/Cardizem, Cardene SR/Cardizem SR

Pharmacokinetics
Absorption	Well absorbed (PO); bioavailability poor
Distribution	Unknown
Metabolism	Liver, extensively
Excretion	Kidneys, minimal
Half-life	2-5 hr

Pharmacodynamics
	PO	PO-SUS REL
Onset	½ hr	Unknown
Peak	1-2 hr	2-6 hr
Duration	8 hr	10-12 hr

Interactions
Individual drugs
Alcohol: ↑ hypotension
Carbamazepine: ↑ risk of toxicity
Cimetidine: ↑ risk of toxicity
Cyclosporine: ↑ risk of toxicity
Digoxin: ↑ digoxin levels, bradycardia, CHF

Phenobarbital: ↓ effectiveness
Phenytoin: ↓ effectiveness
Prazosin: ↑ risk of toxicity
Propranolol: ↑ toxicity
Quinidine: ↑ risk of toxicity
Drug classifications
Antihypertensives: ↑ hypotension
β-Adrenergic blockers: ↑ bradycardia, CHF
Nitrates: ↑ hypotension
NSAIDs: ↓ antihypertensive effect
Food/drug
Grapefruit: ↑ hypotensive effect

NURSING CONSIDERATIONS
Assessment
• Assess fluid volume status (I&O ratio) and record weight, color, quality and sp gr of urine, skin turgor, adequacy of pulses, moist mucous membranes, bilateral lung sounds, peripheral pitting edema; dehydration symptoms of decreasing output, thirst, hypotension, dry mouth, and mucous membranes should be reported
• Monitor B/P and pulse
• Assess anginal pain: intensity, location, duration, alleviating factors
• Monitor potassium, LFTs, renal studies periodically

Nursing diagnoses
☑ Cardiac output, decreased (uses)
☑ Knowledge deficit (teaching)

Implementation
• Give with or without regard to meals
• Store in tight container at room temp
IV **IV route**
• Dilute each 25 mg/240 ml of compatible sol (0.1 mg/ml), give slowly, stable for 24 hr at room temp

Y-*site compatibilities:*
Diltiazem, dobutamine, dopamine, epinephrine, fentanyl, hydromorphone, labetalol, lorazepam, midazolam, milrinone, morphine, nitroglycerin, norepinephrine, ranitidine, vecuronium

Patient/family education
• Advise patient to avoid hazardous activities until stabilized on drug and dizziness is no longer a problem
• Instruct patient to limit caffeine consumption; to avoid alcohol and OTC drugs unless directed by a prescriber
• Instruct patient to comply in all areas of medical regimen: diet, exercise, stress reduction, drug therapy; to notify prescriber of irregular heart beat, shortness of breath, swelling of feet and hands, pronounced dizziness, constipation, nausea, hypotension
• Teach patient to use medication as directed even if feeling better; may be taken with other cardiovascular drugs (nitrates, β-blockers)
• Teach patient to take medication exactly as prescribed
• Advise patient to contact prescriber if anginal attacks continue or become worse

Evaluation
Positive therapeutic outcome
• Decreased angina attacks
• Decreased B/P

Treatment of overdose:
Defibrillation, atropine for AV block, vasopressor for hypotension

---

nicotine polacrilex gum (OTC)
(nik'o-teen)
Nicorette, Nicorette DS
Func. class.: Smoking deterrent
Chem. class.: Ganglionic cholinergic agonist

Pregnancy category D

Action: Agonist at nicotinic receptors in the peripheral and central nervous systems; acts at sympathetic ganglia, on chemoreceptors of the aorta and carotid bodies; also affects adrenalin-releasing catecholamines

Therapeutic Outcome: Decreased withdrawal effects when smoking cessation is attempted

Uses: Deter cigarette smoking

Dosage and routes
Adult: Gum 1 piece chewed × 30 min as needed to abstain from smoking; not to exceed 30/day

Available forms: Gum 2, 4 mg/piece of gum

Adverse effects
CNS: Dizziness, vertigo, insomnia, headache, confusion, convulsions, depression, euphoria, numbness, tinnitus
CV: **Dysrhythmias,** tachycardia, palpitations, edema, flushing, hypertension
EENT: Jaw ache, irritation in buccal cavity
GI: Nausea, vomiting, anorexia, indigestion, diarrhea, abdominal pain, constipation, eructation
RESP: Breathing difficulty, cough, hoarseness, sneezing, wheezing

---

Contraindications: Hypersensitivity, immediate post-MI recovery period, severe angina pectoris, pregnancy **D**

Precautions: Vasospastic disease, dysrhythmias, diabetes mellitus, hyperthyroidism, pheochromocytoma, coronary disease, esophagitis, peptic ulcer, lactation, hepatic/renal disease

Pharmacokinetics
Absorption	Slowly absorbed, buccal cavity
Distribution	Unknown
Metabolism	Liver; some by lungs, kidneys
Excretion	Kidneys, unchanged (20%); breast milk
Half-life	1-2 hr

Pharmacodynamics
Onset	Rapid
Peak	½ hr
Duration	Unknown

Interactions
Individual drugs
Acetaminophen: ↑ effects of acetaminophen
Caffeine: ↑ effects of caffeine
Furosemide: ↑ effects of furosemide
Imipramine: ↑ effects of imipramine
Oxazepam: ↑ effects of oxazepam
Pentazocine: ↑ effects of pentazocine
Propranolol: ↑ effects of propranolol

NURSING CONSIDERATIONS
Assessment
• Assess for adverse reaction to gum: irritation of buccal cavity, dislike of taste, jaw ache
• Assess for withdrawal symptoms: headache, fatigue, drowsiness, restlessness, irritability, severe cravings for nicotine products before, during, and after treatment
• Obtain a nicotine assessment: brand of cigarettes, chewing tobacco, cigars, number of each used per day; what increases need or activities performed when each is used
• Gum should not be used if temporomandibular condition exists
• Assess for nicotine toxicity: GI symptoms (nausea, vomiting, diarrhea), cardiopulmonary symptoms (decreased B/P, dyspnea, change in pulse), weakness, abdominal cramping, headache, blurred vision, tinnitus; drug should be discontinued

Nursing diagnoses
☑ Coping, ineffective individual (uses)
☑ Knowledge deficit (teaching)
☑ Noncompliance (teaching)

Implementation
• Give only prescribed amount, or toxicity may occur
• Protect gum from light and heat

Patient/family education
• Instruct patient to chew gum slowly for 30 min to promote buccal absorption of the drug; do not chew over 45 min
• Advise patient to begin drug withdrawal after 3 mo use; do not exceed 6 mo
• Teach patient all aspects of drug; give package insert to patient and explain; caution patient not to exceed prescribed dose
• Inform patient that gum will not stick to dentures, dental appliances
• Caution patient that gum is as toxic as cigarettes; it is to be used only to deter smoking
• Caution patient not to use

N

during pregnancy; birth defects may occur

Evaluation
Positive therapeutic outcome
- Decrease in urge to smoke
- Decreased need for gum after 3-6 mo

nicotine transdermal/inhaler system (℞, OTC)
Habitrol, Nicoderm, Nicotrol, Prostep
Func. class.: Smoking deterrent
Chem. class.: Ganglionic cholinergic agonist
Pregnancy category   D

Action: Agonist at nicotinic receptors in peripheral, central nervous systems; acts at sympathetic ganglia, on chemoreceptors of aorta, carotid bodies; also affects adrenaline-releasing catecholamines

➡ **Therapeutic Outcome:** Decreased withdrawal efforts when smoking cessation is attempted

Uses: Deter cigarette smoking

Dosage and routes
Nicotrol
Adult: Transdermal 15 mg/day × 12 wk; 10 mg/day × 2 wk; 5 mg/day × 2 wk

Prostep
Adult: Transdermal 22 mg/day × 4-8 wk; 11 mg/day × 2-4 wk

Nicoderm/Habitrol
Adult: Transdermal 21 mg/day × 6 wk; 14 mg/day × 14 days; 7 mg/day × 14 days

Nicotrol inhaler
Delivers 30% of what a smoker receives from an actual cigarette

Available forms: Transdermal patch delivering 7, 14, 21 mg; 15 mg, 10 mg, 5 mg, 22 mg, 11 mg/day patches depending on product; nicotine inhaler

Adverse effects
CNS: Abnormal dreams, *insomnia*, nervousness, *headache*, dizziness, paresthesia, poor concentration, weakness
EENT: Dry mouth, abnormal taste
GI: Diarrhea, dyspepsia, constipation, nausea, abdominal pain, vomiting, dry mouth, abnormal taste
INTEG: Erythema, pruritus, burning at application site, hypersensitivity, sweating, rash
MISC: Chest pain, dysmenorrhea
MS: Arthralgia, myalgia, back pain
RESP: Cough, sinusitis

Contraindications: Hypersensitivity, children, pregnancy **D**, nonsmokers, during immediate post-MI period, life-threatening dysrhythmias, severe or worsening angina pectoris

Precautions: Skin disease, angina pectoris, MI, renal or hepatic insufficiency, peptic ulcer, accelerated hypertension, serious cardiac dysrhythmias, hyperthyroidism, pheochromocytoma, insulin-dependent diabetes, elderly

Pharmacokinetics	
Absorption	Slowly absorbed
Distribution	Unknown
Metabolism	Liver
Excretion	Kidneys, unchanged (20%)
Half-life	1-2 hr

Pharmacodynamics	
Onset	Rapid
Peak	½ hr
Duration	Unknown

Interactions
Individual drugs
Acetaminophen: ↑ effects of acetaminophen
Caffeine: ↑ effects of caffeine
Furosemide: ↑ effects of furosemide
Imipramine: ↑ effects of imipramine
Oxazepam: ↑ effects of oxazepam
Pentazocine: ↑ effects of pentazocine
Propranolol: ↑ effects of propranolol

NURSING CONSIDERATIONS
Assessment
• Monitor for adverse reaction: skin irritation, pruritus, burning at patch site
• Assess for withdrawal symptoms: headache, fatigue, drowsiness, restlessness, irritability, severe cravings for nicotine products before, during, and after treatment
• Obtain a nicotine assessment: brand of cigarettes, chewing tobacco, cigars, number of each used per day; what increases need or activities performed when each is used
• Assess for nicotine toxicity: GI symptoms (nausea, vomiting, diarrhea), cardiopulmonary symptoms (decreased B/P, dyspnea, change in pulse), weakness, abdominal cramping, headache, blurred vision, tinnitus; drug should be discontinued

Nursing diagnoses
☑ Coping, ineffective individual (uses)

☑ Knowledge deficit (teaching)
☑ Noncompliance (teaching)

Implementation
• Protect from heat
• Some patches are worn during the waking hr only (Nicotrol); other patches are worn 24 hr

Patient/family education
• Teach patient all aspects of drug; give package insert to patient and explain
• Caution patient that patch is as toxic as cigarettes; it is to be used only to deter smoking
• Caution patient not to use during pregnancy; birth defects may occur
• Caution patient to keep used and unused system out of reach of children and pets
• Instruct patient to apply once a day to a nonhairy, clean, dry area of skin on upper body or upper outer arm; some products are used during waking hr, some 24 hr/day; to rotate sites to prevent skin irritation
• Instruct patient to stop smoking immediately when beginning treatment with patch
• Teach patient to apply promptly after removing from protective pouch; system may lose strength

Inhaler route
• Puffing on mouthpiece delivers nicotine through the mouth lining

Evaluation
Positive therapeutic outcome
• Decrease in urge to smoke
• Decreased need for patch

N

nifedipine (R)
(nye-fed´i-peen)
Adalat, Adalat CC, Adalat
P.A. ✤, Apo-Nifed ✤, Novo-
Nifedin ✤, NuNifed ✤,
nifedipine, Procardia,
Procardia XL
Func. class.: Calcium
channel blocker, antiangi-
nal, antihypertensive
Chem. class.: Dihydropyri-
dine

Pregnancy category C

Action: Inhibits calcium ion
influx across cell membrane
during cardiac depolarization,
produces relaxation of coronary vascular smooth muscle
and peripheral vascular
smooth muscle, dilates coronary vascular arteries, increases myocardial oxygen
delivery in patients with vasospastic angina

➡ **Therapeutic Outcome:** Decreased angina pectoris, decreased B/P in hyperten-
sion

Uses: Chronic stable angina
pectoris, vasospastic angina,
hypertension

Investigational uses: Hypertension (acute), migraines,
CHF, Raynaud's disease

Dosage and routes
Adult: PO immediate release,
10 mg tid; increase in 10-mg
increments q4-6h, not to
exceed 180 mg/24 hr or single
dose of 30 mg; sus rel, 30-60
mg/day; may increase q7-14
days; doses >120 mg not recommended

P *Child:* PO 0.25-0.5 mg/kg/
dose q4-6h, max 1-2 mg/kg/
day

Available forms: Caps 5 ✤,
10, 20 mg; ext rel tabs 10 ✤,
20 ✤, 30, 60, 90 mg; tabs
10 mg ✤

Adverse effects
CNS: Headache, fatigue,
drowsiness, *dizziness,* anxiety,
depression, weakness, insomnia, *lightheadedness,* paresthesia, tinnitus, blurred vision,
nervousness
CV: **Dysrhythmias,** edema,
CHF, hypotension, palpitations, **MI, pulmonary edema,**
tachycardia
GI: Nausea, vomiting, diarrhea, gastric upset, constipation, increased liver function
studies, dry mouth
GU: Nocturia, polyuria
INTEG: Rash, pruritus, *flushing,* photosensitivity, hair loss
MISC: Sexual difficulties,
cough, fever, chills

Contraindications: Hypersensitivity

Precautions: CHF, hypotension, sick sinus syndrome, 2nd-
or 3rd-degree heart block,
hypotension less than 90 mm
Hg systolic, hepatic injury,
pregnancy **C,** lactation,
P children, renal disease

Pharmacokinetics	
Absorption	Well absorbed (PO)
Distribution	Unknown
Metabolism	Liver, extensively
Excretion	Unknown
Half-life	2-5 hr

Pharmacodynamics		
	PO	PO–SUS REL
Onset	½ hr	Unknown
Peak	Unknown	Unknown
Duration	6-8 hr	24 hr

Interactions
Individual drugs
Alcohol: ↑ hypotension
Carbamazepine: ↑ risk of toxicity
Cimetidine: ↑ risk of toxicity
Cyclosporine: ↑ risk of toxicity
Digoxin: ↑ digoxin levels, bradycardia, CHF
Prazosin: ↑ risk of toxicity
Propranolol: ↑ toxicity
Quinidine: ↑ risk of toxicity
Drug classifications
Antihypertensives: ↑ hypotension
β-Adrenergic blockers: ↑ bradycardia, CHF
Nitrates: ↑ nitrates
NSAIDs: ↓ antihypertensive effect
Food/drug
Grapefruit juice: ↑ nifedipine level
Lab test interferences
Positive: ANA, direct Coombs' test

NURSING CONSIDERATIONS
Assessment
• Assess anginal pain: location, intensity, duration, character, alleviating, aggravating factors
• Monitor potassium, LFTs, renal studies periodically during treatment
• Assess fluid volume status (I&O ratio) and record weight, distended red veins, crackles in lung, color, quality and sp gr of urine, skin turgor, adequacy of pulses, moist mucous membranes, bilateral lung sounds, peripheral pitting edema; dehydration symptoms of decreasing output, thirst, hypotension, dry mouth, and mucous membranes should be reported

• Monitor ALT, AST, bilirubin daily; if these are elevated, hepatotoxicity is suspected
• Monitor cardiac status: B/P, pulse, respirations, ECG
Nursing diagnoses
☑ Cardiac output, decreased (uses)
☑ Pain (uses)
☑ Knowledge deficit (teaching)
Implementation
PO route
• Give without regard to meals
• Store in tight container at room temp
Sublingual route
• Using a sterile needle puncture the cap and squeeze medication in buccal area (not an FDA-approved use)

Patient/family education
• Advise patient to avoid hazardous activities until stabilized on drug and dizziness is no longer a problem
• Instruct patient to limit caffeine consumption; to avoid alcohol and OTC drugs unless directed by prescriber
• Tell patient that ext rel has nonabsorbable shell, may appear in stools
• Instruct patient to comply in all areas of medical regimen: diet, exercise, stress reduction, drug therapy; to notify prescriber of irregular heart beat, shortness of breath, swelling of feet and hands, pronounced dizziness, constipation, nausea, hypotension
• Teach patient to use as directed even if feeling better; may be taken with other cardiovascular drugs (nitrates, β-blockers)

N

Evaluation
Positive therapeutic outcome
• Decreased angina attacks
• Decreased B/P

Treatment of overdose:
Defibrillation, atropine for AV block, vasopressor for hypotension

---

nilutamide (Ᵽ)
(nil-u′ta-mide)
Anandron ✦, Nilandron
Func. class.: Antineoplastic, hormone
Chem. class.: Antiandrogen

Pregnancy category   C

Action: Interferes with testosterone uptake in the nucleus or testosterone activity in target tissues; arrests tumor growth in androgen-sensitive tissue, i.e., prostate gland, prostatic carcinoma is androgen-sensitive, so tumor growth is arrested

➡ **Therapeutic Outcome:**
Decreased tumor size

Uses: Metastatic prostatic carcinoma, stage D2 in combination with surgical castration

Dosage and routes
Adult: PO 300 mg qd × 30 days, then 150 mg qd

Available forms: Tabs 50, 100 mg ✦

Adverse effects
CNS: Hot flashes, drowsiness, insomnia, dizziness, hyperthesia, depression
EENT: Delay in adaptation to dark
GU: Decreased libido, impotence, testicular atrophy, UTI, hematuria, nocturia, gynecomastia

GI: Diarrhea, nausea, vomiting, increased liver function studies, constipation, dyspepsia, **hepatotoxicity**
HEMA: Anemia
INTEG: Rash, sweating, alopecia, dry skin
RESP: Dyspnea, URI, pneumonia, **interstitial pneumonitis**
MISC: Edema

Contraindications: Hypersensitivity, severe hepatic impairment, severe respiratory disease

Precautions: Pregnancy **C**

Pharmacokinetics	
Absorption	Rapidly, completely
Distribution	Unknown
Metabolism	Unknown
Excretion	Urine, feces
Half-life	Unknown

Pharmacodynamics
Unknown

Interactions
Individual drugs
Phenytoin: ↑ toxicity
Theophylline: ↑ toxicity
Vitamin K: ↑ toxicity

NURSING CONSIDERATIONS
Assessment
• Monitor liver function studies: AST, ALT, alk phosphatase, which may be elevated
• Monitor for CNS symptoms: drowsiness, insomnia, dizziness
• Monitor chest x-rays, routinely; dyspnea, cough, which may indicate interstitial pneumonitis, discontinue treatment if this condition is suspected

---

Nursing diagnoses

☑ Infection, risk of (side effects)

☑ Knowledge deficit (teaching)

Implementation

• Administer without regard to meals

Patient/family education

• Advise to report side effects: decreased libido, impotence, breast enlargement, hot flashes, diarrhea, dyspnea, cough; symptoms of hepatotoxicity

• Advise to wear tinted lens to alleviate delay in adapting to the dark

Evaluation

Positive therapeutic outcome

• Decrease in prostatic tumor size, decrease in spread of cancer

Treatment of overdose: Induce vomiting, provide supportive care

---

nimodipine (℞)

(ni-moe′dip-een)

Nimotop

Func. class.: Calcium channel blocker

Chem. class.: Dihydropyridine

Pregnancy category **C**

Action: Unknown, may have greater effect on cerebral arteries

▶**Therapeutic Outcome:** Prevention of vascular spasm (subarachnoid hemorrhage)

Uses: Prevention of cerebral vascular spasm in subarachnoid hemorrhage

Dosage and routes

Adult: PO Begin therapy within 96 hrs, 60 mg q4h ×21 day

Available forms: Caps 30 mg

Adverse effects

CNS: Headache, fatigue, drowsiness, dizziness, anxiety, depression, weakness, insomnia, confusion, paresthesia, somnolence

CV: Dysrhythmia, edema, CHF, bradycardia, hypotension, palpitations, **MI, pulmonary edema**

GI: Nausea, vomiting, diarrhea, gastric upset, constipation, *hepatitis,* abdominal cramps

GU: Nocturia, polyuria, **acute renal failure**

INTEG: Rash, pruritus, urticaria, photosensitivity, hair loss

MISC: Blurred vision, flushing, nasal congestion, sweating, shortness of breath, gynecomastia, hyperglycemia, sexual difficulties

Contraindications: Sick sinus syndrome, 2nd- or 3rd-degree heart block, hypotension less than 90 mm Hg systolic, hypersensitivity

Precautions: CHF, hypotension, hepatic injury, pregnancy 🄿 C, lactation, children, renal 🄶 disease, elderly

Pharmacokinetics	
Absorption	Well absorbed, bioavailability poor
Distribution	Crosses blood-brain barrier
Metabolism	Liver, extensively
Excretion	Kidneys
Half-life	1-2 hr

Pharmacodynamics	
Onset	Unknown
Peak	1 hr
Duration	Unknown

N

Interactions
Individual drugs
Alcohol: ↑ hypotension
Digoxin: ↑ digoxin levels, bradycardia
Phenobarbital: ↓ effectiveness
Phenytoin: ↓ effectiveness
Propranolol: ↑ toxicity
Drug classifications
Antihypertensives: ↑ hypotension
β-Adrenergic blockers: ↑ bradycardia
Nitrates: ↑ nitrates

NURSING CONSIDERATIONS
Assessment
• Assess fluid volume status (I&O ratio) and record weight, distended red veins, crackles in lung, color, quality and sp gr of urine, skin turgor, adequacy of pulses, moist mucous membranes, bilateral lung sounds, peripheral pitting edema; dehydration symptoms of decreasing output, thirst, hypotension, dry mouth and mucous membranes should be reported
• Monitor B/P and pulse; if B/P drops 30 mm Hg, call prescriber
• Monitor ALT, AST, bilirubin daily; if these are elevated, hepatotoxicity is suspected

Nursing diagnoses
✓ Injury, risk for (uses)
✓ Knowledge deficit (teaching)

Implementation
• May puncture cap and dilute in water and give through nasogastric tube; flush tube with 0.9% NaCl
• Store in airtight container at room temp

Evaluation
Positive therapeutic outcome
• Prevention of neurological damage from SAH

---

nisoldipine (℞)
(nye′sol-dye-peen)
Sular
Func. class.: Antihypertensive, calcium channel blocker
Chem. class.: Dihydropyridine

Pregnancy category   C

Action: Inhibits calcium ion influx across cell membrane, resulting in dilation of peripheral arteries

▰**Therapeutic Outcome:** Decreased B/P in hypertension

Uses: Essential hypertension, alone or with other antihypertensives

Dosage and routes
Adult: PO 20 mg qd initially, may increase by 10 mg/wk, usual dose 20-40 mg qd

G *Elderly:* PO 10 mg/day, increase by 10 mg/wk

Available forms: Tabs, ext rel 10, 20, 30, 40 mg

Adverse effects
CNS: Headache, fatigue, drowsiness, dizziness, anxiety, depression, nervousness, insomnia, light-headedness, paresthesia, tinnitus, psychosis, somnolence
CV: **Dysrhythmias,** edema, **CHF,** hypotension, palpitations, **MI, pulmonary edema,** tachycardia, syncope, AV block, angina

---

GI: Nausea, vomiting, diarrhea, gastric upset, constipation, increased liver function studies, dry mouth
HEMA: Anemia
INTEG: Rash, pruritus
MISC: Flushing, sexual difficulties, cough, nasal congestion, shortness of breath, wheezing, epistaxis, respiratory infection, chest pain

Contraindications: Hypersensitivity, sick sinus syndrome, 2nd- or 3rd-degree heart block

Precautions: CHF, hypotension <90 mm Hg systolic, hepatic injury, pregnancy **C**, lactation, children, renal disease, elderly

Pharmacokinetics

Absorption	Well absorbed
Distribution	Unknown
Metabolism	Liver
Excretion	Kidneys
Half-life	Unknown

Pharmacodynamics

Unknown

Interactions
Individual drugs
Alcohol: ↑ hypotension
Carbamazepine: ↑ toxicity
Digoxin: ↑ digoxin levels, ↑ bradycardia, CHF
Phenobarbital: ↓ effectiveness
Phenytoin: ↓ effectiveness
Propranolol: ↑ toxicity
Drug classifications
Antihypertensives: ↑ hypotension
β-Adrenergic blockers: ↑ bradycardia, CHF
Nitrates: ↑ nitrates

Herb/drug
Angelica: ↑ antidysrhythmic effect
Cat's claw: ↑ antidysrhythmic effect
Chicory: ↑ antidysrhythmic effect
Food/drug
High-fat: ↑ nisoldipine level
Grapefruit: ↑ hypotension

NURSING CONSIDERATIONS
Assessment
• Assess fluid volume status: I&O ratio and record; weight; skin turgor; adequacy of pulses; moist mucous membranes; bilateral lung sounds; peripheral pitting edema—dehydration symptoms of decreasing output, thirst, hypotension, dry mouth, and mucous membranes should be reported
• Monitor ALT, AST, bilirubin daily, if these are elevated
• Monitor cardiac status: B/P, pulse, respiration, ECG

Nursing diagnoses
✓ Cardiac output, decreased (uses)
✓ Knowledge deficit (teaching)

Implementation
• Give once a day, with food for GI symptoms, avoid high-fat foods, grapefruit

Patient/family education
• Caution patient to avoid hazardous activities until stabilized on drug, and dizziness is no longer a problem
• Instruct patient to limit caffeine consumption; to avoid alcohol and OTC drugs unless directed by prescriber
• Urge patient to comply in all areas of medical regimen: diet, exercise, stress reduction, drug therapy; to notify prescriber of

N

irregular heart beat, shortness of breath, swelling of feet and hands, pronounced dizziness, constipation, nausea, hypotension

• Teach patient to use as directed even if feeling better; may be taken with other cardiovascular drugs (nitrates, beta blockers)

• Advise patient to rise slowly to prevent orthostatic hypotension

• Teach patient to report nausea, dizziness, edema, shortness of breath, palpitations

Evaluation

Positive therapeutic outcome
• Decreased B/P

---

nitric oxide
See Appendix A, Selected New Drugs

---

nitroglycerin ⚷ (℞)
(nye-troe-gli'ser-in)
Nitro-Bid IV, nitroglycerin, Tridil, Nitrostat, Nitro-Bid Plateau Caps, Nitrocine Timecaps, Nitroglyn, Nitrong, Nitro-Bid, Nitrol, Deponit, Minitran, Nitrek, Nitrodisc, Nitro-Dur, nitroglycerin transdermal, Nitrocine, Transderm-Nitro, Nitrolingual, Nitrogard
Func. class.: Coronary vasodilator, antianginal
Chem. class.: Nitrate
Pregnancy category   C

Action: Decreases preload and afterload, which thus decreases left ventricular end-diastolic pressure and systemic vascular resistance; dilates coronary arteries and improves blood flow

➡ **Therapeutic Outcome:** Prevention of anginal attack

Uses: Chronic stable angina pectoris, prophylaxis of angina pain, CHF associated with acute MI, controlled hypotension in surgical procedures

Dosage and routes
Adult: SL: dissolve tab under tongue when pain begins; may repeat q5 min until relief occurs; take no more than 3 tab/15 min; use 1 tab prophylactically 5-10 min before activities; sus rel cap q6-12h on empty stomach; **top:** 1-2 in q8h; increase to 4 in q4h as needed; **IV:** 5 µg/min, then increase by 5 µg/min q3-5 min; if no response after 20 µg/min, increase by 10-20 µg/min until desired response; **transdermal:** apply a pad qd to a site free from hair; remove patch hs to provide 10-12 hr nitrate-free interval to avoid tolerance; **translingual spray:** 1-2 metered doses onto or under the tongue, max 3 sprays; transmucosal insert between lip and gums above incisors or between gum and cheek 1 mg q3-5 hr during waking hrs

🄿 *Child:* **IV** initial: 0.25-0.5 mg/kg/min, titrate to patient response, usual dose 1-3 mg/kg/min

Available forms: Buccal tab 1, 2, 3 mg; aero 0.4 mg/meter

---

spray; sus rel caps 2.5, 6.5, 9, 13 mg; sus rel tabs 2.6, 6.5, 9 mg; inj 0.5, 5 mg/ml; SL tabs 0.15, 0.3, 0.4, 0.6 mg; trans oint 2%; trans syst 0.1, 0.2, 0.3, 0.4, 0.6 mg/24 hr; inj 25 mg/250 ml, 50 mg/250 ml, 50 mg/500 ml, 100 mg/250 ml, 200 mg/500 ml; patches 22.4, 44.8, 67.2 mg

Adverse effects
CNS: Headache, flushing, dizziness
CV: Postural hypotension, tachycardia, **collapse,** syncope
GI: Nausea, vomiting
INTEG: Pallor, sweating, rash

Contraindications: Hypersensitivity to this drug or nitrites, severe anemia, increased intracranial pressure, cerebral hemorrhage

Precautions: Postural hypotension, pregnancy **C,** lactation

Interactions
Individual drugs
Alcohol: ↑ hypotension
Haloperidol: ↑ hypotension

⬛ Do Not Confuse:
Nitro-Bid/Nicobid

Pharmacokinetics

Absorption	Well absorbed (PO, buccal, SL)
Distribution	Unknown
Metabolism	Liver, extensively
Excretion	Kidney
Half-life	1-4 min

Drug classifications
Antidepressants, tricyclic: ↓ absorption of SL, transmucosal
Antihistamines: ↓ absorption of SL, transmucosal
Antihypertensives: ↑ hypotension
β-Adrenergic blockers: ↑ hypotension
Calcium channel blockers: ↑ hypotension
Phenothiazines: ↓ absorption of SL, transmucosal

NURSING CONSIDERATIONS
Assessment
• Monitor orthostatic B/P, pulse
• Assess pain: duration, time started, activity being performed, character; check for tolerance if taken over long period
• Monitor for headache, lightheadedness, decreased B/P; may indicate a need for decreased dosage

Nursing diagnoses
☑ Cardiac output, decreased (uses)
☑ Poisoning (uses)
☑ Tissue perfusion, decreased (uses)
☑ Knowledge deficit (teaching)
☑ Noncompliance (teaching)

Implementation
IV IV route
• Give **IV** diluted in amount specified D₅W, or 0.9% NaCl or NS for inf; use glass inf

N

Pharmacodynamics

	SUS REL	SL	TRANS	IV	TRANSMU-COSAL	AEROSOL	TOP OINT
Onset	20-45 min	1-3 min	½-1 hr	1-2 min	3 min	2 min	½-1 hr
Peak	Unknown	Unknown	Unknown	Unknown	Unknown	Unknown	Unknown
Duration	3-8 hr	½ hr	12-24 hr	3-5 min	3-5 min	½-1 hr	2-12 hr

---

bottles, non–polyvinyl chloride inf tubing; titrate to patient response; do not use filters

Syringe compatibilities:
Heparin

Y-site compatibilities:
Amiodarone, amphotericin B cholesteryl, amrinone, atracurium, cefmetazole, cisatracurium, diltiazem, dobutamine, dopamine, epinephrine, esmolol, famotidine, fentanyl, fluconazole, furosemide, haloperidol, heparin, hydromorphone, regular insulin, labetalol, lidocaine, lorazepam, midazolam, milrinone, morphine, nicardipine, nitroprusside, norepinephrine, pancuronium, ranitidine, remifentanil, streptokinase, tacrolimus, theophylline, vecuronium

Y-site incompatibilities:
Alteplase

Additive compatibilities:
Alteplase, aminophylline, dobutamine, dopamine, enalaprilat, furosemide, lidocaine, verapamil

Additive incompatibilities:
Manufacturer recommends that nitroglycerin not be admixed with other medications

SL route
• Keep tab in original container
• If 3 SL tab in 15 min do not relieve pain, consider diagnosis of MI
• SL tab should be held under tongue until dissolved (a few min); do not take anything by mouth when SL tab is in place

PO route
• Give 1 hr ac or 2 hr pc with 8 oz of water
• Sus rel tab should not be chewed or crushed

Transmucosal route
• Tab should be placed between cheek and gum line
• Do not take anything PO when tab is in place

Top route
• Apply ointment using dose-measuring papers supplied; apply to an area without hair; ointment should cover 2-3 in area; may apply an occlusive dressing as directed
• Apply trans patches to area without hair; press hard to adhere; if patch becomes dislodged, apply a new one

Patient/family education

• Teach patient to place buccal tab between lip and gum above incisors or between cheek and gum; sus rel tab must be swallowed whole, do not chew; SL should be dissolved under tongue, do not swallow; aerosol should be sprayed under tongue, do not inhale; use inhaler only when lying down; do not inhale spray
• Instruct patient to avoid alcohol
• Advise patient that drug may cause headache; tolerance usually develops; use nonnarcotic analgesic
• Teach patient that drug may be taken before stressful activity, exercise, sexual activity
• Inform patient that SL may sting when drug comes in contact with mucous membranes
• Caution patient to avoid hazardous activities if dizziness occurs
• Instruct patient to comply with complete medical regimen
• Advise patient to make position changes slowly to prevent fainting

Evaluation
Positive therapeutic outcome
• Decreased, prevention of anginal pain

---

nitroprusside (℞)
(nye-troe-pruss'ide)
Nitropress, Sodium nitroprusside
Func. class.: Antihypertensive
Chem. class.: Peripheral vasodilator
Pregnancy category C

Action: Directly relaxes arteriolar, venous smooth muscle, resulting in reduction in cardiac preload, afterload

➡ **Therapeutic Outcome:** Decreased B/P in hypertensive crisis, decreased preload, afterload

Uses: Hypertensive crisis, to decrease bleeding by creating hypotension during surgery, acute CHF, cardiogenic shock

Dosage and routes
Adult: **IV** inf dissolve 50 mg in 2-3 ml of D_5W, then dilute in 250-1000 ml of D_5W; run at 0.5-8 μg/kg/min
P *Child:* **IV** 0.3-0.5 mg/kg/min, titrate to response

Available forms: Inj 50 mg

Adverse effects
CNS: Dizziness, headache, agitation, twitching, decreased reflexes, **coma,** restlessness
CV: Palpitations, severe hypotension, dyspnea
EENT: Tinnitus, blurred vision
GI: Nausea, vomiting, abdominal pain
GU: Impotence

INTEG: Pain, irritation at inj site, sweating
MISC: **Cyanide, thiocyanate toxicity**

Contraindications: Hypersensitivity, hypertension (compensatory)

Precautions: Pregnancy **C,**
P lactation, children, fluid, electrolyte imbalances, hepatic disease, renal disease, hypothy-
G roidism, elderly

Pharmacokinetics	
Absorption	Complete bioavailability
Distribution	Not known
Metabolism	RBCs, tissues
Excretion	Kidneys
Half-life	Unknown

Pharmacodynamics	
Onset	1-2 min
Peak	Rapid
Duration	1-10 min

Interactions
Drug classifications
Antihypertensives: ↑ hypotension
Ganglionic blockers: ↑ hypotension
Herb/drug
Angelica: ↑ nitroprusside effect

NURSING CONSIDERATIONS
Assessment
• Monitor B/P q5 min × 2 hr; then q1h × 2 hr; monitor pulse q4h; monitor jugular venous distention q4h; ECG should be monitored continuously; monitor PCWP
• Monitor electrolytes, blood studies: potassium, sodium, chloride, CO_2, CBC, serum glucose, serum methemoglobin if pulmonary oxygen levels are decreased

N

• Check weight, I&O, edema in feet and legs daily; assess skin turgor, dryness of mucous membranes for hydration status
• Assess for signs of CHF: dyspnea, edema, wet rales
• Monitor for increased lactate, cyanide, thiocyanate levels
• Monitor for decrease in bicarbonate, Pco_2 and blood pH; acidosis may occur with this drug

Nursing diagnoses
☑ Tissue perfusion, altered (uses)
☑ Injury, risk for (adverse reactions)
☑ Knowledge deficit (teaching)

Implementation
• Give by cont inf after diluting 50 mg/2-3 ml of D_5W; further dilute in 250 ml of D_5W; use an inf pump only; wrap bottle with aluminum foil to protect from light; observe for color change in the inf; discard if highly discolored (blue, green, red); titrate to patient response; avoid extravasation

Syringe compatibilities:
Heparin

Y-site compatibilities:
Amrinone, atracurium, diltiazem, dobutamine, dopamine, enalaprilat, famotidine, lidocaine, nitroglycerin, pancuronium, tacrolimus, theophylline, vecuronium

Additive incompatibilities:
Do not give with any other drugs

Patient/family education
• Teach patient to report headache, dizziness, loss of hearing, blurred vision, dyspnea, faintness; may indicate adverse reactions

Evaluation
Positive therapeutic outcome
• Decreased B/P in hypertension
• Absence of bleeding in surgery

Treatment of overdose:
Administer amyl nitrite inh until 3% sodium nitrate sol can be prepared for **IV** administration, then inject sodium thiosulfate **IV**; correct drop in B/P with vasopressor

---

nizatidine (Ŗ, OTC)
(ni-za'ti-deen)
Axid, Axid AR
Func. class.: H_2-Receptor antagonist
Chem. class.: Substituted thiazole

Pregnancy category   C

Action: Blocks H_2 receptors thereby reducing gastric acid output

➡ **Therapeutic Outcome:** Healing of duodenal ulcers or gastric ulcers; prevention of duodenal ulcers; decreases symptoms of GERD

Uses: Benign gastric and duodenal ulceration, prevention of duodenal ulcer recurrence, symptomatic relief of gastroesophageal reflux, heartburn prevention

Dosage and routes
Gastric and duodenal ulcer disease
Adult: PO 300 mg at night or 150 mg bid for 4-8 weeks; maintenance 150 mg at night

Gastroesophageal reflux
Adult: PO 150 mg bid

☑ Herb/drug ⑤ Do Not Crush ◆ Alert ⊶ Key Drug ⑥ Geriatric ⑨ Pediatric

Renal dose

CrCl 20-50 ml/min give 150 mg/day; CrCl <20 ml/min give 150 mg QOD

Available forms: Caps 75, 150, 300 mg

Adverse effects

CNS: Headache, somnolence, confusion, abnormal dreams
ENDO: Gynecomastia
GI: Elevated liver enzymes, hepatitis, jaundice, nausea
HEMA: **Thrombocytopenia**
INTEG: Pruritus, sweating, urticaria, exfoliative dermatitis
METAB: Hyperuricemia
MS: Myalgia
RESP: **Bronchospasm, laryngeal edema**

Contraindications: Hypersensitivity

Precautions: Renal or hepatic impairment (reduce dose in renal impairment), pregnancy **C**, lactation

Pharmacokinetics	
Absorption	PO 70%
Distribution	Breast milk, crosses placenta
Metabolism	Liver, partially
Excretion	Kidney
Half-life	1½ hr

Pharmacodynamics	
Onset	Variable
Peak	½-3 hr
Duration	Unknown

NURSING CONSIDERATIONS
Assessment

• Assess patient with ulcers or suspected ulcers: epigastric or abdominal pain, hematemesis, occult blood in stools, blood or gastric aspirate prior to and throughout treatment, monitor gastric pH (5 should be maintained)

• Monitor I&O ratio, BUN, creatinine, CBC with differential monthly

Nursing diagnoses

☑ Pain (uses)
☑ Knowledge deficit (teaching)

Implementation

• May be given with or without meals
• Give antacids 1 hr before or 1 hr after this drug

Patient/family education

• Caution patient that gynecomastia, impotence may occur and are reversible after treatment is discontinued
• Advise patient to avoid driving, other hazardous activities until stabilized on this medication; drowsiness or dizziness may occur
• Caution patient to avoid black pepper, caffeine, alcohol, harsh spices, extremes in temp of food; tell patient to avoid OTC preparations: aspirin, cough, cold preparations because condition may worsen
• Inform patient that smoking decreases the effectiveness of the drug; that smoking cessation should be considered
• Instruct patient that drug must be continued for prescribed time to be effective and taken exactly as prescribed; doses should not be doubled; a missed dose should be taken as soon as remembered up to 1 hr before next dose
• Advise patient to report bruising, fatigue, malaise; blood dyscrasias may occur
• Advise patient to report diarrhea, black tarry stools, sore throat, rash, dizziness, confusion, or delirium to prescriber immediately

N

Evaluation
Positive therapeutic outcome
- Decreased pain in abdomen
- Healing of ulcers
- Absence of gastroesophageal reflux

---

norfloxacin (℞)
(nor-flox′a-sin)
Chibroxin, Noroxin
Func. class.: Urinary anti-infective
Chem. class.: Fluoroquinolone antibacterial
Pregnancy category   C

Action: Interferes with conversion of intermediate DNA fragments into high-molecular-weight DNA in bacteria

➡ **Therapeutic Outcome:** Bactericidal action against gram-positive *Staphylococcus epidermidis,* methicillin-resistant strains of *Staphylococcus aureus,* group D streptococci; gram-negative *Escherichia coli, Klebsiella pneumoniae, Enterobacter cloacae, Proteus mirabilis, P. vulgaris, Providencia rettgeri, Morganella morganii, Pseudomonas aeruginosa, Citrobacter freundii*

Uses: Adult UTIs (including complicated), uncomplicated gonorrhea, ocular infections

Dosage and routes
Uncomplicated infections
Adult: PO 400 mg bid × 3-10 days 1 hr ac or 2 hr pc

Complicated infections
Adult: PO 400 mg bid × 10-21 days; 400 mg qd × 7-10 days in impaired renal function

Uncomplicated gonorrhea
Adult: PO 800 mg as a single dose

Prostatitis
Adult: PO 400 mg bid × 4 wk

Occular infection
P *Adult and child:* Ophth ɪ̅ gtt qid; may increase to ɪ̅ gtt q2h for severe infections

Renal dose
CrCl ≤30 ml/min 400 mg PO qd

Available forms: Tabs 400 mg; ophth sol 3 mg/ml

Adverse effects
CNS: Headache, dizziness, fatigue, somnolence, depression, insomnia
EENT: Visual disturbances
GI: Nausea, constipation, increased ALT, AST, flatulence, heartburn, vomiting, diarrhea, dry mouth
INTEG: Rash

Contraindications: Hypersensitivity to quinolones

Precautions: Pregnancy **C,**
P lactation, children, renal disease, seizure disorders

Pharmacokinetics

Absorption	30% (PO)
Distribution	Concentration in urinary system
Metabolism	Liver (minimal)
Excretion	Kidneys, unchanged (30%)
Half-life	3-4 hr; increased in renal disease

Pharmacodynamics

	PO
Onset	Unknown
Peak	1 hr

Interactions
Individual drugs
Cyclosporine: ↑ concentrations

Nitrofurantoin: ↓ effectiveness

Probenecid: ↑ blood levels

Sucralfate: ↓ absorption of norfloxacin

Theophylline: ↑ toxicity

Zinc sulfate: ↓ absorption of norfloxacin

Drug classifications
Antacids: ↓ absorption of norfloxacin

Anticoagulants, oral: ↑ effect of anticoagulants

Antineoplastics: ↓ norfloxacin levels

Iron salts: ↓ absorption of norfloxacin

Lab test interferences
↑ AST, ↑ ALT, ↑ BUN, ↑ creatinine, ↑ alkaline phosphatase

NURSING CONSIDERATIONS
Assessment
• Assess patient for previous sensitivity reaction

• Assess patient for signs and symptoms of infection including characteristics of urine, WBC >10,000, temp; obtain baseline information before and during treatment

• Obtain C & S before beginning drug therapy to identify if correct treatment has been initiated

• Assess for allergic reactions: rash, urticaria, pruritus

• Monitor blood studies: AST, ALT, BUN, creatinine, alkaline phosphatase monthly if patient is on long-term therapy

• Assess bowel pattern qd; if severe diarrhea occurs, drug should be discontinued

• Assess for overgrowth of infection: perineal itching, fever, malaise, redness, pain, swelling, drainage, rash, diarrhea, change in cough, sputum

Nursing diagnoses
☑ Infection, risk for (uses)

☑ Diarrhea (adverse reactions)

☑ Injury, risk for (adverse reactions)

☑ Knowledge deficit (teaching)

☑ Noncompliance (teaching)

Implementation
PO route

• Give in equal intervals q12h around the clock to maintain proper blood levels; give with food to increase absorption of drug; do not give within 3 hr of other agents; drug interactions may occur; give with 8 oz of water

• Do not give with iron, zinc products, or antacids, which decrease absorption

Patient/family education
• Instruct patient to take all medication prescribed for the length of time ordered; drug must be taken around the clock to maintain blood levels; do not give medication to others; do not double doses; take any missed dose when remembered

• Advise patient to increase fluids to 2 L/day to prevent crystalluria

• Caution patient to avoid driving and other hazardous activities until response is known; dizziness may occur

• Instruct patient to use sunglasses to prevent photophobia

• Have patient use hard candy, frequent sips of water for dry mouth

• Teach patient correct instillation procedure (ophth)

N

Evaluation
Positive therapeutic outcome
• Reported improvement in symptoms of infection
• Absence of red or itching eyes (ophth)

---

nortriptyline (℞)
(nor-trip'ti-leen)
Aventyl, Pamelor
Func. class.: Antidepressant, tricyclic
Chem. class.: Dibenzocycloheptene, secondary amine
Pregnancy category   C

Action: Blocks reuptake of norepinephrine, serotonin into nerve endings, increasing action of norepinephrine, serotonin in nerve cells; has anticholinergic effects

▶**Therapeutic Outcome:** Decreased symptoms of depression after 2-3 wk

Uses: Major depression

Investigational uses: Chronic pain management

Dosage and routes
Adult: PO 25 mg tid or qid; may increase to 150 mg/day; may give daily dose hs

P G *Adolescents and elderly:* PO 10-25 mg qhs, increase by 10-25 mg at weekly intervals to desired dose; usual maintenance 30-50 mg qd

Available forms: Caps 10, 25, 50, 75 mg; sol 10 mg/5 ml

Adverse effects
CNS: Dizziness, drowsiness, confusion, headache, anxiety, tremors, stimulation, weakness, insomnia, nightmares, EPS **G** (elderly), increased psychiatric symptoms
CV: Orthostatic hypotension, ECG changes, tachycardia, **hypertension,** palpitations
EENT: Blurred vision, tinnitus, mydriasis
GI: Constipation, dry mouth, nausea, vomiting, **paralytic ileus,** increased appetite, cramps, epigastric distress, jaundice, **hepatitis,** stomatitis
GU: Retention, **acute renal failure**
HEMA: **Agranulocytosis, thrombocytopenia, eosinophilia, leukopenia**
INTEG: Rash, urticaria, sweating, pruritus, photosensitivity

Contraindications: Hypersensitivity to tricyclic antidepressants, recovery phase of MI, convulsive disorders, prostatic hypertrophy

Precautions: Suicidal patients, severe depression, increased intraocular pressure, narrow-angle glaucoma, urinary retention, cardiac disease, hepatic disease, hyperthyroidism, electroshock therapy, elective surgery, pregnancy **C**

Ⓝ Do Not Confuse:
nortriptyline/amitriptyline

Pharmacokinetics	
Absorption	Well absorbed
Distribution	Widely distributed; crosses placenta
Metabolism	Liver, extensively
Excretion	Kidneys, breast milk
Half-life	18-28 hr; steady state 4-19 days

Pharmacodynamics	
Unknown	

Interactions
Individual drugs
Alcohol: ↑ CNS depression
Cimetidine: ↑ levels, toxicity
Clonidine: Severe
hypotension; avoid use
Disulfiram: Organic brain
syndrome
Fluoxetine: ↑ levels, toxicity
Guanethidine: ↓ effects
Drug classifications
Analgesics: ↑ CNS depression
Anticholinergics: ↑ side effects
Antihistamines: ↑ CNS depression
Antihypertensives: May block
antihypertensive effect
Barbiturates: ↑ effects
Benzodiazepines: ↑ effects
CNS depressants: ↑ effects
MAOIs: Hypertensive crisis,
convulsions
Oral contraceptives: ↑ effects,
toxicity
Phenothiazines: ↑ toxicity
Sedative/hypnotics: ↑ CNS
depression
**Sympathomimetics, indirect-
acting:** ↓ effects
Smoking
↑ Metabolism, ↓ effects
☑ Herb/drug
Belladonna: ↑ anticholinergic
effect
Henbane: ↑ anticholinergic
effect
Scopolia: ↑ antidepressant
effect
Lab test interferences
↑ Serum bilirubin, ↑ blood
glucose, ↑ alkaline phosphatase
↓ VMA, ↓ 5-HIAA, ↓ blood
glucose
False: ↑ Urinary catechol-
amines

NURSING CONSIDERATIONS
Assessment
• Monitor B/P (with patient
lying, standing), pulse q4h; if
systolic B/P drops 20 mm Hg,
hold drug, notify prescriber;
take VS q4h of patients with
cardiovascular disease
• Monitor blood studies:
CBC, leukocytes, differential,
cardiac enzymes if patient is
receiving long-term therapy
• Monitor hepatic studies:
AST, ALT, bilirubin
• Check weight weekly; appetite may increase with drug
• Assess ECG for flattening of
T wave, bundle branch block,
AV block, dysrhythmias in
cardiac patients
• Assess for EPS primarily in
G elderly: rigidity, dystonia,
akathisia
• Assess mental status: mood,
sensorium, affect, suicidal
tendencies; increase in psychiatric symptoms: depression,
panic
• Monitor urinary retention,
constipation; constipation is
P more likely to occur in children
G or elderly
⊕• Assess for withdrawal
symptoms: headache, nausea,
vomiting, muscle pain, weakness; do not usually occur
unless drug was discontinued
abruptly
• Identify alcohol
consumption; if alcohol is
consumed, hold dose until AM

Nursing diagnoses
☑ Coping, ineffective individual
(uses)
☑ Injury, risk for (adverse reac-
tions)
☑ Knowledge deficit (teaching)
☑ Noncompliance (teaching)

Implementation
• Give with food or milk for
GI symptoms; mix conc with
water, milk, fruit juice to dis-
guise taste
• Give dose hs if oversedation

N

Adverse effects: *italic* = common; **bold** = life-threatening

occurs during day; may take
G entire dose hs; elderly may not
tolerate once/day dosing
• Store at room temp; do not
freeze

Patient/family education
• Teach patient that therapeutic effects may take 2-3 wk
• Teach patient to use caution in driving and other activities requiring alertness because of drowsiness, dizziness, blurred vision; to avoid rising quickly from sitting to standing, espe-
G cially elderly
• Teach patient to avoid alcohol ingestion, other CNS depressants; teach patient not to discontinue medication quickly after long-term use; may cause nausea, headache, malaise
• Teach patient to wear sunscreen or large hat, since photosensitivity occurs
• Teach patient to increase fluids, bulk in diet if constipation, urinary retention occur,
G especially elderly
• Teach patient to take gum, hard sugarless candy, or frequent sips of water for dry mouth

Evaluation
Positive therapeutic outcome
• Decrease in depression
• Absence of suicidal thoughts

Treatment of overdose:
ECG monitoring, induce emesis, lavage, activated charcoal, administer anticonvulsant

---

nystatin (℞, OTC)
(nis′ta-tin)
Mycostatin, Mycostatin Pastilles, Nadostine ✦, Nyaderm ✦, nystatin, Nystex; topical: Mycostatin, Nilstat, Nodostine ✦, Nyoderm ✦, Nystatin, Nystex; vaginal: Mycostatin, Nilstat, Nadostine ✦, Nyoderm ✦, O-V Statin
Func. class.: Antiinfective
Chem. class.: Antifungal

Pregnancy category B; A (vaginal)

Action: Interferes with fungal DNA replication; binds sterols in fungal cell membrane, which increases permeability, resulting in leaking of cell nutrients

▶**Therapeutic Outcome:** Fungistatic/fungicidal against *Candida* organisms

Uses: *Candida* species causing oral, vaginal, intestinal infections; vag: cutaneous vulvovaginal candidiasis, top: mucocutaneous fungal infec-
P tions, infant eczema, pruritus ani and vulvae

Dosage and routes
Oral infection
Adult: Susp 400,000-600,000 U qid, use ½ dose in each side of mouth, swish and swallow

P*Infants:* 200,000 U qid (100,000 U in each side of mouth)

P*Newborn and premature infants:* Susp 100,000 U qid

P*Adult and child:* Troches 200,000-400,000 U qid × up to 2 wks

GI infection
Adult: PO 500,000-1,000,000 U tid

Top

P *Adult and child:* Top apply to affected area bid-tid × 14 days

Vag: 1-2 tabs (100,000 U each) inserted into vagina

Available forms: Tab 500,000 U; powder 50 mill, 150 mill, 500 mill, 1 bill, 2 bill, 5 bill U; troches 200,000 U; susp 100,000 U; cream, oint, powder, spray, vag tab 100,000 U; vag cream, lotion 2%

Adverse effects

GI: Nausea, vomiting, anorexia, diarrhea, cramps
INTEG: Rash, urticaria, stinging, burning

Contraindication: Hypersensitivity

Precautions: Pregnancy **B**, lactation

Pharmacokinetics	
Absorption	Poorly absorbed
Distribution	Unknown
Metabolism	Not metabolized
Excretion	Feces, unchanged
Half-life	Unknown

Pharmacodynamics	
Onset	Rapid
Peak	Unknown
Duration	6-12 hr

Interactions: None

NURSING CONSIDERATIONS
Assessment

• Assess for allergic reaction: rash, urticaria; drug may have to be discontinued
• Assess for predisposing factors for candidal infection: antibiotic therapy, pregnancy, diabetes mellitus, sexual partner infection (vag infections), AIDS

Nursing diagnoses

☑Skin integrity, impaired (uses)
☑Infection, risk for (uses)
☑Knowledge deficit (teaching)

Implementation
PO route

• Give oral susp dose by placing ½ in each cheek, swish for several min, then swallow; shake susp before use
• Store oral susp in refrigerator, tab in tight, light-resistant containers at room temp

Top route

• Administer by moistening lesions with a swab coated with cream or ointment; use enough medication to cover lesions completely; give after cleansing with soap, water before each application; dry well

Vag route

• Insert vag tab high into vagina with applicator provided; administer in gravid client 3-6 wk before term to decrease candidiasis in the **P** newborn
• Store at room temp in dry place; protect from light, air, heat

Patient/family education

• Instruct patient that long-term therapy may be needed to clear infection; to complete entire course of medication
• Teach patient proper hygiene: use no commercial mouthwashes for mouth infection
• Advise patient to avoid getting preparation on hands
• Instruct patient to wear light-day pad for vag preparations to avoid soiling clothing; to avoid sexual contact during treatment to minimize reinfection
• Instruct patient to notify prescriber if irritation occurs;

N

drug may have to be discontinued

• Inform patient that relief from itching may occur after 24-72 hr

Top

• Advise patient to discontinue use and notify prescriber if irritation occurs

• Teach patient to apply with glove to prevent further infection; drug may stain

• Caution patient not to use occlusive dressings; to avoid use of OTC creams, ointments, lotions unless directed by prescriber

Evaluation
Positive therapeutic outcome

• Culture negative for *Candida*

• Decrease in size, number of lesions

• Decreased itching, white patches on vulva (vag)

---

octreotide
See Appendix A,
Selected New Drugs

---

ofloxacin (℞)
(o-flox′a-sin)
Floxin, Floxin IV, Ocuflox
Func. class.: Antiinfective
Chem. class.: Fluoroquinolone

Pregnancy category   C

Action: Interferes with conversion of intermediate DNA fragments into high-molecular-weight DNA in bacteria

▶**Therapeutic Outcome:** Bactericidal action against the following gram-positive pathogens: *Staphylococcus*

epidermidis, methicillin-resistant strains of *S. aureus, Streptococcus pyogenes, S. pneumoniae;* gram-negative pathogens *Escherichia coli, Klebsiella* species, *Enterobacter, Salmonella, Shigella, Proteus vulgaris, P. rettgeri, Providencia stuartii, Morganella morganii, Pseudomonas aeruginosa, Serratia, Haemophilus* species, *Acinetobacter, Neisseria gonorrhoeae, N. meningitidis, Yersinia, Vibrio, Brucella, Campylobacter,* and *Aeromonas* species; anaerobic pathogens: *Bacteroides fragilis intermedius, Clostridium perfrigens, Gardnerella vaginalis, Peptococcus niger, Peptostreptococcus* species; *Chlamydia pneumoniae, C. trachomatis, Legionella pneumoniae, Mycobacterium tuberculosis, Mycoplasma pneumoniae*

Uses: Treatment of lower respiratory tract infections (pneumonia, bronchitis), genitourinary infections (prostatitis, UTIs), skin and skin structure infections, conjunctivitis (ophth)

Dosage and routes
Lower respiratory tract
infection/skin and skin
structure infections
Adult: PO/**IV** 200-400 mg
q12h × 10 days

Cervicitis, urethritis
Adult: PO/**IV** 300 mg
q12h × 7 days

Prostatitis
Adult: PO 300 mg q12h × 6
wk

Acute, uncomplicated
gonorrhea
Adult: PO/**IV** 400 mg as a
single dose

☑ Herb/drug 🚫 Do Not Crush ◆ Alert ⚭ Key Drug 🄶 Geriatric 🄿 Pediatric

Urinary tract infection
Adult: PO/**IV** 200-400 mg
q12h × 3-10 days

Conjunctivitis
P **Adult and child:** Ophth 1-2
gtt q2-4h × 2 days, then
qid × 5 days

Renal dose
CrCl 10-50 ml/min give q24h;
CrCl <10 ml/min give ½ of
dose q24h

Available forms: Tabs 200,
300, 400 mg; inj 200, 400 mg;
ophth sol 0.3%

Adverse effects
CNS: Dizziness, headache,
fatigue, somnolence, depression, insomnia, lethargy, malaise
EENT: Visual disturbances
GI: Diarrhea, nausea, vomiting, anorexia, flatulence, heartburn, dry mouth, increased
AST, ALT, abdominal pain,
constipation
INTEG: Rash, pruritus

Contraindication: Hypersensitivity to quinolones

Precautions: Pregnancy **C**,
P lactation, children, elderly,
G renal disease, seizure disorders,
excessive sunlight

N **Do Not Confuse:**
Ocuflox/Ocufen

Interactions
Individual drugs
Calcium: ↓ ofloxacin effect
Cimetidine: ↑ ofloxacin effect
Nitrofurantoin: ↓ effective-
ness
Probenecid: ↑ blood levels
Procainamide: ↑ procainamide
level
Sucralfate: ↓ absorption of
ofloxacin
Theophylline: ↑ toxicity
Zinc sulfate: ↓ absorption of
ofloxacin
Drug classifications
Antacids: ↓ absorption of
ofloxacin
Anticoagulants, oral: ↑ effect
of anticoagulants
Antidiabetics: Altered blood
glucose levels
Antineoplastics: ↓ ofloxacin
levels
Iron salts: ↓ absorption of
ofloxacin
NSAIDs: ↑ CNS stimulation,
seizures
Theophyllines: ↑ theophylline
effect
Food/drug
↓ Absorption
Lab test interferences
Increase: AST, ALT, BUN,
creatinine, alkaline phosphatase

NURSING CONSIDERATIONS
Assessment
• Assess patient for previous
sensitivity reaction
• Assess patient for signs and
symptoms of infection including characteristics of wounds,
sputum, urine, stool, WBC
>10,000, fever; obtain baseline
information before and during
treatment
• Obtain C&S before beginning drug therapy to identify if
correct treatment has been
initiated

O

Pharmacokinetics	
Absorption	Well absorbed (PO)
Distribution	Widely distributed
Excretion	Kidneys, unchanged; breast milk
Half-life	5-9 hr; increased in renal disease

Pharmacodynamics			
	PO	IV	OPHTH
Onset	Rapid	Rapid	Unknown
Peak	1-2 hr	Inf end	Unknown

- Assess for allergic reactions: rash, urticaria, pruritus
- Monitor blood studies: AST, ALT, CBC, serum glucose monthly if patient is on long-term therapy
- Assess bowel pattern qd; if severe diarrhea occurs, drug should be discontinued
- Assess for overgrowth of infection: perineal itching, fever, malaise, redness, pain, swelling, drainage, rash, diarrhea, change in cough, sputum
- Assess for CNS symptoms: seizures, vertigo, drowsiness, agitation, confusion, tremors

Nursing diagnoses
☑Infection, risk for (uses)
☑Diarrhea (adverse reactions)
☑Injury, risk for (adverse reactions)
☑Knowledge deficit (teaching)
☑Noncompliance (teaching)

Implementation
PO route
- Give in equal intervals q12h around the clock to maintain proper blood levels; do not give within 2 hr of other agents, since drug interactions are possible: give with 8 oz of water
- Do not give with iron, aluminum, zinc products or antacids, which decrease absorption and form insoluble chelate

IV IV route
- For intermittent inf, dilute to 4 mg/ml with D_5W, $D_5/0.9\%$ NaCl, 0.9% NaCl, D_5/LR, sodium bicarbonate, sodium lactate, D_5/Plasmalyte 56; give over 1 hr or more

Syringe compatibilities:
cefotaxime

Y-site compatibilities:
Ampicillin, cisatracurium, granisetron, propofol, remifentanil, thiotepa

Additive compatibilities:
Amoxicillin, ceftazidime, clindamycin, gentamicin, piperacillin, tobramycin, vancomycin

Patient/family education
- Store for 2 wk refrigerated or 6 mo frozen, after reconstitution
- Instruct patient to take all medication prescribed for the length of time ordered; drug must be taken around the clock to maintain blood levels; do not give medication to others
- Teach patient to use sunscreen when outdoors to decrease phototoxicity
- Advise patient to increase fluids to 2 L/day to prevent crystalluria
- Caution patient to avoid driving and other hazardous activities until response is known; dizziness, confusion, drowsiness may occur
- Advise patient to use sunscreen to prevent photosensitivity

Evaluation
Positive therapeutic outcome
- Absence of signs/symptoms of infection (WBC <10,000, temp WNL)
- Reported improvement in symptoms of infection
- Absence of red or itching eyes (ophth)

olanzapine (℞)
(oh-lanz'a-peen)
Zyprexa
Func. class.: Antipsychotic/neuroleptic
Chem. class.: Thienbenzodiazepine
Pregnancy category C

Action: Unknown; may mediate antipsychotic activity by both dopamine and serotonin type 2 (5HT2) antagonism; also, may antagonize muscarinic receptors, histaminic (H_1)- and α-adrenergic receptors

Therapeutic Outcome: Decreased psychotic symptoms

Uses: Psychotic disorders

Dosage and routes
Adult: PO 5-10 mg initially qd, may increase dosage by 5 mg at 1 wk or more intervals

Elderly: PO 5 mg, may increase cautiously at 1 wk intervals

Available forms: Tabs 2.5, 5, 7.5, 10 mg

Adverse effects
CNS: EPS: pseudoparkinsonism, akathisia, dystonia, tardive dyskinesia, **seizures,** headache, **neuroleptic malignant syndrome (rare),** fever, insomnia, somnolence, agitation, nervousness, hostility, dizziness, hypertonia, tremor, euphoria
CV: Orthostatic hypotension, tachycardia, chest pain
EENT: Blurred vision
GI: Dry mouth, nausea, vomiting, anorexia, constipation, abdominal pain, weight gain
GU: Urinary retention, urinary frequency, enuresis, impotence, amenorrhea, gynecomastia, breast engorgement, premenstrual syndrome
INTEG: Rash
MS: Joint pain, twitching
RESP: Dyspnea, rhinitis, cough, pharyngitis

Contraindications: Hypersensitivity

Precautions: Pregnancy **C,** lactation, hypertension, hepatic disease, cardiac disease, elderly

Pharmacokinetics

Absorption	Well
Distribution	93% plasma protein binding
Metabolism	Liver
Excretion	Kidneys
Half-life	Unknown

Pharmacodynamics

Onset	Unknown
Peak	6 hr
Duration	Unknown

Interactions
Individual drugs
Alcohol: ↑ sedation
Bromocriptine: ↓ antiparkinson activity
Carbamazepine: ↓ levels of olanzapine
Levodopa: ↓ antiparkinson activity
Omeprazole: ↓ olanzapine level
Rifampin: ↓ olanzapine level
Drug classifications
Anesthetics, barbiturates: ↑ sedation
Anticholinergics: ↑ anticholinergic effects
Antidepressants: ↑ sedation
Antihistamines: ↑ sedation
Antihypertensives: ↑ hypotension
Lab test interferences
↑ Liver function test, ↑ prolactin, ↑ CPK

NURSING CONSIDERATIONS
Assessment
• Assess mental status, orientation, mood, behavior, presence of hallucinations and type before initial administration and monthly
• Monitor swallowing of PO medication: check for hoarding or giving of medication to other patients
• Monitor I&O ratio; palpate bladder if low urinary output **G** occurs, especially in elderly
• Monitor bilirubin, CBC, liver function studies monthly
• Monitor urinalysis; recommended before, during prolonged therapy
• Assess affect, orientation, LOC, reflexes, gait, coordination, sleep pattern disturbances
• Monitor B/P sitting, standing, lying; take pulse and respirations q4h during initial treatment; establish baseline before starting treatment; report drops of 30 mm Hg; obtain baseline ECG
• Assess dizziness, faintness, palpitations, tachycardia on rising
• Assess for neuroleptic malignant syndrome: hyperpyrexia, muscle rigidity, increased CPK, altered mental status, for acute dystonia (check chewing, swallowing, eyes, pin rolling)
• EPS, including akathisia (inability to sit still, no pattern to movements), tardive dyskinesia (bizarre movements of the jaw, mouth, tongue, extremities), pseudoparkinsonism (rigidity, tremors, pill rolling, shuffling gait)
• Monitor skin turgor daily
• Monitor constipation, urinary retention daily; increase bulk, H_2O in diet

Nursing diagnoses
☑ Thought processes, altered (uses)
☑ Knowledge deficit (teaching)
☑ Noncompliance (teaching)

Implementation
• Give antiparkinsonian agent for EPS
G • Give decreased dose in elderly
• Give PO with full glass of water, milk; or with food to decrease GI upset
• Provide decreased stimuli by dimming light, avoiding loud noises
• Provide supervised ambulation until stabilized on medication; do not involve in strenuous exercise program because fainting is possible; patients should not stand still for long periods
• Give increased fluids to prevent constipation
• Give sips of water, candy, gum for dry mouth
• Store in tight, light-resistant container

Patient/family education
• Teach patient to use good oral hygiene; frequent rinsing of mouth, sugarless gum for dry mouth
• Advise patient to avoid hazardous activities until drug response is determined
• Advise patient that orthostatic hypotension occurs often and to rise from sitting or lying position gradually
• Advise patient to avoid hot tubs, hot showers, tub baths, since hypotension may occur
• Advise patient to avoid abrupt withdrawal of this drug, or EPS may result; drug should be withdrawn slowly
• Advise patient to avoid OTC preparations (cough, hay fever,

---

☑ Herb/drug   ⊘ Do Not Crush   ◆ Alert   ⊶ Key Drug   **G** Geriatric   **P** Pediatric cold) unless approved by prescriber, since serious drug interactions may occur; avoid use with alcohol, CNS depressants, increased drowsiness may occur

• Advise patient that in hot weather, heat stroke may occur; take extra precautions to stay cool

Evaluation

Positive therapeutic outcome

• Decrease in emotional excitement, hallucinations, delusion, paranoia, reorganization of patterns of thought, speech

Treatment of overdose:

Lavage if orally ingested; provide airway; do not induce vomiting or use epinephrine

---

omeprazole (Ŗ)

(oh-mep'ra-zole)
Losec ♣, Prilosec
Func. class.: Proton pump inhibitor
Chem. class.: Benzimidazole

Pregnancy category   C

Action: Suppresses gastric secretion by inhibiting hydrogen/potassium ATPase enzyme system in the gastric parietal cell; characterized as a gastric acid pump inhibitor, since it blocks the final step of acid production

Therapeutic Outcome: Absence of duodenal ulcers; decreased gastroesophageal reflux

Uses: Gastroesophageal reflux disease (GERD), severe erosive esophagitis, poorly responsive systemic GERD, pathologic hypersecretory conditions (Zollinger-Ellison syndrome, systemic mastocytosis, multiple endocrine adenomas); possibly effective for treatment of duodenal ulcers with or without antiinfectives for *Helicobacter pylori*

Investigational uses: Posterior laryngitis, enhancing pancreatin

Dosage and routes
Active duodenal ulcers
Adult: PO 20 mg qd × 4-8 wk; associated with *H. pylori* 40 mg q AM and clarithromycin 500 mg tid on days 1-14, then 20 mg qd days 15-28

Severe erosive esophagitis/ poorly responsive gastroesophageal reflux disease
Adult: PO 20 mg qd × 4-8 wk

Pathologic hypersecretory conditions
Adult: PO 60 mg/day; may increase to 120 mg tid; daily doses >80 mg should be divided

Gastric ulcer
Adult: PO 40 mg qd × 4-8 wk

Available forms: Sus rel cap 20, 40 mg

Adverse effects
CNS: Headache, dizziness, asthenia
CV: Chest pain, angina, tachycardia, bradycardia, palpitations, peripheral edema
EENT: Tinnitus, taste perversion
GI: Diarrhea, abdominal pain, vomiting, nausea, constipation, flatulence, acid regurgitation, abdominal swelling, anorexia, irritable colon, esophageal candidiasis, dry mouth
GU: UTI, frequency, increased creatinine, **proteinuria, hematuria,** testicular pain, glycosuria

---

HEMA: **Pancytopenia, thrombocytopenia, neutropenia, leukocytosis,** anemia
INTEG: Rash, dry skin, urticaria, pruritus, alopecia
META: Hypoglycemia, increased hepatic enzymes, weight gain
MISC: Back pain, fever, fatigue, malaise
RESP: Upper respiratory tract infections, cough, epistaxis

Contraindications: Hypersensitivity

Precautions: Pregnancy **C,**
P lactation, children

N Do Not Confuse:
Prilosec/Prinivil, Prilosec/Prozac, Prilosec/prednisone

Pharmacokinetics

Absorption	Rapidly absorbed
Distribution	Protein binding (95%); gastric parietal cells
Metabolism	Liver, extensively
Excretion	Kidneys, feces
G Half-life	½-1 hr; increased in the elderly, hepatic disease

Pharmacodynamics

Onset	1 hr
Peak	½-3½ hr
Duration	3-4 days

Interactions
Individual drugs
Ampicillin: ↓ absorption of omeprazole
Clarithromycin: ↑ omeprazole level
Diazepam: ↑ serum levels of diazepam
Flurazepam: ↑ omeprazole level
Ketoconazole: ↓ absorption of ketoconazole
Phenytoin: ↑ serum levels of phenytoin
Sucralfate: ↓ absorption

Triazolam: ↑ omeprazole level
Warfarin: ↑ bleeding tendencies
Drug classifications
Iron products: ↓ absorption of iron
☑ Herb/drug
Angelica: ↓ omeprazole effect

NURSING CONSIDERATIONS
Assessment
• Assess GI system: bowel sounds q8h, abdomen for pain and swelling, anorexia
• Monitor hepatic enzymes: AST, ALT, increased alkaline phosphatase during treatment

Nursing diagnoses
☑ Pain (uses)
☑ Knowledge deficit (teaching)

Implementation
• Give before patient eats; patient should swallow cap whole
◯ • Do not open, chew, or crush; may give with antacids

Patient/family education
• Advise patient to report severe diarrhea; drug may have to be discontinued
• Caution patient to avoid driving and other hazardous activities until response to drug is known
• Caution patient to avoid alcohol, salicylates, ibuprofen; may cause GI irritation

Evaluation
Positive therapeutic outcome
• Absence of epigastric pain, swelling, fullness

ondansetron (℞)
(on-dan'sa-tron)
Zofran
Func. class.: Antiemetic
Chem. class.: 5-HT receptor antagonist
Pregnancy category B

Action: Prevents nausea, vomiting by blocking serotonin peripherally, centrally, and in the small intestine

➥Therapeutic Outcome: Control of nausea, vomiting

Uses: Prevention of nausea, vomiting associated with cancer chemotherapy and prevention of postopertive nausea, vomiting

Dosage and routes
Prevention of nausea/vomiting associated with cancer chemotherapy
P *Adult/child 4-18 yr:* **IV** 0.15 mg/kg infused over 15 min, 30 min before start of cancer chemotherapy; 0.15 mg/kg is given 4 hr and 8 hr after first dose or 32 mg as a single dose; dilute in 50 ml of D_5 or 0.9% NaCl before giving

Prevention of nausea/vomiting of radiotherapy
Adult: PO 8 mg tid

Prevention of postoperative nausea/vomiting
Adult: **IV** 4 mg undiluted over >30 sec

P *Child 2-12 yr:* **IV** 0.1 mg/kg (≤40 kg); 4 mg (≥40 kg) give ≥30 secs

Hepatic dose
Max dose 8 mg qd

Available forms: Inj 2 mg/ml, 32 mg/50 ml (premixed); tabs 4, 8 mg; oral sol 4 mg/5 ml

Adverse effects
CNS: Headache, dizziness, drowsiness, fatigue, extrapyramidal syndrome
GI: Diarrhea, constipation, abdominal pain
MISC: Rash, **bronchospasm** (rare), *MS pain, wound problems, shivering, fever, hypoxia, urinary retention*

Contraindications: Hypersensitivity

P Precautions: Pregnancy **B**,
G lactation, children, elderly

Do Not Confuse:
Zofran/Zantac

Pharmacokinetics	
Absorption	Completely absorbed (**IV**)
Distribution	Unknown
Metabolism	Liver, extensively
Excretion	Kidneys
Half-life	3.5-4.7 hr

Pharmacodynamics
Unknown

Interactions: Unknown

O

NURSING CONSIDERATIONS
Assessment
• Assess for absence of nausea, vomiting during chemotherapy
• Assess for hypersensitivity reaction: rash, bronchospasm
• Assess for EPS: shuffling gait, tremors, grimacing, rigidity
Nursing diagnoses
✓ Knowledge deficit (teaching)
✓ Noncompliance (teaching)
Implementation
IV **IV route**
• Give **IV** after diluting a single dose in 50 ml 0.9% NaCl or D_5W, 0.45%; give over 15 min
• Store at room temp for 48-hr after dilution

Y-site compatibilities:
Aldesleukin, amifostine, amikacin, aztreonam, bleomycin, carboplatin, carmustine, cefazolin, ceforanide, cefotazime, cefoxitin, ceftazidime, ceftizoxime, cefuroxime, chlorpromazine, cimetidine, cisatracurium, cisplatin, cladribine, clindamycin, cyclophosphamide, cytarabine, dacarbazine, dactinomycin, daunorubicin, dexamethasone, diphenhydramine, doxorubicin, doxorubicin liposome, doxycycline, droperidol, etoposide, famotidine, filgrastim, floxuridine, fluconazole, fludarabine, gentamicin, haloperidol, heparin, hydrocortisone, hydromorphone, hydroxyzine, ifosfamide, imipenem/cilastatin, magnesium sulfate, mannitol, mechlorethamine, melphalan, meperidine, mesna, methotrexate, metoclopramide, miconazole, mitomycin, mitoxantrone, morphine, paclitaxel, pentostatin, potassium chloride, prochlorperazine, ranitidine, remifentanil, streptozocin, teniposide, thiotepa, ticarcillin, ticarcillin/clavulanate, vancomycin, vinblastine, vincristine, vinorelbine, zidovudine

Y-site incompatibilities:
Acyclovir, aminophylline, amphotericin B, ampicillin, ampicillin/sulbactam, cefoperazone, furosemide, ganciclovir, lorazepam, methylprednisolone, mezlocillin, piperacillin, sargramostim, sodium bicarbonate

Additive compatibilities:
Cisplatin, cyclophosphamide, cytarabine, dacarbazine, dexamethasone, doxorubicin, etoposide, meperidine, methotrexate

Solution compatibilities:
May also be diluted with D_5W, LR, $D_5/0.9\%$ NaCl, $D_5/0.45\%$ NaCl

Patient/family education
• Instruct patient to report diarrhea, constipation, rash, or changes in respirations
• Teach patient reason for medication and expected results

Evaluation
Positive therapeutic outcome
• Absence of nausea, vomiting during cancer chemotherapy

oral contraceptives
(℞)
Func. class.: Hormone
Chem. class.: Estrogen/progestin combinations
Pregnancy category   X

Action: Prevents ovulation by suppressing FSH, LH; **monophasic:** estrogen/progestin (fixed dose) used during a 21-day cycle; ovulation is inhibited by suppression of FSH and LH; thickness of cervical mucus and endometrial lining prevents pregnancy; **biphasic:** ovulation is inhibited by suppression of FSH and LH; alteration of cervical mucus, endometrial lining prevents pregnancy; **triphasic:** ovulation is inhibited by suppression of FSH and LH; change of cervical mucus, endometrial lining prevents pregnancy; variable doses of estrogen/progestin combinations may be similar to natural hormonal fluctuations; **progestin-only pill and**

---

implant: change of cervical mucus and endometrial lining prevents pregnancy; ovulation may be suppressed

⇒ **Therapeutic Outcome:** Prevention of pregnancy, decreased severity of endometriosis, hypermenorrhea

Uses: To prevent pregnancy, endometriosis, hypermenorrhea

Dosage and routes
Adult: PO 1 qd starting on day 5 of menstrual cycle; day 1 is 1st day of period

21-tab packs
Adult: PO 1 qd starting on day 7 of menstrual cycle; day 1 is 1st day of period; then on 20 or 21 days, off 7 days

28-tab packs
Adult: PO 1 qd continuously

Biphasic
Adult: 1 qd × 10 days, then next color 1 qd × 11 days

Triphasic
Adult: 1 qd; check package insert for each brand

Implant
Adult: Subdermal 6 cap implanted during the first wk of menses

Endometriosis
Adult: PO 1 qd × 20 days from day 5 to day 24 of cycle

Adult: PO 1 qd; check package insert for specific instructions

Available forms: Check specific brand

Adverse effects
CNS: Depression, fatigue, dizziness, nervousness, anxiety, headache
CV: Increased B/P, **cerebral hemorrhage, thrombosis,** **pulmonary embolism,** fluid retention, edema
EENT: Optic neuritis, retinal thrombosis, cataracts
ENDO: Decreased glucose tolerance, increased TBG, PBI, T_4, T_3
GI: Nausea, vomiting, cramps, diarrhea, bloating, constipation, change in appetite, **cholestatic jaundice**
GU: Breakthrough bleeding, amenorrhea, spotting, dysmenorrhea, galactorrhea, endocervical hyperplasia, vaginitis, cystitis-like syndrome, breast change
HEMA: Increased fibrinogen, clotting factor
INTEG: Chloasma, melasma, acne, rash, urticaria, erythema, pruritus, hirsutism, alopecia, photosensitivity

Contraindications: Pregnancy **X,** lactation, reproductive cancer, thrombophlebitis, MI, hepatic tumors, hepatic disease, CAD, women 40 yr and over, CVA

Precautions: Depression, hypertension, renal disease, seizure disorders, lupus erythematosus, rheumatic disease, migraine headache, amenorrhea, irregular menses, breast cancer (fibrocystic), gallbladder disease, diabetes mellitus, heavy smoking, acute mononucleosis, sickle cell disease

Pharmacokinetics	
Absorption	Well absorbed
Distribution	Unknown
Metabolism	Liver, extensively
Excretion	Kidneys
Half-life	Unknown

Pharmacodynamics			
	PO	IM	IMPLANT
Onset	1 mo	1 mo	1 mo
Peak	1 mo	1 mo	1 mo
Duration	1 mo	3 mo	5 yr

Interactions
Individual drugs
Aminocaproic acid: ↑ clotting
Bromocriptine: ↓ effectiveness of bromocriptine
Carbamazepine: ↓ effectiveness of oral contraceptive
Chenodiol: ↓ effectiveness of oral contraceptive
Chloramphenicol: ↓ effectiveness of oral contraceptive
Dantrolene: ↑ hepatic toxicity (estrogen only)
Dihydroergotamine: ↓ effectiveness of oral contraceptive
Griseofulvin: ↓ effectiveness of oral contraceptive
Mineral oil: ↓ effectiveness of oral contraceptive
Phenylbutazone: ↓ effectiveness of oral contraceptive
Phenytoin: ↓ effectiveness of oral contraceptive
Primidone: ↓ effectiveness of oral contraceptive
Rifampin: ↓ effectiveness of oral contraceptive
Warfarin: ↑ or ↓ effect of warfarin
Drug classifications
Analgesics: ↓ action of oral contraceptives
Antibiotics: ↓ action of oral contraceptives
Anticonvulsants: ↓ action of oral contraceptives
Antihistamines: ↓ action of oral contraceptives
Glucocorticoids: ↓ action of oral contraceptives
Oral anticoagulants: ↓ action of oral anticoagulants
Tricyclic antidepressants: ↑ toxicity

Food/drug
Grapefruit: ↑ peak level
Lab test interferences
↑ Pro-time; ↑ clotting factors VII, VIII, IX, X; ↑ TBG, ↑ PBI, ↑ T$_4$, ↑ platelet aggregation, ↑ BSP, ↑ triglycerides, ↑ bilirubin, ↑ AST, ↑ ALT ↓ T$_3$, ↓ antithrombin III, ↓ folate, ↓ metyrapone test, ↓ GTT, ↓ 17-OHCS
☑ Herb/drug
St. John's wort: ↓ oral contraceptive effect

NURSING CONSIDERATIONS
Assessment
• Assess for reproductive changes: change in breasts, tumors, positive Pap smear; drug should be discontinued if changes occur
• Monitor glucose, thyroid function, liver function tests, B/P

Nursing diagnoses
☑ Injury, risk for (adverse reactions)
☑ Body image disturbance (adverse reactions)
☑ Knowledge deficit (teaching)
☑ Noncompliance (teaching)

Implementation
PO route
• If GI symptoms occur, medication may be taken with food; take at same time each day
Implant route
• Inject 6 cap subdermally
• Implant is effective for 5 yr, should be removed after that
IM route
• Administer deep in large muscle mass after shaking susp well; ensure pregnancy has not occurred if inj are 2 wk or more apart

Patient/family education
• Teach patient about detection of clots using Homans'

☑ Herb/drug   Ⓢ Do Not Crush   ♦ Alert   ⦿ Key Drug   Ⓖ Geriatric   Ⓟ Pediatric sign; teach monitoring technique for heat, redness, pain, swelling

• Teach patient to use sunscreen or to avoid sunlight; photosensitivity can occur

• Teach patient to take at same time each day to ensure equal drug level; to take another tab as soon as possible if one is missed; teach patient that after drug is discontinued, pregnancy may not occur for several mo

• Instruct patient to report GI symptoms that occur after 4 mo

• Advise patient to use another birth control method during first 3 wk of oral contraceptive use

• Teach patient to report abdominal pain, change in vision, shortness of breath, change in menstrual flow, spotting, breakthrough bleeding, breast lumps, swelling, headache, severe leg pain, mental changes; that continuing medical care is needed: PAP smear and gynecologic examinations q6 mo

• Teach patient to notify physicians and dentist of oral contraceptive use

Evaluation
Positive therapeutic outcome
• Absence of pregnancy
• Decreased severity of endometriosis
• Decreased severity of hypermenorrhea

orlistat
See Appendix A,
Selected New Drugs

oseltamivir
See Appendix A,
Selected New Drugs

oxacillin (℞)
(ox-a-sill'in)
Bactocill, oxacillin sodium, Prostaphilin
Func. class.: Broad-spectrum antiinfective
Chem. class.: Penicillinase-resistant penicillin

Pregnancy category B

Action: Interferes with cell wall replication of susceptible organisms; osmotically unstable cell wall swells, bursts from osmotic pressure

▸**Therapeutic Outcome:** Bactericidal effects for gram-positive cocci *Staphylococcus aureus, Streptococcus pneumoniae,* infections caused by penicillinase-producing *staphylococci*

Uses: Infections caused by penicillinase-producing staphylococci, streptococci; respiratory tract, skin, skin structure, urinary tract, bone, joint infections, sinusitis, endocarditis, septicemia, meningitis

Dosage and routes
Adult: PO 2-6 g/day in divided doses q4-6h; IM/**IV** 2-12 g/day in divided doses q4-6h

▣ *Child:* PO 50-100 mg/kg/day in divided doses q6h; IM/**IV** 50-100 mg/kg/day in divided doses q4-6h

Available forms: Caps 250, 500 mg; powder for oral susp 250 mg/5 ml; powder for inj 250, 500 mg, 1, 2, 4, 10 g

Adverse effects
CNS: Lethargy, hallucinations, anxiety, depression, twitching, **coma, convulsions**
GI: Nausea, vomiting, diarrhea, increased AST, ALT, abdominal pain, glossitis, colitis
GU: **Oliguria, proteinuria, hematuria, vaginitis, moniliasis, glomerulonephritis**
HEMA: Anemia, increased bleeding time, **bone marrow depression, granulocytopenia**

Contraindications: Hypersensitivity to penicillins

Precautions: Pregnancy **B**, hypersensitivity to cephalosporins, neonates

▨ Do Not Confuse:
Bactocill/Pathocil

Pharmacokinetics

Absorption	Rapid, incomplete (PO); well absorbed (IM); completely (**IV**)
Distribution	Widely distributed; crosses placenta
Metabolism	Liver
Excretion	Kidneys, unchanged (51%); breast milk
Half-life	20-50 min; increased in severe hepatic disease

Pharmacodynamics

	PO	IM	IV
Onset	Rapid	Rapid	Rapid
Peak	½-1 hr	½ hr	Inf end

Interactions
Individual drugs
Aspirin: ↑ oxacillin levels, ↓ renal excretion
Chloramphenicol: ↑ half-life of chloramphenicol, ↓ effectiveness of oxacillin
Cholestyramine: ↓ effectiveness of oxacillin
Colestipol: ↓ effectiveness of oxacillin
Disulfiram: ↑ oxacillin effect

Probenecid: ↑ oxacillin levels, ↓ renal excretion
Drug classifications
Erythromycins: ↓ antimicrobial effectiveness
Oral anticoagulants: ↑ anticoagulant effects
Oral contraceptives: ↓ contraceptive effectiveness
Tetracyclines: ↓ antimicrobial effectiveness
Food/drug
Food, carbonated drinks, citrus fruit juices: ↓ absorption
▨ *Herb/drug*
Khat: ↓ absorption
Lab test interferences
False positive: Urine glucose, urine protein

NURSING CONSIDERATIONS
Assessment
• Assess patient for previous sensitivity reaction to penicillins or other cephalosporins; cross-sensitivity between penicillins and cephalosporins is common
• Assess patient for signs and symptoms of infection including characteristics of wounds, sputum, urine, stool, WBC >10,000, fever; obtain baseline information and during treatment
• Obtain C&S before beginning drug therapy to identify if correct treatment has been initiated
• Assess for allergic reactions: rash, urticaria, pruritus, chills, fever, joint pain; angioedema may occur a few days after therapy begins; epinephrine, resuscitation equipment should be available for anaphylactic reaction
◆• Assess urine output; if decreasing, notify prescriber (may indicate nephrotoxicity); also

---

check for increased BUN, creatinine
• Monitor blood studies: AST, ALT, CBC, Hct, bilirubin, LDH, alkaline phosphatase, Coombs' test monthly if patient is on long-term therapy
• Monitor electrolytes: potassium, sodium, chloride monthly if patient is on long-term therapy
• Assess bowel pattern qd; if severe diarrhea occurs, drug should be discontinued; may indicate pseudomembranous colitis
• Monitor for bleeding: ecchymosis, bleeding gums, hematuria, stool guaiac daily if on long-term therapy
• Assess for overgrowth of infection: perineal itching, fever, malaise, redness, pain, swelling, drainage, rash, diarrhea, change in cough, sputum

Nursing diagnoses
☑ Infection, risk for (uses)
☑ Diarrhea (adverse reactions)
☑ Injury, risk for (adverse reactions)
☑ Knowledge deficit (teaching)
☑ Noncompliance (teaching)

Implementation
PO route
• Give in even doses around the clock; if GI upset occurs, give with food; drug must be given for 10-14 days to ensure organism death and prevent superinfection; store in tight container
• Shake susp; store in refrigerator for 2 wk, 1 wk at room temp
IM route
• Reconstitute 250 mg/1.4 ml, 500 mg/2.7-2.8 ml, 1 g/5.7 ml, 2 g/11.4-11.5 ml, 4 g/21.8-23 ml of sterile water for a conc of 250 mg/1.5 ml;

store unused portion in refrigerator for 1 wk or 3 days at room temp
• Inject deeply in large muscle mass
▮ IV route
• Reconstitute 250 mg/1.4 ml, 500 mg/2.7-2.8 ml, 1 g/5.7 ml, 2 g/11.4-11.5 ml, 4 g/21.8-23 ml of sterile water for a conc of 250 mg/1.5 ml; store unused portion in refrigerator for 1 week or 3 days at room temp
• Give direct **IV** by diluting reconstituted sol with 250-500 mg/5 ml, 1 g/10 ml, 2 g/20 ml, 4 g/40 ml of sterile water or 0.9% NaCl, give over 10 min
• Give by intermittent inf by diluting to a conc of 0.5-40 mg/ml with D_5W, 0.9% NaCl, D_5/0.9% NaCl, LR; give over 6 hr or less

Y-site compatibilities:
Acyclovir, cyclophosphamide, diltiazem, famotidine, fluconazole, foscarnet, heparin, hydrocortisone, hydromorphone, labetalol, magnesium sulfate, meperidine, methotrexate, morphine, perphenazine, potassium chloride, tacrolimus, vitamin B with C, zidovudine

Y-site incompatibilities:
Verapamil

Additive compatibilities:
Cephapirin, chloramphenicol, dopamine, potassium chloride, sodium bicarbonate

Additive incompatibilities:
Cytarabine, tetracycline

Patient/family education
• Teach patient to report sore throat, bruising, bleeding, joint pain; may indicate blood dyscrasias (rare)
• Advise patient to contact prescriber if vaginal itching,

O

loose, foul-smelling stools, furry tongue occur; may indicate superinfection
• Instruct patient to take all medication prescribed for the length of time ordered
• Advise patient to notify prescriber of diarrhea with blood or pus, which may indicate pseudomembranous colitis

Evaluation
Positive therapeutic outcome
• Absence of signs/symptoms of infection (WBC <10,000, temp WNL, absence of red, draining wounds)
• Reported improvement in symptoms of infection

Treatment of anaphylaxis: Withdraw drug, maintain airway, administer epinephrine, aminophylline, O_2, **IV** corticosteroids

---

oxaprozin (℞)
(ox-a-proe'zin)
Daypro
Func. class.: Nonsteroidal antiinflammatory
Chem. class.: Propionic acid derivative
Pregnancy category C

Action: Inhibits prostaglandin synthesis by decreasing an enzyme needed for biosynthesis; analgesic, antiinflammatory

➡ **Therapeutic Outcome:** Decreased pain, inflammation

Uses: Acute and long-term management of osteoarthritis, rheumatoid arthritis

Dosage and routes
Adult: PO 600-1200 mg qd; maximum dose 1800 mg/day

or 26 mg/kg, whichever is lower in divided doses

Available forms: Tab 600 mg
Adverse effects
CNS: Dizziness, headache, drowsiness, fatigue, tremors, confusion, insomnia, anxiety, malaise, depression
CV: Tachycardia, peripheral edema, palpitations, dysrhythmias
EENT: Tinnitus, hearing loss, blurred vision
GI: Nausea, *anorexia,* vomiting, *diarrhea,* jaundice, **cholestatic hepatitis,** constipation, flatulence, *cramps,* dry mouth, peptic ulcer, **bleeding,** melena, gastroenteritis
GU: **Nephrotoxicity: dysuria, hematuria, oliguria, azotemia**
HEMA: Increased bleeding time
INTEG: Purpura, rash, pruritus, sweating, photosensitivity
SYST: **Anaphylaxis, angioneurotic edema**

Contraindications: Hypersensitivity, asthma, patients in whom aspirin and iodides have induced symptoms of allergic reactions or asthma

Precautions: Pregnancy **C**, lactation, children, bleeding disorders, GI disorders, cardiac disorders, CHF, hypersensitivity to other antiinflammatory agents, severe renal and hepatic disease, elderly

 Do Not Confuse:
Daypro/Diupres

Pharmacokinetics	
Absorption	Well absorbed
Distribution	Unknown
Metabolism	Liver, extensively
Excretion	Breast milk
Half-life	40-50 hr

Pharmacodynamics	
Onset	Unknown
Peak	2 hr
Duration	Unknown

Interactions
Individual drugs
Acetaminophen (long-term use): ↑ renal reactions
Alcohol: ↑ adverse reactions
Aspirin: ↓ effectiveness, ↑ adverse reactions
Cyclosporine: ↑ toxicity
Digoxin: ↑ toxicity, levels
Insulin: ↑ insulin effect
Lithium: ↑ toxicity
Methotrexate: ↑ toxicity
Phenytoin: ↑ phenytoin level
Radiation: ↑ risk of hematologic toxicity
Sulfonylurea: ↑ toxicity
Drug classifications
Anticoagulants: ↑ risk of bleeding
Antihypertensives: ↓ effect of antihypertensives
Antineoplastics: ↑ risk of hematologic toxicity
β-Adrenergic blockers: ↑ antihypertension
Diuretics: ↓ effectiveness of diuretics
Glucocorticoids: ↑ adverse reactions
NSAIDs: ↑ adverse reactions
Potassium supplements: ↑ adverse reactions
Sulfonamides: ↑ toxicity
Lab test interferences
↑ BUN, ↑ alkaline phosphatase
False: ↑ 5-HIAA, false ↑ 17KS

NURSING CONSIDERATIONS
Assessment
• Assess for pain and ROM: intensity, location, duration
• Monitor blood studies: alkaline phosphatase, LDH, AST, ALT, and bleeding time (may be increased)

• Assess for asthma, aspirin hypersensitivity, nasal polyps; increased hypersensitivity reactions

Nursing diagnoses
☑ Pain (uses)
☑ Mobility, impaired (uses)
☑ Injury, risk for (adverse reactions)
☑ Knowledge deficit (teaching)

Implementation
• Give with food or milk to decrease gastric symptoms

Patient/family education
• Teach patient that drug must be continued for prescribed time to be effective; to avoid aspirin, alcoholic beverages
• Instruct patient to use caution when driving; drowsiness, dizziness may occur
• Teach patient to take with a full glass of water to enhance absorption; patient should sit upright for 30 min to prevent stomach irritation and ulceration
🚫 • Do not crush, break, or chew
• Instruct patient to use sunscreen and protective clothing to prevent burns
• Advise patient to report to prescriber severe abdominal pain, rash, itching, yellowing of skin or eyes, depression

Evaluation
Positive therapeutic outcome
• Decreased pain
• Decreased inflammation
• Increased mobility

oxazepam (℞)
(ox-az′e-pam)
Apo-Oxazepam ✦,
Novoxapam ✦, oxazepam,
Ox-Pam ✦, Serax, Zapex ✦
Func. class.: Sedative/
hypnotic; antianxiety
Chem. class.: Benzodiaze-
pine

Pregnancy category **D**
**Controlled substance
schedule** **IV**

Action: Depresses subcortical
levels of CNS, including limbic
system, reticular formation;
potentiates GABA

➡ **Therapeutic Outcome:** Decreased anxiety, successful
alcohol withdrawal, relaxation

Uses: Anxiety, alcohol withdrawal

Dosage and routes
Anxiety
Adult: PO 10-30 mg tid-qid

Alcohol withdrawal
Adult: PO 15-30 mg tid-qid

Available forms: Caps 10, 15,
30 mg; tab 15 mg

Adverse effects
CNS: Dizziness, drowsiness,
confusion, headache, anxiety,
tremors, fatigue, depression,
insomnia, hallucinations, paradoxic excitement, transient
amnesia
CV: Orthostatic hypotension,
ECG changes, tachycardia,
hypotension
EENT: Blurred vision, tinnitus,
mydriasis
GI: Nausea, vomiting, anorexia
INTEG: Rash, dermatitis,
itching

Contraindications: Hypersensitivity to benzodiazepines,
narrow-angle glaucoma, psy-

P chosis, pregnancy **D,** child
<12 yr

G **Precautions:** Elderly, debilitated, hepatic disease, renal
disease

Pharmacokinetics	
Absorption	Well absorbed
Distribution	Widely distributed; crosses placenta, blood-brain barrier
Metabolism	Liver
Excretion	Kidneys, breast milk
Half-life	5-15 hr

Pharmacodynamics	
Onset	½-1½ hr
Peak	Unknown
Duration	6-12 hr

Interactions
Individual drugs
Alcohol: ↑ CNS depression
Cimetidine: ↑ action
Fluoxetine: ↑ action
Levodopa: ↓ action of levo-
dopa
Metoprolol: ↑ action
Phenytoin: ↓ effect
Propoxyphene: ↑ action
Theophylline: ↓ sedative
effects
Drug classifications
Antidepressants: ↑ CNS
depression
Antihistamines: ↑ CNS de-
pression
Opiates: ↑ CNS depression
Oral contraceptives: ↑ effect
Lab test interferences
↑ AST, ↑ ALT, ↑ serum biliru-
bin
False: ↑ 17-OHCS
↓ RAIU

NURSING CONSIDERATIONS
Assessment
• Assess mental status: mood,
sensorium, anxiety, affect,
sleeping pattern, drowsiness,
G dizziness, especially elderly;

☒ Herb/drug   Ⓢ Do Not Crush   ⬥ Alert   ⬥╥ Key Drug   **G** Geriatric   **P** Pediatric physical dependency, with-drawal symptoms: anxiety, panic attacks, agitation, con-vulsions, headache, nausea, vomiting, muscle pain, weakness; suicidal tendencies; indications of increasing toler-ance and abuse

• Monitor B/P with patient lying, standing, pulse; if sys-tolic B/P drops 20 mm Hg, hold drug, notify prescriber

• Monitor blood studies: CBC during long-term therapy; blood dyscrasias have occurred rarely; decreased hematocrit, neutropenia may occur

• Monitor hepatic studies: AST, ALT, bilirubin, creatinine LDH, alkaline phosphatase

• Monitor I&O; indicate renal dysfunction

Nursing diagnoses
☑ Anxiety (uses)
☑ Depression (uses)
☑ Injury, risk for (adverse reac-tions)
☑ Knowledge deficit (teaching)

Implementation
• Give with food or milk for GI symptoms; tab may be crushed if patient is unable to swallow medication whole; give sugarless gum, hard candy, frequent sips of water for dry mouth

Patient/family education
• Teach patient that drug may be taken with food or fluids; tab may be crushed or swal-lowed whole

• Caution patient not to use for everyday stress or longer than 3 mo unless directed by prescriber; not to take more than prescribed amount; may be habit forming; not to double doses or skip doses

• Advise patient to avoid OTC preparations unless approved

by prescriber; alcohol and CNS depressants will increase CNS depression

• Caution patient to avoid driv-ing and activities that require alertness, since drowsiness may occur; to avoid alcohol and other psychotropic medica-tions; to rise slowly or fainting may occur, especially elderly; that drowsiness may worsen at be-ginning of treatment

• Caution patient not to dis-continue medication abruptly after long-term use; withdrawal symptoms include vomiting, cramping, tremors, seizures

Evaluation
Positive therapeutic outcome
• Decreased anxiety, restless-ness, sleeplessness (short-term treatment only)

Treatment of overdose: Lavage, VS, supportive care

---

oxtriphylline (℞)
(ox-trye′fi-lin)
Apo-Oxtriphylline ✦,
Choledyl, Choledyl SA,
Novotriphyl ✦, oxtriphylline
Func. class.: Bronchodila-tor, spasmolytic
Chem. class.: Choline salt of theophylline
Pregnancy category   C

Action: Relaxes smooth mus-cle of respiratory system by blocking phosphodiesterase, which increases cAMP; 64% theophylline

▸**Therapeutic Outcome:** Bron-chodilatation with ease of breathing

Uses: Acute bronchial asthma, reversible bronchospasm in chronic bronchitis and COPD

✦ Canada Only   Adverse effects: *italic* = common; **bold** = life-threatening

Dosage and routes

P *Adult and child >12 yr:* PO 4.7 mg/kg q8h or sus action q12h

P *Child 9-16 yr and smokers (adult):* 4.7 mg/kg q6h

P *Child 1-9 yr:* 6.2 mg/kg q6h

Available forms: Elix 100 mg/5 ml ✿; syr 50 mg/5 ml; tabs 100, 200 mg; ext rel tabs 400, 600 mg

Adverse effects

CNS: Anxiety, restlessness, insomnia, dizziness, **convulsions,** headache, lightheadedness

CV: **Palpitations, sinus tachycardia,** hypotension

GI: Nausea, vomiting, anorexia, diarrhea, bitter taste, dyspepsia

INTEG: Flushing, urticaria, alopecia

RESP: Increased rate, **respiratory arrest**

Contraindications: Hypersensitivity to xanthines, tachydysrhythmias

G **Precautions:** Elderly, CHF, cor pulmonale, hepatic disease, active peptic ulcer disease, diabetes mellitus, hyperthy-
P roidism, hypertension, children, pregnancy **C,** glaucoma, prostatic hypertrophy

Pharmacokinetics	
Absorption	Well absorbed (PO); slow (PO-SA)
Distribution	Widely distributed; crosses placenta
Metabolism	Liver to caffeine
Excretion	Kidneys, breast milk
Half-life	3-13 hr; increased in renal disease, CHF

Pharmacodynamics		
	PO	PO-SA
Onset	15-60 min	Unknown
Peak	1-5 hr	4-8 hr
Duration	6-8 hr	8-12 hr

Interactions

Individual drugs

Allopurinol: ↓ metabolism, ↑ toxicity

Carbamazepine: ↑ or ↓ oxtriphylline levels

Cimetidine: ↓ metabolism, ↑ toxicity

Disulfiram: ↓ metabolism, ↑ toxicity

Erythromycin: ↓ metabolism, ↑ toxicity

Fluvoxamine: ↑ toxicity

Halothane: ↑ risk of dysrhythmias

Interferon: ↓ metabolism, ↑ toxicity

Isoniazid: ↑ or ↓ oxtriphylline level

Ketoconazole: ↑ metabolism, ↓ effect

Lithium: ↓ effect of lithium

Mexiletine: ↓ metabolism, ↑ toxicity

Phenytoin: ↑ metabolism, ↓ effect

Rifampin: ↑ metabolism, ↓ effect

Thiabendazole: ↓ metabolism, ↑ toxicity

Drug classifications

Barbiturates: ↓ effect of oxtriphylline

β-Adrenergic blockers: ↓ metabolism, ↑ toxicity

Diuretics, loop: ↑ or ↓ oxtriphylline levels

Fluoroquinolones: ↓ metabolism, ↑ toxicity

Glucocorticoids: ↓ metabolism, ↑ toxicity

Oral contraceptives: ↑ toxicity

Sympathomimetics: ↑ CNS, CV adverse reactions

Food/drug
Caffeinated foods (cola, coffee, tea, chocolate):
↑ CNS, CV adverse reactions
Smoking
↑ metabolism, ↓ effect
☑ Herb/drug
Ephedra: ↑ action of both
Lab test interferences
↑ Plasma free fatty acids

NURSING CONSIDERATIONS
Assessment
• Monitor blood levels (therapeutic level is 10-20 µg/ml); toxicity may occur with small increase above 20 µg/ml, **G** especially elderly; check whether theophylline was given recently (24 hr)
• Monitor I&O; diuresis can **G** occur; dehydration may result **P** in elderly or children
• Monitor respiratory rate, rhythm, depth; auscultate lung fields bilaterally; notify prescriber of abnormalities
• Monitor allergic reactions: rash, urticaria; if these occur, drug should be discontinued

Nursing diagnoses
☑ Airway clearance, ineffective (uses)
☑ Activity intolerance (uses)
☑ Injury, risk for (uses, adverse reactions)
☑ Knowledge deficit (teaching)

Implementation
• Give PO pc to decrease GI symptoms; absorption may be affected with a full glass of water; do not crush or chew enteric coated or SA tab

Patient/family education
• Teach patient to take doses as prescribed, not to skip dose; to check OTC medications, current prescription medications for ephedrine, which will increase CNS stimulation; not

to drink alcohol or caffeine products (tea, coffee, chocolate, colas)
• Caution patient to avoid hazardous activities; dizziness may occur
• Instruct patient if GI upset occurs, to take drug with 8 oz water or food
• Teach patient to notify prescriber of change in smoking habit; a change in dosage may be required
• Teach patient to increase fluids to 2L/day to decrease viscosity of secretions

Evaluation
Positive therapeutic outcome
• Decreased dyspnea
• Clear lung fields bilaterally

---

oxybutynin (℞)
(ox-i-byoo'ti-nin)
Ditropan, oxybutynin
Func. class.: Spasmolytic, urinary
Chem. class.: Synthetic tertiary amine
Pregnancy category   B

O

Action: Relaxes smooth muscles in urinary tract by inhibiting acetylcholine at postganglionic sites

➲ Therapeutic Outcome: Decreased symptoms of urgency, nocturia, incontinence

Uses: Antispasmodic for neurogenic bladder

Dosage and routes
Adult: PO 5 mg bid-tid, not to exceed 5 mg qid
G *Elderly:* PO 2.5-5 mg tid, increase by 2.5 mg q several days

---

P *Child >5 yr:* PO 5 mg bid, not to exceed 5 mg tid

P *Child 1-5 yrs:* PO 0.2 mg/kg/dose 2-4 × /day

Available forms: Syrup 5 mg/5 ml; tab 5 mg; tabs ext rel 5, 10 mg

Adverse effects

CNS: Anxiety, restlessness, dizziness, **convulsions,** headache, drowsiness, confusion

CV: Palpitations, sinus tachycardia, hypotension

EENT: Blurred vision, increased intraocular tension, dry mouth, throat

GI: Nausea, vomiting, anorexia, abdominal pain, constipation

GU: Dysuria, retention, hesitancy

Contraindications: Hypersensitivity, GI obstruction, GI hemorrhage, GU obstruction, glaucoma, severe colitis, myasthenia gravis, unstable CV status in acute hemorrhage

Precautions: Pregnancy **B,** **P** lactation, suspected glaucoma, **G** children <12 yr, elderly

Do Not Confuse:
Ditropan/diazepam

Pharmacokinetics	
Absorption	Rapidly absorbed
Distribution	Unknown
Metabolism	Liver
Excretion	Unknown
Half-life	Unknown

Pharmacodynamics	
Onset	½-1 hr
Peak	3-4 hr
Duration	6-10 hr

Interactions
Individual drugs
Acetaminophen: ↓ levels of acetaminophen

Alcohol: ↑ CNS depression

Atenolol: ↑ levels of atenolol

Digoxin: ↑ levels of digoxin

Disopyramide: ↑ anticholinergic effects

Haloperidol: ↑ anticholinergic effects

Levodopa: ↓ levels of levodopa

Nitrofurantoin: ↑ levels of nitrofurantoin

Drug classifications

Antidepressants: ↑ anticholinergic effects

Antihistamines: ↑ CNS depression

Opiates: ↑ CNS depressants

Phenothiazines: ↑ anticholinergic effects

Sedative/hypnotics: ↑ CNS depression

NURSING CONSIDERATIONS
Assessment

• Assess for allergic reactions: rash, urticaria; if these occur, drug should be discontinued

• Assess urinary patterns: distention, nocturia, frequency, urgency, incontinence; catheterization may be required to remove residual urine

Nursing diagnoses

☑ Urinary elimination, altered patterns (uses)

☑ Pain (uses)

☑ Knowledge deficit (teaching)

Implementation

• May be given with meals or fluids or given on an empty stomach

Patient/family education

• Advise patient to avoid hazardous activities until response to drug is known; dizziness may occur

• Caution patient to avoid OTC medication with alcohol or other CNS depressants

• Advise patient to prevent

photophobia by wearing sunglasses
• Caution patient to stay cool, since overheating may occur
• Teach patient to use frequent rinsing of mouth, sips of water
• Teach patient to avoid hot weather, strenuous activity; drug decreases perspiration
• Advise patient to report CNS effects: confusion, anxiety, anticholinergic effect in the elderly

Evaluation
Positive therapeutic outcome
• Absence of dysuria, frequency, nocturia, incontinence

---

oxycodone (℞)
(ox-i-koe′done)
OxyFast, OxyIR, Roxicodone Supeudol ♣;
oxycodone/aspirin:
Endodan ♣, Oxycodan ♣, Percodan, Percodan-Demi, Roxiprin
oxycodone/acetaminophen:
Endocet ♣, Oxycocet ♣, Percocet, Roxicet, Roxilox, Tylox
Func. class.: Opiate analgesic
Chem. class.: Semisynthetic derivative

Pregnancy category **B**
Controlled substance schedule **II**

Action: Inhibits ascending pain pathways in CNS, increases pain threshold, alters pain perception

➡**Therapeutic Outcome:** Decreased pain

Uses: Moderate to severe pain

Dosage and routes
Adult: PO 10-30 mg q4h (5 mg q6h for OxyIR, OxyFast) OxyFast conc sol is extremely concentrated, do not use interchangeably

P *Child:* PO 0.05-0.15 mg/kg/dose up to 5 mg/dose q4-6h; not recommended in children

Available forms: *Oxycodone:* supp 10, 20 mg; tabs 5 mg; caps, immediate rel 5 mg; oral sol conc 20 mg/ml; *oxycodone with acetaminophen:* tab 5 mg/325 mg; cap 5 mg/500 mg; oral sol 5 mg/325 mg/5 ml; *oxycodone with aspirin:* 2.44 mg/325 mg, 4.88 mg/325 mg

Adverse effects
CNS: Drowsiness, dizziness, confusion, headache, sedation, euphoria
CV: Palpitations, bradycardia, change in B/P
EENT: Tinnitus, blurred vision, miosis, diplopia
GI: Nausea, vomiting, anorexia, constipation, cramps
GU: Increased urinary output, dysuria, urinary retention
INTEG: Rash, urticaria, bruising, flushing, diaphoresis, pruritus
RESP: **Respiratory depression**

Contraindications: Hypersensitivity, addiction (opiate)

Precautions: Addictive personality, pregnancy **B,** lactation, increased intracranial pressure, MI (acute), severe heart disease, respiratory depression, hepatic disease, renal **P** disease, child <18 yr

◼ Do Not Confuse:
Percodan/Decadron, Roxicet/Roxanol, Tylox/Xanax, Tylox/Trimox, Tylox/Wymox

O

Pharmacokinetics

Absorption	Well absorbed
Distribution	Widely distributed; crosses placenta
Metabolism	Liver, extensively
Excretion	Kidneys, breast milk
Half-life	2-3 hr

Pharmacodynamics

	PO	REC
Onset	15-30 min	Unknown
Peak	½-1 hr	Unknown
Duration	4-6 hr	4-6 hr

Interactions
Individual drugs
Alcohol: ↑ respiratory depression, hypotension, sedation
Nalbuphine: ↓ analgesia
Pentazocine: ↓ analgesia
Drug classifications
Antihistamines: ↑ respiratory depression, hypotension
CNS depressants: ↑ respiratory depression, hypotension
MAOIs: Do not use 2 wk before oxycodone
Phenothiazines: ↑ respiratory depression, hypotension
Sedative/hypnotics: ↑ respiratory depression, hypotension
Lab test interferences
↑ Amylase

NURSING CONSIDERATIONS
Assessment
• Monitor VS after parenteral route; note muscle rigidity, drug history, liver, kidney function tests, respiratory dysfunction: respiratory depression, character, rate, rhythm; notify prescriber if respirations are <10/min
• Monitor CNS changes: dizziness, drowsiness, hallucinations, euphoria, LOC, pupil reaction
• Monitor allergic reactions: rash, urticaria

Nursing diagnoses
☑ Pain (uses)
☑ Sensory-perceptual alteration: visual, auditory (adverse reactions)
☑ Breathing pattern, ineffective (adverse reactions)
☑ Injury, risk for (adverse reactions)
☑ Knowledge deficit (teaching)

Implementation
• Give with antiemetic if nausea, vomiting occur
• Give when pain is beginning to return; determine dosage interval by patient response; continuous dosing of medication is more effective than when given prn
• Medication should be slowly withdrawn after long-term use to prevent withdrawal symptoms
• Store in light-resistant container at room temp
PO route
• May be given with food or milk to lessen GI upset
Rec route
• Store supp in the refrigerator; run under warm water before insertion

Patient/family education
• Advise patients to avoid CNS depressants: alcohol, sedative/hypnotics
• Discuss with patient that dizziness, drowsiness, and confusion are common; to avoid getting up without assistance
• Discuss in detail all aspects of the drug, including purpose and what to expect
• Advise patient to make position changes slowly to lessen orthostatic hypotension

Evaluation
Positive therapeutic outcome
• Decreased pain

Treatment of overdose: Narcan 0.2-0.8 **IV**, O_2, **IV** fluids, vasopressors

oxymorphone (℞)
(ox-i-mor'fone)
Numorphan
Func. class.: Opiate analgesic
Chem. class.: Semisynthetic phenanthrene derivative

Pregnancy category B
Controlled substance schedule II

Action: Depresses pain impulse transmission at the spinal cord level by interacting with opioid receptors

▶**Therapeutic Outcome:** Decreased pain

Uses: Moderate to severe pain

Dosage and routes
Adult: IM/SC 1-1.5 mg q4-6h prn; **IV** 0.5 mg q4-6h prn; rec 5 mg q4-6h prn

Labor analgesia
Adult: IM 0.5-1 mg

Available forms: Inj 1, 1.5 mg/ml; supp 5 mg

Adverse effects
CNS: Drowsiness, dizziness, confusion, headache, sedation, euphoria
CV: Palpitations, bradycardia, change in B/P
EENT: Tinnitus, blurred vision, miosis, diplopia
GI: Nausea, vomiting, anorexia, constipation, cramps
GU: Increased urinary output, dysuria, urinary retention
INTEG: Rash, urticaria, bruising, flushing, diaphoresis, pruritus

RESP: **Respiratory depression**

Contraindications: Hypersensitivity, addiction (narcotic)

Precautions: Addictive personality, pregnancy **B** (short-term), lactation, increased intracranial pressure, MI (acute), severe heart disease, respiratory depression, hepatic disease, renal disease, child <18 yr

Pharmacokinetics	
Absorption	Well absorbed (rec, IM, SC); completely absorbed (**IV**)
Distribution	Widely distributed; crosses placenta
Metabolism	Liver, extensively
Excretion	Kidneys
Half-life	2½-4 hr

Pharmacodynamics			
	IM/SC	IV	REC
Onset	15 min	10 min	30 min
Peak	1-1½ hr	15-30 min	Unknown
Duration	3-6 hr	3-4 hr	3-6 hr

Interactions
Individual drugs
Alcohol: ↑ respiratory depression, hypotension, sedation
Nalbuphine: ↓ analgesia
Pentazocine: ↓ analgesia
Drug classifications
Antihistamines: ↑ respiratory depression, hypotension
CNS depressants: ↑ respiratory depression, hypotension
MAOIs: Do not use 2 wk before oxymorphone
Sedative/hypnotics: ↑ respiratory depression, hypotension
Lab test interferences
↑ Amylase, ↑ lipase

O

NURSING CONSIDERATIONS
Assessment
• Monitor VS after parenteral route; note muscle rigidity, drug history, liver, kidney function tests, respiratory dysfunction: respiratory depression, character, rate, rhythm; notify prescriber if respirations are <10/min
• Monitor CNS changes: dizziness, drowsiness, hallucinations, euphoria, LOC, pupil reaction
• Monitor allergic reactions: rash, urticaria

Nursing diagnoses
☑ Pain (uses)
☑ Sensory-perceptual alteration: visual, auditory (adverse reactions)
☑ Breathing pattern, ineffective (adverse reactions)
☑ Injury, risk for (adverse reactions)
☑ Knowledge deficit (teaching)

Implementation
• Give with antiemetic if nausea, vomiting occur
• Give when pain is beginning to return; determine dosage interval by patient response; continuous dosing of medication is more effective than when given prn
• Medication should be slowly withdrawn after long-term use to prevent withdrawal symptoms
• Store in light-resistant container at room temp
Rec route
• Store in refrigerator
IV IV route
• Give by direct IV undiluted over 2-3 min

Y-site compatibilities:
Glycopyrrolate, hydroxyzine, ranitidine

Patient/family education
• Advise patients to avoid CNS depressants: alcohol, sedative/hypnotics
• Discuss with patient that dizziness, drowsiness, and confusion are common; to avoid getting up without assistance
• Discuss in detail all aspects of the drug, including purpose and what to expect
• Advise patient to make position changes slowly to lessen orthostatic hypotension

Evaluation
Positive therapeutic outcome
• Decreased pain

Treatment of overdose:
Naloxone (Narcan) 0.2-0.8 mg **IV**, O_2, **IV** fluids, vasopressors

oxytocin ⚷ (℞)
(ox-i-toe'sin)
Pitocin, Syntocinon
Func. class.: Oxytocic hormone
Pregnancy category N/A

Action: Acts directly on myofibrils, producing uterine contraction; stimulates breast milk letdown

▶**Therapeutic Outcome:** Stimulation of labor, control of bleeding; stimulation of milk letdown

Uses: Stimulation, induction of labor; missed or incomplete abortion, postpartum bleeding, postpartum breast engorgement

Dosage and routes
Labor induction
Adult: **IV** 1-2 mU/min, increase by 1-2 mU q15-60 min until regular contractions occur, then decrease dosage

---

☑ Herb/drug 🚫 Do Not Crush ◆ Alert   Key Drug **G** Geriatric **P** Pediatric

Postpartum hemorrhage
Adult: IV 10 U infused at
20-40 mU/min

Adult: IM 10 U after placenta
delivery

Incomplete abortion
Adult: IV 10 U at a rate of
20-40 mU/min

Fetal stress test
Adult: IV 0.5 mU/min; increase q20 min until 3 contractions occur at 10 min; not to
exceed 20 mU only with fetal
monitoring

Available forms: Inj 10 U/ml

Adverse effects
CNS: Hypertension, **convulsions, tetanic contractions**
CV: Hypotension, dysrhythmias, increased pulse, bradycardia, tachycardia, PVC
FETUS: Dysrhythmias, jaundice, hypoxia, **intracranial
hemorrhage**
GI: Anorexia, nausea, vomiting, constipation
GU: **Abruptio placentae,
decreased uterine blood flow**
HEMA: Increased hyperbilirubinemia
INTEG: Rash
RESP: **Asphyxia**

Contraindications: Hypersensitivity, PIH, cephalopelvic
disproportion, fetal distress,
hypertonic uterus

Precautions: Cervical/uterine
surgery, uterine sepsis, primip-
ara >35 yr, 1st, 2nd stage of
labor

Pharmacokinetics

Absorption	Well absorbed (nasal); completely absorbed (**IV**)
Distribution	Widely distributed (extracellular fluid)
Metabolism	Liver, rapidly
Excretion	Kidneys
Half-life	3-12 min

Pharmacodynamics

	NASAL	IV	IM
Onset	5 min	Rapid	3-7 min
Peak	Unknown	Unknown	Unknown
Duration	20 min	1 hr	1 hr

Interactions
Individual drugs
Cyclopropane anesthesia:
↑ hypotension
Drug classifications
Vasopressors: ↑ hypertension
Herb/drug
Ephedra: ↑ hypertension

NURSING CONSIDERATIONS
Assessment
• Assess labor contractions:
fetal heart tones, frequency,
duration, intensity of
contractions; if fetal heart
tones increase or decrease
significantly or if contractions
are longer than 1 min, notify
prescriber; turn patient on left
side to increase oxygen to fetus
• Assess for water intoxication:
confusion, anuria, drowsiness,
headache; notify prescriber
• Watch for fetal distress,
acceleration, deceleration, fetal
presentation, pelvic dimensions
• Monitor B/P, pulse, respiratory rate, rhythm, depth
• Monitor I&O ratio
• Provide an environment
conducive to letdown reflex

Nursing diagnoses
☑ Breastfeeding (uses)
☑ Injury, risk for (uses)
☑ Knowledge deficit (teaching)

Implementation
IV route
• Use an inf pump; rotate sol
for mixing; have magnesium
sulfate available
• For labor induction administer after diluting 10 U/1 L of

D_5W, 0.9% NaCl, 0.45% NaCl, LR, Ringer's for a conc of 10 mU/ml; start at 1-2 mU/min (0.1-0.2 ml); may increase by 1-2 mU/min q15-30 min until labor begins
• For threatened abortion administer after diluting 10 U/500 ml of D_5W, $D_{10}W$, 0.9% NaCl, 0.45% NaCl, LR, Ringer's for a conc of 20 mU/ml; give at 10-40 mU/min
• For postpartum bleeding administer after diluting 10-40 U/L of D_5W, $D_{10}W$, 0.9% NaCl, 0.45% NaCl, LR, Ringer's for a conc of 10-40 mU/ml; may titrate to response

Y-site compatibilities:
Heparin, regular insulin, hydrocortisone, meperidine, morphine, potassium chloride, vit B/C, warfarin

Additive compatibilities:
Chloramphenicol, metaraminol, netilmicin, sodium bicarbonate, thiopental, verapamil

Additive incompatibilities:
Fibrinolysin, warfarin

Patient/family education
• Teach patient to report increased blood loss, abdominal cramps, increased temp or foul-smelling lochia
• Advise patient that contractions will be similar to menstrual cramps, gradually increasing in intensity

Evaluation
Positive therapeutic outcome
• Stimulation of milk letdown (nasal)
• Induction of labor
• Decreased postpartum bleeding

paclitaxel (℞)
(pa-kli-tax'el)
Taxol
Func. class.: Miscellaneous antineoplastic
Chem. class.: Natural diterpene, antimicrotubule
Pregnancy category   D

Action: Inhibits the reorganization of the microtubule network needed for interphase and mitotic cellular functions; also causes abnormal bundles of microtubules during cell cycle and multiple esters of microtubules during mitosis

➡**Therapeutic Outcome:** Prevention of rapidly growing malignant cells

Uses: Metastatic carcinoma of the ovary unresponsive to other treatment, breast; AIDS-related Kaposi's sarcoma (2nd-line), non–small-cell lung cancer

Investigational uses: Advanced head, neck, small-cell lung cancer; non-Hodgkin's lymphoma, adenocarcinoma of the upper GI tract, hormone-refractory prostate cancer

Dosage and routes
Ovarian carcinoma
Adults: IV inf 135 mg/m^2 given over 24 hr q 3 wk or 175 mg/m^2 over 3 hr q3wk

Breast carcinoma
Adult: IV inf 175 mg/m^2 over 3 hr q3wk

AIDS-related Kaposi's sarcoma
Adult: IV inf 135 mg/m^2 over 3 hr q3wk or 100 mg/m^2 over 3 hr q2wk

---

☑ Herb/drug   ⃠ Do Not Crush   ◆ Alert   Key Drug   **G** Geriatric   **P** Pediatric

1st line non–small-cell lung cancer

135 mg/m^2/24 hr infusion with cisplatin

Available forms: Inj 30 mg/5 ml vial

Adverse effects

CV: Bradycardia, hypotension, abnormal ECG
GI: Nausea, vomiting, diarrhea, mucositis; increased bilirubin, alkaline phosphatase, AST
HEMA: Neutropenia, leukopenia, thrombocytopenia, anemia, bleeding, infections
INTEG: Alopecia
MS: Arthralgia, myalgia
NEURO: Peripheral neuropathy
SYST: Hypersensitivity reactions, **anaphylaxis**

Contraindications: Hypersensitivity to paclitaxel or other drugs with polyoxyethylated castor oil, neutropenia of <1500/mm^3, pregnancy **D**

P Precautions: Children, lactation, hepatic disease, cardiovascular disease, CNS disorder

Do Not Confuse:
paclitaxel/paroxetine, paclitaxel/Paxil, Taxol/Paxil

Pharmacokinetics

Absorption	Completely absorbed
Distribution	89%-98% protein binding
Metabolism	Liver, extensively
Excretion	Unknown
Half-life	5-17 hr

Pharmacodynamics

Onset	Unknown
Peak	1-2 wk
Duration	3 wk

Interactions
Individual drugs
Cisplatin: ↑ myelosuppression
Cyclosporine: ↓ metabolism of paclitaxel
Dexamethasone: ↓ metabolism of paclitaxel
Diazepam: ↓ metabolism of paclitaxel
Doxorubicin: ↑ levels of doxorubicin
Etoposide: ↓ metabolism of paclitaxel
Ketoconazole: ↑ toxicity
Quinidine: ↓ metabolism of paclitaxel
Radiation: ↑ myelosuppression
Teniposide: ↓ metabolism of paclitaxel
Testosterone: ↓ metabolism of paclitaxel
Drug classifications
Antineoplastics: ↑ myelosuppression
Live virus vaccines: ↓ immune response

NURSING CONSIDERATIONS
Assessment
• Assess CNS changes: confusion, paresthesias, psychosis, tremors, seizures, neuropathies; drug should be discontinued
• Check buccal cavity q8h for dryness, sores or ulceration, white patches, oral pain, bleeding, dysphagia; obtain prescription for viscous lidocaine (Xylocaine) to use in mouth
• Assess symptoms indicating severe allergic reaction: rash, pruritus, urticaria, purpuric skin lesions, itching, flushing
• Monitor CBC, differential, platelet count weekly; withhold drug if WBC count is <1500/mm^3 or platelet count is <100,000/mm^3, notify prescriber of results

• Monitor renal function studies: BUN, creatinine, serum uric acid, urine CrCl before and during therapy; check I&O ratio; report fall in urine output to <30 ml/hr
• Monitor temp q4h (may indicate beginning of infection)
• Monitor liver function tests before and during therapy (bilirubin, AST, ALT, LDH) as needed or monthly; check for jaundice of skin and sclera, dark urine, clay-colored stools, itchy skin, abdominal pain, fever, diarrhea
• Assess for bleeding: hematuria, stool guaiac, bruising or petechiae, mucosa or orifices q8h; check for inflammation of mucosa, breaks in skin
• Assess effects of alopecia on body image; discuss feelings about body changes

Nursing diagnoses

☑ Injury, risk for (adverse reactions)
☑ Body image disturbance (adverse reactions)
☑ Infection, risk for (adverse reactions)
☑ Knowledge deficit (teaching)

Implementation

IV IV route
• Give after diluting in 0.9% NaCl, D_5, D_5 and 0.9% NaCl, D_5LR to a concentration of 0.3-1.2 mg/ml
• Use an in-line filter ≤0.22 μm
• Give after premedicating with dexamethasone 20 mg PO 12 hr and 6 hr before paclitaxel, diphenhydramine 50 mg **IV** ½-1 hr before paclitaxel and cimetidine 300 mg or ranitidine 50 mg **IV** ½-1 hr before paclitaxel
• Use only glass bottles, poly-propylene, polyolefin bags and administration sets; do not use PVC infusion bags or sets
• Use gloves and cytotoxic handling precautions

Y-site compatiblilities:
Acyclovir, amikacin, aminophylline, bleomycin, butorphanol, calcium chloride, carboplatin, cefepime, cefotetan, ceftazidime, ceftriaxone, cimetidine, cisplatin, cyclophosphamide, cytarabine, dacarbazine, dexamethasone, diphenhydramine, doxorubicin, droperidol, etoposide, famotidine, floxuridine, fluconazole, fluorouracil, furosemide, ganciclovir, gentamicin, haloperidol, heparin, mannitol, meperidine, mesna, methotrexate, metoclopramide, morphine, nalbuphine, ondansetron, pentostatin, potassium chloride, prochlorperazine, propofol, ranitidine, sodium bicarbonate, vancomycin, vinblastine, vincristine, zidovudine
• Give fluids PO before chemotherapy to hydrate patient
• Give antacid before oral agent; give drug after evening meal, before hs; provide antiemetic 30-60 min before giving drug and prn to prevent vomiting; administer antibiotics for prophylaxis of infection
• Give top or syst analgesics for pain to lessen effects of stomatitis
• Give liq diet: carbonated beverages; gelatin may be added if patient is not nauseated or vomiting
• Encourage patient to rinse mouth tid-qid with water, club soda; brush teeth bid-qid with soft brush or cotton-tipped applicators for stomatitis; use unwaxed dental floss

---

☑ Herb/drug ⊘ Do Not Crush ◆ Alert ☙ Key Drug **G** Geriatric **P** Pediatric

Patient/family education
• Inform patient that contraceptive measures are recommended during therapy and >4 mo after; teratogenic effects are possible
• Teach patient to avoid use of products containing aspirin or ibuprofen, razors, commercial mouthwash, since bleeding may occur; to report symptoms of bleeding (hematuria, tarry stools)
• Instruct patient to report signs of anemia (fatigue, headache, irritability, faintness, shortness of breath) and CNS reactions (confusion, psychosis, nightmares, seizures, severe headaches)
• Inform patient that hair may be lost during treatment; a wig or hair piece may make patient feel better; new hair may be different in color, texture
• Inform patient that receiving vaccinations during therapy may cause serious reactions

Evaluation
Positive therapeutic outcome
• Prevention of rapid division of malignant cells

---

palivizumab (℞)
(pal-ih-viz′uh-mab)
Synagis
Func. class.: Monoclonal antibody
Pregnancy category   C

Action: A humanized monoclonal antibody that exhibits neutralizing and fusion-inhibitory activity against respiratory syncytial virus (RSV)

➤**Therapeutic Outcome:** Absence of RSV

Uses: Prevention of serious lower respiratory tract disease caused by RSV in pediatric patients

Dosage and routes
P *Child:* IM 15 mg/kg, those patients who develop RSV should receive monthly doses during RSV season

Available forms: Lyophilized inj 100 mg

Adverse effects
EENT: Otitis media, rhinitis, pharyngitis
GI: Nausea, vomiting, diarrhea, increased AST
INTEG: Rash, inj site reaction
RESP: URI, **apnea**

Contraindications: Hypersensitivity, adults, cyanotic congenital heart disease

Precautions: Thrombocytopenia, coagulation disorders, established RSV, congenital heart disease, chronic lung disease, systemic allergic reactions, pregnancy **C**

Pharmacokinetics	
Absorption	Unknown
Distribution	Unknown
Metabolism	Unknown
Excretion	Unknown
Half-life	20 days

Pharmacodynamics	
Onset	Unknown
Peak	Unknown
Duration	Unknown

Interactions
Unknown

NURSING CONSIDERATIONS
Assessment
• Assess for presence of RSV infection, drug is given to prevent infection
• Assess for side effects and

---

report if allergic reaction is
evident

Nursing diagnoses
☑ Infection, risk for (uses)
☑ Knowledge deficit (teaching)

Implementation
• Give IM only
• Give after adding 1 ml of
sterile water for inj per 100 mg
vial, gently swirl, let stand at
room temperature for 20 min
until sol clarifies; given within
6 hr of reconstitution

Patient/family education
• Teach patient to report
upper respiratory infections,
earaches, rash, sore throat

Evaluation
Positive therapeutic outcome
• Absence of RSV

---

pamidronate (R)
(pam-i-drone′ate)
Aredia
Func. class.: Bone resorption inhibitor
Chem. class.: Bisphospho-
nate

Pregnancy category   C

Action: Absorbs calcium phosphate crystals in bone and may
directly block dissolution of
hydroxyapatite crystals of
bone; inhibits bone resorption,
apparently without inhibiting
bone formation and mineralization

➡ **Therapeutic Outcome:** Serum calcium at normal level

Uses: Moderate to severe
hypercalcemia associated with
malignancy with or without
bone metastases; osteolytic
lesions in breast cancer patients

Dosage and routes
Adult: **IV** inf 60-90 mg in
moderate hypercalcemia, 90
mg in severe hypercalcemia
given over 24 hr

Available forms: Inj 30, 60,
90 mg/vial pamidronate disodium and 470 mg of mannitol

Adverse effects
CNS: Fatigue
*CV: Hypertension, fluid over-
load,* dysrhythmias, tachycardia
*GI: Abdominal pain, anorexia,
constipation, nausea, vomiting*
GU: UTI, fluid overload
INTEG: Redness, swelling,
induration, pain on palpation
at site of catheter insertion
META: Anemia, hypokalemia,
hypomagnesemia, hypophos-
phatemia
MS: Bone pain

Contraindications: Hypersensitivity to bisphosphonates

P **Precautions:** Children, nursing
mothers, pregnancy **C,** renal
dysfunction

⬛ **Do Not Confuse:**
Aredia/Adriamycin

Pharmacokinetics	
Absorption	Rapidly cleared from circulation
Distribution	Mainly to bones
Metabolism	Unknown
Excretion	Kidneys, unchanged (50%)
Half-life	Biphasic 1½ hr; 27 hr; from bone to 300 days

Pharmacodynamics	
Onset	1 day
Peak	1 wk
Duration	Unknown

Interactions: None

NURSING CONSIDERATIONS
Assessment

• Assess for hypocalcemia: Chvostek's, Trousseau's sign, paresthesia, twitching, laryngospasm
• Monitor manifestations of hypocalcemia: personality changes, anxiety, disturbances, depression, psychosis; nausea, vomiting, constipation, abdominal pain from muscle spasm; decreased contractility, decreased cardiac output, hypotension, lengthened ST segment, prolonged QT interval; scaling eczema, alopecia, hyperpigmentation; tetany, muscle twitching, cramping, grimacing, seizure, altered deep tendon reflexes, spasm
• Monitor manifestations of hypomagnesemia: agitation; muscle twitching, paresthesia, hyperactive reflexes, positive Babinski reflex, dysphagia, nystagmus, seizures, tetany; nausea, vomiting, diarrhea, anorexia, abdominal distention; ectopy, tachycardia, broad, flat or inverted T waves, depressed ST segment, prolonged QT, decreased cardiac output, hypotension
• Monitor manifestations of hypokalemia: acidic urine, reduced urine osmolality, nocturia, polyuria, polydipsia; hypotension, broad T wave, U wave, ectopy, tachycardia, weak pulse; muscle weakness, altered LOC, drowsiness, apathy, lethargy, confusion, depression; anorexia, nausea, cramps, constipation, distention, paralytic ileus; hypoventilation, respiratory muscle weakness
• Assess fluid volume status: check I&O ratio and record, assess for distended red veins, crackles in lung, color, quality and sp gr of urine, skin turgor, adequacy of pulses, moist mucous membranes, bilateral lung sounds, peripheral pitting edema
• Monitor electrolytes: phosphorus, potassium, sodium, calcium, magnesium; also include BUN, creatinine, CBC, platelets, hemoglobin
• Assess B/P before and during therapy
• Assess for pain: in joints or on exertion, duration and characteristics; analgesics may be ordered
• Assess for phlebitis at **IV** site: swelling, redness, pain, warmth

Nursing diagnoses

☑ Injury, risk for (uses, adverse reactions)
☑ Fluid excess (side effects)
☑ Knowledge deficit (teaching)

Implementation

• Give by **IV** inf after reconstituting by adding 10 ml of sterile water for inj to each vial, then adding to 1000 ml of sterile 0.45%, 0.9% NaCl, D_5W, run over 24 hr for hypercalcemia or 60 mg ≥4 hr, 90 mg/24 hr
• Store inf sol for up to 24 hr at room temp
• Reconstituted sol with sterile water may be stored under refrigeration for up to 24 hr

Additive incompatibilities:
Calcium products, sol

Evaluation
Positive therapeutic outcome
• Decreased calcium levels to normal

P

pancrelipase (℞)
(pan-kre-li′pase)
Cotazym, Cotazym Capsules, Cotazym-S Capsules, Creon Capsules, Ilozyme, Ku-Zyme HP Capsules, Pancrease Capsules, Pancrease MT 4, Pancrease MT 10, Pancrease MT 16, Ultrase MT 12, Ultrase MT 20, Ultrase MT 24, Viokase Powder, Viokase Tablets, Zymase
Func. class.: Digestant
Chem. class.: Pancreatic enzyme (bovine/porcine)
Pregnancy category   C

Action: Pancreatic enzyme needed for breakdown of substances released from the pancreas

➡**Therapeutic Outcome:** Increases protein, fat, carbohydrate digestion

Uses: Exocrine pancreatic secretion insufficiency, cystic fibrosis (digestive aid), steatorrhea, pancreatic enzyme deficiency

Dosage and routes
P *Adult and child:* PO 1-3 cap/tab ac or with meals, or 1 cap/tab with snack or 1-2 powder packets ac

Available forms: Powder: 16,800 U lipase/ 70,000 U protease and amylase; caps: 8000 U lipase/30,000 U protease and amylase; cap, delayed rel 4000 U lipase/ 12,000 U protease and amylase, 4000 U lipase/25,000 U protease/20,000 U amylase, 5000 U lipase/20,000 U protease and amylase, 10,000 U lipase/30,000 U protease and amylase, 12,000 U lipase/ 24,000 U protease and amylase, 12,000 U lipase/39,000 U protease and amylase, 16,000 U lipase/48,000 U protease and amylase 20,000 U lipase/65,000 U protease and amylase, 24,000 U lipase/ 78,000 U protease and amylase

Adverse effects
GI: Anorexia, nausea, vomiting, diarrhea
GU: Hyperuricuria, hyperuricemia

Contraindications: Allergy to pork

Precautions: Pregnancy **C**

Pharmacokinetics	
Absorption	Unknown
Distribution	Unknown
Metabolism	Unknown
Excretion	Unknown
Half-life	Unknown

Pharmacodynamics
Unknown

Interactions
Individual drugs
Cimetidine: ↓ absorption of pancrelipase
Oral iron: ↓ absorption of pancrelipase
Drug classifications
Antacids: ↓ absorption of pancrelipase
Food/drug
Alkaline foods: ↓ enteric coating

Lab test interferences
↑ Uric acid (serum, urine)

NURSING CONSIDERATIONS
Assessment
• Monitor I&O ratio; watch for increasing urinary output
• Monitor fecal fat, nitrogen, pro-time, during treatment

- Monitor for polyuria, polydipsia, polyphagia (may indicate diabetes mellitus)
- Assess for allergy to pork; patient may also be sensitive to this drug
- Assess for appropriate weight, height, development; there may be a developmental lag
- Check stools for steatorrhea, which signifies undigested fat content

Nursing diagnoses

☑ Nutrition, altered: less than body requirements (uses)

☑ Knowledge deficit (teaching)

Implementation

- Give after antacid or cimetidine; decreased pH inactivates drug
- **P** Give powder mixed in prepared fruit for infants, children
- Administer low-fat diet to decrease GI symptoms
- Store in tight container at room temp

Patient/family education

- Teach patient to take tab with 8 oz or more water, not to let tab sit in mouth; have patient take tab sitting up only
- Advise patient to notify prescriber of allergic reactions, abdominal pain, cramping, or hematuria
- Teach patient not to inhale powder, very irritating to mucous membranes, some powder may irritate skin

Evaluation

Positive therapeutic outcome

- Absence of steatorrhea
- Improved digestion of carbohydrates, proteins, fat

pancuronium (℞)
(pan-cure-oh'nee-yum)
**pancuronium bromide,
Pavulon**
Func. class.: Neuromuscular blocker (nondepolarizing)
Chem. class.: Synthetic curariform

Pregnancy category   C

Action: Inhibits transmission of nerve impulses by binding with cholinergic receptor sites, antagonizing action of acetylcholine; no analgesic response

▶**Therapeutic Outcome:** Paralysis of all skeletal muscles

Uses: Facilitation of endotracheal intubation, skeletal muscle relaxation during mechanical ventilation, surgery, or general anesthesia

Dosage and routes
Adult: **IV** 0.04-0.1 mg/kg, then 0.01 mg/kg q30-60 min

P *Child >10 yr:* **IV** 0.04-0.1 mg/kg, then 1/5 initial dose q30-60 min

Available forms: Inj 1, 2 mg/ml

Adverse effects
CV: Bradycardia, tachycardia, increased, decreased B/P, ventricular extrasystoles
EENT: Increased secretions
INTEG: Rash, flushing, pruritus, urticaria, sweating, salivation
MS: Weakness to prolonged skeletal muscle relaxation
RESP: Prolonged apnea, bronchospasm, cyanosis, respiratory depression

Contraindications: Hypersensitivity to bromide ion

Precautions: Pregnancy C, renal disease, cardiac disease, **P** lactation, children <2 yr, electrolyte imbalances, dehydration, neuromuscular disease, respiratory disease

Pharmacokinetics

Absorption	Complete bioavailability
Distribution	Extracellular space; crosses placenta
Metabolism	Plasma
Excretion	Kidneys, unchanged
Half-life	2 hr

Pharmacodynamics

Onset	30-45 sec
Peak	3-5 min
Duration	35-40 min

Interactions
Individual drugs
Clindamycin: ↑ paralysis length and intensity
Colistin: ↑ paralysis length and intensity
Lidocaine: ↑ paralysis length and intensity
Lithium: ↑ paralysis length and intensity
Magnesium: ↑ paralysis length and intensity
Polymyxin B: ↑ paralysis length and intensity
Procainamide: ↑ paralysis length and intensity
Quinidine: ↑ paralysis length and intensity
Succinylcholine: ↑ paralysis length and intensity
Drug classifications
Aminoglycosides: ↑ paralysis length and intensity
β-Adrenergic blockers: ↑ paralysis length and intensity
Diuretics, potassium-losing: ↑ paralysis length and intensity
General anesthesia: ↑ paralysis length and intensity

NURSING CONSIDERATIONS
Assessment
• Monitor vital signs (B/P, pulse, respirations, airway) until fully recovered; note rate, depth, pattern of respirations, strength of hand grip; patient should be intubated before use
• Monitor for electrolyte imbalances (potassium, magnesium) before drug is used; electrolyte imbalances may lead to increased action of this drug
• Monitor for recovery: decreased paralysis of face, diaphragm, leg, arm, rest of body; residual weakness and respiratory problems may occur during recovery period
• Assess for hypersensitive reactions: rash, fever, respiratory distress, pruritus; drug should be discontinued

Nursing diagnoses
☑ Breathing pattern, ineffective (uses)
☑ Communication, impaired verbal (adverse reactions)
☑ Fear (adverse reactions)
☑ Knowledge deficit (teaching)

Implementation
• Use peripheral nerve stimulator (anesthesiologist) to determine neuromuscular blockade; deep tendon reflexes should be monitored during extended periods
• Give direct **IV** undiluted over 1-2 min, or diluted in D₅W or 0.9% NaCl and give as an inf at prescribed rate; titrate to patient response; should be administered only by qualified person, usually an anesthesiologist; do not administer IM
• Store in light-resistant area
• Give anticholinesterase to reverse neuromuscular blockade

☑ Herb/drug 🚫 Do Not Crush ◆ Alert ☛ Key Drug **G** Geriatric **P** Pediatric

Syringe compatibilities:
Heparin

Y-site compatibilities:
Aminophylline, cefazolin, cefuroxime, cimetidine, dobutamine, dopamine, epinephrine, esmolol, fentanyl, fluconazole, gentamicin, heparin, hydrocortisone, isoproterenol, lorazepam, midazolam, morphine, nitroglycerin, nitroprusside, ranitidine, sulfamethoxazole/trimethoprim, vancomycin

Y-site incompatibilities:
Diazepam

Additive compatibilities:
Verapamil

Additive incompatibilities:
Barbiturates

Patient/family education
• Provide reassurance if communication is difficult during recovery from neuromuscular blockade
• Provide explanation to patients regarding all procedures or treatments; patient will remain conscious if anesthesia is not given also

Evaluation
Positive therapeutic outcome
• Paralysis of jaw, eyelid, head, neck, rest of body as evaluated by peripheral nerve stimulator

Treatment of overdose:
Edrophonium or neostigmine, atropine; monitor VS; may require mechanical ventilation

paricalcitol (℞)
(par-ih-cal'sih-tol)
Zemplar
Func. class.: Vit D analog
Chem. class.: Fat-soluble vitamin

Pregnancy category   C

Action: Reduces parathyroid hormone (PTH) levels; suppresses PTH levels in patients with chronic renal failure with absence of hypercalcemia/hyperphosphatemia. Serum PO_4, Ca, CaXP may increase

⇒ Therapeutic Outcome:
Decreased symptoms of hypoparathyroidism

Uses: Hypoparathyroidism

Dosage and routes
Adult: **IV** BOL 0.04-0.1 μg/kg (2.8-7 μg) no more than qod during dialysis; may increase by 2-4 μg q2-4wk

Available forms: Inj 5 μg/ml

Adverse effects
CNS: Lightheadedness
CV: Palpitations
GI: Nausea, vomiting, anorexia, dry mouth
OTHER: Pneumonia, edema, chills, fever, flu, sepsis

Contraindications: Hypersensitivity, hypercalcemia

Precautions: Cardiovascular disease, renal calculi, pregnancy **C**, elderly, lactation, children

Pharmacokinetics	
Absorption	Unknown
Distribution	Unknown
Metabolism	Unknown
Excretion	Unknown
Half-life	Unknown

P

Pharmacodynamics	
Onset	Unknown
Peak	Unknown
Duration	Unknown

Interactions
Individual drugs
Digitalis: ↑ toxicity

NURSING CONSIDERATIONS
Assessment
• Monitor Ca, PO_4, 2×/wk qwk during initial therapy; after dose is established take calcium and phosphorus qmo

Nursing diagnoses
☑ Knowledge deficit (teaching)

Implementation
IV route
• Give by **IV** bolus only

Patient/family education
• Advise patient to report weakness, lethargy, headache, anorexia, loss of weight
• Teach patient to report nausea, vomiting, palpitations

Evaluation
Positive therapeutic outcome
• Decreased hypoparathyroidism in chronic renal disease

---

paroxetine (℞)
(par-ox′e-teen)
Paxil, Paxil CR
Func. class.: Antidepressant, selective serotonin reuptake inhibitor (SSRI)
Chem. class.: Phenylpiperidine derivative
Pregnancy category   B

Action: Inhibits CNS neuron reuptake of serotonin but not of norepinephrine or dopamine

➤**Therapeutic Outcome:** Relief of depression

Uses: Major depressive disorder, obsessive-compulsive disorder, panic disorder

Investigational uses: Diabetic neuropathy, headache, premature ejaculation

Dosage and routes
Depression
Adult: PO 20 mg qd in AM; after 4 wk if no clinical improvement is noted, dosage may be increased by 10 mg/day weekly to desired response; not to exceed 50 mg/day; cont rel 25 mg/day

G *Elderly:* PO 10 mg qd, ↑ by 10 mg to desired dose, max 40 mg/day; cont rel 12.5 mg/day

Obsessive-compulsive disorder
Adults: PO 40 mg/day in AM; start with 20 mg/day, increase 10 mg/day increments, max 60 mg/day

Panic disorder
Adults: PO 40 mg/day; start with 10 mg/day and increase in 10 mg/day increments, max 60 mg/day

Renal dose
10 mg qd in AM, may ↑ by 10 mg/day qwk, max 40 mg qd

Available forms: Tabs 10, 20, 30, 40 mg; susp 10 mg/5 ml

Adverse effects
CNS: Headache, nervousness, insomnia, drowsiness, anxiety, tremor, dizziness, fatigue, sedation, abnormal dreams, agitation, apathy, euphoria, hallucinations, delusions, psychosis
CV: Vasodilatation, postural hypotension, palpitations
EENT: Visual changes, rhinitis, oropharyngeal disorder
GI: Nausea, diarrhea, constipation, dry mouth, anorexia,

☑ Herb/drug   🚫 Do Not Crush   ◆ Alert   **Key Drug**   **G** Geriatric   **P** Pediatric

dyspepsia, vomiting, taste changes, flatulence, decreased appetite
GU: Dysmenorrhea, decreased libido, urinary frequency, UTI, amenorrhea, cystitis, impotence, *abnormal ejaculation, male genital disorders*
INTEG: Sweating, rash
MS: Pain, arthritis, myalgia, myopathy, myasthenia gravis
RESP: Infection, pharyngitis, nasal congestion, sinus headache, sinusitis, cough, dyspnea
SYST: Asthenia, fever, chills

Contraindications: Hypersensitivity, patients taking MAOIs

Precautions: Pregnancy **B**, lactation, children, elderly, seizure history, patients with history of mania, renal and hepatic disease

Do Not Confuse:
paroxetine/paclitaxel, Paxil/paclitaxel, Paxil/Taxol

Pharmacokinetics	
Absorption	Well absorbed
Distribution	Widely distributed; crosses blood-brain barrier, protein-binding 95%
Metabolism	Liver, mostly
Excretion	Kidneys, unchanged (2%); breast milk
Half-life	21 hrs

Pharmacodynamics	
Onset	Unknown
Peak	5.2 hr
Duration	Unknown

Interactions
Individual drugs
Alcohol: ↑ CNS depression
Digoxin: ↓ effect of digoxin
Phenytoin: ↓ effect of paroxetine
Procycline: ↓ metabolism
Quinidine: ↓ metabolism

Theophylline: ↑ theophylline levels
Warfarin: ↑ warfarin levels
Drug classifications
Antidepressants: ↓ metabolism
Antidysrhythmics, IC: ↓ metabolism
Barbiturates: ↑ effects
Benzodiazepines: ↑ effects
CNS depressants: ↑ effects
MAOIs: Hypertensive crisis, convulsions; do not use together
Phenothiazines: ↓ metabolism
Lab test interferences
↑ Serum bilirubin, ↑ blood glucose, ↑ alkaline phosphatase ↓ VMA, ↓ 5-HIAA, ↓ blood glucose
False: ↑ Urinary catecholamines

NURSING CONSIDERATIONS
Assessment
• Assess mental status: mood, sensorium, affect, suicidal tendencies; increase in psychiatric symptoms: depression, panic
• Assess for withdrawal symptoms: headache, nausea, vomiting, muscle pain, weakness; do not usually occur unless drug was discontinued abruptly
• Monitor B/P (with patient lying, standing), pulse q4h; if systolic B/P drops 20 mm Hg, hold drug, notify prescriber; take VS q4h in patients with cardiovascular disease
• Monitor blood studies: CBC, leukocytes, differential, cardiac enzymes if patient is receiving long-term therapy
• Monitor hepatic studies: AST, ALT, bilirubin
• Check weight weekly; appetite may increase with drug

P

• Assess ECG for flattening of T wave, bundle branch block, AV block, dysrhythmias in cardiac patients

• Assess for EPS primarily in **G** elderly: rigidity, dystonia, akathisia

• Monitor urinary retention, constipation; constipation is **P** more likely to occur in children **G** or elderly

• Identify alcohol consumption; if alcohol is consumed, hold dose until AM

Nursing diagnoses
✓ Coping, ineffective individual (uses)
✓ Injury, risk for (adverse reactions)
✓ Knowledge deficit (teaching)
✓ Noncompliance (teaching)

Implementation
• Give with food or milk for GI symptoms; store at room temp; do not freeze

• Give crushed if patient is unable to swallow whole

Patient/family education
• Advise patient that therapeutic effects may take 1-4 wk

• Teach patient to use caution in driving and other activities requiring alertness because of drowsiness, dizziness, blurred vision; to avoid rising quickly from sitting to standing, espe-**G** cially elderly

• Caution patient to avoid alcohol ingestion, other CNS depressants, and OTC medication unless prescribed

• Caution patient not to discontinue medication quickly after long-term use; may cause nausea, anxiety, headache, malaise; do not double doses if one is missed

• Advise patient to use gum, hard sugarless candy, or fre-

quent sips of water for dry mouth; if dry mouth continues an artificial saliva may be used

Evaluation
Positive therapeutic outcome
• Decrease in depression
• Absence of suicidal thoughts

Treatment of overdose:
Maintain airway, for seizures give diazepam, symptomatic treatment

---

pegaspargase (℞)
(peg-as′per-gase)
Oncaspar, PEG-L-asparaginase
Func. class.: Antineoplastic
Chem. class.: Escherichia coli enzyme

Pregnancy category **D**

Action: Indirectly inhibits protein synthesis in tumor cells; without amino acid, DNA, RNA synthesis is halted; asparagine, protein synthesis is halted; G_1 phase of cell cycle specific; a nonvesicant

→**Therapeutic Outcome:** Prevention of rapidly growing malignant cells

Uses: Acute lymphocytic leukemia in combination with other antineoplastics unresponsive to other agents

Dosage and routes
In combination
P *Adult and child with BSA ≥0.6 m²:* **IV** 1000 IU/kg/day × 10 days given over 30 min; IM 6000 IU/m²/day

P *Child with BSA <0.6 m²:* **IV**/IM 82.5 IU/kg q14 days

Sole induction
Adult: **IV** 200 IU/kg/day × 28 days

☑ Herb/drug 🚫 Do Not Crush ◆ Alert ⚯ Key Drug **G** Geriatric **P** Pediatric

Available forms: Inj 10,000 IU

Adverse effects

CNS: Neuritis, dizziness, headache, **coma,** depression, fatigue, confusion, hallucinations, **seizures**

CV: Chest pain

ENDO: Hyperglycemia

GI: *Nausea, vomiting, anorexia, cramps, stomatitis,* **hepatotoxicity, pancreatitis**

GU: Urinary retention, **renal failure,** glycosuria, polyuria, azotemia, uric acid neuropathy

HEMA: **Thrombocytopenia, leukopenia, myelosuppression, anemia, decreased clotting factors**

INTEG: *Rash,* urticaria, chills, fever

RESP: **Fibrosis, pulmonary infiltrate**

SYST: **Anaphylaxis, hypersensitivity**

Contraindications: Hypersensitivity, infants, pregnancy **D,** lactation, pancreatitis

Precautions: Renal disease, hepatic disease

Pharmacokinetics	
Absorption	Complete bioavailability
Distribution	Intravascular spaces
Metabolism	Unknown
Excretion	Reticuloendothelial system
Half-life	5½ days

Pharmacodynamics	
Onset	Rapid
Peak	Unknown
Duration	2 wks

Interactions

Individual drugs

Methotrexate: Blocking action of methotrexate

Vincristine: ↑ neurotoxicity

Drug classifications

Glucocorticosteroids: ↑ hyperglycemia

Hepatotoxic agents: ↑ hepatotoxic agents

Lab test interferences

↓ Thyroid function tests

↑ BUN

NURSING CONSIDERATIONS

Assessment

• Assess for signs and symptoms of pancreatitis (nausea, vomiting, severe abdominal pain), anaphylaxis (bronchospasm, dyspnea), cyanosis; monitor amylase, glucose

• Assess symptoms indicating severe allergic reaction: rash, pruritus, urticaria, purpuric skin lesions, itching, flushing; monitor for joint pain, bronchospasm, hypotension; epinephrine and crash carts should be nearby

• Monitor for frequency of stools, characteristics: cramping, acidosis; signs of dehydration: rapid respirations, poor skin turgor, decreased urine output, dry skin, restlessness, weakness

• Monitor CBC, differential, platelet count weekly; withhold drug if WBC count is <4000/mm^3 or platelet count is <100,000/mm^3; notify physician of results; also assess PT, PTT and thrombin time, which may be increased

• Monitor renal function studies: BUN, creatinine, serum uric acid, urine CrCl before and during therapy; check I&O ratio; report fall in urine output to <30 ml/hr; patient should be well hydrated with 2-3 L/day to prevent urate deposits

• Monitor temp q4h (may indicate beginning of infection)

P

• Monitor liver function tests before and during therapy (bilirubin, AST, ALT, LDH) as needed or monthly; check for jaundice of skin and sclera, dark urine, clay-colored stools, itchy skin, abdominal pain, fever, diarrhea; also monitor cholesterol, alkaline phosphatase

• Assess for bleeding: hematuria, stool guaiac, bruising or petechiae, mucosa or orifices q8h; check for inflammation of mucosa, breaks in skin

• Identify edema in feet, joint pain, stomach pain, shaking

Nursing diagnoses

☑ Injury, risk for (adverse reactions)

☑ Infection, risk for (adverse reactions)

☑ Knowledge deficit (teaching)

Implementation

• Preparation by trained personnel is required in controlled environment

• Give fluids **IV** or PO before chemotherapy to hydrate patient

• Provide antiemetic 30-60 min before giving drug and PRN to prevent vomiting; administer antibiotics for prophylaxis of infection

• Provide a liq diet: carbonated beverages; gelatin may be added if patient is not nauseated or vomiting

Intradermal route

• After intradermal skin testing and desensitization, give 0.1 ml (2 IU) intradermally after reconstituting with 5 ml sterile water or 0.9% NaCl for inj; then add 0.1 ml of reconstituted drug to 9.9 ml diluent (20 IU/ml); observe for 1 hr, check for wheal; desensitization may be required

• For direct **IV** dilute 10,000 IU/5 ml sterile water for inj or 0.9% NaCl without preservatives; give through 5-μm filter if fibers are present; do not use if cloudy or discolored, give over 30 min through Y-site of full-flowing **IV** of 0.9% NaCl or D₅W; run **IV** sol for at least 2 hr after direct administration

• Give **IV** inf using 21G, 23G, 25G needle; administer by slow **IV** inf via Y-tube or 3-way stopcock of flowing D₅W or NS inf over 30 min after diluting 10,000 IU/5 ml of sterile water or 0.9% NaCl (no preservatives) to 2000 IU/ml; filter may be necessary if fibers are present

• Provide allopurinol or sodium bicarbonate to reduce uric acid levels, alkalinization of urine

IM route

• Dilute 10,000 IU/2 ml 0.9% NaCl with preservatives; give 2 ml or less per site

Patient/family education

• Advise patient that contraceptive measures are recommended during therapy; drug is teratogenic

• Teach patient to avoid use of products containing aspirin or NSAIDs, razors, commercial mouthwash, since bleeding may occur; to report symptoms of bleeding (hematuria, tarry stools)

• Teach patient to report signs of anemia (fatigue, headache, irritability, faintness, shortness of breath)

• Tell patient to avoid crowds and persons with respiratory tract infections to prevent patient infection

• Advise patient to avoid vaccinations, since serious reactions can occur

• Teach patient to report nausea, vomiting, bruising, bleeding, stomatitis, severe diarrhea, jaundice, chest pain, abdominal pain, trouble breathing, rash

Evaluation
Positive therapeutic outcome
• Prevention of rapid division of malignant cells

---

pemoline (℞)
(pem'oh-leen)
Cylert, Cylert Chewable
Func. class.: Cerebral stimulant
Chem. class.: Oxazolidinone derivative

Pregnancy category   **B**
Controlled substance schedule   **IV**

Action: Exact mechanism unknown; may act through dopaminergic mechanisms; produces CNS stimulation and a paradoxic effect in ADHD

➔**Therapeutic Outcome:** Increased alertness, increased attention span, decreased hyperactivity (ADHD)

Uses: Attention deficit hyperactivity disorder for children >6 yr

Investigational uses: Schizophrenia, fatigue, depression

Dosage and routes
Child >6 yr: PO 37.5 mg in AM, increasing by 18.75 mg/wk, not to exceed 112.5 mg/day

Available forms: Tabs 18.75, 37.5, 75 mg; chewable tab 37.5 mg

Adverse effects
CNS: Hyperactivity, insomnia, restlessness, dizziness, depression, headache, stimulation, irritability, aggressiveness, hallucinations, **seizures, masking or worsening of Gilles de la Tourette's syndrome,** drowsiness, dyskinetic movements
CV: Tachycardia
GI: Nausea, *anorexia,* diarrhea, abdominal pain, increased liver enzymes, **hepatitis,** jaundice, weight loss
MISC: Rashes, growth suppression in children

Contraindications: Hypersensitivity, hepatic insufficiency

Precautions: Renal disease, pregnancy **B,** lactation, drug abuse, child <6 yr, psychosis, tics, seizure disorders

Pharmacokinetics
Absorption	Well absorbed
Distribution	Widely distributed; crosses placenta
Metabolism	Liver
Excretion	Kidneys, pH dependent; increased pH, increased reabsorption
Half-life	12 hr; increased when urine is alkaline

Pharmacodynamics
Onset	Unknown
Peak	2-4 hr
Duration	8 hr

Interactions
Drug classifications
Adrenergics: ↑ stimulation
Decongestants: ↑ stimulation
Stimulants, CNS: ↑ stimulation
Food/drug
Caffeine (coffee, teas, chocolate): ↑ stimulation

NURSING CONSIDERATIONS
Assessment
• Monitor VS, B/P, since this drug may reverse antihypertensives; check patients with cardiac disease more often for increased B/P
• Monitor height and weight q3 mo, since growth rate in **P** children may be decreased; appetite is suppressed; weight loss is common during the first few mo of treatment
• Monitor mental status: mood, sensorium, affect, stimulation, insomnia; aggressiveness may occur; depression with crying spells may occur after drug has worn off
• Assess for tolerance; should not be used for extended time except in ADHD; dosage should be diminished gradually to prevent withdrawal symptoms
P • In children or adults with ADHD, monitor for improved organizational skills, attention span, attending to tasks, impulse control, socialization, and ability to get along better with others
• Assess for withdrawal symptoms: headache, nausea, vomiting, muscle pain, weakness; drug tolerance will develop after long-term use; dosage should not be increased if tolerance develops

Nursing diagnoses
☑ Thought processes, altered (uses, adverse reactions)
☑ Coping, impaired individual (uses)
☑ Knowledge deficit (teaching)
☑ Family coping, impaired individual (uses)

Implementation
• Give at least 6 hr before hs to avoid sleeplessness; titrate to patient's response; lowest dosage should be used to control symptoms
• Provide gum, hard candy, frequent sips of water for dry mouth at beginning of treatment; these symptoms tend to lessen with time

Patient/family education
• Teach patient to decrease caffeine consumption (coffee, tea, cola, chocolate), which may increase irritability and stimulation; to avoid OTC preparations unless approved by prescriber; to avoid alcohol ingestion; these may cause serious drug interactions
• Instruct patient to taper off drug over several wk, or depression, increased sleeping, lethargy may occur
• Caution patient to avoid hazardous activities until stabilized on medication
• Instruct patient not to double doses if medication is missed; prescriber may suggest drug holidays (ADHD) during the school year to assess progress and determine continued drug necessity
• Teach patient/family to notify prescriber if significant side effects occur: tremors, insomnia, palpitations, restlessness; drug changes may be needed
• Inform patient that if dry mouth occurs to use frequent sips of water, sugarless gum, hard candy during beginning therapy; dry mouth lessens with continued treatment
• Advise patient to get needed rest; patients will feel more tired at end of day; to take last dose at least 6 hr before hs to avoid insomnia

---

☑ Herb/drug ⓢ Do Not Crush ◆ Alert ⊶ Key Drug �G Geriatric P Pediatric

Evaluation
Positive therapeutic outcome
- Decreased activity in ADHD

Treatment of overdose:
Administer fluids, hemodialysis, peritoneal dialysis, antihypertensives for increased B/P; ammonium chloride for increased excretion

---

PENICILLINS

**penicillin G
benzathine** (℞)
(pen-i-sill'in)
Bicillin L-A, Permapen
**penicillin G
potassium** (℞)
Megacillin ✦, Pfizerpen
**penicillin G
procaine** (℞)
Crysticillin A.S., Duracillin A.S., Pfizerpen-AS, Wycillin
**penicillin G
sodium** (℞)
Crystapen ✦, Pfizerpen ✦
**penicillin V
potassium** (℞)
Apo-Pen-VK ✦, Betapen-VK, Deltapen-VK, Ledercen-VK, Novopen-VK ✦, Penapar-VK, Pen-Vee K ✦, PVFK ✦, Robicillin-VK, Uticillin-VK, V-Cillin K, Veetids
Func. class.: Broad-spectrum antiinfective
Chem. class.: Natural penicillin
Pregnancy category   **B**

Action: Interferes with cell wall replication of susceptible organisms; osmotically unstable cell wall swells and bursts from osmotic pressure, resulting in cell death

⇨**Therapeutic Outcome:** Bactericidal effects on the gram-positive cocci *Staphylococcus, Streptococcus pyogenes, S. viridans, S. faecalis, S. bovis, S. pneumoniae;* gram-negative cocci *Neisseria gonorrhoeae;* gram-positive bacilli *Bacillus anthracis, Clostridium perfringens, C. tetani, Corynebacterium diphtheriae, Listeria monocytogenes;* gram-negative bacilli *Escherichia coli, Proteus mirabilis, Salmonella, Shigella, Enterobacter, Streptobacillus moniliformis,* spirochete *Treponema pallidum; Actinomyces*

Uses: Respiratory tract infections, scarlet fever, erysipelas, otitis media, pneumonia, skin and soft tissue infections, gonorrhea; prevention of rheumatic fever, glomerulonephritis

Dosage and routes
Penicillin G benzathine
Early syphilis
Adult: IM 2.4 million U in single dose

Congenital syphilis
P *Child <2 yr:* IM 50,000 U/kg in single dose

Prophylaxis of rheumatic fever, glomerulonephritis
P *Adult and child >27 kg:* IM 1.2 million U in single dose q mo or 600,000 U q2 wk

P *Child <27 kg:* IM 600,000 U in single dose q mo

Upper respiratory tract infections (group A streptococcal)
Adult: IM 1.2 million U in single dose; PO 400,000-600,000 U q4-6h

P *Child >27 kg:* IM 900,000 U in single dose

P *Child <27 kg:* IM 300,000-600,000 U in single dose

✦ Canada Only   Adverse effects: *italic* = common; **bold** = life-threatening

Available forms: Inj 300,000 U/ml; 600,000; 1,200,000; 2,400,000 U/dose

Penicillin G potassium
Pneumococcal/streptococcal infections (mild to moderate)
Adult: IM/**IV** 2-24 million U in divided doses q4h

P *Child <12 yr:* 100,000-400,000 U/kg/day in 4-6 divided doses

Renal dose
Dosage reduction indicated in renal impairment (CrCl <50 ml/min)

Available forms: Inj 1, 2, 3 million U/50 ml; powder for inj 1, 5, 10, 20 million U/vial

Penicillin G procaine
Moderate to severe infections
P **Adult and child:** IM 600,000-1.2 million U in 1 or 2 doses/day for 10 days to 2 wk

P *Newborn:* 50,000 U/kg IM once daily (avoid use in newborns)

Gonorrhea
P **Adult and child >12 yr:** IM 4.8 million U in two injections given 30 min after probenecid 1 g

Renal dose
CrCl 10-30 ml/min give q8-12h; CrCl <10 ml/min give q12-18h

Available forms: Inj 600,000; 1,200,000; 2,400,000 U/dose

Penicillin G sodium
Moderate to severe infections
Adult: IM/**IV** 2 million-24 million U/day in divided doses q4h

P *Child:* IM/**IV** 50,000-400,000 U/kg/day in divided doses q4-12h

Dental surgery prophylaxis for endocarditis
Adult: IM/**IV** 2 million U ½-1 hr before procedure, then 1 million U 6 hr after procedure

Renal dose
Dosage reduction indicated in renal impairment (CrCl <50 ml/min)

Available forms: Inj 5 million U/vial

Penicillin V potassium
Pneumococcal/staphylococcal infections
Adult: PO 250-500 mg q6h

P *Child <12 yr:* PO 25-50 mg/kg/day in divided doses q6-8h

Streptococcal infections
Adult: PO 125-250 mg q6-8h × 10 days

Prevention of recurrence of rheumatic fever/chorea
Adult: PO 125-250 mg bid continuously

P *Child <5 yr:* PO 125 mg bid

P *Child >5 yr:* PO 250 mg bid

Vincent's gingivitis/pharyngitis
Adult: PO 500 mg q6h

Renal dose
Dosage reduction indicated in renal impairment (CrCl <50 ml/min)

Available forms: Tabs 250, 500 mg; powder for oral sol 125, 250 mg/5 ml

Adverse effects
CNS: Lethargy, hallucinations, anxiety, depression, twitching, **coma, convulsions**
GI: Nausea, vomiting, diar-

rhea, increased AST, ALT, abdominal pain, glossitis, colitis
GU: **Oliguria, proteinuria, hematuria, vaginitis, moniliasis, glomerulonephritis**
HEMA: Anemia, increased bleeding time, **bone marrow depression, granulocytopenia**
META: Hyperkalemia, hypokalemia, alkalosis, hypernatremia
MISC: Local pain, tenderness and fever with IM inj

Contraindications: Hypersensitivity to penicillins; neonates

Precautions: Hypersensitivity to cephalosporins, pregnancy **B,** severe renal disease

Penicillin G benzathine

Pharmacokinetics

Absorption	Delayed; prolonged drug levels
Distribution	Widely distributed; crosses placenta
Metabolism	Liver, minimally
Excretion	Kidneys, unchanged; breast milk
Half-life	½-1 hr

Pharmacodynamics

Onset	Slow
Peak	12-24 hr
Duration	1-4 wk

Penicillin G potassium

Pharmacokinetics

Absorption	Variably absorbed (PO); well absorbed (IM)
Distribution	Widely distributed; crosses placenta
Metabolism	Liver, minimally
Excretion	Kidneys, unchanged; breast milk
Half-life	½-1 hr

Pharmacodynamics

	PO	IM	IV
Onset	Rapid	Rapid	Rapid
Peak	1 hr	¼-½ hr	Immediate

Penicillin G procaine

Pharmacokinetics

Absorption	Delayed; prolonged drug levels
Distribution	Widely distributed; crosses placenta
Metabolism	Liver, minimally
Excretion	Kidneys, unchanged; breast milk
Half-life	½-1 hr

Pharmacodynamics

Onset	Slow
Peak	1-4 hr
Duration	15 hr

Penicillin G sodium

Pharmacokinetics

Absorption	Well absorbed
Distribution	Widely distributed; crosses placenta
Metabolism	Liver, minimally
Excretion	Kidneys, unchanged; breast milk
Half-life	½-1 hr

Pharmacodynamics

	IM	IV
Onset	Rapid	Rapid
Peak	1-3 hr	Rapid

Penicillin V potassium

Pharmacokinetics

Absorption	Widely absorbed
Distribution	Widely distributed; crosses placenta
Metabolism	Liver, minimally
Excretion	Kidneys, unchanged; breast milk
Half-life	½-1 hr

Pharmacodynamics

Onset	Rapid
Peak	½ hr

Interactions
Individual drugs
Aspirin: ↑ penicillin levels, ↓ renal excretion
Chloramphenicol: ↑ half-life

P

of chloramphenicol, ↓ effectiveness of penicillin

Cholestyramine: ↓ effectiveness of penicillin

Colestipol: ↓ effectiveness of penicillin

Probenecid: ↑ penicillin levels, ↓ renal excretion

Drug classifications

Erythromycins: ↓ antimicrobial effectiveness

Oral anticoagulants: ↑ anticoagulant effects

Oral contraceptives: ↓ contraceptive effectiveness

Tetracyclines: ↓ antimicrobial effectiveness

☑ *Herb/drug*

Khat: ↓ absorption of penicillin; separate doses by 2 hr or more

Food/drug

Food, carbonated drinks, citrus fruit juice: ↓ absorption

Lab test interferences

False positive: Urine glucose, urine protein

NURSING CONSIDERATIONS
Assessment

• Assess patient for previous sensitivity reaction to penicillins or cephalosporins; cross-sensitivity between penicillins and cephalosporins is common

• Assess patient for signs and symptoms of infection including characteristics of wounds, sputum, urine, stool, WBC >10,000, earache, fever; obtain baseline information and during treatment

• Obtain C&S before beginning drug therapy to identify if correct treatment has been initiated

• Assess for allergic reactions: rash, urticaria, pruritus, chills, fever, joint pain; angioedema may occur a few days after therapy begins; epinephrine, resuscitation equipment should be available for anaphylactic reaction

◆• Identify urine output; if decreasing, notify prescriber (may indicate nephrotoxicity); also check for increased BUN, creatinine

• Monitor blood studies: AST, ALT, CBC, Hct, bilirubin, LDH, alkaline phosphatase, Coombs' test monthly if patient is on long-term therapy

• Monitor electrolytes: potassium, sodium, chloride monthly if patient is on long-term therapy

• Assess bowel pattern daily; if severe diarrhea occurs, drug should be discontinued; may indicate pseudomembranous colitis

• Monitor for bleeding: ecchymosis, bleeding gums, hematuria, stool guaiac daily if on long-term therapy

• Assess for overgrowth of infection: perineal itching, fever, malaise, redness, pain, swelling, drainage, rash, diarrhea, change in cough, sputum

Nursing diagnoses

☑ Infection, risk for (uses)
☑ Diarrhea (adverse reactions)
☑ Injury, risk for (adverse reactions)
☑ Knowledge deficit (teaching)
☑ Noncompliance (teaching)

Implementation
Penicillin G benzathine
PO route

• Give in even doses around the clock; if GI upset occurs, give with food, avoid acidic juices; carbonated beverages may decrease PO absorption; drug must be given for 10-14 days to ensure organism death and prevent superinfection

• Shake susp

☑ Herb/drug　◎ Do Not Crush　◆ Alert　⊶ Key Drug　🄶 Geriatric　🄿 Pediatric

IM route
- Do not give **IV**
- Give deep in large muscle mass
- Reconstitute with 0.9% NaCl, sterile water for inj, D_5W; refrigerate unused portion

Penicillin G potassium
PO route
- Give in even doses around the clock; if GI upset occurs, give with food; drug must be given for 10-14 days to ensure organism death and prevent superinfection
- Shake susp

IM route
- Reconstitute with D_5W, 0.9% NaCl, sterile water for inj; shake well
- Give deep in large muscle mass; massage
- Do not give SC; may cause severe pain
- If injected near a nerve, loss of function and severe pain may occur

IV IV route
- Change **IV** sites q48h to prevent pain and phlebitis
- Give by intermittent inf by diluting 3 million U or less/50 ml or more; dilute 3 million U or more/100 ml D_5W, $D_{10}W$, 0.45% NaCl, 0.9% NaCl, LR, Ringer's or any combination run over 1-2 hr (adult), 15-30 **P** min (child)
- Give by cont inf by diluting and infusing over 24 hr

Syringe compatibilities:
Heparin
Syringe incompatibilities:
Metoclopramide
Y-site compatibilities:
Acyclovir, amiodarone, cyclophosphamide, diltiazem, enala-

prilat, esmolol, fluconazole, foscarnet, heparin, hydromorphone, labetalol, magnesium sulfate, meperidine, morphine, perphenazine, potassium chloride, tacrolimus, theophylline, verapamil, vit B/C

Additive compatibilities:
Ascorbic acid, calcium chloride, calcium gluconate, cephapirin, chloramphenicol, cimetidine, clindamycin, colistimethate, corticotropin, dimenhydrinate, diphenhydramine, ephedrine, erythromycin, furosemide, hydrocortisone, kanamycin, lidocaine, magnesium sulfate, methicillin, methylprednisolone, metronidazole, polymyxin B, prednisolone, potassium chloride, procaine, prochlorperazine, verapamil

Additive incompatibilities:
Aminoglycosides, aminophylline, amphotericin B, chlorpromazine, dopamine, floxacillin, hydroxyzine, metaraminol, oxytetracycline, pentobarbital, prochlorperazine mesylate, promazine, tetracycline, thiopental

Penicillin G procaine
- Do not give **IV**
- Give deeply in large muscle mass
- Reconstitute with 0.9% NaCl, sterile water for inj, D_5W; refrigerate unused portion
- Shake medication before administering
- IM route may include procaine reactions: fear of death, depression, convulsions, anxiety, confusion, hallucinations

Penicillin G sodium
IM route
- Reconstitute with 0.9% NaCl, D_5W, sterile water

P

- May be diluted with lidocaine (1%, 2%) to prevent pain from inj (IM only); use lidocaine without epinephrine only
- Shake after reconstitution; give deep in large muscle mass; massage
- Do not give SC; severe pain may occur
- Inj near nerves can result in severe pain and loss of function of nerve that was injected

IV IV route
- Change **IV** sites q48h to prevent phlebitis and pain at site
- Give by intermittent inf by diluting 3 million U or less/50 ml or more; or doses of 73 million U/100 ml D₅W, 0.9% NaCl; give over 1-2 hr (adult) or 30 min (child)
- Give by cont inf by diluting in compatible sol and run over 24 hr

Syringe compatibilities:
Aminoglycosides, chloramphenicol, cimetidine, colistimethate, gentamicin, heparin, kanamycin, lincomycin, polymyxin B, streptomycin

Syringe incompatibilities:
Oxytetracycline, tetracycline

Additive compatibilities:
Calcium chloride, calcium gluconate, chloramphenicol, clindamycin, colistimethate, diphenhydramine, erythromycin, furosemide, gentamicin, hydrocortisone, kanamycin, methicillin, polymyxin B, prednisolone, procaine, ranitidine, verapamil, vit B/C

Additive incompatibilities:
Amphotericin B, bleomycin, cephalothin, chlorpromazine, cytarabine, floxacillin, hydroxyzine, methylprednisolone, oxytetracycline, prochlorperazine, promethazine

Penicillin V potassium
- Give in even doses around the clock; if GI upset occurs, give with food; drug must be given for 10-14 days to ensure organism death and prevent superinfection; store in tight container
- Shake susp; store in refrigerator for 2 wk or for 1 wk at room temp

Patient/family education
- Teach patient to report sore throat, bruising, bleeding, joint pain; may indicate blood dyscrasias (rare)
- Advise patient to contact prescriber if vaginal itching, loose, foul-smelling stools, furry tongue occur; may indicate superinfection
- Instruct patient to take all medication prescribed for the length of time ordered
- Advise patient to notify prescriber of diarrhea with blood or pus, which may indicate pseudomembranous colitis

Evaluation
Positive therapeutic outcome
- Absence of signs/symptoms of infection (WBC <10,000, temp WNL, absence of red, draining wounds, earache)
- Reported improvement in symptoms of infection

Treatment of anaphylaxis:
Withdraw drug, maintain airway, administer epinephrine, aminophylline, O₂, **IV** corticosteroids

---

☑ Herb/drug   ⊗ Do Not Crush   ◆ Alert   ⚷ Key Drug   **G** Geriatric   **P** Pediatric

pentamidine (℞)
(pen-tam′i-deen)
Nebupent, Pentam 300,
Pentacarinat ✤,
Pneumopent ✤
Func. class.: Antiprotozoal
Chem. class.: Aromatic
diamide derivative
Pregnancy category **C**

Action: Interferes with DNA/
RNA synthesis in protozoa; has
direct effect on islet cells in the
pancreas

➡ **Therapeutic Outcome:** Protozoa death

Uses: Treatment/prevention
of *Pneumocystis carinii* infections

Investigational uses: Babesi-
osis, leishmaniasis, African
trypanosomiasis

Dosage and routes
Ｐ *Adult and child:* **IV**/IM 4
mg/kg/day × 2-3 wk; neb 300
mg via specific nebulizer given
q4wk for prevention

Available forms: Inj; aerosol
300 mg/vial; sol for aerosol 60
mg/vial ✤

Adverse effects
CNS: Disorientation, hallucinations, dizziness, confusion
CV: Hypotension, ventricular
tachycardia, ECG abnormalities; **dysrhythmias**
*GI: Nausea, vomiting, an-
orexia,* increased AST, ALT,
acute pancreatitis, metallic
taste
GU: **Acute renal failure,**
increased serum creatinine,
renal toxicity
HEMA: Anemia, **leukopenia,**
thrombocytopenia
INTEG: Sterile abscess, pain at
inj site, pruritus, urticaria, rash
META: Hyperkalemia, hypo-

calcemia, *hypoglycemia, hyperglycemia*
MISC: Fatigue, chills, night
sweats, **anaphylaxis, Stevens-
Johnson syndrome**
RESP: Cough, shortness of
breath, **bronchospasm** (with
aerosol)

Precautions: Blood dyscrasias,
hepatic disease, renal disease,
diabetes mellitus, cardiac disease, hypocalcemia, pregnancy
C, hypertension, hypotension,
Ｐ lactation, children

Pharmacokinetics	
Absorption	Well absorbed (IM); minimally absorbed (inh); completely absorbed (**IV**)
Distribution	Widely distributed; does not appear in CSF
Metabolism	Not known
Excretion	Kidneys, unchanged (up to 30%)
Half-life	6½-9½ hr; increased in renal disease

Pharmacodynamics			
	IM	IV	INH
Onset	Un-known	Un-known	Un-known
Peak	½-1 hr	Inf end	Unknown

Ｐ

Interactions
Individual drugs
Amphotericin B: ↑ nephro-
toxicity
Cisplatin: ↑ bone marrow
depression
Colistin: ↑ nephrotoxicity
Erythromycin IV: fatal dys-
rhythmias
Foscarnet: ↑ nephrotoxicity
Methoxyflurane: ↑ bone
marrow depression
Polymyxin B: ↑ bone marrow
depression
Radiation: ↑ nephrotoxicity,
bone marrow depression

✤ Canada Only   Adverse effects: *italic* = common; **bold** = life-threatening

Vancomycin: ↑ bone marrow depression

Drug classifications
Aminoglycosides: ↑ nephrotoxicity
Antineoplastics: ↑ nephrotoxicity, bone marrow depression

NURSING CONSIDERATIONS
Assessment
⬥• Assess any patient with compromised renal system: drug is excreted slowly in poor renal system function; toxicity may occur rapidly
• Assess patient for infection including increased temp, thick sputum, WBC >10,000; monitor these signs of infection throughout treatment; obtain C&S before beginning therapy; treatment may begin after culture is obtained
• Assess respiratory system including rate, rhythm, bilateral lung sounds, shortness of breath, wheezing, dyspnea
• Monitor ECG for cardiac dysrhythmias; ECG and pulse should be checked frequently during treatment, since cardiotoxicity can occur
• Assess for hypoglycemia including nausea, tremors, anxiety, chills, diaphoresis, headache, hunger, cold, pale skin; this side effect can last for several mo after treatment is completed
• Monitor for hyperglycemia including flushed, dry skin, acetone breath, thirst, anorexia, drowsiness, polyuria; this side effect can last for several mo after treatment is completed
• Monitor renal studies including BUN, urinalysis, creatinine; obtain at baseline and frequently during treatment; nephrotoxicity may occur;

check I&O, report hematuria, oliguria
• Monitor blood studies including blood glucose, CBC, platelets; blood glucose fluctuations are common; anemia, leukopenia, thrombocytopenia can occur
• Monitor liver studies including AST, ALT, alkaline phosphatase, bilirubin before beginning treatment and every 3 days during therapy
• Monitor calcium and magnesium before beginning treatment and every 3 days during therapy; hypocalcemia may occur

Nursing diagnoses
☑ Infection, risk for (uses)
☑ Knowledge deficit (teaching)

Implementation
IM route
• Reconstitute 300 mg/3 ml sterile water for inj; give deep in large muscle mass by Z-track; IM is a painful route
• Do not mix in normal saline
Ⅳ **IV route**
• For intermittent inf reconstitute 300 mg/3-5 ml sterile water for inj, D₅W; withdraw dose and further dilute in 50-250 ml D₅W; diluted sol is stable for 48 hr; discard unused sol; give over 1 hr or more

Y-site compatibilities:
Zidovudine

Y-site incompatibilities:
Foscarnet, fluconazole
Inh route
• Dilute 300 mg/600 ml sterile water for inj; put reconstituted sol into nebulizer; do not use with other drugs or sol precipitate may occur; stable for 48 hr at room temp; protect from light; administer over 30-45 min

Patient/family education

• Teach patient to report sore throat, fever, fatigue; could indicate superinfection

• Advise patient not to drink alcohol or take aspirin, since gastric bleeding may occur

• Teach patient to make position changes slowly to prevent orthostatic hypotension

• Advise patient to maintain adequate fluid intake

Evaluation

Positive therapeutic outcome

• Decreased signs and symptoms of protozoan infections

• Decreased signs and symptoms of *Pneumocystis carinii* pneumonia in HIV infections

---

pentazocine (℞)

(pen-taz′oh-seen)

Talwin, Talwin NX

Func. class.: Opiate analgesic

Chem. class.: Synthetic benzomorphan (agonist/antagonist)

Pregnancy category **C**

Controlled substance schedule **IV**

Action: Inhibits ascending pain pathways in limbic system, thalamus, midbrain, hypothalamus by binding to opiate receptor sites, altering pain perception and response

⇒**Therapeutic Outcome:** Relief of pain

Uses: Moderate to severe pain

Dosage and routes

Adult: PO 50-100 mg q3-4h prn, not to exceed 600 mg/day; **IV**/IM/SC 30 mg q3-4h prn, not to exceed 360 mg/day

Labor

Adult: IM 60 mg; **IV** 30 mg q2-3h when contractions are regular

Renal dose

CrCl 10-50 ml/min give q24-36h; CrCl <10 ml/min give q48h

Available forms: SC, IM, **IV** 30 mg/ml; tab 50 mg

Adverse effects

CNS: Drowsiness, dizziness, confusion, headache, sedation, euphoria, hallucinations, dreaming

CV: Palpitations, bradycardia, change in B/P, tachycardia, increased B/P (high doses)

EENT: Tinnitus, blurred vision, miosis (high doses), diplopia

GI: Nausea, vomiting, anorexia, constipation, cramps

GU: Urinary retention

INTEG: Rash, urticaria, bruising, flushing, diaphoresis, pruritus, severe irritation at inj sites

RESP: Respiratory depression

Contraindications: Hypersensitivity, addiction (narcotic)

Precautions: Addictive personality, pregnancy **C,** lactation, increased intracranial pressure, MI (acute), severe heart disease, respiratory depression, hepatic disease, renal disease, seizure disorder, child <18 yr, head trauma

Pharmacokinetics

Absorption	Well absorbed (PO, SC, IM); completely absorbed (**IV**)
Distribution	Widely distributed; crosses placenta
Metabolism	Liver, extensively
Excretion	Kidneys, small amounts (unchanged)
Half-life	2-3 hr

Pharmacodynamics

	PO	SC/IM	IV
Onset	15-30 min	15-30 min	Rapid
Peak	1-3 hr	1-2 hr	15 min
Duration	3 hr	2-4 hr	1 hr

Interactions
Individual drugs
Alcohol: ↑ respiratory depression, hypotension, sedation
Drug classifications
Antihistamines: ↑ respiratory depression, hypotension
CNS depressants: ↑ respiratory depression, hypotension
MAOIs: Use cautiously; results are unpredictable
Opiates: ↑ opioid withdrawals (dependency)
Phenothiazines: ↑ respiratory depression, hypotension
Sedative/hypnotics: ↑ respiratory depression, hypotension
Lab test interferences
↑ Amylase, ↑ lipase

NURSING CONSIDERATIONS
Assessment
• Assess pain characteristics: location, intensity, type of pain before medication administration and following treatment
• Monitor VS after parenteral route; note muscle rigidity, drug history, liver, kidney function tests, respiratory dysfunction: respiratory depression, character, rate, rhythm; notify prescriber if respirations are <10/min
• Monitor CNS changes: dizziness, drowsiness, hallucinations, euphoria, LOC, pupil reaction
• Monitor allergic reactions: rash, urticaria
• Assess for withdrawal symptoms in opiate-dependent patients

Nursing diagnoses
☑ Pain (uses)
☑ Sensory-perceptual alteration: visual, auditory (adverse reactions)
☑ Breathing pattern, ineffective (adverse reactions)
☑ Knowledge deficit (teaching)

Implementation
• Give by inj (IM, **IV**), only when resuscitative equipment available; give slowly to prevent rigidity
• Store in light-resistant area at room temp
PO route
• Tabs made in the United States contain naloxone 0.5 mg to prevent abuse if the PO preparation is used **IV**
IM route
• Give deeply in large muscle mass; rotate inj sites
IV route
• Give by direct **IV** after diluting 5 mg/ml of sterile water for inj; give 5 mg or less over 1 min

Syrinige compatibilities:
Atropine, benzquinamide, butorphanol, chlorpromazine, cimetidine, dimenhydrinate, diphenhydramine, droperidol, fentanyl, hydromorphone, hydroxyzine, meperidine, metoclopramide, morphine, perphenazine, prochlorperazine, promazine, prometha-

---

zine, propiomazine, ranitidine, scopolamine

Syringe incompatibilities:
Glycopyrrolate, heparin, pentobarbital, other barbiturates

Y-site compatibilities:
Heparin, hydrocortisone, potassium chloride, vit B/C

Y-site incompatibilities:
Nafcillin

Additive incompatibilities:
Aminophylline, amobarbital, pentobarbital, phenobarbital, secobarbital, sodium bicarbonate

Patient/family education
• Teach patient to report any symptoms of CNS changes, allergic reactions
• Advise patients to avoid CNS depressants: alcohol, sedative/hypnotics for at least 24 hr after taking this drug
• Discuss with patient that dizziness, drowsiness, and confusion are common; to avoid getting up without assistance
• Discuss in detail all aspects of the drug
• Instruct patient to change position slowly to prevent orthostatic hypotension
• Teach patient to turn, cough, deep breathe after surgery to prevent atelectasis

Evaluation
Positive therapeutic outcome
• Relief of pain

Treatment of overdose:
Naloxone (Narcan) 0.2-0.8 mg **IV**, O_2, **IV** fluids, vasopressors

---

pentobarbital (℞)
(pen-toe-bar′bi-tal)
Nembutal, Nova-Rectal ✦,
**pentobarbital sodium,
Pentogen** ✦
Func. class.: Sedative/hypnotic barbiturate
Chem. class.: Barbitone, short acting
Pregnancy category **D**
**Controlled substance
schedule** **II** (USA),
schedule **G** (Canada)

Action: Depresses activity in brain cells, primarily in reticular activating system in brainstem; also selectively depresses neurons in posterior hypothalamus, limbic structures; may decrease cerebral blood flow, intracranial pressure (**IV**) and cerebral edema; may potentiate GABA, an inhibitory neurotransmitter

⇒**Therapeutic Outcome:** Sedation, sleep

Uses: Insomnia, sedation, preoperative medication, increased intracranial pressure, dental anesthetic

Dosage and routes
Adult: PO 100-200 mg hs; IM 150-200 mg hs; **IV** 100 mg initially, then up to 500 mg; REC 120-200 mg hs

P *Child:* IM 2-6 mg/kg, not to exceed 100 mg; PO 2-6 mg/kg/day in divided doses; PO preoperatively 2-6 mg/kg, max 100 mg/dose; **IV** 50 mg (hypnotic/anticonvulsant)

Available forms: Caps 50, 100 mg; elix 18.2 mg/5 ml; rec supp 25 ✦, 30, 50 ✦, 60, 120, 200 mg; inj 50 mg/ml

---

Adverse effects
CNS: Lethargy, drowsiness, hangover, dizziness, paradoxic **G P** stimulation in elderly and children, lightheadedness, dependence, **CNS depression,** mental depression, slurred speech
CV: Hypotension, bradycardia
GI: Nausea, vomiting, diarrhea, constipation
HEMA: **Agranulocytosis, thrombocytopenia, megaloblastic anemia** (long-term treatment)
INTEG: Rash, urticaria, pain, abscesses at inj site, angioedema, thrombophlebitis, **Stevens-Johnson syndrome**
RESP: **Depression, apnea, laryngospasm, bronchospasm**

Contraindications: Hypersensitivity to barbiturates, respiratory depression, addiction to barbiturates, severe liver, renal impairment, porphyria, uncontrolled pain, pregnancy **D**

Precautions: Anemia, lactation, hepatic disease, renal **G** disease, hypertension, elderly, acute/chronic pain

N Do Not Confuse:
pentobarbital/phenobarbital

Pharmacokinetics	
Absorption	Well absorbed
Distribution	Widely distributed; crosses placenta, enters breast milk
Metabolism	Liver
Excretion	Kidneys, unchanged (minimally)
Half-life	15-48 hr

Pharmacodynamics				
	PO	IM	IV	REC
Onset	15-30 min	10-25 min	Immediate	Slow
Peak	3-4 hr	Unknown	1 min	Unknown
Duration	4-6 hr	1-4 hr	15 min	4-6 hr

Interactions:
Individual drugs
Alcohol: ↑ CNS depression
Chloramphenicol: ↓ effectiveness
Cyclophosphamide: ↑ hematologic toxicity
Cyclosporine: ↓ effectiveness
Dacarbazine: ↓ effectiveness
Quinidine: ↓ effectiveness
Valproic acid: ↑ sedation
Drug classifications
Anticoagulants: ↓ effectiveness
Antidepressants: ↑ CNS depression
Antihistamines: ↑ CNS depression
Glucocorticoids: ↓ effectiveness
MAOIs: ↑ CNS depression
Opiates: ↑ CNS depression
Oral contraceptives: ↓ effectiveness
Sedative/hypnotics: ↑ CNS depression
Tricyclic antidepressants: ↓ effectiveness
☑ Herb/drug
Quinine: ↑ pentobarbital level

NURSING CONSIDERATIONS
Assessment
• Assess mental status: mood, sensorium, affect, memory **G** (long, short), especially elderly; if using as a hypnotic, assess sleep patterns during therapy; drug suppresses REM sleep with dreaming; withdrawal insomnia may occur after short-term use; do not start using drug again; insomnia will improve in 1-3 nights; may experience increased dreaming
• Monitor for respiratory dysfunction: respiratory depression, character, rate, rhythm (when using **IV**); hold drug if respirations are <10/ min or if pupils are dilated; also

check VS q30 min after parenteral route for 2 hr
• Assess for blood dyscrasias: fever, sore throat, bruising, rash, jaundice, epistaxis (long-term treatment only)
• Assess seizure activity including type, location, duration, and character; provide seizure precaution
• Assess for pain in postoperative patients; pain threshold is lowered when patients are taking this medication

Nursing diagnoses
☑ Injury, risk for (side effects)
☑ Knowledge deficit (teaching)

Implementation
• Administer only after removal of cigarettes, to prevent fires
• Reserve use until after trying conservative measures for insomnia

PO route
• Give 30 min before hs for expected sleeplessness
• May dilute elixir in juice, milk, or water if needed
• Give on empty stomach for best absorption

IM route
• Give deeply in muscle mass (gluteal) to minimize irritation to tissues; split inj of >5 ml into two since irritation to tissues may occur; do not administer SC

IV route
• Use large vein to prevent extravasation; if extravasation occurs, use moist heat to the area and 5% procaine sol injected into area; give at 50 mg/1 min or more
• Give **IV** only with resuscitative equipment available (and only by qualified personnel)

Syringe compatibilities:
Aminophylline, ephedrine, hydromorphone, neostigmine, scopolamine, sodium bicarbonate, thiopental

Syringe incompatibilities:
Benzquinamide, butorphanol, chlorpromazine, cimetidine, dimenhydrinate, diphenhydramine, droperidol, fentanyl, glycopyrrolate, hydroxyzine, meperidine, midazolam, nalbuphine, pentazocine, perphenazine, prochlorperazine, promazine, promethazine, ranitidine

Y-site compatibilities:
Acyclovir, regular insulin, propofol

Additive compatibilities:
Amikacin, aminophylline, calcium chloride, cephapirin, chloramphenicol, dimenhydrinate, erythromycin, lidocaine, thiopental, verapamil

Additive incompatibilities:
Chlorpheniramine, codeine, ephedrine, erythromycin gluceptate, regular insulin, levorphanol, hydrocortisone, sodium succinate, hydroxyzine, methadone, norepinephrine, pentazocine, penicillin G potassium, phenytoin, promazine, promethazine, streptomycin, triflupromazine, vancomycin

Patient/family education
• Teach patient to carry ID card or Medic Alert bracelet stating name, drugs taken, condition, prescriber's name, phone number
• Caution patient to avoid driving and other activities that require alertness
• Caution patient to avoid alcohol ingestion and CNS depressants; increased sedation may occur
• Teach patient not to discontinue medication quickly after

long-term use; taper off over several wk

Evaluation
Positive therapeutic outcome
- Improved sleeping patterns
- Decreased seizure activity
- Improved energy

Treatment of overdose:
Lavage, activated charcoal, warming blanket, vital signs, hemodialysis

---

pentostatin (℞)
(pen'toe-sta-tin)
Nipent
Func. class.: Antineoplastic, enzyme inhibitor
Chem. class.: Streptomyces antibioticus derivative

Pregnancy category   D

Action: Inhibits the enzyme adenosine deaminase (ADA), which is able to block DNA synthesis and some RNA synthesis

➡ **Therapeutic Outcome:** Prevention of rapidly growing malignant cells

Uses: α-Interferon–refractory hairy cell leukemia, chronic lymphocytic leukemia

Dosage and routes
Adult: **IV** 4 mg/m² every other wk; may be given **IV** bol or diluted in a larger volume and given over 20-30 min

Available forms: Inj 10 mg/vial

Adverse effects
CNS: Headache, anxiety, confusion, depression, dizziness, insomnia, nervousness, paresthesia
GI: Nausea, vomiting, anorexia, diarrhea, constipation, flatulence, stomatitis, elevated liver function tests
GU: **Hematuria,** dysuria, increased BUN/creatinine
HEMA: **Leukopenia, anemia, thrombocytopenia, ecchymosis, lymphadenopathy,** petechiae
INTEG: Rash, eczema, dry skin, pruritus, sweating, herpes simplex/zoster
RESP: Cough, upper respiratory tract infection, bronchitis, dyspnea, epistaxis, pneumonia, pharyngitis, rhinitis, sinusitis
SYST: Fever, infection, fatigue, pain, allergic reaction, chills, **death, sepsis,** chest pain, flu syndrome

Contraindications: Hypersensitivity to this drug or mannitol, pregnancy **D**

Precautions: Renal disease, ℗ lactation, children, bone marrow depression

Pharmacokinetics

Absorption	Completely absorbed
Distribution	Unknown; low protein binding
Metabolism	Unknown
Excretion	Kidneys
Half-life	5-7 hr; increased in renal disease

Pharmacodynamics

Onset	4-5 mo
Peak	Unknown
Duration	1½-34 mo

Interactions
Individual drugs
Fludarabine: Fatal pulmonary reaction
Vidarabine: ↑ adverse reactions

NURSING CONSIDERATIONS
Assessment
- Assess CNS changes: confusion, paresthesias, psychosis,

tremors, seizures, neuropathies; drug should be discontinued
• Assess for toxicity: facial flushing, epistaxis, increased pro-time, thrombocytopenia; drug should be discontinued
• Assess acidosis, signs of dehydration: rapid respirations, poor skin turgor, decreased urine output, dry skin, restlessness, weakness
• Check buccal cavity q8h for dryness, sores or ulceration, white patches, oral pain, bleeding, dysphagia; obtain prescription for viscous lidocaine (Xylocaine) to use in mouth
• Assess symptoms indicating severe allergic reaction: rash, pruritus, urticaria, purpuric skin lesions, itching, flushing
• Assess tachypnea, ECG changes, dyspnea, edema, fatigue; respiratory and cardiovascular reaction can be severe
• Monitor CBC, differential, platelet count weekly; withhold drug if WBC count is <2000/mm^3 or platelet count is <100,000/mm^3, notify prescriber of results
• Monitor renal function studies: BUN, creatinine, serum uric acid, urine CrCl before and during therapy; I&O ratio; report fall in urine output to <30 ml/hr
• Monitor temp q4h (may indicate beginning of infection)
• Monitor liver function tests before and during therapy (bilirubin, AST, ALT, LDH) as needed or monthly; check for jaundice of skin and sclera, dark urine, clay-colored stools, itchy skin, abdominal pain, fever, diarrhea
• Assess for bleeding: hematuria, stool guaiac, bruising or petechiae, mucosa or orifices q8h; check for inflammation of mucosa, breaks in skin
• Assess effects of alopecia on body image; discuss feelings about body changes

Nursing diagnoses
☑ Injury, risk for (adverse reactions)
☑ Body image disturbance (adverse reactions)
☑ Infection, risk for (adverse reactions)
☑ Knowledge deficit (teaching)

Implementation
• Give fluids **IV** or PO before chemotherapy to hydrate patient
• Give antacid before oral agent, antiemetic 30-60 min before giving drug and prn to prevent vomiting; administer antibiotics for prophylaxis of infection
• Give top or syst analgesics for pain to lessen effects from stomatitis
• Give liq diet: carbonated beverages; gelatin may be added if patient is not nauseated or vomiting
• Encourage patient to rinse mouth tid-qid with water, club soda; brush teeth bid-qid with soft brush or cotton-tipped applicators for stomatitis; use unwaxed dental floss
• Preparation should be done by personnel knowledgeable in preparing antineoplastics wearing gloves, gown, mask in biologic cabinet
• Give by direct **IV** by reconstituting 10 mg/5 ml of sterile water for inj (2 mg/ml); shake well
• Give over 5 min
• Give by intermittent inf after diluting 10 mg/25-50 ml of

P

0.9% NaCl, D$_5$W; give over 30 min
• Diluted sol should be used within 8 hr at room temp

Y-site compatibilities:
Fludarabine, melphalan, ondansetron, paclitaxel, sargramostim

Solution compatibilities:
D$_5$W, 0.9% NaCl, LR

Patient/family education
• Teach patient to avoid use of products containing aspirin or NSAIDs, razors, commercial mouthwash, since bleeding may occur; to report symptoms of bleeding (hematuria, tarry stools)
• Advise patient to report signs of anemia (fatigue, headache, irritability, faintness, shortness of breath); CNS reactions including confusion, psychosis, nightmares, seizures, severe headaches
• Inform patient that hair may be lost during treatment; a wig or hair piece may make patient feel better; new hair may be different in color, texture
• Advise patient to use sunscreen and protective clothing to prevent photosensitive reactions

Evaluation
Positive therapeutic outcome
• Prevention of rapid division of malignant cells
• Decreased bone marrow hairy cells

---

pentoxifylline (R)
(pen-tox-if′i-lin)
Trental
Func. class.: Hemorheologic agent
Chem. class.: Dimethylxanthine derivative
Pregnancy category C

Action: Decreases blood viscosity, stimulates prostacyclin formation, increases blood flow by increasing flexibility of RBCs; decreases RBC hyperaggregation; reduces platelet aggregation, decreases fibrinogen concentration

▶**Therapeutic Outcome:** Decreased claudication and improved blood flow

Uses: Intermittent claudication related to chronic occlusive vascular disease

Investigational uses: Cerebrovascular insufficiency, diabetic neuropathies, TIAs, leg ulcers, strokes

Dosage and routes
Adult: PO 400 mg tid with meals

Available forms: Ext rel tab 400 mg

Adverse effects
CNS: Headache, anxiety, *tremors,* confusion, *dizziness*
CV: Angina, dysrhythmias, palpitations, hypotension, chest pain, dyspnea, edema
EENT: Blurred vision, earache, increased salivation, sore throat, conjunctivitis
GI: Dyspepsia, nausea, vomiting, anorexia, bloating, belching, constipation, cholecystitis, dry mouth, thirst, bad taste
INTEG: Rash, pruritus, urticaria, brittle fingernails

🗗 Herb/drug 🚫 Do Not Crush ◆ Alert ⛐ Key Drug ᴳ Geriatric ᴾ Pediatric

MISC: Epistaxis, flulike symptoms, laryngitis, nasal congestion, *leukopenia,* malaise, weight changes

Contraindications: Hypersensitivity to this drug or xanthines, retinal/cerebral hemorrhage

Precautions: Pregnancy **C,** angina pectoris, cardiac disease, lactation, children, impaired renal function, recent surgery, peptic ulcer

Pharmacokinetics
Absorption	Well absorbed
Distribution	Unknown
Metabolism	Liver, degradation
Excretion	Kidneys
Half-life	½-1 hr

Pharmacodynamics
Onset	Unknown
Peak	1 hr
Duration	Unknown

Interactions
Individual drugs
Plicamycin: ↑ risk of bleeding
Theophylline: ↑ theophylline level
Valproic acid: ↑ risk of bleeding
Drug classifications
Antihypertensives: ↑ hypotension
Nitrates: ↑ hypotension
NSAIDs: ↑ risk of bleeding
Salicylates: ↑ risk of bleeding
Thrombolytics: ↑ risk of bleeding

NURSING CONSIDERATIONS
Assessment
• Monitor B/P, respirations in patient taking antihypertensives
• Assess for intermittent claudication during treatment

Nursing diagnoses
☑ Pain (uses)
☑ Activity intolerance (uses)
☑ Knowledge deficit (teaching)
☑ Noncompliance (teaching)

Implementation
• Give with meals to prevent GI upset
🚫• Tab should not be crushed or chewed

Patient/family education
• Teach patient that therapeutic response may take 2-4 wk
• Advise patient that decreased fats, cholesterol, increased exercise, decreased smoking are necessary to correct condition
• Instruct patient to observe feet for arterial insufficiency
• Instruct patient to use cotton socks, well-fitted shoes; not to go barefoot
• Advise patient to watch for bleeding, bruises, petechiae, epistaxis

Evaluation
Positive therapeutic outcome
• Decreased pain, cramping
• Increased ambulation

---

perindopril
See Appendix A, Selected New Drugs

---

perphenazine (℞)
(per-fen′a-zeen)
Apo-Perphenazine ✦, Trilafon, perphenazine, Phenazine ✦, PMS Perphenazine ✦
Func. class.: Antipsychotic/neuroleptic
Chem. class.: Phenothiazine piperidine
Pregnancy category   C

Action: Depresses cerebral cortex, hypothalamus, limbic system, which control activity,

---

aggression; blocks neurotransmission produced by dopamine at synapse; exhibits strong α-adrenergic, anticholinergic blocking action; as antiemetic inhibits medullary chemoreceptor trigger zone; mechanism for antipsychotic effects is unclear

⇒ **Therapeutic Outcome:** Decreased signs and symptoms of psychosis; decreased nausea and vomiting

Uses: Psychotic disorders, schizophrenia, nausea, vomiting

Dosage and routes
G *Elderly:* PO 2-4 mg qd-bid, increase by 2-4 mg/wk to desired dose

Nausea/vomiting/alcoholism
P *Adult and child >12 yr:* IM 5-10 mg prn, max 15 mg in ambulatory patients; 30 mg in hospitalized patients; PO 8-16 mg/day in divided doses, up to 24 mg; **IV** not to exceed 5 mg; give diluted or slow **IV** drip

Psychiatric use in hospitalized patients
Adults: PO 8-16 mg bid-qid, gradually increased to desired dose, not to exceed 64 mg/day; IM 5 mg q6h, not to exceed 30 mg/day

P *Child >12 yr:* PO 6-12 mg in divided doses

Nonhospitalized patients
Adult: PO 4-8 mg tid

Available forms: Tabs 2, 4, 8, 16 mg; oral sol 16 mg/5ml; inj 5 mg/ml; syrup 2 mg/5 ml ✦

Adverse effects
CNS: EPS: pseudoparkinsonism, **neuroleptic malignant syndrome,** *akathisia, dystonia,*

tardive dyskinesia, **seizures,** *headache*
CV: Orthostatic hypotension, **cardiac arrest,** ECG changes, **tachycardia**
EENT: Blurred vision, glaucoma
GI: Dry mouth, nausea, vomiting, anorexia, constipation, diarrhea, jaundice, weight gain
GU: Urinary retention, urinary frequency, enuresis, impotence, amenorrhea, gynecomastia
HEMA: Anemia, **leukopenia, leukocytosis, agranulocytosis**
INTEG: Rash, photosensitivity, dermatitis
RESP: **Laryngospasm,** dyspnea, **respiratory depression**

Contraindications: Hypersensitivity, blood dyscrasias, coma, **P** child <12 yr, brain damage, bone marrow depression

Precautions: Pregnancy **C**, lactation, seizure disorders, hypertension, hepatic disease, **G** cardiac disease, elderly

Pharmacokinetics	
Absorption	Variably absorbed (PO); well absorbed (IM)
Distribution	Widely distributed; high concentrations in CNS; crosses placenta
Metabolism	Liver, extensively; GI mucosa
Excretion	Kidneys

Pharmacodynamics			
	PO	IM	IV
Onset	Erratic	10 min	Rapid
Peak	2-4 hr	1-2 hr	Unknown
Duration	6-12 hr	6-12 hr	Unknown

Interactions
Individual drugs
Alcohol: ↑ effects of both drugs, oversedation

Aluminum hydroxide: ↓ absorption

Bromocriptine: ↓ antiparkinson activity

Disopyramide: ↑ anticholinergic effects

Epinephrine: ↑ toxicity

Guanethidine: ↓ antihypertensive response

Levodopa: ↓ antiparkinson activity

Lithium: ↓ perphenazine levels, ↑ EPS, masking of lithium toxicity

Magnesium hydroxide: ↓ absorption

Norepinephrine: ↓ vasoresponse, ↑ toxicity

Phenobarbital: ↓ effectiveness, ↑ metabolism

Drug classifications

Antacids: ↓ absorption

Anticholinergics: ↑ anticholinergic effects

Antidepressants: ↑ CNS depression

Antidiarrheals, adsorbent: ↓ absorption

Antihistamines: ↑ CNS depression

Antihypertensives: ↑ hypotension

Antithyroid agents: ↑ agranulocytosis

Barbiturate anesthetics: ↑ CNS depression

β-Adrenergics: ↑ effects of both drugs

General anesthetics: ↑ CNS depression

MAOIs: ↑ CNS depression

Opiates: ↑ CNS depression

Sedative/hypnotics: ↑ CNS depression

Herb/drug

Henbane: ↑ anticholinergic effect

Lab test interferences

↑ Liver function tests, ↑ cardiac enzymes, ↑ cholesterol, ↑ blood glucose, ↑ prolactin, ↑ bilirubin, ↑ PBI, ↑ cholinesterase, ↑ iodine, ↑ alkaline phosphatase, ↑ leukocytes, ↑ granulocytes, ↑ platelets

↓ Hormones (blood and urine)

False positive: Pregnancy tests, PKU

False negative: Urinary steroids, 17-OHCS

NURSING CONSIDERATIONS
Assessment

• Assess mental status: orientation, mood, behavior, presence and type of hallucinations before initial administration and monthly; this drug should significantly reduce psychotic behavior

• Check for swallowing of PO medication; check for hoarding or giving medication to other patients

• Monitor I&O ratio; palpate bladder if low urinary output occurs, especially in elderly; urinalysis recommended before, during prolonged therapy

• Monitor bilirubin, CBC, liver function studies monthly

• Assess affect, orientation, LOC, reflexes, gait, coordination, sleep pattern disturbances

• Monitor B/P with patient sitting, standing, and lying; take pulse and respirations q4h during initial treatment; establish baseline before starting treatment; report drops of 30 mm Hg; obtain baseline ECG, Q wave and T wave changes

• Check for dizziness, faintness, palpitations, tachycardia on rising; severe orthostatic hypotension is common

• Identify for neuroleptic malignant syndrome: hyperpyrexia, muscle rigidity, increased CPK, altered mental status; drug should be discontinued

• Assess for EPS including

---

akathisia (inability to sit still, no pattern to movements), tardive dyskinesia (bizarre movements of the jaw, mouth, tongue, extremities), pseudoparkinsonism (ragged tremors, pill rolling, shuffling gait); an antiparkinsonian drug should be prescribed

• Assess for constipation, urinary retention daily; if these occur, increase bulk, water in diet

Nursing diagnoses
☑ Thought processes, altered (uses)
☑ Coping, ineffective individual (uses)
☑ Knowledge deficit (teaching)
☑ Noncompliance (teaching)

Implementation
PO route
• Administer drug in liq form mixed in glass of juice or cola if hoarding is suspected; do not mix in caffeine drinks, tannics, pectins
• Administer decreased dose in **G** elderly, in whom metabolism is slowed
• Administer PO with full glass of water, milk; or give with food to decrease GI upset
• Store in airtight, light-resistant container; oral sol in amber bottle

IM route
• Inject in deep muscle mass; do not give SC; do not administer sol with a precipitate

IV IV route
• Give by direct **IV** after diluting with 0.9% NaCl to a conc of 0.5 mg/1 ml; administer at 1 mg/min; may be further diluted and given as an inf

Syringe compatibilities:
Atropine, benztropine, butorphanol, chlorpromazine, cimetidine, dimenhydrinate, diphenhydramine, droperidol, fentanyl, hydroxyzine, meperidine, methotrimeprazine, metoclopramide, morphine, pentazocine, prochlorperazine, promethazine, ranitidine, scopolamine

Syringe incompatibilities:
Midazolam, opium alkaloids, pentobarbital, thiethylperazine

Y-site compatibilities:
Acyclovir, amikacin, ampicillin, azlocillin, cefamandole, cefazolin, cefotaxime, cefoxitin, cefuroxime, cephalothin, cephapirin, chloramphenicol, clindamycin, co-trimoxazole, doxycycline, erythromycin, famotidine, gentamicin, kanamycin, metronidazole, mezlocillin, minocycline, moxalactam, nafcillin, oxacillin, penicillin G potassium, piperacillin, sulfamethoxazole, tacrolimus, ticarcillin, ticarcillin/clavulanate, tobramycin, trimethoprim, vancomycin

Additive compatibilities:
Ascorbic acid, ethacrynate, netilmicin

Additive incompatibilities:
Cefoperazone

Patient/family education
• Teach patient to use good oral hygiene; frequent rinsing of mouth, sugarless gum for dry mouth
• Advise patient to avoid hazardous activities until drug response is determined, dizziness, blurred vision may occur
• Inform patient that orthostatic hypotension occurs often and to rise from sitting or lying position gradually; to remain lying down after IM inj for at least 30 min; tell patient to avoid hot tubs, hot showers, tub baths, since hypotension

may occur; teach patient that in hot weather heat stroke may occur; take extra precautions to stay cool
• Teach patient to avoid abrupt withdrawal of this drug, or EPS may result; drug should be withdrawn slowly
• Teach patient to avoid OTC preparations (cough, hay fever, cold) unless approved by prescriber, since serious drug interactions may occur; avoid use with alcohol, CNS depressants; increased drowsiness may result
• Caution patient to use a sunscreen and sunglasses to prevent burns
• Teach patient about EPS and necessity of meticulous oral hygiene, since oral candidiasis may occur
• Instruct patient to take antacids 2 hr before or after taking this drug
• Teach patient to report sore throat, malaise, fever, bleeding, mouth sores; if these occur, CBC should be drawn and drug discontinued
• Teach patient that urine may turn pink or red

Evaluation
Positive therapeutic outcome
• Decrease in emotional excitement, hallucinations, delusions, paranoia
• Reorganization of patterns of thought, speech

Treatment of overdose:
Lavage if orally ingested; provide airway; *do not induce vomiting or use epinephrine*

phenazopyridine
(℞/OTC)
(fen-az-o-peer'i-deen)
AZO-Standard, Baridium, Eridium, Geridium, Phenazo ✤, Phenazodine, phenazopyridine HCl, Prodium, Pyridate, Pyridiate, Pyridium, Urodine, Urogesic, Viridium
Func. class.: Nonopioid analgesic
Chem. class.: Azodye
Pregnancy category B

Action: Exerts analgesic, anesthetic action on the urinary tract mucosa

Uses: Urinary tract irritation, infection (for symptoms only of pain, burning, itching) used with urinary antiinfectives

Dosage and routes
Adult: PO 200 mg tid × 2 days or less when used with antibacterial for UTI
Child 6-12 yr: PO 4 mg/kg tid × 2 days
Renal dose
Do not use in CrCl <50 ml/min

Available forms: Tabs 95, 100, 200 mg

Adverse effects
CNS: Headache
GI: Nausea, vomiting, diarrhea, heartburn, anorexia, **hepatic toxicity**
GU: **Renal toxicity,** *orange-red urine*
HEMA: **Thrombocytopenia, agranulocytosis, leukopenia, neutropenia, hemolytic anemia, methemoglobinemia**
INTEG: Rash, pruritus, skin pigmentation

Contraindications: Hypersensitivity, renal insufficiency

Precautions: Pregnancy **B**, P renal disease, lactation, children <12 yr

Pharmacokinetics

Absorption	Well absorbed
Distribution	Unknown; crosses placenta
Metabolism	Unknown
Excretion	Kidneys, unchanged
Half-life	Unknown

Pharmacodynamics

Onset	Unknown
Peak	5-6 hr
Duration	8 hr

Interactions: None
Lab test interferences
Interference: Urinalysis

NURSING CONSIDERATIONS
Assessment
• Assess urinary status: burning, pain, itching, urgency, frequency, hematuria before, during and after completion of drug therapy
• Monitor liver function studies: AST, ALT, bilirubin if patient is on long-term therapy
✦• Assess for hepatotoxicity: dark urine, clay-colored stools, yellowing of skin and sclera, itching, abdominal pain, fever, diarrhea if patient is on long-term therapy
• Assess for allergic reactions: rash, urticaria; if these occur, drug may have to be discontinued

Nursing diagnoses
☑ Pain (uses)
☑ Urinary elimination, altered patterns (uses)
☑ Knowledge deficit (teaching)

Implementation
• Give to patient crushed or

whole; chew tab may be chewed
• Give with food or milk to decrease gastric symptoms

Patient/family education
• Advise patient to report any symptoms of hepatotoxicity
• Caution patient not to exceed recommended dosage and to take with meals; to read label on other OTC drugs
• Teach patient not to discontinue after pain is relieved but continue to take concurrent prescribed antiinfective until finished
• Inform patient urine may turn red-orange, may stain clothing or contact lens

Evaluation
Positive therapeutic outcome
• Decrease in pain, burning, itching when urinating

Treatment of overdose:
Methylene blue 1-2 mg/kg **IV** or 100-200 mg vitamin C PO

---

phenelzine (℞)
(fen′el-zeen)
Nardil
Func. class.: Antidepressant, MAOI
Chem. class.: Hydrazine
Pregnancy category C

Action: Increases concentrations of endogenous epinephrine, norepinephrine, serotonin, dopamine in storage sites in CNS by inhibition of MAO; increased concentration reduces depression

➡**Therapeutic Outcome:** Decreased symptoms of depression after 2-3 wk

Uses: Depression, when uncontrolled by other means

Investigational uses: Bulimia, cocaine addiction, migraines, seasonal affective disorder, panic disorder

Dosage and routes
Adult: PO 45 mg/day in divided doses; may increase to 60 mg/day

G *Elderly:* PO 7.5 mg qd, increase by 7.5-15 mg q3-4 days

Available forms: Tab 15 mg

Adverse effects
CNS: Dizziness, drowsiness, confusion, headache, anxiety, tremors, stimulation, weakness, hyperreflexia, mania, insomnia, fatigue, weight gain
CV: Orthostatic hypotension, hypertension, **dysrhythmias, hypertensive crisis**
EENT: Blurred vision
ENDO: **SIADH-like syndrome**
GI: Constipation, dry mouth, nausea, vomiting, *anorexia,* diarrhea, weight gain
GU: Change in libido, frequency of urination
HEMA: Anemia
INTEG: Rash, flushing, increased perspiration

Contraindications: Hypersensitivity to MAOIs, elderly, hypertension, CHF, severe hepatic disease, pheochromocytoma, severe renal disease, severe cardiac disease

Precautions: Suicidal patients, convulsive disorders, severe depression, schizophrenia, hyperactivity, diabetes mellitus, pregnancy **C**

Pharmacokinetics

Absorption	Well absorbed
Distribution	Crosses placenta
Metabolism	Liver, extensively
Excretion	Kidneys, breast milk
Half-life	Unknown

Pharmacodynamics
Unknown

Interactions
Individual drugs
Alcohol: ↑ CNS depression
Clonidine: Severe hypotension; avoid use
Guanethidine: ↓ effects
L-**tryptophan:** ↑ confusion, shivering, hyperreflexia
Methylphenidate: Hypertensive crisis, convulsions, do not use together
Sumatriptan: ↑ toxicity
Drug classifications
Analgesics: ↑ CNS depression
Anticholinergics: ↑ side effects
Antidiabetics: ↑ hypoglycemia
Antihistamines: ↑ CNS depression
Antihypertensives: May block antihypertensive effect
Barbiturates: ↑ effects of barbiturates
Benzodiazepines: ↑ effects of benzodiazepines
CNS depressants: ↑ effects of CNS depressants
Diuretics, thiazide: ↑ hypotension
Oral contraceptives: ↑ effects, toxicity
Phenothiazines: ↑ toxicity
Rauwolfias: ↓ seratonin, norepinephrine
Sedative/hypnotics: ↑ CNS depression
SSRIs: ↑ Hyperpyrectic crisis, convulsions, hypertensive episode
Sulfonamides: ↑ toxicity
Sympathomimetics, indirect-acting or mixed: ↑ pressor effect
Food/drug
Caffeine: ↑ hypertension
Tyramine-containing foods: Hypertensive crisis

P

⬚ *Herb/drug*

Brewer's yeast: ↑ hypertension

Ephedra: ↑ sympathomimetic effect

Ginseng: ↑ tension headache, irritability, visual hallucinations

NURSING CONSIDERATIONS
Assessment

• Monitor B/P (with patient lying, standing), pulse q4h; if systolic B/P drops 20 mm Hg, hold drug, notify prescriber; take VS q4h in patients with cardiovascular disease

• Monitor hepatic studies: AST, ALT, bilirubin if patient is on long-term therapy

• Check weight weekly; appetite may increase with drug

• Assess ECG for flattening of T wave, bundle branch block, AV block, dysrhythmias in cardiac patients

• Assess mental status: mood, sensorium, affect, suicidal tendencies; increase in psychiatric symptoms: depression, panic

• Monitor urinary retention, constipation; constipation is **G** more likely to occur in elderly

• Assess for withdrawal symptoms: headache, nausea, vomiting, muscle pain, weakness; do not usually occur unless drug was discontinued abruptly

• Identify alcohol consumption; if alcohol is consumed, hold dose until AM

Nursing diagnoses

☑ Coping, ineffective individual (uses)

☑ Injury, risk for (adverse reactions)

☑ Knowledge deficit (teaching)

☑ Noncompliance (teaching)

Implementation

• Give with food or milk for GI symptoms; crush if patient is unable to swallow medication whole and mix with food or fluids

• Store at room temp; do not freeze

Patient/family education

• Teach patient that therapeutic effects may take 2-3 wk

• Advise patient to use caution in driving and other activities requiring alertness because of drowsiness, dizziness, blurred vision; to avoid rising quickly from sitting to standing, especially elderly **G**

• Caution patient to avoid alcohol ingestion, other CNS depressants; serious reaction can occur

• Advise patient not to discontinue medication quickly after long-term use: may cause nausea, headache, malaise, sweating, hallucinations

• Instruct patient to increase fluids, bulk in diet if constipation, urinary retention occur, **G** especially elderly; a stool softener may be ordered

• Teach patient to take gum, hard sugarless candy, or frequent sips of water for dry mouth

• Teach patient that therapeutic effects may take 1-4 wk

• Teach patient to avoid alcohol ingestion, CNS depressants, OTC medications: cold, weight loss, hay fever, cough syrup

• Teach patient not to discontinue medication quickly after long-term use

• Teach patient to avoid high-tyramine foods: cheese (aged), sour cream, beer, wine, pickled products, liver, raisins, bananas,

---

⬚ Herb/drug 🚫 Do Not Crush ◆ Alert ⚕ Key Drug **G** Geriatric **P** Pediatric

figs, avocados, meat tenderizers, chocolate, yogurt; increased caffeine
• Teach patient to report headache, palpitations, neck stiffness, dizziness, constriction in chest, throat

Evaluation
Positive therapeutic outcome
• Decrease in depression
• Absence of suicidal thoughts

Treatment of overdose: Lavage, activated charcoal, monitor electrolytes, VS, diazepam **IV**, sodium bicarbonate

---

phenobarbital ⚷ (℞)
(fee-noe-bar'bit-tal)
Ancalixir ✦, Barbita, Luminal, phenobarbital sodium, Solfoton
Func. class.: Anticonvulsant, sedative/hypnotic
Chem. class.: Barbiturate
Pregnancy category D
Controlled substance schedule IV

Action: Depresses activity in brain cells primarily in reticular activating system in brainstem; also selectively depresses neurons in posterior hypothalamus, limbic structures; able to decrease seizure activity by inhibition of impulses in CNS; decreases motor activity

Therapeutic Outcome: Sedation, anticonvulsant, improved energy

Uses: All forms of epilepsy, status epilepticus, febrile seizures in children, sedation, insomnia

Investigational uses: Hyperbilirubinemia, chronic cholestasis

Dosage and routes
Seizures
Adult: PO 60-200 mg/day in divided doses tid or total dose hs
Child: PO 4-6 mg/kg/day in divided doses q12h; may be given as single dose

Status epilepticus
Adult: **IV** inf 10 mg/kg; run no faster than 50 mg/min; may give up to 20 mg/kg
Child: **IV** inf 5-10 mg/kg; may repeat q10-15 min up to 20 mg/kg; run no faster than 50 mg/min

Insomnia
Adult: PO/IM 100-320 mg
Child: PO/IM 3-5 mg/kg

Sedation
Adult: PO 30-120 mg/day in 2-3 divided doses
Child: PO 3-5 mg/kg/day in 3 divided doses

Preoperative sedation
Adult: IM 100-200 mg 1-1½ hr before surgery
Child: IM 16-100 mg or PO/IM/**IV** 1-3 mg/kg 1-1½ hr before surgery

Available forms: Cap 16 mg; elix 15 ✦, 20 mg/5 ml; tabs 8, 15, 30, 60, 100 mg; inj 30, 60, 130 mg/ml

Adverse effects
CNS: Paradoxic excitement (elderly), drowsiness, lethargy, *hangover headache*, flushing, hallucinations, **coma**
GI: Nausea, vomiting, diarrhea, constipation
INTEG: Rash, urticaria, **Stevens-Johnson syndrome, angioedema,** local pain, swelling, necrosis, **thrombophlebitis**

Contraindications: Hypersensitivity to barbitures, porphyria, hepatic disease, respiratory disease, nephritis, hyperthyroidism, diabetes **G** mellitus, elderly, lactation, pregnancy **D**

Precautions: Anemia

N Do Not Confuse:
phenobarbital/pentobarbital

Pharmacokinetics

Absorption	Slow (70%-90%) (PO/IM/**IV**)
Distribution	Not known; crosses placenta
Metabolism	Liver (75%)
Excretion	Kidneys (25% unchanged)
Half-life	2-6 days

Pharmacodynamics

	PO	IM	IV
Onset	30-60 min	10-30 min	5 min
Peak	Unknown	Unknown	30 min
Duration	6-8 hr	4-6 hr	4-6 hr

Interactions
Individual drugs
Alcohol: ↑ CNS depression
Chloramphenicol: ↓ effectiveness
Cyclophosphamide: ↑ hematologic toxicity
Cyclosporine: ↓ effectiveness
Dacarbazine: ↓ effectiveness
Quinidine: ↓ effectiveness
Valproic acid: ↑ sedation
Drug classifications
Anticoagulants: ↓ effectiveness
Antidepressants: ↑ CNS depression
Antihistamines: ↑ CNS depression
Glucocorticoids: ↓ effectiveness
MAOIs: ↑ CNS depression
Opiates: ↑ CNS depression

Oral contraceptives: ↓ effectiveness
Sedative/hypnotics: ↑ CNS depression
Tricyclic antidepressants: ↓ effectiveness
☑ Herb/drug
Quinine: ↑ phenobarbital level

NURSING CONSIDERATIONS
Assessment
• Assess mental status: mood, sensorium, affect, memory **G** (long, short), especially elderly; if using as a hypnotic, assess sleep patterns during therapy; drug suppresses REM sleep with dreaming
• Withdrawal insomnia may occur after short-term use; do not start using drug again; insomnia improves in 1-3 nights; may experience increased dreaming
• Assess respiratory dysfunction: respiratory depression, character, rate, rhythm when using **IV**; hold drug if respirations are <10/min or if pupils are dilated; also check VS q30 min after parenteral route for 2 hr
• Assess for barbiturate toxicity: hypotension, pulmonary constriction, cold, clammy skin, cyanosis of lips, CNS depression, nausea, vomiting, hallucinations, delirium, weakness, coma, pupillary constriction; mild symptoms occur in 8-12 hr without drug
• Assess for pain in postoperative patients; pain threshold is lowered when patients are taking this medication
• Assess for blood dyscrasias: fever, sore throat, bruising, rash, jaundice, epistaxis (long-term treatment only)
• Assess seizure activity including type, location, duration,

and character; provide seizure precaution

Nursing diagnoses

☑ Sleep pattern disturbance (uses)

☑ Injury, risk for (adverse reactions)

☑ Knowledge deficit (teaching)

Implementation

• Give medication after removal of cigarettes to prevent fires

• Give medication after trying conservative measures for insomnia

PO route

• Tab may be crushed and mixed with food if swallowing is difficult; also may be mixed with other fluids 30-60 min before hs for expected sleeplessness; on empty stomach for best absorption

IM route

• Give in deep muscle mass (gluteal) to minimize irritation to tissues

• Split inj of >5 ml into two, since irritation to tissues may occur

IV Direct IV route

• Use large vein to prevent extravasation; if extravasation occurs, use moist heat to the area and 5% procaine sol injected into area; give at 65 mg or less/min; titrate to patient response

Syringe compatibilities:
Heparin

Syringe incompatibilities:
Benzquinamide, ranitidine

Y-site compatibilities:
Enalaprilat, meropenem, propofol, sufentanil

Y-site incompatibilities:
Hydromorphone

Additive compatibilities:
Amikacin, aminophylline, calcium chloride, calcium gluceptate, cephapirin, colistimethate, dimenhydrinate, meropenem, polymyxin B, sodium bicarbonate, thiopental, verapamil

Additive incompatibilities:
Cephalothin, chlorpromazine, codeine, ephedrine, hydralazine, hydrocortisone sodium succinate, hydroxyzine, insulin, levorphanol, meperidine, methadone, morphine, norepinephrine, pentazocine, procaine, prochlorazine mesylate, promazine, promethazine, streptomycin, vancomycin

Solution compatibilities:
D_5W, $D_{10}W$, 0.45% NaCl, 0.9% NaCl, Ringer's, dextrose/saline combinations, dextrose/Ringer's, dextrose/LR combinations, sodium lactate

Patient/family education

• Teach patient that hangover is common

• Instruct patient that drug is indicated only for short-term treatment of insomnia and is probably ineffective after 2 wk

• Inform patient that physical dependency may result when used for extended time (45-90 days depending on dosage)

• Teach patient to avoid driving and other activities requiring alertness

• Caution patient to avoid alcohol ingestion and CNS depressants; serious CNS depression may result

• Instruct patient not to discontinue medication quickly after long-term use; may cause seizures; drug should be tapered over 1 wk; take exactly as prescribed

P

✦ Canada Only   Adverse effects: *italic* = common; **bold** = life-threatening

- Emphasize the need to tell all prescribers that a barbiturate is being taken
- Teach the patient to make position changes slowly; orthostatic hypotension may occur
- Teach patient that response may take from 4 days to 2 wk of therapy
- Instruct patient to notify prescriber immediately if bruising, bleeding occur, which may indicate blood dyscrasias

Evaluation
Positive therapeutic outcome
- Improved sleeping patterns
- Decreased seizure activity
- Sedative preoperatively

Treatment of overdose: Lavage, activated charcoal, warming blanket, VS, hemodialysis, alkalinize urine, give **IV** volume expanders, **IV** fluids

phenolphthalein (OTC)
(fee-nol-thay'leen)
Alophen, Correctol, Espotabs, Evac-U-Gen, Evac-U-Lax, Ex-Lax, Feen-A-Mint, Lax-Pills, Modane, Medilax, Phenolax, Prulet
Func. class.: Laxative, stimulant/irritant
Chem. class.: Diphenylmethane

Pregnancy category   C

Action: Directly acts on intestinal smooth muscle by increasing motor activity; thought to irritate colonic intramural plexus; increases fluid in small intestine; alters fluid and electrolytes; action requires presence of bile

➡ **Therapeutic Outcome:** Decreased constipation

Uses: Constipation, preparation for bowel surgery or examination

Dosage and routes
Adult: PO 30-270 mg hs
P *Child >6 yr:* 30-60 mg/day
P *Child 2-5 yr:* 15-20 mg/day

Available forms: Tabs 60, 90, 97.2, 130 mg; chew tabs 65, 90, 97.2 mg; chew gum 97.2 mg; wafers 64.8 mg; chew wafers 80 mg

Adverse effects
GI: Nausea, vomiting, anorexia, diarrhea, abdominal cramps, rectal burning
INTEG: Rash, urticaria, **Stevens-Johnson syndrome**
META: Hypokalemia, electrolyte and fluid imbalances

Contraindications: Hypersensitivity, GI obstructions, abdominal pain, nausea/vomiting, fecal impaction, rectal fissures, hemorrhoids (ulcerated)

Precautions: Pregnancy **C**, lactation

Pharmacokinetics	
Absorption	Minimally absorbed (15%)
Distribution	Unknown
Metabolism	Not metabolized
Excretion	Kidneys, feces
Half-life	Unknown

Pharmacodynamics	
Onset	6-8 hr
Peak	Unknown
Duration	3-4 days

Interactions
Drug classifications
Oral drugs (any): ↓ absorption
Lab test interferences
Interference: BSP test

NURSING CONSIDERATIONS
Assessment
• Monitor blood, urine electrolytes if used often by patient; check I&O ratio to identify fluid loss
• Assess for cramping, rec bleeding, nausea, vomiting; if these symptoms occur, drug should be discontinued; identify cause of constipation; identify whether fluids, bulk, or exercise is missing from lifestyle
• Assess stool for color, consistency, amount, presence of flatulence

Nursing diagnoses
☑ Constipation (uses)
☑ Diarrhea (adverse reaction)
☑ Knowledge deficit (teaching)
☑ Noncompliance (teaching)

Implementation
• Chew well before swallowing; follow with 4 oz of water to prevent undissolved tab entering small intestine
• Give with 8 oz water (tab); administer on empty stomach for more rapid results; do not give at hs

Patient/family education
• Discuss with the patient that adequate fluid consumption is necessary
• Teach patient that normal bowel movements do not always occur daily
• Caution patient not to use in presence of abdominal pain, nausea, vomiting; tell patient to notify prescriber if constipation is unrelieved or if symptoms of electrolyte imbalance occur (muscle cramps, pain, weakness, dizziness, excessive thirst)
• Teach patient not to use laxatives for long-term therapy; bowel tone will be lost
• Shake susp well as needed
• Teach patient not to take at hs as a laxative; may interfere with sleep; also can cause problems with lipid pneumonia
• Teach patient not to use with food or vitamin preparations; delays digestion and absorption of fat-soluble vitamins

Evaluation
Positive therapeutic outcome
• Decreased constipation in 8-10 hr

---

phentolamine (℞)
(fen-tole´a-meen)
Regitine, Rogitine ✦
Func. class.: Antihypertensive
Chem. class.: α-Adrenergic blocker
Pregnancy category   C

Action: α-Adrenergic blocker, binds to α-adrenergic receptors, dilating peripheral blood vessels, lowering peripheral resistances, lowering blood pressure

Therapeutic Outcome: Decreased B/P, reversal of vasoconstriction (dermal necrosis)

Uses: Hypertension, pheochromocytoma, prevention, treatment of dermal necrosis following extravasation of norepinephrine or dopamine, impotence

Dosage and routes
Treatment of hypertensive episodes in pheochromocytoma
Adult: **IV**/IM 5 mg; repeat if necessary

P *Child:* **IV**/IM 1 mg; repeat if necessary

Diagnosis of pheochromocytoma
Adult: **IV** 2.5 mg; if negative, repeat with 5 mg **IV**

P *Child:* **IV** 0.5 mg; if negative, repeat with 1 mg **IV**

Prevention of dermal necrosis
Adult: **IV** 10 mg/100 ml of **IV** fluids with norepinephrine

P *Child:* 0.1-0.2 mg/kg, max 10 mg

Impotence (adjunct)
Adult: Intracavernosal 0.5-1 mg with 30 mg papaverine given 1, 2, or 3 treatments/wk

Available forms: Inj 5 mg/ml

Adverse effects
CNS: Dizziness, flushing, weakness, **cerebrovascular spasm**
CV: Hypotension, **tachycardia,** *angina,* **dysrhythmias, MI**
EENT: Nasal congestion
GI: Dry mouth, nausea, vomiting, diarrhea, abdominal pain

Contraindications: Hypersensitivity, MI, coronary insufficiency, angina

Precautions: Pregnancy C, lactation

Pharmacokinetics	
Absorption	Well absorbed (IM); completely absorbed (**IV**)
Distribution	Unknown
Metabolism	Unknown
Excretion	Kidneys, unchanged (10%)
Half-life	Unknown

Pharmacodynamics			
	IM	IV	INTRA-CAVER-NOSAL
Onset	Unknown	Rapid	Unknown
Peak	20 min	2 min	5-10 min
Duration	½-1 hr	½ hr	4 hr

Interactions
Individual drugs
Dopamine: ↓ peripheral vasoconstriction
Ephedrine: ↓ pressor effect
Epinephrine: ↑ effects of epinephrine, hypotension
Guanadrel: ↑ hypotension, bradycardia
Guanethidine: ↑ hypotension, bradycardia
Metaraminol: ↓ pressor effect
Methoxamine: ↑ effects of methoxamine, hypotension
Phenylephrine: ↓ pressor effect
Drug classifications
α-**Adrenergics:** Antagonistic effect
Antihypertensives: ↑ effects of antihypertensives

NURSING CONSIDERATIONS
Assessment
• Monitor B/P, orthostatic hypotension, syncope, pulse and ECG until stable
Nursing diagnoses
✓ Cardiac output, decreased (uses)
✓ Injury, potential for (adverse reactions)
✓ Knowledge deficit (teaching)
✓ Noncompliance (teaching)
Implementation
• Give with vasopressor nearby
IV **IV route**
• Give by direct **IV** after diluting 5 mg/1 ml sterile water for

---

inj or 0.9% NaCl; give 5 mg or less/min
• Give by cont inf by further diluting 5-10 mg/500 ml D_5W, titrate to patient response

Syringe compatibilities:
Papaverine

Y-site compatibilities:
Amiodarone

Additive compatibilities:
Dobutamine, verapamil
Prevention of dermal necrosis
• Add 10 mg/L to norepinephrine in **IV** sol

Patient/family education
• Caution patient not to discontinue drug abruptly
• Teach patient not to use OTC products (cough, cold, allergy) unless directed by prescriber
• Teach patient the importance of complying with dosage schedule, even if feeling better
• Emphasize the need to rise slowly to sitting or standing position to minimize orthostatic hypotension
• Teach patient to notify prescriber of mouth sores, sore throat, fever, swelling of hands or feet, irregular heartbeat, chest pain
• Caution patient to report excessive perspiration, dehydration, vomiting, diarrhea; may lead to fall in B/P
• Caution patient that drug may cause dizziness, fainting, lightheadedness; may occur during 1st few days of therapy
• Teach patient how to take B/P, and normal readings for age group

Evaluation
Positive therapeutic outcome
• Decreased B/P in hypertension

• Resolution of impotence
• Prevention of dermal necrosis

Treatment of overdose:
Administer norepinephrine; discontinue drug

phenylephrine (℞)
(fen-ill-ef′rin)
Neo-Synephrine
Func. class.: Adrenergic, direct acting
Chem. class.: Direct sympathomimetic amine (α-agonist)
Pregnancy category **C**

Action: Powerful and selective receptor agonist causing contraction of blood vessels, vasoconstriction of eye arterioles; decreases eye engorgement by stimulation of α-adrenergic receptors

Therapeutic Outcome: Increased B/P, decreased nasal-congestion, decreased eye irritation

Uses: Hypotension, paroxysmal supraventricular tachycardia, shock, B/P maintenance during spinal anesthesia, top ocular vasoconstrictor in uveitis, open-angle glaucoma, preoperatively, diagnostic procedures, refraction without cycloplegia, nasal congestion

Dosage and routes
Hypotension
Adult: SC/IM 2-5 mg; may repeat q10-15 min if needed, do not exceed initial dose; **IV** 0.1-0.5 mg; may repeat q10-15 min if needed, do not exceed initial dose
P *Child:* IM/SC 0.1 mg/kg/dose q1-2 h PRN

P

PVCs
Adult: **IV** bol 0.5 mg given rapidly, not to exceed prior dose by >0.1 mg; total dose >1 mg

Shock
Adult: **IV** inf 10 mg/500 ml D$_5$W given 100-180 µg/min (if 20 gtt/ml device is used), then maint of 40-60 µg/min (if 20 gtt/ml device is used)

P *Child:* **IV** bol 5-20 µg/kg/dose q10-15 min; **IV** inf 0.1-0.5 mg/kg/min

Available forms: inj 1% (10 mg/ml)

Adverse effects
CNS: Headache, dizziness, weakness, anxiety, tremor, insomnia
CV: Reflex bradycardia, **dysrhythmias,** *hypertension,* **tachycardia,** CV collapse, palpitations, ectopic beats, angina
EENT: Stinging, lacrimation, blurred vision, conjunctival allergy
GI: Nausea, vomiting
INTEG: Necrosis, tissue sloughing with extravasation, **gangrene**
MISC: Anaphylaxis

Contraindications: Hypersensitivity, narrow-angle glaucoma, ventricular fibrillation, tachydysrhythmias, pheochromocytoma

Precautions: Severe hypertension, diabetes, hyperthyroidism, elderly, severe arteriosclerosis, cardiac disease, infants, pregnancy **C,** lactation, arterial embolism, peripheral vascular disease, bradycardia, myocardial disease

Pharmacokinetics	
Absorption	Well absorbed (IM); completely absorbed (**IV**); minimally absorbed (nasal, ophth)
Distribution	Unknown
Metabolism	Liver
Excretion	Unknown
Half-life	Unknown

Pharmacodynamics		
	IV	SC/IM
Onset	Rapid	15 min
Peak	Unknown	Unknown
Duration	20-30 min	45-60 min

Interactions
Individual drugs
Bretylium: ↑ dysrhythmias
Guanethidine: ↑ pressor effect
Mecamylamine: ↑ hypotension
Methyldopa: ↑ hypotension
Reserpine: ↑ hypotension
Drug classifications
Antidepressants, tricyclic: ↑ pressor effect
β-Adrenergic blockers: ↑ pressor effect
General anesthetics: ↑ dysrhythmias
H$_1$ antihistamines: ↑ pressor effect
MAOIs: ↑ pressor effect
Oxytocics: ↑ B/P

NURSING CONSIDERATIONS
Assessment
• Monitor I&O ratio, notify prescriber if output <30 ml/hr
• Monitor ECG during administration continuously; if B/P increases, drug is decreased
• Monitor B/P and pulse q5 min after parenteral route; CVP or PWP during inf if possible
• Assess for paresthesias and coldness of extremities; peripheral blood flow may decrease

Nursing diagnoses
☑ Tissue perfusion, altered (uses)
☑ Cardiac output, decreased (uses)
☑ Knowledge deficit (teaching)

Implementation

IV **IV route**
- Give plasma expanders for hypovolemia
- Give **IV** after diluting 1 mg/9 ml sterile water for inj; give dose over 30-60 sec; may be diluted 10 mg/500 ml of D_5W or NS; titrate to patient response; low normal B/P; check for extravasation; check site for infiltration; use inf pump
- Store reconstituted sol in refrigerator for no longer than 24 hr
- Do not use discolored sol

Y-*site compatibilities:*
Amrinone, famotidine, haloperidol, zidovudine

Additive compatibilities:
Chloramphenicol, dobutamine, lidocaine, potassium chloride, sodium bicarbonate

Patient/family education
- Inform patient of reason for drug administration and expected result
- Advise patient to report pain at inf site immediately
- Instruct patient to report change in vision, blurring, loss of sight; breathing trouble, sweating, flushing

Evaluation
Positive therapeutic outcome
- Increased B/P with stabilization

---

phenytoin ⚷ (℞)
(fen′i-toyn)
Diphenylhydantoin, Dilantin, Dilantin Capsules, Diphenylan, Phenytoin Oral Suspension
Func. class.: Anticonvulsant/antidysrhythmic (**IB**)
Chem. class.: Hydantoin
Pregnancy category   D

Action: Inhibits spread of seizure activity in motor cortex by altering ion transport; increases AV conduction to decrease dysrhythmias

→Therapeutic Outcome: Decreased seizures, absence of dysrhythmias

Uses: Generalized tonic-clonic seizures, status epilepticus, non-epileptic seizures associated with Reye's syndrome or after head trauma, migraines, trigeminal neuralgia, Bell's palsy, ventricular dysrhythmias uncontrolled by antidysrhythmics

Dosage and routes
Seizures
Adult: PO 1 g or 20 mg/kg (ext rel) in 3-4 divided doses given q2h or 400 mg, then 300 mg q2h × 2 doses, maintenance 300-400 mg/day; max 600 mg/day; **IV** 15-20 mg/kg, max 25-50 mg/min then 100 mg q6-8h

P **Child:** PO 5 mg/kg/day in 2-3 divided doses, maintenance 4-8 mg/kg/day in 2-3 divided doses, max 300 mg/day; **IV** 15-20 mg/kg at 1-3 mg/kg/min

P

Status epilepticus
Adult: **IV** 15-20 mg/kg, max 25-50 mg/min; may give 100 mg q6-8h thereafter
P *Child:* **IV** 15-20 mg/kg given 1-3 mg/kg/min

Neuritic pain
Adult: PO 200-400 mg/day in divided doses

Ventricular dysrhythmias
Adult: PO loading dose 1 g divided over 24 hr, then 500 mg/day × 2 days; **IV** 250 mg given over 5 min until dysrhythmias subside or 1 g is given, or 100 mg q15 min until dysrhythmias subside or 1 g is given

P *Child:* PO 3-8 mg/kg or 250 mg/m^2/day as single dose or divided in 2 doses; **IV** 3-8 mg/kg given over several min, or 250 mg/m^2/day as single dose or divided in 2 doses

Renal dose
CrCl <10 ml/min do not use loading dose

Available forms: Susp 30, 125 mg/5 ml; chew tab 50 mg; inj 50 mg/ml; ext rel cap 100 mg; prompt caps 30 ♣, 100 mg

Adverse effects
CNS: Drowsiness, dizziness, insomnia, paresthesias, depression, suicidal tendencies, aggression, headache, confusion, slurred speech
CV: Hypotension, **ventricular fibrillation**
EENT: Nystagmus, diplopia, blurred vision
GI: Nausea, vomiting, constipation, anorexia, weight loss, **hepatitis,** jaundice, gingival hyperplasia
GU: **Nephritis,** urine discoloration

HEMA: **Agranulocytosis, leukopenia, aplastic anemia, thrombocytopenia, megaloblastic anemia**
INTEG: Rash, **lupus erythematosus, Stevens-Johnson syndrome,** hirsutism
SYST: Hypocalcemia

Contraindications: Hypersensitivity, psychiatric condition, pregnancy **D**, bradycardia, SA and AV block, Stokes-Adams syndrome, hepatic failure

Precautions: Allergies, hepatic **G** disease, renal disease, elderly, petit mal seizures

Pharmacokinetics	
Absorption	Slowly absorbed from GI tract; erratic (IM)
Distribution	Crosses placenta, highly protein bound
Metabolism	Liver, extensively
Excretion	Kidneys, minimally; enters breast milk
Half-life	22 hr

Pharmacodynamics				
	PO	PO-EXT REL	IM	IV
Onset	2-24 hr	2-24 hr	Erratic	1-2 hr
Peak	1.5-3 hr	4-12 hr	Erratic	Unknown
Duration	6-12 hr	12-36 hr	12-24 hr	12-24 hr

Interactions
Individual drugs
Alcohol: ↑ CNS depression
Carbamazepine: ↓ effectiveness
Chloramphenicol: ↑ blood level
Cimetidine: ↓ metabolism, ↑ action, blood level
Disulfiram: ↓ metabolism, ↑ action
Felbamate: ↑ blood level
Fluconazole: ↑ blood level
Isoniazid: ↓ metabolism, ↑ action

☑ Herb/drug ◐ Do Not Crush ◆ Alert ☊ Key Drug **G** Geriatric **P** Pediatric

Ketoconazole: ↓ metabolism, ↑ action
Metronidazole: ↑ blood level
Miconazole: ↑ blood level
Omeprazole: ↑ blood level
Phenylbutazone: ↑ blood level
Valproic acid: ↑ seizures
Warfarin: ↓ blood level of phenytoin

Drug classifications
Anticonvulsants: ↑ CNS depression
Antidepressants: ↑ CNS depression
Antihistamines: ↑ CNS depression
Barbiturates: ↑ CNS depression, ↓ effect of phenytoin
Benzodiazepines: ↑ blood levels
General anesthetics: ↑ CNS depression
Hypnotics: ↑ CNS depression
Opiates: ↑ CNS depression
Oral contraceptives: ↓ metabolism, ↑ action
Sedatives: ↑ CNS depression
Sulfonamides: ↑ blood levels

Herb/drug
Aloe: ↑ hypokalemia
Buckthorn: ↑ hypokalemia
Cascara sagrada: ↑ hypokalemia
Senna: ↑ hypokalemia

Lab test interferences
↓ Dexamethasone, ↓ metyrapone test serum, ↓ PBI, ↓ urinary steroids
↑ Glucose, ↑ alkaline phosphatase, ↑ BSP

NURSING CONSIDERATIONS
Assessment
• Assess drug level: toxic level 30-50 µg/ml; therapeutic level 7.5-20 µg/ml, wait ≥1 wk to draw level
• Assess mental status: mood, sensorium, affect, memory (long, short), especially elderly

• Assess for blood dyscrasias: fever, sore throat, bruising, rash, jaundice, epistaxis (long-term treatment only)
• Assess seizure activity including type, location, duration, and character; provide seizure precaution
• Assess renal studies: urinalysis, BUN, urine creatinine
• Monitor blood studies: RBC, Hct, Hgb, reticulocyte counts weekly for 4 wk then monthly; also check thyroid function tests, serum calcium
• Monitor hepatic studies: ALT, AST, bilirubin, creatinine
• Assess for signs of physical withdrawal if medication suddenly discontinued
• Assess eye problems: need for ophth examinations before, during, after treatment (slit lamp, fundoscopy, tonometry)
• Assess allergic reaction: red raised rash, increased temp, lymphadenopathy; if this occurs, drug should be discontinued
• Monitor for toxicity: bone marrow depression, nausea, vomiting, ataxia, diplopia, cardiovascular collapse, slurred speech, confusion

Nursing diagnoses
☑ Injury, risk for (uses, adverse reactions)
☑ Knowledge deficit (teaching)
☑ Noncompliance (teaching)

Implementation
PO route
• Give with meals to decrease GI upset
• Chew tab can be crushed or chewed; cap can be opened and mixed with foods or fluids; cap and tab are not interchangeable
• Give by G tube/NG tube: dilute susp prior to administra-

tion, flush tube with 20 ml H₂O after dose
• Shake oral susp well; use measuring device for correct dose

IV IV route
• Administer by direct **IV** after diluting with special diluent provided (1 ml/50 mg, 2.2 ml/100 mg, 5.2 ml/250 mg); shake; place vial in warm water to dissolve powder; give through Y-tube or 3-way stopcock; inject slowly <50 mg/min
• Give intermittent **IV** after diluting to a conc of 1-10 mg/ml
• Clear **IV** tubing first with 0.9% NaCl sol; use in-line filter; discard 4 hr after preparation; inject into large veins to prevent purple glove syndrome

Additive compatibilities:
Bleomycin, verapamil

Y-site compatibilities:
Esmolol, famotidine, fluconazole, foscarnet, tacrolimus

Y-site incompatibilities:
Enalaprilat, potassium chloride, vit B/C

Patient/family education
• Teach patient to carry ID card or Medic Alert bracelet stating name, drugs taken, condition, prescriber's name and phone number
• Advise patient to avoid driving and other activities that require alertness until drug response is known; dizziness, drowsiness can occur
• Advise patient to avoid alcohol ingestion and CNS depressants unless approved by prescriber; increased sedation may occur
• Teach patient not to discon-

tinue medication quickly after long-term use; taper off over several wk
• Advise patient that urine may turn pink, red, or brown, which is normal
• Caution patient to avoid antacids within 2-3 hr of taking phenytoin
• To prevent gingival hyperplasia, instruct patient in proper oral hygiene; a dentist should be seen routinely

Evaluation
Positive therapeutic outcome
• Decreased seizure activity
• Decreased dysrhythmias
• Relief of pain

---

phytonadione (℞)
(fye-toe-na-dye′one)
**AquaMEPHYTON,
Konakion, Mephyton,
vitamin K₁**
Func. class.: Vitamin K₁,
fat-soluble vitamin
Pregnancy category   C

Action: Needed for adequate blood clotting (factors II, VII, IX, X)

➲Therapeutic Outcome: Prevention of bleeding

Uses: Vitamin K malabsorption, hypoprothrombinemia, prevention of hypoprothrombinemia caused by oral anticoagulants, prevention of hemorrhagic disease of the newborn

Dosage and routes
*Hypoprothrombinemia
caused by vitamin K
malabsorption*
Adult: PO/IM 2.5-25 mg; may repeat or increase to 50 mg

P *Child:* PO/IM 5-10 mg

P *Infants:* PO/IM 2 mg

Prevention of hemorrhagic disease of the newborn

P *Neonate:* IM 0.5-1 mg within 1 hr after birth; repeat in 2-3 wks if required

Hypoprothrombinemia caused by oral anticoagulants

P *Adult and child:* PO/SC/IM 2.5-10 mg, may repeat 12-48 hr after PO dose or 6-8 hr after SC/IM dose, based on PT

Available forms: Tab 5 mg; inj 2 mg/ml; aqueous colloidal (IM, **IV**); inj aqueous dispersion 10 mg/ml (IM)

Adverse effects
CNS: Headache, **brain damage** (large doses)
GI: Nausea, decreased liver function tests
HEMA: **Hemolytic anemia, hemoglobinuria, hyperbilirubinemia**
INTEG: Rash, urticaria

Contraindications: Hypersensitivity, severe hepatic disease, last few wk of pregnancy

Precautions: Pregnancy **C**,
P neonates

Pharmacokinetics	
Absorption	Well absorbed (PO, IM, SC)
Distribution	Crosses placenta
Metabolism	Liver, rapidly
Excretion	Breast milk
Half-life	Unknown

Pharmacodynamics		
	PO	SC/IM
Onset	6-12 hr	1-2 hr
Peak	Unknown	6 hr
Duration	Unknown	14 hr

Interactions
Individual drugs
Cholestyramine: ↓ action of phytonadione
Mineral oil: ↓ action of phytonadione
Sucralfate: ↓ phytonadione absorption
Drug classifications
Antiinfectives: ↑ phytonadione need
Oral anticoagulants: ↓ action of phytonadione
Salicylates: ↑ phytonadione need

NURSING CONSIDERATIONS
Assessment
• Monitor pro-time during treatment (2-sec deviation from control time, bleeding time, and clotting time); monitor for bleeding, pulse, and BP
• Assess nutritional status: liver (beef), spinach, tomatoes, coffee, asparagus, broccoli, cabbage, lettuce, greens
• Assess for bleeding or bruising: hematuria, black tarry stools, hematemesis

Nursing diagnoses
☑ Nutrition, altered: less than body requirements (uses)
☑ Tissue perfusion, altered (uses)
☑ Knowledge deficit (teaching)

Implementation
IV **IV route**
• Give **IV** after diluting with D₅ NS 10 ml or more; give 1 mg/min or more
• Give **IV** only when other routes not possible (deaths have occurred)
• Store in tight, light-resistant container

Syringe compatibilities:
Doxapram

Y-site compatibilities:
Ampicillin, epinephrine, famotidine, heparin, hydrocorti-

P

sone, potassium chloride, tolazoline, vit B/C

Additive compatibilities:
Amikacin, calcium gluceptate, cephapirin, chloramphenicol, cimetidine, netilmicin, sodium bicarbonate

Patient/family education
• Teach patient not to take other supplements, unless directed by prescriber; to take this medication as directed
• Teach patient necessary foods to be included in diet high in vitamin K
• Advise patient to avoid IM inj, hard toothbrush, flossing; use electric razor until treatment is terminated
• Instruct patient to report symptoms of bleeding, bruising, nosebleeds, blood in urine, heavy menstruation, black tarry stools
• Caution patient not to use OTC medications unless approved by prescriber
• Stress the need for periodic lab tests to monitor coagulation levels
• Stress the need for patient to wear identification with condition, treatment, and medication taken

Evaluation
Positive therapeutic outcome
• Decreased bleeding tendencies
• Decreased pro-time
• Decreased clotting time

---

pindolol (℞)
(pin′doe-lole)
Novo-Pindol ✦, **Syn-Pindol** ✦, **Visken**
Func. class.: Antihypertensive
Chem. class.: Nonselective β-blocker

Pregnancy category **B**

Action: Competitively blocks stimulation of β-adrenergic receptor within vascular smooth muscle; produces chronotropic, inotropic activity (decreases rate of SA node discharge, increases recovery time), slows conduction of AV node, decreases heart rate, which decreases O_2 consumption in myocardium; also decreases renin-aldosterone-angiotensin system and at high doses inhibits $β_2$ receptors in bronchial system

➡ **Therapeutic Outcome:** Increased B/P in hypertension, heart rate

Uses: Mild to moderate hypertension

Investigational uses: Mitral valve prolapse, hypertrophic cardiomyopathy, angina pectoris, ventricular dysrhythmias, anxiety

Dosage and routes
Adult: PO 5 mg bid; usual dose 15 mg/day (5 mg tid); may increase by 10 mg/day q3-4 wk to a max of 60 mg/day

G *Elderly:* PO 5 mg qd increase by 5 mg q3-4 wk

Available forms: Tabs 5, 10 mg

Adverse effects
CNS: Insomnia, dizziness, hallucinations, anxiety, fatigue
CV: Hypotension, bradycardia, **CHF,** edema, chest pain, palpitations, claudication, tachycardia, **AV block**
EENT: Visual changes, sore throat, *double vision,* dry burning eyes
GI: Nausea, vomiting, **ischemic colitis,** diarrhea, *abdominal pain,* **mesenteric arterial thrombosis**
GU: Impotence, frequency
HEMA: **Agranulocytosis, thrombocytopenia, purpura**
INTEG: Rash, alopecia, pruritus, fever
MISC: Joint pain, muscle pain
RESP: **Bronchospasm,** *dyspnea,* cough, rales

Contraindications: Hypersensitivity to β-blockers, cardiogenic shock, 2nd-, 3rd-degree heart block, sinus bradycardia, CHF, cardiac failure, bronchial asthma

Precautions: Major surgery, pregnancy **B,** lactation, diabetes mellitus, renal disease, thyroid disease, COPD, well-compensated heart failure, CAD, nonallergic bronchospasm

◼ Do Not Confuse:
pindolol/Parlodel, pindolol/Plendil

Pharmacokinetics

Absorption	Well absorbed
Distribution	Crosses placenta; some penetration in CNS
Metabolism	Liver, moderately (60%-65%)
Excretion	Kidneys, unchanged (30%-45%)
Half-life	3-4 hr

Pharmacodynamics

Onset	Unknown
Peak	2-4 hr
Duration	8-24 hr

Interactions
Individual drugs
Alcohol: ↑ hypotension (large amounts)
Epinephrine: α-Adrenergic stimulation
Hydralazine: ↑ hypotension, bradycardia
Insulin: ↑ hypoglycemia
Methyldopa: ↑ hypotension, bradycardia
Prazosin: ↑ hypotension, bradycardia
Reserpine: ↑ hypotension, bradycardia
Thyroid: ↓ effect of β-blockers
Verapamil: ↑ cardiac depression
Drug classifications
Antihypertensives: ↑ hypertension
β₂-Agonist: ↓ bronchodilatation
Cardiac glycosides: ↑ bradycardia
Nitrates: ↑ hypotension
NSAIDs: ↓ antihypertensive effect
Oral hypoglycemics: ↑ hypoglycemia
Theophyllines: ↓ bronchodilatation
Lab test interferences
False: ↑ Urinary catecholamines

NURSING CONSIDERATIONS
Assessment
• Monitor B/P during beginning treatment, periodically thereafter; pulse q4h; note rate, rhythm, quality: apical/radial pulse before administration; notify prescriber of any significant changes (pulse <50 bpm)

P

• Check for baselines in renal, liver function tests before therapy begins
• Assess for edema in feet, legs daily; monitor I&O, daily weight; check for jugular vein distention, rales bilaterally, dyspnea (CHF)
• Monitor skin turgor, dryness of mucous membranes for hydration status, especially **G** elderly

Nursing diagnoses
☑ Cardiac output, decreased (uses)
☑ Injury, potential for (adverse reactions)
☑ Knowledge deficit (teaching)
☑ Noncompliance (teaching)

Implementation
• Given ac, hs, tab may be crushed or swallowed whole; give with food to prevent GI upset; reduced dosage in renal impairment
• Store protected from light, moisture; place in cool environment

Patient/family education
• Teach patient not to discontinue drug abruptly; taper over 2 wk; may cause precipitate angina if stopped abruptly
• Teach patient not to use OTC products containing α-adrenergic stimulants (such as nasal decongestants, cold preparations); to avoid alcohol, smoking, and to limit sodium intake as prescribed
• Teach patient how to take pulse and B/P at home; advise when to notify prescriber
• Instruct patient to comply with weight control, dietary adjustments, modified exercise program
• Tell patient to carry/wear Medic Alert ID to identify drug being taken, allergies; tell patient drug controls symptoms but does not cure
• Caution patient to avoid hazardous activities if dizziness, drowsiness present
• Teach patient to report symptoms of CHF: difficult breathing, especially on exertion or when lying down, night cough, swelling of extremities or bradycardia, dizziness, confusion, depression, fever
• Teach patient to take drug as prescribed, not to double doses, skip doses; take any missed doses as soon as remembered if at least 4 hr until next dose

Evaluation
Positive therapeutic outcome
• Decreased B/P in hypertension (after 1-2 wk)

Treatment of overdose:
Lavage, **IV** atropine for bradycardia, **IV** theophylline for bronchospasm, digitalis, O_2, diuretic for cardiac failure, hemodialysis, **IV** glucose for hyperglycemia, **IV** diazepam (or phenytoin) for seizures

---

pioglitazone
See Appendix A,
Selected New Drugs

---

pipecuronium (℞)
(pip-e-kyoor′oh′nee-um)
Arduran
Func. class.: Neuromuscular blocker (nondepolarizing)
Chem. class.: Synthetic curariform

Pregnancy category   C

Action: Inhibits transmission of nerve impulses by binding with cholinergic receptor sites,

---

☑ Herb/drug   🚫 Do Not Crush   ◆ Alert   ✦☞ Key Drug   **G** Geriatric   **P** Pediatric antagonizing action of acetylcholine; no analgesic response

→ **Therapeutic Outcome:** Paralysis of all skeletal muscles

Uses: Facilitation of endotracheal intubation, skeletal muscle relaxation during mechanical ventilation, surgery, or general anesthesia

Dosage and routes
Adult: **IV** dosage is individualized; in patients with normal renal function who are not obese, initial dose is 70-85 µg/kg; maintenance dose ranges from 10-15 µg/kg

P *Child 1-14 yr:* **IV** 57 µg/kg

P *Child 3 mo-1 yr:* **IV** 40 µg/kg

Available forms: Inj 10-mg vials

Adverse effects
CNS: Hypesthesia, CNS depression
CV: Bradycardia, tachycardia, increased or decreased B/P, ventricular extrasystole, **myocardial ischemia, cardiovascular accident, thrombosis, atrial fibrillation**
EENT: Increased secretions
GU: Anuria
INTEG: Rash, urticaria
META: Hypoglycemia, hyperkalemia, increased creatinine
MS: Weakness to prolonged skeletal muscle relaxation
RESP: **Prolonged apnea, bronchospasm, cyanosis, respiratory depression**

Contraindications: Hypersensitivity to bromide ion

Precautions: Pregnancy **C**, renal disease, cardiac disease, **P** lactation, children <3 mo, fluid and electrolyte imbalances, neuromuscular diseases, respiratory disease, obesity

Pharmacokinetics

Absorption	Complete bioavailability
Distribution	Unknown
Metabolism	Unknown
Excretion	Kidneys, unchanged (>75%)
Half-life	1½ hr; increased in renal disease

Pharmacodynamics

Onset	30-45 sec
Peak	3-5 min
Duration	1-2 hr

Interactions
Individual drugs
Clindamycin: ↑ paralysis length and intensity
Colistin: ↑ paralysis length and intensity
Lidocaine: ↑ paralysis length and intensity
Lithium: ↑ paralysis length and intensity
Magnesium: ↑ paralysis length and intensity
Polymyxin B: ↑ paralysis length and intensity
Procainamide: ↑ paralysis length and intensity
Quinidine: ↑ paralysis length and intensity
Succinylcholine: ↑ paralysis length and intensity
Drug classifications
Aminoglycosides: ↑ paralysis length and intensity
β-Adrenergic blockers: ↑ paralysis length and intensity
Diuretics, potassium-losing: ↑ paralysis length and intensity
General anesthesia: ↑ paralysis length and intensity

NURSING CONSIDERATIONS
Assessment
• Monitor vital signs (B/P, pulse, respirations, airway) until fully recovered; rate, depth, pattern of respirations, strength of hand grip; pa-

P

tient should be intubated before use

• Monitor for electrolyte imbalances (potassium, magnesium) before drug is used; electrolyte imbalances may lead to increased action of this drug

• Monitor for recovery: decreased paralysis of face, diaphragm, leg, arm, rest of body; residual weakness and respiratory problems may occur during recovery period

• Assess for hypersensitive reactions: rash, fever, respiratory distress, pruritus; drug should be discontinued

Nursing diagnoses

☑ Breathing pattern, ineffective (uses)

☑ Communication, impaired verbal (adverse reactions)

☑ Fear (adverse reactions)

☑ Knowledge deficit (teaching)

Implementation

• Use peripheral nerve stimulator (anesthesiologist) to determine neuromuscular blockade; deep tendon reflexes should be monitored during extended periods

• Give **IV** after reconstituting with 0.9% NaCl, D₅W, D₅/ 0.9% NaCl, LR, sterile water for inj; sol with benzyl alcohol should not be used for

P newborns; should be administered only by qualified person, usually an anesthesiologist; do not administer IM

• Store in light-resistant area (powder); refrigerate unused portions (sterile water); use within 24 hr

Patient/family education

• Provide reassurance if communication is difficult during recovery from neuromuscular blockade

• Provide explanation to patients regarding all procedures or treatments; patient will remain conscious if anesthesia is not given also

Evaluation

Positive therapeutic outcome

• Paralysis of jaw, eyelid, head, neck, rest of body as evaluated by peripheral nerve stimulator

Treatment of overdose:

Edrophonium or neostigmine, atropine, monitor VS; may require mechanical ventilation

---

piperacillin (℞)

(pi-per'a-sill-in)

Pipracil

Func. class.: Broad-spectrum antiinfective

Chem. class.: Extended-spectrum penicillin

Pregnancy category **B**

Action: Interferes with cell wall replication of susceptible organisms; osmotically unstable cell wall swells and bursts from osmotic pressure

➡**Therapeutic Outcome:** Bactericidal effects for gram-positive cocci *Staphylococcus aureus, Streptococcus pyogenes, S. viridans, S. faecalis, S. bovis, S. pneumoniae;* gram-negative cocci *Neisseria gonorrhoeae, N. meningitidis;* gram-positive bacilli *Clostridium perfringens, C. tetani;* gram-negative bacilli *Bacteroides, Fusobacterium nucleatum, Escherichia coli, Klebsiella, Proteus mirabilis, P. vulgaris, P. rettgeri, Morganella morganii, Enterobacter, Citrobacter, Pseudomonas aeruginosa, Serratia, Acinetobacter, Peptococcus, Peptostreptococcus, Eubacterium*

☑ Herb/drug ◎ Do Not Crush ◆ Alert ⚷ Key Drug ᴳ Geriatric ᴾ Pediatric

Uses: Respiratory tract, skin, skin structure, urinary tract, bone, and joint infections; gonorrhea, pneumonia, endocarditis, septicemia, meningitis, sinusitis; infections caused by penicillinase-producing staphylococci, streptococci; may be combined with an aminoglycoside for *Pseudomonas* infection

Dosage and routes
Urinary tract infections
Adult: IV 8-16 g/day (125-200 mg/kg/day) in divided doses q6-8h

Serious systemic infections
P Adult and child >12 yr:
IM/IV 100-300 mg/kg/day in divided doses q4-6h

P Child <12 yr: IM/IV 200-300 mg/kg/day in divided doses q4-6h

P Neonates <36 wks: IV 75 mg/kg q12h in the 1st wk of life, then q8h in 2nd wk

P Full term infants: IV 75 mg/kg q8h in 1st wk of life, then q6h thereafter

Prophylaxis of surgical infections
Adult: IV 2 g 30-60 min before procedure; may be repeated during or after surgery

Renal dose
CrCl 20-40 ml/min give q8h; CrCl <20 ml/min give q12h

Available forms: Powder for inj 2, 3, 4, 40 g

Adverse effects
CNS: Lethargy, hallucinations, anxiety, depression, twitching, **coma, convulsions**
GI: Nausea, vomiting, diarrhea, increased AST, ALT, abdominal pain, glossitis, colitis

GU: **Oliguria, proteinuria, hematuria, vaginitis, moniliasis, glomerulonephritis**
HEMA: Anemia, increased bleeding time, **bone marrow depression, thrombocytopenia**
META: Hypokalemia, hypernatremia

Contraindications: Hypersensitivity to penicillins; neonates

Precautions: Pregnancy **B**, hypersensitivity to cephalosporins, CHF, renal disease

Pharmacokinetics

Absorption	Well absorbed (80%)
Distribution	Widely distributed; crosses placenta
Metabolism	Not metabolized
Excretion	Kidneys, unchanged (90%); bile (10%); breast milk
Half-life	0.7-1.3 hr

Pharmacodynamics

	IM	IV
Onset	Rapid	Rapid
Peak	30-50 min	Inf end

Interactions
Individual drugs
Aminoglycosides: ↓ half-life in renal disease
Amphotericin B: ↑ hypokalemia
Aspirin: ↑ piperacillin levels, ↓ renal excretion
Chloramphenicol: ↑ half-life of chloramphenicol, ↓ effectiveness of piperacillin
Cholestyramine: ↓ effectiveness of piperacillin
Colestipol: ↓ effectiveness of piperacillin
Erythromycin: ↓ antimicrobial effectiveness
Lithium: ↓ excretion, ↑ toxicity

Probenecid: ↑ piperacillin levels, ↓ renal excretion
Drug classifications
Diuretics: ↑ hypokalemia
Glucocorticoids: ↑ hypokalemia
Hepatotoxic agents: ↑ hepatotoxicity
Oral anticoagulants: ↑ anticoagulant effects
Oral contraceptives: ↓ contraceptive effectiveness
Tetracyclines: ↓ antimicrobial effectiveness
Food/drug
Food, carbonated drinks, citrus fruit juices: ↓ absorption
☑ *Herb/drug*
Khat: ↓ absorption
Lab test interferences
False positive: Urine glucose, urine protein

NURSING CONSIDERATIONS
Assessment
• Assess patient for previous sensitivity reaction to penicillins or other cephalosporins; cross-sensitivity between penicillins and cephalosporins is common
• Assess patient for signs and symptoms of infection including characteristics of wounds, sputum, urine, stool, WBC >10,000, fever; obtain baseline information and during treatment
• Obtain C&S before beginning drug therapy to identify if correct treatment has been initiated
• Assess for allergic reactions: rash, urticaria, pruritus, chills, fever, joint pain; angioedema may occur a few days after therapy begins; epinephrine, resuscitation equipment should be available for anaphylactic reaction

◆• Identify urine output; if decreasing, notify prescriber (may indicate nephrotoxicity); also check for increased BUN, creatinine
• Monitor blood studies: AST, ALT, CBC, Hct, bilirubin, LDH, alkaline phosphatase, Coombs' test monthly if patient is on long-term therapy
• Monitor electrolytes: potassium, sodium, chloride monthly if patient is on long-term therapy
• Assess bowel pattern daily; if severe diarrhea occurs, drug should be discontinued; may indicate pseudomembranous colitis
• Monitor for bleeding: ecchymosis, bleeding gums, hematuria, stool guaiac daily if on long-term therapy
• Assess for overgrowth of infection: perineal itching, fever, malaise, redness, pain, swelling, drainage, rash, diarrhea, change in cough, sputum

Nursing diagnoses
☑ Infection, risk for (uses)
☑ Diarrhea (adverse reactions)
☑ Injury, risk for (adverse reactions)
☑ Knowledge deficit (teaching)
☑ Noncompliance (teaching)

Implementation
IM route
• Reconstitute 2 g/4 ml, 3 g/6 ml, 4 g/7.8 ml with sterile water, 0.9% NaCl, bacteriostatic water, 0.5% or 1% lidocaine without epinephrine
• Inject deep in large muscle mass, massage; split inj over 2 g into 2 inj
Ⅳ IV route
• Reconstitute with 5 ml or more 0.9% NaCl, bacteriostatic water; shake sol to dissolve

---

☑ Herb/drug   🚫 Do Not Crush   ◆ Alert   ☛ Key Drug   🄶 Geriatric   🄿 Pediatric

- Change **IV** sites q48h to prevent phlebitis and pain
- Give direct **IV** over 3-5 min
- Give by intermittent inf by diluting in 50 ml or more D_5W, 0.9% NaCl, D_5/0.9% NaCl, LR, give over 20-30 min by Y-site; discontinue primary inf during intermittent inf

Syringe compatibilities:
Heparin

Y-site compatibilities:
Acyclovir, aldesleukin, allopurinol, amifostine, aztreonam, ciprofloxacin, cyclophosphamide, diltiazem, enalaprilat, esmolol, famotidine, fludarabine, foscarnet, heparin, hydromorphone, IL-2, labetalol, lorazepam, magnesium sulfate, melphalan, meperidine, midazolam, morphine, perphenazine, propofol, ranitidine, tacrolimus, teniposide, theophylline, thiotepa, verapamil, zidovudine

Y-site incompatibilities:
Ondansetron, fluconazole, sargramostim, vinorelbine

Additive compatibilities:
Ciprofloxacin, clindamycin, flucloxacillin, fluconazole, hydrocortisone sodium succinate, ofloxacin, potassium chloride, verapamil

Additive incompatibilities:
Aminoglycosides

Patient/family education
- Teach patient to report sore throat, bruising, bleeding, joint pain; may indicate blood dyscrasias (rare)
- Advise patient to contact prescriber if vaginal itching, loose, foul-smelling stools, furry tongue occur; may indicate superinfection
- Advise patient to notify prescriber of diarrhea with blood or pus, which may indicate pseudomembranous colitis

Evaluation
Positive therapeutic outcome
- Absence of signs/symptoms of infection (WBC <10,000, temp WNL, absence of red, draining wounds)
- Reported improvement in symptoms of infection

Treatment of anaphylaxis:
Withdraw drug, maintain airway, administer epinephrine, aminophylline, O_2, **IV** corticosteroids

piperacillin/ tazobactam (R)
Pipracil
Func. class.: Broad-spectrum antiinfective
Chem. class.: Extended-spectrum penicillin
Pregnancy category   B

Action: Interferes with cell wall replication of susceptible organisms; osmotically unstable cell wall swells and bursts from osmotic pressure

Therapeutic Outcome: Bactericidal effects for piperacillin-resistant β-lactamase, *Escherichia coli, Staphylococcus aureus, Bacteroides fragilis, Haemophilus influenzae*

Uses: Respiratory tract, skin, skin structure, urinary tract, bone, and joint infections; gonorrhea, pneumonia, infections from penicillinase-producing staphylococci, streptococci

Dosage and routes
Nosocomial pneumonia
Adult: **IV** 3.375 g q4h with an aminoglycoside × 1-2 wk;

continue aminoglycoside only if *P. aeruginosa* is isolated

Other infections
Adult: **IV** 6-12 g/day, given 3.375 g q6h × 7-10 days

Renal dose
CrCl 20-40 ml/min give 2.25 g q6h; CrCl <20 ml/min give 2.25 g q8h

Available forms: Powder for inj 2 g piperacillin/0.25 g tazobactam; 3 g piperacillin/ 0.375 g tazobactam, 4 g piperacillin/0.5 g tazobactam, 36 g piperacillin/4.5 g tazobactam

Adverse effects
CNS: Headache, insomnia, agitation, dizziness, fever
CV: Chest pain, edema, hypertension
EENT: Rhinitis
GI: Nausea, vomiting, diarrhea, increased AST, ALT, abdominal pain, glossitis, colitis, constipation
INTEG: Rash, pruritus
MISC: Fever, superinfection
RESP: Dyspnea

Contraindications: Hypersensitivity to penicillins, cephalosporins, tazobactam; **P** neonates

Precautions: Pregnancy **B**, CHF, renal disease, lactation, sodium restriction

Pharmacokinetics	
Absorption	Well absorbed (80%)
Distribution	Widely distributed; crosses placenta
Metabolism	Not metabolized
Excretion	Kidneys, unchanged (90%); bile (10%); breast milk
Half-life	0.7-1.3 hr

Pharmacodynamics	
Onset	Rapid
Peak	Inf end

Interactions
Individual drugs
Aminoglycosides: ↓ half-life in renal disease
Amphotericin B: ↑ hypokalemia
Aspirin: ↑ piperacillin levels, ↑ renal excretion
Chloramphenicol: ↑ half-life of chloramphenicol, ↓ effectiveness of piperacillin
Cholestyramine: ↓ effectiveness of piperacillin
Colestipol: ↓ effectiveness of piperacillin
Diuretics: ↑ hypokalemia
Glucocorticoids: ↑ hypokalemia
Hepatotoxic agents: ↑ hepatotoxicity
Probenecid: ↑ piperacillin levels, ↓ renal excretion
Drug classifications
Erythromycins: ↓ antimicrobial effectiveness
Lithium: ↓ excretion, ↑ toxicity
Oral anticoagulants: ↑ anticoagulant effects
Oral contraceptives: ↓ contraceptive effectiveness
Tetracyclines: ↓ antimicrobial effectiveness
Food/drug
Food, carbonated drinks, citrus fruit juices: ↓ absorption
Herb/drug
Khat: ↓ absorption
Lab test interferences
False positive: Urine glucose, urine protein

NURSING CONSIDERATIONS
Assessment
• Assess patient for previous sensitivity reaction to penicillins or other cephalosporins, cross-sensitivity between penicillins and cephalosporins is common

• Assess patient for signs and symptoms of infection including characteristics of wounds, sputum, urine, stool, WBC >10,000, fever; obtain baseline information and during treatment

• Obtain C&S before beginning drug therapy to identify if correct treatment has been initiated

• Assess for allergic reactions: rash, urticaria, pruritus, chills, fever, joint pain; angioedema may occur a few days after therapy begins; epinephrine, resuscitation equipment should be available for anaphylactic reaction

◆• Identify urine output; if decreasing, notify prescriber (may indicate nephrotoxicity); also check for increased BUN, creatinine

• Monitor blood studies: AST, ALT, CBC, Hct, bilirubin, LDH, alkaline phosphatase, Coombs' test monthly if patient is on long-term therapy

• Monitor electrolytes: potassium, sodium, chloride monthly if patient is on long-term therapy

• Assess bowel pattern daily; if severe diarrhea occurs, drug should be discontinued; may indicate pseudomembranous colitis

• Monitor for bleeding: ecchymosis, bleeding gums, hematuria, stool guaiac daily if on long-term therapy

• Assess for overgrowth of infection: perineal itching, fever, malaise, redness, pain, swelling, drainage, rash, diarrhea, change in cough, sputum

Nursing diagnoses
✓ Infection, risk for (uses)
✓ Diarrhea (adverse reactions)
✓ Injury, risk for (adverse reactions)
✓ Knowledge deficit (teaching)
✓ Noncompliance (teaching)

Implementation
• Reconstitute with 5 ml or more 0.9% NaCl, bacteriostatic water; shake sol to dissolve

• Give by intermittent inf by diluting in 50 ml or more D_5W, 0.9% NaCl, D_5/0.9% NaCl, LR; give over 20-30 min by Y-site; discontinue primary inf during intermittent inf

• Change **IV** sites q48h to prevent phlebitis and pain

• Give direct **IV** over 3-5 min

Y-site compatibilities:
Aminophylline, aztreonam, bleomycin, bumetanide, buprenorphine, butorphanol, calcium gluconate, carboplatin, carmustine, cefepime, cimetidine, clindamycin, cyclophosphamide, cytarabine, dexamethasone, diphenhydramine, dopamine, enalaprilat, etoposide, floxuridine, fluconazole, fludarabine, fluorouracil, furosemide, gallium, granisetron, heparin, hydrocortisone, hydromorphone, ifosfamide, leucovorin, lorazepam, magnesium sulfate, mannitol, meperidine, mesna, methotrexate, methylprednisolone, metoclopramide, metronidazole, morphine, ondansetron, plicomycin, potassium chloride, ranitidine, sargramostim, sodium bicarbonate, thiotepa, trimethoprim/sulfamethoxazole, vinblastine, vincristine, zidovudine

Y-site incompatibilities:
Fluconazole, ondansetron, sargramostim, vinorelbine

P

Patient/family education

• Teach patient to report sore throat, bruising, bleeding, joint pain; may indicate blood dyscrasias (rare)

• Advise patient to contact prescriber if vaginal itching, loose, foul-smelling stools, furry tongue occur; may indicate superinfection

• Advise patient to notify prescriber of diarrhea with blood or pus, which may indicate pseudomembranous colitis

Evaluation

Positive therapeutic outcome

• Absence of signs/symptoms of infection (WBC <10,000, temp WNL, absence of red, draining wounds)

• Reported improvement in symptoms of infection

Treatment of anaphylaxis: Withdraw drug, maintain airway, administer epinephrine, aminophylline, O_2, **IV** corticosteroids

---

pirbuterol (℞)

(peer-byoo'ter-ole)

Maxair

Func. class.: Bronchodilator

Chem. class.: β-Adrenergic agonist

Pregnancy category   C

Action: Relaxes bronchial smooth muscle by direct action on $β_2$-adrenergic receptors, with increased levels of cAMP and increased bronchodilatation, diuresis, and cardiac and CNS stimulation

▶ **Therapeutic Outcome:** Bronchodilatation with ease of breathing

Uses: Reversible bronchospasm (prevention, treatment), including asthma, may be given with theophylline or steroids

Dosage and routes

P *Adult and child >12 yr:* Inh 1-2 (0.4 mg) q4-6h; max 12 inh/day

Available forms: Aerosol delivers 0.2 mg pirbuterol/actuation

Adverse effects

CNS: Tremors, anxiety, insomnia, headache, dizziness, stimulation, restlessness, hallucinations, drowsiness, irritability

CV: Palpitations, tachycardia, hypertension, angina, hypotension, **dysrhythmias**

EENT: Dry nose and mouth, irritation of nose, throat

GI: Gastritis, nausea, vomiting, anorexia

MS: Muscle cramps

RESP: **Paradoxical bronchospasm,** dyspnea, coughing

Contraindications: Hypersensitivity to sympathomimetics, tachycardia

Precautions: Lactation, pregnancy **C**, cardiac disorders, hyperthyroidism, diabetes mellitus, prostatic hypertrophy

Pharmacokinetics	
Absorption	Minimally absorbed
Distribution	Unknown
Metabolism	Liver
Excretion	Unknown
Half-life	2 hr

Pharmacodynamics	
Onset	5-15 min
Peak	1-1½ hr
Duration	5 hr

☑ Herb/drug   ⊘ Do Not Crush   ◆ Alert   ⊶ Key Drug   **G** Geriatric   **P** Pediatric

Interactions
Drug classifications
β-Adrenergic blockers: Block therapeutic effect
Bronchodilators, aerosol: ↑ action of bronchodilator
MAOIs: ↑ chance of hypertensive crisis
Sympathomimetics: ↑ adrenergic side effects
Herb/drug
Ephedra: ↑ action of both

NURSING CONSIDERATIONS
Assessment
• Monitor respiratory function: vital capacity, FEV, ABGs, lung sounds, heart rate, rhythm (baseline)
• Monitor for evidence of allergic reactions; paradoxic bronchospasm; withhold dose; notify prescriber

Nursing diagnoses
✓ Airway clearance, ineffective (uses)
✓ Gas exchange, impaired (uses)
✓ Knowledge deficit (teaching)

Implementation
• Give after shaking; have patient exhale, place mouthpiece in mouth, inhale slowly, hold breath, remove, exhale slowly; allow at least 1 min between inh
• Store in light-resistant container; do not expose to temp over 86° F (30° C)

Patient/family education
• Advise patient not to use OTC medications; extra stimulation may occur; to use this medication before other medications and allow at least 1 min between each to prevent overstimulation
• Teach patient use of inhaler; review package insert with patient; to avoid getting aerosol in eyes; blurring may result; to wash inhaler in warm water and dry daily; to avoid smoking, smoke-filled rooms, persons with respiratory tract infections
• Teach patient that paradoxic bronchospasm may occur and to stop drug immediately and notify prescriber; to limit caffeine products such as chocolate, coffee, tea, and colas
• Instruct patient on administration of dose; not to use more than prescribed; serious side effects may occur

Evaluation
Positive therapeutic outcome
• Absence of dyspnea, wheezing after 1 hr
• Improved airway exchange
• Improved ABGs

Treatment of overdose: Administer a β₂-adrenergic blocker

---

piroxicam (℞)
(peer-ox′i-kam)
Apo-Piroxicam ✦, **Feldene, Novopirocam** ✦, **Nu-Pirox, PMS-Piroxicam**
Func. class.: Nonsteroidal antiinflammatory
Chem. class.: Oxicam derivative

Pregnancy category   C

Action: Inhibits prostaglandin synthesis by decreasing an enzyme needed for biosynthesis; analgesic, antiinflammatory

Therapeutic Outcome: Decreased pain, inflammation

Uses: Mild to moderate pain, osteoarthritis, rheumatoid arthritis

P

✦ Canada Only   Adverse effects: *italic* = common; **bold** = life-threatening

Dosage and routes
Adult: PO 20 mg qd or 10 mg bid

Available forms: Caps 10, 20 mg

Adverse effects
CNS: Dizziness, *drowsiness,* fatigue, tremors, confusion, insomnia, anxiety, depression, *headache*

CV: Tachycardia, peripheral edema, palpitations, **dysrhythmias**

EENT: Tinnitus, hearing loss, blurred vision

GI: Nausea, anorexia, vomiting, diarrhea, jaundice, **cholestatic hepatitis,** constipation, flatulence, cramps, dry mouth, peptic ulcer, **bleeding, ulceration, perforation**

GU: **Nephrotoxicity: dysuria, hematuria, oliguria, azotemia**

HEMA: **Blood dyscrasias**

INTEG: Purpura, rash, pruritus, sweating, photosensitivity

Contraindications: Hypersensitivity, asthma, severe renal disease, severe hepatic disease, ulcer disease, cardiac disease

Precautions: Pregnancy C, **P** lactation, children, bleeding disorders, GI disorders, cardiac disorders, hypersensitivity to other antiinflammatory agents, CHF

Pharmacokinetics
Absorption	Well absorbed
Distribution	Unknown
Metabolism	Liver, extensively
Excretion	Kidneys, minimal; breast milk
Half-life	30-80 hr

Pharmacodynamics
Onset	1 hr
Peak	Unknown
Duration	48-72 hr

Interactions
Individual drugs

Acetaminophen (long-term use): ↑ renal reactions

Alcohol: ↑ adverse reactions

Aspirin: ↓ effectiveness, ↑ adverse reactions

Coumadin: ↑ anticoagulant effects

Digoxin: ↑ toxicity, levels

Insulin: ↓ insulin effect

Lithium: ↑ toxicity

Methotrexate: ↑ toxicity

Phenytoin: ↑ toxicity

Probenecid: ↑ toxicity

Radiation: ↑ risk of hematologic toxicity

Sulfonylurea: ↑ toxicity

Drug classifications

Anticoagulants: ↑ risk of bleeding

Antihypertensives: ↓ effect of antihypertensives

Antineoplastics: ↑ risk of hematologic toxicity

β-Adrenergic blockers: ↑ antihypertension

Cephalosporins: ↑ risk of bleeding

Diuretics: ↓ effectiveness of diuretics

Glucocorticoids: ↑ adverse reactions

Hypoglycemics: ↓ hypoglycemic effect

NSAIDs: ↑ adverse reactions

Potassium supplements: ↑ adverse reactions

Sulfonamides: ↑ toxicity

Lab test interferences

↑ Serum potassium, ↑ liver function studies

↓ Hct, ↓ Hgb, ↓ blood glucose

NURSING CONSIDERATIONS
Assessment
• Monitor blood counts during therapy; watch for decreasing platelets; if low, therapy may need to be discontinued, restarted after hematologic

---

recovery; check for blood dyscrasia (thrombocytopenia): bruising, fatigue, bleeding, poor healing
• Assess for pain: location, duration, ROM, before and 1-2 hr after administration
• Assess for aspirin sensitivity, asthma, nasal polyps; these may develop allergic reactions

Nursing diagnoses
✓ Pain (uses)
✓ Mobility, impaired (uses)
✓ Knowledge deficit (teaching)
✓ Injury, risk for (adverse reactions)

Implementation
• Administer to patient whole; give with food or milk to decrease gastric symptoms
🚫• Do not crush, chew caps

Patient/family education
• Teach patient that drug must be continued for prescribed time to be effective; to avoid aspirin, alcoholic beverages and other OTC medications unless approved by prescriber
• Caution patient to report bleeding, bruising, fatigue, malaise, since blood dyscrasias do occur
• Instruct patient to use caution when driving; drowsiness, dizziness may occur
• Teach patient to take with a full glass of water to enhance absorption; do not crush, break, or chew

Evaluation
Positive therapeutic outcome
• Decreased pain
• Decreased inflammation
• Increased mobility

---

plasma protein fraction (R)
Plasmanate, Plasma Plex, Plasmatein, Protenate
Func. class.: Blood derivative
Chem. class.: Human plasma in sodium chloride
Pregnancy category C

Action: Exerts similar oncotic pressure as human plasma, expands blood volume, shifts water from extravascular space to intravascular space

▶**Therapeutic Outcome:** Shift of fluid from extravascular into intravascular space

Uses: Hypovolemic shock, hypoproteinemia, ARDS, preoperative cardiopulmonary bypass, acute liver failure, nephrotic syndrome

Dosage and routes
Hypovolemia
Adult: **IV** inf 250-500 ml (12.5-25 g protein), not to exceed 10 ml/min
P *Child:* **IV** inf 22-33 ml/kg at 5-10 ml/min

Hypoproteinemia
Adult: **IV** inf 1000-1500 ml qd, not to exceed 8 ml/min

Available forms: Inj 5%

Adverse effects
CNS: Fever, chills, headache, paresthesias, flushing
CV: Fluid overload, hypotension, erratic pulse
GI: Nausea, vomiting, increased salivation
INTEG: Rash, urticaria, cyanosis
RESP: Altered respirations, dyspnea, pulmonary edema

P

Contraindications: Hypersensitivity, CHF, severe anemia, renal insufficiency

Precautions: Decreased salt intake, decreased cardiac reserve, lack of albumin deficiency, hepatic disease, renal disease, pregnancy **C**

Pharmacokinetics

Absorption	Completely absorbed
Distribution	Intravascular space
Metabolism	Unknown
Excretion	Unknown
Half-life	Unknown

Pharmacodynamics

Onset	15-30 min
Peak	Unknown
Duration	Unknown

Interactions: None
Lab test interferences
False: ↑ Alkaline phosphatase

NURSING CONSIDERATIONS
Assessment
• Monitor blood studies: Hct, Hgb; electrolytes, serum protein, if serum protein declines, dyspnea, hypoxemia can result
• Monitor B/P (decreased), pulse (erratic), respiration during inf; CVP, jugular vein distention, pulmonary wedge pressure (increases if overload occurs); SOB, anxiety, insomnia, expiratory rales, frothy blood-tinged cough, cyanosis indicate pulmonary overload
• Monitor I&O ratio; urinary output may decrease
• Assess for allergy: fever, rash, itching, chills, flushing, urticaria, nausea, vomiting, or hypotension requires discontinuation of inf; use new lot if therapy reinstituted

Nursing diagnoses
☑ Fluid volume deficit (uses)
☑ Cardiac output, decreased (uses)
☑ Fluid volume excess (adverse reactions)

Implementation
• Give by **IV**; no dilution required; use inf pump, large-gauge needle (≥20 G); discard unused portion; infuse slowly within 4 hr of opening
• Provide adequate hydration before administration
• When storing, check type of albumin, date; may have to refrigerate

Additive compatibilities:
Carbohydrate and electrolyte sol, whole blood, packed red blood cells, chloramphenicol, tetracycline

Additive incompatibilities:
Protein hydrolysate sol, amino acids solution, alcohol, norepinephrine

Patient/family education
• Explain reason for and expected result of medication

Evaluation
Positive therapeutic outcome
• Increased B/P
• Decreased edema
• Increased serum albumin

---

plicamycin (℞)
(plik-a-mi′cin)
Mithramycin, Mithracin
Func. class.: Antineoplastic, antibiotic; hypocalcemic
Chem. class.: Crystalline aglycone

Pregnancy category   X

Action: Inhibits DNA, RNA, protein synthesis; derived from *Streptomyces plicatus;* replication is decreased by binding to DNA; demonstrates calcium-lowering effect not related to

---

its tumoricidal activity; also acts on osteoclasts and blocks action of parathyroid hormone; a vesicant

→ **Therapeutic Outcome:** Prevention of rapidly growing malignant cells, decreased calcium levels

Uses: Testicular cancer, hypercalcemia, hypercalciuria, symptomatic treatment of advanced neoplasms

Dosage and routes
Testicular tumors
Adult: IV 25-30 µg/kg/day × 8-10 days, not to exceed 30 µg/kg/day

Hypercalcemia/hypercalciuria
Adult: IV 25 µg/kg/day × 3-4 days; repeat at intervals of 1 wk

Available forms: Inj 2500 µg/vial powder

Adverse effects
CNS: Drowsiness, weakness, lethargy, headache, flushing, fever, depression
GI: Nausea, vomiting, anorexia, diarrhea, stomatitis, increased liver enzymes
GU: Increased BUN, creatinine, **proteinuria**
HEMA: **Hemorrhage, thrombocytopenia,** decreased protime, WBC count
INTEG: Rash, cellulitis, **extravasation,** facial flushing
META: Decreased serum calcium, potassium, phosphorus

Contraindications: Hypersensitivity, thrombocytopenia, bone marrow depression, bleeding disorders, pregnancy **X**

Precautions: Renal disease, hepatic disease, electrolyte imbalances

Pharmacokinetics

Absorption	Completely absorbed
Distribution	Crosses blood-brain barrier; concentration in bone, liver, renal system
Metabolism	Unknown
Excretion	Kidneys
Half-life	Unknown

Pharmacodynamics
Unknown

Interactions
Individual drugs
Aspirin: ↑ risk of bleeding
Dextran: ↑ risk of bleeding
Heparin: ↑ risk of bleeding
Radiation: ↑ toxicity, bone marrow suppression
Sulfinpyrazone: ↑ risk of bleeding
Valproic acid: ↑ risk of bleeding
Drug classifications
Anticoagulants, oral: ↑ risk of bleeding
Antineoplastics: ↑ toxicity, bone marrow suppression
Cephalosporins: ↑ risk of bleeding
Hepatotoxic agents: ↑ hepatotoxicity
Neurotoxic agents: ↑ neurotoxicity
NSAIDs: ↑ risk of bleeding
Thrombolytics: ↑ risk of bleeding

NURSING CONSIDERATIONS
Assessment
• Assess buccal cavity q8h for dryness, sores or ulceration, white patches, oral pain, bleeding, dysphagia; obtain prescription for viscous lidocaine (Xylocaine)
• Assess symptoms indicating severe allergic reaction: rash, pruritus, urticaria, purpuric skin lesions, itching, flushing

P

• Monitor CBC, differential, platelet count weekly; withhold drug if WBC count is <4000/mm^3 or platelet count is <100,000/mm^3; notify prescriber of results if WBC <20,000/mm^3, platelets <150,000/mm^3

• Monitor renal function studies: BUN, creatinine, serum uric acid, urine CrCl before and during therapy; I&O ratio; report fall in urine output to <30 ml/hr

• Monitor temp q4h (may indicate beginning of infection)

• Monitor liver function tests before and during therapy (bilirubin, AST, ALT, LDH) as needed or monthly; check for jaundice of skin and sclera, dark urine, clay-colored stools, itchy skin, abdominal pain, fever, diarrhea

• Assess for bleeding: hematuria, stool guaiac, bruising or petechiae, mucosa or orifices q8h; check for inflammation of mucosa, breaks in skin

Nursing diagnoses

☑ Injury, risk for (adverse reactions)

☑ Body image disturbance (adverse reactions)

☑ Infection, risk for (adverse reactions)

☑ Knowledge deficit (teaching)

Implementation

• Avoid contact with skin; very irritating; wash completely to remove

• Give fluids **IV** or PO before chemotherapy to hydrate patient

• Give antacid before oral agent; give drug after evening meal, before hs; provide antiemetic 30-60 min before giving drug and prn to prevent vomiting; administer antibiotics for prophylaxis of infection

• Give top or syst analgesics for pain

• Give in AM so drug can be eliminated before hs

• Provide liq diet: carbonated beverages; gelatin may be added if patient is not nauseated or vomiting

• Encourage patient to rinse mouth tid-qid with water, club soda; brush teeth bid-qid with soft brush or cotton-tipped applicators for stomatitis; use unwaxed dental floss

• Make sure drug is prepared by experienced personnel using proper precautions

• Give **IV** intermittent inf by diluting 2.5 mg/4.9 ml of sterile water; (1 ml = 500 μg); dilute single dose in 1000 ml of D$_5$W run over 4-6 hr; give slow **IV** inf using 20 G, 21 G needle

• Administer EDTA for extravasation; apply ice compress

Y-site compatibilities:
Allopurinol, amifostine, aztreonam, filgrastim, melphalan, piperacillin/tazobactam, teniposide, thiotepa, vinorelbine

Patient/family education

• Teach patient to avoid use of products containing aspirin or NSAIDs, razors, commercial mouthwash, since bleeding may occur; to report symptoms of bleeding (hematuria, tarry stools)

• Caution patient to report signs of anemia (fatigue, headache, irritability, faintness, shortness of breath)

• Advise patient to report any changes in breathing or coughing even several mo after treatment; to avoid crowds or persons with respiratory tract and other infections

• Advise patient that hair may be lost during treatment; a wig or hair piece may make patient feel better; new hair may be different in color, texture

• Caution patient not to have any vaccinations without the advice of the prescriber; serious reactions can occur

• Advise patient that contraception is needed during treatment and for several mo after completion of therapy

Evaluation

Positive therapeutic outcome

• Prevention of rapid division of malignant cells

---

poractant alpha
See Appendix A, Selected New Drugs

---

porfirmer (℞)
(pour'fur-meer)
Photofrin
Func. class.: Antineoplastic-misc.
Chem. class.: Photosensitizing agent
Pregnancy category C

Action: Used in photodynamic treatment of tumors (PDT); antitumor and cytotoxic actions are light and O_2 dependent; used with 630 nm laser light

➡ Therapeutic Outcome: Prevention of growth of tumor

Uses: Esophageal cancer (completely obstructing), endobronchial non–small-cell lung cancer

Dosage and routes
Refer to guide for complete instructions

Adult: **IV** 2 mg/kg, then illumination with laser light 40-50 hr after inj; a second laser light application may be given 96-120 hr after inj; may repeat q 30 days × 3

Endobronchial cancer
Adult: 200 joules/cm of tumor length

Available forms: Cake/powder for inj 75 mg

Adverse effects
CNS: Anxiety, confusion, insomnia
CV: Hypotension, hypertension, **atrial fibrillation, cardiac failure,** *tachycardia*
GI: Abdominal pain, constipation, diarrhea, dyspepsia, dysphagia, eructation, esophageal edema/bleeding, hematemesis, melena, nausea, vomiting, anorexia
MISC: Dehydration, weight decrease, anemia, photosensitivity reaction, UTI, moniliasis
RESP: **Pleural effusion,** pneumonia, dyspnea, resp insufficiency, **tracheoesophageal fistula**

Contraindications: Porphyria, porphyrin allergy (porfirmer); tracheoesophageal, bronchoesophageal fistula; major blood vessels with eroding tumors (PDT)

Precautions: Elderly, pregnancy C, lactation, children

Pharmacokinetics	
Absorption	Unknown
Distribution	Unknown
Metabolism	Unknown
Excretion	Unknown
Half-life	250 hr

Pharmacodynamics
Unknown

Interactions
Drug classifications
Phenothiazines: ↑ photosensitivity
Sulfonamides: ↑ photosensitivity
Sulfonylureas: ↑ photosensitivity
Thiazides: ↑ photosensitivity

NURSING CONSIDERATIONS
Assessment
• Assess for ocular sensitivity; sensitivity to sun, bright lights, car headlights; patients should wear dark sunglasses with an average white light transmittance of <4%
• Assess for chest pain: may be so severe as to necessitate opiate analgesics
• Assess for extravasation at inj site: take care to protect from light

Nursing diagnoses
☑ Infection, risk for (adverse reactions)
☑ Knowledge deficit (teaching)

Implementation
• Give porfirmer as a single slow **IV** inj over 3-5 min at 2mg/kg; reconstitute each vial with 31.8 ml D5 or 0.9% NaCl (2.5 mg/ml), shake well, do not mix with other drugs or sol, protect from light, and use immediately
• Laser light is initiated 630 nm wave length laser light
• Wipe spills with damp cloth, avoid skin/eye contact, use rubber gloves, eye protection; dispose of material in polyethylene bag according to policy

Patient/family education
• Advise patient to report chest pain, eye sensitivity
• Advise patient to wear sunglasses with average white light transmittance of <4%

**potassium acetate/
potassium
bicarbonate** (Ⅸ)
K+Care ET, K-Electrolyte, K-Ide, Klor-Con/EF, K-Lyte, K-Vescent
**potassium
bicarbonate/
potassium chloride** (Ⅸ)
Klorvess, Klorvess Effervescent Granules, K-Lyte/Cl, Neo-K ✤
**potassium
bicarbonate/
potassium citrate** (Ⅸ)
Effer-K, K-Lyte DS
potassium chloride (Ⅸ)
Apo-K ✤, Cena-K, Gen-K, K+care, K+10, Kalium Durules ✤, Kaochlor, Kaochlor S-F, Kaon-Cl, Kay Ciel, KCl, K-Dur, K-Lease, K-Long ✤, K-Lor, Klor-Con, Klorvess, Klotrix, K-Lyte/Cl powder, K-med, K-Norm, K-Sol, K-Tab, Micro-K, Micro-LS, Potasalan, Roychlor, Rum-K, Slow-K, Ten-K
**potassium chloride/
potassium bicarbonate/potassium citrate**
Kaochlor Eff
potassium gluconate
Kaon, Kaylixir, K-G Elixir, Potassium-Rougier ✤
**potassium gluconate/
potassium chloride**
Kolyum
**potassium gluconate/
potassium citrate**
Twin-K
Func. class.: Electrolyte
Chem. class.: Potassium
Pregnancy category   C

Action: Needed for adequate transmission of nerve impulses

☑ Herb/drug 🚫 Do Not Crush ◆ Alert ⊶ Key Drug Ⓖ Geriatric Ⓟ Pediatric and cardiac contraction, renal function, intracellular ion maintenance

➡️ **Therapeutic Outcome:** Potassium level 3.0-5.0 mg/dl

Uses: Prevention and treatment of hypokalemia

Dosage and routes
Potassium bicarbonate
Adult: PO dissolve 25-50 mEq in water qd-qid

Potassium acetate—hypokalemia
🅿 *Adult and child:* PO 40-100 mEq/day in divided doses × 2-4 days

Hypokalemia (prevention)
🅿 *Adult and child:* PO 20 mEq/day in 2-4 divided doses

Potassium chloride
Adult: PO 40-100 mEq in divided doses tid-qid; **IV** 20 mEq/hr when diluted as 40 mEq/1000 ml, not to exceed 150 mEq/day

🅿 *Child:* PO 2-4 mEq/kg/day

Potassium gluconate
Adult: PO 40-100 mEq in divided doses tid-qid

Potassium phosphate
Adult: **IV** 1 mEq/hr in sol of 60 mEq/L, not to exceed 150 mEq/day; PO 40-100 mEq/day in divided doses

🅿 *Child:* **IV** max rate of infusion 1 mEq/kg/min

Available forms: Tabs for sol 6.5, 25 mEq; inj for prep of **IV** 2, 4 mEq; ext rel caps 8, 10 mEq; powder for sol 3.3, 5, 6.7, 10, 13.3 mEq/5 ml; tabs 4, 13.4 mEq; ext rel tabs 6.7, 8, 10 mEq; inj for prep of **IV** 1.5, 2, 2.4, 3, 3.2 mEq/ml; elix 6.7 mEq/5 ml; tabs 2, 5 mEq; oral sol 2.375 mEq/5 ml; inj for prep of **IV** 4.4, 4.7 mEq/ml

Adverse effects
CNS: Confusion
CV: Bradycardia, *cardiac depression,* **dysrhythmias, arrest, peaking T waves, lowered R and depressed RST, prolonged PR interval, widened QRS complex**
GI: Nausea, vomiting, cramps, pain, *diarrhea,* ulceration of small bowel
GU: Oliguria
INTEG: Cold extremities, rash

Contraindications: Renal disease (severe), severe hemolytic disease, Addison's disease, hyperkalemia, acute dehydration, extensive tissue breakdown

Precautions: Cardiac disease, potassium-sparing diuretic therapy, systemic acidosis, pregnancy **C**

Pharmacokinetics and pharmacodynamics unavailable.

Interactions
Drug classifications
Angiotensin converting enzyme inhibitors: ↑ hyperkalemia
Potassium-sparing diuretics: ↑ hyperkalemia

NURSING CONSIDERATIONS
Assessment
• Assess ECG for peaking T waves, lowered R, depressed RST, prolonged PR interval, widening QRS complex, hyperkalemia; drug should be reduced or discontinued
• Monitor potassium level during treatment (3.5-5.0 mg/dl is normal level)
• Monitor I&O ratio; watch for decreased urinary output;

notify prescriber immediately; check urinary pH in patients receiving the drug as a urinary acidifier

• Assess cardiac status: rate, rhythm, CVP, PWP, PAWP if being monitored directly

Nursing diagnoses

☑ Nutrition, altered: less than body requirements (uses)

☑ Knowledge deficit (teaching)

Implementation

IV **IV route**

• Give through large-bore needle to decrease vein inflammation; check for extravasation; administer in large vein, avoiding scalp vein

P in child

• After diluting in large volume of **IV** sol give as an **IV** inf slowly to prevent toxicity; never give **IV** bolus or IM

Potassium acetate
Additive compatibilities:
Metoclopramide

Potassium chloride
Y-site compatibilities:
Acyclovir, aldesleukin, allopurinol, amifostine, aminophylline, amiodarone, ampicillin, amrinone, atropine, aztreonam, betamethasone, calcium gluconate, cefmetazole, cephalothin, cephapirin, chlordiazepoxide, chlorpromazine, ciprofloxacin, cladribine, cyanocobalamin, dexamethasone, digoxin, diltiazem, diphenhydramine, dobutamine, dopamine, droperidol, edrophonium, enalaprilat, epinephrine, esmolol, estrogens, ethacrynate, famotidine, fentanyl, filgrastim, fludarabine, fluorouracil, furosemide, gallium, granisetron, heparin, hydralazine, idarubicin, indomethacin, insulin, regular, isoproterenol, kana-

mycin, labetalol, lidocaine, lorazepam, magnesium sulfate, melphalan, meperidine, methicillin, methoxamine, methylergonovine, midazolam, minocycline, morphine, neostigmine, norepinephrine, ondansetron, oxacillin, oxytocin, paclitaxel, penicillin G potassium, pentazocine, phytonadione, piperacillin/tazobactam, prednisolone, procainamide, prochlorperazine, propofol, propranolol, pyridostigmine, sargramostim, scopolamine, sodium bicarbonate, succinylcholine, tacrolimus, teniposide, theophylline, thiotepa, trimethaphan, trimethobenzamide, vinorelbine, zidovudine

Additive compatibilities:
Aminophylline, amiodarone, atracurium, bretylium, calcium chloride, cefepime, cephalothin, cephapirin, chloramphenicol, cimetidine, ciprofloxacin, clindamycin, cloxacillin, corticotropin, cytarabine, dimenhydrinate, dopamine, enalaprilat, erythromycin, floxacillin, fluconazole, furosemide, heparin, hydrocortisone, isoproterenol, lidocaine, metaraminol, methicillin, methyldopa, metoclopramide, mitoxantrone, nafcillin, netilmicin, norepinephrine, oxacillin, penicillin G potassium or sodium, phenylephrine, piperacillin, ranitidine, sodium bicarbonate, thiopental, vancomycin, verapamil, vit B/C

Potassium chloride
Y-site compatibilities:
Aldesleukin, amifostine, granisetron, lorazepam, midazolam, thiotepa

---

☑ Herb/drug   ⊘ Do Not Crush   ◆ Alert   ☛ Key Drug   **G** Geriatric   **P** Pediatric

PO route

• Give with meal or pc; dissolve effervescent tab, powder in 8 oz cold water or juice; do not give IM, SC
• Store at room temp

Patient/family education

• Teach patient to eat foods rich in potassium after medication is discontinued
• Advise patient to avoid OTC products: antacids, salt substitutes, analgesics, vitamin preparations, unless specifically directed by prescriber
• Advise patient to report hyperkalemia symptoms or continued hypokalemia symptoms
• Tell patient to take cap with full glass of liq; to dissolve powder or tab completely in at least 120 ml water or juice; not to chew time rel or ext rel preparations
• Emphasize importance of regular follow-up

Evaluation
Positive therapeutic outcome
• Absence of fatigue, muscle weakness, and decreased thirst and urinary output, cardiac changes
• Potassium level normal

---

pramipexole (℞)
(pra-mi-pex′ol)
Mirapex
Func. class.: Antiparkinsonian agent
Chem. class.: Dopamine-receptor agonist, nonergot
Pregnancy category **C**

Action: Selective agonist for D_2 receptors (presynaptic/postsynaptic sites); binding at D_3 receptor contributes to antiparkinson effects

⮕**Therapeutic Outcome:** Decreased symptoms of Parkinson's disease (involuntary movements)

Uses: Parkinsonism

Dosage and routes
Initial treatment
Adult: PO from a starting dose of 0.375 mg/day given in 3 divided doses; increase gradually at 5-7 day intervals until total daily dose of 4.5 mg is reached

Maintenance treatment
Adult: PO 1.5-4.5 mg qd in 3 divided doses

Available forms: Tabs 0.125, 0.25, 1.5 mg

Adverse effects
CNS: Agitation, insomnia, psychosis, hallucinations, depression, dizziness
CV: Orthostatic hypotension
EENT: Blurred vision
GI: Nausea, anorexia, constipation
GU: Impotence

Contraindications: Hypersensitivity

Precautions: Renal disease, cardiac disease, MI with dysrhythmias, affective disorders, psychosis, pregnancy **C**

Pharmacokinetics	
Absorption	Well absorbed
Distribution	Widely distributed
Metabolism	Liver, minimally
Excretion	Kidneys, unchanged
Half-life	8-14 hr

Pharmacodynamics
Unknown

Interactions
Individual drugs
Cimetidine: ↑ pramipexole levels

Diltiazem: ↑ pramipexole levels

Levodopa: ↑ pramipexole levels

Metoclopramide: ↓ pramipexole effect

Quinidine: ↑ pramipexole levels

Ranitidine: ↑ pramipexole levels

Triamterene: ↑ pramipexole levels

Drug classifications
Butyrophenones: ↓ pramipexole effect

Dopamine antagonists: ↓ pramipexole levels

Phenothiazines: ↓ pramipexole effect

☑ Herb/drug
Chaste tree fruit: ↓ pramipexole effect

NURSING CONSIDERATIONS
Assessment
• Monitor B/P, respiration during initial treatment; hypotension or hypertension should be reported
• Assess mental status: affect, mood, behavioral changes, depression; complete suicide assessment
• Monitor renal function studies
• Assess for involuntary movements in parkinsonism: akinesia, tremors, staggering gait, muscle rigidity, drooling; these symptoms should improve with therapy

Nursing diagnoses
✓ Mobility, impaired (uses)
✓ Injury, risk for (uses)
✓ Knowledge deficit (teaching)
✓ Noncompliance (teaching)

Implementation
PO route
• Give drug until NPO before surgery
• Adjust dosage to patient response
• Give with meals to decrease GI upset

Patient/family education
• Advise patient that therapeutic effects may take several wk to a few mo
• Caution patient to change positions slowly to prevent orthostatic hypotension
• Instruct patient to use drug exactly as prescribed; if drug is discontinued abruptly, parkinsonian crisis may occur; if treatment is to be discontinued, taper over 1 wk

Evaluation
Positive therapeutic outcome
• Decreased akathisia, other involuntary movements
• Increased mood

---

pravastatin (℞)
(pra'va-sta-tin)
Pravachol
Func. class.: Antilipidemic

Pregnancy category X

Action: Inhibits biosynthesis of VLDL, LDL, which are responsible for cholesterol development, by inhibiting the enzyme HMG-CoA reductase

▶ **Therapeutic Outcome:** Decreasing cholesterol levels and LDL, increased HDLD

Uses: As an adjunct in primary hypercholesterolemia types IIa, IIb, artherosclerosis, to reduce the risk of recurrent MI, atherosclerosis

---

Dosage and routes
Adult: PO 10-20 mg qd at hs (range 10-40 mg qd)
G *Elderly/renal/hepatic dose:* PO 10 mg/day

Available forms: Tabs 10, 20, 40 mg

Adverse effects
CNS: Headache, dizziness, psychic disturbances
EENT: Lens opacities, common cold, rhinitis, cough
GI: Nausea, constipation, diarrhea, dyspepsia, flatus, abdominal pain, heartburn, **liver dysfunction, pancreatitis, hepatitis**
INTEG: Rash, pruritus, photosensitivity
MS: Muscle cramps, myalgia, **myositis, rhabdomyolysis**

Contraindications: Hypersensitivity, pregnancy **X,** lactation, active liver disease

Precautions: Past liver disease, alcoholism, severe acute infections, trauma, hypotension, uncontrolled seizure disorders, severe metabolic disorders, electrolyte imbalances, renal disease

Do Not Confuse:
Pravachol/Prevacid

Pharmacokinetics	
Absorption	Poorly absorbed, erratic
Distribution	Unknown
Metabolism	Liver, extensively
Excretion	Feces (70%-75%); kidneys, unchanged (10%), breast milk (minimal)
Half-life	2 hr

Pharmacodynamics	
Onset	Unknown
Peak	1-1½ hr
Duration	Unknown

Interactions
Individual drugs
Cholestyramine: ↓ action of pravastatin
Clarithromycin: ↑ risk for myopathy
Clofibrate: ↑ risk for myopathy
Colestipol: ↓ action of pravastatin
Cyclosporine: ↑ risk of myopathy, rhabdomyolysis
Erythromycin: ↑ risk of myopathy, rhabdomyolysis
Gemfibrozil: ↑ risk of myopathy, rhabdomyolysis
Itraconazole: ↑ risk for myopathy
Niacin: ↑ risk of myopathy, rhabdomyolysis
Propranolol: ↓ effect of pravastatin
Warfarin: ↑ bleeding
Drug classifications
Protease inhibitors: ↑ risk of myopathy
Lab test interferences
↑ CPK, ↑ liver function tests

NURSING CONSIDERATIONS
Assessment
• Assess nutrition: fat, protein, carbohydrates; nutritional analysis should be completed by dietician before treatment
• Monitor triglycerides, esterol, cholesterol at baseline and throughout treatment; LDL and HDL should be watched closely; if increased, drug should be discontinued

Nursing diagnoses
✓ Knowledge deficit (teaching)
✓ Noncompliance (teaching)

Implementation
• Give at hs only; give 1 hr before or 4 hr after bile acid sequestrants
• Store in cool environment in tight, light-resistant container

P

Patient/family education
• Inform patient that compliance is needed for positive results to occur; not to double doses or skip doses
• Teach patient that risk factors should be decreased: high-fat diet, smoking, alcohol consumption, absence of exercise
• Advise patient to notify prescriber of weakness, tenderness, or limited mobility
• Explain to patient that contraception is necessary, since drug produces teratogenic effects

Evaluation
Positive therapeutic outcome
• Decreased cholesterol serum triglyceride levels and improved ratio with HDL

---

prazosin ⛗ (℞)
(pra′zoe-sin)
Minipress, prazosin
Func. class.: Antihypertensive
Chem. class.: α_1-Adrenergic blocker
Pregnancy category   C

Action: Peripheral blood vessels dilate, peripheral resistance drops; reduction in blood pressure results from α-adrenergic receptors being blocked

➤**Therapeutic Outcome:** Decreased B/P in hypertension; decreased cardiac preload, afterload

Uses: Hypertension

Investigational uses: Benign prostatic hypertrophy to decreased urine outflow obstruction

Dosage and routes
Hypertension
Adult: PO 1 mg bid or tid, increasing to 20 mg qd in divided doses if required, usual range 6-15 mg/day, not to exceed 1 mg initially; max 20-40 mg/day
[P] *Child:* PO 0.5-7 mg bid

Benign prostatic hypertrophy
Adult: PO 1-5 mg bid

Available forms: Caps 1, 2, 5 mg

Adverse effects
CNS: Dizziness, headache, drowsiness, anxiety, depression, vertigo, weakness, fatigue
CV: Palpitations, orthostatic hypotension, tachycardia, edema, rebound hypertension
EENT: Blurred vision, epistaxis, tinnitus, dry mouth, red sclera
GI: Nausea, vomiting, diarrhea, constipation, abdominal pain
GU: Urinary frequency, incontinence, impotence, priapism, water and sodium retention

Contraindications: Hypersensitivity

Precautions: Pregnancy **C**,
[P] children

Pharmacokinetics	
Absorption	60%
Distribution	Widely distributed
Metabolism	Liver, extensively
Excretion	Kidneys, unchanged (10%), bile (90%)
Half-life	2-3 hr

Pharmacodynamics	
Onset	2 hr
Peak	1-3 hr
Duration	6-12 hr

Interactions
Individual drugs
Alcohol: ↑ hypotension
Indomethacin: ↓ effect
Nitroglycerin: ↑ hypotension
Drug classifications
Antihypertensives: ↑ hypotension
β-Adrenergic blockers: ↑ hypotension
Nitrates: ↑ hypotension
Lab test interferences
↑ Urinary norepinephrine, ↑ VMA

NURSING CONSIDERATIONS
Assessment
• Monitor B/P, orthostatic hypotension, syncope; check for edema in feet, legs daily; monitor I&O, weight daily; notify prescriber of changes
• Assess for allergic reactions: rash, fever, pruritus, urticaria; drug should be discontinued if antihistamines fail to help
• Assess for orthostatic hypotension; tell patient to rise slowly from sitting or lying position

Nursing diagnoses
☑ Cardiac output, decreased (uses)
☑ Injury, risk for (adverse reactions)
☑ Knowledge deficit (teaching)
☑ Noncompliance (teaching)

Implementation
• Severe hypotension may occur after 1st dose of this medication; hypotension may be prevented by reducing or discontinuing diuretic therapy 3 days before beginning prazosin therapy
• Store in airtight container at 86° F (30° C) or less

Patient/family education
• Instruct patient not to discontinue drug abruptly; stress the importance of complying with dosage schedule, even if feeling better; if dose is missed, take as soon as remembered; take at same time each day
• Advise patient not to use OTC products (cough, cold, allergy) unless directed by prescriber; also to avoid large amounts of caffeine
• Emphasize the need to rise slowly to sitting or standing position to minimize orthostatic hypotension
• Teach patient to notify prescriber of mouth sores, sore throat, fever, swelling of hands or feet, irregular heartbeat, chest pain
• Caution patient to report excessive perspiration, dehydration, vomiting, diarrhea; may lead to fall in B/P
• Caution patient that drug may cause dizziness, fainting, lightheadedness; may occur during 1st few days of therapy; to avoid hazardous activities
• Teach patient how to take B/P and normal readings for age group; instruct to take B/P q7 days

Evaluation
Positive therapeutic outcome
• Decreased B/P in hypertension

Treatment of overdose:
Administer volume expanders or vasopressors, discontinue drug, place in supine position

---

prednisolone (R)
(pred-niss'oh-lone)
Articulose-50, Delta-Cortef,
Prednisolone, Prelone, Key-
Pred 25, Key-Pred 50,
Predaject-50, Predalone 50,
Predcor-25, Predcor-50,
Prednisolone Acetate,
Hydeltrasol, Key-Pred-SP,
Pediapred, Hydeltra-T.B.A.,
Predalone-T.B.A., Prednisol
TBA
Func. class.: Corticoste-
roid
Chem. class.: Intermediate-
acting glucocorticoid
Pregnancy category   C

Action: Decreases inflammation by suppressing migration
of polymorphonuclear leukocytes, fibroblasts; reversal to
increase capillary permeability
and lysosomal stabilization,
minimal mineralocorticoid

Therapeutic Outcome: Decreased inflammation, de-
creased adrenal insufficiency

Uses: Severe inflammation,
immunosuppression, neo-
plasms

Dosage and routes
Adult: PO 2.5-15 mg bid-qid;
IM 2-30 mg (acetate, phosphate) q12h; **IV** 2-30 mg
(phosphate) q12h, 2-30 mg in
joint or soft tissue (phosphate),
4-40 mg in joint of lesion
(tebutate)

Asthma/antiinflammatory
P *Child:* PO 1-2 mg/kg/day; **IV**
2-4 mg/kg/day

Available forms: *Predniso-*
lone: tab 5 mg, syrup 5 mg/
5 ml, 15 mg/5 ml; *predniso-*
lone acetate: inj 25, 50 mg/ml;
prednisolone tebutate: inj 20

mg/ml; *prednisolone phosphate:*
inj 20 mg/ml, oral liquid
5 mg/5 ml

Adverse effects
CNS: Depression, flushing,
sweating, headache, mood
changes
CV: Hypertension, **circulatory**
collapse, thrombophlebitis,
embolism, tachycardia
EENT: Fungal infections,
increased intraocular pressure,
blurred vision
GI: Diarrhea, nausea, abdomi-
nal distention, **GI hemor-**
rhage, increased appetite,
pancreatitis
HEMA: **Thrombocytopenia**
INTEG: Acne, poor wound
healing, ecchymosis, petechiae
MS: Fractures, osteoporosis,
weakness

Contraindications: Psychosis,
hypersensitivity, idiopathic
thrombocytopenia, acute glomerulonephritis, amebiasis,
fungal infections, nonasthmatic
P bronchial disease, child <2 yr

Precautions: Pregnancy **C,**
diabetes mellitus, glaucoma,
osteoporosis, seizure disorders,
ulcerative colitis, CHF, myasthenia gravis

Do Not Confuse:
prednisolone/prednisone

Pharmacokinetics	
Absorption	Well absorbed (PO, IM), completely absorbed (**IV**)
Distribution	Widely distributed; crosses placenta
Metabolism	Liver, extensively
Excretion	Kidney, breast milk
Half-life	2-4 hr

Pharmacodynamics

	PO	IM (phosphate)	IV	IA/IL
Onset	1 hr	Rapid	Rapid	Slow
Peak	2 hr	1 hr	Unknown	Unknown
Duration	1½ days	Unknown	Unknown	Up to 1 mo

Interactions
Individual drugs
Alcohol: ↑ GI effects
Amphotericin B: ↑ hypokalemia
Aspirin: ↑ GI effects
Insulin: ↑ need for insulin
Mezlocillin: ↑ hypokalemia
Phenytoin: ↓ action, ↑ metabolism
Piperacillin: ↑ hypokalemia
Rifampin: ↓ action, ↑ metabolism
Ticarcillin: ↑ hypokalemia
Drug classifications
Barbiturates: ↓ action, ↑ metabolism
Diuretics: ↑ hypokalemia
Hypoglycemic agents: ↑ need for hypoglycemic agents
Herb/drug
Aloe: ↑ hypokalemia
Buckthorn: ↑ hypokalemia
Cascara sagrada: ↑ hypokalemia
Senna: ↑ hypokalemia
Lab test interferences
↑ Cholesterol, ↑ sodium, ↑ blood glucose, ↑ uric acid, ↑ calcium, ↑ urine glucose
↓ Calcium, ↓ potassium, ↓ T$_4$, ↓ T$_3$, ↓ thyroid ^{131}I uptake test, ↓ urine 17-OHCS, ↓ 17-KS, ↓ PBI
False negative: Skin allergy tests

NURSING CONSIDERATIONS
Assessment
• Monitor potassium, blood sugar, urine glucose while patient is on long-term therapy; hypokalemia and hyperglycemia may occur
• Monitor weight daily; notify prescriber of weekly gain >5 lb; monitor I&O ratio; be alert for decreasing urinary output and increasing edema
• Monitor B/P q4h, pulse; notify prescriber if chest pain occurs
• Monitor plasma cortisol levels during long-term therapy (normal level; 138-635 nmol/L SI units when drawn at 8 AM)
• Assess adrenal function periodically for HPA axis suppression
• Assess infection: increased temp, WBC even after withdrawal of medication; drug masks infection symptoms
• Assess for potassium depletion: paresthesias, fatigue, nausea, vomiting, depression, polyuria, dysrhythmias, weakness, edema, hypertension, cardiac symptoms
• Assess mental status: affect, mood, behavioral changes, aggression
• Monitor temp; if fever develops, drug should be discontinued
• Assess for systemic absorption: increased temp, inflammation, irritation (top)

Nursing diagnoses
☑ Infection, risk for (adverse reactions)
☑ Knowledge deficit (teaching)
☑ Noncompliance (teaching)

Implementation
☑ **IV route**
• Give by direct **IV** only sodium phosphate product; give over >1 min; may be given by **IV** inf in D$_5$W, 0.9% NaCl
• Give after shaking susp (parenteral)

• Give titrated dose; use lowest effective dosage

Y-site compatibilities:
Ciprofloxacin, potassium chloride, vit B/C

Additive compatibilities:
Ascorbic acid, cephalothin, cytarabine, erythromycin, fluorouracil, heparin, methicillin, penicillin G potassium, penicillin G sodium, vit B/C

Additive incompatibilities:
Calcium gluceptate, methotrexate, polymyxin B sulfate

IM route
• Give IM inj deep in large muscle mass; rotate sites; avoid deltoid; use 21 G needle
• Give in one dose in AM to prevent adrenal suppression; avoid SC administration; may damage tissue

PO route
• Give with food or milk to decrease GI symptoms

Patient/family education
• Advise patient that ID as steroid user should be carried
• Advise patient to notify prescriber if therapeutic response decreases; dosage adjustment may be needed
• Caution patient not to discontinue abruptly; adrenal crisis can result
• Caution patient to avoid OTC products: salicylates, alcohol in cough products, cold preparations unless directed by prescriber
• Teach patient all aspects of drug usage including cushingoid symptoms
• Teach patient symptoms of adrenal insufficiency: nausea, anorexia, fatigue, dizziness, dyspnea, weakness, joint pain
• Advise patient that long-term therapy may be needed to clear infection (1-2 mo depending on type of infection)

Evaluation
Positive therapeutic outcome
• Decreased inflammation

---

prednisone ♦▅ (Ŗ)
(pred′ni-sone)
Apo-Prednisone ✦,
Deltasone, Liquid Pred,
Meticorten, Orasone,
Panasol-S, Prednicen-M,
Prednisone, Sterapred,
Winpred
Func. class.: Corticosteroid
Chem. class.: Intermediate-acting glucocorticoid
Pregnancy category   C

Action: Decreases inflammation by suppressing migration of polymorphonuclear leukocytes, fibroblasts; reversal to increase capillary permeability and lysosomal stabilization

⮕**Therapeutic Outcome:** Decreased inflammation, decreased adrenal insufficiency

Uses: Severe inflammation, immunosuppression, neoplasms, multiple sclerosis, collagen disorders, dermatologic disorders

Dosage and routes
Adult: PO 1.5-2.5 mg bid-qid, then qd or qod; maintenance up to 250 mg/day
P *Child:* PO 0.05-2 mg/kg/day divided 1-4 ×/day

Nephrosis
P *Child 18 mo-4 yr:* 7.5-10 mg qid initially
P *Child 4-10 yr:* 15 mg qid initially

☑ Herb/drug   🚫 Do Not Crush   ◆ Alert   ♦▅ Key Drug   G Geriatric   P Pediatric

P *Child >10 yr:* 20 mg qid initially

Multiple sclerosis
Adult: PO 200 mg/day × 1 wk, then 80 mg qod × 1 mo

Available forms: Tabs 1, 2.5, 5, 10, 20, 25, 50 mg; oral sol 5 mg/5 ml; syr 5 mg/5 ml

Adverse effects
CNS: Depression, flushing, sweating, headache, mood changes
CV: Hypertension, **circulatory collapse, thrombophlebitis, embolism,** tachycardia
EENT: Fungal infections, increased intraocular pressure, blurred vision
GI: Diarrhea, nausea, abdominal distention, **GI hemorrhage,** increased appetite, **pancreatitis**
HEMA: **Thrombocytopenia**
INTEG: Acne, poor wound healing, ecchymosis, petechiae
MS: Fractures, osteoporosis, weakness

Contraindications: Psychosis, hypersensitivity, idiopathic thrombocytopenia, acute glomerulonephritis, amebiasis, fungal infections, nonasthmatic
P bronchial disease, child <2 yr, AIDS, TB

Precautions: Pregnancy **C,** diabetes mellitus, glaucoma, osteoporosis, seizure disorders, ulcerative colitis, CHF, myasthenia gravis, renal disease, esophagitis, peptic ulcer

Do Not Confuse:
prednisone/methylprednisolone, prednisone/prednisolone, prednisone/Prilosec

Pharmacokinetics	
Absorption	Well absorbed
Distribution	Widely distributed; crosses placenta
Metabolism	Liver, extensively
Excretion	Kidney, breast milk
Half-life	3-4 hr

Pharmacodynamics	
Onset	Unknown
Peak	1-2 hr
Duration	1½ days

Interactions
Individual drugs
Alcohol: ↑ GI effects
Amphotericin B: ↑ hypokalemia
Aspirin: ↑ GI effects
Insulin: ↑ need for insulin
Mezlocillin: ↑ hypokalemia
Ticarcillin: ↑ hypokalemia
Drug classifications
Diuretics: ↑ hypokalemia
Hypoglycemic agents: ↑ need for hypoglycemic agents
Herb/drug
Aloe: ↑ hypokalemia
Buckthorn: ↑ hypokalemia
Rhubarb: ↑ hypokalemia
Senna: ↑ hypokalemia
Lab test interferences
↑ Cholesterol, ↑ sodium, ↑ blood glucose, ↑ uric acid, ↑ calcium, ↑ urine glucose
↓ Calcium, ↓ potassium, ↓ T_4, ↓ T_3, ↓ thyroid ^{131}I uptake test, ↓ urine 17-OHCS, ↓ 17-KS, ↓ PBI
False negative: Skin allergy tests

NURSING CONSIDERATIONS
Assessment
• Monitor potassium, blood sugar, urine glucose while on long-term therapy; hypokalemia and hyperglycemia may occur
• Monitor weight daily; notify prescriber of weekly gain >5 lb;

P

monitor I&O ratio; be alert for decreasing urinary output and increasing edema
• Monitor B/P q4h, pulse; notify prescriber if chest pain occurs
• Monitor plasma cortisol levels during long-term therapy (normal level 138-635 nmol/L when drawn at 8 AM)
• Assess adrenal function periodically for HPA axis suppression
• Assess infection: increased temp, WBC even after withdrawal of medication; drug masks infection symptoms
• Assess for potassium depletion: paresthesias, fatigue, nausea, vomiting, depression, polyuria, dysrhythmias, weakness, edema, hypertension, cardiac symptoms
• Assess mental status: affect, mood, behavioral changes, aggression
• Monitor temp; if fever develops, drug should be discontinued
• Assess for systemic absorption: increased temp, inflammation, irritation (top)

Nursing diagnoses
☑ Infection, risk for (adverse reactions)
☑ Knowledge deficit (teaching)
☑ Noncompliance (teaching)

Implementation
• Give with food or milk to decrease GI symptoms; use measuring device for liq route

Patient/family education
• Advise patient that ID as steroid user should be carried
• Advise patient to notify prescriber if therapeutic response decreases; dosage adjustment may be needed
• Caution patient not to discontinue abruptly; adrenal crisis can result
• Caution patient to avoid OTC products: salicylates, alcohol in cough products, cold preparations unless directed by prescriber
• Teach patient all aspects of drug usage including cushingoid symptoms
• Teach patient symptoms of adrenal insufficiency: nausea, anorexia, fatigue, dizziness, dyspnea, weakness, joint pain
• Advise patient that long-term therapy may be needed to clear infection (1-2 mo depending on type of infection)

Evaluation
Positive therapeutic outcome
• Decreased inflammation

---

primidone (℞)
(pri′mi-done)
Apo-Primidone ✦,
Mysoline, PMS-Primidone ✦, **primidone,
Sertan** ✦
Func. class.: Anticonvulsant
Chem. class.: Barbiturate derivative
Pregnancy category **D**

Action: Raises seizure threshold by conversion of drug to phenobarbital; decreases neuron firing

➡ **Therapeutic Outcome:** Reduction in seizure activity

Uses: Generalized tonic-clonic (grand mal), complex-partial, psychomotor seizures

Dosage and routes
P *Adult and child >8 yr:* PO 100-125 mg hs on days 1, 2, 3; then 100-125 mg bid on

---

days 4, 5, 6; then 100-125 mg tid on days 7, 8, 9; then maintenance 250 mg tid-qid, max 2 g/day in divided doses

P *Child <8 yr:* PO 50 mg hs on days 1, 2, 3; then 50 mg bid on days 4, 5, 6; then 100 mg bid on days 7, 8, 9; maintenance 125-250 mg tid

Available forms: Tabs 50, 250 mg; susp 250 mg/5 ml; chew tab 125 mg ♣

Adverse effects
CNS: Stimulation, drowsiness, dizziness, confusion, sedation, headache, flushing, hallucinations, **coma,** psychosis, ataxia, *vertigo*
EENT: Diplopia, nystagmus, edema of eyelids
GI: Nausea, vomiting, anorexia, **hepatitis**
GU: Impotence
HEMA: **Thrombocytopenia, leukopenia, neutropenia, eosinophilia, megaloblastic anemia,** decreased serum folate level, lymphadenopathy
INTEG: Rash, edema, alopecia, lupuslike syndrome

Contraindications: Hypersensitivity, porphyria, pregnancy **D**

Precautions: COPD, hepatic disease, renal disease, hyperac-**P** tive children

Pharmacokinetics	
Absorption	60%-80%
Distribution	Widely distributed; crosses placenta
Metabolism	Liver, converted to phenobarbital + PEMA
Excretion	Kidneys, breast milk
Half-life	3-24 hr

Pharmacodynamics	
Onset	Unknown
Peak	4 hr
Duration	Unknown

Interactions
Individual drugs
Acebutolol: ↓ effectiveness
Acetazolamide: ↓ primidone levels
Alcohol: ↑ CNS depression
Carbamazepine: ↓ primidone levels
Chloramphenicol: ↓ effectiveness
Doxycycline: ↑ half-life
Griseofulvin: ↓ effectiveness
Isoniazide: ↑ primidone levels
Metoprolol: ↓ effectiveness
Nicotinamide: ↑ primidone levels
Phenobarbital: ↑ toxicity
Propranolol: ↓ effectiveness
Quinidine: ↓ effectiveness
Timolol: ↓ effectiveness
Drug classifications
Antidepressants, tricyclic: ↑ CNS depression
Antihistamines: ↑ CNS depression
Glucocorticoids: ↓ effectiveness
Hydantoins: ↑ primidone levels
Opiates: ↑ CNS depression
Oral contraceptives: ↓ effectiveness
Phenothiazines: ↓ CNS depression
Sedative/hypnotics: ↑ CNS depression
Succinimides: ↓ primidone levels
Lab test interferences
False: ↑ Sulfobromophthalein

NURSING CONSIDERATIONS
Assessment
• Assess mental status: mood, sensorium, affect, memory (long, short), especially elderly
• Assess for blood dyscrasias: fever, sore throat, bruising, rash, jaundice, epistaxis (long-term treatment only)
• Assess seizure activity includ-

ing type, location, duration, and character; provide seizure precaution

• Assess renal studies: urinalysis, BUN, urine creatinine

• Monitor blood studies: RBC, Hct, Hgb, reticulocyte counts weekly for 4 wk then monthly

• Monitor hepatic studies: ALT, AST, bilirubin, creatinine

• Monitor drug levels during initial treatment

• Assess for signs of physical withdrawal if medication suddenly discontinued

• Assess eye problems: need for ophthalmic examinations before, during, after treatment (slit lamp, fundoscopy, tonometry)

• Assess allergic reaction: red raised rash; if this occurs, drug should be discontinued

• Monitor for toxicity: bone marrow depression, nausea, vomiting, ataxia, diplopia, cardiovascular collapse

Nursing diagnoses
☑ Injury, risk for (side effects)
☑ Knowledge deficit (teaching)

Implementation
• May give with food to decrease gastric irritation
• May crush tab and mix with food or fluid

Patient/family education
• Teach patient to carry ID card or Medic Alert bracelet stating name, drugs taken, condition, prescriber's name, phone number

• Advise patient to avoid driving and other activities that require alertness

• Caution patient to avoid alcohol and CNS depressants; increased sedation may occur

• Teach patient not to discontinue medication quickly after

long-term use; taper off over several wk

Evaluation
Positive therapeutic outcome
• Decreased seizure activity

---

probenecid (℞)
(proe-ben′e-sid)
Benemid, Benuryl ✦,
Probalan, probenecid
Func. class.: Uricosuric;
antigout
Chem. class.: Sulfonamide
derivative

Pregnancy category **B**

Action: Inhibits tubular reabsorption of urates, with increased excretion of uric acids

➡**Therapeutic Outcome:** Decreased uric acid levels

Uses: Hyperuricemia in gout, gouty arthritis; adjunct to cephalosporin or penicillin treatment (gonorrhea)

Dosage and routes
Gonorrhea
Adult: PO 1 g with 3.5 g ampicillin or 1 g 30 min before 4.8 million U of aqueous penicillin G procaine injected into 2 sites IM

Gout/gouty arthritis
Adult: PO 250 mg bid for 1 wk, then 500 mg bid, not to exceed 2 g/day; maintenance 500 mg/day × 6 mo

Adjunct in penicillin/ cephalosporin treatment
🅟*Adult and child >50 kg:* PO 500 mg qid

🅟*Child <50 kg:* PO 25 mg/kg, then 40 mg/kg in divided doses qid

Renal dose
Avoid use in CrCl <30 ml/min

Available forms: Tab 0.5 g

Adverse effects

CNS: Drowsiness, headache

CV: Bradycardia

GI: Gastric irritation, nausea, vomiting, anorexia, **hepatic necrosis**

GU: Glycosuria, thirst, frequency, **nephrotic syndrome**

INTEG: Rash, dermatitis, pruritus, fever

META: Acidosis, hypokalemia, hyperchloremia, hyperglycemia

RESP: **Apnea,** irregular respirations

Contraindications: Hypersensitivity, severe hepatic disease, severe renal disease, CrCl <50 mg/min, history of uric acid calculus

Precautions: Pregnancy **B,** child <2 yr

Pharmacokinetics	
Absorption	Well absorbed
Distribution	Crosses placenta
Metabolism	Liver
Excretion	Kidneys
Half-life	5-8 hr

Pharmacodynamics	
Onset	½ hr
Peak	2-4 hr
Duration	8 hr

Interactions

Individual drugs

Acyclovir: ↑ toxicity

Allopurinol: ↑ effect

Aspirin: ↑ uricosuric effect

Clofibrate: ↑ effect

Dapsone: ↑ effect

Dyphylline: ↑ effect

Heparin: ↑ effect

Methotrexate: ↑ toxicity

Nitrofurantoin: ↑ toxicity

Penicillamine: ↑ effect

Zidovudine: ↑ effect

Drug classifications

Barbiturates: ↑ effect

Benzodiazepine: ↑ effect

Cephalosporins: ↑ levels

Fluoroquinolones: ↑ levels

NSAIDs: ↑ toxicity

Penicillins: ↑ levels

Herb/drug

Henbane: ↑ anticholinergic effect

Lab test interferences

↑ BSP/urinary PSP, ↑ theophylline levels

False positive: Urine glucose with copper sulfate test

NURSING CONSIDERATIONS

Assessment

• Monitor I&O ratio; observe for decrease in urinary output; increase fluids to 2-3 L/day; urine may be alkalized with sodium bicarbonate acetazolamide

• Assess mobility, joint pain, and swelling in the joints

• Monitor CBC, urine pH, uric acid and BUN, creatinine before and periodically during treatment

Nursing diagnoses

Pain, chronic (uses)

Mobility, impaired (uses)

Knowledge deficit (teaching)

Implementation

• Give with food or antacid to decrease GI upset

• Reduce dosage gradually if uric acid levels are normal after 6 mo

Patient/family education

• Advise patient to increase fluids to 2-3 L/day

• Caution patient to avoid salicylates; probenecid levels will be decreased

• Advise patient to report any pain, redness, or hard area, usually in legs

• Instruct patient in importance of complying with medical regimen including weight loss program, diet restrictions, and alcohol intake

Evaluation
Positive therapeutic outcome
- Decreased pain in joints
- Normal serum uric acid levels
- Increased duration of antiinfectives

---

procainamide ⚷ (℞)
(proe'kane-ah-mide)
Procan SR, Promine, procainamide, Procanbid, Pronestyl, Pronestyl-SR
Func. class.: Antidysrhythmic (Class IA)
Chem. class.: Procaine HCl amide analog
Pregnancy category **C**

Action: Prolongs action potential duration and effective refractory period; reduces disparity in refractory between normal and infarcted myocardium; prevents increased myocardial excitability and conduction contractility

➤**Therapeutic Outcome:** Prevention of dysrhythmias

Uses: PVCs, atrial fibrillation, PAT, ventricular tachycardia, atrial dysrhythmias, ventricular tachycardia

Dosage and routes
Atrial fibrillation/PAT
Adult: PO 1-1.25 g; may give another 750 mg if needed; if no response, 500 mg-1g q2h until desired response; maintenance 50 mg/kg in divided doses q6h

Ventricular tachycardia
Adult: PO 1 g; maintenance 50 mg/kg/day given in 3-hr intervals; sus rel tab 500 mg-1.25 g q6h

Other dysrhythmias
Adult: **IV** bol 100 mg q5 min, given 25-50 mg/min, not to exceed 500 mg; or 17 mg/kg total, then **IV** inf 2-6 mg/min

Available forms: Caps 250, 375, 500 mg; tabs 250, 375, 500 mg; sus rel tabs 250, 500, 750, 1000 mg; inj **IV** 100, 500 mg/ml

Adverse effects
CNS: Headache, dizziness, confusion, psychosis, restlessness, irritability, weakness
*CV: Hypotension, **heart block**, **cardiovascular collapse**, **arrest***
GI: Nausea, vomiting, anorexia, diarrhea, hepatomegaly
HEMA: SLE syndrome, ***agranulocytosis, thrombocytopenia, neutropenia, hemolytic anemia***
INTEG: Rash, urticaria, edema, swelling (rare), pruritus

Contraindications: Hypersensitivity, myasthenia gravis, severe heart block

Precautions: Pregnancy **C**,
Ⓟ lactation, children, renal disease, liver disease, CHF, respiratory depression

Pharmacokinetics	
Absorption	Well absorbed
Distribution	Rapidly distributed
Metabolism	Liver
Excretion	Kidneys, unchanged (50%-70%)
Half-life	2½-4½ hr; increased in renal disease

Pharmacodynamics			
	PO	PO–ext rel	IV
Onset	½ hr	Unknown	Rapid
Peak	1-1½ hr	Unknown	½-1 hr
Duration	3 hr	Up to 8 hr	3-4 hr

Interactions
Individual drugs
Atropine: ↑ anticholinergic effect
Digoxin: ↑ blood levels, toxicity
Disopyramide: ↑ levels, toxicity
Flecainide: ↑ levels, toxicity
Lidocaine: Bradycardia, arrest
Haloperidol: ↑ anticholinergic effect
Mexiletine: ↑ levels, toxicity
Phenytoin: ↑ blood levels
Quinidine: ↑ levels, toxicity
Warfarin: ↑ level, bleeding
Drug classifications
β-Adrenergic blockers: ↑ dysrhythmias, arrest
Calcium channel blockers: ↑ dysrhythmias, arrest
Phenothiazines: ↑ anticholinergic effect
Lab test interferences
↑ CPK

NURSING CONSIDERATIONS
Assessment
• Assess for oxygenation or perfusion deficit: decreased B/P, chest pain, dizziness, loss of consciousness
• Assess respiratory status: auscultate lung fields for bibasilar crackles in patients with advanced CHF
• Monitor I&O ratio; electrolytes: potassium, sodium, chloride; watch for decreasing urinary output, possible retention
• Monitor liver function studies: AST, ALT, bilirubin, alkaline phosphatase
• Monitor ECG continuously to determine drug effectiveness; measure PR, QRS, QT intervals; check for PVCs, other dysrhythmias; check B/P continuously for hypotension, hypertension; for rebound hypertension after 1-2 hr; prolonged PR/QT intervals, QRS complex; if QT or QRS increases by 50% or more, withhold next dose, notify prescriber
• Monitor for dehydration or hypovolemia
• Monitor for CNS symptoms: confusion, psychosis, numbness, depression, involuntary movements; if these occur, drug should be discontinued
• Monitor blood levels (therapeutic level 3-10 µg/ml), ANA titer or NAPA levels; notify prescriber of abnormal results
• Assess cardiac rate, respiration: rate, rhythm, character, chest pain, ventricular tachycardia, supraventricular tachycardia or fibrillation

P

Nursing diagnoses
☑ Cardiac output, decreased (uses)
☑ Impaired gas exchange (adverse reactions)
☑ Knowledge deficit (teaching)

Implementation
PO route
• Give on an empty stomach with a full glass of water
• May be given with meals if GI irritation occurs; absorption will be decreased
• Tab may be crushed and mixed with fluid or foods for patients with swallowing difficulties; do not break, chew, or crush sus-rel tab

---

IV **IV route**
- Give by direct **IV** after diluting 100 mg/10 ml of D_5W or sterile water for inj; give 50 mg/min or less
- Give by intermittent inf after diluting to a conc of 2-4 mg/ml, 200 mg up to 1 g/50-500 ml D_5W; give over 30 min (2-6 mg/min maintenance); use inf pump for correct dosage
- Do not use dark sol or if precipitate is present

Y-site compatibilities:
Amiodarone, famotidine, heparin, hydrocortisone, potassium chloride, ranitidine, vit B/C

Y-site incompatibilities:
Milrinone

Additive compatibilities:
Amiodarone, dobutamine, flumazenil, lidocaine, netilmicin, verapamil

Additive incompatibilities:
Esmolol, ethacrynate, milrinone

Solution compatibilities:
D_5W, D_5/0.9% NaCl, 0.45% NaCl, 0.9% NaCl, water for inj

Patient/family education
- Advise patient to report side effects immediately to prescriber; to take exactly as prescribed; if dose is missed take when remembered if within 3-4 hr of next dose, do not double doses
- Caution patient that dark glasses may be needed for photophobia; to use sunscreen or stay out of sun to prevent burns; avoid temp extremes; impairment of heat-regulating mechanism can occur
- Advise patient to complete follow-up appointment with prescriber including pulmonary function studies, chest x-ray
- Instruct patient that dry mouth may be relieved by frequent sips of water, hard candy, sugarless gum
- Caution patient to make position changes from lying to standing slowly to prevent orthostatic hypotension

Evaluation
Positive therapeutic outcome
- Decreased PVCs, ventricular tachycardia

Treatment of overdose: O_2, artificial ventilation, ECG, administer dopamine for circulatory depression, administer diazepam or thiopental for convulsions, isoproterenol

---

procarbazine (℞)
(proe-kar'ba-zeen)
Matulane, Natulan ✦
Func. class.: Antineoplastic, alkylating agent
Chem. class.: Hydrazine derivative
Pregnancy category　D

Action: Inhibits DNA, RNA, protein synthesis, cell cycle S phase specific; has multiple sites of action; a nonvesicant

▶**Therapeutic Outcome:** Prevention of rapidly growing malignant cells

Uses: Lymphoma, Hodgkin's disease, cancers resistant to other therapy

Investigational uses: Brain, lung malignancies, other lymphomas, multiple myeloma, malignant melanoma, polycythemia vera

---

Dosage and routes
Adult: PO 2-4 mg/kg/day for first wk; maintain dosage of 4-6 mg/kg/day until platelets and WBC fall; after recovery, 1-2 mg/kg/day

P *Child:* PO 50 mg/m²/day for 7 days, then 100 mg/m² until desired response, leukopenia, or thrombocytopenia occurs; 50 mg/day is maintenance after bone marrow recovery

Available forms: Cap 50 mg

Adverse effects
CNS: Headache, dizziness, **seizures,** insomnia, hallucinations, confusion, **coma,** pain, chills, fever, sweating, paresthesias
EENT: Retinal hemorrhage, nystagmus, photophobia, diplopia
GI: Nausea, vomiting, anorexia, diarrhea, constipation, dry mouth, stomatitis
GU: Azoospermia, cessation of menses
HEMA: **Thrombocytopenia, anemia, leukopenia, myelosuppression, bleeding tendencies,** purpura, petechiae, epistaxis
INTEG: Rash, pruritus, dermatitis, alopecia, herpes, hyperpigmentation
MS: Arthralgias, myalgias
RESP: Cough, pneumonitis

Contraindications: Hypersensitivity, thrombocytopenia, bone marrow depression, pregnancy **D**

Precautions: Renal disease, hepatic disease, radiation therapy

Pharmacokinetics

Absorption	Well absorbed
Distribution	Widely distributed; crosses blood-brain barrier
Metabolism	Liver
Excretion	Kidneys
Half-life	1 hr

Pharmacodynamics
Unknown

Interactions
Individual drugs
Alcohol: ↑ CNS depressant, disulfiram reaction
Guanadrel: ↑ hypertensive crisis
Guanethidine: ↑ hypertensive crisis
Levodopa: ↑ hypertensive crisis
Meperidine: Avoid use; paradoxic reactions
Radiation: ↑ toxicity, bone marrow suppression
Reserpine: ↑ hypertensive crisis
Drug classifications
Antidepressants: ↑ hypertensive crisis
Antihistamines: ↑ CNS depression
Antineoplastics: ↑ toxicity bone marrow suppression
CNS depressants: ↑ CNS depression
Local anesthetics: ↑ hypertensive crisis
MAOIs: ↑ seizures, temperature
Opiates: ↑ CNS depression
Sedative/hypnotics: ↑ CNS depression
Sympathomimetic amines: ↑ hypertensive crisis
Vasoconstrictors: ↑ hypertensive crisis

P

NURSING CONSIDERATIONS
Assessment
• Monitor CBC, differential, platelet count weekly; withhold drug if WBC is <4000 or platelet count is <75,000; notify prescriber of results if WBC <20,000/mm³, platelets <150,000/mm³
• Monitor pulmonary function tests, chest x-ray films before, during therapy; chest film should be obtained q2 wk during treatment; check for dyspnea, rales, unproductive cough, chest pain, tachypnea
• Monitor renal function studies: BUN, serum uric acid, urine CrCl before, during therapy; I&O ratio; report fall in urine output of 30 ml/hr; for decreased hyperuricemia
• Monitor for cold, fever, sore throat (may indicate beginning infection); identify edema in feet, joint and stomach pain, shaking; prescriber should be notified
• Assess for bleeding: hematuria, guaiac, bruising or petechiae, mucosa or orifices q8h, no rectal temp
• Assess for tyramine foods in the diet, hypertensive crisis can occur

Nursing diagnoses
☑ Injury, risk for (adverse reactions)
☑ Body image disturbance (adverse reactions)
☑ Infection, risk for (adverse reactions)
☑ Knowledge deficit (teaching)

Implementation
• Give with foods, fluids for GI upset; open cap and give with food/fluids for swallowing difficulty; administer as directed

Patient/family education
• Teach patient to avoid use of products containing aspirin or NSAIDs, razors, commercial mouthwash, since bleeding may occur; to report symptoms of bleeding (hematuria, tarry stools)
• Caution patient to report signs of anemia (fatigue, headache, irritability, faintness, shortness of breath)
• Advise patient to report any changes in breathing or coughing even several mo after treatment; to avoid crowds and persons with respiratory tract or other infections
• Inform patient hair loss is common; discuss the use of wigs or hair pieces
• Caution patient not to have any vaccinations without the advice of the prescriber; serious reactions can occur
• Advise patient that contraception is needed during treatment and for several mo after the completion of therapy

Evaluation
Positive therapeutic outcome
• Absence of swelling at night
• Increased appetite, increased weight

---

prochlorperazine (℞)
(proe-klor-pair′a-zeen)
Chlorpazine, Compa-Z, Compazine, Contranzine, Provazin ♣, Stemetil ♣, Ultrazine
Func. class.: Antiemetic/antipsychotic
Chem. class.: Phenothiazine, piperazine derivative
Pregnancy category   C

Action: Depresses cerebral cortex, hypothalamus, limbic system, which control activity aggression; blocks neurotransmission produced by dopamine at synapse; exhibits a strong α-adrenergic, anticholinergic blocking action; mechanism for antipsychotic effects is unclear; acts centrally by blocking chemoreceptor trigger zone, which in turn acts on vomiting center

▸**Therapeutic Outcome:** Decreased nausea, vomiting, decreased signs and symptoms of psychosis

Uses: Nausea, vomiting, psychosis

Dosage and routes
Postoperative nausea/vomiting
Adult: IM 5-10 mg 1-2 hr before anesthesia; may repeat in 30 min; **IV** 5-10 mg 15-30 min before anesthesia; **IV** inf 20 mg/L D₅W or NS 15-30 min before anesthesia, not to exceed 40 mg/day

Severe nausea/vomiting
Adult: PO 5-10 mg tid-qid; sus rel 15 mg qd in AM or 10 mg q12h; rec 25 mg/bid; IM 5-10 mg; may repeat q4h, not to exceed 40 mg/day

P *Child 18-39 kg:* PO 2.5 mg tid or 5 mg bid; do not exceed 15 mg/day; IM 0.132 mg/kg

P *Child 14-17 kg:* PO/rec 2.5 mg bid-tid, not to exceed 10 mg/day; IM 0.132 mg/kg

P *Child 9-13 kg:* PO/rec 2.5 mg qd-bid, not to exceed 7.5 mg/day; IM 0.132 mg/kg

Antipsychotic
P *Adult and child ≥12 yr:* PO 5-10 mg tid-qid; may increase q2-3 day, max 150 mg/day; IM 10-20 mg q2-4h up to 4 doses, then 10-20 mg q4-6h, max 200 mg/day; rec 10 mg tid-qid may increase by 5-10 mg q2-3 days as needed

P *Child 2-12 yr:* PO 2.5 mg bid-tid; IM 132 μg/kg, max 10 mg/dose

Antianxiety
P *Adult and child ≥12 yr:* 5 mg tid-qid, max 20 mg/day or >12 wk; IM 5-10 mg q3-4h, max 40 mg/day; **IV** 2.5-10 mg; max 40 mg/day

P *Child 2-12 yr:* IM 132 μg/kg

Available forms: Syr 5 mg/ml; inj 5 mg/ml; tabs 5, 10, 25 mg; sus rel caps 10, 15, 30 mg; supp 2.5, 5, 25 mg

Adverse effects
CNS: Tardive dyskinesia, *euphoria,* **depression,** *EPS,* restlessness, tremor, dizziness, **neuroleptic malignant syndrome**
CV: **Circulatory failure, tachycardia**
GI: Nausea, vomiting, anorexia, dry mouth, diarrhea, constipation, weight loss, metallic taste, cramps, hepatitis
RESP: **Respiratory depression**

Contraindications: Hypersensitivity to phenothiazines,

P

coma, seizure, encephalopathy, bone marrow depression

P **Precautions:** Children <2 yr,
G pregnancy **C**, elderly

N **Do Not Confuse:**
Compazine/Coumadin, prochlorperazine/ chlorpromazine

Pharmacokinetics	
Absorption	Variably absorbed (PO); well absorbed (IM)
Distribution	Widely distributed; high concentration in CNS; crosses placenta
Metabolism	Liver, extensively; GI mucosa
Excretion	Kidneys, breast milk
Half-life	Unknown

Pharmacodynamics					
	PO	PO-EXT REL	REC	IM	IV
Onset	½ hr	½ hr	1 hr	10-20 min	4-5 min
Peak	Unkn	Unkn	Unkn	Unkn	Unkn
Duration	3-4 hr	10-12 hr	3-4 hr	3-4 hr	3-4 hr

Interactions
Individual drugs
Alcohol: ↑ effects of both drugs, oversedation
Aluminum hydroxide: ↓ absorption
Bromocriptine: ↓ antiparkinsonian activity
Disopyramide: ↑ anticholinergic effects
Epinephrine: ↑ toxicity
Guanethidine: ↓ antihypertensive response
Levodopa: ↓ antiparkinsonian activity
Lithium: ↓ prochlorperizine levels, ↑ extrapyramidal symptoms, masking of lithium toxicity
Magnesium hydroxide: ↓ absorption

Norepinephrine: ↓ vasoresponse, ↑ toxicity
Phenobarbital: ↓ effectiveness, ↑ metabolism
Drug classifications
Antacids: ↓ absorption
Anticholinergics: ↑ anticholinergic effects
Antidepressants: ↑ CNS depression
Antidiarrheals, adsorbent: ↓ absorption
Antihistamines: ↑ CNS depression
Antihypertensives: ↑ hypotension
Antithyroid agents: ↑ agranulocytosis
Barbiturate anesthetics: ↑ CNS depression
β-Adrenergics: ↑ effects of both drugs
General anesthetics: ↑ CNS depression
MAOIs: ↑ CNS depression
Opiates: ↑ CNS depression
Sedative/hypnotics: ↑ CNS depression
Herb/drug
Henbane: ↑ anticholinergic effect
Lab test interferences
↑ Liver function tests, ↑ cardiac enzymes, ↑ cholesterol, ↑ blood glucose, ↑ prolactin, ↑ bilirubin, ↑ PBI, ↑ cholinesterase, ↑ ^{131}I, ↑ alkaline phosphatase, ↑ leukocytes, ↑ granulocytes, ↑ platelets
↓ Hormones (blood and urine)
False positive: Pregnancy tests, PKU, urine bilirubin
False negative: Urinary steroids, 17-OHCS, pregnancy tests

NURSING CONSIDERATIONS
Assessment
• Assess mental status: orientation, mood, behavior, presence and type of hallucinations

before initial administration and monthly; this drug should significantly reduce psychotic behavior

• Check for swallowing of PO medication; check for hoarding or giving of medication to other patients

G • Monitor I&O ratio; palpate bladder if low urinary output occurs, especially in elderly; urinalysis recommended before, during prolonged therapy

• Monitor bilirubin, CBC, liver function studies monthly

• Assess affect, orientation, LOC, reflexes, gait, coordination, sleep pattern disturbances

• Monitor B/P with patient sitting, standing, and lying; take pulse and respirations q4h during initial treatment; establish baseline before starting treatment; report drops of 30 mm Hg; obtain baseline ECG, Q wave and T wave changes

• Check for dizziness, faintness, palpitations, tachycardia on rising; severe orthostatic hypotension is common

• Identify neuroleptic malignant syndrome: hyperpyrexia, muscle rigidity, increased CPK, altered mental status; drug should be discontinued

• Assess for EPS including akathisia (inability to sit still, no pattern to movements), tardive dyskinesia (bizarre movements of the jaw, mouth, tongue, extremities), pseudoparkinsonism (ragged tremors, pill rolling, shuffling gait); an antiparkinsonism drug should be prescribed

• Assess for constipation, urinary retention daily; if these occur, increase bulk, water in diet

Nursing diagnoses

☑ Thought processes, altered (uses)
☑ Coping, ineffective individual (uses)
☑ Knowledge deficit (teaching)
☑ Noncompliance (teaching)

Implementation
PO route

• Give drug in liq form mixed in glass of juice or cola if hoarding is suspected; do not mix in caffeine drinks, tannics, pectins

G • Give decreased dosage in elderly since metabolism is slowed

• Give PO with full glass of water, milk; or give with food to decrease GI upset

• Store in airtight, light-resistant container; oral sol in amber bottle

• Do not crush or chew sus rel cap

IM route

• Inject slowly in deep muscle mass; do not give SC; aspirate to avoid **IV** administration; do not administer sol with a precipitate; have patient lie down afterward for at least 30 min

IV IV route

• Give by direct **IV** after diluting **IV** using 0.9% NaCl to 1 mg/1 ml; administer at 1 mg/min or less

• Administer by intermittent inf after diluting 20 mg/L or less LR, Ringer's, dextrose, saline, or any combination

Syringe compatibilities:

Atropine, butorphanol, chlorpromazine, cimetidine, diamorphine, diphenhydramine, droperidol, fentanyl, glycopyrrolate, hydroxyzine, meperidine, metoclopramide, nalbuphine, pentazocine, perphenazine, promazine,

P

---

promethazine, ranitidine, scopolamine, sufentanil

Syringe incompatibilities:
Dimenhydrinate, midazolam, pentobarbital, thiopental

Y-site compatibilities:
Amsacrine, calcium gluconate, cisplatin, cladribine, cyclophosphamide, cytarabine, doxorubicin, fluconazole, granisetron, heparin, hydrocortisone, melphalan, methotrexate, ondansetron, paclitaxel, potassium chloride, propofol, sargramostim, sufentanil, teniposide, thiotepa, vinorelbine, vit B/C

Y-site incompatibilities:
Foscarnet

Additive compatibilities:
Amikacin, ascorbic acid, dexamethasone, dimenhydrinate, erythromycin, ethacrynate, lidocaine, nafcillin, netilmicin, sodium bicarbonate, vit B/C

Additive incompatibilities:
Aminophylline, amphotericin B, ampicillin, calcium gluceptate, cefoperazone, cephalothin, chloramphenicol, chlorothiazide, floxacillin, furosemide, hydrocortisone sodium succinate, methohexital sodium, penicillin G sodium, phenobarbital, thiopental

Patient/family education
• Teach patient to use good oral hygiene; frequent rinsing of mouth, sugarless gum for dry mouth
• Caution patient to avoid hazardous activities until drug response is determined; dizziness, blurred vision may occur
• Inform patient that orthostatic hypotension occurs often and to rise from sitting or lying position gradually; to remain lying down after IM inj for at least 30 min; tell patient to avoid hot tubs, hot showers, tub baths, since hypotension may occur; tell patient that in hot weather heat stroke may occur; take extra precautions to stay cool
• Advise patient to avoid abrupt withdrawal of this drug, or EPS may result; drug should be withdrawn slowly
• Teach patient to avoid OTC preparations (cough, hay fever, cold) unless approved by prescriber, since serious drug interactions may occur; avoid use with alcohol, CNS depressants; increased drowsiness may occur; avoid activities requiring mental alertness
• Instruct patient to use a sunscreen and sunglasses to prevent burns
• Teach patient about EPS and necessity of meticulous oral hygiene, since oral candidiasis may occur
• Advise patient to take antacids 2 hr before or after taking this drug
• Advise patient to report sore throat, malaise, fever, bleeding, mouth sores; if these occur, CBC should be drawn and drug discontinued
• Teach patient not to double or skip doses
• Teach patient urine may turn pink to reddish brown
• Instruct patient to report dark urine, clay-colored stools, bleeding, bruising, rash, blurred vision

Evaluation
Positive therapeutic outcome
• Relief of nausea and vomiting
• Decrease in emotional excitement, hallucinations, delusions, paranoia

- Reorganization of patterns of thought, speech

Treatment of overdose: Lavage if orally ingested; provide airway; *do not induce vomiting or use epinephrine*

---

progesterone ♀ (Ŗ)
(proe-jess'ter-one)
Crinone, progesterone,
Progesterone in Oil
Func. class.: Progestogen
Chem. class.: Progesterone derivative

Pregnancy category **X**

Action: Inhibits secretion of pituitary gonadotropins, which prevents follicular maturation, ovulation; stimulates growth of mammary tissue; antineoplastic action against endometrial cancer

Therapeutic Outcome: Decreased abnormal uterine bleeding, absence of amenorrhea

Uses: Contraception, amenorrhea, premenstrual syndrome, abnormal uterine bleeding

Dosage and routes
Infertility
Adult: Vag 90 mg qd

Amenorrhea/uterine bleeding
Adult: IM 5-10 mg qd × 6-8 doses

Available forms: Cap 100 mg; inj 50 mg/ml; powder micronized, vag gel 8%

Adverse effects
CNS: Dizziness, headache, migraines, depression, fatigue
CV: Hypotension, thrombophlebitis, edema, **thromboembolism, stroke, pulmonary embolism, MI**
EENT: Diplopia
GI: *Nausea*, vomiting, anorexia, cramps, increased weight, **cholestatic jaundice**
GU: Amenorrhea, cervical erosion, breakthrough bleeding, dysmenorrhea, vaginal candidiasis, breast changes, *gynecomastia, testicular atrophy, impotence,* endometriosis, **spontaneous abortion**
INTEG: Rash, urticaria, acne, hirsutism, alopecia, oily skin, seborrhea, purpura, melasma
META: Hyperglycemia

Contraindications: Breast cancer, hypersensitivity, thromboembolic disorders, reproductive cancer, genital bleeding (abnormal, undiagnosed), cerebral hemorrhage, pregnancy **X**

Precautions: Lactation, hypertension, asthma, blood dyscrasias, gallbladder disease, CHF, diabetes mellitus, bone disease, depression, migraine headache, convulsive disorders, hepatic disease, renal disease, family history of breast or reproductive tract cancer

Pharmacokinetics	
Absorption	Unknown
Distribution	Unknown
Metabolism	Unknown
Excretion	Breast milk
Half-life	Unknown

Pharmacodynamics			
	IM	REC	VAG
Onset	Unknown	Unknown	Unknown
Peak	Unknown	Unknown	Unknown
Duration	24 hr	24 hr	24 hr

P

Interactions
Individual drugs
Bromocriptine: ↓ effectiveness of bromocriptine
☑ *Herb/drug*
Alfalfa: ↑ hormonal effect
Lab test interferences
↑ Alkaline phosphatase, ↑ nitrogen (urine), ↑ pregnanediol, ↑ amino acids, ↑ factors VII, VIII, IX, X
↓ GTT, ↓ HDL

NURSING CONSIDERATIONS
Assessment
• Monitor B/P at beginning of treatment and periodically; check weight daily; notify prescriber of weekly weight gain >5 lb
• Monitor I&O ratio: be alert for decreasing urinary output, increasing edema, hypertension
• Assess liver function studies: ALT, AST, bilirubin periodically during long-term therapy
• Assess edema, hypertension, cardiac symptoms, jaundice
• Assess mental status: affect, mood, behavioral changes, depression
• Assess hypercalcemia

Nursing diagnoses
☑ Sexual dysfunction (uses)
☑ Tissue perfusion, altered (adverse reactions)
☑ Injury, risk for (adverse reactions)
☑ Knowledge deficit (teaching)

Implementation
IM route
• Store in dark area
• Give titrated dose; use lowest effective dosage; give oil sol deep in large muscle mass; rotate sites; use after warming to dissolve crystals

Patient/family education
• Teach patient to report breast lumps, vaginal bleeding, edema, jaundice, dark urine, clay-colored stools, dyspnea, headache, blurred vision, abdominal pain, numbness or stiffness in legs, chest pain
• Teach patient to report suspected pregnancy

Evaluation
Positive therapeutic outcome
• Decreased abnormal uterine bleeding
• Absence of amenorrhea
• Prevented pregnancy

---

promazine (Ŗ)
(proe′ma-zeen)
promazine, Sparine
Func. class.: Antipsychotic/neuroleptic
Chem. class.: Phenothiazine, aliphatic
Pregnancy category　C

Action: Depresses cerebral cortex, hypothalamus, limbic system, which control activity, aggression; blocks neurotransmission produced by dopamine at synapse; exhibits a strong α-adrenergic, anticholinergic blocking action; as antiemetic, inhibits medullary chemoreceptor trigger zone; mechanism for antipsychotic effects is unclear

▶ **Therapeutic Outcome:** Decreased signs and symptoms of psychosis, absence of nausea, vomiting

Uses: Psychotic disorders, schizophrenia, nausea, vomiting, alcohol withdrawal

Dosage and routes
Psychosis
Adult: PO 10-200 mg q4-6h; max dose 1000 mg/day; IM 50-150 mg, followed in 30

---

min with additional dose up to a total dose of 300 mg

G *Elderly:* PO 25 mg qd-bid, increase by 25 mg q4-7 days

P *Child >12 yr:* PO 10-25 mg q4-6h

Available forms: Tabs 25, 50 mg; inj 25, 50 mg/ml

Adverse effects

CNS: Extrapyramidal symptoms: pseudoparkinsonism, akathisia, dystonia, tardive dyskinesia, drowsiness, headache, **seizures, neuroleptic malignant syndrome**

CV: Orthostatic hypotension, **cardiac arrest,** ECG changes, **tachycardia**

EENT: Blurred vision, glaucoma, dry eyes

GI: Dry mouth, nausea, vomiting, anorexia, constipation, diarrhea, jaundice, weight gain

GU: Urinary retention, urinary frequency, enuresis, impotence, amenorrhea, gynecomastia

HEMA: Anemia, **leukopenia, leukocytosis, agranulocytosis**

INTEG: Rash, photosensitivity, dermatitis

RESP: **Laryngospasm,** dyspnea, **respiratory depression**

Contraindications: Hypersensitivity, blood dyscrasias, coma, **P** child <12 yr, brain damage, bone marrow depression, glaucoma

Precautions: Pregnancy **C,** lactation, seizure disorders, hypertension, hepatic disease, cardiac disease

Pharmacokinetics

Absorption	Variably absorbed (PO); well absorbed (IM); completely absorbed (**IV**)
Distribution	Widely distributed; high concentrations in CNS; crosses placenta
Metabolism	Liver, extensively
Excretion	Kidneys, breast milk
Half-life	Unknown

Pharmacodynamics

	PO	IM
Onset	½ hr	Up to ½ hr
Peak	2-4 hr	Unknown
Duration	4-6 hr	4-6 hr

Interactions

Individual drugs

Alcohol: ↑ effects of both drugs, oversedation

Aluminum hydroxide: ↓ absorption

Bromocriptine: ↓ antiparkinsonian activity

Disopyramide: ↑ anticholinergic effects

Epinephrine: ↑ toxicity

Guanethidine: ↓ antihypertensive response

Levodopa: ↓ antiparkinsonian activity

Lithium: ↓ promazine levels, ↑ EPS, masking of lithium toxicity

Magnesium hydroxide: ↓ absorption

Norepinephrine: ↓ vasoresponse, ↑ toxicity

Phenobarbital: ↓ effectiveness, ↑ metabolism

Drug classifications

Antacids: ↓ absorption

Anticholinergics: ↑ anticholinergic effects

Antidepressants: ↑ CNS depression

Antidiarrheals, adsorbent: ↓ absorption

Antihistamines: ↑ CNS depression

P

Antihypertensives: ↑ hypotension

Antithyroid agents: ↑ agranulocytosis

Barbiturate anesthetics: ↑ CNS depression

β-Adrenergics: ↑ effects of both drugs

General anesthetics: ↑ CNS depression

MAOIs: ↑ CNS depression

Opiates: ↑ CNS depression

Sedative/hypnotics: ↑ CNS depression

☑ *Herb/drug*

Henbane: ↑ anticholinergic effect

Lab test interferences

↑ Liver function tests, ↑ cardiac enzymes, ↑ cholesterol, ↑ blood glucose, ↑ prolactin, ↑ bilirubin, ↑ PBI, ↑ cholinesterase, ↑ iodine, ↑ alkaline phosphatase, ↑ leukocytes, ↑ granulocytes, ↑ platelets ↓ Hormones (blood and urine)

False positive: Pregnancy tests, PKU, urine bilirubin

False negative: Urinary steroids, 17-OHCS

NURSING CONSIDERATIONS
Assessment

• Assess mental status: orientation, mood, behavior, presence and type of hallucinations before initial administration and monthly; this drug should significantly reduce psychotic behavior

• Check for swallowing of PO medication; check for hoarding or giving of medication to other patients

• Monitor I&O ratio; palpate bladder if low urinary output ☐ occurs, especially in elderly; urinalysis recommended before, during prolonged therapy

• Monitor bilirubin, CBC, liver function studies monthly

• Assess affect, orientation, LOC, reflexes, gait, coordination, sleep pattern disturbances

• Monitor B/P with patient sitting, standing and lying, take pulse and respirations q4h during initial treatment; establish baseline before starting treatment; report drops of 30 mm Hg; obtain baseline ECG, Q wave and T wave changes

• Check for dizziness, faintness, palpitations, tachycardia on rising; severe orthostatic hypotension is common

◆• Identify for neuroleptic malignant syndrome: hyperpyrexia, muscle rigidity, increased CPK, altered mental status; drug should be discontinued

• Assess for EPS including akathisia (inability to sit still, no pattern to movements), tardive dyskinesia (bizarre movements of the jaw, mouth, tongue, extremities), pseudoparkinsonism (ragged tremors, pill rolling, shuffling gait); an antiparkinsonian drug should be prescribed

• Assess for constipation, urinary retention daily; if these occur, increase bulk, water in diet

Nursing diagnoses
☑ Thought processes, altered (uses)
☑ Coping, ineffective individual (uses)
☑ Knowledge deficit (teaching)
☑ Noncompliance (teaching)

Implementation
PO route
• Give decreased dosage in ☐ elderly since metabolism is slowed

• Give PO with full glass of water, milk; or give with food to decrease GI upset

---

☑ Herb/drug ⊘ Do Not Crush ◆ Alert ⟿ Key Drug ☐ Geriatric ☐ Pediatric

- Store in airtight, light-resistant container

IM route

- Inject in deep muscle mass; do not give SC; do not administer sol with a precipitate; patient should remain recumbent for at least 30 min to prevent severe hypotension

Patient/family education

- Teach patient to use good oral hygiene; frequent rinsing of mouth, sugarless gum for dry mouth
- Advise patient to avoid hazardous activities until drug response is determined; dizziness, blurred vision may occur
- Inform patient that orthostatic hypotension occurs often and to rise from sitting or lying position gradually; to remain lying down after IM injection for at least 30 min; tell patient to avoid hot tubs, hot showers, tub baths, since hypotension may occur; tell patient that in hot weather heat stroke may occur; take extra precautions to stay cool
- Caution patient to avoid abrupt withdrawal of this drug, or EPS may result; drug should be withdrawn slowly
- Teach patient to avoid OTC preparations (cough, hay fever, cold) unless approved by prescriber, since serious drug interactions may occur; avoid use with alcohol, CNS depressants; increased drowsiness may occur
- Caution patient to use a sunscreen and sunglasses to prevent burns
- Teach patient about EPS and necessity of meticulous oral hygiene, since oral candidiasis may occur
- Instruct patient to take

antacids 2 hr before or after taking this drug

- Teach patient to report sore throat, malaise, fever, bleeding, mouth sores; if these occur, CBC should be drawn and drug discontinued
- Teach patient that urine may turn pink or red

Evaluation

Positive therapeutic outcome

- Decrease in emotional excitement, hallucinations, delusions, paranoia
- Reorganization of patterns of thought, speech

Treatment of overdose:
Lavage if orally ingested; provide airway; *do not induce vomiting or use epinephrine*

---

promethazine (R)
(proe-meth′a-zeen)
Anergan 50, Phenergan, Phenergan Fortis, Phenergan Plain, promethazine HCl
Func. class.: Antihistamine, H_1-receptor antagonist; antiemetic; sedative/hypnotic
Chem. class.: Phenothiazine derivative

Pregnancy category   C

Action: Acts on blood vessels, GI, respiratory system by competing with histamine for H_1-receptor site; decreases allergic response by blocking histamine; also acts on chemoreceptor trigger zone to decrease vomiting; increases CNS stimulation, has anticholinergic response

➡**Therapeutic Outcome:** Absence of allergy symptoms and

P

rhinitis, absence of nausea/vomiting, sedation

Uses: Motion sickness, rhinitis, allergy symptoms, sedation, nausea, preoperative and postoperative sedation

Dosage and routes
Nausea
Adult: PO/IM/**IV**/rec 10-25 mg; may repeat 12.5-25 mg q4-6h
P *Child >2 yr:* PO/IM/**IV**/rec 0.25-0.5 mg/kg q4-6h
Motion sickness
Adult: PO 25 mg bid; give 30-60 min before departure
P *Child >2 yr:* PO/IM/rec 12.5-25 mg bid; give 30-60 min before departure
Allergy/rhinitis
Adult: PO 12.5 mg qid, or 25 mg hs
P *Child >2 yr:* PO 6.25-12.5 mg tid or 25 mg hs
Sedation
Adult: PO/IM/**IV**/rec 25-50 mg hs
P *Child >2 yr:* PO/IM/rec/**IV** 12.5-25 mg hs
Sedation (preoperative/postoperative)
Adult: PO/IM/**IV** 25-50 mg
P *Child >2 yr:* PO/IM/**IV** 12.5-25 mg

Available forms: Tabs 12.5, 25, 50 mg; supp 12.5, 25, 50 mg; inj 25, 50 mg/ml; syrup 6.25, 10, 25 mg/5 ml

Adverse effects
CNS: Dizziness, drowsiness, poor coordination, fatigue, anxiety, euphoria, confusion, paresthesia, neuritis, EPS
CV: Hypotension, palpitations, tachycardia

EENT: Blurred vision, dilated pupils, tinnitus, nasal stuffiness, dry nose, throat, mouth, photosensitivity
GI: Constipation, dry mouth, nausea, vomiting, anorexia, diarrhea
GU: Retention, dysuria, frequency
HEMA: **Thrombocytopenia, agranulocytosis, hemolytic anemia**
INTEG: Rash, urticaria, photosensitivity
RESP: Increased thick secretions, wheezing, chest
P tightness, **apnea in pediatric patients**

Contraindications: Hypersensitivity to H_1-receptor antagonist, acute asthma attack, lower respiratory tract disease

Precautions: Increased intraocular pressure, renal disease, cardiac disease, hypertension, bronchial asthma, seizure disorder, stenosed peptic ulcers, hyperthyroidism, prostatic hypertrophy, bladder neck obstruction, pregnancy **C**

Do Not Confuse:
Phenergan/Theragran

Pharmacokinetics	
Absorption	Well absorbed (PO, IM); erratically absorbed (rec)
Distribution	Widely distributed; crosses the blood-brain barrier, placenta
Metabolism	Liver
Excretion	Kidneys, breast milk
Half-life	Unknown

Pharmacodynamics		
	PO/IM/REC	IV
Onset	20 min	3-5 min
Peak	Unknown	Unknown
Duration	4-6 hr	4-6 hr

Interactions
Individual drugs
Alcohol: ↑ CNS depression
Atropine: ↑ anticholinergic reactions
Disopyramide: ↑ anticholinergic reactions
Haloperidol: ↑ anticholinergic reactions
Quinidine: ↑ anticholinergic reactions
Drug classifications
Antidepressants: ↑ anticholinergic reactions
Antihistamines: ↑ anticholinergic reactions
CNS depressants: ↑ CNS depression
MAOIs: ↑ anticholinergic effect
Opiates: ↑ CNS depression
Phenothiazines: ↑ anticholinergic reactions
Sedative/hypnotics: ↑ CNS depression
☑ Herb/drug
Henbane: ↑ anticholinergic effect
Lab test interferences
False negative: Skin allergy tests (discontinue antihistamines 3 days before testing)
↑ Serum glucose

NURSING CONSIDERATIONS
Assessment
• Assess respiratory status: rate, rhythm, increase in bronchial secretions, wheezing, chest tightness; provide fluids to 2 L/day to decrease secretion thickness
• Monitor I&O ratio: be alert for urinary retention, frequency, dysuria, especially
G elderly; drug should be discontinued if these occur
• Monitor CBC during long-term therapy; blood dyscrasias may occur but are rare

Nursing diagnoses
☑ Airway clearance, ineffective (uses)
☑ Injury, risk for (adverse reactions)
☑ Knowledge deficit (teaching)
☑ Noncompliance (teaching, overuse)

Implementation
PO route
• Give with meals to decrease GI upset
• Store in tight, light-resistant container
IM route
• Give IM inj in large muscle mass; aspirate to avoid **IV** administration; do not give SC; necrosis may occur
IV IV route
• Give **IV** directly; give 25 mg or less over 1 min; rapid drop in B/P may occur with rapid administration

Syringe compatibilities:
Atropine, butorphanol, chlorpromazine, cimetidine, diphenhydramine, droperidol, fentanyl, glycopyrrolate, hydromorphone, hydroxyzine, meperidine, metoclopramide, midazolam, pentazocine, perphenazine, prochlorperazine, promazine, ranitidine, scopolamine

Syringe incompatibilities:
Dimenhydrinate, heparin, pentobarbital, thiopental

Y-site compatibilities:
Amifostine, amsacrine, aztreonam, ciprofloxacin, cisplatin, cladribine, cyclophosphamide, cytarabine, doxorubicin, filgrastim, fluconazole, fludarabine, granisetron, melphalan, ondansetron, sargramostim, teniposide, thiotepa, vinorelbine

P

Y-site incompatibilities:
Cefoperazone, foscarnet,
heparin

Additive compatibilities:
Amikacin, ascorbic acid, chloroquine, hydromorphone,
netilmicin, vit B/C

Additive incompatibilities:
Aminophylline, carbenicillin,
chloramphenicol, chlorothiazide, floxacillin, furosemide,
heparin, hydrocortisone sodium succinate, methicillin,
methohexital, penicillin G,
pentobarbital, phenobarbital,
thiopental

Patient/family education
• Inform patient that a false
negative result may occur
with skin testing; these procedures should not be scheduled
until 3 days after discontinuing use
• Advise patient to take 30
min before departure to prevent motion sickness
• Caution patient to avoid
hazardous activities, activities
requiring alertness, since dizziness may occur; instruct patient to request assistance with
ambulation
• Advise patient to avoid alcohol, other depressants; serious
CNS depression may occur
• Teach all aspects of drug use;
to notify prescriber if confusion, sedation, hypotension
occur; to avoid driving and
other hazardous activity if
drowsiness occurs; to avoid
alcohol and other CNS depressants that may potentiate effect
• Advise patient to take 1 hr ac
or 2 hr pc to facilitate absorption
• Caution patient not to exceed recommended dosage;
dysrhythmias may occur
• Inform patient hard candy,

gum, frequent rinsing of
mouth may be used for dryness

Evaluation
Positive therapeutic outcome
• Absence of motion sickness
• Absence of nausea, vomiting

Treatment of overdose:
Administer ipecac syrup or
lavage, diazepam, vasopressors,
barbiturates (short-acting)

---

propantheline (℞)
(proe-pan'the-leen)
Pro-Banthine,
Propanthel ✦,
propantheline bromide
Func. class.: GI anticholinergic; antimuscarinic
Chem. class.: Synthetic
quaternary ammonium
compound
Pregnancy category C

Action: Inhibits muscarinic
actions of acetylcholine at
postganglionic parasympathetic
neuroeffector sites

Therapeutic Outcome: Absence of peptic ulcer disease
symptoms

Uses: Treatment of peptic
ulcer disease, irritable bowel
syndrome, duodenography,
urinary incontinence

Investigational uses: Antispasmodic uses

Dosage and routes
Adult: PO 15 mg tid ac, 30
mg hs

G *Elderly:* PO 7.5 mg tid ac

Antispasmodic
P *Child:* PO 2-3 mg/kg/day

Antisecretory
P *Child:* PO 1.5 mg/kg/day in
3-4 divided doses

Available forms: Tabs 7.5, 15 mg

Adverse effects

CNS: *Confusion, stimulation in* **G** *elderly,* headache, insomnia, dizziness, drowsiness, anxiety, weakness, hallucinations

CV: Palpitations, tachycardia, **G** orthostatic hypotension (elderly)

EENT: *Blurred vision,* photophobia, mydriasis, cycloplegia, increased ocular tension

GI: *Dry mouth, constipation,* **paralytic ileus,** heartburn, nausea, vomiting, dysphagia, absence of taste

GU: Hesitancy, retention, impotence

INTEG: Urticaria, rash, pruritus, anhidrosis, fever, allergic reactions

Contraindications: Hypersensitivity to anticholinergics, narrow-angle glaucoma, GI obstruction, myasthenia gravis, paralytic ileus, GI atony, toxic megacolon

Precautions: Hyperthyroidism, CAD, dysrhythmias, CHF, ulcerative colitis, hypertension, hiatal hernia, hepatic disease, renal disease, pregnancy **C,** urinary retention, prostatic hypertrophy

Pharmacokinetics	
Absorption	Moderately absorbed
Distribution	Unknown
Metabolism	Unknown
Excretion	Unknown
Half-life	Unknown

Pharmacodynamics	
Onset	½ hr
Peak	2-6 hr
Duration	4-6 hr

Interactions

Individual drugs

Amantadine: ↑ anticholinergic effect

Atropine: ↑ anticholinergic effect

Disopyramide: ↑ anticholinergic effect

Haloperidol: ↑ anticholinergic effect

Potassium chloride, oral: ↑ GI lesions

Quinidine: ↑ anticholinergic effect

Drug classifications

Antacids: ↓ absorption of propantheline

Anticholinergics: ↑ anticholinergic effect

Antidepressants, tricyclic: ↑ anticholinergic effect

Antihistamines: ↑ anticholinergic effect

Phenothiazines: ↑ anticholinergic effect

NURSING CONSIDERATIONS

Assessment

• Assess for the pain of peptic ulcer disease before, during, and after treatment

Nursing diagnoses

☑ Pain (uses)

☑ Constipation (adverse reactions)

☑ Thought processes, impaired (adverse reactions)

☑ Knowledge deficit (teaching)

Implementation

• Give 30 min ac and at hs; do not give with antacids; separate by at least 1 hr

Patient/family education

• Teach patient to report blurred vision, chest pain, allergic reactions

• Advise patient not to perform strenuous activity in high temp; heat stroke may result due to decreased perspiration

P

- Instruct patient to take as prescribed; not to skip doses
- Instruct patient to report change in vision; blurring or loss of sight; drug should be discontinued
- Advise patient not to operate machinery or drive if dizziness occurs
- Caution patient not to take OTC products without approval of prescriber

Evaluation
Positive therapeutic outcome
- Decreased pain in peptic ulcer disease

---

propoxyphene (℞)
(proe-pox'i-feen)
Darvin, Darvon-N, Dolene, Novapropoxyn ✿, propoxyphene HCl
Func. class.: Opiate analgesics
Chem. class.: Synthetic opiate

Pregnancy category C
Controlled substance schedule IV

Action: Depresses pain impulse transmission at the spinal cord level by interacting with opioid receptors

➤**Therapeutic Outcome:** Decreased pain

Uses: Mild to moderate pain

Dosage and routes
Adult: PO 65 mg q4h prn (HCl)

Adult: PO 100 mg q4h prn (napsylate)

Available forms: Propoxyphene HCl: cap 32, 65 mg; propoxyphene napsylate: tabs 100 mg; oral susp 50 mg/5 ml

Adverse effects
CNS: *Drowsiness, dizziness, confusion, headache, sedation,* euphoria, **convulsions, hyperthermia**
CV: Palpitations, bradycardia, change in B/P, **dysrhythmias**
EENT: Tinnitus, blurred vision, miosis, diplopia
GI: *Nausea, vomiting, anorexia, constipation, cramps*
GU: Urinary retention, dysuria
INTEG: *Rash,* urticaria, bruising, flushing, diaphoresis, pruritus
RESP: **Respiratory depression**

Contraindications: Hypersensitivity to ASA products (some preparations), addiction (narcotic)

Precautions: Addictive personality, pregnancy **C,** lactation, increased intracranial pressure, MI (acute), severe heart disease, respiratory depression, **P** hepatic disease, renal **G** disease, child <18 yr, elderly

Pharmacokinetics	
Absorption	Well absorbed
Distribution	Widely distributed; crosses placenta
Metabolism	Liver, extensively
Excretion	Kidneys, breast milk
Half-life	6-12 hr

Pharmacodynamics	
Onset	½-1 hr
Peak	2-2½ hr
Duration	4-6 hr

Interactions
Individual drugs
Alcohol: ↑ respiratory depression, hypotension, sedation
Nalbuphine: ↓ analgesia
Pentazocine: ↓ analgesia

Drug classifications
Antihistamines: ↑ respiratory depression, hypotension
CNS depressants: ↑ respiratory depression, hypotension
MAOIs: Use ↓ dosage; reaction is unpredictable
Sedative/hypnotics: ↑ respiratory depression, hypotension
Smoking
↓ analgesic effect
Lab test interferences
↑ Amylase

NURSING CONSIDERATIONS
Assessment
• Assess pain: location, duration, intensity before and 1 hr after administration
• Monitor CNS changes: dizziness, drowsiness, euphoria, LOC, pupil reaction
• Monitor allergic reactions: rash, urticaria

Nursing diagnoses
✓ Pain (uses)
✓ Sensory-perceptual alteration: visual, auditory (adverse reactions)
✓ Breathing pattern, ineffective (adverse reactions)
✓ Injury, risk for (adverse reactions)
✓ Knowledge deficit (teaching)

Implementation
• Give with antiemetic if nausea, vomiting occur
• Give when pain is beginning to return; determine dosage interval by patient response; continuous dosing of medication is more effective than when given prn
• Withdraw medication slowly after long-term use to prevent withdrawal symptoms
• Store in light-resistant container at room temp
• May be given with food or milk to lessen GI upset

Patient/family education
• Teach patient to avoid CNS depressants: alcohol, sedative/hypnotics for at least 24 hr after taking this drug
• Discuss with patient that dizziness, drowsiness, and confusion are common; to avoid getting up without assistance
• Discuss in detail all aspects of the drug, including purpose and what to expect after anesthesia
• Advise patient to make position changes slowly to lessen orthostatic hypotension

Evaluation
Positive therapeutic outcome
• Decreased pain

Treatment of overdose:
Narcan 0.2-0.8 mg **IV**, O_2, **IV** fluids, vasopressors

---

propranolol ⚬π (℞)
(proe-pran'oh-lole)
Apo-Propranolol ✢, Detensol ✢, Inderal, Inderal LA, propranolol HCl, Propranolol Intensol, Novopranol ✢
Func. class.: Antihypertensive, antianginal
Chem. class.: β-Adrenergic blocker
Pregnancy category C

Action: Competitively blocks stimulation of β-adrenergic receptor within vascular smooth muscle; produces chronotropic, inotropic activity (decreases rate of SA node discharge, increases recovery time), slows conduction of AV node, decreased heart rate, which decreases O_2 consumption in myocardium; also suppresses renin-aldosterone-angiotensin system at high doses, inhibits β_2-receptors in bronchial system (high doses)

⇒**Therapeutic Outcome:** Decreased B/P, heart rate

Uses: Chronic stable angina pectoris, hypertension, supraventricular dysrhythmias, migraine, prophylaxis, MI, pheochromocytoma, essential tremor, tetralogy of Fallot, cyanotic spells

Investigational uses: Mitral valve prolapse, anxiety, dysrhythmias associated with thyrotoxicosis

Dosage and routes
Dysrhythmias
Adult: PO 10-30 mg tid-qid; **IV** bol 0.5-3 mg over 1 mg/min; may repeat in 2 min; may repeat q4h thereafter

P *Child:* PO 0.5-1 mg/kg/day divided q6-8h, **IV** 0.01-0.1 mg/kg

Hypertension
Adult: PO 40 mg bid or 80 mg qd (ext rel) initially; usual dosage 120-240 mg/day bid-tid or 120-160 mg qd (ext rel)

P *Child:* PO 0.5-1 mg/kg/day divided q6-12h

Angina
Adult: PO 80-320 mg in divided doses bid-qid or 80 mg qd (ext rel); usual dosage 160 mg qd (ext rel)

MI prophylaxis
Adult: PO 180-240 mg/day tid-qid starting 5 days to 3 wk after MI

Pheochromocytoma
Adult: PO 60 mg/day × 3 days preoperatively in divided doses or 30 mg/day in divided doses (inoperable tumor)

Migraine
Adult: PO 80 mg/day (ext rel) or in divided doses; may increase to 160-240 mg/day in divided doses

P *Child:* PO 0.6-1.5 mg/kg/day divided q8h

Essential tremor
Adult: PO 40 mg bid; usual dosage 120 mg/day

Tetralogy of Fallot
P *Child:* PO 1-2 mg/kg/dose q6h

Available forms: Sus rel caps 60, 80, 120, 160 mg; caps ext rel 60 mg; tabs 10, 20, 40, 60, 90 mg; inj 1 mg/ml; oral sol 4 mg, 8 mg/ml; conc oral sol 80 mg/ml

Adverse effects
CNS: Depression, hallucinations, dizziness, fatigue, lethargy, paresthesia, bizarre dreams, disorientation
CV: Bradycardia, hypotension, **CHF,** palpitations, AV block, peripheral vascular insufficiency, vasodilatation
EENT: Sore throat, **laryngospasm,** blurred vision, dry eyes
GI: Nausea, vomiting, diarrhea, colitis, constipation, cramps, dry mouth, hepatomegaly, gastric pain, acute pancreatitis
GU: Impotence, decreased libido, UTIs
HEMA: **Agranulocytosis, thrombocytopenia**
INTEG: Rash, pruritus, fever
META: Hyperglycemia, hypoglycemia
MISC: Facial swelling, weight change, Raynaud's phenomenon
MS: Joint pain, arthralgia, muscle cramps, pain
RESP: Dyspnea, respiratory dysfunction, **bronchospasm**

Contraindications: Hypersensitivity to this drug, cardiac failure, cardiogenic shock, 2nd- or 3rd-degree heart block, bronchospastic disease, sinus bradycardia, CHF

Precautions: Diabetes mellitus, pregnancy **C,** renal disease, lactation, hyperthyroidism, COPD, hepatic disease, ▣ children, myasthenia gravis, peripheral vascular disease, hypotension, CHF

▶ **Do Not Confuse:**
Inderal/Toradol, Inderal LA/ IMDUR

Pharmacokinetics	
Absorption	Well absorbed (PO); slowly absorbed (ext rel); completely absorbed (**IV**)
Distribution	Widely distributed; crosses blood-brain barrier
Metabolism	Liver, extensively
Excretion	Kidneys
Half-life	3-5 hr; ext rel 8-11 hr

Pharmacodynamics			
	PO	PO–Ext Rel	IV
Onset	½ hr	Unknown	Rapid
Peak	1-1½ hr	6 hr	1 min
Duration	6-12 hr	24 hr	4-6 hr

Interactions
Individual drugs
Alcohol: ↑ hypotension (large amounts)
Epinephrine: α-Adrenergic stimulation
Hydralazine: ↑ hypotension, bradycardia
Indomethacin: ↓ antihypertensive effect
Insulin: ↑ hypoglycemia
Methyldopa: ↑ hypotension, bradycardia
Prazosin: ↑ hypotension, bradycardia

Reserpine: ↑ hypotension, bradycardia
Thyroid: ↓ effect of propranolol
Verapamil: ↑ myocardial depression
Drug classifications
Antihypertensive: ↑ hypertension
Cardiac glycosides: ↑ bradycardia
Nitrates: ↑ hypotension
Sulfonylureas: ↓ hypoglycemic effect
Theophyllines: ↓ bronchodilatation
Lab test interferences
False: ↑ Urinary catecholamines

NURSING CONSIDERATIONS
Assessment
• Monitor B/P during beginning treatment, periodically thereafter; pulse q4h; note rate, rhythm, quality; check apical/radial pulse before administration; notify prescriber of any significant changes (pulse <50 bpm)
• Check for baselines in renal, liver function tests before therapy begins and periodically thereafter
• Assess for edema in feet, legs daily; monitor I&O, weight daily; check for jugular vein distention, rales bilaterally; dyspnea (CHF)
• Monitor skin turgor, dryness of mucous membranes for hydration status, especially ▣ elderly

Nursing diagnoses
✓ Cardiac output, decreased (uses)
✓ Injury, potential for (adverse reactions)
✓ Knowledge deficit (teaching)
✓ Noncompliance (teaching)

Implementation
PO route
• Given ac, hs, tab may be crushed or swallowed whole; do not crush or chew ext rel cap; give with food to prevent GI upset; reduce dosage in renal dysfunction
• Store protected from light, moisture; placed in cool environment

IV **IV route**
• Give by direct **IV** undiluted or diluted 1 mg/10 ml D_5W for inj; administer over 1 min or more
• Give by intermittent inf after diluting in 50 ml D_5W, 0.9% NaCl, D_5/0.45% NaCl, D_5/0.9% NaCl, LR; administer over 15 min

Syringe compatibilities:
Amrinone, benzquinamide, milrinone

Y-site compatibilities:
Amrinone, heparin, hydrocortisone, meperidine, milrinone, morphine, potassium chloride, tacrolimus, vit B/C

Y-site incompatibilities:
Diazoxide

Additive compatibilities:
Dobutamine, verapamil

Solution compatibilities:
0.9% NaCl, 0.45% NaCl, Ringer's, D_5W, D_5/0.9% NaCl, D_5/0.45% NaCl

Patient/family education
• Teach patient not to discontinue drug abruptly, taper over 2 wk; may cause precipitate angina if stopped abruptly
• Teach patient not to use OTC products containing α-adrenergic stimulants (such as nasal decongestants, cold preparations); to avoid alcohol, smoking and to limit sodium intake as prescribed
• Teach patient how to take pulse and B/P at home; advise when to notify prescriber
• Instruct patient to comply with weight control, dietary adjustments, modified exercise program
• Instruct patient to carry/wear Medic Alert ID to identify drug being taken, allergies; tell patient drug controls symptoms but does not cure
• Caution patient to avoid hazardous activities if dizziness, drowsiness is present
• Teach patient to report symptoms of CHF: difficult breathing, especially on exertion or when lying down, night cough, swelling of extremities or bradycardia, dizziness, confusion, depression, fever
• Teach patient to take drug as prescribed, not to double doses, skip doses; take any missed doses as soon as remembered if at least 8 hr until next dose

Evaluation
Positive therapeutic outcome
• Decreased B/P in hypertension (after 1-2 wk)
• Decreased tremors
• Absence of dysrhythmias
• Decreased migraine headaches

Treatment of overdose:
Lavage, **IV** atropine for bradycardia, **IV** theophylline for bronchospasm, digitalis, O_2, diuretic for cardiac failure, hemodialysis, **IV** glucose for hyperglycemia, **IV** diazepam (or phenytoin) for seizures

---

propylthiouracil (℞)
(proe-pill-thye-oh-yoor'a-sill)
propylthiouracil, Propyl-
Thyracil ✦, PTU
Func. class.: Thyroid
hormone antagonist
(antithyroid)
Chem. class.: Thioamide
Pregnancy category D

Action: Blocks synthesis peripherally of T_3, T_4, inhibits
organification of iodine

➡ **Therapeutic Outcome:** Decreased T_3, T_4 levels, hyperthyroid symptoms

Uses: Preparation for thyroidectomy, thyrotoxic crisis, hyperthyroidism, thyroid storm

Dosage and routes
Thyrotoxic crisis
🅟 *Adult and child:* PO same as
hyperthyroidism with iodine
and propranolol

*Preparation for
thyroidectomy*
Adult: PO 600-1200 mg/day
🅟 *Child:* PO 10 mg/kg/day in
divided doses

Hyperthyroidism
Adult: PO 100 mg tid increasing to 300 mg q8h if condition
is severe; continue to euthyroid
state, then 100 mg qd-tid
🅟 *Child >10 yr:* PO 100 mg tid;
continue to euthyroid state,
then 25 mg tid to 100 mg bid
🅟 *Child 6-10 yr:* PO 50-150 mg
in divided doses q8h
🅟 *Neonates:* PO 10 mg/kg/
day in divided doses
Available forms: Tab 50 mg
Adverse effects
CNS: Drowsiness, headache,

vertigo, fever, paresthesias,
neuritis
*GI: Nausea, diarrhea, vomit-
ing, jaundice, hepatitis,* loss of
taste
GU: **Nephritis**
HEMA: **Agranulocytosis,
leukopenia, thrombocytopenia, hypothrombinemia,
lymphadenopathy,** bleeding,
vasculitis, periarteritis
*INTEG: Rash, urticaria, pru-
ritus, alopecia, hyperpigmentation,* lupuslike syndrome
MS: Myalgia, arthralgia, nocturnal muscle cramps, osteoporosis

Contraindications: Hypersensitivity, pregnancy **D**, lactation

Precautions: Infection, bone
marrow depression, hepatic
disease

Pharmacokinetics	
Absorption	Rapidly absorbed
Distribution	Crosses placenta; concentration in thyroid gland
Metabolism	Liver
Excretion	Urine, bile, breast milk
Half-life	1-2 hr

Pharmacodynamics	
Onset	30-40 min
Peak	Unknown
Duration	2-4 hr

Interactions
Individual drugs
Heparin: ↑ anticoagulant
effect
Lithium: ↑ antithyroid effect
Radiation: ↑ bone marrow
depression
Drug classifications
Antineoplastics: ↑ bone mar-
row depression
Oral anticoagulants: ↑ antico-
agulant effect

Phenothiazines: ↑ agranulocytosis

Lab test interferences
↑ Pro-time, ↑ AST, ↑ ALT, ↑ alkaline phosphatase

NURSING CONSIDERATIONS
Assessment
• Monitor pulse, B/P, temp; I&O ratio; check for edema (puffy hands, feet, periorbits); indicates hypothyroidism
• Check weight daily with same clothing, scale, time of day
• Monitor T_3, T_4, which are increased; check serum TSH, which is decreased; assess free thyroxine index, which is increased if dosage is too low; discontinue drug 3-4 wk before RAIU
• Monitor blood work: CBC for blood dyscrasias (leukopenia, thrombocytopenia, agranulocytosis); liver function tests
◆• Assess overdose (peripheral edema, heat intolerance, diaphoresis, palpitations, dysrhythmias, severe tachycardia, increased temp, delirium, CNS irritability); drug should be discontinued
• Assess for hypersensitivity (rash, enlarged cervical lymph nodes); drug may have to be discontinued
• Assess for hypoprothrombinemia (bleeding, petechiae, ecchymosis)
• Monitor clinical response: after 3 wk should include increased weight, decreased pulse, decreased T_4
• Assess for bone marrow depression: sore throat, fever, fatigue

Nursing diagnoses
☑ Knowledge deficit (teaching)
☑ Noncompliance (teaching)

Implementation
• Give with meals to decrease GI upset
• Give at same time each day to maintain drug level
• Give lowest dosage that relieves symptoms
• Store in light-resistant container
• Increase fluids to 3-4 L/day, unless contraindicated

Patient/family education
• Advise patient to abstain from breastfeeding after delivery; drug appears in breast milk
• Teach patient to take pulse daily and to keep graph of weight, pulse, mood
• Advise patient to report redness, swelling, sore throat, mouth lesions, which indicate blood dyscrasias
• Caution patient to avoid OTC products that contain iodine; that seafood, other iodine-containing foods may be restricted by prescriber
• Caution patient not to discontinue this medication abruptly; thyroid crisis may occur; stress patient compliance
• Teach patient that response may take several mo if thyroid is large
• Teach patient symptoms/signs of overdose: periorbital edema, cold intolerance, mental depression; notify prescriber at once
• Teach patient symptoms of inadequate dose: tachycardia, diarrhea, fever, irritability; prescriber should be notified to adjust dosage
• Teach patient to take medication exactly as prescribed, not to skip or double doses; missed doses should be taken when remembered up to 1 hr before next dose

☑ Herb/drug ⑤ Do Not Crush ◆ Alert ⟳ Key Drug ⑥ Geriatric ℗ Pediatric

• Instruct patient to carry identification (Medic Alert) indicating medication taken and condition being treated

Evaluation
Positive therapeutic outcome
• Weight gain
• Decreased pulse
• Decreased T_4
• Decreased B/P

---

protamine (℞)
(proe'ta-meen)
Func. class.: Heparin antagonist
Chem. class.: Low-molecular-weight protein
Pregnancy category **C**

Action: Binds heparin, making it ineffective

➔ Therapeutic Outcome: Prevention of heparin overdose

Uses: Heparin overdose; neutralizes heparin in procedures

Dosage and routes
P *Adult and child:* **IV** 1 mg of protamine/90-115 U heparin given; administer slowly over 1-3 min; not to exceed 50 mg/10 min

Available forms: Inj 10 mg/ml

Adverse effects
CNS: Lassitude
CV: Hypotension, bradycardia, **circulatory collapse**
GI: Nausea, vomiting, anorexia
INTEG: Rash, dermatitis, urticaria
HEMA: Bleeding, **anaphylaxis**
RESP: Dyspnea, **pulmonary edema, severe respiratory distress**

Contraindication: Hypersensitivity

Precautions: Pregnancy **C**, **P** lactation, children, allergy to fish

Pharmacokinetics
Absorption	Completely absorbed
Distribution	Unknown
Metabolism	Unknown
Excretion	Unknown
Half-life	Unknown

Pharmacodynamics
Onset	5 min
Peak	Unknown
Duration	2 hr

Interactions: None

NURSING CONSIDERATIONS
Assessment
• Monitor blood studies (Hct, platelets, occult blood stools) q3 mo
• Monitor coagulation tests (APTT, ACT) 15 min after dose, then in several hr
• Monitor VS, B/P, pulse q 30 min, plus 3 hr after dose
• Assess for skin rash, urticaria, dermatitis
• Assess for allergy to fish; use with caution in these patients

Nursing diagnoses
✓ Injury, risk for (uses)
✓ Tissue perfusion, altered (uses)
✓ Knowledge deficit (teaching)

Implementation
• Give by direct **IV** after diluting 50 mg/5 ml sterile bacteriostatic water for inj; shake; give 20 mg or less over 1-3 min
• Give by intermittent inf after further diluting with equal volume of NaCl or D_5W and run over 2-3 min; titrate to APTT, ACT; use inf pump
• Store at 36° to 46° F (2°-8° C)

P

♣ Canada Only   Adverse effects: *italic* = common; **bold** = life-threatening

Additive compatibilities:
Cimetidine, ranitidine, verapamil

Additive incompatibilities:
Penicillins, cephalosporins

Patient/family education
• Explain reason for medication and expected results
• Caution patient to avoid contact activities that may result in bleeding

Evaluation
Positive therapeutic outcome
• Reversal of heparin overdose

---

pseudoephedrine (OTC)
(soo-doe-e-fed′rin)
Afrin, Allermed, Canafed, Cenafed, Children's Congestion Relief, Children's Silfedrine, Congestion Relief, Decofed Syrup, DeFed-60, Dorcol Children's Decongestant, Drixoral Non-Drowsy Formula, Dynafed, Eltor ♦, Efidac/24, Genaphed, Halofed, Mini Thin Pseudo, Pedia Care Infant's Decongestant, pseudoephedrine HCl, Pseudogest, Seudotabs, Sinustop Pro, Sudafed, Sudafed 12 hour, Sudex, Triaminic AM Decongestant Formula
Func. class.: Adrenergic
Chem. class.: Substituted phenylethylamine

Pregnancy category   B

Action: Primary activity through α-adrenergic effects on respiratory mucosal membranes reducing congestion, hyperemia, edema; minimal bronchodilatation secondary to β-adrenergic effects

▷**Therapeutic Outcome:** Decreased nasal congestion, swelling

Uses: Nasal decongestant, otitis media adjustment, adjunct with antihistamines

Dosage and routes
P *Adult and child >12 yr:* PO 60 mg q6h; ext rel 60-120 mg q12h or q24h

G *Elderly:* PO 30-60 mg q6h prn

P *Child 6-12 yr:* PO 30 mg q6h, not to exceed 120 mg/day

P *Child 2-6 yr:* PO 15 mg q6h, not to exceed 60 mg/day

Available forms: Ext rel caps 120, 240 mg; oral sol 15 mg, 30 mg/5 ml; drops 7.5 mg/ 0.8 ml; tabs 30, 60 mg; cap 60 mg; ext rel tabs 120 mg

Adverse effects
CNS: Tremors, anxiety, insomnia, headache, dizziness, anxiety, hallucinations, **seizures**
CV: Palpitations, tachycardia, hypertension, chest pain, **dysrhythmias**
EENT: Dry nose, irritation of nose and throat
GI: Anorexia, nausea, vomiting, dry mouth
GU: Dysuria

Contraindications: Hypersensitivity to sympathomimetics, narrow-angle glaucoma

Precautions: Pregnancy **B,** cardiac disorders, hyperthyroidism, diabetes mellitus, prostatic hypertrophy

---

Pharmacokinetics

Absorption	Well absorbed
Distribution	Enters CSF, crosses placenta
Metabolism	Liver, partially
Excretion	Kidneys, unchanged (75%); breast milk
Half-life	7 hr

Pharmacodynamics

	PO	PO-EXT REL
Onset	15-30 min	1 hr
Peak	Unknown	Unknown
Duration	4-6 hr	12 hr

Interactions
Individual drugs
Methyldopa: ↓ effect of pseudoephedrine
Rauwolfia: ↓ effect of pseudoephedrine
Drug classifications
β-Adrenergic blockers: Hypertensive crisis
MAOIs: Hypertensive crisis
Urinary acidifiers: ↓ effect of pseudoephedrine
Urinary alkalizers: ↑ effect of pseudoephedrine

NURSING CONSIDERATIONS
Assessment
G • Assess for CNS side effects in the elderly: excitation, seizures, hallucinations
• Monitor for nasal congestion; auscultate lung sounds; check for tenacious
P bronchial secretions; children with otitis media should be assessed for eustachian tube congestion
• Monitor B/P and pulse throughout treatment

Nursing diagnoses
✓ Airway clearance, ineffective (uses)
✓ Knowledge deficit (teaching)

Implementation
• Give ext rel cap and tab whole
🚫 • Do not crush, break or chew
• Give several hr before hs if insomnia occurs
• Store at room temp

Patient/family education
• Teach patient reason for drug administration and expected results
• Instruct patient not to use continuously, or more than recommended dose; rebound congestion may occur
• Advise patient to check with prescriber before using other drugs, as drug interactions may occur
• Advise patient to avoid taking near bedtime; stimulation can occur
• Caution patient not to use if stimulation, restlessness, tremors occur
P • Notify parents of possible excessive agitation in children

Evaluation
Positive therapeutic outcome
• Decreased nasal congestion

P

psyllium (OTC)
(sill'i-um)
Alramucil, Fiberall, Fiberall
Natural Flavor and Orange
Flavor, Genifiber, Hydrocil
Instant, Karacil ✦, Konsyl,
Konsyl Orange, Maalox Daily
Fiber Therapy, Metamucil,
Metamucil Lemon Lime,
Metamucil Orange Flavor,
Metamucil Sugar Free,
Metamucil Sugar Free
Orange Flavor, Modane
Bulk, Mylanta Natural Fiber
Supplement, Natural Fiber
Laxative, Natural Fiber
Laxative Sugar Free, Natural
Vegetable Reguloid,
Perdiem, Prodiem Plain ✦,
Reguloid Natural, Reguloid
Orange, Reguloid Sugar Free
Orange, Reguloid Sugar Free
Regular, Restore, Restore
Sugar Free, Serutan, Syllact,
V-Lax
Func. class.: Laxative,
bulk-forming
Chem. class.: Psyllium
colloid

Pregnancy category   C

Action: Promotes peristalsis by
combining with water in the
intestine to form a gel-like
substance that is easily evacuated

⇒**Therapeutic Outcome:** Decreased constipation, decreased
diarrhea in colitis

Uses: Chronic constipation,
ulcerative colitis, irritable
bowel syndrome

Dosage and routes
Adult: PO 1-2 tsp in 8 oz
water bid or tid, then 8 oz
water or 1 premeasured packet
in 8 oz water bid or tid, then 8
oz water

P *Child >6 yr:* 1 tsp in 4 oz
water hs

Available forms: Chew pieces
1.7, 3.4 g/piece; powder
effervescent 3.4, 3.7 g/packet;
granules 2.5, 4.03 g/tsp;
powder 3.3, 3.4, 3.5, 4.94
g/tsp; wafers 3.4 g/wafer

Adverse effects
*GI: Nausea, vomiting, an-
orexia, diarrhea,* cramps,
intestinal/esophageal blockage

Contraindications: Hypersensitivity, intestinal obstruction,
abdominal pain, nausea/
vomiting, fecal impaction

Precautions: Pregnancy **C**

Pharmacokinetics	
Absorption	None
Distribution	None
Excretion	Feces
Half-life	Unknown

Pharmacodynamics	
Onset	12-24 hr
Peak	2-4 days
Duration	Unknown

Interactions
Drug classifications
Cardiac glycosides: ↓ absorp-
tion of cardiac glycosides
Oral anticoagulants: ↓ ab-
sorption of oral anticoagu-
lants
Salicylates: ↓ absorption of
salicylates
Lab test interferences
↑ Blood glucose

NURSING CONSIDERATIONS
Assessment
• Monitor blood, urine electrolytes if used often by
patient; check I&O ratio to
identify fluid loss
• Assess for cramping, rec

bleeding, nausea, vomiting; if these symptoms occur, drug should be discontinued; identify cause of constipation; identify whether fluids, bulk, or exercise is missing from lifestyle
• Assess stool for color, consistency, amount, presence of flatulence

Nursing diagnoses
☑ Constipation (uses)
☑ Knowledge deficit (teaching)
☑ Noncompliance (teaching)

Implementation
• Give alone for better absorption; give after mixing with water immediately before use; administer with 8 oz water or juice followed by another 8 oz of fluid
• Administer in AM or PM (oral dose)

Patient/family education
• Discuss with patient that adequate fluid consumption is necessary
• Teach patient that normal bowel movements do not always occur daily
• Caution patient not to use in presence of abdominal pain, nausea, vomiting; tell patient to notify prescriber if constipation is unrelieved or if symptoms of electrolyte imbalance occur (muscle cramps, pain, weakness, dizziness, excessive thirst)
• Teach patient not to use laxatives for long-term therapy; bowel tone will be lost and will decrease
• Teach patient to shake susp well as needed
• Teach patient not to take at hs as a laxative; may interfere with sleep; also problems with lipid pneumonia

• Teach patient not to use with food or vitamin preparations; delays digestion and absorption of fat-soluble vitamins

Evaluation
Positive therapeutic outcome
• Decreased constipation in 12-24 hr

---

pyrazinamide (℞)
(peer-a-zin'a-mide)
PMS Pyrazinamide ✤, pyrazinamide, Tebrazid ✤
Func. class.: Antitubercular agent
Chem. class.: Pyrazinoic acid amine/nicoturimide analog
Pregnancy category   C

Action: Bactericidal interference with lipid; nucleic acid biosynthesis is possible

▶**Therapeutic Outcome:** Bactericidal for *Mycobacterium* species

Uses: Tuberculosis, as an adjunct when other drugs are not feasible

Dosage and routes
▣*Adult and child:* PO 15-30 mg/kg qd, not to exceed 3 g/day

Available forms: Tab 500 mg

Adverse effects
CNS: Headache
GI: Hepatotoxicity, abnormal liver function tests, peptic ulcer, nausea, vomiting, anorexia
GU: Urinary difficulty, increased uric acid
HEMA: Hemolytic anemia
INTEG: Photosensitivity, urticaria

Contraindications: Hypersensitivity, severe hepatic damage

Precautions: Pregnancy **C**, **P** child <13 yr

Pharmacokinetics

Absorption	Well absorbed
Distribution	Widely distributed
Metabolism	Liver, extensively
Excretion	Kidneys, breast milk
Half-life	9-10 hr

Pharmacodynamics

Onset	Unknown
Peak	2 hr
Duration	9½ hr; metabolites 12 hr

Interactions: None

NURSING CONSIDERATIONS
Assessment
• C&S studies should be taken before treatment begins, and periodically during treatment
• Monitor serum uric acid, which may be elevated and cause gout symptoms
• Monitor liver studies weekly: ALT, AST, bilirubin; hepatic status: decreased appetite, jaundice, dark urine, fatigue
• Monitor renal status: before treatment and monthly thereafter: BUN, creatinine, output, sp gr, urinalysis, uric acid
• Monitor mental status often: affect, mood, behavioral changes; psychosis may occur

Nursing diagnoses
☑ Infection, risk for (uses)
☑ Diarrhea (adverse reactions)
☑ Injury, risk for (adverse reactions)
☑ Knowledge deficit (teaching)
☑ Noncompliance (teaching)

Implementation
• Give with meals to decrease GI symptoms
• Give antiemetic if vomiting occurs

• May be given with other antituberculars

Patient/family education
• Instruct patient that compliance with dosage schedule, duration is necessary; that scheduled appointments must be kept or relapse may occur
• Advise diabetic patient to use blood glucose monitor to obtain correct result
• Advise patient to report weakness, fatigue, loss of appetite, nausea, vomiting, yellowing of skin or eyes, tingling/numbness of hands/feet

Evaluation
Positive therapeutic outcome
• Decreased symptoms of TB
• Sputum culture negative × 3

---

pyridostigmine (℞)
(peer-id-oh-stig′meen)
Regonol
Func. class.: Cholinergic, anticholinesterase
Chem. class.: Tertiary amine carbamate

Pregnancy category   C

Action: Inhibits destruction of acetylcholine, which increases concentration at sites where acetylcholine is released; this facilitates transmission of impulses across myoneural junction

Therapeutic Outcome: Decreased action of nondepolarizing muscle relaxant; increased muscle strength in myasthenia gravis

Uses: Nondepolarizing muscle relaxant antagonist, myasthenia gravis

---

Dosage and routes
Myasthenia gravis
Adult: PO 60-180 mg bid-qid, not to exceed 1.5 g/day; IM/**IV** 1/30 of PO dose; sus rel 180-540 mg qd or bid at intervals of at least 6 hr

P *Child:* 7 mg/kg/day in 5-6 divided doses

Nondepolarizing neuromuscular blocker antagonist
Adult: 0.6-1.2 mg **IV** atropine, then 10-30 mg

P *Child:* 0.1-0.25 mg/kg/dose

Available forms: Tab 60 mg; sus rel tab 180 mg; syr 60 mg/5 ml; inj 5 mg/ml

Adverse effects
CNS: Dizziness, headache, sweating, weakness, **convulsions,** uncoordination, paralysis, drowsiness, LOC
CV: Tachycardia, dysrhythmias, bradycardia, AV block, hypotension, ECG changes, **cardiac arrest,** syncope
EENT: Miosis, blurred vision, lacrimation, visual changes
GI: Nausea, diarrhea, vomiting, cramps, increased salivary and gastric secretions, peristalsis
GU: Frequency, incontinence, urgency
INTEG: Rash, urticaria, flushing
RESP: **Respiratory depression, bronchospasm, constriction, laryngospasm, respiratory arrest**

Contraindications: Bradycardia, hypotension, obstruction of intestine, or renal system, bromide sensitivity

Precautions: Seizure disorders, bronchial asthma, coronary occlusion, hyperthyroidism, dysrhythmias, peptic ulcer, megacolon, poor GI motility, pregnancy **C**

Pharmacokinetics
Absorption	Poorly absorbed (PO)
Distribution	Widely distributed; crosses placenta
Metabolism	Liver, plasma cholinesterase
Excretion	Kidneys
Half-life	2 hr (**IV**); 4 hr (PO)

Pharmacodynamics
	PO	IM/IV	PO-SUS REL
Onset	20-30 min	2-15 min	½-1 hr
Peak	Unknown	Unknown	Unknown
Duration	3-6 hr	2-4 hr	3-6 hr

Interactions
Individual drugs
Digitalis: Bradycardia
Magnesium: ↓ action of pyridostigmine
Mecamylamine: ↓ action of pyridostigmine
Polymyxin: ↓ action of pyridostigmine
Procainamide: ↓ action of pyridostigmine
Quinidine: ↓ action of pyridostigmine
Drug classifications
Antidepressants: ↑ antagonism
Antihistamines: ↑ antagonism
Cholinesterase inhibitors: ↑ toxicity
Muscle relaxants, depolarizing: ↑ action of muscle relaxants
Phenothiazines: ↑ antagonism

NURSING CONSIDERATIONS
Assessment
• Monitor VS, respiration; ↑ B/P during test and at baseline

P

• Monitor diabetic patient carefully, since this drug lowers blood glucose

Nursing diagnoses

☑ Breathing pattern, ineffective (uses)

☑ Knowledge deficit (teaching)

Implementation

IV IV route

• Give **IV** undiluted, give through Y-tube or 3-way stopcock; give 0.5 mg or less/min

• Give only when atropine sulfate available for cholinergic crisis

Syringe compatibilities:
Glycopyrrolate

Y-site compatibilities:
Heparin, hydrocortisone, potassium chloride, vit B/C

PO route

• Give only after all other cholinergics have been discontinued

• Give increased doses if tolerance occurs

• Give larger doses after exercise or fatigue

• Give on empty stomach for better absorption

• Store at room temp

Patient/family education

• Advise patient to wear Medic Alert ID specifying myasthenia gravis, drugs taken

Evaluation

Positive therapeutic outcome

• Increased muscle strength, hand grasp

• Improved gait

• Absence of labored breathing (if severe)

Treatment of overdose:
Discontinue drug, atropine 1-4 mg **IV**

---

pyridoxine (vitamin B₆)
(OTC, ℞)
(peer-i-dox′een)
Nestrex, pyridoxine HCl, Vitamin B₆
Func. class.: Vitamin B₆, water soluble

Pregnancy category **A**

Action: Needed for fat, protein, carbohydrate metabolism; enhances glycogen release from liver and muscle tissue; needed as coenzyme for metabolic transformations of a variety of amino acids

▶ **Therapeutic Outcome:** Absence of vitamin B₆ deficiency

Uses: Vitamin B₆ deficiency associated with the following: inborn errors of metabolism, seizures, cycloserine, hydralazine penicillamine, isoniazid therapy, oral contraceptives, alcoholism, polyneuritis

Dosage and routes
RDA
Adult: Male 1.7-2 mg; female 1.4-1.6 mg

Vitamin B₆ deficiency
Adult: PO/IM/**IV** 10-20 mg qd × 3 wk

P *Child:* PO/IM/**IV** 100 mg until desired response

Deficiency caused by isoniazid, cycloserine, hydralazine, penicillamine
Adult: PO 6-100 mg qd

P *Child:* PO 5-25 mg/day

Prevention of deficiency caused by isoniazid, cycloserine, hydralazine, penicillamine
Adult: PO 6-50 mg qd

P *Child:* PO 0.5-1.5 mg qd

☑ Herb/drug 🚫 Do Not Crush ◆ Alert ⌐ Key Drug **G** Geriatric **P** Pediatric

P *Infant:* PO 0.1-0.5 mg qd

Available forms: Tabs 10, 25, 50, 100 mg; time rel tabs 100 mg; inj 100 mg/ml; time rel caps 100 mg

Adverse effects
CNS: Paresthesia
INTEG: Pain at inj site

Contraindication: Hypersensitivity

Precautions: Pregnancy **A,** **P** lactation, children, Parkinson's disease

Pharmacokinetics	
Absorption	Well absorbed (PO)
Distribution	Stored in liver, muscle, brain; crosses placenta
Metabolism	Unknown
Excretion	Kidneys, unchanged (not used)
Half-life	Unknown

Pharmacodynamics
Unknown

Interactions
Individual drugs
Chloramphenicol: ↓ effects of pyridoxine
Cycloserine: ↓ effects of pyridoxine
Hydralazine: ↓ effects of pyridoxine
Isoniazid: ↓ effects of pyridoxine
Levodopa: ↓ effects of levodopa
Penicillamine: ↓ effects of pyridoxine
Drug classifications
Immunosuppressants: ↓ effects of pyridoxine
Oral contraceptives: ↓ effects of pyridoxine
Lab Test Interferences
False: ↑ Urobilinogen

NURSING CONSIDERATIONS
Assessment
• Monitor pyridoxine levels throughout treatment
• Assess nutritional status: yeast, liver, legumes, bananas, green vegetables, whole grains
• Assess for pyridoxine (B₆) deficiency: nausea, vomiting, dermatitis, cheilosis, seizures, irritability, dermatitis before and during treatment

Nursing diagnoses
✓ Nutrition: less then body requirements (uses)
✓ Knowledge deficit (teaching)
✓ Noncompliance (teaching, overuse)

Implementation
IV route
• Give **IV** undiluted or added to most **IV** sol; give 50 mg or less/1 min if undiluted
IM route
• Rotate sites; burning or stinging at site may occur; give by Z-track to minimize pain
• Store in tight, light-resistant container

Syringe compatibilities: Doxapram

Additive incompatibilities: Erythromycin, iron salts, kanamycin, riboflavin, streptomycin
PO route
⊘ • Ext rel cap and tab should be swallowed whole; do not break, crush, or chew
IM/SC route
• Administer in different site each time to avoid pain

Patient/family education
• Teach patient to avoid other vitamin supplements unless directed by prescriber
• Advise patient to increase meat, bananas, potatoes, lima beans, whole grain cereals in

P

diet which are high in vitamin B_6

• Caution patient not to increase dosage, since serious reactions may occur

Evaluation
Positive therapeutic outcome
• Absence of nausea, vomiting, anorexia, skin lesions, glossitis, stomatitis, edema, convulsions, restlessness, paresthesia

---

pyrimethamine (℞)
(peer-i-meth'a-meen)
Daraprim, Fansidar (with sulfadoxine)
Func. class.: Antimalarial, antiprotozoal
Chem. class.: Folic acid antagonist
Pregnancy category C

Action: Inhibits folic acid metabolism in parasite; prevents transmission by stopping growth of fertilized gametes

▶**Therapeutic Outcome:** Prevention of malaria

Uses: Malaria prophylaxis, antiprotozoal action against *Plasmodium vivax*

Investigational uses: *Pneumocystis carinii* pneumonia as an adjunct

Dosage and routes
Prophylaxis of malaria
P **Adult and child >10 yr:** PO 25 mg qwk

P **Child 4-10 yr:** PO 12.5 mg qwk

P **Child <4 yr:** PO 6.25 mg qwk

Toxoplasmosis
Adult: PO 100 mg, then 25 mg qd × 4-5 wk, with 1 g sulfadiazine q6h

P **Child:** PO 1 mg/kg/day in 2 divided doses or 2 mg/kg/day × 3 days, then 1 mg/kg/day or divided twice qd × 4 wk, max 25 mg/day

Toxoplasmosis in AIDS patients
Adult: PO 100-200 mg/day × 1-2 days, then 50-100 mg/day × 3-6 wk, then 25-50 mg/day for life (given with clindamycin or sulfadiazine)

Available forms: Tab 25 mg; combo tab 500 mg sulfadoxine/25 mg pyrimethamine

Adverse effects
CNS: Stimulation, irritability, **convulsions,** tremors, ataxia, fatigue
GI: Nausea, vomiting, cramps, anorexia, diarrhea, atrophic glossitis, gastritis
HEMA: **Thrombocytopenia, leukopenia, pancytopenia, megaloblastic anemia,** decreased folic acid, **agranulocytosis**
INTEG: Skin eruptions, photosensitivity
RESP: **Respiratory failure**

Contraindications: Hypersensitivity, chloroquine-resistant malaria, megaloblastic anemia caused by folate deficiency

Precautions: Blood dyscrasias, seizure disorder, pregnancy **C,** lactation, G6PD disease, renal/hepatic disease

Pharmacokinetics	
Absorption	Well absorbed
Distribution	Widely; crosses placenta
Metabolism	Liver, extensively
Excretion	Kidneys, unchanged (30%); breast milk
Half-life	4 days

Pharmacodynamics	
Onset	Unknown
Peak	2 hr
Duration	Unknown

Interactions
Individual drugs
Folic acid: ↑ synergistic action
Drug classifications
Antiinfectives: ↑ bone marrow suppression

NURSING CONSIDERATIONS
Assessment
• C&S studies should be taken before treatment begins and periodically during treatment
• Monitor serum uric acid, which may be elevated and cause gout symptoms
• Monitor liver studies weekly: ALT, AST, bilirubin; hepatic status: decreased appetite, jaundice, dark urine, fatigue
• Monitor renal status: before therapy and monthly thereafter: BUN, creatinine, output, sp gr, urinalysis
• Monitor mental status often: affect, mood, behavioral changes; psychosis may occur

Nursing diagnoses
☑ Infection, risk for (uses)
☑ Diarrhea (adverse reactions)
☑ Injury, risk for (adverse reactions)
☑ Knowledge deficit (teaching)
☑ Noncompliance (teaching)

Implementation
• Give with meals to decrease GI symptoms
• Give antiemetic if vomiting occurs

Patient/family education
• Instruct patient that compliance with dosage schedule, duration is necessary; that scheduled appointments must be kept or relapse may occur
• Advise diabetic patient to use blood glucose monitor to obtain correct result
• Advise patient to report weakness, fatigue, loss of appetite, nausea, vomiting, yellowing of skin or eyes, sore throat, glossitis

Evaluation
Positive therapeutic outcome
• Decreased symptoms of toxoplasmosis
• Decreased symptoms of *Pneumocystis carinii* pneumonia

---

quetiapine (℞)
(kwe-tie'a-peen)
Seroquel
Func. class.: Antipsychotic/neuroleptic
Pregnancy category C

Action: Functions as an antagonist at multiple neurotransmitter receptors in the brain including $5HT_{1A}$, $5HT_2$, dopamine D_1, D_2, H_1, adrenergic α_{-1}, α_{-2} receptors

→ **Therapeutic Outcome:** Decreased hallucination and disorganized thought

Uses: Psychotic disorders

Dosage and routes
Adult: PO 25 mg bid, with incremental increases of 25-50 mg bid-tid on days 2 and 3 to a dose of 300-400 mg qd given bid-tid

Available forms: Tabs 25, 100, 200 mg

Adverse effects
CNS: Extrapyrimidal symptoms, pseudoparkinsonism,

Q

akathisia, dystonia, tardive dyskinesia, drowsiness, insomnia, agitation, anxiety, *headache,* **neuroleptic malignant syndrome,** dizziness
CV: Orthostatic hypotension, **tachycardia**
GI: Nausea, anorexia, constipation, abdominal pain, dry mouth
INTEG: Rash
MISC: Asthenia, back pain, fever, ear pain
RESP: Rhinitis

Contraindications: Hypersensitivity

P **Precautions:** Children, lactation, long-term use, seizures, dementia, pregnancy **C,** hepatic disease, elderly, breast cancer

Pharmacokinetics	
Absorption	Rapidly
Distribution	Widely
Metabolism	Liver, extensively
Excretion	Urine, feces
Half-life	≥6 hr

Pharmacodynamics	
Onset	Unknown
Peak	1.5 hr
Duration	Up to 12 hr

Interactions
Individual drugs
Cimetidine: ↓ clearance of quetiapine
Levodopa: ↓ effect of levodopa
Lorazepam: ↓ clearance of lorazepam
Phenytoin: ↑ clearance of quetiapine
Thioridazine: ↑ clearance of quetiapine

Drug classifications
Barbiturates: ↑ clearance of quetiapine

Dopamine agonists: ↓ effects of dopamine agonists
Glucocorticoids: ↑ clearance of quetiapine

NURSING CONSIDERATIONS
Assessment
• Assess mental status: orientation, mood, behavior, presence and type of hallucinations before initial administration and monthly; this drug should significantly reduce psychotic behavior
• Check that patient swallows all PO medication; check for hoarding or giving of medication to other patients
• Monitor I&O ratio, palpate bladder if low urinary output **G** occurs, especially in elderly; urinalysis recommended before, during prolonged therapy
• Monitor bilirubin, CBC, liver function studies monthly
• Assess affect, orientation, LOC, reflexes, gait, coordination, sleep pattern disturbances
• Monitor B/P with patient in sitting, standing, and lying positions; take pulse and respirations q4h during initial treatment; establish baseline before starting treatment; report drops of 30 mm Hg; obtain baseline ECG; and Q-wave and T-wave changes
• Check for dizziness, faintness, palpitations, tachycardia on rising; severe orthostatic hypotension is common
• Identify for neuroleptic malignant syndrome: hyperpyrexia, muscle rigidity, increased CPK, altered mental status; drug should be discontinued

---

☑ Herb/drug   ⊘ Do Not Crush   ◆ Alert   ☛ Key Drug   **G** Geriatric   **P** Pediatric

• Assess for extrapyramidal symptoms including akathisia (inability to sit still, no pattern to movements), tardive dyskinesia (bizarre movements of the jaw, mouth, tongue, extremities) pseudoparkinsonism (rigidity, tremors, pill rolling, shuffling gait); an antiparkinson drug should be prescribed

• Assess for constipation, urinary retention daily; if these occur, increase bulk, water in diet

Nursing diagnoses

✓ Thought processes, altered (uses)
✓ Coping, ineffective individual (uses)
✓ Knowledge deficit (teaching)
✓ Noncompliance (teaching)

Implementation

• PO with full glass of water, milk; or give with food to decrease GI upset
• Store in airtight, light-resistant container

Patient/family education

• Teach patient to use good oral hygiene; frequent rinsing of mouth, sugarless gum for dry mouth
• Caution patient to avoid hazardous activities until drug response is determined—dizziness, blurred vision may occur
• Inform patient that orthostatic hypotension occurs often—patient should rise from sitting or lying position gradually
• Instruct patient to avoid hot tubs, hot showers, tub baths—hypotension may occur
• Inform patient that heat stroke may occur in hot

weather, and to take extra precautions to stay cool
• Advise patient to avoid abrupt withdrawal of this drug, or extrapyramidal symptoms may result; drug should be withdrawn slowly
• Teach patient to avoid OTC preparations (cough, hayfever, cold) unless approved by prescriber—serious drug interactions may occur; avoid use with alcohol, CNS depressants because increased drowsiness may occur

Evaluation

Positive therapeutic outcome

• Decrease in emotional excitement, hallucinations, delusions, paranoia
• Reorganization of patterns of thought, speech

Treatment of overdose: Lavage, provide airway

---

quinapril (℞)
(kwin′a-pril)
Accupril
Func. class.: Antihypertensive
Chem. class.: Angiotensin-converting enzyme (ACE) inhibitor

Pregnancy category **D** (2nd/3rd trimesters); **C** (1st trimester)

Q

Action: Selectively suppresses renin-angiotensin-aldosterone system; inhibits ACE, prevents conversion of angiotensin I to angiotensin II; results in dilation of arterial, venous vessels

➔ **Therapeutic Outcome:** Decreased B/P in hypertension

Uses: Hypertension, alone or in combination with thiazide diuretics, systolic CHF

Dosage and routes
Hypertension
Adult: PO 10-20 mg qd initially, then 20-80 mg/day divided bid or qd

G *Elderly:* PO 10 mg qd, titrate to desired response

Congestive heart failure
Adult: PO 2.5 mg initially, then 5-40 mg/day maintenance dose given qd or in 2 divided doses

Renal dose
CrCl 30-60 ml/min 5 mg/day initially; CrCl <30 ml/min 2.5 mg/day initially

Available forms: Tabs 5, 10, 20, 40 mg

Adverse effects
CNS: Headache, dizziness, fatigue, somnolence, depression, malaise, nervousness, vertigo
CV: Hypotension, postural hypotension, syncope, palpitations, angina pectoris, MI, tachycardia, vasodilation
GI: Nausea, constipation, vomiting, gastritis, GI hemorrhage, dry mouth
GU: Increased BUN, creatinine, decreased libido, impotence, urinary tract infection
HEMA: **Thrombocytopenia, agranulocytosis**
INTEG: **Angioedema,** rash, sweating, photosensitivity, pruritus
META: Hyperkalemia
MISC: Back pain, amblyopia, pharyngitis
MS: Arthralgia, arthritis, myalgia
RESP: Cough, bronchitis

Contraindications: Hypersensitivity to ACE inhibitors, pregnancy **D** (2nd/3rd trimesters), children **P**

Precautions: Impaired renal and liver function, dialysis patients, hypovolemia, blood dyscrasias, COPD, asthma, elderly, lactation, pregnancy **C** **G** (1st trimester)

Pharmacokinetics	
Absorption	Well absorbed
Distribution	Unknown, crosses placenta
Metabolism	Unknown
Excretion	Unknown
Half-life	2 hr

Pharmacodynamics	
Onset	½-1 hr
Peak	2-6 hr
Duration	12-24 hr

Interactions
Individual drugs
Alcohol: ↑ hypotension (large amounts)
Allopurinol: ↑ hypersensitivity
Hydralazine: ↑ toxicity
Indomethacin: ↓ antihypertensive effect
Lithium: ↑ serum levels
Prazosin: ↑ toxicity
Drug classifications
Adrenergic blockers: ↑ hypotension
Antacids: ↓ absorption
Antihypertensives: ↑ hypotension
Diuretics: ↑ hypotension
Diuretics, potassium-sparing: ↑ toxicity
Ganglionic blockers: ↑ hypotension
Potassium supplements: ↑ toxicity
Sympathomimetics: ↑ toxicity

Lab test interferences
False positive: Urine acetone

NURSING CONSIDERATIONS
Assessment
• Monitor blood studies: neutrophils, decreased platelets
• Monitor B/P, check for orthostatic hypotension, syncope; if changes occur dosage change may be required
• Monitor renal studies: protein, BUN, creatinine; watch for increased levels that may indicate nephrotic syndrome and renal failure; monitor renal symptoms: polyuria, oliguria, frequency, dysuria
• Establish baselines in renal, liver function tests before therapy begins
• Check potassium levels throughout treatment, although hyperkalemia rarely occurs
• Check for edema in feet, legs daily
• Assess for allergic reactions: rash, fever, pruritus, urticaria; drug should be discontinued if antihistamines fail to help

Nursing diagnoses
☑ Cardiac output, decreased (uses)
☑ Injury, risk for physical (adverse reactions)
☑ Knowledge deficit (teaching)
☑ Noncompliance (teaching)

Implementation
• Store in airtight container at 86° F (30° C) or less
• Severe hypotension may occur after 1st dose of this medication; may be prevented by reducing or discontinuing diuretic therapy 3 days before beginning quinapril therapy

Patient/family education
• Advise patient not to discontinue drug abruptly; advise patient to tell all persons associated with care
• Teach patient not to use OTC products (cough, cold, allergy) unless directed by physician; serious side effects can occur
• Inform patient that xanthines such as coffee, tea, chocolate, cola can prevent action of drug
• Caution patient on the importance of complying with dosage schedule, even if feeling better; to continue with medical regimen to decrease B/P: exercise, cessation of smoking, decreasing stress, diet modifications
• Emphasize the need to rise slowly to sitting or standing position to minimize orthostatic hypotension; not to exercise in hot weather or increased hypotension can occur
• Teach patient to notify prescriber of mouth sores, sore throat, fever, swelling of hands or feet, irregular heartbeat, chest pain, coughing, shortness of breath
• Caution patient to report excessive perspiration, dehydration, vomiting, diarrhea; may lead to fall in B/P
• Caution patient that drug may cause dizziness, fainting, lightheadedness; may occur during 1st few days of therapy; to avoid activities that may be hazardous
• Teach patient how to take B/P, and normal readings for age group

Q

Evaluation

Positive therapeutic outcome
• Decreased B/P in hypertension

Treatment of overdose: 0.9% NaCl **IV** inf, hemodialysis

---

quinidine ⚏ₙ (℞)
(kwin'i-deen)
Apo-Quinidine ✦, Cin-Quin, Duraquin, Novoquinidin ✦, Quinaglute, Quinalan, quinidine gluconate; Cardioquin; Quinidex Extentabs, quinidine sulfate
Func. class.: Antidysrhythmic (Class IA)
Chem. class.: Quinine dextro isomer
Pregnancy category   C

Action: Prolongs action, potential duration, and effective refractory period, thus decreasing myocardial excitability; anticholinergic properties

⮞ **Therapeutic Outcome:** Treatment of dysrhythmias

Uses: PVCs, atrial fibrillation, PAT, ventricular tachycardia, atrial dysrhythmias

Investigational uses: Malaria/**IV** quinidine gluconate

Dosage and routes
Quinidine sulfate
Atrial fibrillation/flutter
Adult: PO 200 mg q2-3h × 5-8 doses; may increase qd until sinus rhythm is restored; max 4 g/day given only after digitalization

Paroxysmal supraventricular tachycardia
Adult: PO 400-600 mg q2-3h, then 200-300 mg q6-8h or 300-600 mg q8-12h (sus rel)

Premature atrial/ventricular contraction
Adult: PO 200-300 mg q6-8h or 300-600 mg (sus rel) q8-12h, not to exceed 4 g/day
🅟 *Child:* PO 30 mg/kg/day or 900 mg/m²/day in 5 divided doses

Quinidine gluconate
Adult: PO 324-660 mg q6-12h (sus rel); IM 600 mg, then 400 mg q2h; **IV** give 16 mg/min

Quinidine polygalacteronate
Adult: PO 275-825 mg q3-4h × 4 doses, then increase by 137.5-275 mg; repeat up to 4 × until dysrhythmia decreases
🅟 *Child:* PO 8.25 mg/kg (247.5 mg/m²) 5/day

Available forms: (Gluconate) tabs sus rel 324, 330 mg; inj gluconate 80 mg/ml; (sulfate) tabs 200, 300 mg; tabs sus rel 300 mg; (polygalacturonase) tab 275 mg

Adverse effects
CNS: Headache, dizziness, involuntary movement, confusion, psychosis, restlessness, irritability, syncope, excitement
CV: Hypotension, bradycardia, PVCs, **heart block, cardiovascular collapse, arrest, Torsades de pointes**
EENT: Cinchonism: tinnitus, blurred vision, hearing loss, mydriasis, disturbed color vision

---

GI: Nausea, vomiting, anorexia, *diarrhea*, **hepatotoxicity**

HEMA: **Thrombocytopenia**, hemolytic anemia, agranulocytosis, hypoprothrombinemia

INTEG: Rash, urticaria, angioedema, swelling, photosensitivity

RESP: Dyspnea, **respiratory depression**

Contraindications: Hypersensitivity, blood dyscrasias, severe heart block, myasthenia gravis

Precautions: Pregnancy **C**, lactation, children, renal disease, K imbalance, liver disease, CHF, respiratory depression

Interactions
Individual drugs
Amiodarone: ↑ toxicity
Cimetidine: ↑ effects of quinidine
Coumadin: ↑ levels of coumadin
Digoxin: ↑ blood levels, ↑ toxicity
Nifedipine: ↓ effects of quinidine
Phenytoin: ↓ effects of quinidine
Propranolol: ↑ effects of quinidine
Rifampin: ↓ effects of quinidine
Verapamil: ↑ effects of quinidine

Drug classifications
Antacids: ↑ effects of quinidine
Anticholinergics: ↑ vagolytic effects
Anticoagulants (oral): ↑ levels of anticoagulant
Antidysrhythmics: ↑ cardiac depression
Barbiturates: ↓ effects of quinidine
Phenothiazines: ↑ cardiac depression
Thiazide diuretics: ↑ effects of quinidine

Herb/drug
Aloe: ↑ hypokalemia
Buckthorn: ↑ hypokalemia
Cascara sagrada: ↑ hypokalemia
Senna: ↑ hypokalemia

Food/drug
Grapefruit: ↓ absorption

Lab test interferences
↑ CPK

NURSING CONSIDERATIONS
Assessment
• Monitor ECG continuously to determine drug effectiveness, measure PR, QRS, QT intervals, check for PVCs, other dysrhythmias; monitor B/P continuously for hypotension, hypertension; for rebound hypertension after 1-2

Pharmacokinetics
Absorption	Well absorbed (PO, IM), slowly absorbed (sus-rel)
Distribution	Widely distributed, crosses placenta
Metabolism	Liver
Excretion	Kidney unchanged, breast milk
Half-life	6-8 hr

Pharmacodynamics
	PO (SULFATE)	PO-SR	PO (GLUCONATE)	PO (POLY-GALACTU-RONASE)	IM	IV
Onset	½ hr	Unknown	Unknown	Unknown	½ hr	5 min
Peak	1-1½ hr	4 hr	4 hr	6 hr	½-1½ hr	Unknown
Duration	6-8 hr	8-12 hr	6-8 hr	8-12 hr	6-8 hr	6-8 hr

♣ Canada Only   Adverse effects: *italic* = common; **bold** = life-threatening

hr; check for dehydration or hypovolemia

• Monitor I&O ratio; electrolytes: [K, Na, Cl]; check weight daily; check for signs of CHG or pulmonary toxicity: dyspnea, fatigue, cough, fever, chest pain; if these occur, drug should be discontinued

• Monitor liver function studies: AST, ALT, bilirubin, alk phosphatase

• Assess for CNS symptoms: confusion, psychosis, numbness, depression, involuntary movements; if these occur, drug should be discontinued

• Monitor cardiac rate, respiration: rate, rhythm, character, chest pain; watch for ventricular tachycardia, supraventricular tachycardia, or fibrillation that indicates toxicity

Nursing diagnoses

☑Cardiac output, decreased (uses)

☑Impaired gas exchange (adverse reactions)

☑Knowledge deficit (teaching)

Implementation

PO route

• Give on an empty stomach with a full glass of water

• May be given with meals if GI irritation occurs, absorption will be decreased

• Tab may be crushed and mixed with fluid or foods for patients with swallowing

Ⓢdifficulties; do not break, chew or crush sus rel tab

Ⅳ IV route

• Give by intermittent inf after diluting 800 mg/50 ml D_5W (gluconate) (16 mg/ml) give at 1 ml/min or less using an inf pump for correct dose

• Do not use colored sol or sol with precipitate

• Diluted quinidine is stable for 24 hr at room temp

Y-site compatibilities: Diazepam, milrinone

Y-site incompatibilities: Furosemide

Additive compatibilities: Bretylium, cimetidine, milrinone, ranitidine, verapamil

Additive incompatibilities: Amiodarone

Patient/family education

• Instruct patient to report adverse effects immediately to prescriber

• Caution patient that dark glasses may be needed for photophobia; to use sunscreen, protective clothing, or stay out of sun to prevent burns

• Instruct patient to complete follow-up appointments with health care provider including pulmonary function studies, chest x-ray, ophth and otoscopic examinations

Treatment of overdose: O_2, artificial ventilation, ECG, administer dopamine for circulatory depression, administer diazepam or thiopental for convulsions, isoproterenol

---

raloxifene (℞)

(ral-ox′ih-feen)

Evista

Func. class.: Selective estrogen receptor modulator (SERM)

Chem. class.: Benzthiophene

Pregnancy category   X

Action: Reduces resorption of bone and decreases bone turnover; mediated through estrogen receptor binding

---

☑ Herb/drug   Ⓢ Do Not Crush   ◆ Alert   ⊶ Key Drug   Ⓖ Geriatric   Ⓟ Pediatric

⇒Therapeutic Outcome:
Absence of osteoporosis in postmenopausal women

Uses: Prevention of osteoporosis in postmenopausal women

Dosage and routes
Hormone replacement
Adult: PO 60 mg qd

Available forms: Tabs 60 mg

Adverse effects
CNS: Insomnia, migraines, depression
CV: Hot flashes
GI: Nausea, vomiting, diarrhea, anorexia, cramps
GU: Vaginitis, UTI, leukorrhea, endometrial disorder, breast pain
INTEG: Rash, sweating
META: Weight gain, peripheral edema
MS: Arthralgia, myalgia, leg cramps, arthritis
RESP: Sinusitis, pharyngitis, increased cough, pneumonia, laryngitis

Contraindications: Hypersensitivity, pregnancy **X,** lactation

Precautions: Lactation, venous thromboembolic events, hepatic disease

Pharmacokinetics	
Absorption	Unknown
Distribution	Highly protein bound
Metabolism	Unknown
Excretion	Feces, breast milk
Half-life	28 hr (elimination)

Pharmacodynamics	
Onset	Unknown
Peak	Unknown
Duration	Unknown

Interactions
Individual drugs
Ampicillin: ↓ action of raloxifene

Cholestyramine: ↓ action of raloxifene
Drug classifications
Anticoagulants: ↓ action of anticoagulants
Highly protein-bound drugs: Administer cautiously
Lab test interferences
↑ Apolipoproteins A_1 and B, ↑ lipoprotein, ↑ fibrinogen, ↑ LDL cholesterol, ↑ total cholesterol, ↑ total cholesterol, ↑ corticosteroid-binding globulin, ↑ thyroxine-binding globulin (TBG) ↓ calcium, ↓ total protein, ↓ albumin, ↓ platelets

NURSING CONSIDERATIONS
Assessment
• Monitor blood glucose of diabetic patients
• Monitor weight daily, notify prescriber of weekly weight gain >5 lb
• Monitor B/P q4h, watch for increase caused by H_2O and Na retention
• Monitor liver function studies, including AST, ALT, bilirubin, alk phosphatase
• Monitor I&O ratio; decreasing urinary output, increasing edema

Nursing diagnoses
☑Immobility, risk for (uses)
☑Knowledge deficit (teaching)

R

Implementation
PO route
• Administer without regard to meals

Patient/family education
• Teach patient to weigh weekly, report gain >5 lb
• Teach patients to discontinue drug 72 hr before prolonged bedrest
• Advise patient to avoid maintaining one position for long periods

---

• Advise patient to take calcium supplements, vit D if intake is inadequate
• Advise patient to increase exercise using weights
• Advise patient to stop smoking and to decrease alcohol consumption
• Inform patient that this drug does not help control hot flashes
• Teach patient to report fever, acute migraine, insomnia, emotional distress; urinary tract infection or vaginal burning/itching; swelling, warmth, or pain in calves

Evaluation
Positive therapeutic outcome
• Prevention of osteoporosis

---

ramipril (℞)
(ra-mi′pril)
Altace
Func. class.: Antihypertensive
Chem. class.: Angiotensin-converting enzyme (ACE) inhibitor

Pregnancy category D
(2nd/3rd trimesters), C (1st trimester)

Action: Selectively suppresses renin-angiotensin-aldosterone system; inhibits ACE; prevents conversion of angiotensin I to angiotensin II; results in dilation of arterial, venous vessels

➡**Therapeutic Outcome:** Decreased B/P in hypertension

Uses: Hypertension, alone or in combination with thiazide diuretics; CHF (post MI)

Dosage and routes
Adult: PO 2.5 mg qd initially, then 2.5-20 mg/day divided bid or qd; renal impairment: 1.25 mg qd with CrCl <40 ml/min/1.73 m², increase as needed to max or 5 mg/day
CHF
Adult: PO 1.25-2.5 mg bid may increase to 5 mg bid

Available forms: Caps 1.25, 2.5, 5, 10 mg

Adverse effects
CNS: Headache, dizziness, anxiety, insomnia, paresthesia, fatigue, depression, malaise, vertigo, **convulsions,** hearing loss
CV: Hypotension, chest pain, palpitations, angina, syncope, **dysrhythmia**
GI: Nausea, constipation, vomiting, dyspepsia, dysphagia, anorexia, diarrhea, abdominal pain
GU: **Proteinuria,** increased BUN, creatinine, impotence
HEMA: Decreased Hct, Hgb, **eosinophilia, leukopenia**
INTEG: **Angioedema,** rash, sweating, photosensitivity, pruritus
META: Hyperkalemia
MS: Arthralgia, arthritis, myalgia
RESP: Cough, dyspnea

Contraindications: Hypersensitivity to ACE inhibitors, pregnancy **D** (2nd/3rd trimesters), lactation, children

Precautions: Impaired renal and liver function, dialysis patients, hypovolemia, blood dyscrasias, COPD, asthma, elderly, renal artery stenosis, pregnancy **C** (1st trimester)

Do Not Confuse:
Altace/alteplase, Altace/Artane, ramipril/enalapril

Pharmacokinetics	
Absorption	Well absorbed
Distribution	Not known, crosses placenta
Metabolism	Liver, extensively
Excretion	Urine
Half-life	Ramipril (5 hr), ramiprilat (24 hr)

Pharmacodynamics	
Onset	½-1 hr
Peak	6-8 hr
Duration	24-72 hr

Interactions
Individual drugs
Alcohol: ↑ hypotension (large amounts)
Allopurinol: ↑ hypersensitivity
Digoxin: ↑ serum levels
Hydralazine: ↑ toxicity
Indomethacin: ↓ antihypertensive effect
Lithium: ↑ serum levels
Prazosin: ↑ toxicity
Drug classifications
Adrenergic blockers: ↑ hypotension
Antacids: ↓ absorption
Antihypertensives: ↑ hypotension
Diuretics: ↑ hypotension
Diuretics, potassium sparing: ↑ toxicity
Ganglionic blockers: ↑ hypotension
Potassium supplements: ↑ toxicity
Sympathomimetics: ↑ toxicity
Lab test interferences
False positive: Urine acetone

NURSING CONSIDERATIONS
Assessment
• Monitor blood studies: neutrophils, decreased platelets
• Monitor B/P, check for orthostatic hypotension, syncope; if changes occur, dosage may need to be changed
• Monitor renal studies: protein, BUN, creatinine; watch for increased levels that may indicate nephrotic syndrome and renal failure; monitor renal symptoms: polyuria, oliguria, frequency, dysuria
• Establish baselines in renal, liver function tests before therapy begins
• Check potassium levels throughout treatment, although hyperkalemia rarely occurs
• Check for edema in feet, legs daily
• Assess for allergic reactions: rash, fever, pruritus, urticaria; drug should be discontinued if antihistamines fail to help

Nursing diagnoses
☑ Cardiac output, decreased (uses)
☑ Injury, risk for (side effects)
☑ Knowledge deficit (teaching)
☑ Noncompliance (teaching)

Implementation
• Caps can be opened and added to food
• Store in air-tight container at 86° F (30° C) or less
• Severe hypotension may occur after 1st dose of this medication; decreased hypotension may be prevented by reducing or discontinuing diuretic therapy 3 days before beginning benazepril therapy
• Give **IV** inf of 0.9% NaCl (as ordered) to expand fluid volume if severe hypotension occurs

Patient/family education
• Caution patient not to discontinue drug abruptly; advise patient to tell all persons associated with care
• Teach patient not to use OTC products (cough, cold, allergy) unless directed by

R

physician; serious side effects can occur—xanthines such as coffee, tea, chocolate, cola can prevent action of drug

• Instruct patient on the importance of complying with dosage schedule, even if feeling better; to continue with medical regimen to decrease B/P: exercise, cessation of smoking, decreasing stress, diet modifications

• Emphasize the need to rise slowly to sitting or standing position to minimize orthostatic hypotension; not to exercise in hot weather because increased hypotension can occur

• Teach patient to notify prescriber of mouth sores, sore throat, fever, swelling of hands or feet, irregular heartbeat, chest pain, coughing, shortness of breath

• Caution patient to report excessive perspiration, dehydration, vomiting, diarrhea; may lead to fall in B/P

• Caution patient that drug may cause dizziness, fainting, lightheadedness; may occur during 1st few days of therapy; to avoid activities that may be hazardous

• Teach patient how to take B/P, and normal readings for age group

Evaluation

Positive therapeutic outcome

• Decreased B/P in hypertension

Treatment of overdose: 0.9% NaCl **IV** inf, hemodialysis

---

ranitidine (Ⓡ)
(ra-nit′i-deen)
Apo-Ranitidine ✦, Tritec, Zantac, Zantac-C ✦
Func. class.: H₂ histamine receptor antagonist
Pregnancy category **B**

Action: Inhibits histamine at H₂ receptor site in the gastric parietal cells, which inhibits gastric acid secretion

▶**Therapeutic Outcome:** Healing of duodenal ulcers or gastric ulcers; prevention of duodenal ulcers; decreases symptoms of GERD or Zollinger-Ellison syndrome

Uses: Short-term treatment of duodenal and gastric ulcers and maintenance; management of gastroesophageal reflux disease (GERD), Zollinger-Ellison syndrome, active duodenal ulcers with *Helicobacter pylori* in combination with clarithromycin

Investigational uses: Prevention of aspiration pneumonitis, stress ulcers, upper GI bleeding

Dosage and routes
Renal dose
CrCl <50 ml/min give PO q24h, give IM/**IV** q8-24h

Adult: PO 150 mg bid, 300 mg hs; IM 50 mg q6-8h; **IV** bol 50 mg diluted to 20 ml over 5 min q6-8h; **IV** int inf 50 mg/100 ml D₅ over 15-20 min, q6-8h

Ⓟ *Child:* PO 4-5 mg/kg/day divided q8-12h, max 6 mg/kg/day or 300 mg; **IV** 2-4 mg/kg/day divided q6-8h

Duodenal ulcer
Adult: PO 150 mg bid, maintenance 150 mg hs

Zollinger-Ellison syndrome
Adult: PO 150 mg bid, may increase if needed

Gastric ulcer
Adult: PO 150 mg bid × 6 wk, then 150 mg hs

GERD
Adult: PO 150 mg bid

Erosive esophagitis
Adult: PO 150 mg qid

Available forms: Tabs 75, 150, 300 mg; inj 0.5, 25 mg/ml; caps ✤ 150, 300 mg; syr 15 mg/ml

Adverse effects
CNS: Headache, sleeplessness, dizziness, confusion, agitation, depression, hallucination
CV: Tachycardia, bradycardia, PVCs
EENT: Blurred vision, increased ocular pressure
GI: Constipation, abdominal pain, diarrhea, nausea, vomiting, **hepatotoxicity**
GU: Impotence, gynecomastia
INTEG: Urticaria, rash, fever

Contraindications: Hypersensitivity

Precautions: Pregnancy **B**, lactation, child <12 yr, hepatic disease, renal disease

Do Not Confuse:
Zantac/Xanax, Zantac/ Zofran, ranitidine/amantadine

Pharmacokinetics	
Absorption	Well absorbed (PO, IM), completely absorbed (**IV**)
Distribution	Widely distributed, crosses placenta
Metabolism	Liver (30%)
Excretion	Kidneys unchanged (70%)
Half-life	2-3 hr, ↑ renal disease

Pharmacodynamics		
	PO	IV/IM
Onset	Unknown	Unknown
Peak	2-3 hr	15 min
Duration	8-12 hr	8-12 hr

Interactions
Individual drugs
Ketoconazole: ↓ absorption of ranitidine
Drug classifications
Antacids: ↓ absorption of ranitidine
Smoking
↓ effectiveness
Lab test interferences
↑ Alk phosphatase, ↑ AST, ↑ creatinine
False positive: Gastric bleeding test

NURSING CONSIDERATIONS
Assessment
• Assess patient with ulcers or suspected ulcers: epigastric or abdominal pain, hematemesis, occult blood in stools, blood in gastric aspirate prior to and throughout treatment, monitor gastric pH (5 should be maintained)
• Monitor I&O ratio, BUN, creatinine, CBC with differential monthly

Nursing diagnoses
☑ Pain (uses)
☑ Knowledge deficit (teaching)

Implementation
PO route
• May be given with or without meals
• Give antacids 1 hr before or 1 hr after this drug
IV IV route
Direct **IV**
• Give by direct **IV** after diluting 50 mg/20 ml of 0.9% D_5W, NaCl given over 5 min or more

R

Intermittent inf
- Give by intermittent inf over 15 min after diluting 50 mg/100 ml D$_5$W, 0.9% NaCl

Continuous inf
- Give by continuous inf for a concentration 150 mg/250 ml, give 6.25 mg/hr
- Give Zollinger-Ellison patients up to a conc of 2.5 mg/ml at 1 mg/kg/hr initially

Syringe compatibilities:
Atropine, cyclizine, dexamethasone, dimenhydrinate, diphenhydramine, dobutamine, dopamine, fentanyl, glycopyrrolate, hydromorphone, meperidine, metoclopramide, morphine, nalbuphine, oxymorphone, pentazocine, perphenazine, prochlorperazine, promethazine, scopolamine

Syringe incompatibilities:
Hydroxyzine, methotrimeprazine, midazolam, pentobarbital, phenobarbital

Y-site compatibilities: Acyclovir, aldesleukin, allopurinol, amifostine, aminophylline, atracurium, aztreonam, bretylium, dobutamine, dopamine, doxorubicin, enalaprilat, epinephrine, esmolol, fentanyl, filgrastim, fluconazole, fludarabine, foscarnet, furosemide, gallium, granisetron, heparin, hydromorphone, idarubicin, labetalol, lorazepam, melphalan, meperidine, methotrexate, midazolam, milrinone, morphine, nicardipine, nitroglycerin, norepinephrine, ondansetron, paclitaxel, pancuronium, piperacillin, piperacillin/tazobactam, procainamide, propofol, sargramostim, vecuronium, zidovudine

Additive compatibilities:
Acetazolamide, amikacin, aminophylline, chloramphenicol, chlorothiazide, ciprofloxacin, colistimethate, dexamethasone, digoxin, dobutamine, dopamine, doxycycline, furosemide, gentamicin, heparin, lidocaine, penicillin G sodium, potassium chloride, ticarcillin, tobramycin, vancomycin

Additive incompatibilities:
Amphotericin B, clindamycin

Patient/family education
- Caution patient that gynecomastia, impotence may occur and are reversible after treatment is discontinued
- Advise patient to avoid driving, other hazardous activities until stabilized on this medication; drowsiness or dizziness may occur
- Caution patient to avoid black pepper, caffeine, alcohol, harsh spices, extremes in temp of food; tell patient to avoid OTC preparations: aspirin, cough, cold preparations because condition may worsen
- Inform patient that smoking decreases the effectiveness of the drug; that smoking cessation should be considered
- Instruct patient that drug must be continued for prescribed time to be effective and taken exactly as prescribed; doses should not be doubled; a missed dose should be taken when remembered up to 1 hr before next dose
- Advise patient to report bruising, fatigue, malaise; blood dyscrasias may occur
- Inform patient to report diarrhea, black tarry stools, sore throat, rash, dizziness, confusion, rash or delirium to prescriber immediately

☑ Herb/drug Ⓢ Do Not Crush ✦ Alert ⚷ Key Drug Ⓖ Geriatric Ⓟ Pediatric

Evaluation
Positive therapeutic outcome
- Decreased pain in abdomen
- Healing of ulcers
- Absence of gastroesophageal reflux

---

rapacuronium
See Appendix A,
Selected New Drugs

---

rapeprazole
See Appendix A,
Selected New Drugs

---

remifentanil (℞)
(re-me-fin'ta-nill)
Ultiva
Func. class.: Opiate agonist analgesic
Chem. class.: Mu-opioid agonist

Pregnancy category **C**
Controlled substance schedule **II**

Action: Inhibits ascending pain pathways in limbic system, thalamus, midbrain, hypothalamus

Therapeutic Outcome: Maintenance of anesthesia

Uses: In combination with other drugs in general anesthesia, as a primary anesthetic in general surgery

Dosage and routes
Adult: Induction **IV** 0.5-1 µg/kg/min with a hypnotic or volatile agent; maintenance with isoflurane (0.4-1.5 MAC) or propofol (100-200 µg/kg/min) 0.25 µg/kg/min

Available forms: Powder for inj—lyophilized 1 mg/ml after reconstitution

Adverse effects
CNS: Drowsiness, *dizziness,* confusion, *headache,* sedation, euphoria, delirium, agitation, anxiety
CV: Palpitations, **bradycardia,** change in B/P; facial flushing, syncope, **asystole**
EENT: Tinnitus, blurred vision, miosis, diplopia
GI: Nausea, vomiting, anorexia, constipation, cramps, dry mouth
GU: Urinary retention, dysuria
INTEG: Rash, urticaria, bruising, flushing, diaphoresis, pruritus
MS: Rigidity
RESP: **Respiratory depression, apnea**

Contraindications: Child <12 yr, hypersensitivity

Precautions: Pregnancy C, lactation, increased intracranial pressure, acute MI, severe heart disease; renal disease, hepatic disease, asthma, respiratory conditions, convulsive disorders, elderly

Pharmacokinetics

Absorption	Complete
Distribution	Unknown
Metabolism	Unknown
Excretion	Unknown
Half-life	Unknown

Pharmacodynamics

Onset	Immediate
Peak	Unknown
Duration	Unknown

Interactions
Individual drugs
Alcohol: ↑ respiratory depression, hypotension, profound sedation

---

Drug classifications
Antihistamines: ↑ respiratory depression, hypotension, profound sedation
Phenothiazine: ↑ respiratory depression, hypotension, profound sedation
Sedative/hypnotics: ↑ respiratory depression, hypotension, profound sedative

NURSING CONSIDERATIONS
Assessment
• Monitor I&O ratio, check for decreasing output; may indicate urinary retention, **G** especially in elderly
• Assess CNS changes: dizziness, drowsiness, hallucinations, euphoria, LOC pupil reaction
• Assess allergic reactions: rash, urticaria
• Assess respiratory dysfunction: respiratory depression, character, rate, rhythm; notify prescriber if respirations are <12/min; CV status, bradycardia, syncope
• Use pain scoring to determine pain perception

Nursing diagnoses
☑ Knowledge deficit (teaching)

Implementation
• Give by direct **IV** over 1½-3 min; use tuberculin syringe
• Store in light-resistant area at room temperature

Y-site compatibilities: Acyclovir, alfentanil, amikacin, aminophylline, ampicillin, ampicillin/sulbactam, amrinone, aztreonam, bretylium, bumetanide, buprenorphine, butorphanol, calcium gluconate, cefazolin, cefotaxime, cefotetan, cefoxitin, ceftazidime, ceftizoxime, ceftriaxone, cefuroxime, cimetidine, ciprofloxacin, cisatracurium, clinda-mycin, dexamethasone, digoxin, diphenhydramine, dobutamine, dopamine, doxycycline, droperidol, enalaprilat, epinephrine, esmolol, famotidine, fentanyl, fluconazole, furosemide, ganciclovir, gentamicin, haloperidol, heparin, hydrocortisone sodium succinate, hydromorphone, hydroxyzine, imipenem/cilastatin, isoproterenol, ketorolac, lidocaine, lorazepam, magnesium sulfate, mannitol, meperidine, methlyprednisolone sodium succinate, metoclopramide, metronidazole, mezlocillin, midazolam, minocycline, morphine, nalbuphine, netilmicin, nitroglycerin, norepinephrine, ofloxacin, ondansetron

Patient/family education
• Advise to call for assistance when ambulating or smoking; drowsiness, dizziness may occur
• Advise patient to make position changes slowly to prevent orthostatic hypotension

Evaluation
Positive therapeutic outcome
• Maintenance of anesthesia

---

repaglinide (℞)
(re-pag'lih-nide)
Prandin
Func. class.: Antidiabetic
Chem. class.: Meglitinides
Pregnancy category   C

Action: Causes functioning β-cells in pancreas to release insulin, leading to drop in blood glucose levels; closes ATP-dependent potassium channels in the β-cell membrane; this leads to open-

---

ing of calcium channels; increased calcium influx induces insulin secretion

→ **Therapeutic Outcome:** Blood glucose controlled

Uses: Stable adult-onset diabetes mellitus (type II) NIDDM

Dosage and routes
Adult: PO 0.5-4 mg ac

Available forms: Tabs 0.5, 1, 2 mg

Adverse effects
CNS: Headache, weakness, paresthesia
ENDO: Hypoglycemia
GI: Nausea, vomiting, diarrhea, constipation, dyspepsia
INTEG: Rash, allergic reactions
MS: Back pains, arthralgia
RESP: URI, sinusitis, rhinitis, bronchitis

Contraindications: Hypersensitivity to meglitinides, diabetic ketoacidosis, type I diabetes

Precautions: Pregnancy **C,** [G] elderly, cardiac disease, severe renal disease, severe hepatic disease, thyroid disease, severe hypoglycemic reactions, [P] lactation, children

Pharmacokinetics	
Absorption	Complete
Distribution	98% protein binding, crosses placenta
Metabolism	Liver
Excretion	Urine/feces
Half-life	1 hr

Pharmacodynamics	
Onset	2-4 hr
Peak	2-8 hr
Duration	24 hr

Interactions
Individual drugs
Carbamazepine: ↑ repaglinide metabolism
Chloramphenicol: ↑ effect of repaglinide
Erythromycin: ↓ repaglinide metabolism
Isoniazid: ↓ action of repaglinide
Phenobarbital: ↓ action of repaglinide
Phenytoin: ↓ action of repaglinide
Probenecid: ↑ effect of repaglinide
Rifampin: ↓ action of repaglinide
Drug classifications
Antifungals: ↓ repaglinide metabolism
Barbiturates: ↑ repaglinide metabolism
β-Adrenergic blockers: ↑ repaglinide effect
Calcium channel blockers: ↓ repaglinide effect
Corticosteroids: ↓ repaglinide effect
Coumarins: ↑ repaglinide effect
Diuretics, thiazide: ↓ repaglinide effect
Estrogens: ↓ repaglinide effect
NSAIDs: ↑ repaglinide effect
Oral contraceptives: ↓ repaglinide effect
Phenothiazines ↓ repaglinide effect
Salicylates: ↑ repaglinide effect
Sulfonamides: ↑ repaglinide effect
Sympathomimetics: ↓ repaglinide effect
Thyroid preparations: ↓ repaglinide effect
Herb/drug
Broom: ↓ hypoglycemia
Buchu: ↓ hypoglycemia
Chromium: ↑ or ↓ hypoglycemia

R

Dandelion: ↓ hypoglycemia
Fenugreek: ↑ or ↓ hypoglycemia
Ginseng: ↑ or ↓ hypoglycemia
Juniper: ↓ hypoglycemia
Karela: ↑ glucose tolerance

NURSING CONSIDERATIONS
Assessment
• Assess for hypoglycemic or hyperglycemic reaction, which can occur soon after meals

Nursing diagnoses
☑ Nutrition, altered (more than body requirements) (uses)
☑ Knowledge deficit (teaching)
☑ Noncompliance (teaching)

Implementation
PO route
• 15 min before meals: 2, 3, or 4 ×/day preprandially
• Skip dose if meal is skipped; add dose if meal is added
• Store in tight container in cool environment

Patient/family education
• Advise patient to avoid alcohol; explain disulfiram reaction
• Teach patient to use a capillary blood glucose test while on this drug
• Teach patient the symptoms of hypoglycemia and hyperglycemia; what to do about each
• Teach patient that drug must be continued on daily basis; explain consequence of discontinuing drug abruptly
• Advise patient to avoid OTC medications unless ordered by prescriber
• Advise patient that diabetes is a lifelong illness; drug will not cure disease
• Advise patient to eat all food included in diet plan to prevent hypoglycemia; to have glucagon emergency kit available
• Instruct patient to carry a Medic Alert ID for emergency purposes

Evaluation
Positive therapeutic outcome
• Decrease in polyuria, polydipsia, polyphagia, clear sensorium, absence of dizziness, stable gait

Treatment of overdose:
Glucose 25 g **IV** via dextrose 50% solution, 50 ml or 1 mg glucagon

---

reserpine (℞)
(re-ser′peen)
Novoreserpine ✦,
Reserfia ✦, reserpine
Func. class.: Antihypertensive
Chem. class.: Antiadrenergic agent (peripherally acting)

Pregnancy category   D

Action: Inhibits norepinephrine release, depleting norepinephrine stores in adrenergic nerve endings

➡ **Therapeutic Outcome:** Decreased B/P

Uses: Hypertension

Dosage and routes
Hypertension
Adult: PO 0.25-0.5 mg qd × 1-2 wk, then 0.1-0.25 mg qd for maintenance

G *Elderly:* PO 0.05 mg qd, increase by 0.05 weekly to desired dose

Psychiatric disorders
Adult: PO 0.5 mg qd, may range from 0.1-1 mg

Available forms: Tabs 0.1, 0.25 mg

☑ Herb/drug   🚫 Do Not Crush   ◆ Alert   ⟐ Key Drug   **G** Geriatric   **P** Pediatric

Adverse effects

CNS: Drowsiness, fatigue, lethargy, dizziness, depression, anxiety, headache, increased dreaming, nightmares, convulsions, parkinsonism, EPS (high doses)

CV: Bradycardia, chest pain, dysrhythmias, prolonged bleeding time, **thrombocytopenia,** purpura

EENT: Lacrimation, miosis, blurred vision, ptosis, dry mouth, epistaxis

GI: Nausea, vomiting, cramps, peptic ulcer, dry mouth, increased appetite, anorexia

GU: Impotence, dysuria, nocturia, Na and H_2O retention, edema, breast engorgement, galactorrhea, gynecomastia

INTEG: Rash, purpura, alopecia, flushing, warm feeling, pruritus, ecchymosis

RESP: **Bronchospasm,** dyspnea, cough, rales

Contraindications: Hypersensitivity, depression, suicidal patients, active peptic ulcer disease, ulcerative colitis, pregnancy **D,** Parkinson's disease

Precautions: Lactation, seizure disorders, renal disease, P children

N **Do Not Confuse:** reserpine/Risperdal

Pharmacokinetics

Absorption	40%-50%
Distribution	Widely distributed, crosses placenta
Metabolism	Liver
Excretion	Feces 50% unabsorbed drug, kidneys small amounts
Half-life	11 days

Pharmacodynamics

Onset	Unknown
Peak	4 hr
Duration	1-6 wk

Interactions

Individual drugs
Alcohol: ↑ CNS depression
Drug classifications
Amphetamines: ↓ hypotensive effects
Anesthetics: ↑ CNS depression
Antidepressants, tricyclic: ↓ hypotensive effects
β-Adrenergic blockers: ↑ bradycardia
Cardiac glycosides: ↑ bradycardia
Diuretics: ↑ hypotensive effects
Hypnotics: ↑ CNS depression
MAOIs: avoid use
Nitrates: ↑ hypotensive effects
Opiates: ↑ CNS depression
Sedatives: ↑ CNS depression
Lab test interferences
↑ VMA excretion, ↑ 5-HIAA excretion, ↑ prolactin
Interference: 17-OHCS, 17-KS

NURSING CONSIDERATIONS
Assessment

• Monitor B/P, orthostatic hypotension, syncope; check for edema in feet, legs daily; check I&O; monitor for weight daily; notify prescriber of changes

• Assess for allergic reactions: rash, fever, pruritus, urticaria; drug should be discontinued if antihistamines fail to help

• Assess for orthostatic hypotension, tell patient to rise slowly from sitting or lying position

Nursing diagnoses

☑ Cardiac output, decreased (uses)
☑ Injury, risk for (adverse reactions)
☑ Knowledge deficit (teaching)
☑ Noncompliance (teaching)

R

Implementation

• Store in tight container at 86° F (30° C) or less
• May be used in combination with other antihypertensives
• May be given with food to prevent GI symptoms

Patient/family education

• Caution patient not to discontinue drug abruptly and about the importance of complying with dosage schedule, even if feeling better; if dose is missed take as soon as remembered; take dose at same time each day
• Teach patient not to use OTC products (cough, cold, allergy) unless directed by prescriber and to avoid large amounts of caffeine
• Emphasize the need to rise slowly to sitting or standing position to minimize orthostatic hypotension
• Teach patient to notify prescriber of swelling of hands or feet, irregular heartbeat, chest pain
• Caution patient to report excessive perspiration, dehydration, vomiting, diarrhea; may lead to fall in B/P
• Caution patient that drug may cause dizziness, fainting, lightheadedness; may occur during 1st few days of therapy; to avoid hazardous activities
• Teach patient how to take B/P, and normal readings for age group; to take B/P q7 days

Evaluation

Positive therapeutic outcome
• Decreased B/P in hypertension, decrease in psychiatric symptoms

Treatment of overdose:

Administer volume expanders or vasopressors; discontinue drug; place patient in supine position

---

respiratory syncytial virus immune globulin (RSV-IGIV) (℞)

RespiGam
Func. class.: Immune serums
Chem. class.: Immunoglobulin G (IgG)
Pregnancy category C

Action: High titer of neutralizing antibody against RSV (respiratory syncytial virus)

➡**Therapeutic Outcome:** Resolution of infection

Uses: Prevention of serious lower respiratory tract infection caused by RSV in children <2 yr with bronchopulmonary dysplasia, or premature birth

Dosage and routes

P *Child <2 yr:* IV INF 1.5 ml/kg/hr × 15 min, then 3 ml/kg/hr 15-30 min; then 6 ml/kg/hr from 30 min to end of inf given monthly

Available forms: Inj 2500 mg RSV immunoglobulin

Adverse effects

CNS: Fever
CV: Hypertension, tachycardia, fluid overload
GI: Diarrhea, gastroenteritis, vomiting
OTHER: Rash, overdose effect, inj-site inflammation, **anaphylaxis, angioneurotic edema**
RESP: **Respiratory distress, hypoxia,** tachypnea, rales, wheezing

Contraindications: Hypersensitivity to this drug or other

---

human immunoglobulin preparations; IgA deficiency

Precautions: Pregnancy **C**, fluid overload

Pharmacokinetics

Absorption	Unknown
Distribution	Unknown
Metabolism	Unknown
Excretion	Unknown
Half-life	Unknown

Pharmacodynamics
Unknown

Interactions
Individual drugs
DPT: ↓ immune response
Haemophilus: ↓ immune response
Influenza B: ↓ immune response
MMR: ↓ immune response

NURSING CONSIDERATIONS
Assessment
• Monitor VS for increase in heart rate, respiratory rate, retractions, rales; a loop diuretic may be needed for fluid overload
• Assess for aseptic meningitis syndrome (AMS): severe headache, drowsiness, photophobia, fever, painful eye movements, nausea, vomiting, muscle rigidity; discontinue RSV-IGIV if these occur

Nursing diagnoses
✓ Infection, risk for (uses)
✓ Knowledge deficit (teaching)

Implementation
• Give by infusion: do not admix; begin infusion within 6 hr and complete within 12 hr after the single-use vial is entered
• Store refrigerated, do not freeze, do not shake vial; discard after use

Patient/family education
• Teach patient the reason for **IV** infusion and expected results

---

Rh$_o$ (D) immune globulin, human (℞)
Gamulin Rh, HypoRho-D, MICRhoGAM, Mini-Gamulin RH, Hypo Rho-D Mini-Dose, Rhesonatin, RhoGAM
Rh$_o$ (D) immune globulin intravenous, human (℞)
WinRho SD
Func. class.: IgG, immunizing agent

Pregnancy category   C

Action: Suppresses immune response of nonsensitized Rh$_o$ (D or D^u)-negative patients who are exposed to Rh$_o$ (D or D^u)-positive blood

⇒**Therapeutic Outcome:** Absence of Rh factor and transfusion error

Uses: Prevention of isoimmunization in Rh-negative women exposed to Rh-positive blood given after abortions, miscarriages, amniocentesis

Dosage and routes
Rh$_o$(D) immune globulin, human
After delivery
Adult: IM 1 vial of fetal packed RBCs <15 ml, or 2 vials of fetal packed RBCs >15 ml; given within 72 hr of delivery or miscarriage

Before delivery
Adult: IM 1 vial (standard dose) at 26-28 wk, 1 vial (standard dose) 72 hr after delivery

R

Pregnancy termination
<13 wk
Adult: IM 1 vial (micro dose) within 72 hr

Pregnancy termination
>13 wk
Adult: IM 1 vial (standard dose) within 72 hr

Fetal-maternal hemorrhage
Adult: IM packed RBCs volume of hemorrhage/15 = needed vials (standard dose)

Transfusion error
Adult: IM—give within 72 hr

Rh$_o$(D) immune globulin IV human
After 34 wk gestation
Adult: IM/**IV** 120 μg, give within 72 hr

Available forms: Inj single-dose vial (50 μg/vial-microdose, 300 μg/vial-standard); inj 120, 300 μg Rh$_o$(D) immune globulin **IV**, human

Adverse effects
CNS: Lethargy
INTEG: Irritation at inj site, fever
MS: Myalgia

Contraindications: Previous immunization with this drug, Rh$_o$ (O)-positive/D^u-positive patient

Precautions: Pregnancy **C**

▧ **Do Not Confuse:**
Gamulin Rh/MICRh$_o$GAM

Pharmacokinetics	
Absorption	Well absorbed
Distribution	Unknown
Metabolism	Unknown
Excretion	Unknown
Half-life	Unknown

Pharmacodynamics	
Onset	Rapid
Peak	Unknown
Duration	Unknown

Interactions
Drug classifications
Live virus vaccines: ↓ antibody response to vaccine

NURSING CONSIDERATIONS
Assessment
• Assess for allergies, reactions to immunizations; previous immunization with this drug
• Obtain type and cross-match of mother's blood and of neonate's cord blood; neonate must be Rh$_o$(D)-positive, mother must be Rh$_o$(D)-negative and (D^u)-negative, medication should be given if there is a doubt

Nursing diagnoses
☑ Knowledge deficit (teaching)

Implementation
• Give after sending newborn's cord blood to lab after delivery for cross, match, type
• Give IM in deltoid; aspirate to prevent **IV** administration
• Give only equal lot numbers of drug, cross match
• Give only MICRhoGAM for abortions or miscarriages <13 wk unless fetus or father is Rh-negative
• Store in refrigerator

Patient/family education
• Teach patient how drug works; that drug must be given after subsequent deliveries if subsequent babies are Rh-positive

Evaluation
Positive therapeutic outcome
• Prevention of Rh$_o$(D) sensitization in transfusion error
• Prevention of erythroblastosis fetalis in subsequent Rh$_o$(D)-positive neonates

---

☑ Herb/drug 🚫 Do Not Crush ◆ Alert ⟜ Key Drug **G** Geriatric **P** Pediatric

ribavarin (Ŗ)
(rye-ba-vye′rin)
Virazole
Func. class.: Synthetic antiviral
Chem. class.: Tricyclic amine

Pregnancy category X

Action: Prevents replication of DNA and RNA synthesis

Therapeutic Outcome: Resolution of severe lower respiratory tract infections

Uses: Severe lower respiratory tract infections in infants and children

Investigational uses: Influenza A or B (early)

Dosage and routes
Infants and young children:
Inh 20 mg/ml × 12-18 hrs/day × 3-7 days

Available forms: Powder for reconstitution for aerosol: 6 g/vial

Adverse effects
CNS: Dizziness, faintness
CV: Hypotension, **cardiac arrest**
EENT: Eye irritation, conjunctivitis, blurred vision, photosensitivity
INTEG: Rash

Contraindications: Hypersensitivity, lactation, child <1 yr, pregnancy **X**

Precautions: Epilepsy, hepatic disease, renal disease

Pharmacokinetics
Absorption	Inh (systemic)
Distribution	To respiratory tract
Metabolism	Liver
Excretion	Respiratory tract
Half-life	9½ hr

Pharmacodynamics
Onset	Unknown
Peak	Inh end
Duration	Unknown

Interactions
Individual drugs
Zidovudine: ↓ antiviral action, ↑ toxicity
Drug classification
Cardiac glycosides: ↑ toxicity

NURSING CONSIDERATIONS
Assessment
• Assess allergies before initiation of treatment, reaction of each medication; list allergies on chart in bright red letters
• Monitor respiratory status: rate, character, wheezing, tightness in chest
• Obtain C&S test results before starting treatment

Nursing diagnoses
✓ Infection, risk for (uses)
✓ Gas exchange, impaired (uses)
✓ Knowledge deficit (teaching)

Implementation
• Give by the viratek SPAG (SPAG-2), do not use other inh equipment
• May be given by an oxygen hood for infants, or a face mask may be attached to the SPAG-2
• Reconstitute 6 g sterile water for inj or inh, place sol in the Erlenmeyer flask and dilute further to 20 mg/ml

Patient/family education
• Teach patient and parents aspects of drug therapy

Evaluation
Positive therapeutic outcome
• Absence of RSV (respiratory syncytial virus)

R

**riboflavin
(vitamin B₂)** (OTC)
(rye′boo-flay-vin)
Func. class.: Vitamin B₂,
water soluble
Pregnancy category   A

Action: Needed for respiratory
reactions (catalyzes proteins)
and for normal vision

Therapeutic Outcome: Prevention or treatment of riboflavin deficiency

Uses: Vit B₂ deficiency or
polyneuritis; cheilosis adjunct
with thiamine

Dosage and routes
P *Adult and child >12 yr:* PO
5-25 mg qd
P *Child <12 yr:* PO 2-10 mg qd,
then 0.6 mg/1000 calories
ingested
RDA
Adult: males 1.4-1.8 mg;
females 1.2-1.3 mg

Available forms: Tabs 25, 50,
100 mg

Adverse effects
GU: Yellow discoloration of
urine (large doses)

P **Contraindications:** Child
<12 yr

Precautions: Pregnancy **A**

Pharmacokinetics	
Absorption	Well absorbed (by active transport)
Distribution	60% protein bound, widely distributed, crosses placenta
Metabolism	Unknown
Excretion	Kidneys (unchanged), excess amounts
Half-life	1-1½ hr

Pharmacodynamics

Unknown

Interactions
Individual drugs
Alcohol: ↑ riboflavin need
Probenecid: ↑ riboflavin need
Tetracycline: ↓ action of tetra-
cycline
Drug classifications
Antidepressants, tricyclic:
↑ riboflavin need
Phenothiazines: ↑ riboflavin
need
Lab test interferences
False: ↑ Urinary catechol-
amines, ↑ urobilinogen

**NURSING CONSIDERATIONS
Assessment**
• Assess patient's nutritional
status: liver, eggs, dairy prod-
ucts, yeast, whole grain, green
vegetables
• Assess for vitamin B₂
deficiency: photophobia, chei-
losis, stomatitis, ocular swelling
Nursing diagnoses
☑ Nutrition: less than body re-
quirements (uses)
☑ Knowledge deficit (teaching)
Implementation
• Give with food for better
absorption
• Store in tight, light-resistant
container
Patient/family education
• Inform patient that urine
may turn bright yellow
• Instruct patient about addition of needed foods that are
rich in riboflavin
Evaluation
Positive therapeutic outcome
• Absence of headache, GI
problems, cheilosis, skin le-
sions, depression, burning,
itchy eyes, anemia

rifabutin (℞)
(riff'a-byoo-tin)
Mycobutin
Func. class.: Antimycobacterial
Chem. class.: Rifamycin S derivative
Pregnancy category **B**

Action: Inhibits DNA-dependent RNA polymerase in susceptible strains

→ **Therapeutic Outcome:** Antimycobacterial death of *E. coli, B. subtilis,* and *M. avium*

Uses: Prevention of *M. avium* complex (MAC) in patients with advanced HIV infection

Dosage and routes
Adult: PO 300 mg qd (may take as 150 mg bid)

Available forms: Cap 150 mg

Adverse effects
CNS: Headache, fatigue, anxiety, confusion, insomnia
GI: Nausea, vomiting, anorexia, diarrhea, heartburn, **hepatitis**
GU: Hematuria
HEMA: **Hemolytic anemia, eosinophilia, thrombocytopenia, leukopenia**
INTEG: Rash
MISC: Flulike syndrome, shortness of breath, chest pressure
MS: Asthenia, arthralgia, myalgia

Contraindications: Hypersensitivity, active TB, WBC <1000, platelets <50,000

Precautions: Pregnancy **B**, lactation, hepatic disease, blood dyscrasias, children

⬛ **Do Not Confuse:**
rifabutin/rifampin

Pharmacokinetics
Absorption	Well absorbed
Distribution	Widely distributed
Metabolism	Liver
Excretion	Kidney
Half-life	45 hr

Pharmacodynamics
Onset	Unknown
Peak	2-3 hr

Interactions
Individual drugs
Alcohol: ↑ toxicity
Carbamazepine: ↑ toxicity
Cycloserine: ↑ toxicity
Ethionamide: ↑ toxicity
Rifampin: ↑ toxicity
Drug classifications
Antacids, aluminum: ↓ absorption
Food/drug
High fat: ↓ absorption

NURSING CONSIDERATIONS
Assessment
• Assess for active tuberculosis: chest x-ray, sputum culture, blood culture, biopsy of lymph nodes, obtain PPD test; drug should be given only for Mycobacterium avium complex (MAC) and never for TB
• Monitor CBC for neutropenia, thrombocytopenia, eosinophilia

Nursing diagnoses
☑ Infection, risk for (uses)
☑ Diarrhea (adverse reaction)
☑ Injury, risk for (adverse reaction)
☑ Knowledge deficit (teaching)
☑ Noncompliance (teaching)

Implementation
• Give with meals to decrease GI symptoms; better to take on empty stomach 1 hr ac or 2 hr pc; high fat food slows absorption

R

🍁 Canada Only   Adverse effects: *italic* = common; **bold** = life-threatening

• Give antiemetic if vomiting occurs

Patient/family education
• Caution patient that compliance with dosage schedule and duration is necessary
• Instruct patient that scheduled appointments must be kept or relapse may occur
• Instruct patient to notify prescriber if hepatitis, neutropenia, or thrombocytopenia occurs: sore throat, fever, bleeding, bruising, yellow sclera, anorexia, nausea, vomiting, fatigue, weakness
• Advise patient that urine, feces, saliva, sputum, sweat, tears may be colored redorange; soft contact lens may become permanently stained
• Caution patients using oral contraceptives to use a nonhormonal method of birth control because rifabutin may decrease efficiency of oral contraceptives

Evaluation
Positive therapeutic outcome
• Decreased symptoms of *M. avium* in patients with HIV

---

rifampin (℞)
(rif'am-pin)
Rifadin, Rimactane,
Rofact ✦
Func. class.: Antitubercular
Chem. class.: Rifamycin B derivative
Pregnancy category   C

Action: Inhibits DNA-dependent polymerase, decreases replication

⇒**Therapeutic Outcome:** Bactericidal against the following organisms: mycobacteria, *Staphylococcus aureus, Hemophilus influenzae, Neisseria men-* *ingitides, Legionella pneumophilia*

Uses: Pulmonary tuberculosis, meningococcal carriers (prevention)

Dosage and routes
Tuberculosis
Adult: PO/**IV** 600 mg/day as single dose 1 hr ac or 2 hr pc or 10 mg/kg/day

6 month regimen: 2 mo treatment of isoniazid, rifampin, pyrazinamide, and possibly streptomycin or ethambutol; then rifampin and isoniazid × 4 mo

9 month regimen: Rifampin and isoniazid supplemented with pyrazinamide, or streptomycin or ethambutol

P *Child >5 yr:* PO/**IV** 10-20 mg/kg/day as single dose 1 hr ac or 2 hr pc, not to exceed 600 mg/day, with other antituberculars

Meningococcal carriers
Adult: PO/**IV** 600 mg bid × 2 days

P *Child >5 yr:* PO/**IV** 10 mg/kg bid × 2 days, not to exceed 600 mg/dose

P *Infant 3 mo-1 yr:* PO 5 mg/kg bid for 2 days

Available forms: Caps 150, 300 mg; powder for inj 600 mg/vial

Adverse effects
CNS: Headache, fatigue, anxiety, drowsiness, confusion
EENT: Visual disturbances
GI: Nausea, vomiting, anorexia, diarrhea, **pseudomembranous colitis,** *heartburn,* sore mouth and tongue, pancreatitis
GU: **Hematuria, acute renal failure, hemoglobinuria**

HEMA: **Hemolytic anemia, eosinophilia, thrombocytopenia, leukopenia**
INTEG: Rash, pruritus, urticaria
MISC: Flulike syndrome, menstrual disturbances, edema, shortness of breath
MS: Ataxia, weakness

Contraindications: Hypersensitivity

Precautions: Pregnancy **C**, lactation, hepatic disease, blood dyscrasias

▧ Do Not Confuse:
rifampin/rifabutin

Pharmacokinetics

Absorption	Well absorbed (PO), completely absorbed (**IV**)
Distribution	Widely distributed, crosses placenta
Metabolism	Liver—extensively
Excretion	Feces
Half-life	3 hr

Pharmacodynamics

	PO	IV
Onset	Rapid	Rapid
Peak	2-3 hr	Inf end

Interactions
Individual drugs
Alcohol: ↑ toxicity
Chloramphenicol: ↓ effect of chloramphenicol
Disopyramide: ↓ effect of disopyramide
Fluconazole: ↓ effect of fluconazole
Isoniazid: ↑ toxicity
Ketoconazole: ↑ toxicity
Lithium: ↑ lithium toxicity
Miconazole: ↑ toxicity
Phenytoin: ↓ effect of phenytoin
Quinidine: ↓ effect of quinidine

Theophylline: ↓ effect of theophylline
Tocainide: ↓ effect of tocainide
Verapamil: ↓ effect of verapamil
Drug classifications
Glucocorticoids: ↓ effect
Opiates: ↓ effect
Oral contraceptives: ↓ effect

NURSING CONSIDERATIONS
Assessment
• Monitor liver studies qwk: ALT, AST, bilirubin
• Monitor renal status: before, qmo: BUN, creatinine, output, sp gr, urinalysis
• Monitor mental status often: affect, mood, behavioral changes; psychosis may occur
• Monitor hepatic status: decreased appetite, jaundice, dark urine, fatigue
• Assess for infection: sputum culture, lung sounds
• C&S tests should be performed prior to beginning treatment, during, and after therapy is completed

Nursing diagnoses
☑ Infection, risk for (uses)
☑ Diarrhea (adverse reactions)
☑ Injury, risk for (adverse reactions)
☑ Knowledge deficit (teaching)
☑ Noncompliance (teaching)

Implementation
PO route
• Administer with meals to decrease GI symptoms; better to take on empty stomach 1 hr ac or 2 hr pc
▧ IV route
Intermittent **IV**
• Give by intermittent inf after reconstituting 600 mg/10 ml of sterile water for inj, agitate gently; dilute further in 100 or 500 ml 0.9% NaCl or D_5W;

R

give 100 ml/30 min or 500 ml/3 hr
• Do not mix with other drugs or sols

Patient/family education
• Instruct patient that compliance with dosage schedule, duration is necessary
• Instruct patient that scheduled appointments must be kept or relapse may occur
• Instruct patient to notify prescriber if hepatitis, neutropenia, or thrombocytopenia occurs: sore throat, fever, bleeding, bruising, yellow sclera, anorexia, nausea, vomiting, fatigue, weakness
• Advise patient that urine, feces, saliva, sputum, sweat, tears may be colored red-orange; soft contact lens may be permanently stained
• Caution patients using oral contraceptives to use a nonhormonal method of birth control because rifabutin may decrease the efficiency of oral contraceptives

Evaluation
Positive therapeutic outcome
• Decreased symptoms of TB

---

rifapentine (℞)
(riff'ah-pen-teen)
Priftin
Func. class.: Antitubercular
Chem. class.: Rifamycin derivative

Pregnancy category   C

Action: Inhibits DNA-dependent polymerase, decreases tubercule bacilli replication

➔**Therapeutic Outcome:** Resolution of pulmonary TB

Uses: Pulmonary tuberculosis; must be used with at least one other antitubercular

Dosage and routes
Intensive phase
Adult: **PO** 600 mg (four 150 mg tabs 2×/wk), with an interval of 72 hr between doses × 2 mo; must be given with at least one other antitubercular

Continuation phase
Adult: **PO** continue with 1×/wk × 4 mo in combination with isoniazid or other appropriate antitubercular

Available forms: Tabs 150 mg

Adverse effects
CNS: Headache, fatigue, anxiety, dizziness
EENT: Visual disturbances
GI: Nausea, vomiting, anorexia, diarrhea, bilirubinemia, hepatitis, increased ALT, AST, *heartburn,* **pancreatitis**
GU: **Hematuria,** pyuria, proteinuria, urinary casts
HEMA: **Thrombocytopenia, leukopenia, neutropenia, lymphopenia,** anemia, **leukocytosis,** purpura, hematoma
INTEG: Rash, pruritis, urticaria, acne
MISC: Edema, aggressive reaction
MS: Gout, arthrosis

Contraindications: Hypersensitivity to rifamycins

Precautions: Pregnancy **C,** lactation, hepatic disease, ▣blood dyscrasias, children <12 yr

Pharmacokinetics	
Absorption	Unknown
Distribution	Unknown
Metabolism	Unknown
Excretion	Unknown
Half-life	Unknown

Pharmacodynamics	
Onset	Unknown
Peak	Unknown
Duration	Unknown

Interactions
Individual drugs
Amitriptyline: ↓ action of amitriptyline

Chloramphenicol: ↓ action of chloramphenicol

Clarithromycin: ↓ action of chloramphenicol

Clofibrate: ↓ action of clofibrate

Cyclosporine: ↓ action of cyclosporine

Dapsone: ↓ action of dapsone

Delaviridine: ↓ action of delaviridine

Diazepam: ↓ action of diazepam

Digoxin: ↓ action of digoxin

Diltiazem: ↓ action of diltiazem

Disopyramide: ↓ action of disopyramide

Doxycycline: ↓ action of doxycycline

Fluconazole: ↓ action of fluconazole

Haloperidol: ↓ action of haloperidol

Indinavir: ↓ action of indinavir

Itraconazole: ↓ action of itraconazole

Ketoconazole: ↓ action of ketoconazole

Methadone: ↓ action of methadone

Mexiletine: ↓ action of mexiletine

Nelfinavir: ↓ action of nelfinavir

Nifedipine: ↓ action of nifedipine

Nortriptyline: ↓ action of nortriptyline

Phenytoin: ↓ action of phenytoin

Quinidine: ↓ action of quinidine

Quinine: ↓ action of quinine

Ritonavir: ↓ action of ritonavir

Saquinavir: ↓ action of saquinavir

Sildenafil: ↓ action of sildenafil

Tacrolimus: ↓ action of tacrolimus

Theophylline: ↓ action of theophylline

Tocainide: ↓ action of tocainide

Verapamil: ↓ action of verapamil

Zidovudine: ↓ action of zidovudine

Drug classifications
Anticoagulants: ↓ action of anticoagulants

Antidiabetics: ↓ action of antidiabetics

Barbiturates: ↓ action of barbiturates

Corticosteroids: ↓ action of corticosteroids

Fluoroquinolones: ↓ action of fluoroquinolones

Oral contraceptives ↓ action of oral contraceptives

Protease inhibitors: Use extreme caution

Thyroid preparations: ↓ action of thyroid preparations

Food/drug
Food: ↑ drug concentration by 44%

Lab test interferences:
Interference: Folate level, vit B_{12}

NURSING CONSIDERATIONS
Assessment
• Monitor baselines in CBC, AST, ALT, bilirubin, platelets

• Assess for infection: sputum culture, lung sounds
• Assess signs of anemia: Hct, Hgb, fatigue
• Monitor liver studies qmo: ALT, AST, bilirubin
• Monitor renal status qmo: BUN, creatinine, output, specific gravity, urinalysis
• Assess hepatic status: decreased appetite, jaundice, dark urine, fatigue

Nursing diagnoses
☑ Infection, risk for (uses)
☑ Diarrhea (side effects)
☑ Knowledge deficit (teaching)
☑ Noncompliance (teaching)

Implementation
PO route
• Give PO, may be given with food for GI upset
• Give antiemetic if vomiting occurs
• Administer after C&S is completed; qmo to detect resistance

Patient/family education
• Advise patient that compliance with dosage schedule, duration is necessary
• Instruct patient that scheduled appointments must be kept; relapse may occur
• Teach patient that urine, feces, saliva, sputum, sweat, tears may be colored red-orange; soft contact lenses may be permanently stained
• Teach patient to use alternate method of contraception, oral contraceptive action may be decreased
• Teach patient to report flulike symptoms: excessive fatigue, anorexia, vomiting, sore throat; unusual bleeding, jaundice of skin, eyes

Evaluation
Positive therapeutic outcome
• Decreased symptoms of TB
• Culture-negative

riluzole (℞)
(ri-loo′zole)
Rilutek
Func. class.: ALS agent
Chem. class.: Benzathiazole
Pregnancy category   C

Action: Unknown; may act by inhibiting glutamate, interfering with binding of amino acid receptors, inactivation of voltage-dependent sodium channels

⮞ **Therapeutic Outcome:** Decreased symptoms of ALS

Uses: Amyotropic lateral sclerosis (ALS)

Dosage and routes
Adult: PO 50 mg q12h, take 1 hr ac or 2 hr pc

Available forms: Tab 50 mg

Adverse effects
CNS: Hypertonia, depression, dizziness, insomnia, somnolence, vertigo
CV: Hypertension, tachycardia, phlebitis, palpitation, postural hypertension
GI: Nausea, vomiting, dyspepsia, anorexia, diarrhea, flatulence, stomatitis, dry mouth
GU: UTI, dysuria
HEMA: **Neutropenia**
INTEG: Pruritus, eczema, alopecia, **exfoliative dermatitis**
RESP: Decreased lung function; rhinitis, increased cough

Contraindications: Hypersensitivity

☑ Herb/drug 🚫 Do Not Crush ◆ Alert ⛒ Key Drug **G** Geriatric **P** Pediatric

Precautions: Neutropenia, renal disease, hepatic disease, **G** elderly, pregnancy **C**, lactation, **P** children

Pharmacokinetics

Absorption	Well
Distribution	Unknown
Metabolism	Extensively-live
Excretion	Urine, feces
Half-life	Unknown

Pharmacodynamics

Unknown

Interactions
Individual drugs
Amitriptyline: ↓ elimination of riluzole
Caffeine: ↓ elimination of riluzole
Cigarette smoke: ↑ elimination of riluzole
Omeprazole: ↑ elimination of riluzole
Rifampin: ↑ elimination of riluzole
Theophylline: ↓ elimination of riluzole
Drug classifications
Quinolones: ↓ elimination of riluzole
Food/drug
Charcoal-broiled foods: ↑ elimination of riluzole

NURSING CONSIDERATIONS
Assessment
• Monitor LFTs: AST, ALT, bilirubin, GGT, baseline and q mo × 3 mo, then q3 mo; monitor liver chemistries
• Assess for neutropenia <500/mm³
Nursing diagnoses
☑ Physical mobility, impaired (uses)
☑ Knowledge deficit (teaching)

Implementation
• Give 1 hr ac or 2 hr pc; a high-fat meal decreases absorption

Patient/family education
• Advise to report febrile illness, may indicate neutropenia
• Teach reason for drug and expected results

---

rimantadine (℞)
(ri-man′ti-deen)
Flumadine
Func. class.: Synthetic antiviral
Chem. class.: Tricyclic amine
Pregnancy category   C

Action: Prevents uncoating of nucleic acid in viral cell, preventing penetration of virus to host; causes release of dopamine from neurons

➡ **Therapeutic Outcome:** Prevention of influenza type A

Uses: Prophylaxis or treatment of influenza type A

Dosage and routes
Renal/hepatic dose
Reduce as needed
Influenza type A prophylaxis
Adult: PO 100 mg bid; in renal hepatic disease, lower dose to 100 mg/day
P *Child: <10 yr:* PO 5 mg/kg/day, not to exceed 150 mg
Treatment
P *Adult and child >10 yr:* PO 100 mg bid; in renal or hepatic disease, lower dose to 100 mg/day; start treatment at onset of symptoms, continue for at least 1 wk

R

G *Elderly:* PO 100 mg/day

Available forms: Tab 100 mg; syr 50 mg/5 ml

Adverse effects

CNS: Headache, dizziness, fatigue, depression, hallucinations, tremors, **convulsions,** insomnia, *poor concentration,* asthenia, gait abnormalities

CV: Pallor, palpitations, hypertension

EENT: Tinnitus, taste abnormality, eye pain

GI: Nausea, vomiting, constipation, dry mouth, anorexia, abdominal pain, diarrhea, dyspepsia

INTEG: Rash

Contraindications: Hypersensitivity, lactation, child <1 yr **P**

Precautions: Epilepsy, hepatic disease, renal disease, pregnancy **C**

N Do Not Confuse:
rimantadine/amantadine

Pharmacokinetics	
Absorption	Minimally absorbed (PO)
Distribution	Widely distributed, crosses placenta, CSF concentration 50% plasma
Metabolism	Liver
Excretion	95% unchanged—kidneys
Half-life	2-3.5 hr, increased in renal disease

Pharmacodynamics	
	PO
Onset	Unknown
Peak	1½-2½

Interactions
Individual drugs
Amphotericin B: ↑ neurotoxicity, nephrotoxicity
Interferon: ↑ neurotoxicity, nephrotoxicity

Methotrexate: ↑ neurotoxicity, nephrotoxicity
Probenecid: ↑ neurotoxicity, nephrotoxicity
Drug classification
Aminoglycosides: ↑ neurotoxicity, nephrotoxicity

NURSING CONSIDERATIONS
Assessment
• Assess allergies before initiation of treatment, patient's reaction to each medication; list allergies on chart in bright red letters
• Monitor respiratory status: rate, character, wheezing, tightness in chest

Nursing diagnoses
☑ Infection, risk for (uses)
☑ Knowledge deficit (teaching)

Implementation
• Give before exposure to influenza; continue for 10 days after contact
• Give at least 4 hr before hs to prevent insomnia
• Administer pc for better absorption, to decrease GI symptoms; cap may be opened and mixed with food for easy swallowing
• Give in divided doses to prevent CNS disturbances: headache, dizziness, fatigue, drowsiness
• Store in tight, dry container

Patient/family education
• Instruct patient about aspects of drug therapy: need to report dyspnea, dizziness, poor concentration, behavioral changes
• Advise patient to avoid hazardous activities if dizziness occurs
• Caution patient to discuss with prescriber before taking OTC medications, or

---

☑ Herb/drug ⬯ Do Not Crush ◆ Alert ☋ Key Drug **G** Geriatric **P** Pediatric alcohol—serious drug interactions may result

Evaluation
Positive therapeutic outcome
• Absence of fever, malaise, cough, dyspnea

Treatment of overdose: Withdraw drug, maintain airway, administer epinephrine, aminophylline, O₂, **IV** corticosteroids, physostigmine

---

risedronate (℞)
(rih-sed'roh-nate)
Actonel
Func. class: Bone resorption inhibitor
Chem. class.: Biphosphonate
Pregnancy category   C

Action: Absorbs calcium phosphate crystal in bone and may directly block dissolution of hydroxyapatite crystals of bone; inhibits bone resorption, apparently without inhibiting bone formation, mineralization

➔**Therapeutic Outcome:** Increased bone mass, activity without fractures

Uses: Paget's disease

Investigational uses: Osteoporosis in postmenopausal women

Dosage and routes
Adult: PO 30 mg qd × 2 mo; patients with Paget's disease should receive calcium and vit D if dietary intake is lacking; if relapse occurs, retreatment is advised

Available forms: Tabs 30 mg

Adverse effects
CNS: Dizziness, headache
CV: Chest pain

GI: Abdominal pain, anorexia, diarrhea, *nausea*
MS: Bone pain, arthralgia

Contraindications: Hypersensitivity to biphosphonates

P Precautions: Children, lactation, pregnancy **C**, renal disease

Pharmacokinetics	
Absorption	Unknown
Distribution	To bones
Metabolism	Unknown
Excretion	Kidneys
Half-life	Unknown

Pharmacodynamics	
Onset	Unknown
Peak	Unknown
Duration	Unknown

Interactions
Drug classifications
Antacids: ↓ absorption of risedronate
Calcium supplement: ↓ absorption of risedronate
Food/drug
Food: ↓ bioavailability: take ½ hr before food or drinks

NURSING CONSIDERATIONS
Assessment
• Monitor electrolytes: renal function studies; Ca, P, Mg, K
• Assess for hypercalcemia: paresthesia, twitching, laryngospasm, Chvostek's/Trousseau's signs

Nursing diagnoses
✓Immobility, impaired (uses)
✓Nutrition, altered, less than body requirements (uses)
✓Knowledge deficit (teaching)

Implementation
• Give PO for 2 months to be effective in Paget's disease
• Give with a full glass of water; patient should be in upright position

R

- Administer supplemental calcium and vit D in Paget's disease
- Store in cool environment, out of direct sunlight

Evaluation
Positive therapeutic outcome
- Increased bone mass, absence of fractures

---

risperidone (℞)
(res-pare′a-done)
Risperdal
Func. class: Antipsychotic/neuroleptic
Chem. class.: Benzisoxazole derivative
Pregnancy category C

Action: Unknown; may be mediated through both dopamine type 2 (D_2) and serotinin type 2 ($5-HT_2$) antagonism

Therapeutic Outcome: Decreased hallucination and disorganized thought

Uses: Psychotic disorders

Dosage and routes
Adult: PO 1 mg bid, with incremental increases of 1 mg bid on days 2 and 3 to a dose of 3 mg bid by day 3; then do not increase dose for at least 1 wk

G *Elderly:* PO 0.5 mg qd-bid increase by 1 mg qwk

Available forms: Tabs 1, 2, 3, 4 mg; oral sol 1 mg/ml

Adverse effects
CNS: Extrapyrimidal symptoms, pseudoparkinsonism, akathisia, dystonia, tardive dyskinesia, drowsiness, insomnia, agitation, anxiety, headache, **neuroleptic malignant syndrome**

CV: Orthostatic hypotension, **tachycardia**
EENT: Blurred vision
GI: Nausea, vomiting, *anorexia, constipation,* jaundice, weight gain
RESP: Rhinitis

Contraindications: Hypersensitivity, lactation, seizure disorders

P Precautions: Children, renal disease, pregnancy **C**, hepatic
G disease, elderly, breast cancer

N Do Not Confuse:
Risperdal/reserpine

Pharmacokinetics	
Absorption	Unknown
Distribution	Unknown
Metabolism	Liver, extensively
Excretion	Unknown
Half-life	Unknown

Pharmacodynamics	
Onset	Unknown
Peak	Unknown
Duration	Up to 12 hr

Interactions
Individual drugs
Alcohol: ↑ effects of both drugs, oversedation
Lithium: ↑ extrapyramidal symptoms, masking of lithium toxicity
Tegretol: ↑ excretion of risperidone
Drug classifications
Antidepressants: ↑ CNS depression
Antihistamines: ↑ CNS depression
Barbiturate anesthetics: ↑ CNS depression
General anesthetics: ↑ CNS depression
MAOIs: ↑ CNS depression
Opiates: ↑ CNS depression
Sedative/hypnotics: ↑ CNS depression

☑ *Herb/drug*
Kava: ↑ CNS depression
Lab test interferences
↑ Liver function tests, ↑ cardiac enzymes, ↑ cholesterol, ↑ blood glucose, ↑ prolactin, ↑ bilirubin, ↑ PBI, ↑ cholinesterase; ↑ I, ↑ alk phosphatase, ↑ leukocytes, ↑ granulocytes, ↑ platelets
↓ Hormones (blood and urine)
False positive: Pregnancy tests, PKU, urine bilirubin
False negative: Urinary steroids, 17-OCHS

NURSING CONSIDERATIONS
Assessment
• Assess mental status: orientation, mood, behavior, presence and type of hallucinations before initial administration and monthly; this drug should significantly reduce psychotic behavior
• Check that patient swallows all PO medication; check for hoarding or giving of medication to other patients
• Monitor I&O ratio, palpate bladder if low urinary output
🄶 occurs, especially in elderly; urinalysis recommended before, during prolonged therapy
• Monitor bilirubin, CBC, liver function studies monthly
• Assess affect, orientation, LOC, reflexes, gait, coordination, sleep pattern disturbances
• Monitor B/P with patient in sitting, standing, and lying positions; take pulse and respirations q4h during initial treatment; establish baseline before starting treatment; report drops of 30 mm Hg; obtain baseline ECG; and Q-wave and T-wave changes
• Check for dizziness, faintness, palpitations, tachycardia

on rising; severe orthostatic hypotension is common
◀◆• Identify for neuroleptic malignant syndrome: hyperpyrexia, muscle rigidity, increased CPK, altered mental status; drug should be discontinued
• Assess for extrapyramidal symptoms including akathisia (inability to sit still, no pattern to movements), tardive dyskinesia (bizarre movements of the jaw, mouth, tongue, extremities) pseudoparkinsonism (rigidity, tremors, pill rolling, shufling gait); an antiparkinsonian drug should be prescribed
• Assess for constipation, urinary retention daily; if these occur, increase bulk, water in diet

Nursing diagnoses
☑ Thought processes, altered (uses)
☑ Coping, ineffective individual (uses)
☑ Knowledge deficit (teaching)
☑ Noncompliance (teaching)

Implementation
• PO with full glass of water, milk; or give with food to decrease GI upset
• Store in airtight, light-resistant container

Patient/family education
• Teach patient to use good oral hygiene; frequent rinsing of mouth, sugarless gum for dry mouth
• Caution patient to avoid hazardous activities until drug response is determined—dizziness, blurred vision may occur
• Inform patient that orthostatic hypotension occurs often—patient should rise from sitting or lying position gradually and remain lying down for at least 30 min after IM inj

R

• Instruct patient to avoid hot tubs, hot showers, tub baths—hypotension may occur

• Inform patient that heat stroke may occur in hot weather, and to take extra precautions to stay cool

• Advise patient to avoid abrupt withdrawal of this drug, or extrapyramidal symptoms may result; drug should be withdrawn slowly

• Teach patient to avoid OTC preparations (cough, hay fever, cold) unless approved by prescriber—serious drug interactions may occur; avoid use with alcohol, CNS depressants because increased drowsiness may occur

Evaluation
Positive therapeutic outcome
• Decrease in emotional excitement, hallucinations, delusions, paranoia
• Reorganization of patterns of thought, speech

Treatment of overdose: Lavage, provide airway

---

ritonavir (℞)
(ri-toe'na-veer)
Norvir
Func. class.: Antiviral
Chem. class.: Petidomimetic inhibitor

Pregnancy category   B

Action: Inhibits human immunodeficiency virus (HIV) protease and prevents maturation of the infectious virus

Therapeutic Outcome: Improvement of HIV infection

Uses: HIV in combination with AZT, ddc, or alone

Dosage and routes
Adult: PO 600 mg bid; if nausea occurs, begin dose at ½ and gradually increase

P *Child:* PO 250 mg/m^2 bid, titrate upward to 400 mg/m^2 bid

Available forms: Caps 100 mg; oral sol 80 mg/ml

Adverse effects
CNS: Paresthesia, headache
GI: Diarrhea, buccal mucosa ulceration, abdominal pain, nausea, taste perversion, dry mouth
INTEG: Rash
MS: Pain
OTHER: Asthenia

Contraindications: Hypersensitivity

Precautions: Liver disease, **P** pregnancy **B,** lactation, children

Pharmacokinetics	
Absorption	Unknown
Distribution	Unknown
Metabolism	Unknown
Excretion	Unknown
Half-life	Unknown

Pharmacodynamics
Unknown

Interactions
Individual drugs
Clarithromycin: ↑ level of both drugs
ddc: ↑ level of both drugs
Desipramine: ↑ level
Disulfiram: ↑ level
Fluconazole: ↑ level
Metronidazole: ↑ level
Sulfamethoxazole: ↓ level
Theophylline: ↓ level
Zidovudine: ↓ level

⊘ Herb/drug   ⊘ Do Not Crush   ◆ Alert   ⬥┰ Key Drug   **G** Geriatric   **P** Pediatric

Lab test interferences
↑ ALT, ↑ GGT, ↑ PT, triglyc-
erides
↓ HCT, ↓ RBC

NURSING CONSIDERATIONS
Assessment
• Assess for signs of infection,
anemia
• Assess for liver studies: ALT,
AST
• Assess for C&S before drug
therapy; drug may be taken as
soon as culture is taken; repeat
C&S after treatment; determine the presence of other
sexually transmitted disease
• Assess for bowel pattern
before, during treatment; if
severe abdominal pain with
bleeding occurs, drug should
be discontinued; monitor
hydration
• Assess for skin eruptions,
rash
• Assess for allergies before
treatment, reaction to each
medication; place allergies on
chart
Nursing diagnoses
☑ Infection, risk for (uses)
☑ Knowledge deficit (teaching)
Patient/family education
• Teach patient to take as
prescribed; if dose is missed,
take as soon as remembered up
to 1 hr before next dose; do
not double dose
• Teach patient that drug must
be taken in equal intervals
around the clock to maintain
blood levels for duration of
therapy

rituximab (℞)
(rih-tuks′ih-mab)
Rituxan
Func. class.: Misc. antineoplastic
Chem. class.: Murine/
human monoclonal anti-
body
Pregnancy category   C

Action: Directed against the
CD20 antigen that is found
on malignant B lymphocytes;
CD20 regulates a portion of
cell-cycle initiation/
differentiation

➡**Therapeutic Outcome:** Decreased tumor size, prevention
of spread of cancer

Uses: Non-Hodgkin's lymphoma (CD20 positive, B-cell)

Dosage and routes
Adult: **IV inf** 375 mg/m² qwk
× 4 doses; give at 50 mg/hr
for 1st inf; if hypersensitivity
does not occur, increase rate by
50 mg/hr q½h, max 400
mg/hr; slow/interrupt inf if
hypersensitivity occurs; other
inf can be given at 100 mg/hr
and increased by 100 mg/hr,
max 400 mg/hr

Available forms: Inj 10
mg/ml

Adverse effects
GI: Nausea, vomiting, anorexia
**HEMA: Leukopenia, neutro-
penia, thrombocytopenia**
INTEG: Irrigation at site, rash
OTHER: Fever, chills, asthenia, headache, angioedema,
hypotension, myalgia, bronchospasm

Contraindications: Hypersensitivity, murine proteins

🅿**Precautions:** Lactation, children,
🅖 elderly, pregnancy **C**

R

Pharmacokinetics

Absorption	Unknown
Distribution	Unknown
Metabolism	Unknown
Excretion	Unknown
Half-life	42-79 min

Pharmacodynamics

Onset	Unknown
Peak	Unknown
Duration	Unknown

Interactions
Unknown

NURSING CONSIDERATIONS
Assessment
• Monitor CBC, differential, platelet count weekly; withhold drug if WBC is <3500/mm^3, or platelet count <100,000/mm^3; notify prescriber of these results; drug should be discontinued
• Assess food preferences: list likes, dislikes
• Assess GI symptoms: frequency of stools
• Assess signs of dehydration: rapid respirations, poor skin turgor, decreased urine output, dry skin, restlessness, weakness

Nursing diagnoses
☑ Injury, risk for (side effects)
☑ Knowledge deficit (teaching)

Implementation
IV IV infusion
• Administer after diluting to a final conc of 1-4 mg/ml; use 0.9% NaCl, D$_5$W, gently invert bag to mix; do not mix with other drugs
• Increase fluid intake to 2-3 L/day to prevent dehydration, unless contraindicated
• Change **IV** site q48h
• Provide nutritious diet with iron, vitamin supplement, low fiber, few dairy products
• Store vials at 36°-40° F, protect vials from direct sunlight, inf sol is stable at 36°-46° F × 24 hr and room temp for another 12 hr

Patient/family education
• Teach patient to report adverse reactions

Evaluation
Positive therapeutic outcome
• Decrease in tumor size, decrease in spread of cancer

---

rizatriptan (℞)
(rye-zah-trip′tan)
Maxalt, Maxalt-MLT
Func. class.: Migraine agent
Chem. class.: 5-HT$_1$-like receptor agonist
Pregnancy category C

Action: Binds selectively to the vascular 5-HT$_1$ receptor subtype, exerts antimigraine effect; causes vasoconstriction in cranial arteries

➡ **Therapeutic Outcome:** After treatment, relief of migraine

Uses: Acute treatment of migraine

Dosage and routes
Adult: **PO** 5-10 mg single dose, redosing separate by 2 hr or more; max 30 mg/24 hr

Available forms: Maxalt: tabs 5, 10 mg; Maxalt-MLT: tabs, orally disintegrating 5, 10 mg

Adverse effects
CNS: Dizziness, headache, fatigue
GI: Nausea, dry mouth
RESP: Chest tightness, pressure

Contraindications: Angina pectoris, history of MI, docu-

---

mented silent ischemia, Prinzmetal's angina, ischemic heart disease, concurrent ergotamine-containing preparations, uncontrolled hypertension, hypersensitivity, basilar or hemiplegic migraine

Precautions: Postmenopausal women, men >40 yr, risk factors for CAD, hypercholesterolemia, obesity, diabetes, impaired hepatic or renal **P** function, pregnancy **C**, **G** lactation, children, elderly

Pharmacokinetics

Absorption	Unknown
Distribution	Unknown
Metabolism	Liver (metabolite)
Excretion	Urine/feces
Half-life	2-3 hr

Pharmacodynamics

Onset	10 min-2 hr
Peak	Unknown
Duration	Unknown

Interactions
Individual drugs
Cimetidine: ↑ action of rizatriptan
Ergot: ↑ vasospastic effects
Propranolol: ↑ action of rizatriptan
Drug classifications
Ergot derivatives: ↑ vasospastic effects
MAOIs: ↑ action of rizatriptan
5-HT$_1$ receptor agonist: ↑ vasospastic effects
SSRIs: ↑ weakness, hyperreflexia, incoordination

NURSING CONSIDERATIONS
Assessment
• Assess for tingling, hot sensations, burning, feeling of pressure, numbness, flushing, injection site reaction
• Assess for stress level, activity, recreation, coping mechanisms
• Assess neurologic status: LOC, blurring vision, nausea, vomiting, tingling in extremities preceding headache
• Monitor for ingestion of tyramine foods (pickled products, beer, wine, aged cheese), food additives, preservatives, colorings, artificial sweeteners, chocolate, caffeine, which may precipitate these types of headaches

Nursing diagnoses
☑ Pain (uses)
☑ Knowledge deficit (teaching)

Implementation
• Provide quiet, calm environment with decreased stimulation for noise, bright light, excessive talking

Patient/family education
• Teach patient use of orally disintegrating tab: instruct patient not to open blister until use, to peel blister open with dry hands, to place tab on tongue, where it will dissolve, and to swallow with saliva (contains phenylalanine)
• Advise patient to report any side effects to prescriber
• Advise patient to use alternate contraception while taking **R** drug if oral contraceptives are being used

Evaluation
Positive therapeutic outcome
• Decrease in frequency, severity of headache

---

rofecoxib
See Appendix A, Selected New Drugs

---

ropinirole (℞)
(roe-pin'e-role)
Requip
Func. class.: Antiparkinsonian agent
Chem. class.: Dopamine-receptor agonist, nonergot
Pregnancy category C

Pharmacokinetics

Absorption	Well absorbed
Distribution	Widely distributed
Metabolism	Liver, extensively
Excretion	Kidneys
Half-life	6 hr

Pharmacodynamics
Unknown

Action: Selective agonist for D_2 receptors (presynaptic/postsynaptic sites); binding at D_3 receptor contributes to antiparkinson effects

Therapeutic Outcome: Decreased symptoms of Parkinson's disease (involuntary movements)

Uses: Parkinsonism

Dosage and routes
Adult: PO 0.25 mg tid, titrate weekly to a max of 24 mg/day

Available forms: Tabs 0.25, 0.5, 1, 2, 5 mg

Adverse effects
CNS: Dystonia, *agitation, insomnia,* dizziness, psychosis, hallucinations, depression
CV: Orthostatic hypotension, hypotension, syncope, palpitations, **tachycardia,** hypertension
EENT: Blurred vision
GI: Nausea, vomiting, anorexia, dry mouth, constipation, dyspepsia, flatulence
GU: Impotence, urinary frequency
INTEG: Rash, sweating
RESP: Pharyngitis, rhinitis, sinusitis, bronchitis, dyspnea

Contraindications: Hypersensitivity

Precautions: Renal disease, cardiac disease, dysrhythmias, affective disorders, psychosis, pregnancy **C**

Interactions
Individual drugs
Cimetidine: ↑ effect of ropinirole
Ciprofloxacin: ↑ ropinirole effect
Diltiazem: ↑ ropinirole effect
Enoxacin: ↑ ropinirole effect
Erythromycin: ↑ ropinirole effect
Estrogen: ↓ oral clearance of ropinirole
Fluvoxamine: ↑ ropinirole effect
Levodopa: ↑ effect of levodopa
Mexiletine: ↑ ropinirole effect
Norfloxacin: ↑ ropinirole effect
Tacrine: ↑ ropinirole effect
Herb/drug
Chaste tree fruit: ↓ ropinirole action

NURSING CONSIDERATIONS
Assessment
• Monitor B/P, respiration during initial treatment; hypotension or hypertension should be reported
• Assess mental status: affect, mood, behavioral changes, depression; complete suicide assessment
• Assess for involuntary movements in parkinsonism: akinesia, tremors, staggering gait, muscle rigidity, drooling; these symptoms should improve with therapy

---

🗷 Herb/drug 🛇 Do Not Crush ◆ Alert ⚏ Key Drug �G Geriatric 🅟 Pediatric

Nursing diagnoses
- ✓ Mobility, impaired (uses)
- ✓ Injury, risk for (uses)
- ✓ Knowledge deficit (teaching)
- ✓ Noncompliance (teaching)

Implementation
- Give drug until NPO before surgery
- Adjust dosage to patient response
- Give with meals to decrease GI upset

Patient/family education
- Advise patient that therapeutic effects may take several wk to a few mo
- Caution patient to change positions slowly to prevent orthostatic hypotension
- Instruct patient to use drug exactly as prescribed; if drug is discontinued abruptly, parkinsonian crisis may occur

Evaluation
Positive therapeutic outcome
- Decreased akathisia, other involuntary movements
- Increased mood

---

ropivacaine (℞)
(roe-pi'va-kane)
Naropin
Func. class.: Local anesthetic
Chem. class.: Amide
Pregnancy category **B**

Action: Competes with calcium for sites in nerve membrane that control sodium transport across cell membrane; decreases rise of depolarization phase of action potential

➥**Therapeutic Outcome:** Maintenance of local anesthesia

Uses: Peripheral nerve block, caudal anesthesia, central neural block, vaginal block

Dosage and routes
Varies with route of anesthesia

Available forms: Inj 2, 5, 7.5 mg/ml

Adverse effects
CNS: Anxiety, restlessness, **convulsions, loss of consciousness,** drowsiness, disorientation, tremors, shivering
CV: **Myocardial depression, cardiac arrest, dysrhythmias,** bradycardia, hypotension, hypertension, **fetal bradycardia**
EENT: Blurred vision, tinnitus, pupil constriction
GI: Nausea, vomiting
INTEG: Rash, urticaria, allergic reactions, edema, burning, skin discoloration at injection site, tissue necrosis
RESP: **Status asthmaticus, respiratory arrest, anaphylaxis**

Contraindications: Hypersensitivity, child <12 yr, elderly, severe liver disease

Precautions: Severe drug allergies, pregnancy **B**

Pharmacokinetics

Absorption	Complete
Distribution	Unknown
Metabolism	Liver
Excretion	Kidneys
Half-life	Unknown

Pharmacodynamics

Onset	2-8 min
Peak	Unknown
Duration	3-6 hr

Interactions
Individual drugs
Chloroprocaine: ↓ action of ropivacaine
Enflurane: ↑ dysrhythmias
Epinephrine: ↑ dysrhythmias
Halothane: ↑ dysrhythmias

Drug classifications
Antidepressants, tricyclic:
↑ hypertension
MAOIs: ↑ hypertension
Phenothiazines: ↑ hypertension

NURSING CONSIDERATIONS
Assessment
• Assess B/P, pulse, respiration during treatment
• Assess fetal heart tones during labor
• Assess allergic reactions: rash, urticaria, itching
• Assess cardiac status: ECG for dysrhythmias, pulse, B/P during anesthesia

Nursing diagnoses
☑ Knowledge deficit (teaching)

Implementation
• Give only with crash cart, resuscitative equipment nearby
• Give only drugs without preservaties for epidural or caudal anesthesia
• Use new sol; discard unused portions

Evaluation
Positive therapeutic outcome
• Anesthesia necessary for procedure

Treatment of overdose:
Airway, O₂, vasopressor, **IV** fluids, anticonvulsants for seizures

---

rosiglitazone
See Appendix A,
Selected New Drugs

---

salmeterol (℞)
(sal-met'er-ole)
Serevent
Func. class.: Adrenergic β₂ agonist

Pregnancy category   C

Action: Causes bronchodilatation by action on β₂ (pulmonary) receptors by increasing levels of cAMP, which relaxes smooth muscle; with very little effect on heart rate, maintains improvement in FEV from 3 to 12 hr; prevents nocturnal asthma symptoms

▸**Therapeutic Outcome:** Ease of breathing

Uses: Prevention of exercise-induced asthma, bronchospasm, COPD

Dosage and routes
Adult: Inh 2 puffs bid (AM and PM)

Available forms: Aerosol 25 µg/actuation; inhalation powder 50 µg

Adverse effects
CNS: Tremors, anxiety, insomnia, headache, dizziness, stimulation, restlessness, hallucinations, flushing, irritability
CV: Palpitations, **tachycardia,** hypertension, angina, hypotension, **dysrhythmias**
EENT: Dry nose, irritation of nose and throat
GI: Heartburn, nausea, vomiting
MS: Muscle cramps
RESP: **Bronchospasm**

Contraindications: Hypersensitivity to sympathomimetics, tachydysrhythmias, severe cardiac disease

Precautions: Lactation, pregnancy **C,** cardiac disorders,

☑ Herb/drug   ⊘ Do Not Crush   ◆ Alert   ⌒ᴛᴛ Key Drug   ⑤ Geriatric   ⑨ Pediatric hyperthyroidism, diabetes mellitus, hypertension, prostatic hypertrophy, narrow-angle glaucoma, seizures

Pharmacokinetics

Absorption	Unknown
Distribution	Unknown
Metabolism	Unknown
Excretion	Unknown
Half-life	Unknown

Pharmacodynamics

Onset	5-15 min
Peak	4 hr
Duration	12 hr

Interactions
Drug classifications
β-Adrenergic blockers: Block therapeutic effect
Bronchodilators, aerosol: ↑ action of bronchodilator
MAOIs: ↑ chance of hypertensive crisis
Sympathomimetics: ↑ adrenergic side effects

NURSING CONSIDERATIONS
Assessment
• Monitor respiratory function: vital capacity, forced expiratory volume, ABGs, lung sounds, heart rate, rhythm (baseline)

Nursing diagnoses
☑ Airway clearance, ineffective (uses)
☑ Impaired gas exchange (uses)
☑ Knowledge deficit (teaching)

Implementation
• Shake aerosol container, ask patient to exhale, then place mouthpiece in mouth, inhale slowly, hold breath, remove, exhale slowly; allow at least 1 min between inh
P • Use spacing device for
G pediatric/geriatric patients
• Store in light-resistant container, do not expose to temp over 86° F (30° C)

Patient/family education
• Caution patient not to use OTC medications because extra stimulation may occur
• Instruct patient to use this medication before other medications and to allow at least 1 min between each, to prevent overstimulation
• Teach patient how to use inhaler; review package insert with patient; to avoid getting aerosol in eyes; blurring may result; to wash inhaler in warm water qd and dry; to avoid smoking, smoke-filled rooms, and persons with respiratory infections
• Instruct patient on administration of dose, not to use more than prescribed; serious side effects may occur

Evaluation
Positive therapeutic outcome
• Absence of dyspnea, wheezing
• Improved airway exchange
• Improved ABGs

Treatment of overdose: Administer a β₂-adrenergic blocker

---

salsalate (℞)
(sal-sa'late)
Amigesic, Argesic-SA, Arthra-G, Disalcid, Marthritic, Mono-Gesic, Salflex, Salsalate, Salsitab
Func. class.: Nonnarcotic analgesic; nonsteroidal antiinflammatory agent
Chem. class.: Salicylate
Pregnancy category   C

S

Action: Blocks formation of peripheral prostaglandins, which cause pain and inflammation; antipyretic action results from inhibition of hypothalamic heat-regulating center; does not inhibit platelet aggregation

➡**Therapeutic Outcome:** Decreased pain, inflammation

Uses: Mild to moderate pain or fever, including arthritis, juvenile rheumatoid arthritis

Dosage and routes
Adult: PO 3 g/day in divided doses

Available forms: Cap 500 mg; tabs 500, 750 mg

Adverse effects
CNS: Stimulation, drowsiness, dizziness, confusion, **convulsions,** headache, flushing, hallucinations, coma
CV: Rapid pulse, **pulmonary edema**
EENT: Tinnitus, hearing loss
ENDO: Hypoglycemia, hyponatremia, hypokalemia, alteration in acid-base balance
GI: Nausea, vomiting, GI bleeding, diarrhea, heartburn, anorexia, **hepatotoxicity**
HEMA: **Thrombocytopenia, agranulocytosis, leukopenia, neutropenia, hemolytic anemia,** increased pro-time
INTEG: Rash, urticaria, bruising
RESP: Wheezing, hyperpnea

Contraindications: Hypersensitivity to salicylates, NSAIDs, GI bleeding, bleeding disorders, children <3 yr, vitamin K deficiency

Precautions: Anemia, hepatic disease, renal disease, Hodgkin's disease, pregnancy **C,** lactation, elderly

Pharmacokinetics

Absorption	Absorbed in small intestine
Distribution	Rapidly and widely distributed, crosses placenta
Metabolism	Not metabolized
Excretion	Unchanged—kidneys
Half-life	2-3 hr (low doses), 15-30 hr (high doses)

Pharmacodynamics

Onset	30 min
Peak	1-3 hr
Duration	3-6 hr

Interactions
Individual drugs
Alcohol: ↑ bleeding
Cefamandole: ↑ bleeding
Furosemide: ↑ toxic effects
Heparin: ↑ bleeding
Insulin: ↑ effects
Methotrexate: ↑ effects
PABA: ↑ toxic effects
Phenytoin: ↑ effects
Plicamycin: ↑ bleeding
Probenecid: ↓ effects
Spironolactone: ↓ effects
Sulfinpyrazone: ↓ effects
Valproic acid: ↑ effects, ↑ bleeding
Vancomycin: ↑ ototoxicity
Drug classifications
Antacids: ↓ effects of aspirin
Anticoagulants: ↑ effects
Carbonic anhydrase inhibitors: ↑ toxic effects
NSAIDs: ↑ gastric ulcers
Penicillins: ↑ effects
Salicylates: ↓ blood sugar levels
Steroids: ↓ effects of aspirin, ↑ gastric ulcers
Sulfonylamides: ↓ effects
Urinary acidifiers: ↑ salicylate levels
Urinary alkalizers: ↓ effects of aspirin
Food/drug
Foods causing acidic urine may ↑ level

☑ *Herb/drug*
Alfalfa: ↑ risk of bleeding
Angelica: ↑ risk of bleeding
Lab test interferences
↑ Coagulation studies, ↑ liver
function studies, ↑ serum uric
acid, ↑ amylase, ↑ CO_2, ↑ urinary protein
↓ Serum potassium, ↓ PBI,
↓ cholesterol, ↓ blood glucose
Interference: Urine catecholamines, pregnancy test

NURSING CONSIDERATIONS
Assessment
• Monitor liver function
studies: AST, ALT, bilirubin,
creatinine if patient is on long-term therapy
• Monitor renal function
studies: BUN, urine creatinine
if patient is on long-term therapy
• Monitor blood studies:
CBC, Hct, Hgb, pro-time if
patient is on long-term therapy
• Check I&O ratio; decreasing
output may indicate renal
failure if patient is on long-term therapy
• Assess hepatotoxicity: dark
urine, clay-colored stools,
yellowing of the skin and
sclera, itching, abdominal pain,
fever, diarrhea if patient is on
long-term therapy
• Assess for allergic reactions:
rash, urticaria; if these occur,
drug may have to be discontinued; assess for asthma, aspirin sensitivity, nasal polyps, may
develop hypersensitivity
• Assess for ototoxicity: tinnitus, ringing, roaring in ears;
audiometric testing needed
before, after long-term therapy
• Assess for visual changes:
blurring, halos; corneal, retinal
damage
• Check edema in feet, ankles,
legs

• Identify prior drug history;
many drug interactions are
possible
• Monitor pain: location,
duration, type, intensity, prior
to dose and 1 hr after
• Monitor musculoskeletal
status: ROM prior to dose
• Identify fever, length of time,
and related symptoms

Nursing diagnoses
☑ Pain (uses)
☑ Mobility, impaired physical
mobility (uses)
☑ Knowledge deficit (teaching)
☑ Injury, risk for (side effects)

Implementation
• Administer to patient
crushed or whole; chewable
tab may be chewed
• Give with food or milk to
decrease gastric symptoms;
give 30 min ac or 2 hr pc;
absorption may be slowed
• Give antacids 1-2 hr after
enteric products

Patient/family education
• Advise patient to report any
symptoms of hepatotoxicity,
renal toxicity, visual changes,
ototoxicity, allergic reactions,
bleeding (long-term therapy)
• Instruct patient to take with
8 oz of water and sit upright
for ½ hr after dose
• Caution patient not to exceed recommended dosage;
acute poisoning may result
• Advise patient to read label
on other OTC drugs; many
contain aspirin
• Inform patient that the
therapeutic response takes 2
wk (arthritis)
• Teach patient to report
tinnitus, confusion, diarrhea,
sweating, hyperventilation
• Caution patient to avoid
alcohol ingestion; GI bleeding
may occur

S

- Inform patient that patients who have allergies may develop allergic reactions

Evaluation
Positive therapeutic outcome
- Decreased pain
- Decreased inflammation

Treatment of overdose: Lavage, activated charcoal, monitor electrolytes, VS

---

saquinavir (℞)
(sa-quen'a-ver)
Invirase, Fortovase
Func. class.: Antiviral
Chem. class.: Synthetic peptide-like substrate analog
Pregnancy category **B**

Action: Inhibits human immunodeficiency virus (HIV) protease

➔ **Therapeutic Outcome:** Prevents maturation of the infectious virus

Uses: HIV in combination with AZT, zalcitabine, ddc

Dosage and routes
Adult: PO 600 mg (hard cap) or 1200 mg (soft cap) tid within 2 hr after a full meal; given with either zalcitabine 0.75 mg tid or AZT 200 mg tid

Available forms: Cap 200 mg (soft); 200 mg (hard)

Adverse effects
CNS: Paresthesia, headache
GI: Diarrhea, buccal mucosa ulceration, *abdominal pain, nausea*
INTEG: Rash
MS: Pain
OTHER: Asthenia, *hyperglycemia*

Contraindications: Hypersensitivity

Precautions: Liver disease, **P** pregnancy **B,** lactation, children

Pharmacokinetics

Absorption	↑ with food
Distribution	Protein-binding 98%
Metabolism	Extensively
Excretion	Unknown
Half-life	Unknown

Pharmacodynamics
Unknown

Interactions
Individual drugs
Carbamazepine: ↓ saquinavir levels
Clindamycin: ↑ toxicity
Dapsone: ↑ toxicity
Dexamethasone: ↓ saquinavir levels
Midazolam: ↑ toxicity
Phenobarbital: ↓ saquinavir levels
Quinidine: ↑ toxicity
Rifamycin: ↓ saquinavir levels
Triazolam: ↑ toxicity
Drug classifications
Calcium channel blockers: ↑ toxicity
Lab test interferences
Interference: CPK, glucose (low)

NURSING CONSIDERATIONS
Assessment
- Assess signs of infection, anemia
- Monitor liver studies: ALT, AST
- Monitor C&S before drug therapy; drug may be taken as soon as culture is taken; repeat C&S after treatment; determine the presence of other sexually transmitted diseases
- Assess bowel pattern before,

---

during treatment; if severe abdominal pain with bleeding occurs, drug should be discontinued; monitor hydration
• Assess skin eruptions, rash, urticaria, itching
• Assess allergies before treatment, reaction of each medication; place allergies on chart

Nursing diagnoses
☑ Infection, risk for (uses)
☑ Knowledge deficit (teaching)

Patient/family education
• Advise patient to take as prescribed within 2 hr of a full meal; if dose is missed, take as soon as remembered up to 1 hr before next dose; do not double dose
• Advise patient that drug must be taken in equal intervals around the clock to maintain blood levels for duration of therapy

sargramostim (R)
(sar-gram'oh-stim)
Leukine, rhu GM-CSF recombinant human
Func. class.: Biologic modifier: cytokine
Chem. class.: Granulocyte/ macrophage colony stimulating factor
Pregnancy category   C

Action: Stimulates proliferation and differentiation of hematopoietic progenitor cells (granulocyte, macrophage)

Uses: Acceleration of myeloid recovery in patients with non-Hodgkin's lymphoma, acute lymphoblastic leukemia, autologous bone marrow transplantation in Hodgkin's disease; bone marrow transplantation failure or engraftment delay

Dosage and routes
Myeloid reconstitution after autologous bone marrow transplantation
Adult: **IV** 250 μg/m^2/day × 3 wk; give over 2 hr, 2-4 hr after autologous bone marrow inf, and not less than 24 hr after last dose of antineoplastics and 12 hr after last dose of radiotherapy, bone marrow transplantation failure, or engraftment delay

Acceleration of myeloid recovery
Adult: **IV** 250 μg/m^2/day × 14 days; give over 2 hr; may repeat in 7 days, may repeat 500 μg/m^2/day × 14 days after another 7 days if no improvement

Available forms: Powder for inj lyophilized 250, 500 μg; liquid 500 μg/ml

Adverse effects
CNS: Fever, malaise, CNS disorder, weakness, chills
CV: Supraventricular tachycardia, peripheral edema, pericardial effusion
GI: Nausea, vomiting, diarrhea, anorexia, **GI hemorrhage,** stomatitis, **liver damage**
GU: Urinary tract disorder, abnormal kidney function
HEMA: **Blood dyscrasias, hemorrhage**
INTEG: Alopecia, rash, peripheral edema
MS: Bone pain
RESP: Dyspnea

Contraindications: Hypersensitivity to GM-CSF, yeast products; excessive leukemic myeloid blast in the bone marrow or peripheral blood

S

Precautions: Pregnancy **C**, lactation, children; renal, hepatic, lung disease; cardiac disease; pleural, pericardial effusions

Do Not Confuse:
Leukine/leucovorin, Leukine/Leukeran

Pharmacokinetics

Absorption	Completely absorbed
Distribution	Unknown
Metabolism	Unknown
Excretion	Unknown
Half-life	2 hr

Pharmacodynamics

Onset	Rapid
Peak	2 hr
Duration	Unknown

Interactions
Individual drugs
Lithium: ↑ myeloproliferation
Drug classifications
Antineoplastics: Do not use together
Corticosteroids: ↑ myeloproliferation

NURSING CONSIDERATIONS
Assessment
• Monitor blood studies: CBC, differential count before treatment and twice weekly; leukocytosis may occur (WBC >50,000 cells/mm^3, ANC >20,000 cells/mm^3)
• Monitor renal and hepatic studies before treatment: BUN, creatinine, urinalysis; AST, ALT, alk phosphatase; monitoring is needed twice a week in renal, hepatic disease
• Assess for hypersensitive reactions/rashes, and local inj site reactions; usually transient
• Assess for increased fluid retention in cardiac disease
Nursing diagnoses
☑ Infection, risk for (uses)
☑ Knowledge deficit (teaching)

Implementation
• Reconstitute with 1 ml sterile water for inj without preservative; do not reenter vial; discard unused portion; direct reconstitution sol at side of vial; rotate contents; do not shake
• Give by intermittent inf after diluting in 0.9% NaCl inj to prepare **IV** inf; if final conc is <10 μg/ml, add human albumin to make a final conc of 0.1% to the NaCl before adding sargramostim to prevent absorption; for a final conc of 0.1% albumin, add 1 mg human albumin/1 ml 0.9% NaCl inj; run over 2 hr; give within 6 hr after reconstitution
• Store in refrigerator; do not freeze

Y-site compatibilities:
Amikacin, aminophylline, aztreonam, bleomycin, butorphanol, calcium gluconate, carboplatin, carmustine, cefazolin, cefepime, cefotaxime, cefotetan, ceftizoxime, ceftriaxone, cefuroxime, cimetidine, cisplatin, clindamycin, cyclophosphamide, cyclosporine, cytarabine, dacarbazine, dactinomycin, dexamethasone, diphenhydramine, dopamine, doxorubicin, doxycycline, droperidol, etoposide, famotidine, fentanyl, floxuridine, fluconazole, fluorouracil, furosemide, gentamicin, granisetron, heparin, idarubicin, ifosfamide, immune globulin, magnesium sulfate, mannitol, mechlorethamine, meperidine, mesna, methotrexate, metoclopramide, metronidazole, mezlocillin, miconazole, minocycline, mitoxantrone, netilmicin, pentostatin, piperacillin/tazobactam, potassium chloride, prochlorperazine,

---

☑ Herb/drug   ⊘ Do Not Crush   ◆ Alert   ☋ Key Drug   ᴳ Geriatric   ᴾ Pediatric promethazine, ranitidine, teniposide, ticarcillin, ticarcillin/clavulanate, trimethoprim/sulfamethoxazole, vinblastine, vincristine, zidovudine

Y-site incompatibilities: Acyclovir, ampicillin, ampicillin/sulbactam, cefonicid, cefoperazine, ceftazidime, chlorpromazine, ganciclovir, haloperidol, hydrocortisone, hydromorphone, hydroxyzine, idarubicin, imipenem/cilastatin, lorazepam, methylprednisolone sodium succinate, mitomycin, morphine, nalbuphine, ondansetron, piperacillin, sodium bicarbonate, tobramycin

Patient/family education
• Teach patient reason for medication and expected results
• Advise patient to notify nurse or prescriber of side effects

Evaluation
Positive therapeutic outcome
• WBC and differential recovery
• Absence of infection

---

scopolamine (℞)
(skoe-pol′a-meen)
Transderm-Scop, Isopoto-Hyoscine, Transderm-V ✦, Triptol
Func. class.: Antiemetic, anticholinergic, mydriatic
Chem. class.: Belladonna alkaloid
Pregnancy category   C

Action: Inhibits acetylcholine at receptor sites in autonomic nervous system, which controls secretions, free acids in stomach; blocks central muscarinic receptors, which decreases involuntary movements; blocks response of iris sphincter muscle, muscle of accommodation of ciliary body to cholinergic stimulation, resulting in dilation, paralysis of accommodation

▶**Therapeutic Outcome:** Absence of vomiting, secretions (preop), involuntary movements

Uses: Reduction of secretions before surgery, calm delirium, motion sickness, uveitis, iritis, cycloplegia, mydriasis; prevention of motion sickness, parkinson symptoms

Dosage and routes
Ophth
Adult: Instill 1-2 gtt before refraction or 1-2 gtt qd-tid for iritis or uveitis
▣ *Child:* Instill 1 gtt bid × 2 days before refraction

Prevention of motion sickness
Adult: 1 patch placed behind ear 4-5 hr before travel
▣ Not recommended for children

Parkinson symptoms
Adult: IM/SC/**IV** 0.3-0.6 mg tid-qid diluted using dilution provided

Preoperatively
Adult: SC 0.4-0.6 mg
▣ *Child:* SC 0.006 mg/kg or 0.2 mg/m²

Available forms: Sol 0.25%; patch 0.5 mg delivered in 72 hr; inj 0.3, 0.4, 0.86, 1 mg/ml
Adverse effects
CNS: Confusion, anxiety, restlessness, irritability, delusions, hallucinations, headache, sedation, depression, incoher-

S

---

ence, dizziness, excitement, delirium, flushing, weakness
CV: Palpitations, **tachycardia,** postural hypotension, paradoxical bradycardia
EENT: Blurred vision, photophobia, dilated pupils, difficulty swallowing, mydriasis, cycloplegia
GI: Dryness of mouth, constipation, nausea, vomiting, abdominal distress, **paralytic ileus**
GU: Hesitancy, retention
INTEG: Urticaria
MISC: Suppression of lactation, nasal congestion, decreased sweating

Contraindications: Hypersensitivity, narrow-angle glaucoma, myasthenia gravis, GI/GU obstruction, hypersensitivity to belladonna, barbiturates

Precautions: Pregnancy **C,**
G elderly, lactation, prostatic hypertrophy, CHF, hypertension, dysrhythmia,
P children, gastric ulcer

Pharmacokinetics

Absorption	Well absorbed (IM, SC, Trans)
Distribution	Crosses placenta, blood-brain barrier
Metabolism	Liver
Excretion	Unknown
Half-life	8 hr

Pharmacodynamics

	SC/IM	IV	TRANS	OPHTH
Onset	30-45 min	10-15 min	4-5 hr	Unknown
Peak	1 hr	1 hr	Unknown	20-30 min
Duration	6 hr	4 hr	72 hr	3-7 days

Interactions
Individual drugs
Alcohol: ↑ CNS depression
Quinidine: ↑ anticholinergic effect

Drug classifications
Antidepressants: ↑ anticholinergic effect
Antihistamines: ↑ anticholinergic effect
Narcotics: ↑ anticholinergic effect
Phenothiazines: ↑ anticholinergic effect
Tricyclic antidepressants: ↑ anticholinergic effect

NURSING CONSIDERATIONS
Assessment
• Assess for eye pain; discontinue use (opticue)
• Monitor I&O ratio; retention commonly causes decreased urinary output
• Assess for parkinsonism, extrapyramidal symptoms: shuffling gait, muscle rigidity, involuntary movements
• Assess for urinary hesitancy, retention; palpate bladder if retention occurs
• Assess for constipation; increase fluids, bulk, exercise if this occurs
• Assess for tolerance over long-term therapy; dose may have to be increased or changed
• Assess mental status: affect, mood, CNS depression, worsening of mental symptoms during early therapy

Nursing diagnoses
☑ Fluid volume deficit (uses)
☑ Knowledge deficit (teaching)

Implementation
IV **SC/IM/IV route**
• Administer parenteral dose with patient recumbent to prevent postural hypotension
IV **IV route**
• Give by direct **IV** after diluting with sterile water; give slowly

---

☑ Herb/drug ⊗ Do Not Crush ◆ Alert ⟶ Key Drug **G** Geriatric **P** Pediatric

Syringe compatibilities:
Atropine, benzquinamide, butorphanol, chlorpromazine, cimetidine, dimenhydrinate, diphenhydramine, droperidol, fentanyl, glycopyrrolate, hydromorphone, hydroxyzine, meperidine, metoclopramide, midazolam, morphine, nalbuphine, pentazocine, pentobarbital, perphenazine, prochlorperazine, promazine, promethazine, ranitidine, sufentanil, thiopental

Y-site compatibilities:
Heparin, hydrocortisone, potassium chloride, propofol, sufentanil, vit B/C

Additive compatibilities:
Floxacillin, furosemide, meperidine, succinylcholine

Patient/family education
• Tell patient to avoid hazardous activities, activities requiring alertness; dizziness may occur
Trans route
• Instruct patient to wash, dry hands before and after applying to surface behind ear; to change patch q72h; to apply at least 4 hr before traveling
• Advise patient to discontinue use if blurred vision, severe dizziness, drowsiness occurs—another type of antiemetic may be used
• Instruct patient to read labels of all OTC medications; if any scopolamine is found in product, avoid use
• Advise patient to keep medication out of children's reach
• Caution patient to report change in vision; blurring or loss of sight; trouble breathing; inhibition of sweating; flushing
Ophth route
• Teach patient method of instill: pressure on lacrimal sac

for 1 min; do not touch dropper to eye
• Inform patient that blurred vision will decrease with repeated use of drug
• Advise patient to wait 5 min to use other drops; blink more than usual
• Caution patient not to discontinue this drug abruptly; to taper off over 1 wk

Evaluation
Positive therapeutic outcome
• Decrease in inflammation, cycloplegic refraction
• Decreased secretions
• Absence of motion sickness

---

secobarbital (℞)
(see-koe-bar'bi-tal)
Secogen Sodium ✦, Seconal Sodium Pulvules, Seral ✦
Func. class.: Sedative/hypnotic-barbiturate
Chem. class.: Barbitone (short-acting)

Pregnancy category D
Controlled substance schedule II (USA), schedule G (Canada)

Action: Depresses activity in brain cells primarily in reticular activating system in brainstem; selectively depresses neurons in posterior hypothalamus, limbic structures; decreases seizure activity by inhibition of epileptic activity in CNS

⮚**Therapeutic Outcome:** Sedation, anticonvulsant, improved energy

Uses: Insomnia, sedation, preoperative medication, status epilepticus, acute tetanus convulsions

S

✦ Canada Only   Adverse effects: *italic* = common; **bold** = life-threatening

Dosage and routes
Insomnia
Adult: PO/IM 100-200 mg hs

P *Child:* IM 3-5 mg/kg, not to exceed 100 mg, not to inject >5 ml in one site

Sedation/preoperatively
Adult: PO 200-300 mg 1-2 hr preoperatively

P *Child:* PO 50-100 mg 1-2 hr preoperatively

Status epilepticus
P *Adult and child:* IM/**IV** 250-350 mg

Acute psychotic agitation
P *Adult and child:* IM/**IV** 5.5 mg/kg q3-4h

Available forms: Caps 50, 100 mg; tab 100 mg; inj 50 mg/ml

Adverse effects
CNS: Lethargy, drowsiness, hangover, dizziness, paradoxical
G stimulation in the elderly and
P children, lightheadedness, dependency, CNS depression, mental depression, slurred speech
CV: Hypotension, bradycardia
GI: Nausea, vomiting, diarrhea, constipation
HEMA: **Agranulocytosis, thrombocytopenia, megaloblastic anemia** (long-term treatment)
INTEG: Rash, urticaria, pain, abscesses at inj site, angioedema, thrombophlebitis, **Stevens-Johnson syndrome**
RESP: Depression, **apnea, laryngospasm, bronchospasm**

Contraindications: Hypersensitivity to barbiturates, respiratory depression, pregnancy **D**, addiction to barbiturates, severe liver impairment, por-

phyria, uncontrolled severe pain

Precautions: Anemia, lactation, hepatic disease, renal
G disease, hypertension, elderly, acute/chronic pain

Pharmacokinetics	
Absorption	Slow (70%-90%) (PO), **IV** complete
Distribution	Not known, crosses placenta
Metabolism	Liver (75%)
Excretion	Kidneys (25% unchanged)
Half-life	2-6 days

Pharmacodynamics			
	PO	IM	IV
Onset	30-60 min	10-30 min	5 min
Peak	Unknown	Unknown	30 min
Duration	6-8 hr	4-6 hr	4-6 hr

Interactions
Individual drugs
Alcohol: ↑ CNS depression
Chloramphenicol: ↓ effectiveness
Cyclophosphamide: ↑ hematologic toxicity
Cyclosporine: ↓ effectiveness
Dacarbazine: ↓ effectiveness
Quinidine: ↓ effectiveness
Valproic acid: ↑ sedation
Drug classifications
Anticoagulants: ↓ effectiveness
Antidepressants: ↑ CNS depression
Antihistamines: ↑ CNS depression
Glucocorticoids: ↓ effectiveness
MAOIs: ↑ CNS depression
Opiates: ↑ CNS depression
Oral contraceptives: ↓ effectiveness
Sedatives/hypnotics: ↑ CNS depression

Tricyclics: ↓ effectiveness
🗌 *Herb/drug*
Kava: ↑ CNS depression

NURSING CONSIDERATIONS
Assessment
• Assess patient's mental status: mood, sensorium, affect, memory (long, short), 🄖 especially in elderly patients; if using as a hypnotic, assess sleep patterns during therapy; drug suppresses REM sleep with dreaming; withdrawal insomnia may occur after short-term use; do not start using drug again—insomnia will improve in 1-3 nights; patient may experience increased dreaming
• Monitor patient for respiratory dysfunction: respiratory depression, character, rate, 🄸🄥 rhythm (when using **IV**); hold drug if resp are <10/min or if pupils are dilated. Also check VS q30 min after parenteral route for 2 hr
🄸🄥• Assess patient for barbiturate toxicity: hypotension; pulmonary constriction; cold, clammy skin; cyanosis of lips; CNS depression; nausea; vomiting; hallucinations; delirium; weakness; coma; pupillary constriction, mild symptoms may occur in 8-12 hr without drug
• Assess patient for blood dyscrasias: fever, sore throat, bruising, rash, jaundice, epistaxis (long-term treatment only)
• Assess for pain in postoperative patients; pain threshold is lowered when patients are taking this medication
Nursing diagnoses
☑ Sleep pattern disturbance (uses)
☑ Injury, risk for (adverse reactions)
☑ Knowledge deficit (teaching)

Implementation
• Administer after removal of cigarettes, to prevent fires
• Administer after trying conservative measures for insomnia
PO route
• Tab may be crushed and mixed with food if swallowing is difficult. Also may be mixed with other fluids ½-1 hr before hs for expected sleeplessness; on empty stomach for best absorption
IM route
• Give in deep muscle mass (gluteal) to minimize irritation to tissues
• Split inj of >5 ml into two because irritation to tissues may occur
🄸🄥 **Direct IV route**
• Use large vein to prevent extravasation; if extravasation occurs, use moist heat to the area and procaine sol 5% inj into area
• Give at rate of 65 mg or less/min; titrate to patient response

Syringe incompatibilities:
Benzquinamide, dimenhydrinate, diphenhydramine, erythromycin gluceptate, hydroxyzine, kanamycin, oxytetracycline, phenytoin, prochlorperazine, promazine, promethazine, ranitidine, tetracycline

Additive compatibilities:
Amikacin, aminophylline

Additive incompatibilities:
Cephalothin, chlorpromazine, codeine, ephedrine, hydralazine, hydrocortisone sodium succinate, hydroxyzine, insulin, levorphanol, meperidine, methadone, morphine, norepinephrine, pentazocine, procaine, prochlorazine mesylate, promazine,

S

promethazine, streptomycin, vancomycin

Solution compatibilities:
D_5W, $D_{10}W$, 0.45% NaCl, 0.9% NaCl, Ringer's sol, dextrose/saline combinations, dextrose/Ringer's or dextrose/lactated Ringer's combinations

Patient/family education

• Teach patient that hangover is common
• Instruct patient that drug is indicated only for short-term treatment of insomnia and is probably ineffective after 2 wk
• Inform patient that physical dependency may result when used for extended time (45-90 days depending on dose)
• Caution patient to avoid driving or other activities requiring alertness
• Caution patient to avoid alcohol ingestion or CNS depressants; serious CNS depression may result
• Instruct patient not to discontinue medication quickly after long-term use; drug should be tapered over 1 wk
• Emphasize the need to tell all prescribers that a barbiturate is being taken
• Inform patient that withdrawal insomnia may occur after short-term use; patient should not start using drug again—insomnia will improve in 1-3 nights; patient may experience increased dreaming
• Inform patient that effects may take 2 nights for benefits to be noticed; teach patient alternate measures to improve sleep: reading, exercise several hours before hs, warm bath, warm milk, TV, self-hypnosis, deep breathing
• Teach patient to make posi-

tion changes slowly; orthostatic hypotension may occur
• Instruct patient to notify prescriber immediately if bruising or bleeding occur, which may indicate blood dycrasias

Evaluation
Positive therapeutic outcome
• Improved sleeping patterns
• Decreased seizure activity
• Improved energy

Treatment of overdose:
Lavage, activated charcoal, warming blanket, vital signs, hemodialysis, alkalinize urine; give **IV** volume expanders, **IV** fluids

---

selegiline (R)
(se-le'ji-leen)
Carbex, Eldepryl, Novo-Selegiline ✦, SD-Deprenyl
Func. class.: Antiparkinson agent
Chem. class.: Levorotatory acetylenic derivative of phenethylamine
Pregnancy category   C

Action: Increased dopaminergic activity by inhibition of MAO type B activity; not fully understood

Therapeutic Outcome: Decreased symptoms of Parkinson's disease

Uses: Adjunct management of Parkinson's disease in patients being treated with levodopa/carbidopa who have responded poorly to therapy

Investigational use: Alzheimer's disease

Dosage and routes
Adult: PO 10 mg/day in divided doses 5 mg at breakfast and lunch with levodopa/

---

carbidopa; after 2-3 days begin
to reduce the dose of
levodopa/carbidopa 10%-30%
Available forms: Tab 5 mg
Adverse effects
CNS: Increased tremors, chorea, restlessness, blepharospasm, increased bradykinesia, grimacing, tardive dyskinesia, dystonic symptoms, involuntary movements, increased apraxia, hallucinations, dizziness, mood changes, nightmares, delusions, lethargy, apathy, overstimulation, sleep disturbances, headache, migraine, numbness, muscle cramps, confusion, anxiety, tiredness, vertigo, personality change, back/leg pain
CV: Orthostatic hypotension, hypertension, **dysrhythmia,** palpitations; angina pectoris, hypotension, tachycardia, edema, sinus bradycardia, syncope
EENT: Diploplia, dry mouth, blurred vision, tinnitus
GI: Nausea, vomiting, constipation, weight loss, anorexia, diarrhea, heartburn, rectal bleeding, poor appetite, dysphagia
GU: Slow urination, nocturia, prostatic hypertrophy, hesitation, retention, frequency, sexual dysfunction
INTEG: Increased sweating, alopecia, hematoma, rash, photosensitivity, facial hair
RESP: Asthma, shortness of breath

Contraindications: Hypersensitivity

Precautions: Pregnancy **C,** lactation, children

Do Not Confuse:
Eldepryl/enalapril

Pharmacokinetics
Absorption	Well absorbed
Distribution	Widely distributed
Metabolism	Rapidly, liver
Excretion	Metabolites-N-desmethyldeprenyl, amphetamine, meth-amphetamine
Half-life	Unknown

Pharmacodynamics
Onset	Unknown
Peak	½-2 hr
Duration	Unknown

Interactions
Individual drugs
Fluoxetine: ↑ serotonin syndrome (confusion, seizures, fever, hypertension, agitation) discontinue 5 wk prior to selegiline
Fluvoxamine: ↑ serotonin syndrome (confusion, seizures, fever, hypertension, agitation) discontinue 5 wk prior to selegiline
Levodopa/carbidopa: ↑ side effects
Meperidine: Do not use—fatal reaction
Paroxetine: ↑ serotonin syndrome (confusion, seizures, fever, hypertension, agitation) discontinue 5 wk prior to selegiline
Sertraline: ↑ serotonin syndrome (confusion, seizures, fever, hypertension, agitation) discontinue 5 wk prior to selegiline
Drug classifications
Opioids: Do not use—fatal reaction
Food/drug
Tyramine foods: ↑ hypertension
Herb/drug
Chaste tree fruit: ↓ selegiline action

S

Lab test interferences
False positive: Urine ketones, urine glucose
False negative: Urine glucose (glucose oxidase)
False: ↑ Uric acid, false ↑ urine protein
↓ VMA

NURSING CONSIDERATIONS
Assessment
• Monitor B/P, respiration throughout treatment
• Assess mental status: affect, mood, behavioral changes, depression; perform suicide assessment
• Assess for decreased Parkinson's symptoms: rigidity, unsteady gait, weakness, tremors; these should decrease in severity

Nursing diagnoses
☑ Physical mobility, impaired (uses)
☑ Knowledge deficit (teaching)

Implementation
• Adjust dosage to patient response
• Give with meals; limit protein taken with drug
• Give at doses <10 mg/day because of risks associated with nonselective inhibition of MAO

Patient/family education
• Caution patient to change positions slowly to prevent orthostatic hypotension
• Advise patient to report side effects: twitching, eye spasms —may indicate overdose
• Caution patient to use drug exactly as prescribed; if drug is discontinued abruptly, parkinsonian crisis may occur
• Instruct patient to avoid foods high in tyramine: cheese, pickled products, wine, beer, large amounts of caffeine

• Instruct patient not to exceed recommended dose of 10 mg—might precipitate a hypertensive crisis; report severe headache or other unusual symptoms

Evaluation
Positive therapeutic outcome
• Decreased symptoms of Parkinson's disease

Treatment of overdose: IV fluids for hypertension, **IV** dilute pressure agent for B/P titration

---

senna (OTC)
(sin'na)
Black Draught, Dr. Caldwell Dosalax, Fletcher's Castoria, Gentlax, Senexon, Senna-Gen, Senokot, Senokotxtra
Func. class.: Laxative-stimulant
Chem. class.: Anthraquinone
Pregnancy category C

Action: Stimulates peristalsis by action on Auerbach's plexus; softens feces by increasing water and electrolytes in large intestine

➡ **Therapeutic Outcome:** Decreased constipation

Uses: Acute constipation; bowel preparation for surgery or examination

Dosage and routes
Adult: PO 1-8 tab (Senokot)/day or 1/2 to 4 tsp of granules added to water or juice; rec supp 1-2 hs; syr 1-4 tsp hs (1 tsp = 4 ml), 7.5-15 ml; (Black Draught) 3/4 oz dissolved in 2.5 oz liq given between 2-4 PM the day before procedure (X-Prep)

P *Child >27 kg:* ½ adult dose; do not use Black Draught for children

P *Child 1 mo-1 yr:* Syr 1.25-2.5 ml (Senokot) hs

Available forms: Supp 625 mg, 30 mg sennosides; powder 662 mg/g, 6, 15 mg sennosides/3 g; tab 8.6 sennosides, 180 mg; oral sol 3 mg senosides/ml

Adverse effects
GI: Nausea, vomiting, anorexia, abdominal cramps, diarrhea, flatulence
GU: Pink-red or brown-black discoloration of urine
META: Hypocalcemia, enteropathy, alkalosis, hypokalemia, **tetany**

Contraindications: Hypersensitivity, GI bleeding, intestinal obstruction, CHF, lactation, abdominal pain, nausea/vomiting, appendicitis, acute surgical abdomen

Precautions: Pregnancy **C**

Pharmacokinetics	
Absorption	Minimally absorbed (PO)
Distribution	Unknown
Metabolism	Not metabolized
Excretion	Kidneys, feces
Half-life	Unknown

Pharmacodynamics		
	PO	REC
Onset	6-24 hr	Unknown
Peak	Unknown	Unknown
Duration	3-4 days	Unknown

Interactions
Individual drugs
Disulfiram: Do not use together
Drug classifications
Oral drugs: ↓ absorption

NURSING CONSIDERATIONS
Assessment
• Monitor blood, urine electrolytes if used often by patient; check I&O ratio to identify fluid loss
• Assess cramping, rec bleeding, nausea, vomiting; if these symptoms occur, drug should be discontinued; identify cause of constipation; identify whether fluids, bulk, or exercise is missing from lifestyle
• Assess for Mg toxicity: thirst, confusion, decrease in reflexes
• Monitor blood ammonia level (30-70 mg/100 ml); monitor for clearing of confusion, lethargy, restlessness, irritability (hepatic encephalopathy)
• Monitor blood, urine electrolytes if drug is used often by patient

Nursing diagnoses
☑ Bowel elimination, altered: constipation (uses)
☑ Bowel elimination, altered; diarrhea (side effects)
☑ Knowledge deficit (teaching)
☑ Noncompliance (teaching)

Implementation
PO route
• Administration on empty stomach produces more rapid results
• Give with a full glass of water in AM or PM (oral dose); evacuation occurs 6-12 hr later
• Dissolve granules in water or juice before administration
• Shake oral sol before giving

Patient/family education
• Discuss with the patient that adequate fluid consumption is necessary
• Inform patient that normal bowel movements do not always occur daily

S

• Teach patient not to use in presence of abdominal pain, nausea, vomiting; tell patient to notify prescriber if constipation is unrelieved or if symptoms of electrolyte imbalance occur: muscle cramps, pain, weakness, dizziness, excessive thirst

Evaluation
Positive therapeutic outcome
• Decreased constipation in 8-10 hr

---

sertraline (℞)
(ser'tra-leen)
Zoloft
Func. class.: Antidepressant
Chem. class.: SSRI
Pregnancy category   B

Action: Inhibits serotonin reuptake in the CNS, thus increasing action of serotonin; does not affect dopamine, norepinephrine

➡ **Therapeutic Outcome:** Relief of depression, OCD

Uses: Major depression, obsessive-compulsive disorder (OCD)

Dosage and routes
Adult: PO 50 mg qd; may increase to a maximum of 200 mg/day, do not change dose at intervals of <1 wk; administer qd in AM or PM
ⓖ *Elderly:* PO 25 mg qd, increase by 25 mg q3 days to desired dose
ⓟ *Child 6-12 yr:* PO 25 mg qd
ⓟ *Child 13-17 yr:* PO 50 mg qd
Available forms: Tabs 25, 50, 100 mg

Adverse effects
CNS: Insomnia, agitation, somnolence, dizziness, headache, tremor, fatigue, paresthesia, twitching, confusion, ataxia, fever, gait abnormality
ⓖ (elderly)
CV: Palpitations, chest pain
EENT: Vision abnormalities
ⓖ *ENDO:* SIADH (elderly)
GI: Diarrhea, nausea, constipation, anorexia, dry mouth, dyspepsia, *vomiting, flatulence*
GU: Male sexual dysfunction, micturition disorder
INTEG: Increased sweating, rash, hot flashes

Contraindications: Hypersensitivity to this drug or SSRIs

Precautions: Pregnancy **B,**
ⓖ lactation, elderly, hepatic, renal disease, epilepsy

🚫 **Do Not Confuse:**
Zoloft/Zocor

Pharmacokinetics	
Absorption	Well absorbed
Distribution	Unknown, steady state 1 wk
Metabolism	Liver, extensively
Excretion	Feces (14%)
Half-life	26-104 hr

Pharmacodynamics	
Onset	Unknown
Peak	4.5-8.4 hr
Duration	Unknown

Interactions
Individual drugs
Cimetidine: ↑ sertraline
Warfarin: ↑ effect of warfarin
Drug classifications
Antidepressants, tricyclics: ↑ effect
Benzodiazepines: ↑ effect
MAOIs: Hypertensive crisis, convulsions, do not use together

☑ *Herb/drug*
St. John's Wort: ↑ effect of SSRIs, do not use together
Lab test interferences
↑ AST, ↑ ALT

NURSING CONSIDERATIONS
Assessment
• Assess mental status: mood, sensorium, affect, suicidal tendencies; increase in psychiatric symptoms: depression, panic
• Identify alcohol consumption; if alcohol is consumed, hold dose until AM

Nursing diagnoses
☑ Coping, ineffective individual (uses)
☑ Injury, risk for (adverse reactions)
☑ Knowledge deficit (teaching)
☑ Noncompliance (teaching)

Implementation
• Administer dosage hs if oversedation occurs during day; may take entire dose hs; may crush
• Store at room temp; do not freeze

Patient/family education
• Teach patient that therapeutic effects may take 1 wk
• Instruct patient to use caution in driving or other activities requiring alertness because of drowsiness, dizziness, blurred vision; to avoid rising quickly from sitting to standing, especially elderly
• Advise patient to avoid alcohol ingestion, other CNS depressants
◆• Teach patient not to discontinue medication quickly after long-term use: may cause nausea, headache, malaise
• Caution patient to wear sunscreen or large hat because photosensitivity can occur

• Teach patient to increase fluids, bulk in diet if constipation, urinary retention occur, especially elderly
• Instruct patient to take gum, hard sugarless candy, or frequent sips of water for dry mouth

Evaluation
Positive therapeutic outcome
• Decrease in depression, OCD
• Absence of suicidal thoughts

Treatment of overdose: ECG monitoring, induce emesis, lavage, activated charcoal, administer anticonvulsant

---

sibutramine (℞)
(si-byoo'tra-meen)
Meridia
Func. class.: Appetite suppressant
Pregnancy category   UK

Action: Inhibits reuptake of serotonin, norepinephrine, dopamine

▶**Therapeutic Outcome:** Weight loss with B/P in normal range

Uses: Obesity in conjunction with other treatments

Dosage and routes
Adult: PO 10 mg qd; may be increased to 15 mg qd after 4 wk, or lowered to 5 mg qd depending on response

Available forms: Caps 5, 10, 15 mg

Adverse effects
CNS: Headache, insomnia, seizures, stimulation, drowsiness, dizziness, nervousness, emotional lability
CV: Hypotension, palpitations, vasodilation, tachycardia

EENT: Laryngitis, pharyngitis, rhinitis, sinusitis
GI: Anorexia, constipation, dry mouth, taste aberration, nausea, increased appetite
GU: Dysmenorrhea
INTEG: Rash, sweating

Contraindications: Hypersensitivity, hypothyroidism, anorexia nervosa, severe hepatic/renal disease, uncontrolled hypertension, history of CAD, CHF, dysrhythmias, pregnancy, lactation

Precautions: History of seizures, elderly, children <16 yr, **G** narrow-angle glaucoma **P**

Pharmacokinetics

Absorption	Unknown
Distribution	Widely
Metabolism	Liver (extensively)
Excretion	Unknown
Half-life	14 hr (metabolites)

Pharmacodynamics

Onset	Unknown
Peak	3-4 hr
Duration	Unknown

Interactions
Individual drugs
Dextromethorphan: Fatal serotonin syndrome, do not use together
Dihydroergotamine: Fatal serotonin syndrome, do not use together
Fentanyl: Fatal serotonin syndrome, do not use together
Ketoconazole: ↑ levels of sibutramine
Lithium: Fatal serotonin syndrome, do not use together
Meperidine: Fatal serotonin syndrome, do not use together
Naratriptan: Fatal serotonin syndrome, do not use together

Pentazocine: Fatal serotonin syndrome, do not use together
Sumatriptan: Fatal serotonin syndrome, do not use together
Tryptophan: Fatal serotonin syndrome, do not use together
Zolmitriptan: Fatal serotonin syndrome, do not use together

Drug classifications
Appetite suppressants, centrally acting: Fatal serotonin syndrome, do not use together
Decongestants: Hypertension
MAOIs: Fatal serotonin syndrome, do not use together
SSRIs: Fatal serotonin syndrome, do not use together

NURSING CONSIDERATIONS
Assessment
• Monitor B/P, pulse during treatment; if B/P or pulse rises or if palpitations, tachycardia occur, drug may need to be discontinued
• Assess patient's current dosage of antihypertensives, antidiabetics; these may need to be adjusted
• Assess need for medication and results when combined with other weight-loss strategies

Nursing diagnoses
✓ Knowledge deficit (teaching)
✓ Noncompliance (teaching)

Implementation
• Give PO with or without meals qd

Patient/family education
• Instruct patient to discuss all other medications taken (including OTC) with health care provider; serious—even fatal—interactions can occur
• Advise patient to take exactly as prescribed, and not to exceed recommended dose

---

☑ Herb/drug   Ⓢ Do Not Crush   ✦ Alert   ☌ Key Drug   **G** Geriatric   **P** Pediatric

Evaluation
Positive therapeutic outcome
• Decrease in weight over time

---

sildenafil (℞)
(sil-den'a-fill)
Viagra
Func. class.: Erectile agent
Chem. class.: Selective inhibitor of cGMP-PDE5

Pregnancy category B

Action: Enhances the effect of nitric oxide (NO) by inhibiting phosphodiesterase type 5 (PDE5), which is necessary for degrading cGMP in the carpus cavernosum

▶**Therapeutic Outcome:** Ability to achieve and maintain erection

Uses: Treatment of erectile dysfunction

Dosage and routes
Adult: PO 50 mg 1 hr before sexual activity or may be taken ½-4 hr before sexual activity; may be increased to 100 mg or decreased to 25 mg; max once/day

Available forms: Tabs 25, 50, 100 mg

Adverse effects
CNS: Headache, flushing, dizziness
OTHER: Dyspepsia, nasal congestion, UTI, abnormal vision, diarrhea, rash

Contraindications: Hypersensitivity

Precautions: Anatomical penile deformities, sickle cell anemia, leukemia, multiple myeloma, pregnancy **B**

Pharmacokinetics

Absorption	Rapidly, bioavailability (40%)
Distribution	Unknown
Metabolism	Liver (active metabolites)
Excretion	Feces, urine
Half-life	4 hr

Pharmacodynamics

Onset	Unknown
Peak	½-1½ hr
Duration	Unknown

Interactions
Individual drugs
Amlodipine: ↓ B/P
Cimetidine: ↑ sildenafil levels
Erythromycin: ↑ sildenafil levels
Itraconazole: ↑ sildenafil levels
Ketoconazole: ↑ sildenafil levels
Nitrates: Fatal reaction, do not use together
Rifampin: ↓ sildenafil levels

NURSING CONSIDERATIONS
Assessment
• Identify organic nitrates that should not be used with this drug

Nursing diagnoses
✓ Noncompliance (teaching)
✓ Knowledge deficit (teaching)

Implementation
• Give approximately 1 hr before sexual activity, do not use more than once a day

Patient/family education
• Teach patient that drug does not protect against sexually transmitted diseases, including HIV
• Teach patient that drug absorption is reduced with a high fat meal
• Teach patient that drug should not be used with nitrates in any form

S

Evaluation
Positive therapeutic outcome
• Ability to achieve and maintain an erection

---

simethicone (OTC)
(si-meth′i-kone)
Extra Strength Gas-X, Flatulex, Gas-X, Major Con, Mylanta Gas, Mylicon, Ovol ✦, Phazyme, Phazyme 95, Phazyme 125
Func. class.: Antiflatulent
Pregnancy category **C**

Action: Disperses, prevents gas pockets in GI system; does not decrease gas production

▶ **Therapeutic Outcome:** Belching or flatus

Uses: Flatulence

Dosage and routes
P *Adult and child >12 yr:* PO 40-100 mg pc, hs
P *Child <2 yr:* PO 20 mg qid

Available forms: Chew tabs 40, 80, 125 mg; tabs 60, 95 mg; drops 40 mg/0.6 ml; cap 125 mg; caps, soft gel 125 mg

Adverse effects
GI: Belching, rectal flatus

Contraindications: Hypersensitivity

Precautions: Pregnancy **C**

◨ **Do Not Confuse:**
Mylicon/Mylanta Gas

Pharmacokinetics

Absorption	None
Distribution	None
Metabolism	None
Excretion	None
Half-life	Unknown

Pharmacodynamics

Onset	Rapid
Peak	Unknown
Duration	3 hr

Interactions: None

NURSING CONSIDERATIONS
Assessment
• Identify the reason for excess gas production; decreased bowel sounds, recent surgery, other GI conditions

Nursing diagnoses
☑ Pain (uses)
☑ Knowledge deficit (teaching)

Implementation
• Give pc and hs
• Shake suspension well before administration
• Chewable tab should be chewed and not swallowed whole

Patient/family education
• Caution patient that tab must be chewed; to shake suspension well before pouring

Evaluation
Positive therapeutic outcome
• Absence of flatulence

---

simvastatin (℞)
(sim-va-stat′in)
Zocor
Func. class.: Antilipidemic
Chem. class.: HMG-CoA reductase inhibitor
Pregnancy category **X**

Action: Inhibits HMG-COA reductase enzyme, which reduces cholesterol synthesis; this enzyme is needed for cholesterol production

▶ **Therapeutic Outcome:** Decreasing cholesterol levels and low-density lipoproteins, increased high-density lipoproteins

Uses: As an adjunct in primary hypercholesterolemia (types IIa, IIb), mixed hyperlipidemia, coronary artery disease

Dosage and routes
Adult: PO 5-10 mg qd in PM initially, usual range 5-40 mg/day qd in PM, not to exceed 40 mg/day; dosage adjustments may be made at 4-wk intervals or more

🅖 *Elderly/renal dose*
PO 5 mg/day

Available forms: Tabs 5, 10, 20, 40, 80 mg

Adverse effects
CNS: Headache, tremor, vertigo, peripheral neuropathy
EENT: Lens opacities
GI: Nausea, constipation, diarrhea, dyspepsia, flatus, abdominal pain, heartburn, **liver dysfunction**
INTEG: Rash, pruritus, alopecia, photosensitivity
MS: Muscle cramps, myalgia, **myositis, rhabdomyolysis**

Contraindications: Hypersensitivity, pregnancy **X,** lactation, active liver disease

Precautions: Past liver disease, alcoholism, severe acute infections, trauma, hypotension, uncontrolled seizure disorders, severe metabolic disorders, 🅔electrolyte imbalances, elderly, renal disease

🅝 **Do Not Confuse:**
Zocor/Cozaar, Zocor/Zoloft

Pharmacokinetics	
Absorption	85%
Distribution	Unknown
Metabolism	Liver—extensively
Excretion	70% feces, 20% kidneys
Half-life	3 hr

Pharmacodynamics	
Onset	Unknown
Peak	1-2½ hr
Duration	Unknown

Interactions
Individual drugs
Cholestyramine: ↓ action of simvastatin
Colestipol: ↓ action of simvastatin
Cyclosporine: ↑ risk of myopathy, rhabdomyolysis
Erythromycin: ↑ risk of myopathy
Gemfibrozil: ↑ risk of myopathy, rhabdomyolysis
Niacin: ↑ risk of myopathy
Warfarin: ↑ risk of bleeding
Food/drug
↑ levels of lovastatin
Lab test interferences
↑ CPK, ↑ liver function tests

NURSING CONSIDERATIONS
Assessment
• Assess nutrition: fat, protein, carbohydrates; nutritional analysis should be completed by dietician before treatment is initiated
• Monitor bowel pattern daily; diarrhea may be a problem
• Monitor triglycerides, cholesterol baseline and throughout treatment; LDL, ADL, TG and cholesterol at 6-8 wk and q6 mo should be watched closely; if it increases, drug should be discontinued

Nursing diagnoses
☑Diarrhea (adverse reactions)
☑Knowledge deficit (teaching)
☑Noncompliance (teaching)

Implementation
• Give 30 min before AM and PM meals

S

✦ Canada Only   Adverse effects: *italic* = common; **bold** = life-threatening

Patient/family education
• Inform patient that compliance is needed for positive results to occur; not to double doses
• Advise patient to lower risk factors: high-fat diet, smoking, alcohol consumption, absence of exercise
• Advise patient to notify health care prescriber if the GI symptoms of diarrhea, abdominal or epigastric pain, nausea, vomiting occur; or if chills, fever, sore throat occur

Evaluation
Positive therapeutic outcome
• Decreased cholesterol levels, serum triglycerides and improved ratio with high-density lipoproteins (HDLs)

---

sirolimus
See Appendix A,
Selected New Drugs

---

sodium bicarbonate (OTC)
Arm and Hammer Pure Baking Soda, Bell/ans, Citrocarbonate, Neut, Soda Mint
Func. class.: Alkalinizer; antacid
Pregnancy category **C**

Action: Orally neutralizes gastric acid, which forms water, NaCl, CO_2; increases plasma bicarbonate, which buffers H^+ ion concentration; reverses acidosis **IV**

➡**Therapeutic Outcome:** Correction of acidosis, gastric acid neutralization

Uses: Acidosis (metabolic), cardiac arrest, alkalinization (systemic/urinary); antacid (PO)

Dosage and routes
Acidosis, metabolic
P *Adult and child:* **IV** inf 2-5 mEq/kg over 4-8 hr depending on CO_2, pH
Cardiac arrest
P *Adult and child:* **IV** bol 1 mEq/kg of 7.5% or 8.4% sol, then 0.5 mEq/kg q10 min, then doses based on ABGs
P *Infant:* **IV** inf not to exceed 8 mEq/kg/day based on ABGs (4.2% sol)
Alkalinization of urine
Adult: PO 325 mg-2 g qid or 48 mEq/kg (4 g), then 12-24 mEq q4hr
P *Child:* PO 12-120 mg/kg/day (1-10 mEq/kg)
Antacid
Adult: PO 300 mg-2 g chewed, taken with water qd-qid

Available forms: Tabs 300, 325, 600, 650 mg; inj 4.2%, 5%, 7.5%, 8.4%

Adverse effects
CNS: Irritability, headache, confusion, stimulation, tremors, *twitching, hyperreflexia,* **tetany,** weakness, **convulsions** caused by alkalosis
CV: Irregular pulse, **cardiac arrest,** water retention, edema, weight gain
GI: Flatulence, *belching, distention,* **paralytic ileus,** acid rebound
GU: Calculi
META: Alkalosis
RESP: Shallow, slow respirations, cyanosis, **apnea**

Contraindications: Hypertension, peptic ulcer, renal disease, hypocalcemia

---

Precautions: CHF, cirrhosis, toxemia, renal disease, pregnancy **C**

Pharmacokinetics

Absorption	Unknown
Distribution	Widely distributed—extracellular fluids
Metabolism	Unknown
Excretion	Kidneys
Half-life	Unknown

Pharmacodynamics

	PO	IV
Onset	2 min	Rapid
Peak	½ hr	Rapid
Duration	1-3 hr	Unknown

Interactions
Individual drugs
Flecainide: ↑ effects
Ketoconazole: ↓ absorption of ketoconazole
Methenamine: ↓ effect of methenamine
Mexiletine: ↑ blood level of mexiletine
Quinidine: ↑ effects
Drug classifications
Amphetamines: ↑ effects
Anorexiants: ↑ effects
Barbiturates: ↓ effects of barbiturates
Corticosteroids: ↑ sodium, potassium
Fluoroquinolones: ↑ crystalluria
Salicylates: ↓ effect of salicylates
▨*Herb/drug*
Oak bark: ↓ action of sodium bicarbonate
Lab test interferences
↑ Urinary urobilinogen
False positive: Urinary protein, blood lactate

NURSING CONSIDERATIONS
Assessment
• Assess respiratory and pulse rate, rhythm, depth, lung sounds; notify prescriber of abnormalities
• Assess for GI perforation secondary to CO_2 in GI tract; may lead to perforation if ulcer is severe
• Monitor fluid balance (I&O, weight qd, edema); notify prescriber of fluid overload
• Monitor electrolytes: blood pH, PO_2, HCO_3, during beginning treatment; ABGs frequently during emergencies
• Monitor urine pH, urinary output, during beginning treatment
• Monitor extravasation with **IV** administration (tissue sloughing, ulceration, and necrosis)
• Assess for alkalosis: irritability, confusion, twitching, hyperreflexia, stimulation, slow respirations, cyanosis, irregular pulse
• Monitor manifestations of hypokalemia: *Renal:* acidic urine, reduced urine osmolality, nocturia, polyuria, polydipsia; *Cardiac:* hypotension, broad T wave, U wave, ectopy, tachycardia, weak pulse; *Neurologic:* muscle weakness, altered LOC, drowsiness, apathy, lethargy, confusion, depression; *GI:* anorexia, nausea, cramps, constipation, distension, paralytic ileus; *Respiratory:* hypoventilation, respiratory muscle weakness
• Monitor for manifestations of hyponatremia: *CV:* ↑ B/P, cold, clammy skin, hypo or hypervolemia; *GI:* anorexia, nausea, vomiting, diarrhea, abdominal cramps; *Neuro:* lethargy, increased ICP, confusion, headache, seizures, coma, fatigue, tremors, hyperreflexia
• Assess for milk-alkali syndrome: confusion, head-

S

Adverse effects: *italic* = common; **bold** = life-threatening

ache, nausea, vomiting, anorexia, urinary stones, hypercalcemia

Nursing diagnoses

☑ Gas exchange, impaired (uses)
☑ Fluid volume excess (adverse reactions)
☑ Knowledge deficit (teaching)

Implementation

PO route

• Tab must be chewed and taken with 8 oz of water
• Dissolve effervescent tab in water
• May be used to neutralize gastric acid in peptic ulcer disease, given 1 and 3 hr pc and hs

Ⅳ IV route

• Give **IV** bol in cardiac arrest, may be repeated q10min
• Give by intermittent or continuous inf in prepared sol or diluted in an equal amount of any dextrose/saline combination; administer 2-5mEq/kg over 4-8 hr, not to exceed 50mEq/hr; slower
Ｐ rate in children

Syringe compatibilities:
Milrinone, pentobarbital

Syringe incompatibilities:
Glycopyrrolate, metoclopramide, thiopental

Y-site compatibilities:
Acyclovir, amifostine, asparaginase, aztreonam, cefepime, cefmetazole, ceftriaxone, cladribine, cyclophosphamide, cytarabine, daunorubicin, dexamethasone, dexchlorpheniramine, doxorubicin, etoposide, famotidine, filgrastim, fludarabine, gallium, granisetron, heparin, ifosfamide, indomethacin, insulin, melphalan, mesna, methylprednisolone, morphine, paclitaxel, piperacillin/tazobactam, potassium

chloride, propofol, tacrolimus, teniposide, thiotepa, tolazoline, vancomycin, vit B/C

Y-site incompatibilities:
Amrinone, calcium chloride, idarubicin, sargramostim, verapamil, vinorelbine

Additive compatibilities:
Amikacin, aminophylline, amobarbital, amphotericin B, atropine, bretylium, calcium chloride, calcium gluceptate, cefoxitin, ceftazidime, cephalothin, cephapirin, chloramphenicol, chlorothiazide, cimetidine, clindamycin, cytarabine, droperidol/fentanyl, ergonovine, erythromycin, esmolol, floxacillin, furosemide, heparin, hyaluronidase, hydrocortisone, kanamycin, lidocaine, mannitol, metaraminol, methotrexate, methyldopate, multivitamins, nafcillin, nalmefene, netilmicin, nizatidine, ofloxacin, oxacillin, oxytocin, phenobarbital, phenylephrine, phenytoin, phytonadione, potassium chloride, prochlorperazine, thiopental, verapamil

Additive incompatibilities:
Amoxicillin, ascorbic acid, carboplatin, carmustine, cefotaxime, cisplatin, codeine, dobutamine, epinephrine, hydromorphone, imipenem/cilastatin, insulin, isoproterenol, labetalol, levorphanol, magnesium sulfate, methadone, morphine, norepinephrine, pentazocine, pentobarbital, procaine, secobarbital, streptomycin, succinylcholine, tetracycline, vit B/C

Patient/family education

• Instruct patient to chew antacid tab and drink 8 oz water; not to take antacid with

---

milk because milk-alkali syndrome may result; not to use antacid for more than 2 wk
• Advise patient to notify prescriber if indigestion is accompanied by chest pain; dyspnea; diarrhea; dark, tarry stools
• Teach patient about sodium-restricted diet; to avoid use of baking soda for indigestion

Evaluation
Positive therapeutic outcome
• ABGs, electrolytes, blood pH, HCO_3 normal levels
• Decreased gastric pain

---

sodium biphosphate (OTC)

Fleet Enema, Phospho-Soda
Func. class.: Laxative, saline
Pregnancy category   C

Action: Increases water absorption in the small intestine by osmotic action; laxative effect occurs by increased peristalsis and water retention

▶**Therapeutic Outcome:** Absence of constipation

Uses: Constipation, bowel or rectal preparation for surgery, examination

Dosage and routes
Adult: PO 20-30 ml (phospho-soda)
P *Child:* PO 5-15 ml (phospho-soda)
P *Adult and child >12 yr:* Rec enema (118 ml)
P *Child 2-12 yr:* Rec ½ enema (59 ml)

Available forms: Enema 7 g/phosphate and 19 g/biphosphate/118 ml; oral sol 18 g phosphate/48 g biphosphate/100 ml

Adverse effects
GI: Nausea, cramps, diarrhea
META: Electrolyte, fluid imbalances

Contraindications: Hypersensitivity, rectal fissures, abdominal pain, nausea/vomiting, appendicitis, acute surgical abdomen, ulcerated hemorrhoids, Na-restricted diets (Sal-Hepatica, PhosphoSoda)

Precautions: Pregnancy **C**

Pharmacokinetics	
Absorption	Up to 20% (Rec)
Distribution	Unknown
Metabolism	Unknown
Excretion	Kidneys
Half-life	Unknown

Pharmacodynamics		
	PO	REC
Onset	½-3 hr	5 min
Peak	Unknown	Unknown
Duration	Unknown	Unknown

Interactions: None

NURSING CONSIDERATIONS
Assessment
• Assess stools: color, amount, consistency
• Assess for bowel pattern, bowel sounds (frequency, intensity), flatulence, distention, increased temp, dietary patterns (fluid, bulk), exercise
• Assess for cramping, rec bleeding, nausea, vomiting; if these symptoms occur, drug should be discontinued

Nursing diagnoses
☑ Constipation (uses)
☑ Knowledge deficit (teaching)

Implementation
PO route
• Give on empty stomach
• Mix oral sol in cold water

S

• Alone for better absorption; do not take within 1 hr of other drugs

Patient/family education
• Advise patient not to use laxatives or enema for long-term therapy; bowel tone will be lost
• Teach patient that normal bowel movements do not always occur daily
• Caution patient not to use in presence of abdominal pain, nausea, vomiting
• Caution patient to notify prescriber if constipation is unrelieved or if symptoms of electrolyte imbalance occur: muscle cramps, pain, weakness, dizziness, excessive thirst
• Instruct patient to maintain adequate fluid consumption to help prevent constipation

Evaluation
Positive therapeutic outcome
• Decrease in constipation

---

sodium polystyrene sulfonate (℞)
(po-lee-stye′reen)
Kayexalate, SPS
Func. class.: Potassium-removing resin
Chem. class.: Cation exchange resin

Pregnancy category C

Action: Removes potassium by exchanging sodium for potassium in body; occurs primarily in large intestine

▶**Therapeutic Outcome:** Potassium levels within accepted range

Uses: Hyperkalemia in conjunction with other measures

Dosage and routes
Adult: PO 15 g qd-qid; rec enema 30-50 g/100 ml of sorbitol warmed to body temp q6h

P *Child:* PO/rec 1 mEq of K exchanged/g of resin, approximate dose 1g/kg q6hr

Available forms: Susp, 15 g polystyrene sulfonate, 21.5 ml sorbitol, 15 g (65 mEq) sodium/60 ml; powder 15 g/4 level tsp

Adverse effects
GI: *Constipation,* anorexia, nausea, vomiting, diarrhea (sorbitol), *fecal impaction,* gastric irritation
META: Hypocalcemia, hypokalemia, hypomagnesemia, sodium retention

Precautions: Pregnancy **C**, renal failure, CHF, severe edema, severe hypertension

---

Pharmacokinetics	
Absorption	None
Distribution	None
Metabolism	None
Excretion	Feces
Half-life	Unknown

Pharmacodynamics		
	PO	REC
Onset	2-12 hr	2-12 hr
Peak	Unknown	Unknown
Duration	6-24 hr	4-6 hr

Interactions
Drug classifications
Antacids, calcium or magnesium: ↓ effect of sodium polystyrene
Laxatives: ↓ effect of sodium polystyrene

NURSING CONSIDERATIONS
Assessment
• Assess bowel function daily: amount of stool, color, characteristics

---

• Assess hypotension: confusion, irritability, muscular pain, weakness

• Monitor for manifestations of hypokalemia: *Renal:* acidic urine, reduced urine osmolality, nocturia, polyuria, polydipsia; *Cardiac:* hypotension, broad T wave, U wave, ectopy, tachycardia, weak pulse; *Neuro:* muscle weakness, altered LOC, drowsiness, apathy, lethargy, confusion, depression; *GI:* anorexia, nausea, cramps, constipation, distension, paralytic ileus; *Respiratory:* hypoventilation, respiratory muscle weakness

• Monitor for manifestations of hypocalcemia: *CNS:* personality changes, anxiety, disturbances, depression, psychosis, nausea, vomiting, *GI:* constipation, abdominal pain from muscle spasm; *CV:* decreased contractility, decreased cardiac output, hypotension, lengthened ST segment, prolonged QT interval; *Integ:* scaling eczema, alopecia, hyperpigmentation; *Neuro:* tetany, muscle twitching, cramping grimacing, seizure, altered deep tendon reflexes, spasm

• Monitor for manifestations of hypomagnesemia; *CNS:* agitation; *Neuro:* muscle twitching, paresthesias, hyperactive reflexes, positive Babinski reflex, dysphagia, nystagmus, seizures, tetany; *GI:* nausea, vomiting, diarrhea, anorexia, abdominal distention; *Cardiac:* ectopy; tachycardia, broad, flat, or inverted T waves; depressed ST segment; prolonged QT; decreased cardiac output; hypotension

• Monitor electrolytes: potassium, sodium, calcium, magnesium

Nursing diagnoses
☑ Constipation (adverse reactions)
☑ Diarrhea (adverse reactions)
☑ Knowledge deficit (teaching)

Implementation
PO route
• Give oral dose as susp mixed with H_2O or syr (20-100 ml)
• Give mild laxative as ordered to prevent constipation and fecal impaction; sorbitol as ordered to prevent constipation
Rec route
• Give by retention enema after mixing with warm water; introduce by gravity, continue stirring, flush with 100 ml of fluid, clamp, and leave in place for at least ½-1 hr
• Complete irrigation of colon after enema with 1-2 qt of nonsodium sol, drain
• Store freshly prepared sol for 24 hr at room temp

Patient/family education
• Explain reason for medication and expected results

Evaluation
Positive therapeutic outcome
• Potassium level normal

---

somatropin (℞)
(soe-ma-troe′pin)
Genotropin, Humatrope, Norditropin, Nutropin, Nutropin AQ, Saizen, Serostim
Func. class.: Pituitary hormone
Chem. class.: Growth hormone
Pregnancy category   C

Action: Stimulates growth; similar to natural growth hormone—both preparations

S

are developed by recombinant DNA technique

Therapeutic Outcome: Increase in height as a result of skeletal growth in pituitary growth hormone deficiency

Uses: Pituitary growth hormone deficiency (hypopituitary dwarfism), children with human growth hormone deficiency, AIDs wasting syndrome, cachexia, adults with somatropin deficiency syndrome (SDS)

Dosage and routes
Genotropin: SC 0.16-0.24 mg/kg 1 wk, divided into 6 or 7 inj, give in abdomen, thigh, buttocks

Humatrope: SC/IM 0.18 mg/kg divided into equal doses either on 3 alternate days or 6×/wk, max wk dose is 0.3 mg/kg

Growth Hormone Deficiency Nutropin/Nutropin AQ: SC 0.2 mg/kg/wk

Serostim: SC at hs >55 kg 6 mg, 45-55 kg 5 mg, 35-45 kg 4 mg

Norditropin: SC 0.024-0.034 mg/kg 6-7×/wk

Available forms: Powder for inj (lyophilized) 1.5 mg (4IU/ml), 4 mg (12IU/vial), 5 mg (13IU/vial), 5 mg (15IU/vial), 5 mg (15IU/ml) rDNA origin, 5.8 mg (15IU/ml), 6 mg (18IU.ml), 8 mg (24IU/vial), 10 mg (26IU/vial), inj 10 mg (30IU/vial)

Adverse effects
CNS: Headache, **growth of intracranial tumor**
ENDO: Hyperglycemia, ketosis, hypothyroidism
GU: Hypercalciuria

INTEG: Rash, urticaria, pain, inflammation at injection site
MS: Tissue swelling, joint and muscle pain
SYST: Antibodies to growth hormone

Contraindications: Hypersensitivity to benzyl alcohol, closed epiphyses, intracranial lesions

Precautions: Diabetes mellitus, hypothyroidism, pregnancy **C**

Pharmacokinetics	
Absorption	Well absorbed (SC/IM)
Distribution	Unknown
Metabolism	Unknown
Half-life	15-60 min

Pharmacodynamics	
	IM/SC (GROWTH)
Onset	Unknown
Peak	Unknown
Duration	7 days

Interactions
Drug classifications
Androgens: ↑ epiphyseal closure
Glucocorticosteroids: ↓ growth, ↓ somatotropin response
Thyroid hormones: ↑ epiphyseal closure

NURSING CONSIDERATIONS
Assessment
• Identify growth hormone antibodies if patient fails to respond to therapy
• Monitor thyroid function tests: T_3, T_4, T_7, TSH to identify hypothyroidism
• Assess for allergic reaction: rash, itching, fever, nausea, wheezing
• Assess for hypercalciuria: urinary stones; groin, flank

---

pain; nausea, vomiting, frequency, hematuria, chills
P • Monitor growth rate of child at intervals during treatment

Nursing diagnoses
✓ Body image disturbance (uses)
✓ Knowledge deficit (teaching)

Implementation
• Store in refrigerator for <1 mo; if reconstituted, <1 wk; do not use discolored or cloudy sol

IM route
• Norditropin: After reconstituting 4-8 mg/2 ml diluent
• Humetrope: 5 mg/1.5-5 ml dilute, do not shake
• Nutropin/Nutropin AQ: Reconstitute 5 mg/1-5 ml or 10 mg/1-10 ml bacteriostatic water for inj (benzyl alcohol preserved)

Patient/family education
• Explain reason for medication and expected results; that treatment may continue for yrs
• Advise patient that routine follow-up is needed to monitor growth rate
• Instruct parents on procedure for medication preparation and inj use—request demonstration, return demonstration; provide written instructions

Evaluation
Positive therapeutic outcome
• Growth in children until epiphyseal plates close

---

sotalol (R)
(soe-ta'lole)
Betapace, Sotacar ✤
Func. class.: Antidysrhythmic, group II, III
Chem. class.: Nonselective β-blocker

Pregnancy category B

Action: Competitively blocks stimulation of β-adrenergic receptor within vascular smooth muscle; produces chronotropic, inotropic activity (decreases rate of SA node discharge, increases recovery time), slows conduction of AV node, decreases heart rate, which decreases O_2 consumption in myocardium; also decreases renin-aldosterone-angiotensin system at high doses, inhibits β-2 receptors in bronchial system (high doses)

➡ Therapeutic Outcome: Decreased B/P, heart rate, AV conduction

Uses: Life-threatening ventricular dysrhythmias

Dosage and routes
Adult: PO initial 80 mg bid, may increase to total of 240-320 mg/day

Renal dose
CrCl 30-60 ml/min give q24h; CrCl 10-29 ml/min give q36-48 h; CrCl <10 ml/min individualize dose

Available forms: Tabs 80, 120, 160, 240 mg

Adverse effects
CNS: Dizziness, mental changes, drowsiness, fatigue, headache, catatonia, depression, anxiety, nightmares, paresthesia, lethargy, insomnia, decreased concentration

S

CV: Orthostatic hypotension, bradycardia, **CHF,** chest pain, **ventricular dysrhythmias,** AV block, peripheral vascular insufficiency, palpitations, prodysrhythmia, **torsades de pointes**

EENT: Tinnitus, visual changes, sore throat, double vision, dry, burning eyes

GI: Nausea, vomiting, diarrhea, dry mouth, flatulence, constipation, anorexia

HEMA: **Agranulocytosis, thrombocytopenic purpura (rare), thrombocytopenia,** leukopenia

INTEG: Rash, alopecia, urticaria, pruritus, fever

MS: Joint pain, arthralgia, muscle cramps, pain

RESP: **Bronchospasm,** dyspnea, wheezing, nasal stuffiness, pharyngitis

OTHER: Facial swelling, decreased exercise tolerance, weight change, Raynaud's disease

Contraindications: Hypersensitivity to β-blockers, cardiogenic shock, heart block (2nd or 3rd degree), sinus bradycardia, CHF, bronchial asthma, congenital or acquired long QT syndrome

Precautions: Major surgery, pregnancy **B,** lactation, diabetes mellitus, renal disease, thyroid disease, COPD, well-compensated heart failure, CAD, nonallergic bronchospasm, electrolyte disturbances, bradycardia, cardiac dysrhythmias, peripheral vascular disease

Pharmacokinetics

Absorption	Variable (30%)
Distribution	Crosses placenta, minimal penetration in CNS
Metabolism	Liver
Excretion	70% unchanged—kidneys
Half-life	10-24 hr, ↑ in renal disease

Pharmacodynamics

Onset	Several hr
Peak	Unknown
Duration	Unknown

Interactions
Individual drugs
Digoxin: ↑ blood levels, ↑ toxicity
Disopyramide: ↑ levels, ↑ toxicity
Flecainide: ↑ levels, ↑ toxicity
Lidocaine: Bradycardia, arrest
Mexiletine: ↑ levels, ↑ toxicity
Phenytoin: ↑ blood levels
Procainamide: ↑ levels, ↑ toxicity
Quinidine: ↑ levels, ↑ toxicity
Warfarin: ↑ level, ↑ bleeding
Drug classifications
Calcium channel blockers: ↑ dysrhythmias, arrest
☑ Herb/drug
Aloe: ↑ hypokalemia
Buckthorn: ↑ hypokalemia
Cascara sagrada: ↑ hypokalemia
Senna: ↑ hypokalemia
Lab test interferences
False: ↑ Urinary catecholamines

NURSING CONSIDERATIONS
Assessment
• Monitor B/P during beginning treatment, periodically thereafter; pulse q4hr; note rate, rhythm, quality: apical/radial pulse before administration; notify prescriber of

---

any significant changes (pulse <50 bpm)

• Check for baselines in renal, liver function tests before therapy begins

• Assess for edema in feet, legs daily, monitor I&O, daily weight; check for jugular vein distention, rales, bilaterally, dyspnea (CHF)

• Monitor skin turgor, dryness of mucous membranes for hydration status, especially in 🄖 elderly

Nursing diagnoses

☑ Cardiac output, decreased (uses)

☑ Injury, risk for (adverse reactions)

☑ Knowledge deficit (teaching)

☑ Noncompliance (teaching)

Implementation

• Given ac, hs, tab may be crushed or swallowed whole; give with food to prevent GI upset; reduce dosage in renal dysfunction

• Store protected from light, moisture; place in cool environment

Patient/family education

• Teach patient not to discontinue drug abruptly, taper over 2 wk; may cause precipitate angina if stopped abruptly

• Teach patient not to use OTC products containing α-adrenergic stimulants (such as nasal decongestants, cold preparations); to avoid alcohol and smoking and to limit sodium intake as prescribed

• Teach patient how to take pulse and B/P at home, advise when to notify prescriber

• Instruct patient to comply with weight control, dietary adjustments, modified exercise program

• Caution patient to carry/ wear Medic Alert ID to identify drug being taken, allergies

• Inform patient that drug controls symptoms but does not cure

• Caution patient to avoid hazardous activities if dizziness, drowsiness is present

• Teach patient to report symptoms of CHF: difficulty breathing, especially on exertion or when lying down; night cough; swelling of extremities; bradycardia; dizziness; confusion; depression; fever

• Teach patient to take drug as prescribed, not to double or skip doses; take any missed doses as soon as remembered if at least 4 hr until next dose

Evaluation

Positive therapeutic outcome

• Absence of dysrhythmias

Treatment of overdose:

Lavage; **IV** atropine for bradycardia; **IV** theophylline for bronchospasm; digitalis, O_2, diuretic for cardiac failure; hemodialysis; **IV** glucose for hyperglycemia; **IV** diazepam (or phenytoin) for seizures

---

sparfloxacin (℞)

(spare-floks'a-sin)

Zagam

Func. class.: Antiinfective

Chem. class.: Fluoroquinolone antibacterial

Pregnancy category   C

Action: Interferes with conversion of intermediate DNA fragments into high-molecular-weight DNA in bacteria; DNA gyrase inhibitor

➡ **Therapeutic Outcome:** Bactericidal action against the following organisms: *Chla-*

mydia pneumoniae, Haemophilus influenzae, H. parainfluenzae, Moraxella catarrhalis

Uses: Adult infections (including complicated): lower respiratory, community-acquired pneumonia, chronic bronchitis

Dosage and routes
Adult: PO 400 mg loading dose, then 200 mg q24h × 10 days

Renal dose
400 mg on day 1 if CrCl <50 ml/min; then 200 mg qod on days 2-10

Available forms: Tabs 200 mg

Adverse effects
CNS: Headache, dizziness, insomnia
CV: QT interval prolongation, vasodilation
GI: Nausea, flatulence, abdominal pain, **pseudomembranous colitis,** *vomiting,* diarrhea
HEMA: **Leukopenia,** eosinophilia, anemia
INTEG: Pruritus, photosensitivity

Contraindications: Hypersensitivity to quinolones

Precautions: Pregnancy **C,** lactation, children, renal disease, seizure disorder

Pharmacokinetics	
Absorption	Slow-erratic
Distribution	Widely distributed
Metabolism	Liver
Excretion	Kidneys, feces
Half-life	20 hr

Pharmacodynamics	
Unknown	

Interactions
Individual drugs
Amiodarone: ↑ torsades de pointes
Bepridil: ↑ torsades de pointes
Caffeine: ↑ toxicity
Cimetidine: ↑ sparfloxacin
Cyclosporine: ↑ toxicity
Disopyramide: ↑ torsades de pointes
Erythromycin: ↑ torsades de pointes
Pentamine: ↑ torsades de pointes
Phenytoin: ↓ effect
Probenecid: ↑ sparfloxacin
Sucralfate: ↓ absorption
Zinc sulfate: ↓ absorption of sparfloxacin
Drug classifications
Antacids: ↓ absorption of sparfloxacin
Antidysrhythmics Class Ia/ III: ↑ torsades de pointes
Phenothiazines: ↑ torsades de pointes
Tricyclic antidepressants: ↑ torsades de pointes
Lab test interferences
↑ AST, ↑ ALT

NURSING CONSIDERATIONS
Assessment
• Assess patient for previous sensitivity reaction
• Assess patient for signs and symptoms of infection including characteristics of wounds, sputum, urine, stool, WBC >10,000, fever; obtain baseline information before and during treatment
• Obtain C&S before beginning drug therapy to identify if correct treatment has been initiated
• Assess for allergic reactions: rash, urticaria, pruritus, chills, fever, joint pain; may occur a few days after therapy begins;

epinephrine and resuscitation equipment should be available for anaphylactic reaction
• Identify urine output; if decreasing, notify prescriber (may indicate nephrotoxicity); also check for increased BUN, creatinine
• Monitor blood studies: AST, ALT, CBC, Hct, bilirubin, LDH, alkaline phosphatase, Coombs' test monthly if patient is on long-term therapy
• Assess bowel pattern qd; if severe diarrhea occurs, drug should be discontinued
• Monitor for bleeding; ecchymosis, bleeding gums, hematuria, stool guaiac daily if on long-term therapy
• Assess for overgrowth of infection: perineal itching, fever, malaise, redness, pain, swelling, drainage, rash, diarrhea, change in cough, sputum

Nursing diagnoses
✓ Infection, risk for (uses)
✓ Diarrhea (side effects)
✓ Injury, risk for (side effects)
✓ Knowledge deficit (teaching)
✓ Noncompliance (teaching)

Implementation
PO route
• Give around the clock to maintain proper blood levels
• Give 4 hrs before or after antacids/calcium

IV IV route
• Check for irritation, extravasation, phlebitis daily
• For intermittent inf, dilute to 1-2 mg/ml of D_5W, 0.9% NaCl; give over 60 min; it will remain stable under refrigeration for 2 wks

Patient/family education
• Advise patient to contact prescriber if vaginal itching, loose foul-smelling stools,

furry tongue occur; may indicate superinfection; report itching, rash, pruritus, urticaria
• Instruct patient to take all medication prescribed for the length of time ordered; drug must be taken around the clock to maintain blood levels; do not give medication to others
• Teach patient to avoid direct sunlight
• Advise patient to drink plenty of fluids, take 4 hrs before or after antacids/calcium
• Advise patient to notify prescriber of diarrhea with blood or pus

Evaluation
Positive therapeutic outcome
• Absence of signs/symptoms of infection (WBC <10,000, temp WNL)
• Reported improvement in symptoms of infection

---

spectinomycin (℞)
(spek-ti-noe-mye'sin)
Trobicin
Func. class.: Antiinfective
Chem. class.: Amino-cyclitol
Pregnancy category   B

Action: Inhibits bacterial synthesis by binding to 30S subunit on ribosome

Therapeutic Outcome: Treatment and resolution of gonococcal infection

Uses: Gonorrhea, gonococcal urethritis, cervicitis, proctitis

Dosage and routes
Adult and child >45 kg: IM 2-4 g as single dose
Child <45 kg: IM 40 mg/kg as single dose

S

Gonococcal infections in pregnancy
Adult: IM 2 g, to treat those allergic to cephalosporins

Available forms: Powder for inj 400 mg/ml when reconstituted

Adverse effects
CNS: Dizziness, chills, fever, insomnia, headache, anxiety
GI: Nausea, vomiting, increased BUN
GU: Decreased urine output
HEMA: Anemia
INTEG: Pain at injection site, urticaria, rash, pruritus, fever

Contraindications: Hypersensitivity, syphilis

Precautions: Pregnancy **B**, 🅿 infants, children, lactation

Pharmacokinetics	
Absorption	Well absorbed
Distribution	Unknown
Metabolism	Liver
Excretion	Kidneys
Half-life	1⅕-2½ hr

Pharmacodynamics	
Onset	Rapid
Peak	1 hr

NURSING CONSIDERATIONS
Assessment
• Monitor gonorrhea culture after treatment
• Monitor I&O ratio; report decreased output
• Monitor liver studies: AST, ALT, serum alk phosphatase following multiple doses
• Monitor blood studies: Hct, Hgb, BUN if multiple diagnoses given
• Monitor serologic test for gonorrhea 3 mo after treatment
• Assess for allergies before

treatment, reaction of each medication

Nursing diagnoses
☑ Infection, risk for (uses)
☑ Knowledge deficit (teaching)

Implementation
• Give after shaking vial; IM in deep muscle mass (glutens only); with 20-gauge needle; no more than 5 ml per site
• Store at room temp; reconstituted sol should be discarded after 24 hr

Evaluation
Positive therapeutic outcome
• Negative gonorrhea culture after treatment

spironolactone (℞)
(speer'on-oh-lak'tone)
Aldactone, Novospiroton ✦
Func. class: Potassium-sparing diuretic
Chem. class.: Aldosterone antagonist
Pregnancy category D

Action: Competes with aldosterone at receptor sites in the distal tubule in the renal system, resulting in excretion of sodium, chloride, water, bicarbonate, and calcium; potassium, phosphate, and hydrogen are retained

➔**Therapeutic Outcome:** Diuretic and antihypertensive effect while retaining potassium; lowered aldosterone levels

Uses: Edema of CHF, hypertension, diuretic-induced hypokalemia, primary hyperaldosteronism (diagnosis, short-term treatment, long-term treatment), edema of nephrotic syndrome, cirrhosis of the liver with ascites

Dosage and routes
Edema/hypertension
Adult: PO 25-200 mg/qd in single or divided doses

Edema
P *Child:* PO 3.3 mg/kg/day in single or divided doses

Hypertension
P *Child:* PO 1-2 mg/kg bid

Hypokalemia
Adult: PO 25-100 mg/day; if PO, K supplements are unable to be used

Primary hyperaldosteronism diagnosis
Adult: PO 400 mg/day × 4 days depending on the test, then 100-400 mg/day maintenance

Available forms: Tabs 25, 50, 100 mg

Adverse effects
CNS: Headache, confusion, drowsiness, lethargy, ataxia
ELECT: Hyperchloremic metabolic acidosis, **hyperkalemia,** hyponatremia
ENDO: Impotence, gynecomastia, irregular menses, amenorrhea, postmenopausal bleeding, hirsutism, deepening voice
GI: Diarrhea, cramps, bleeding, gastritis, vomiting
HEMA: **Agranulocytosis**

Contraindications: Hypersensitivity, anuria, severe renal disease, hyperkalemia, pregnancy **D**

Precautions: Dehydration, hepatic disease, lactation, **G** elderly, renal disease

Pharmacokinetics

Absorption	GI tract; well absorbed
Distribution	Crosses placenta
Metabolism	Liver to canrenone (active metabolite)
Excretion	Renal; breast milk
Half-life	12-24 hr (canrenone)

Pharmacodynamics

Onset	24-48 hr
Peak	48-72 hr
Duration	Unknown

Interactions
Individual drugs
Aspirin: ↓ action of spironolactone
Lithium: ↑ action, toxicity
Drug classifications
ACE inhibitors: ↑ hyperkalemia
Anticoagulants: ↓ effects of anticoagulants
Antihypertensives: ↑ action
Diuretics, potassium-sparing: ↑ hyperkalemia
Potassium products: ↑ hyperkalemia
Salt substitutes: ↑ hyperkalemia
Food/drug
Potassium foods: ↑ hyperkalemia
Herb/drug
Licorice: Hypokalemic alkalosis
Lab test interferences
False: ↑ Urinary catecholamines
Interference: Glucose, insulin tolerance tests

NURSING CONSIDERATIONS
Assessment
• Monitor for manifestations of hyperkalemia: *MS:* fatigue, muscle weakness; *Cardiac:* arrhythmias, hypotension, *Neuro:* paresthesias, confusion, *Resp:* dyspnea

S

• Monitor for manifestations of hyponatremia: *CV:* ↑ B/P, cold, clammy skin, hypo or hypervolemia; *GI:* anorexia, nausea, vomiting, diarrhea, abdominal cramps; *Neuro:* lethargy, increased ICP, confusion headache, seizures, coma, fatigue, tremors, hyperreflexia

• Monitor for manifestations of hyperchloremia: *Neuro:* weakness, lethargy, coma; *Resp:* deep rapid breathing

• Assess fluid volume status: I&O ratios and record, count or weigh diapers as appropriate, weight, distended red veins, crackles in lung, color, quality and sp gr of urine, skin turgor, adequacy of pulses, moist mucous membranes, bilateral lung sounds, peripheral pitting edema; dehydration symptoms of decreasing output, thirst, hypotension, dry mouth and mucous membranes should be reported

• Monitor electrolytes: potassium, sodium, calcium, magnesium; also include BUN, ABGs, uric acid, CBC, blood sugar

Associated nursing diagnoses

☑ Urinary elmination, altered (adverse reactions)
☑ Fluid volume deficit (adverse reactions)
☑ Fluid volume excess (uses)
☑ Knowledge deficit (teaching)

Implementation

• Give in AM to avoid interference with sleep

• With food, if nausea occurs, absorption may be increased; take at same time each day

Patient/family education

• Teach patient to take the medication early in the day to prevent nocturia

• Instruct patient to take with food or milk if GI symptoms of nausea and anorexia occur

• Teach patient to maintain a record of weight on a weekly basis and notify prescriber of weight loss of >5 lbs

• Caution patient that this drug causes an increase in potassium levels, that foods high in potassium should be avoided; refer to dietician for assistance planning

• Teach patient not to use alcohol, or any over-the-counter medications without prescriber's approval; serious drug reactions may occur

• Emphasize the need to contact prescriber immediately if muscle cramps, weakness, nausea, dizziness, or numbness occurs

• Teach patient to take own B/P and pulse and record

• Advise patient that dizziness and confusion may occur; avoid driving or other hazardous activities if alertness is decreased

• Teach patient to continue taking medication even if feeling better; this drug controls symptoms but does not cure the condition

• Advise patient with hypertension to continue other treatment (exercise, weight loss, relaxation techniques, cessation of smoking)

Evaluation

Positive therapeutic outcome

• Prevention of hypokalemia (diuretic use)

• Decreased edema

• Decreased B/P

• Decreased aldosterone levels

• Increased diuresis

Treatment of overdose:
• Lavage if taken orally, monitor electrolytes
• Administer sodium bicarbonate for K² 6.5 mEq/L
• Monitor hydration, CV, renal status

stavudine (℞)
(sta'vu-deen)
Zerit
Func. class.: Antiviral
Chem. class.: Primidone nucleoside

Pregnancy category   C

Action: Prevents replication of HIV by the inhibition of the enzyme reverse transcriptase

Therapeutic Outcome: Decreasing diarrhea, fatigue, night sweats; increased body weight

Uses: Treatment of advanced HIV infection for patients who have not responded to other antivirals

Dosage and routes
Adult >60 kg: PO 40 mg q12h up to 2 mg/kg/day

Adult <60 kg: 30 mg q12h

P *Child:* PO 2 mg/kg/day divided q12h

Renal dose
Adult >60 kg: CrCl 26-50 ml/min 20 mg q12h; CrCl 10-25 ml/min 20 mg q24h

Adult <60 kg: CrCl 26-50 ml/min 15 mg q12h; CrCl 10-25 ml/min 15 mg q24h

Available forms: Caps 15, 20, 30, 40 mg; PO powder for sol 1 mg/ml

Adverse effects
CNS: Peripheral neuropathy, headache, chills/fever, malaise

GI: **Hepatotoxicity**
HEMA: **Bone marrow suppression,** anemia
INTEG: Rash
MS: Myalgia

Contraindications: Hypersensitivity to this drug or zidovudine, didanosine, zalcitabine; severe peripheral neuropathy

Precautions: Advanced HIV infections, pregnancy **C**, lactation, bone marrow suppression, renal disease, liver disease, folic acid or B$_{12}$ deficiency, peripheral neuropathy

Pharmacokinetics	
Absorption	Rapidly absorbed, 82% bioavailability
Distribution	Cerebrospinal fluid
Metabolism	Unknown
Excretion	Kidneys, breast milk
Half-life	Elimination: 1-1.6 hr, intracellular: 3-3.5 hr

Pharmacodynamics	
Onset	Unknown
Peak	1 hr
Duration	Unknown

Interactions
Drug classifications
Myelosuppressants: ↑ myelosuppressor

NURSING CONSIDERATIONS
Assessment
• Monitor liver studies: AST, ALT
• Monitor blood studies: WBC, diff, RBC, Hct, Hgb, platelets
• Monitor renal studies: urinalysis, protein, blood
• Obtain C&S before drug therapy; drug may be taken as soon as culture is taken; C&S may be taken after therapy
• Monitor bowel pattern before, during treatment

• Monitor fluid overload; drug requires large volume to stay in sol

• Assess for weakness, tremors, confusion, dizziness, psychosis; if these occur, drug may have to be decreased or discontinued

Nursing diagnoses
☑ Infection, risk for (uses)
☑ Knowledge deficit (teaching)

Implementation
• Give with or without meals; absorption does not appear to be lowered when taken with food

Patient/family education
• Teach patient signs of peripheral neuropathy: burning, weakness, pain, pricking feeling in the extremities
• Caution patient that this drug should not be given with antineoplastics
• Inform patient that GI complaints and insomnia resolve after 3-4 wk of treatment
• Inform patient that drug is not a cure for AIDS, but will control symptoms
• Advise patient to call prescriber if sore throat, swollen lymph nodes, malaise, fever occur—may indicate presence of other infections
• Caution patient that even with drug administration, patient is still infective and may pass AIDS virus on to others
• Caution patient that follow-up visits must be continued because serious toxicity may occur; blood counts must be done q2wk
• Teach patient that drug must be taken q4hr around clock even during night
• Caution patient that serious drug interactions may occur if

OTC products are ingested; check with prescriber first if taking aspirin, acetaminophen, indomethacin
• Inform patient that other drugs may be necessary to prevent other infections
• Inform patient that drug may cause fainting or dizziness

Evaluation
Positive therapeutic outcome
• Decreased symptoms of HIV

---

streptokinase ⚓ (℞)
(strep-toe-kye′nase)
Kabikinase, Streptase
Func. class.: Thrombolytic enzyme
Chem. class.: β-Hemolytic streptococcus filtrate (purified)

Pregnancy category **C**

Action: Activates conversion of plasminogen to plasmin (fibrinolysin): plasmin breaks down clots (fibrin), fibrinogen, factors V, VII; occlusion of venous access lines

➡**Therapeutic Outcome:** Lysis of emboli, or thrombosis in various parts of the body

Uses: Deep vein thrombosis, pulmonary embolism, arterial thrombosis, arterial embolism, arteriovenous cannula occlusion, lysis of coronary artery thrombi after MI, acute evolving transmural MI

Dosage and routes
Lysis of coronary artery thrombi
Adult: CC 20,000 IU, then 2000 IU/min over 1 hr as **IV** inf

---

☑ Herb/drug   🚫 Do Not Crush   ◆ Alert   ⚓ Key Drug   🅖 Geriatric   🅟 Pediatric

Arteriovenous cannula occlusion
Adult: IV inf 250,000 IU/2 ml sol into occluded limb of cannula run over ½ hr; clamp for 2 hr; aspirate contents; flush with NaCl sol and reconnect

Thrombosis/embolism /DVT/ pulmonary embolism
Adult: IV inf 250,000 IU over ½ hr, then 100,000 IU/hr for 72 hr for deep thrombosis; 100,000 IU/hr over 24-72 hr for pulmonary embolism; 100,000 IU/hr x 24-72 hr for arterial thrombosis or embolism

Acute evolving transmural MI
Adult: IV inf 1,500,000 IU diluted to a volume of 45 ml; give within 1 hr; intracoronary inf 20,000 IU by bol, then 2,000 IU/min x 1 hr, total dose 140,000 IU

Available forms: Powder for inj, lyophilized 250,000, 600,000, 750,000, 1,500,000 IU vial

Adverse effects
CNS: Headache, fever
CV: **Dysrrhythmias,** hypotension, non-cardiogenic pulmonary edema, **pulmonary embolism**
EENT: Periorbital edema
GI: Nausea
HEMA: Decreased Hct, **bleeding**
INTEG: Rash, urticaria, phlebitis at IV inf site, itching, flushing
MS: Low back pain
RESP: Altered respirations, SOB, **bronchospasm**
SYST: GI, GU, intracranial retroperitoneal bleeding, surface bleeding, **anaphylaxis**

Contraindications: Hypersensitivity, active bleeding, intraspinal surgery, neoplasms of the CNS, ulcerative colitis, enteritis, severe hypertension, severe renal disease, hepatic disease, hypocoagulation, COPD, subacute bacterial endocarditis, rheumatic valvular disease, cerebral embolism/thrombosis/hemorrhage, intraarterial diagnostic procedure or surgery (10 days), recent major surgery

Precautions: Arterial emboli from left side of heart, pregnancy **C**

Pharmacokinetics

Absorption	Completely absorbed
Distribution	Unknown
Metabolism	>80%—liver, rapidly cleared by reticuloendothelial system
Excretion	Kidneys
Half-life	35 min

Pharmacodynamics

Onset	Immediate
Peak	Rapid
Duration	<12 hr

Interaction
Individual drugs
Aspirin: ↑ bleeding
Dipyridamole: ↑ bleeding
Heparin: ↑ bleeding
Plicamycin: ↑ bleeding
Valproic acid: ↑ bleeding
Drug classifications
Anticoagulants, oral: ↑ bleeding
Cephalosporins: ↑ bleeding
NSAIDs: ↑ bleeding
Lab test interferences
↑ PT, ↑ APTT, ↑ TT
↓ Plasminogen, ↓ fibrinogen

NURSING CONSIDERATIONS
Assessment
• Monitor VS, B/P, pulse, respirations (including periph-

S

---

eral), neurologic signs, temp at least q4h; temp >104° F (40° C) indicates internal bleeding; monitor rhythm closely; ventricular dysrhythmias may occur with hyperfusion; monitor heart, breath sounds, neuro status, peripheral pulses

◆• Assess for bleeding during first hr of treatment: hematuria, hematemesis, bleeding from mucous membranes, epistaxis, ecchymosis; guaiac, all body fluids, stools; may require transfusion (rare); blood studies (Hct, platelets, PTT, PT, TT, APTT) before starting therapy; PT or APTT must be less than 2 × control before starting therapy TT or PT q3-4h during treatment

• Assess allergy: fever, rash, itching, chills; mild reaction may be treated with antihistamines; report to prescriber

• Monitor ECG on monitor, watch for segment changes, changes in rhythm; sinus bradycardia, ventricular tachycardia, accelerated idioventricular rhythm may occur as a result of reperfusion (coronary thrombosis)

• Monitor ABGs, respiratory rate, (depth, characteristics), pulse, B/P, hemodynamics (pulmonary embolism)

• Monitor peripheral pulses, assess Homan's sign, check for redness, swelling q hr; notify health care prescriber of changes; B/P should not be taken in extremities (deep vein thrombosis)

• Check catheter for ability to aspirate blood from port; patient must exhale and hold breath when inserting and removing syringe to prevent air embolism (catheter/cannula occlusion)

• Assess for Guillain-Barré syndrome that may occur after treatment with this drug

• Assess for respiratory depression

Nursing diagnoses
☑ Tissue perfusion, altered (uses)
☑ Injury, risk for (adverse reactions)
☑ Impaired gas exchange (uses)
☑ Knowledge deficit (teaching)

Implementation
• Give after reconstituting with provided diluent; add appropriate amount of sterile water for inj (no preservatives) 20 mg vial/20 ml or 50 mg vial/50 ml to make 1 mg/ml, mix by slow inversion or dilute with NaCl, D_5W to a concentration of 0.5 mg/ml; further dilution, 1.5 to <0.5 mg/ml may result in precipitation of drug; use 18-gauge needle; flush line with NaCl after administration; reconstituted **IV** solution within 8 hr; within 6 hr of coronary occlusion for best results

• Give **IV** loading dose over 30 min to avoid hypotension

• **IV** after dilution with 4-5 g/250 ml NS, D_5W, LR, give over 1 hr; may give by continuous inf after loading dose(s) of 1 g/hr diluted in 50-100 ml of compatible sol; use inf pump; do not give by direct **IV**

• Give heparin therapy after thrombolytic therapy is discontinued, TT, ACT, or APTT less than 2 × control (about 3-4 hr); **IV** heparin with loading dose is recommended after discontinuing streptokinase to prevent redevelopment of thrombis

• Avoid invasive procedures, injection, taking temp via rec route

---

• Apply pressure for 30 sec to minor bleeding sites; 30 min to sites of atrial puncture, followed by pressure dressing; inform prescriber if this does not attain hemostasis; apply pressure dressing
• Store powder at room temp or refrigerate; protect from excessive light

Y-site compatibilities:
Dobutamine, dopamine, heparin, lidocaine, nitroglycerin

Additive incompatibilities:
Do not mix with other medications

Patient/family education
• Teach patient reason for medication, signs and symptoms of bleeding, allergic reactions, when to notify prescriber
• Explain that patient is to remain on bed rest to avoid injury

Evaluation
Positive therapeutic outcome
• Lysis of thrombi or emboli

---

streptomycin (℞)
(strep-toe-mye'sin)
Func. class.: Antiinfective, antitubercular
Chem. class.: Aminoglycoside
Pregnancy category **B**

Action: Interferes with protein synthesis in bacterial cell by binding to ribosomal subunit, causing inaccurate peptide sequence to form in protein chain, resulting in bacterial death

➤**Therapeutic Outcome:** Bactericidal effects for the following organisms: sensitive strains

of *Mycobacterium tuberculosis,* nontuberculous infections caused by sensitive strains of *Yersinia pestis, Brucella, Haemophilus influenzae, Klebsiella pneumoniae, Escherichia coli, E. aerogenes, Streptococcus viridans, F. tularensis, Proteus*

Uses: Active TB; used in combination for streptococcal and enterococcal infections; endocarditis, tularemia, plague

Dosage and routes
Tuberculosis
Adult: IM 15 mg/kg (max 1 g) qd × 2-3 mo, then 1 g 2-3 ×/week given with other antitubercular drugs

P *Child:* IM 20-40 mg/kg/day in divided doses given with other antitubercular drugs; max 15 mg/kg/day

Streptococcal endocarditis
Adult: IM 1 g q12h × 1 wk with penicillin, then 500 mg bid × 1 wk

Enterococcal endocarditis
Adult: IM 1 g q12h × 2 wk, then 500 mg q12h × 4 wk with penicillin max 15 mg/kg/day

Available forms: Inj 400 mg/ml

Adverse effects
CNS: Confusion, depression, numbness, tremors, **convulsions,** muscle twitching, **neurotoxicity**
CV: Hypotension, myocarditis, palpitations
EENT: Ototoxicity, deafness, visual disturbances
GI: Nausea, vomiting, anorexia, increased ALT, AST, bilirubin, hepatomegaly, **hepatic necrosis,** splenomegaly
GU: **Oliguria, hematuria, renal damage, azotemia, renal failure, nephrotoxicity**

S

HEMA: **Agranulocytosis, thrombocytopenia, leukopenia, eosinophilia, anemia**
INTEG: Rash, burning urticaria, dermatitis, alopecia

Contraindications: Severe renal disease, hypersensitivity

Precautions: Neonates, mild renal disease, pregnancy **B,** myasthenia gravis, lactation, **G** hearing deficits, elderly, Parkinson's disease

Pharmacokinetics

Absorption:	Well absorbed
Distribution	Widely distributed in extracellular fluids, poorly distributed in CSF; crosses placenta
Metabolism	Minimal—liver
Excretion	Mostly unchanged (>90%) kidneys
Half-life	2-2½ hr, increase in renal disease

Pharmacodynamics

Onset	Rapid
Peak	1-2 hr

Interactions
Individual drugs
Amphotericin B: ↑ Ototoxicity, neurotoxicity, nephrotoxicity
Cisplatin: ↑ Ototoxicity, neurotoxicity, nephrotoxicity
Ethacrynic acid: ↑ Ototoxicity, neurotoxicity, nephrotoxicity
Furosemide: ↑ Ototoxicity, neurotoxicity, nephrotoxicity
Mannitol: ↑ Ototoxicity, neurotoxicity, nephrotoxicity
Methoxyflurane: ↑ Ototoxicity, neurotoxicity, nephrotoxicity
Polymyxin: ↑ Ototoxicity, neurotoxicity, nephrotoxicity
Succinylcholine: ↑ Neuromuscular blockade, respiratory depression

Vancomycin: ↑ Ototoxicity, neurotoxicity, nephrotoxicity
Drug classifications
Aminoglycosides: ↑ Ototoxicity, neurotoxicity, nephrotoxicity
Anesthetics: ↑ Neuromuscular blockade, respiratory depression
Nondepolarizing neuromuscular blockers: ↑ Neuromuscular blockade, respiratory depression
Penicillins: Inactivated in renal disease

NURSING CONSIDERATIONS
Assessment
• Assess patient for previous sensitivity reaction
• Assess patient for signs and symptoms of infection including characteristics of sputum, urine, stool WBC >10,000, temp
• Obtain baseline information before and during treatment
• Complete C&S testing before and beginning drug therapy—this will identify if correct treatment has been initiated
• Assess for allergic reactions: rash, urticaria, pruritus, chills, fever, joint pain; angioedema may occur a few days after therapy begins—epinephrine, resuscitation equipment should be on unit for anaphylactic reaction
• Identify urine output; if decreasing, notify prescriber (may indicate nephrotoxicity); also, increased BUN, creatinine, urine CrCl <80 ml/min
• Monitor blood studies: AST, ALT, CBC, Hct, bilirubin, LDH, alk phosphatase, Coombs' test monthly if patient is on long-term therapy
• Monitor electrolytes: potas-

sium, sodium, chloride, magnesium monthly if patient is on long-term therapy

• Monitor for bleeding: ecchymosis, bleeding gums, hematuria, stool guaiac daily if on long-term therapy

• Assess for overgrowth of infection: perineal itching, fever, malaise, redness, pain, swelling, drainage, rash, diarrhea, change in cough, sputum

• Obtain weight before treatment; calculation of dosage is usually based on ideal body weight, but may be calculated on actual body weight

• Monitor I&O ratio; urinalysis daily for proteinuria, cells, casts; report sudden change in urine output

• Obtain serum peak 60 min after IM inj, trough level drawn just before next dose; blood level should be 2-4 times bacteriostatic level

• Monitor for deafness by audiometric testing, ringing, roaring in ears, vertigo; assess hearing before, during, after treatment

• Monitor for dehydration: high sp gr, decrease in skin turgor, dry mucous membranes, dark urine

• Monitor for overgrowth of infection including increased temp, malaise, redness, pain, swelling, perineal itching, diarrhea, stomatitis, change in cough, sputum

Nursing diagnoses

☑ Infection, risk for (uses)
☑ Diarrhea (adverse reactions)
☑ Injury, risk for (adverse reactions)
☑ Knowledge deficit (teaching)
☑ Noncompliance (teaching)

Implementation

• Give deeply in large muscle mass

• Reconstitute with 4.2-4.5 ml sterile water for inj or 0.9% NaCl/1 g (200 mg/ml); 3.2-3.5 ml/1 g (250 mg/ml); 17 ml/5 g (250 mg/ml) (500 mg/ml); give at 500 mg/ml or less

Syringe compatibilities:
Penicillin G sodium

Syringe incompatibilities:
Heparin

Y-site compatibilities:
Esmolol

Additive compatibilities:
Bleomycin

Patient/family education

• Teach patient to report sore throat, bruising, bleeding, joint pain, (may indicate blood dyscrasias—rare), ringing, roaring in the ears

• Advise patient to contact prescriber if vaginal itching, loose, foul-smelling stools, furry tongue occur—may indicate superimposed infection

Evaluation

Positive therapeutic outcome

• Absence of signs/symptoms of infection

• Reported improvement in symptoms of infection

Treatment of overdose:
Withdraw drug, hemodialysis, monitor serum levels of drug, may give ticarcillin or carbenicillin

S

streptozocin (℞)
(strep-toe-zoe′sin)
Zanosar
Func. class.: Antineoplastic
alkylating agent
Chem. class.: Nitrosourea
Pregnancy category   C

Action: Alkylates DNA, RNA;
inhibits enzymes that allow
synthesis of amino acids in
proteins; is also responsible for
cross-linking DNA strands;
activity is not specific to phase
of cell cycle

▶ **Therapeutic Outcome:** Prevention of rapidly growing
malignant cells, decreased
calcium levels

Uses: Metastatic islet cell
carcinoma of pancreas

Investigational uses: Prevention of spread of Hodgkin's
disease, metastatic carcinoid
tumor, pancreatic adenocarcinoma colon malignancies

Dosage and routes
Adult: **IV** 500 mg/m² × 5
days q6 wk until desired
response; or 1 g/m² qwk × 2
wk, not to exceed 1.5 g/m² in
1 dose

Available forms: Powder for
inj 1 g

Adverse effects
CNS: Confusion, depression,
lethargy
*GI: Nausea, vomiting, diar-
rhea, weight loss,* **hepatotoxicity**
GU: **Nephrogenic diabetes
insipidus**
HEMA: **Thrombocytopenia,
leukopenia, pancytopenia**

Contraindications: Hypersensitivity

Precautions: Radiation ther-
Ⓟ apy, children, lactation, pregnancy **C,** hepatic disease, renal
disease

Pharmacokinetics	
Absorption	Complete bioavail-ability
Distribution	Rapid, crosses placenta
Metabolism	Liver, kidneys—exten-sively
Excretion	<20% kidneys un-changed
Half-life	35-40 min

Pharmacodynamics	
Onset	Unknown
Peak	Unknown
Duration	Unknown

Interactions
Individual drugs
Doxorubicin: ↑ toxicity
Phenytoin: ↑ toxicity
Radiation: ↑ toxicity, bone
marrow suppression
Drug classifications
Aminoglycosides: ↑ risk of
nephrotoxicity
Antineoplastics: ↑ toxicity,
bone marrow suppression
Live virus vaccines: ↓ anti-
body response

NURSING CONSIDERATIONS
Assessment
• Assess symptoms indicating
severe allergic reaction: rash,
pruritus, urticaria, purpuric
skin lesions, itching, flushing
• Monitor CBC, differential,
platelet count weekly; withhold
drug if WBC count is <4000/
mm³ or platelet count is
<100,000/mm³; notify pre-
scriber of results if WBC
<20,000/mm³, platelets
<50,800/mm³
• Monitor renal function
studies: BUN, creatinine,
serum uric acid, urine CrCl

---

before and during therapy; I&O ratio; report fall in urine output to <30 ml/hr

• Monitor temp q4hr (may indicate beginning of infection)

• Monitor liver function tests before and during therapy [bilirubin, AST, ALT, LDH] as needed or monthly; yellowing of skin, sclera, dark urine, clay-colored stools, itchy skin, abdominal pain, fever, diarrhea

• Assess for bleeding: hematuria, stool guaiac, bruising or petechiae, mucosa or orifices q8hr; inflammation of mucosa, breaks in skin

• Identify edema in feet, joint pain, stomach pain, shaking; health care prescriber should be notified

• Identify inflammation of mucosa, breaks in skin

Nursing diagnoses

✓Injury, risk for (adverse reactions)

✓Body image disturbance (adverse reactions)

✓Infection, risk for (adverse reactions)

✓Knowledge deficit (teaching)

Implementation

• Hypoglycemia may occur, have **IV** dextrose available

• Give fluids **IV** or PO before chemotherapy to hydrate patient

• Give antiemetic 30-60 min before giving drug to prevent vomiting, and prn

• Give antibiotics for prophylaxis of infection

• Give topical or systemic analgesics for pain

• Provide liq diet: carbonated beverages; gelatin may be added if patient is not nauseated or vomiting

• Provide rinsing of mouth

tid-qid with water, club soda; brushing of teeth bid-qid with soft brush or cotton-tipped applicators for stomatitis; use unwaxed dental floss

• Give **IV** after diluting 1 g/9.5 ml 0.9% NaCl or D_5 (100 mg/ml)

• May be further diluted with 10-200 ml 0.9% NaCl, D_5W give over prescribed rate, usually 15 min

Y-*site compatibilities:*

Filgrastim, melphalan, ondansetron, teniposide, vinorelbine

Patient/family education

• Inform patient that contraceptive measures are recommended during therapy

• Caution patient to avoid use of products containing aspirin or ibuprofen, razors, commercial mouthwash—bleeding may occur; to report symptoms of bleeding (hematuria, tarry stools)

• Instruct patient to report signs of anemia, (fatigue, headache, irritability, faintness, shortness of breath)

• Caution patient not to have any vaccinations without the advice of the prescriber, serious reactions can occur

Evaluation

Positive therapeutic outcome

• Prevention of rapid division of malignant cells

S

succimer (R̲)
(sux'i-mer)
Chemet
Func. class: Heavy metal
antagonist
Chem. class.: Chelating
agent
Pregnancy category C

Action: Binds with ions of lead
to form a water-soluble complex that is excreted by kidneys

➡ **Therapeutic Outcome:** Removal of lead from the body

P **Uses:** Lead poisoning in children with lead levels above 45
µg/dl; may be beneficial in
mercury, arsenic poisoning

Dosage and routes
P *Child:* PO 10 mg/kg or 350
mg/m² q8h × 5 days, then 10
mg/kg or 350 mg/m² q12h ×
2 wk; another course may be
required depending on lead
levels; allow 2 wk between
courses

Available forms: Cap 100 mg
Adverse effects
CNS: Drowsiness, dizziness,
paresthesia, sensorimotor
neuropathy
EENT: Otitis media, watery
eyes, film in eyes, plugged ears
*GI: Nausea, vomiting, diar-
rhea, metallic taste, anorexia*
GU: Proteinuria, decreased
urination, voiding difficulties
*HEMA: Increased platelets,
intermittent eosinophilia*
INTEG: Rash, urticaria, pruritus
META: Increased AST, ALT,
alk phosphatase, cholesterol
RESP: Sore throat, rhinorrhea,
nasal congestion, cough
SYST: Back, stomach, head,
rib, flank pain; abdominal

cramps; chills; fever; flulike
symptoms, head cold; headache

Contraindications: Hypersensitivity

Precautions: Pregnancy **C**,
P lactation, children <1 yr

Pharmacokinetics	
Absorption	Rapidly absorbed
Distribution	Unknown
Metabolism	Liver—extensively
Excretion	Kidneys—unchanged
Half-life	2 days

Pharmacodynamics	
Onset	Up to 2 hr
Peak	2-4 hr
Duration	8-12 hr

Interactions
Drug classifications
**Heavy metal antagonist,
others:** Do not use together

NURSING CONSIDERATIONS
Assessment
• Assess VS, B/P, pulse, respirations, weigh daily
• Monitor I&O, kidney function studies, BUN, creatinine,
CrCl; watch for decreasing
urine output
• Assess neuro status: watch
for paresthesias, beginning
convulsions
• Monitor urine: pH, albumin,
casts, blood, coproporphyrins,
calcium
• Assess for febrile reactions
that may occur 4-8 hr following drug therapy
• Monitor for cardiac abnormalities: dysrhythmias, hypotension, tachycardia
• Assess for allergic reactions
(rash, urticaria); if these occur,
drug should be discontinued

Nursing diagnoses

☑ Poisoning, risk for (uses)
☑ Injury, risk for (uses, adverse reactions)
☑ Knowledge deficit (teaching)

Implementation

• Give PO whole or cap contents mixed with food or fluid

Patient/family education

• Explain reason for medication and expected results
• Provide a referral to health department to assess lead levels in home or workplace

Evaluation

Positive therapeutic outcome

• Decreased symptoms of lead intoxication
• Decreased lead level <50 µg/dl

---

succinylcholine (℞)

(suk-sin-ill-koe'leen)
Anectine, Anectine Flo-Pack, Quelicin, succinylcholine chloride, Sucostrin, Suxamethonium
Func. class.: Neuromuscular blocker (depolarizing—ultra short)

Pregnancy category   C

Action: Inhibits transmission of nerve impulses by binding with cholinergic receptor sites, antagonizing action of acetylcholine; causes release of histamine

➡ **Therapeutic Outcome:** Paralysis of skeletal muscles

Uses: Facilitation of endotracheal intubation, skeletal muscle relaxation during orthopedic manipulations

Dosage and routes

Adult: **IV** 0.6 mg/kg, then 2.5 mg/min as needed; IM 2.5 mg/kg, not to exceed 150 mg

P *Child:* **IV**/IM 1-2 mg/kg, not to exceed 150 mg IM

Available forms: Inj 20, 50, 100 mg/ml; powder for inj 100/vial; powder for inf 500 mg/vial, 1 g/vial

Adverse effects

CV: Bradycardia, tachycardia; increased, decreased B/P, **sinus arrest, dysrhythmias**
EENT: Increased secretions, increased IOP
HEMA: Myoglobulinemia
INTEG: Rash, flushing, pruritus, urticaria
MS: Weakness, muscle pain, fasciculation, prolonged relaxation
RESP: **Prolonged apnea, bronchospasm, cyanosis, respiratory depression**

Contraindications: Hypersensitivity, malignant hyperthermia, decreased plasma pseudocholinesterase, penetrating eye injuries, acute narrow-angle glaucoma

Precautions: Pregnancy **C**, cardiac disease, severe burns, fractures—fasciculation may increase damage—lactation,
P children <2 yr, electrolyte imbalances, dehydration, neuromuscular disease, respiratory disease, collagen diseases, glaucoma, eye surgery, pene-
G trating eye wounds, elderly or debilitated patients

S

Pharmacokinetics

Absorption	Well absorbed (IM)
Distribution	Widely distributed, crosses placenta
Metabolism	Plasma (90%)
Excretion	Hydrolyzed in urine (active/inactive metabolites)
Half-life	Unknown

Pharmacodynamics

	IV	IM
Onset	1 min	2-3 min
Peak	2-3 min	Unknown
Duration	6-10 min	10-30 min

Interactions
Individual drugs
Clindamycin: ↑ neuromuscular blockade
Enflurane: ↑ neuromuscular blockade
Isofluorophate: ↑ paralysis
Isoflurane: ↑ neuromuscular blockade
Lincomycin: ↑ neuromuscular blockade
Quinidine: ↑ neuromuscular blockade
Drug classifications
Aminoglycosides: ↑ neuromuscular blockade
β-Adrenergic blockers: ↑ neuromuscular blockade
Diuretics, potassium-losing: ↑ neuromuscular blockade
Local anesthetics: ↑ neuromuscular blockade
Magnesium salts: ↑ neuromuscular blockade
Polymyxin antibiotics: ↑ neuromuscular blockade

NURSING CONSIDERATIONS
Assessment
• Assess for electrolyte imbalances (potassium, magnesium); may lead to increased action of this drug
• Monitor vital signs (B/P, pulse, respirations, airway) until fully recovered; rate, depth, pattern of respirations, strength of hand grip
• Monitor I&O ratio; check for urinary retention, frequency, hesitancy
• Assess for recovery: decreased paralysis of face, diaphragm, leg, arm, rest of body
• Assess for allergic reactions: rash, fever, respiratory distress, pruritus; drug should be discontinued if these occur

Nursing diagnoses
☑ Communication, impaired verbal (adverse reactions)
☑ Breathing pattern, ineffective (uses)

Implementation
IV IV route
• Use nerve stimulator by anesthesiologist to determine neuromuscular blockade
• Give anticholinesterase to reverse neuromuscular blockade
• Give by **IV** inf; dilute 1-2 mg/ml in D_5, isotonic saline sol, give 0.5-10 mg/min, titrate to patient response; may be given directly over 1 min

Syringe compatibilities:
Heparin

Y-site compatibilities:
Etomidate, heparin, potassium chloride, propofol, vit B/C

Additive compatibilities:
Amikacin, cephapirin, isoproterenol, meperidine, methyldopate, morphine, norepinephrine, scopolamine

Additive incompatibilities:
Barbiturates, nafcillin, sodium bicarbonate
IM route
• Give deep IM, preferably high in deltoid muscle
• Store in refrigerator; store powder at room temp; close container tightly

---

Patient/family education
• Explain reason for medication and expected results
• Provide reassurance if communication is difficult during recovery from neuromuscular blockade; postoperative stiffness is normal, soon subsides

Evaluation
Positive therapeutic outcome
• Paralysis of jaw, eyelid, head, neck, rest of body

Treatment of overdose:
Edrophonium or neostigmine, atropine, monitor VS; may require mechanical ventilation

---

sucralfate (℞)
(soo-kral′fate)
Carafate, Sulcrate ♣
Func. class.: Protectant; antiulcer
Chem. class.: Aluminum hydroxide/sulfated sucrose

Pregnancy category   B

Action: Forms a complex that adheres to ulcer site, adsorbs pepsin

▷**Therapeutic Outcome:** Healing of ulcers

Uses: Duodenal ulcer, oral mucositis, stomatitis after radiation of head and neck

Investigational uses: Gastric ulcers, gastroesophageal reflux

Dosage and routes
Adult: PO 1 g qid 1 hr ac, hs
🄿 *Child:* PO 40-80 mg/kg/day

Available forms: Tab 1 g; oral susp 500 mg/5 ml ♣

Adverse effects
CNS: Drowsiness, dizziness
GI: Dry mouth, constipa-tion, nausea, gastric pain, vomiting
INTEG: Urticaria, rash, pruritus

Contraindications: Hypersensitivity

Precautions: Pregnancy **B**,
🄿 lactation, children, renal failure

◣**Do Not Confuse:**
Carafate/Cafergot

Pharmacokinetics	
Absorption	Minimally absorbed
Distribution	Unknown
Metabolism	Not metabolized
Excretion	Feces (90%)
Half-life	6-20 hr

Pharmacodynamics	
Onset	½ hr
Peak	Unknown
Duration	5 hr

Interactions
Individual drugs
Phenytoin: ↓ absorption
Tetracycline: ↓ absorption
Drug classifications
Antacids: ↓ absorption of sucralfate
Fat-soluble vitamins: ↓ absorption
Fluoroquinolones: ↓ absorption

NURSING CONSIDERATIONS
Assessment
• Monitor gastric pH (>5 should be maintained)

Nursing diagnoses
☑ Pain, chronic (uses)
☑ Pain (uses)
☑ Constipation (adverse reactions)
☑ Knowledge deficit (teaching)

Implementation
• Give on empty stomach 1 hr ac and hs
• Store at room temp

S

Patient/family education
• Advise patient to avoid black pepper, caffeine, alcohol, harsh spices, extremes in temp of food—may aggravate condition
• Instruct patient to take medication on empty stomach
• Caution patient to take full course of therapy
• Caution patient to avoid antacids within ½ hr of drug or 1 hr after this drug

Evaluation
Positive therapeutic outcome
• Absence of pain or GI complaints

---

sufentanil (℞)
(soo-fen′ta-nil)
Sufenta
Func. class.: Opiate analgesic

Pregnancy category C
Controlled substance schedule II

Action: Inhibits ascending pain pathways in CNS, increases pain threshold, alters pain perception

➡ **Therapeutic Outcome:** Anesthesia, decreased pain

Uses: Primary anesthetic, adjunct to general anesthetic

Dosage and routes
Primary anesthetic
Adult: **IV** 8-30 μg/kg given with 100% O_2, a muscle relaxant

Adjunct
Adult: **IV** 1-8 μg/kg given with nitrous oxide/O_2

Available forms: Inj 50 μg/ml

Adverse effects
CNS: Drowsiness, dizziness, confusion, headache, sedation, euphoria
CV: Palpitations, bradycardia, change in B/P
EENT: Tinnitus, blurred vision, miosis, diplopia
GI: Nausea, vomiting, anorexia, constipation, abdominal cramps
GU: Increased urinary output, dysuria, urinary retention
INTEG: Rash, urticaria, bruising, flushing, diaphoresis, pruritus
RESP: **Respiratory depression**

Contraindications: Hypersensitivity, addiction (opiate)

Precautions: Addictive personality, pregnancy **C**, lactation, increased intracranial pressure, MI (acute), severe heart disease, respiratory depression, hepatic disease, renal **P** disease, child <18 yr

Pharmacokinetics	
Absorption	Completely absorbed
Distribution	Crosses placenta
Metabolism	Liver—extensively, small intestines—small amount
Excretion	Kidneys, breast milk
Half-life	2½ hr

Pharmacodynamics	
Onset	1½-3 hr
Peak	Unknown
Duration	5 min

Interactions
Individual drugs
Alcohol: ↑ respiratory depression, hypotension, ↑ sedation
Cimetidine: ↑ recovery
Erythromycin: ↑ recovery
Nalbuphine: ↓ analgesia
Pentazocine: ↓ analgesia
Drug classifications
Antihistamines: ↑ respiratory depression, hypotension

CNS depressants: ↑ respiratory depression, hypotension
MAOIs: Do not use 2 wk before alfentanil
Phenothiazines: ↑ respiratory depression, hypotension
Sedative/hypnotics: ↑ respiratory depression, hypotension
⬚ *Herb/drug*
Kava: ↑ CNS depression
Lab test interferences
↑ Amylase

NURSING CONSIDERATIONS
Assessment
• Monitor VS after parenteral route; note muscle rigidity, drug history, liver, kidney function tests
• Monitor respiratory dysfunction: respiratory depression, character, rate, rhythm; notify prescriber if respirations are <10/min
• Monitor for CNS changes: dizziness, drowsiness, hallucinations, euphoria, LOC, pupil reaction
• Monitor allergic reactions: rash, urticaria

Nursing diagnoses
☑ Pain (uses)
☑ Sensory perceptual alteration: visual, auditory (adverse reactions)
☑ Breathing pattern, ineffective (adverse reactions)
☑ Knowledge deficit (teaching)

Implementation
• Give by inj (IM, **IV**), only with resuscitative equipment available; give slowly to prevent rigidity
• Give **IV** undiluted by anesthesiologist or diluted as an inf in 0.9% NaCl

Y site compatibilities:
Amphotericin B cholesteryl, cisatracurium, remifentanil

• Store in light-resistant area at room temp

Patient/family education
• Advise patient to report any symptoms of CNS changes, allergic reactions
• Caution patient to avoid CNS depressants: alcohol, sedative/hypnotics for at least 24 hr after this drug
• Discuss with patient that dizziness, drowsiness, and confusion are common, to avoid getting up without assistance
• Discuss in detail all aspects of the drug

Evaluation
Positive therapeutic outcome
• Maintenance of anesthesia
Treatment of overdose: Narcan 0.2-0.8 **IV**, O₂, **IV** fluids, vasopressors

---

sulfamethoxazole (℞)
(sul-fa-meth-ox′a-zole)
Apo-Sulfamethoxazole ✦,
Gantanol
Func. class.: Antiinfective
Chem. class.: Sulfonamide, intermediate-acting
Pregnancy category **B**

Action: Interferes with bacterial biosynthesis of proteins by competitive antagonism of PABA

➡ **Therapeutic Outcome:** Bactericidal action against susceptible organisms: Streptococci and staphylococci, *Clostridium perfringens, Clostridium tetani, Nocardia asteroides;* active against gram-negative pathogens, including *Enterobacter, Escherichia coli, Klebsiella,*

S

Proteus mirabilis, Proteus vulgaris, Salmonella, Shigella

Uses: UTIs, chancroid, inclusion conjunctivitis, malaria, meningococcal meningitis, nocardiosis, acute otitis media, toxoplasmosis, trachoma

Dosage and routes
Adult: PO 2 g, then 1 g bid or tid for 7-10 days

🅿 *Child >2 mo:* PO 50-60 mg/kg then 25-30 mg/kg × 1 dose bid, not to exceed 75 mg/kg/day

Lymphogranuloma venereum
Adult: PO 1 g bid × 14 days

Renal dose
CrCl <50 ml/min give 50% of dose

Available forms: Tab 500 mg

Adverse effects
CNS: Headache, insomnia, hallucinations, depression, vertigo, fatigue, anxiety, convulsions, drug fever, chills, drowsiness
CV: Allergic myocarditis
GI: Nausea, vomiting, abdominal pain, stomatitis, **hepatitis,** glossitis, **pancreatitis,** diarrhea, **enterocolitis,** anorexia
GU: Renal failure, toxic nephrosis, increased BUN, creatinine, crystalluria, hematuria, proteinuria
HEMA: Leukopenia, thrombocytopenia, agranulocytosis, hemolytic anemia, aplastic anemia
INTEG: Rash, dermatitis, urticaria, **Stevens-Johnson syndrome,** erythema, photosensitivity, alopecia
SYST: Anaphylaxis

Contraindications: Hypersensitivity to sulfonamides, sulfonylureas, thiazide and loop diuretics, salicylates, sunscreen 🅿 with PABA, lactation, infants <2 mo (except congenital toxoplasmosis), pregnancy at term, porphyria

Precautions: Pregnancy **B,** lactation, impaired hepatic/renal function, severe allergy, bronchial asthma

Pharmacokinetics	
Absorption	Well absorbed
Distribution	Widely distributed, crosses placenta
Metabolism	Liver, large amounts
Excretion	Unchanged kidneys (20%), enters breast milk
Half-life	7-12 hr

Pharmacodynamics	
Onset	1 hr
Peak	3-4 hr

Interactions
Individual drugs
Cyclosporine: ↑ nephrotoxicity
Indomethacin: ↑ drug-free concentrations
Methotrexate: ↑ toxicity
Phenytoin: ↑ folic acid deficiency
Probenecid: ↑ drug-free concentrations
Drug classifications
Anticoagulants, oral: ↑ effects of anticoagulant
Barbiturates: ↑ effects
Hypoglycemics, oral: ↑ effects of hypoglycemics
Salicylates: ↑ drug-free concentrations
Thiazide diuretics: ↑ thrombocytopenia
Uricosurics: ↑ effect
Lab test interferences
False positive: Urinary glucose test

☑ Herb/drug 🚫 Do Not Crush ◆ Alert ☾ Key Drug 🅖 Geriatric 🅿 Pediatric

NURSING CONSIDERATIONS
Assessment
- Assess patient for previous sensitivity reaction
- Assess patient for signs and symptoms of infection including characteristics of wounds, sputum, urine, stool, WBC >10,000, elevated temp; obtain baseline information before and during treatment
- Complete C & S studies before beginning drug therapy to identify if correct treatment has been initiated
- Assess for allergic reactions: rash, urticaria, pruritus, chills, fever, joint pain; angioedema may occur a few days after therapy begins; epinephrine, resuscitation equipment should be on unit for anaphylactic reaction—AIDS patients are more susceptible
- Monitor blood studies: CBC, Hct, bilirubin, alk phosphatase, monthly if patient is on long-term therapy
- Monitor for bleeding: ecchymosis, bleeding gums, hematuria, stool guaiac daily if patient is on long-term therapy
- Assess for overgrowth of infection: perineal itching, fever, malaise, redness, pain, swelling, drainage, rash, diarrhea, change in cough, sputum

Nursing diagnoses
- ✓ Infection, risk for (uses)
- ✓ Diarrhea (adverse reactions)
- ✓ Injury, risk for (adverse reactions)
- ✓ Knowledge deficit (teaching)
- ✓ Noncompliance (teaching)

Implementation
- Give around the clock to maintain proper blood levels; give on empty stomach to increase absorption of drug; do not give within 3 hr of other agents, drug actions may occur
- Give with 8 oz of water to prevent crystalluria

Patient/family education
- Teach patient to report sore throat, bruising, bleeding, joint pain—may indicate blood dyscrasias (rare)
- Advise patient to contact prescriber if vaginal itching, loose, foul-smelling stools, furry tongue occur—may indicate superinfection; report itching, rash, pruritus, urticaria
- Instruct patient to take all medication prescribed for the length of time ordered; drug must be taken around the clock to maintain blood levels; do not give medication to others

Evaluation
Positive therapeutic outcome
- Absence of signs/symptoms of infection (WBC <10,000, temp WNL, absence of urinary pain, hematuria)
- Reported improvement in symptoms of infection
- Negative C&S

---

sulfasalazine (℞)
(sul-fa-sal′a-zeen)
Azulfidine, Azulfidine EN-Tabs, PMS-Sulfasalazine ✦, S.A.S. ✦, Salazopyrin ✦, sulfasalazine
Func. class.: Antiinflammatory
Chem. class.: Sulfonamide
Pregnancy category   **C**

Action: Prodrug to deliver sulfapyridine and 5-aminosalicylic acid to colon; antinflammatory in connective tissue

S

➡️**Therapeutic Outcome:** Treatment of ulcerative colitis, rheumatoid arthritis

Uses: Ulcerative colitis, rheumatoid arthritis (delayed rel tab) in patients who inadequately respond to or are intolerant of analgesics/NSAIDs

Investigational uses: Ankylosing spondylitis, collagenous colitis, Crohn's disease, psoriasis

Dosage and routes
Adult: PO 3-4 g/day in divided doses; maintenance 1.5-2 g/day in divided doses q6h

🅿️ *Child >2 yr:* PO 40-60 mg/kg/day in 4-6 divided doses, then 20-30 mg/kg/day in 4 doses, max 2 g/day

Rheumatoid arthritis
Adult: PO 2 g/day in evenly divided doses, initiate treatment with a lower dose of enteric-coated tab

Renal dose
CrCl 10-30 ml/min give bid; CrCl <10 ml/min give qd

Available forms: Tab 500 mg

Adverse effects
CNS: Headache, confusion, insomnia, hallucinations, depression, vertigo, fatigue, anxiety, **convulsions,** drug fever, chills
CV: **Allergic myocarditis**
GI: *Nausea, vomiting, abdominal pain,* stomatitis, **hepatitis,** glossitis, **pancreatitis,** diarrhea, anorexia
GU: **Renal failure, toxic nephrosis,** increased BUN, creatinine, crystalluria

Contraindications: Hypersensitivity to sulfonamides or salicylates, pregnancy at term, 🅿️ child <2 yr, intestinal, urinary obstruction

Precautions: Pregnancy **C,** lactation, impaired hepatic function, severe allergy, bronchial asthma, impaired renal function

🔽 **Do Not Confuse:**
sulfasalazine/sulfisoxazole

Pharmacokinetics	
Absorption	Partially absorbed
Distribution	Crosses placenta
Metabolism	Liver
Excretion	Kidneys, breast milk
Half-life	6 hr

Pharmacodynamics	
Onset	1 hr
Peak	1½-6 hr
Duration	6-12 hr

Interactions
Individual drugs
Digoxin: ↓ effectiveness
Methotrexate: ↓ renal excretion
Phenytoin: ↓ hepatic clearance
Drug classifications
Anticoagulants, oral: ↑ toxicity
Hypoglycemics, oral: ↑ toxicity
Food/drug
Iron, folic acid will be poorly absorbed
Lab test interferences
False positive: Urinary glucose test

NURSING CONSIDERATIONS
Assessment
• Monitor I&O ratio; note color, amount, character, pH of urine if drug administered for urinary tract infections; output should be 800 ml less than intake; if urine is highly acidic, alkalization may be needed
• Monitor kidney function studies: BUN, creatinine,

urinalysis if on long-term therapy
• Monitor blood dyscrasias: skin rash, fever, sore throat, bruising, bleeding, fatigue, joint pain; monitor CBC before and q3mo
• Assess for allergic reaction: rash, dermatitis, urticaria, pruritus, dyspnea, bronchospasm

Nursing diagnoses
☑ Injury, risk for (uses)
☑ Knowledge deficit (teaching)

Implementation
• Give with full glass of water to maintain adequate hydration; increase fluids to 2 L/day to decrease crystallization in kidneys; contact lens, urine, skin may be yellow-orange
• Give total daily dose in evenly spaced doses and after meals to help minimize GI intolerance
• Store in tight, light-resistant container at room temp

Patient/family education
• Advise patient to take each oral dose with full glass of H₂O to prevent crystalluria
• Teach patient to avoid sunlight or to use sunscreen to prevent burns
• Teach patient to avoid OTC medication (aspirin, vit C) unless directed by prescriber
• Advise patient to notify prescriber if skin rash, sore throat, fever, mouth sores, unusual bruising, bleeding occur
• Advise patient to use rectal susp at hs and retain all night

Evaluation
Positive therapeutic outcome
• Absence of fever, mucus in stools or pain in joints

---

sulfinpyrazone (℞)
(sul-fin-peer′a-zone)
Anturane, sulfinpyrazone
Func. class.: Uricosuric
Chem. class.: Pyrazolone
Pregnancy category   C

Action: Inhibits tubular reabsorption of urates, with increased excretion of uric acid; inhibits prostaglandin synthesis, which decreases platelet aggregation

➔ **Therapeutic Outcome:** Decreased uric acid levels, absence of platelet aggregation

Uses: Inhibition of platelet aggregation, gout

Dosage and routes
Inhibition of platelet aggregation
Adult: PO 200 mg qid

Gout/gouty arthritis
Adult: PO 100-200 mg bid × 1 wk, then 200-400 mg bid, not to exceed 800 mg/day

Available forms: Tab 100 mg; cap 200 mg

Adverse effects
CNS: Dizziness, **convulsions, coma**
EENT: Tinnitus
GI: Gastric irritation, nausea, vomiting, anorexia, **hepatic necrosis,** GI bleeding
GU: Renal calculi, hypoglycemia
HEMA: **Agranulocytosis** (rare)
INTEG: Rash, dermatitis, pruritus, fever, photosensitivity
RESP: **Apnea,** irregular respirations

Contraindications: Hypersensitivity to pyrazolone derivatives, blood dyscrasias, CrCl

S

<50 ml/min, active peptic ulcer, GI inflammation

Precautions: Pregnancy **C**

Pharmacokinetics

Absorption	Well absorbed
Distribution	Unknown
Metabolism	Liver
Excretion	Feces (metabolites/active drug)
Half-life	4 hr

Pharmacodynamics

Onset	Unknown
Peak	1-2 hr
Duration	4-6 hr

Interactions
Individual drugs:

Acetaminophen: ↑ toxicity
Aspirin: ↑ risk of bleeding
Cefamandole: ↑ risk of bleeding
Cefoperazone: ↑ risk of bleeding
Cefotetan: ↑ risk of bleeding
Niacin: ↓ effect of sulfinpyrazone
Nitrofurantoin: ↑ effect of sulfinpyrazone
Plicamycin: ↑ risk of bleeding
Theophylline: ↓ effect of sulfinpyrazone
Tolbutamide: ↑ effect of tolbutamide
Warfarin: ↑ effect of warfarin
Valproic acid: ↑ risk of bleeding
Verapamil: ↓ effect of sulfinpyrazone

Drug classifications

Anticoagulants: ↑ risk of bleeding
Antiinflammatories: ↑ risk of bleeding
Salicylates: ↓ effect of sulfinpyrazone
Thrombolytics: ↑ risk of bleeding

Lab test interferences
↑ Alk phosphatase, ↑ AST/ALT
False positive: RBC, Hgb

NURSING CONSIDERATIONS
Assessment
• Monitor I&O ratio; observe for decrease in urinary output; increase fluids to 2-3 L/day
• Monitor CBC, platelets, reticulocytes before, during therapy (q3mo)
• Assess mobility, joint pain, and swelling in the joints

Nursing diagnoses
☑ Pain, chronic (uses)
☑ Immobility, impaired physical (uses)
☑ Knowledge deficit (teaching)

Implementation
• Give with food or antacid to decrease GI upset
• Reduce dose gradually if uric acid levels are normal after 6 mo

Patient/family education
• Advise patient to increase fluids to 3-4 L/day
• Caution patient to avoid alcohol, OTC preparations that contain alcohol—skin rashes may occur
• Advise patient to report any pain, redness, or hard area, usually in legs
• Instruct patient on importance of complying with medical regimen; bone marrow depression may occur

Evaluation
Positive therapeutic outcome
• Decreased pain in joints
• Normal serum uric acid levels
• Increased duration of antiinfectives

☑ Herb/drug 🚫 Do Not Crush ◆ Alert ☛ Key Drug **G** Geriatric **P** Pediatric

sulfisoxazole (R)
(sul-fi-sox′a-zole)
Gantrisin, Novosoxazole ✦,
sulfisoxazole
Func. class.: Antiinfective
Chem. class.: Sulfonamide,
short-acting
Pregnancy category **B**

Action: Interferes with bacterial biosynthesis of proteins by competitive antagonism of PABA

⇒**Therapeutic Outcome:** Bactericidal action against susceptible organisms; gram-positive pathogens, including *Streptococci* and *Staphylococci, Clostridium perfringens, Clostridium tetani, Nocardia asteroides;* active against gram-negative pathogens, including *Enterobacter, Escherichia coli, Klebsiella, Proteus mirabilis, Proteus vulgaris, Salmonella, Shigella*

Uses: Urinary tract; chancroid; trachoma; toxoplasmosis; acute otitis media; malaria, *H. influenzae,* meningitis, meningococcal meningitis, nocardiosis

Dosage and routes
Renal dose
CrCl 10-50 ml/min give q8-12h; CrCl <10 ml/min give q12-24h

Adult: PO 2-4 g loading dose, then 1-2 g qid × 7-10 days

P *Child >2 mo:* PO 75 mg/kg or 2 g/m^2 loading dose, then 120-150 mg/kg/day or 4 g/m^2/day in divided doses q6h, not to exceed 6 g/day

Available forms: Tab 500 mg

Adverse effects
CNS: Headache, insomnia, hallucinations, depression, vertigo, fatigue, anxiety, **convulsions,** drug fever, chills, drowsiness
CV: **Allergic myocarditis**
GI: *Nausea, vomiting, abdominal pain,* stomatitis, **hepatitis,** glossitis, pancreatitis, diarrhea, **enterocolitis,** anorexia
GU: **Renal failure, toxic nephrosis,** increased BUN, creatinine, crystalluria, hematuria, proteinuria
HEMA: **Leukopenia, thrombocytopenia, agranulocytosis, hemolytic anemia, aplastic anemia**
INTEG: Rash, dermatitis, urticaria, **Stevens-Johnson syndrome,** erythema, photosensitivity, alopecia
SYST: **Anaphylaxis**

Contraindications: Hypersensitivity to sulfonamides and sulfonylureas, thiazide and loop diuretics, salicylates; sunscreen with PABA,
P lactation, infants <2 mo (except congenital toxoplasmosis); pregnancy at term, porphyria

Precautions: Pregnancy **B,** lactation, impaired hepatic/renal function, severe allergy, bronchial asthma

◨ Do Not Confuse:
sulfisoxazole/sulfasalazine

S

Pharmacokinetics	
Absorption	Well absorbed
Distribution	Widely distributed, crosses placenta
Metabolism	Liver, mostly
Excretion	Breast milk
Half-life	4-7 hr

Pharmacodynamics	
Onset	Unknown
Peak	2-4 hr

Interactions
Individual drugs
Cyclosporine: ↑ nephrotoxicity
Indomethacin: ↑ drug-free concentrations
Methotrexate: ↑ toxicity
Phenytoin: ↑ folic acid deficiency
Probenecid: ↑ drug-free concentrations
Drug classifications
Anticoagulants, oral: ↑ effects of anticoagulant
Barbiturates: ↑ effects of barbiturates
Hypoglycemics, oral: ↑ effects of hypoglycemics
Salicylates: ↑ drug-free concentrations
Thiazide diuretics: ↑ thrombocytopenia
Uricosurics: ↑ effects of uricosurics
Lab test interferences
False positive: Urinary glucose test

NURSING CONSIDERATIONS
Assessment
• Assess patient for previous sensitivity reaction
• Assess patient for signs and symptoms of infection including characteristics of wounds, sputum, urine, stool, WBC >10,000, temp; obtain baseline information before and during treatment
• Complete C&S testing before beginning drug therapy to identify if correct treatment has been initiated
• Assess for allergic reactions: rash, urticaria, pruritus, chills, fever, joint pain; angioedema may occur a few days after therapy begins; epinephrine, resuscitation equipment should be on unit for anaphylactic reaction

• Monitor blood studies: CBC, Hct, bilirubin, alk phosphatase monthly if patient is on long-term therapy
• Monitor for bleeding: ecchymosis, bleeding gums, hematuria, stool guaiac daily if on long-term therapy
• Assess for overgrowth of infection: perineal itching, fever, malaise, redness, pain, swelling, drainage, rash, diarrhea, change in cough, sputum

Nursing diagnoses
☑ Infection, risk for (uses)
☑ Diarrhea (adverse reactions)
☑ Injury, risk for (adverse reactions)
☑ Knowledge deficit (teaching)
☑ Noncompliance (teaching)

Implementation
• Give around the clock to maintain proper blood levels; give on an empty stomach to increase absorption of drug; do not give within 3 hr of other agents—drug interactions may occur
• Give with 8 oz of water

Patient/family education
• Teach patient to report sore throat, bruising, bleeding, joint pain—may indicate blood dyscrasias (rare)
• Advise patient to contact prescriber if vaginal itching; loose, foul-smelling stools; or furry tongue occur—may indicate superinfection; report itching, rash, pruritus, urticaria
• Instruct patient to take all medication prescribed for the length of time ordered; drug must be taken around the clock to maintain blood levels; medication should not be shared with others

---

☑ Herb/drug   Ⓢ Do Not Crush   ◆ Alert   ☯ Key Drug   Ⓖ Geriatric   Ⓟ Pediatric

Evaluation
Positive therapeutic outcome
- Absence of signs/symptoms of infection (WBC <10,000, temp WNL, absence of urinary pain, hematuria)
- Reported improvement in symptoms of infection
- Negative C&S

---

sulindac (℞)
(sul-in'dak)
Apo-Sulin ✲, Clinoril, Novosundac ✲, sulindac
Func. class.: Nonsteroidal antiinflammatory
Chem. class.: Indeneacetic acid derivative
Pregnancy category C

Action: Inhibits prostaglandin synthesis by decreasing an enzyme needed for biosynthesis; analgesic, antiinflammatory, antipyretic

➔**Therapeutic Outcome:** Decreased pain, inflammation

Uses: Mild to moderate pain, osteoarthritis, rheumatoid, gouty arthritis, ankylosing spondylitis

Dosage and routes
Arthritis
Adult: PO 150 mg bid, may increase to 200 mg bid
Bursitis/acute arthritis
Adult: PO 200 mg bid × 1-2 wk, then reduce dose

Available forms: Tabs 150, 200 mg

Adverse effects
CNS: Dizziness, drowsiness, fatigue, tremors, confusion, insomnia, anxiety, depression, *headache*
CV: Tachycardia, peripheral edema, palpitations, dysrhythmias
EENT: Tinnitus, hearing loss, blurred vision
GI: Nausea, anorexia, vomiting, diarrhea, jaundice, **cholestatic hepatitis,** constipation, flatulence, cramps, dry mouth, peptic ulcer, **bleeding, ulceration, perforation**
GU: **Nephrotoxicity: dysuria, hematuria, oliguria, azotemia**
HEMA: **Blood dyscrasias with prolonged use**
INTEG: Purpura, *rash, pruritus,* sweating, photosensitivity

Contraindications: Hypersensitivity, asthma, severe renal disease, severe hepatic disease, active ulcers

Precautions: Pregnancy C, lactation, children, bleeding disorders, GI disorders, cardiac, renal disorders, hypersensitivity to other antiinflammatory agents

Do Not Confuse:
Clinoril/Clozaril, Clinoril/Oruvail

Pharmacokinetics	
Absorption	Well absorbed
Distribution	Not known
Metabolism	Converted to active drug—liver
Excretion	Minimal unchanged kidneys, breast milk
Half-life	7.8 hr; 16.4-hr active metabolite

Pharmacodynamics	
Onset	Unknown
Peak	2 hr
Duration	Unknown

Interactions
Individual drugs
Acetaminophen (long-term use): ↑ renal reactions
Alcohol: ↑ adverse reactions

S

Aspirin: ↓ effectiveness, ↑ adverse reactions
Cyclosporine: ↑ nephrotoxicity
Diflunisal: ↓ sulindac effect
Digoxin: ↑ toxicity, ↑ levels
Insulin: ↓ insulin effect
Lithium: ↑ toxicity
Methotrexate: ↑ toxicity
Phenytoin: ↑ toxicity
Probenecid: ↑ toxicity
Radiation: ↑ risk of hematologic toxicity
Sulfonylurea: ↑ toxicity
Drug classifications
Anticoagulants: ↑ risk of bleeding
Antihypertensives: ↓ effect of antihypertensives
Antineoplastics: ↑ risk of hematologic toxicity
β-Adrenergic blockers: ↑ antihypertension
Cephalosporins: ↑ risk of bleeding
Diuretics: ↓ effectiveness of diuretics
Glucocorticoids: ↑ adverse reactions
Hypoglycemics: ↓ hypoglycemic effect
NSAIDs: ↑ adverse reactions
Potassium supplements: ↑ adverse reactions
Sulfonamides: ↑ toxicity
Lab test interferences
↑ Liver function studies, ↑ serum potassium, ↑ glucose, ↑ alk phosphatase

NURSING CONSIDERATIONS
Assessment

• Monitor blood counts during therapy; watch for decreasing platelets; if low, therapy may need to be discontinued, restarted after hematologic recovery; and for blood dyscrasia (thrombocytopenia): bruising, fatigue, bleeding, poor healing

• Assess pain: frequency, intensity, characteristics, relief 1-2 hr after medication
• Assess for asthma, aspirin hypersensitivity, nasal polyps; hypersensitivity may develop

Nursing diagnoses
☑ Pain (uses)
☑ Mobility, impaired physical (uses)
☑ Knowledge deficit (teaching)
☑ Injury, risk for (adverse reactions)

Implementation
• Administer with food or milk to decrease gastric symptoms—food slows absorption slightly, does not decrease absorption

Patient/family education
• Advise patient that drug must be continued for prescribed time to be effective; to avoid aspirin, alcoholic beverages
• Caution patient to report bleeding, bruising, fatigue, malaise because blood dyscrasias do occur
• Instruct patient to use caution when driving; drowsiness, dizziness may occur
• Teach patient to take with a full glass of water to enhance
◎ absorption; do not crush, break or chew

Evaluation
Positive therapeutic outcome
• Decreased pain
• Decreased inflammation
• Increased mobility

---

sumatriptan (R)
(soo-ma-trip′tan)
Imitrex
Func. class.: Migraine agent
Chem. class.: 5HT–1 receptor agonist
Pregnancy category C

Action: Binds selectively to the vascular 5-HT-1 receptor subtype and exerts antimigraine effect; causes vasoconstriction in cranial arteries

➤**Therapeutic Outcome:** Absence of migraines

Uses: Acute treatment of migraine with or without aura and cluster headache

Dosage and routes
Adult: SC 6 mg or less; may repeat in 1 hr; not to exceed 12 mg/24 hr; PO 25 mg with fluids, max 100 mg; nasal: 1 dose of 5, 10 or 20 mg in one nostril, may repeat in 2 hrs, max 40 mg/24 hr

Available forms: Inj 6 mg (12 mg/ml); tabs 25, 50 mg; nasal spray 5 mg/100 mcl-U dose spray device 20 mg/100 mcl-U

Adverse effects
CV: Flushing
EENT: Throat, mouth, nasal discomfort, vision changes
GI: Abdominal discomfort
INTEG: Injection site reaction, sweating
MS: Weakness, neck stiffness, myalgia
NEURO: Tingling, hot sensation, burning, feeling of pressure, tightness, numbness, dizziness, sedation, headache, anxiety, fatigue
RESP: Chest tightness, pressure

Contraindications: Angina pectoris, history of MI, documented silent ischemia, Prinzmetal's angina, ischemic heart disease, **IV** use, concurrent ergotamine-containing preparations, uncontrolled hypertension, hypersensitivity, basilar or hemiplegic migraine

Precautions: Postmenopausal women, men >40 yr, risk factors for CAD, hypercholesterolemia, obesity, diabetes, impaired hepatic or renal
P function, pregnancy **C,** lacta-
G tion, children, elderly

Pharmacokinetics	
Absorption	Well absorbed (SC)
Distribution	10%-20% plasma protein binding
Metabolism	Liver (metabolite)
Excretion	Urine, feces
Half-life	2 hr

Pharmacodynamics	
	SC
Onset	10-20 min
Peak	10 min-2 hr
Duration	Up to 24 hr (pain relief)

Interactions
Individual drugs
Ergotamine: ↑ risk of vasospastic reaction
Drug classifications
MAOIs: ↑ sumatriptan levels

NURSING CONSIDERATIONS
Assessment
• Assess for tingling, hot sensation, burning, feeling of pressure, numbness, flushing, infection site reaction
• Assess B/P; signs/symptoms of coronary vasospasm
• Monitor stress level, activity, reaction, coping mechanisms of patient
• Assess neurologic status: LOC, blurring vision, nausea,

S

vomiting, tingling in extremities preceding headache
• Assess for ingestion of tyramine-containing foods (pickled products, beer, wine, aged cheese), food additives, preservatives, colorings, artificial sweeteners, chocolate, caffeine, which may precipitate these types of headaches

Nursing diagnoses
☑ Pain (uses)
☑ Knowledge deficit (teaching)

Implementation
PO route
• Swallow whole
SC route
• Give by SC route only, avoid IM or **IV** administration

Patient/family education
• Teach patient to use the self-dosing system as soon as pain begins, do not use before a migraine is beginning, may repeat dose if migraine returns
• Caution patient not to take more than 2 dose/day or 12 mg/day; allow at least 1 hr between doses
• Caution patient to avoid driving or hazardous activities if dizziness or drowsiness occurs
• Teach patient to report chest tightness, heat, flushing, drowsiness, dizziness, fatigue, or any allergic reactions that occur
• Inform patient to report any side effects to prescriber
• Caution patient to use contraception when taking drug, to notify prescriber if pregnancy is suspected or planned

Nasal spray
• Teach patient to spray once in 1 nostril, may repeat if headache returns, do not repeat if pain continues after 1st dose

Evaluation
Positive therapeutic outcome
• Decrease in frequency, severity of headache

tacrine (℞)
(tack'rin)
Cognex
Func. class.: Reversible cholinesterase
Pregnancy category   C

Action: Elevates acetylcholine concentrations (cerebral cortex) by slowing degrading of acetylcholine released in cholinergic neurons; does not alter underlying dementia

▶**Therapeutic Outcome:** Improvement in symptoms of dementia in Alzheimer's disease

Uses: Treatment of mild to moderate dementia in Alzheimer's disease

Dosage and routes
Adult: PO 10 mg qid × 6 wk, then 20 mg qid × 6 wk, increase at 6-wk intervals if patient tolerates drug well and if transaminase is within normal limits

Available forms: Caps 10, 20, 30, 40 mg

Adverse effects
CNS: Dizziness, confusion, insomnia, tremor, *ataxia, somnolence, anxiety, agitation, depression, hallucinations, hostility, abnormal thinking,* chills, fever
CV: Hypotension or hypertension
GI: Nausea, vomiting, anorexia, abdominal pain, constipation, dyspepsia, flatulence

GU: Frequency, UTI, incontinence
INTEG: Rash, flushing
RESP: Rhinitis, URI, cough, pharyngitis

Contraindications: Hypersensitivity to this drug or acridine derivatives, patients treated with this drug who developed jaundice with a total bilirubin of >3 mg/dL

Precautions: Sick sinus syndrome, history of ulcers, GI bleeding, hepatic disease, bladder obstruction, asthma, pregnancy **C**, lactation, **P** children, seizure disorder

◣ Do Not Confuse:
Cognex/Corgard

Pharmacokinetics	
Absorption	Rapidly absorbed, low
Distribution	55% plasma protein bound
Metabolism	Liver, extensively
Excretion	Unknown
Half-life	2-4 hr

Pharmacodynamics
Unknown

Interactions
Individual drugs
Bethanechol: ↑ effect
Cimetidine: ↑ tacrine level
Succinylcholine: ↑ effect
Theophylline: ↑ toxicity

NURSING CONSIDERATIONS
Assessment
• Monitor ALT qo wk × 4-16 wks, then q3mo; weekly ALT × 6 wks if dose is increased
• Monitor B/P for hypotension or hypertension
• Assess mental status: affect, mood, behavioral changes, depression, hallucinations, confusion; conduct suicide assessment
• Assess GI status: nausea, vomiting, anorexia, constipation, abdominal pain; add bulk and increase fluids for constipation
• Assess GU status: urinary frequency, incontinence

Nursing diagnoses
✓ Injury, risk for (uses)
✓ Thought processes, altered (uses)
✓ Knowledge deficit (teaching)

Implementation
• Give dosage adjusted to patient's response no more than q6wk
• Provide assistance with ambulation if needed during beginning therapy; dizziness, ataxia may occur
• Give between meals; if GI symptoms occur, may be given with meals

Patient/family education
• Advise patient to report side effects: twitching, eye spasms; may indicate overdose
• Instruct patient to use drug exactly as prescribed at regular intervals, preferably between meals; may be taken with meals for GI upset; drug is not a cure
• Advise patient to notify prescriber of nausea, vomiting, diarrhea (dose increased or beginning treatment) or rash, very dark or very light stools, jaundice (delayed onset)
• Caution patient not to increase or abruptly decrease dose; serious consequences may result

Evaluation
Positive therapeutic outcome
• Decrease in confusion, improved mood

T

Treatment of overdose:
Withdraw drug, administer
tertiary anticholinergics, provide supportive care

---

tacrolimus (℞)
(tak-roe′li-mus)
Prograf
Func. class.: Immunosup-
pressant
Chem. clas.: Macrolide
Pregnancy category   C

Action: Produces immunosuppression by inhibiting lymphocytes (T)

➡ **Therapeutic Outcome:** Prevention of rejection in organ
transplant

Uses: Organ transplants— to
prevent rejection

Dosage and routes
🅿 *Adult and child:* **IV** 0.03-0.05
mg/kg/day × 3 days then PO
0.15 mg/kg bid; adjust dose in
renal impairment

Available forms: Inj **IV**

Adverse effects
CNS: Tremors, headache, insomnia, paresthesia, anxiety,
hyperesthesia, numbness,
dizziness, fatigue
CV: Hypertension
EENT: Blurred vision, photophobia
GI: Nausea, vomiting, diarrhea, *oral Candida, gum hyperplasia,* **hepatotoxicity,** constipation
GU: Urinary tract infections,
**albuminuria, hematuria,
proteinuria, renal failure**
HEMA: Anemia, **leukocytosis,
thrombocytopenia purpura**
INTEG: Rash, flushing, itching, alopecia
META: Hirsutism, hypergly-

cemia, hyperkalemia, hyperuricemia, hypokalemia, hypomagnesemia
RESP: Pleural effusion, atelectasis, dyspnea

Contraindications: Hypersensitivity

Precautions: Severe renal
disease, severe hepatic disease,
pregnancy **C**, diabetes mellitus,
hyperkalemia, hyperuricemia

Pharmacokinetics	
Absorption	Erractically absorbed (PO), completely absorbed (**IV**)
Distribution	Crosses placenta, 75% protein binding
Metabolism	Liver to metabolite
Excretion	Kidney—minimal, breast milk, bile
Half-life	10 hr

Pharmacodynamics		
	PO	IV
Onset	Unknown	Unknown
Peak	1-4 hr	Unknown
Duration	12 hr	12 hr

Interactions
Individual drugs
Cyclosporine: ↑ nephrotoxi-
city, do not use together
Danazol: ↑ toxicity
Erthromycin: ↑ toxicity
Ibuprofen: ↑ oliguria

NURSING CONSIDERATIONS
Assessment
• Monitor blood studies: Hgb,
WBC, platelets during treatment monthly; if leukocytes are
<3000/mm³, or platelets
<100,000/mm³, drug should
be discontinued or reduced;
decreased hemoglobulin level
may indicate bone marrow
suppression
• Monitor liver function
studies: alk phosphatase, AST,
ALT, amylase, bilirubin, and
for hepatotoxicity: dark urine,

jaundice, itching, light-colored stools; drug should be discontinued

Nursing diagnoses

☑ Infection, risk for (uses)

☑ Knowledge deficit (teaching)

Implementation

PO route

• Give all medications PO if possible; avoid IM inj because bleeding may occur

• Give with meals to reduce GI upset; nausea is common

• Give for several days before transplant surgery; patients should be placed in protective isolation

Ⅳ IV route

• Give after diluting in 0.9% NaCl or D$_5$W to a concentration of 0.004 mg/ml to 0.02 mg/ml as a continuous inf

Y-site compatibilities:

Acyclovir, aminophylline, amphotericin B, ampicillin, ampicillin/sulbactam, benztropine, calcium gluconate, cefazolin, cefotetan, ceftazidime, ceftriaxone, cefuroxime, chloramphenicol, cimetidine, ciprofloxacin, clindamycin, dexamethasone, digoxin, diphenhydramine, dobutamine, dopamine, doxycycline, erythromycin, esmolol, fluconazole, furosemide, ganciclovir, gentamicin, haloperidol, heparin, hydrocortisone, imipenem/cilastatin, regular insulin, isoproterenol, leucovorin, lorazepam, methylprednisolone, metoclopramide, metronidazole, mezlocillin, multivitamins, nitroglycerin, nitroprusside, oxacillin, penicillin C potassium, perphenazine, phenytoin, piperacillin, potassium chloride, propranolol, ranitidine, sodium bicarbonate, trimethoprim/sulfamethoxazole, vancomycin

Patient/family education

• Instruct patient to report fever, rash, severe diarrhea, chills, sore throat, fatigue because serious infections may occur; clay-colored stools, cramping may indicate hepatotoxicity

• Caution patient to avoid crowds or persons with known infections to reduce risk of infection

Evaluation

Positive therapeutic outcome

• Absence of graft rejection

• Immunosuppression in autoimmune disorders

---

tamoxifen (℞)

(ta-mox'i-fen)

Nolvadex, Nolvadex-D ✤, Novo-Tamoxifen ✤, Tamofen ✤, Tamone ✤

Func. class.: Antineoplastic

Chem. class.: Antiestrogen hormone

Pregnancy category **D**

Action: Inhibits cell division by binding to cytoplasmic estrogen receptors; resembles normal cell complex but inhibits DNA synthesis and estrogen response of target tissue

Ⅾ Therapeutic Outcome: Prevention of rapidly growing malignant cells

Uses: Advanced breast carcinoma that has not responded to other therapy in estrogen-receptor-positive patients (usually postmenopausal), prevention of breast cancer

T

Dosage and routes
Adult: PO 10-20 mg bid

Available forms: Tab 10, 20 mg

Adverse effects
CNS: Hot flashes, headache, lightheadedness, depression
CV: Chest pain
EENT: Ocular lesions, retinopathy, corneal opacity, blurred vision (high doses)
GI: Nausea, vomiting, altered taste (anorexia)
GU: Vaginal bleeding, pruritus vulvae
HEMA: Thrombocytopenia, leukopenia, DVT, PE
INTEG: Rash, alopecia
META: Hypercalcemia

Contraindications: Hypersensitivity, pregnancy **D**

Precautions: Leukopenia, thrombocytopenia, lactation, cataracts

Pharmacokinetics	
Absorption	Adequately absorbed
Distribution	Unknown
Metabolism	Liver—extensively
Excretion	Feces—slowly, small amounts (kidneys)
Half-life	1 wk

Pharmacodynamics	
Onset	Unknown
Peak	4-7 hr
Duration	Unknown

Interactions
Individual drugs
Bromocriptine: ↑ tamoxifen level
Radiation: ↑ myelosuppression
Drug classifications
Anticoagulants: ↑ risk of bleeding
Antineoplastics: ↑ thromboembolic action

Lab test interferences
↑ Serum Ca

NURSING CONSIDERATIONS
Assessment
• Monitor CBC, differential, platelet count weekly; withhold drug if WBC is <4000 or platelet count is <75,000; notify prescriber of results; monitor calcium levels (hypercalcemia is common)
◆• Assess for tumor flare: increase in bone, tumor pain during beginning treatment; give analgesics as ordered to decrease pain
• Assess for bleeding: hematuria, guaiac, bruising or petechiae, mucosa or orifices q8h, no rec temp

Nursing diagnoses
☑ Injury, risk for (adverse reactions)
☑ Knowledge deficit (teaching)

Implementation
• Give with food or fluids for
🚫 GI upset; do not break, crush, or chew enteric products; repeat dose may be needed if vomiting occurs
• Store in light-resistant container at room temp

Patient/family education
• Instruct patient to report any complaints, side effects to health care prescriber; if dose is missed, do not double next dose
• Advise patient that vaginal bleeding, pruritus, hot flashes, can occur, and are reversible after discontinuing treatment
• Instruct patient to report immediately decreased visual acuity, which may be irreversible; stress need for routine eye exams
• Inform patient about who

☑ Herb/drug   🚫 Do Not Crush   ◆ Alert   ☙ Key Drug   **G** Geriatric   **P** Pediatric should be told about tamoxifen therapy

• Advise patient to report vaginal bleeding immediately; that tumor flare—increase in size or tumor, increased bone pain—may occur and will subside rapidly; may take analgesics for pain; that premenopausal women must use mechanical birth control method because ovulation may be induced (teratogenic drug)

• Caution patient to use sunscreen and protective clothing to prevent burns because photosensitivity is common

• Teach patient that hair loss may occur during treatment; a wig or hairpiece may make patient feel better; new hair may be different in color, texture

• Inform patient rash or lesions are temporary and may become large during beginning therapy

Evaluation
Positive therapeutic outcome
• Decreased spread of malignant cells in breast cancer

---

tamsulosin (℞)
(tam-sue-lo'sen)
Flomax
Func. class.: Selective α-adrenergic blocker
Chem. class.: Sulfamoyl phenethylamine derivative
Pregnancy category   B

▷ **Therapeutic Outcome:** Decreased symptoms of BPH

Uses: Symptoms of benign prostatic hyperplasia

Dosage and routes
Adult: PO 0.4 mg qd, increas-

ing up to 0.8 mg qd if required after 2 wk

Available forms: Caps 0.4 mg

Adverse effects
CNS: Dizziness, headache, asthenia
CV: Chest pain
EENT: Amblyopia
GI: Nausea, diarrhea
GU: Decreased libido, abnormal ejaculation
MS: Back pain
RESP: Rhinitis, pharyngitis, cough

Contraindications: Hypersensitivity

Precautions: Pregnancy **B,** children, lactation, hepatic disease, coronary artery disease, severe renal disease

Pharmacokinetics	
Absorption	Well absorbed
Distribution	Not known; 98% plasma protein bound
Metabolism	Liver, extensively
Excretion	Kidneys
Half-life	9-15 hr

Pharmacodynamics
Unknown

Interactions
Drug classifications
α₁**-Adrenergic blockers:** Do not use together

NURSING CONSIDERATIONS
Assessment
• Monitor CBC with diff and liver function studies; B/P and heart rate
• Monitor urodynamic studies/urinary flow rates, residual volume

Nursing diagnoses
✓ Cardiac output, decreased (uses)
✓ Injury, potential for physical (side effects)

✓ Knowledge deficit (teaching)
✓ Noncompliance (teaching)

Implementation
• Store in tight container at 86° F (30° C) or less
• May be given with food to prevent GI symptoms

Patient/family education
• Teach patient not to discontinue drug abruptly; emphasize the importance of complying with dosage schedule, even if feeling better; if dose is missed take as soon as remembered; take at same time each day
• Teach patient not to use OTC products (cough, cold, allergy) unless directed by prescriber; also to avoid large amounts of caffeine
• Caution patient that drug may cause dizziness, may occur during 1st few days of therapy; to avoid hazardous activities

Evaluation
Positive therapeutic outcome
• Decreased symptoms of benign prostatic hyperplasia

---

telmisartan (℞)
(tel-mih-sar'tan)
Micardis
Func. class.: Antihypertensive
Chem. class.: Angiotensin II receptor (Type AT_1)
**Pregnancy category C (1st trimester)
D (2nd/3rd trimesters)**

Action: Blocks the vasoconstrictor and aldosterone-secreting effects of angiotensin II; selectively blocks the binding of angiotensin II to the AT_1 receptor found in tissues

▶**Therapeutic Outcome:** ↓ B/P

Uses: Hypertension, alone or in combination

Investigational uses: Heart failure

Dosage and routes
Adult: PO 40 mg qd; range 20-80 mg

Available forms: Tabs 40, 80 mg

Adverse effects
CNS: Dizziness, insomnia, anxiety
GI: Diarrhea, dypepsia, *anorexia, vomiting*
MS: Myalgia, pain
RESP: Cough, *upper respiratory infection*

Contraindications: Hypersensitivity, pregnancy **D** (2nd and 3rd trimesters)

Precautions: Hypersensitivity to ACE inhibitors; pregnancy **C** (1st trimester); lactation, **G** children, elderly

Pharmacokinetics	
Absorption	Unknown
Distribution	Highly protein bound
Metabolism	Liver (extensively)
Excretion	Urine/feces
Half-life	Terminal 24 hr

Pharmacodynamics	
Onset	Unknown
Peak	Unknown
Duration	Unknown

Interactions
Digoxin: ↑ digoxin peak, trough concentrations

NURSING CONSIDERATIONS
Assessment
• Monitor B/P, pulse q4h; note rate, rhythm, quality
• Monitor electrolytes: K, Na, Cl

- Monitor baselines in renal, liver function tests before therapy begins
- Assess edema in feet, legs qd
- Assess skin turgor, dryness of mucous membranes for hydration status

Nursing diagnoses

☑ Tissue perfusion, altered (uses)
☑ Knowledge deficit (teaching)
☑ Noncompliance (teaching)

Implementation

- Give without regard to meals
- Give increased dose to black patients, B/P response may be reduced

Patient/family education

- Instruct patient to comply with dosage schedule, even if feeling better
- Advise patient to notify prescriber of mouth sores, fever, swelling of hands or feet, irregular heartbeat, chest pain
- Teach patient that excessive perspiration, dehydration, vomiting, diarrhea may lead to fall in blood pressure; consult prescriber if these occur
- Teach patient that drug may cause dizziness, fainting; lightheadedness may occur

Evaluation

Positive therapeutic outcome

- Decreased B/P

temazepam (℞)
(tem-az′a-pam)
Razepam, Restoril, Temazepam
Func. class.: Sedative/hypnotic
Chem. class.: Benzodiazepine

Pregnancy category X

Controlled substance schedule IV (USA)
schedule F (Canada)

Action: Produces CNS depression at limbic, thalamic, hypothalamic levels of the CNS; may be mediated by neurotransmitter γ-aminobutyric acid (GABA); results are sedation, hypnosis, skeletal muscle relaxation, anticonvulsant activity, anxiolytic action

⇒ **Therapeutic Outcome:** Decreased insomnia

Uses: Insomnia (short-term)

Dosage and routes
Adult: PO 15-30 mg hs

Available forms: Caps 7.5, 15, 30 mg

Adverse effects
CNS: Lethargy, drowsiness, daytime sedation, dizziness, confusion, lightheadedness, headache, anxiety, irritability
CV: Chest pain, pulse changes
GI: Nausea, vomiting, diarrhea, heartburn, abdominal pain, constipation, anorexia
HEMA: **Leukopenia, granulocytopenia** (rare)

Contraindications: Hypersensitivity to benzodiazepines, pregnancy **X,** lactation, intermittent porphyria

Precautions: Anemia, hepatic disease, renal disease, suicidal individuals, drug abuse, elderly,

P psychosis, child <15 yr, acute narrow-angle glaucoma, seizure disorders

Pharmacokinetics

Absorption	Well absorbed
Distribution	Widely distributed, crosses placenta, crosses blood-brain barrier
Metabolism	Liver
Excretion	Kidneys, breast milk
Half-life	10-20 hr

Pharmacodynamics

Onset	½ hr
Peak	2-3 hr
Duration	6-8 hr

Interactions
Individual drugs
Alcohol: ↑ CNS depression
Cimetidine: ↑ action
Disulfiram: ↑ action
Fluoxetine: ↑ action
Isoniazid: ↑ action
Ketoconazole: ↑ action
Levodopa: ↓ action of levodopa
Metoprolol: ↑ action
Propoxyphene: ↑ action
Propranolol: ↑ action
Rifampin: ↓ action of temazepam
Theophylline: ↓ sedative effects
Valproic acid: ↑ action
Drug classifications
Antidepressants: ↑ CNS depression
Antihistamines: ↑ CNS depression
Barbiturates: ↓ effect of temazepam
Contraceptives: ↑ effect
Opiates: ↑ CNS depression
Herb/drug
Kava: ↑ CNS depression
Lab test interferences
↑ AST/ALT, ↑ serum bilirubin
False: ↑ 17-OHCS
↓ RAIU

NURSING CONSIDERATIONS
Assessment
• Assess mental status: mood, sensorium, anxiety, affect, sleeping pattern, drowsiness, **G** dizziness, especially elderly; physical dependency, withdrawal symptoms: anxiety, panic attacks, agitation, convulsions, headache, nausea, vomiting, muscle pain, weakness; suicidal tendencies; for indications of increasing tolerance and abuse
• Monitor B/P (lying, standing), pulse; if systolic B/P drops 20 mm Hg, hold drug, notify prescriber
• Monitor blood studies: CBC during long-term therapy; blood dycrasias have occurred rarely; decreased hematocrit, neutropenia may occur
• Monitor hepatic studies: AST, ALT, bilirubin, creatinine LDH, alk phosphatase
• Monitor I&O; indicate renal dysfunction

Nursing diagnoses
☑ Anxiety (uses)
☑ Depression (uses)
☑ Injury, risk for (adverse reactions)
☑ Knowledge deficit (teaching)

Implementation
• Give with food or milk for GI symptoms; if patient is unable to swallow medication whole, tab may be crushed and mixed with foods or fluids
• Give sugarless gum, hard candy, frequent sips of water for dry mouth

Patient/family education
• Inform patient that drug may be taken with food, and that fluids and tab may be crushed or swallowed whole
• Advise patient not to use for everyday stress or longer than

3 mo unless directed by prescriber; not to take more than prescribed amount; may be habit forming; not to double doses or skip doses

• Caution patient to avoid OTC preparations unless approved by health care prescriber; alcohol and CNS depressants will increase CNS depression

• Advise patient to avoid driving, activities that require alertness, because drowsiness may occur; to avoid alcohol ingestion or other psychotropic medications; to rise slowly or fainting may occur, especially in elderly; that drowsiness may worsen at beginning of treatment

• Caution patient not to discontinue medication abruptly after long-term use; withdrawal symptoms include vomiting, cramping, tremors, seizures

Evaluation
Positive therapeutic outcome
• Decreased anxiety, restlessness, sleeplessness (short-term treatment only)

Treatment of overdose: Lavage, VS, supportive care

temozolomide
See Appendix A, Selected New Drugs

---

terazosin (℞)
(ter-ay'zoe-sin)
Hytrin, terazosin
Func. class.: Antihypertensive
Chem. class.: Adrenergic blocker (peripherally acting)
Pregnancy category **C**

Action: Peripheral blood vessels are dilated, peripheral resistance lowered; reduction in blood pressure results from α-adrenergic receptors being blocked

Therapeutic Outcome: Decreased B/P in hypertension, decreased symptoms of BPH

Uses: Hypertension, as a single agent or in combination with diuretics or β-blockers, BPH

Dosage and routes
Adult: PO 1 mg hs, may increase doses slowly to desired response; not to exceed 20 mg/day

Available forms: Caps 1, 2, 5, 10 mg

Adverse effects
CNS: Dizziness, headache, drowsiness, anxiety, depression, vertigo, weakness, fatigue
CV: Palpitations, orthostatic hypotension, tachycardia, edema, rebound hypertension
EENT: Blurred vision, epistaxis, tinnitus, dry mouth, red sclera, nasal congestion, sinusitis
GI: Nausea, vomiting, diarrhea, constipation, abdominal pain
GU: Urinary frequency, incontinence, impotence, priapism
RESP: Dyspnea

T

Contraindications: Hypersensitivity

Precautions: Pregnancy **C**, 🅿 children, lactation

Pharmacokinetics

Absorption	Well absorbed
Distribution	Not known
Metabolism	Liver—50%
Excretion	Kidneys unchanged—10%, feces unchanged—20%
Half-life	9-12 hr

Pharmacodynamics

Onset	15 min
Peak	1 hr
Duration	24 hr

Interactions
Individual drugs
Alcohol: ↑ CNS depression
Drug classifications
Antihypertensives: ↑ hypotension
Estrogens: ↓ antihypertensive effect
Nitrates: ↑ hypotensive effects
NSAIDs: ↓ antihypertensive effect
Sympathomimetics: ↓ antihypertensive effect
☑ *Herb/drug*
Angelica: ↑ terazosin effect
Lab test interferences
↑ VMA excretion, ↑ 5-HIAA excretion
Interference: 17-OHCS, 17-KS

NURSING CONSIDERATIONS
Assessment
• Monitor B/P, orthostatic hypotension, syncope; check for edema in feet, legs daily; I&O; monitor for weight daily; notify prescriber of changes
• Assess for allergic reactions: rash, fever, pruritus, urticaria; drug should be discontinued if antihistamines fail to help

Nursing diagnoses
☑ Cardiac output, decreased (uses)
☑ Injury, risk for (adverse reactions)
☑ Knowledge deficit (teaching)
☑ Noncompliance (teaching)

Implementation
• Store in tight container at 86° F (30° C) or less
• May be used in combination with other antihypertensives
• May be given with food to prevent GI symptoms

Patient/family education
• Caution patient not to discontinue drug abruptly; the importance of complying with dosage schedule, even if feeling better; if dose is missed take as soon as remembered; take medication at same time each day
• Teach patient not to use OTC products (cough, cold, allergy) unless directed by prescriber; also to avoid large amounts of caffeine
• Emphasize the need to rise slowly to sitting or standing position to minimize orthostatic hypotension
• Teach patient to notify prescriber of mouth sores, sore throat, fever, swelling of hands or feet, irregular heartbeat, chest pain
• Caution patient to report excessive perspiration, dehydration, vomiting, diarrhea; may lead to fall in B/P
• Caution patient that drug may cause dizziness, fainting, lightheadedness; may occur during 1st few days of therapy; to avoid hazardous activities
• Teach patient how to take B/P, and normal readings for age group; to take B/P q7 days

---

Evaluation
Positive therapeutic outcome
- Decreased B/P in hypertension
- Decreased symptoms of BPH

Treatment of overdose: Administer volume expanders or vasopressors; discontinue drug; place patient in supine position

---

terbutaline (℞)
(ter-byoo′te-leen)
Brethaire, Brethine, Bricanyl
Func. class.: Selective β_2-agonist; bronchodilator
Chem. class.: Catecholamine
Pregnancy category **B**

Action: Relaxes bronchial smooth muscle by direct action on β_2-adrenergic receptors through accumulation of cAMP at β-adrenergic receptor sites; results are bronchodilation, diuresis, and CNS and cardiac stimulation; relaxes uterine smooth muscle

Therapeutic Outcome: Bronchodilation with ease of breathing

Uses: Bronchospasm

Investigational uses: Premature labor, hyperkalemia

Dosage and routes
Bronchospasm
Adult and child >12 yr: Inh 2 puffs q1min, then q4-6h; PO 2.5-5 mg q8h; SC 0.25 mg q8h

Available forms: Tabs 2.5, 5 mg; aerosol 0.2 mg/actuation; inj 1 mg/ml

Adverse effects
CNS: Tremors, anxiety, insom-

nia, headache, dizziness, stimulation
CV: Palpitations, tachycardia, hypertension, dysrhythmias, **cardiac arrest**
GI: Nausea, vomiting

Contraindications: Hypersensitivity to sympathomimetics, narrow-angle glaucoma, tachydysrhythmias

Precautions: Pregnancy **B,** cardiac disorders, hyperthyroidism, diabetes mellitus, prostatic hypertension, lactation, elderly, hypertension, glaucoma

Pharmacokinetics

Absorption	Well absorbed (SC), partially absorbed (PO)
Distribution	Unknown
Metabolism	Liver—partially
Excretion	Unknown
Half-life	Unknown

Pharmacodynamics

	PO	INH	SC	IV
Onset	½ hr	5-15 min	10-15 min	Rapid
Peak	1-2 hr	1-2 hr	½-1 hr	Unknown
Duration	4-8 hr	4-6 hr	1½-4 hr	Unknown

Interactions
Drug classifications
β-Adrenergic blockers: Block therapeutic effect
Bronchodilators, aerosol: ↑ action of bronchodilator
MAOIs: ↑ chance of hypertensive crisis
Sympathomimetics: ↑ adrenergic side effects

NURSING CONSIDERATIONS
Assessment
- Monitor respiratory function: vital capacity, forced expiratory volume, ABGs, lung

---

Adverse effects: *italic* = common; **bold** = life-threatening

sounds, heart rate, rhythm (baseline)

• Determine that patient has not received theophylline therapy before giving dose; assess client's ability to self-medicate

• Monitor for evidence of allergic reactions; paradoxical bronchospasm; withhold dose; notify prescriber

Nursing diagnoses

☑ Airway clearance, ineffective (uses)

☑ Impaired gas exchange (uses)

☑ Knowledge deficit (teaching)

☑ Noncompliance (teaching)

Implementation

Aerosol route

• Give after shaking; ask patient to exhale, place mouthpiece in mouth, then inhale slowly; hold breath, remove, exhale slowly; allow at least 1 min between inh

• Store in light-resistant container, do not expose to temp over 86° F (30° C)

PO route

• Give PO with meals to decrease gastric irritation; tab may be crushed and mixed with foods and fluids

SC route

• Do not give by IM route

IV **IV route**

• Give at 5 μg q 10 min until contractions are stopped, use inf pump for correct dose; after ½-1 hr with no contraction decrease dose by 5 μg; switch to PO dose when possible

Syringe compatibilities:
Doxapram

Y-site compatibilities:
Regular insulin

Additive compatibilities:
Aminophylline

Additive incompatibilities:
Bleomycin

Patient/family education

• Advise patient not to use OTC medications; extra stimulation may occur; to use this medication before other medications and allow at least 5 min between each to prevent overstimulation

• Teach patient how to use inhaler; review package insert with patient; to avoid getting aerosol in eyes because blurring may result; to wash inhaler in warm water qd and dry; to avoid smoking, smoke-filled rooms, persons with respiratory infections

• Teach patient that paradoxical bronchospasm may occur and to stop drug immediately and notify health care prescriber; to limit caffeine products such as chocolate, coffee, tea, and colas

• Instruct patient on administration of dose, not to use more than prescribed; serious side effects may occur; if taking PO regularly and dose is missed, take when remembered; space other doses on new time schedule

Evaluation

Positive therapeutic outcome

• Absence of dyspnea, wheezing after 1 hr

• Improved airway exchange

• Improved ABGs

Treatment of overdose:
Administer a β_2-adrenergic blocker

---

testosterone ⊶ (R)
(tess-toss′te-rone)
Andro L.A. 200, Delatest, Delatestryl, Durathate-200, Everone 100, Everone 200, Testone LA 100, Testone LA 200, testosterone enanthate, Testrin PA, Andro-Cyp 100, Andro-Cyp 200, Andronate 100, Andronate 200, depAndro 100, depAndro 200, Depotest 100, Depotest 200, Depo-Testosterone, Duratest-100, Duratest-200, testosterone cypionate, Testred Cypionate, Testex, testosterone propionate, Testoderm Transdermal
Func. class.: Androgenic anabolic steroid
Chem. class.: Halogenated testosterone derivative

Pregnancy category **X**

Action: Increases weight by building body tissue; increases potassium, phosphorus, chloride, nitrogen levels; increases bone development; responsible for maintenance of secondary sex characteristics (male)

➡ **Therapeutic Outcome:** Increased hormone levels in eunuchoidism, decreased tumor growth in female breast cancer, onset of male puberty

Uses: Female breast cancer, eunuchoidism, male climacteric, oligospermia, impotence, osteoporosis, weight loss in AIDS patients, vulvar dystrophies

Dosage and routes
Replacement
Adult: **IM** 25-50 mg 2-3 ×/wk (base or propionate) or 50-400 mg q2-4wk (enanthate or cypionate); adult trans testo-derm 4-6 mg applied q24h; Androderm-5 mg applied q24h

Breast cancer
Adult: **IM** 50-100 mg 3 ×/wk (propionate) or 200-400 mg q2-4 wk (cypionate or enanthate)

Delayed male puberty
P *Child >12 yr:* **IM** up to 100 mg/mo for up to 6 mo

Available forms: Propionate inj 25, 50, 100 mg/ml; enanthate inj 100, 200 mg/ml; cypionate inj 50, 100, 200 mg/ml; patches 4, 6 mg/day, transdermal patches: Testoderm 4 mg/day (30 patches), 6 mg/day (30 patches), Androderm 2.5 mg/day (60 patches), 5 mg/day (60 patches)

Adverse effects
CNS: Dizziness, headache, fatigue, tremors, paresthesias, flushing, sweating, anxiety, lability, insomnia, carpal tunnel syndrome
CV: Increased B/P
EENT: Conjunctival edema, nasal congestion
ENDO: Abnormal GTT
GI: Nausea, vomiting, constipation, weight gain, **cholestatic jaundice**
GU: Hematuria, amenorrhea, vaginitis, decreased libido, decreased breast size, clitoral hypertrophy, testicular atrophy
INTEG: Rash, acneiform lesions, oily hair and skin, flushing, sweating, acne vulgaris, alopecia, hirsutism
MS: Cramps, spasms

Contraindications: Severe renal disease, severe cardiac disease, severe hepatic disease, hypersensitivity, pregnancy **X**, lactation, genital bleeding (abnormal)

T

Precautions: Diabetes mellitus, CV disease, MI

Pharmacokinetics	
Absorption	Well but slowly absorbed
Distribution	Crosses placenta
Metabolism	Liver
Excretion	Kidneys, breast milk
Half-life	8 days (cypionate) 10-100 min (Base)

Pharmacodynamics

	IM (base)	IM (cypionate)	IM (enanthate)	IM (propionate)
Onset	Unknown	Unknown	Unknown	Unknown
Peak	Unknown	Unknown	Unknown	Unknown
Duration	1-3 days	2-4 wk	2-4 wk	1-3 days

Interactions
Individual drugs
ACTH: ↑ edema
Insulin: ↓ effects of insulin
Oxyphenbutazone: ↑ effects of oxyphenbutazone
Drug classifications
Adrenal steroids: ↑ edema
Anticoagulants: ↑ pro-time
Oral antidiabetics: ↑ effects of oral antidiabetics
Lab test interferences
↑ Serum cholesterol, ↑ blood glucose, ↑ urine glucose
↓ Serum Ca, ↓ serum K, ↓ T_4, ↓ T_3, ↓ thyroid ^{131}I uptake test, ↓ urine 17-OHCS, ↓ 17-KS, ↓ PBI

NURSING CONSIDERATIONS
Assessment
• Monitor patient's weight daily; notify prescriber if weekly weight gain is >5 lb; assess I&O ratio; be alert for decreasing urinary output, increasing edema
• Monitor B/P q4h
P• Assess growth rate in adolescent because growth rate may be uneven (linear/bone growth) if used for extended periods
• Monitor electrolytes: potassium, sodium, chloride, calcium; cholesterol
• Monitor liver function studies: ALT, AST, bilirubin
• Assess edema, hypertension, cardiac symptoms, jaundice
• Assess mental status: affect, mood, behavioral changes, aggression
• Assess signs of masculinization in female: increased libido, deepening of voice, decreased breast tissue, enlarged clitoris, menstrual irregularities; male: gynecomastia, impotence, testicular atrophy
• Assess hypercalcemia: lethargy, polyuria, polydipsia, nausea, vomiting, constipation; drug may have to be decreased
• Assess hypoglycemia in diabetics because oral antidiabetic action is increased

Nursing diagnoses
☑ Infection, risk for (adverse reactions)
☑ Injury, risk for (adverse reactions)
☑ Knowledge deficit (teaching)

Implementation
• Administer diet with increased calories, protein; decreased sodium if edema occurs
• Administer supportive drug if anemia occurs
• Give titrated dose; use lowest effective dose
• Give IM deep into upper outer quadrant of gluteal muscle; route can be painful

Patient/family education
• Inform patient that drug needs to be combined with complete health plan: diet, rest, exercise
• Caution patient to notify

prescriber if therapeutic response decreases; not to discontinue this medication abruptly
• Inform women patients to report menstrual irregularities; about changes in sex characteristics
• Discuss that 1-3 mo course is necessary for response in breast cancer
• Transdermal patches: testoderm to skin of scrotum, Androderm to skin of back, upper arms, thighs, abdomen; area must be dry and free of hair; may be reapplied after bathing, swimming

Evaluation
Positive therapeutic outcome
• Decrease size of tumor in breast cancer
• Increased androgen levels

---

tetracycline (℞)
(tet-ra-sye'kleen)
Achromycin V, Alatel, Apo-Tetra ✦, Novotetra ✦, Nu-Tetra ✦, Panmycin, Robitet, Sumycin, Teline, Tetracap, tetracycline HCl, Tetracyn, Tetralan, Tetralean ✦, Tetram
Func. class.: Broad-spectrum antiinfective
Chem. class.: Tetracycline
Pregnancy category   D

Action: Inhibits protein synthesis and phosphorylation in microorganisms; bacteriostatic

▷**Therapeutic Outcome:** Bactericidal action against susceptible organisms; gram-positive pathogens: *Bacillus antracis, Clostridium perfringens, Clos-*

tridium tetani, Listeria monocytogenes, Nocardia, Propionibacterium acnes, Actinomyces isrealii; gram-negative pathogens *Haemophilus influenzae, Legionella pneumophila, Yersinia entercolitica, Yersinia pestis, Neisseria gonorrhoeae, Neisseria meningitidis*

Uses: Syphilis, chlamydia trachomatis, gonorrhea, lymphogranuloma venereum, uncommon gram-positive, gram-negative organisms, rickettsial infections

Dosage and routes
Adult: PO 250-500 mg q6h

▣ *Child >8 yr:* PO 25-50 mg/kg/day in divided doses q6h

Gonorrhea
Adult: PO 1.5 g, then 500 mg qid for a total of 9 g over 7 days

Chlamydia trachomatis
Adult: PO 500 mg qid × 7 days

Syphilis
Adult: PO 2-3 g in divided doses × 10-15 days; if syphilis duration >1 yr, must treat 30 days

Brucellosis
Adult: PO 500 mg qid × 3 wk with 1 g streptomycin IM 2 ×/day × 1 wk, and 1 ×/day the second wk

Urethral syndrome in women
Adult: PO 500 mg qid × 7 days

Acne
Adult: 1 g/day in divided doses; maintenance 125-500 mg/day

Available forms: Oral susp 125 mg/5 ml, caps 100, 200,

T

---

500 mg; tabs 100, 250,
500 mg

Adverse effects

CNS: Fever, headache, paresthesia

CV: **Pericarditis**

EENT: Dysphagia, glossitis, decreased calcification (permanent discoloration) of deciduous teeth, oral candidiasis

GI: Nausea, abdominal pain, *vomiting, diarrhea,* anorexia, enterocolitis, **hepatotoxicity,** flatulence, abdominal cramps, epigastric burning, stomatitis

GU: Increased BUN

HEMA: **Eosinophilia, neutropenia, thrombocytopenia, leukocytosis, hemolytic anemia**

INTEG: Rash, urticaria, photosensitivity, increased pigmentation, **exfoliative dermatitis,** pruritus, **angioedema**

Contraindications: Hypersensitivity to tetracyclines, children <8 yr, pregnancy **D,** lactation

Precautions: Renal disease, hepatic disease

Pharmacokinetics	
Absorption	60%-80% (PO), lower (IM)
Distribution	Widely distributed, some in CSF; crosses placenta
Metabolism	Not metabolized
Excretion	Unchanged—kidneys
Half-life	6-10 hr

Pharmacodynamics	
Onset	1-2 hr
Peak	2-3 hr

Interactions
Individual drugs
Calcium: Forms chelates, ↓ absorption

Carbamazepine: ↑ effect of carbamazepine

Cholestyramine: ↓ absorption of tetracycline

Colestipol: ↓ absorption of tetracycline

Iron: Forms chelates, ↓ absorption

Magnesium: Forms chelates, ↓ absorption

Phenytoin: ↓ effect of tetracycline

Sucralfate: Prevents absorption of tetracycline

Drug classifications
Anticoagulants, oral: ↑ effect of anticoagulants

Barbiturates: ↓ effect of tetracycline

Contraceptives, oral: ↓ effect of oral contraception

Food/drug
↓ absorption with dairy products; forms insoluble chelate

☑ *Herb/drug*
Dong Quai: ↑ photosensitivity

Lab test interferences
False: ↑ Urinary catecholamines

False negative: Urine glucose with Clinistix, Tes-Tape

NURSING CONSIDERATIONS
Assessment
• Assess patient for previous sensitivity reaction

• Assess patient for signs and symptoms of infection including characteristics of wounds, sputum, urine, stool, WBC >10,000, temp; obtain baseline information before and during treatment

• Complete C&S testing before beginning drug therapy to identify if correct treatment has been initiated

• Assess for allergic reactions: rash, urticaria, pruritus, chills, fever, joint pain; angioedema

☑ Herb/drug   ⬡ Do Not Crush   ◆ Alert   ⦿ᴛ Key Drug   Ɠ Geriatric   ᴘ Pediatric may occur a few days after therapy begins—epinephrine, resuscitation equipment should be on unit for anaphylactic reaction

• Identify urine output; if decreasing, notify prescriber (may indicate nephrotoxicity); also, increased BUN, creatinine

• Monitor blood studies: AST, ALT, CBC, Hct, bilirubin, LDH, alk phosphatase, monthly if patient is on long-term therapy

• Assess bowel pattern qd; if severe diarrhea occurs, drug should be discontinued

• Monitor for bleeding: ecchymosis, bleeding gums, hematuria, stool guaiac daily if on long-term therapy; blood dyscrasias may occur

• Assess for overgrowth of infection: perineal itching, fever, malaise, redness, pain, swelling, drainage, rash, diarrhea, change in cough, sputum

Nursing diagnoses
☑ Infection, risk for (uses)
☑ Diarrhea (adverse reactions)
☑ Injury, risk for (adverse reactions)
☑ Knowledge deficit (teaching)
☑ Noncompliance (teaching)

Implementation
PO route
• Give around the clock to maintain proper blood levels; give with food to increase absorption of drug; do not give within 3 hr of other agents—drug actions may occur

• Give with 8 oz of water

• Shake liq preparation well before giving; use calibrated device for proper dosing

Patient/family education
• Teach patient to report sore throat, bruising, bleeding,

joint pain—may indicate blood dyscrasias (rare)

• Advise patient to use a sunscreen when outdoors to decrease photosensitivity reaction

• Advise patient to contact prescriber if vaginal itching; loose, foul-smelling stools; furry tongue occur that may indicate superimposed infection; report itching, rash, pruritus, urticaria

• Instruct patient to take all medication prescribed for the length of time ordered; drug must be taken around the clock to maintain blood levels; do not give medication to others

Evaluation
Positive therapeutic outcome
• Absence of signs/symptoms of infection (WBC <10,000, temp WNL, absence of red, draining wounds)

• Reported improvement in symptoms of infection

theophylline ⚏ (℞)

(thee-off'i-lin)

Accurbron, Aquaphyllin, Asmalix, Bronkodyl, Elixomin, Elixophyllin, Lanophyllin, Quibron-T Dividose, Quibron-T/SR, Respbid, Slo-bid Gyrocaps, Slo-Phyllin, Sustaire, Theo-24, Theobid Duracaps, Theochron, Theoclear-80, Theoclear L.A., Theo-Dur, Theolair-SR, Theo-Sav, Theospan-SR, Theostat 80, Theovent, Theo-X, T-Phy, Uni-Dur, Uniphyl

Func. class.: Spasmolytic, bronchodilator

Chem. class.: Xanthine, ethylenediamine

Pregnancy category C

Action: Relaxes smooth muscle of respiratory system by blocking phosphodiesterase, which increases cAMP, which increases bronchodilation, diuresis, circulation, CNS stimulation

➡ **Therapeutic Outcome:** Ability to breathe without difficulty

Uses: Bronchial asthma, bronchospasm of COPD, chronic bronchitis

Dosage and routes
Bronchospasm, bronchial asthma
Adult: PO 100-200 mg q6h; dosage must be individualized; rec 250-500 mg q9-12h

P *Child:* PO 50-100 mg q6h, not to exceed 12 mg/kg/24 h

COPD, chronic bronchitis
Adult: PO 30-660 q6-8h pc (sodium glycinate)

P *Child 1-9 yr:* PO 5 mg/kg loading dose, then 4 mg/kg q6h

P *Child 9-16 yr:* PO 5 mg/kg losding dose, then 3 mg/kg q6h

Apnea of prematurity
P *Neonate:* 2-10 mg/kg/day divided q8-12h (usual loading dose is 4 mg/kg)

Available forms: Caps 50, 100, 200, 250 mg; tabs 100, 125, 200, 225, 250, 300 mg; time-release tabs 100, 200, 250, 300, 400, 500 mg; time-release caps 50, 65, 100, 125, 130, 200, 250, 260, 300, 400, 500 mg; elix 80, 11.25 mg/15 mg; sol 80 mg/15 ml; liq 80, 150, 160 mg/15 ml; susp 300 mg/15 ml

Adverse effects
CNS: Anxiety, restlessness, insomnia, dizziness, convulsions, headache, lightheadedness, muscle twitching, tremors
CV: Palpitations, sinus tachycardia, hypotension, other dysrhythmias, fluid retention with tachycardia
ENDO: Hyperglycemia
GI: Nausea, vomiting, anorexia, diarrhea, bitter taste, dyspepsia, gastric distress
INTEG: Flushing, urticaria
RESP: Increased rate

Contraindications: Hypersensitivity to xanthines, tachydysrhythmias

G **Precautions:** Elderly, CHF, cor pulmonale, hepatic disease, active peptic ulcer disease, diabetes mellitus, hyperthyroidism, hypertension,
P children, pregnancy **C**

Pharmacokinetics

Absorption	Well absorbed (PO), slowly absorbed (ext rel)
Distribution	Crosses placenta, widely distributed
Metabolism	Liver
Excretion	Kidneys, breast milk
Half-life	3-13, increased in liver disease, CHF, elderly

Pharmacodynamics

	PO	PO-ER	IV
Onset	Rapid	Slow	Immediate
Peak	1 hr	4-8 hr	Inf end
Duration	6 hr	12-24 hr	6-8 hr

Interactions
Individual drugs
Carbamazepine: ↓ theophylline level
Cimetidine: ↑ action of theophylline
Ciprofloxacin: ↑ theophylline action
Erythromycin: ↑ action of theophylline
Lithium: ↓ effect of lithium
Phenobarbital: ↓ theophylline
Phenytoin: ↓ theophylline
Propranolol: ↑ action of theophylline
Rifampin: ↓ theophylline
Drug classifications
β-Adrenergic blockers: cardiotoxicity
Oral contraceptives: ↑ theophylline action
Herb/drug
Ma Huang: ↑ toxicity

NURSING CONSIDERATIONS
Assessment
• Monitor theophylline blood levels (therapeutic level is 5-15 µg/ml); toxicity may occur with small increase above 15 µg/ml
• Monitor I&O; diuresis occurs; dehydration may result in elderly or children
• Assess for signs of toxicity: irritability, insomnia, restlessness, tremors, nausea, vomiting
• Monitor respiratory rate, rhythm, depth; auscultate lung fields bilaterally; notify prescriber of abnormalities
• Assess for allergic reactions: rash, urticaria; if these occur, drug should be discontinued

Nursing diagnoses
☑ Airway clearance, ineffective (uses)
☑ Knowledge deficit (teaching)

Implementation
PO route
• Give PO pc to decrease GI symptoms; absorption may be affected
IV route

Y-site compatibilities:
Acyclovir, ampicillin, aztreonam, cefazolin, cefotetan, ceftazidime, ceftriaxone, cimetidine, clindamycin, dexamethasone, diltiazem, dobutamine, dopamine, doxycycline, erythromycin, famotidine, fluconazole, gentamicin, haloperidol, heparin, hydrocortisone, lidocaine, methyldopate, methylprednisolone, metronidazole, midazolam, nafcillin, nitroglycerin, nitroprusside, penicillin G potassium, piperacillin, potassium chloride, ranitidine, ticarcillin, ticarcillin/clavulanate, tobramycin, vancomycin

Additive compatibilities:
Cefepime, chlorpromazine, fluconazole, methylprednisolone, verapamil

Patient/family education
• Advise patient to check OTC medications, current prescription medications for ephedrine, which will increase stimulation, and to avoid alcohol, caffeine

T

- Caution patient to avoid hazardous activities; dizziness may occur
- Inform patient that if GI upset occurs, to take drug with 8 oz water; avoid food; absorption may be decreased
- Teach patient not to crush, dissolve, or chew slow-release products
- Teach patient that contents of bead-filled cap may be sprinkled over food for children's use
- Advise patient to notify prescriber of toxicity: nausea, vomiting, anxiety, insomnia, convulsions
- Advise patient to notify prescriber of change in smoking habit; dosage may have to be changed

Evaluation
Positive therapeutic outcome
- Ability to breathe more easily

---

thiamine (vitamin B₁) (PO, OTC; IV ℞)
Betaxin ✦, Betalin S, Biamine, Revitonus, Thiamilate, thiamine HCl, vitamin B
Func. class.: Vitamin B₁
Chem. class.: Water soluble

Pregnancy category   A

Action: Needed for pyruvate metabolism, carbohydrate metabolism

→**Therapeutic Outcome:** Prevention and treatment of thiamine deficiency

Uses: Vitamin B₁ deficiency or polyneuritis, cheilosis adjunct with thiamine beriberi, Wernicke-Korsakoff syndrome, pellagra, metabolic disorders

Dosage and routes
RDA
Adult: Male 1.2-1.5 mg; females 1.1 mg; pregnancy 1.5 mg; lactation 1.6 mg
P *Child 7-10 yr:* 1.3 mg
P *Child 4-6 yr:* 0.9 mg
P *Child 1-3 yr:* 0.7 mg
P *Infants 6 mo-1 yr:* 0.4 mg
P *Neonates and infants to 6 mo:* 0.3 mg

Beriberi
Adult: IM 10-20 mg tid × 2 wk, then 5-10 mg qd × 1 mo

Beriberi with cardiac failure
P *Adult and child:* IV 10-30 mg tid

Available forms: Tab 50, 100, 250, 500 mg; inj 100 mg/ml; enteric-coated tab 20 mg

Adverse effects
CNS: Weakness, restlessness
CV: **Collapse, pulmonary edema,** hypotension
EENT: Tightness of throat
GI: Hemorrhage, *nausea, diarrhea*
INTEG: **Angioneurotic edema,** cyanosis, sweating, warmth
SYST: Anaphylaxis

Contraindications: Hypersensitivity

Precautions: Pregnancy A

⊠ **Do Not Confuse:** thiamine/Tenormin

Pharmacokinetics	
Absorption	Well absorbed (PO, IM) completely absorbed (**IV**)
Distribution	Widely distributed
Metabolism	Liver
Excretion	Kidneys (unchanged—excess amounts)
Half-life	Unknown

Pharmacodynamics
Unknown

Interactions
Drug classifications
Neuromuscular blockers:
↑ effect

NURSING CONSIDERATIONS
Assessment
• Monitor thiamine levels throughout treatment
• Assess nutritional status: yeast, beef, liver, whole or enriched grains, legumes

Nursing diagnoses
✓ Nutrition: less than body requirements (uses)
✓ Knowledge deficit (teaching)

Implementation
IV **IV route**
• **IV** undiluted given over 5 min or diluted with **IV** sol and given as an inf at a rate of 100 mg or less/5 min or more

Syringe compatibilities:
Doxapram

Y-site compatibilities:
Famotidine

Additive incompatibilities:
Barbiturates; sol with neutral or alkaline pH, such as carbonates, bicarbonates, citrates and acetates; erythromycin, kanamycin, or streptomycin
IM route
• Give by IM inj; rotate sites if pain and inflammation occur; do not mix with alkaline sol; z-track to minimize pain
• Application of cold may decrease pain
• Store in tight, light-resistant container

Patient/family education
• Teach patient necessary foods to be included in diet:
yeast, beef, liver, legumes, whole grains

Evaluation
Positive therapeutic outcome
• Absence of nausea, vomiting, anorexia, insomnia, tachycardia, paresthesias, depression, muscle weakness

thiethylperazine (℞)
(thye-eth-il-per'a-zeen)
Norzine, Torecan
Func. class.: Antiemetic
Chem. class.: Phenothiazine, piperazine derivative
Pregnancy category   X

Action: Acts centrally by blocking chemoreceptor trigger zone, which in turn acts on vomiting center

➡**Therapeutic Outcome:** Control of nausea, vomiting

Uses: Nausea, vomiting

Dosage and routes
Adult: PO/IM 10 mg/qd-tid

Available forms: Tab 10 mg; inj 5 mg/ml

Adverse effects
CNS: Euphoria, depression, restlessness, tremor, extrapyramidal symptoms, **convulsions,** drowsiness
CV: **Circulatory failure, tachycardia,** postural hypotension, ECG changes
GI: Nausea, vomiting, anorexia, dry mouth, diarrhea, constipation, weight loss, metallic taste, cramps
GU: Urinary retention, dark urine
RESP: **Respiratory depression**

Contraindications: Hypersensitivity to phenothiazines,

T

---

coma, seizure, encephalopathy, bone marrow depression, pregnancy **X**

P G Precautions: Children <2 yr, elderly

N Do Not Confuse:
Torecan/Toradol

Pharmacokinetics

Absorption	Readily absorbed
Distribution	Crosses placenta
Metabolism	Liver
Excretion	Kidneys, breast milk
Half-life	Unknown

Pharmacodynamics

	PO	REC	IM
Onset	45-60 min	45-60 min	Unknown
Peak	Unknown	Unknown	Unknown
Duration	4 hr	Unknown	Unknown

Interactions
Drug classifications
Antacids: ↓ absorption
Anticholinergics: ↑ anticholinergic effects
Antidepressants: ↑ CNS depression
Antidiarrheals, adsorbent: ↓ absorption
Antihistamines: ↑ CNS depression
Antihypertensives: ↑ hypotension
Antithyroid agents: ↑ agranulocytosis
Barbiturate anesthetics: ↑ CNS depression
β-Adrenergics: ↑ effects of both drugs
General anesthetics: ↑ CNS depression
MAOIs: ↑ CNS depression
Opiates: ↑ CNS depression
Sedative/hypnotics: ↑ CNS depression

NURSING CONSIDERATIONS
Assessment
• Monitor I&O ratio, palpate bladder if low urinary output **G** occurs, especially in elderly; urinalysis recommended before, during prolonged therapy
• Monitor bilirubin, CBC, liver function studies monthly
• Assess affect, orientation, LOC, reflexes, gait, coordination, sleep pattern disturbances
• Monitor B/P with patient in sitting, standing, and lying positions; take pulse and respirations q4h during initial treatment; establish baseline before starting treatment; report drops of 30 mm Hg
• Check for dizziness, faintness, palpitations, tachycardia on rising; severe orthostatic hypotension is common
• Identify for neuroleptic malignant syndrome: hyperpyrexia, muscle rigidity, increased CPK, altered mental status; drug should be discontinued
• Assess for extrapyramidal symptoms including akathisia (inability to sit still, no pattern to movements), tardive dyskinesia (bizarre movements of the jaw, mouth, tongue, extremities), pseudoparkinsonism (tremors, pill rolling, shuffling gait); antiparkinsonian drug should be prescribed
• Assess for constipation, urinary retention daily; if these occur, increase bulk, water in diet

Nursing diagnoses
☑ Thought processes, altered (uses)
☑ Coping, ineffective individual (uses)
☑ Knowledge deficit (teaching)
☑ Noncompliance (teaching)

☑ Herb/drug ☒ Do Not Crush ◆ Alert ☮ Key Drug **G** Geriatric **P** Pediatric

Implementation
IM route
- Give IM inj in large muscle mass; aspirate to avoid **IV** administration; give slowly; have patient remain supine for 1 hr after administration

Syringe compatibilities:
Butorphanol, hydromorphone, midazolam, ranitidine

Y-site compatibilities:
Aldesleukin

Patient/family education
- Teach patient to use good oral hygiene; frequent rinsing of mouth, sugarless gum for dry mouth
- Caution patient to avoid hazardous activities until drug response is determined— dizziness, blurred vision may occur
- Inform patient that orthostatic hypotension occurs often and to rise from sitting or lying position gradually
- Instruct patient to remain lying down after IM inj for at least 30 min
- Advise patient to avoid hot tubs, hot showers, tub baths, since hypotension may occur
- Inform patient that heat stroke may occur in hot weather, and to take extra precautions to stay cool
- Teach patient to avoid OTC preparations (cough, hay fever, cold) unless approved by prescriber because serious drug interactions may occur; avoid use with alcohol, CNS depressants because increased drowsiness may occur
- Inform patient to use a sunscreen and sunglasses to prevent burns
- Teach patient about extrapyramidal symptoms
- Instruct patient to report sore throat, malaise, fever, bleeding, mouth sores; if these occur, CBC should be drawn and drug discontinued

Evaluation
Positive therapeutic outcome
- Absence of nausea, vomiting

---

thioguanine (6-TG) (℞)
(thye-oh-gwah'neen)
thioguanine, Lanvis ♣
Func. class.: Antineoplastic-antimetabolite
Chem. class.: Purine analog
Pregnancy category **D**

Action: Interferes with synthesis, utilization of purine nucleotides; S phase of cell cycle specific

Therapeutic Outcome: Prevention of rapidly growing malignant cells

Uses: Acute leukemias, chronic granulocytic leukemia, lymphomas, multiple myeloma, solid tumors

Dosage and routes
Adult and child: PO 2 mg/kg/day, then increase slowly to 3 mg/kg/day after 4 wk

Available forms: Tab 40 mg

Adverse effects
GI: Nausea, vomiting, anorexia, diarrhea, stomatitis, **hepatotoxicity,** gastritis, jaundice

GU: **Renal failure,** hyperuricemia, oliguria

HEMA: **Thrombocytopenia, leukopenia, myelosuppression, anemia**

INTEG: Rash, dermatitis, dry skin

Contraindications: Prior drug resistance, leukopenia (2500/

T

mm^3), thrombocytopenia
(<100,000/mm^3), anemia,
pregnancy **D**
Precautions: Liver disease

Pharmacokinetics

Absorption	Variably absorbed, 30%
Distribution	Crosses placenta
Metabolism	Liver—extensively
Excretion	Kidneys
Half-life	11 hr

Pharmacodynamics

Unknown

Interactions
Individual drugs
Radiation: ↑ toxicity, bone
marrow suppression
Drug classifications
Antineoplastics: ↑ toxicity,
bone marrow suppression
Lab test interferences
↑ Uric acid (blood, urine)

NURSING CONSIDERATIONS
Assessment
• Assess buccal cavity q8h for
dryness, sores or ulceration,
white patches, oral pain, bleeding, dysphagia; obtain prescription for viscous lidocaine (Xylocaine)
◆• Assess symptoms indicating
severe allergic reaction: rash,
pruritus, urticaria, purpuric
skin lesions, itching, flushing
• Monitor CBC, differential,
platelet count weekly; withhold
drug if WBC count is <4000/
mm^3 or platelet count is
<100,000/mm^3, notify pre-
scriber of results if WBC
<20,000/mm^3, platelets
</50,000/mm^3
• Assess for increased uric acid
levels, swelling, joint pain
(primarily in extremities);
patient should be well hydrated
to prevent urate deposits

• Monitor renal function
studies: BUN, creatinine,
serum uric acid, urine CrCl
before and during therapy;
I&O ratio; report fall in urine
output to <30 ml/hr
• Monitor temp q4h (may indicate beginning of infection)
• Monitor liver function tests
before and during therapy
(bilirubin, AST, ALT, LDH) as
needed or monthly; jaundice,
sclera, dark urine, clay-colored
stools, itchy skin, abdominal
pain, fever, diarrhea
• Assess for bleeding: hematuria, stool guaiac, bruising or
petechiae, mucosa or orifices
q8h; inflammation of mucosa,
breaks in skin
• Identify edema in feet, joint
pain, stomach pain, shaking;
prescriber should be notified
Nursing diagnoses
☑ Injury, risk for (adverse reactions)
☑ Body image disturbance (adverse reactions)
☑ Infection, risk for (adverse
reactions)
☑ Knowledge deficit (teaching)
Implementation
• Avoid contact with skin (very
irritating), wash completely to
remove
• Give fluids **IV** or PO before
chemotherapy to hydrate patient
• Give antiemetic 30-60 min
before giving drug to prevent
vomiting, and prn; antibiotics
for prophylaxis of infection
• Give top or syst analgesics
for pain
• Provide liq diet: carbonated
beverages; gelatin may be
added if patient is not nauseated or vomiting
• Provide rinsing of mouth
tid-qid with water, club soda;

---

brushing of teeth bid-qid with soft brush or cotton-tipped applicators for stomatitis; use unwaxed dental floss
• Give 1 hr ac or 2 hr pc to prevent vomiting

Patient/family education
• Inform patient that contraceptive measures are recommended during therapy
• Caution patient to avoid use of products containing aspirin or NSAIDs, razors, commercial mouthwash, bleeding may occur; to report symptoms of bleeding (hematuria, tarry stools)
• Advise patient to report signs of anemia, (fatigue, headache, irritability, faintness, shortness of breath)
• Caution patient not to have any vaccinations without the advice of the prescriber— serious reactions can occur

Evaluation
Positive therapeutic outcome
• Prevention of rapid division of malignant cells

---

thioridazine (℞)
(thye-or-rid′a-zeen)
Apo-Thioridazine ✦, Mellaril, Mellaril Concentrate, Mellaril-5, Novo-Ridazine ✦, PMS-Thioridazine ✦, thioridazine HCl
Func. class.: Antipsychotic/neuroleptic
Chem. class.: Phenothiazine, piperidine
Pregnancy category   C

Action: Depresses cerebral cortex, hypothalamus, limbic system, which control activity, aggression; blocks neurotransmission produced by dopamine at synapse; exhibits strong α-adrenergic, anticholinergic blocking action; mechanism for antipsychotic effects is unclear

▷**Therapeutic Outcome:** Decreased signs and symptoms of psychosis

Uses: Psychotic disorders, schizophrenia, behavioral problems in children, alcohol withdrawal as adjunct, anxiety, major depressive disorders, organic brain syndrome

Dosage and routes
Psychosis
Adult: PO 25-100 mg tid, max dose 800 mg/day; dose is gradually increased to desired response, then reduced to minimum maintenance

Depression/behavioral problems/organic brain syndrome
Adult: PO 25 tid, range from 10 mg bid-qid to 50 mg tid-qid

G *Geriatric:* PO 10-25 mg qd-bid, increase 4-7 days by 10-25 mg to desired dose

P *Child 2-12 yr:* PO 0.5-3 mg/kg/day in divided doses

Available forms: Tabs 10, 15, 25, 50, 100, 150, 200 mg; conc 30, 100 mg/ml; susp 25, 100 mg/5 ml; syrup 10 mg/15 ml

Adverse effects
CNS: Extrapyramidal symptoms (rare): pseudoparkinsonism, akathisia, dystonia, tardive dyskinesia, **seizures,** *headache,* confusion, **neuroleptic malignant syndrome**
CV: Orthostatic hypotension, **cardiac arrest,** ECG changes, **tachycardia**

✦ Canada Only   Adverse effects: *italic* = common; **bold** = life-threatening

EENT: Blurred vision, glaucoma, dry eyes

GI: *Dry mouth, nausea, vomiting, anorexia, constipation,* diarrhea, jaundice, weight gain

GU: Urinary retention, urinary frequency, enuresis, impotence, amenorrhea, gynecomastia

HEMA: Anemia, **leukopenia, leukocytosis, agranulocytosis**

INTEG: *Rash,* photosensitivity, dermatitis

RESP: **Laryngospasm,** dyspnea, **respiratory depression**

Contraindications: Hypersensitivity, blood dyscrasias, coma, child <2 yr, brain damage, bone marrow depression

Precautions: Pregnancy **C,** lactation, seizure disorders, hypertension, hepatic disease, cardiac disease

▧ Do Not Confuse:
Mellaril/Elavil

Pharmacokinetics	
Absorption	Variably absorbed (tab)
Distribution	Widely distributed, high concentrations in CNS, crosses placenta
Metabolism	Liver, extensively, GI mucosa
Excretion	Kidneys, breast milk
Half-life	26-36 hr

Pharmacodynamics	
Onset	Erratic
Peak	2-4 hr
Duration	8-12 hr

Interactions
Individual drugs
Alcohol: ↑ effects of both drugs, oversedation
Aluminum hydroxide: ↓ absorption
Bromocriptine: ↓ antiparkinson activity
Disopyramide: ↑ anticholinergic effects

Epinephrine: ↑ toxicity
Guanethidine: ↓ antihypertensive response
Levodopa: ↓ antiparkinson activity
Lithium: ↓ thioridazine levels, ↑ extrapyramidal symptoms, masking of lithium toxicity
Magnesium hydroxide: ↓ absorption
Norepinephrine: ↓ vasoresponse, ↑ toxicity
Phenobarbital: ↓ effectiveness, ↑ metabolism
Drug classifications
Antacids: ↓ absorption
Anticholinergics: ↑ anticholinergic effects
Antidepressants: ↑ CNS depression
Antidiarrheals, adsorbent: ↓ absorption
Antihistamines: ↑ CNS depression
Antihypertensives: ↑ hypotension
Antithyroid agents: ↑ agranulocytosis
Barbiturate anesthetics: ↑ CNS depression
β-Adrenergic blockers: ↑ effects of both drugs
General anesthetics: ↑ CNS depression
MAOIs: ↑ CNS depression
Opiates: ↑ CNS depression
Sedative/hypnotics: ↑ CNS depression
▨ *Herb/drug*
Kava: ↑ CNS depression
Lab test interferences
↑ Liver function tests, ↑ cardiac enzymes, ↑ cholesterol, ↑ blood glucose, ↑ prolactin, ↑ bilirubin, ↑ PBI, ↑ cholinesterase, ↑ ^{131}I, ↑ alk phosphatase, ↑ leukocytes, ↑ granulocytes, ↑ platelets
↓ Hormones (blood and urine)
False positive: Pregnancy tests, PKU, urine bilirubin

False negative: Urinary steroids, 17-OHCS

NURSING CONSIDERATIONS
Assessment
• Assess mental status: orientation, mood, behavior, presence of hallucinations, and type before initial administration and monthly; this drug should significantly reduce psychotic behavior
• Check for swallowing of PO medication; check for hoarding or giving of medication to other patients
• Monitor I&O ratio, palpate bladder if low urinary output occurs, especially in elderly; urinalysis recommended before, during prolonged therapy
• Monitor bilirubin, CBC, liver function studies monthly
• Assess affect, orientation, LOC, reflexes, gait, coordination, sleep pattern disturbances
• Monitor B/P sitting, standing and lying, take pulse and respirations q4h during initial treatment; establish baseline before starting treatment; report drops of 30 mm Hg; obtain baseline ECG, Q-wave and T-wave changes
• Check for dizziness, faintness, palpitations, tachycardia on rising; severe orthostatic hypotension is common
• Identify for neuroleptic malignant syndrome: hyperpyrexia, muscle rigidity, increased CPK, altered mental status; drug should be discontinued
• Assess for extrapyramidal symptoms including akathisia (inability to sit still, no pattern to movements), tardive dyskinesia (bizarre movements of the jaw, mouth, tongue, extremities), pseudoparkinsonism (ragged tremors, pill rolling, shuffling gate)—an antiparkinsonian drug should be prescribed
• Assess for constipation, urinary retention daily; if these occur, increase bulk, water in diet

Nursing diagnoses
☑ Thought processes, altered (uses)
☑ Coping, ineffective individual (uses)
☑ Knowledge deficit (teaching)
☑ Noncompliance (teaching)

Implementation
• Administer drug in liq form mixed in glass of juice or cola if hoarding is suspected; do not mix in caffeine drinks, tannics, pectins
G • Decrease dose in elderly; metabolism is slowed in the elderly
• Administer PO with full glass of water, milk; or give with food to decrease GI upset
• Store in tight, light-resistant container, oral sol in amber bottle

Patient/family education
• Teach patient to use good oral hygiene; frequent rinsing of mouth, sugarless gum for dry mouth
• Advise patient to avoid hazardous activities until drug response is determined; dizziness, blurred vision are common
• Inform patient that orthostatic hypotension occurs often and to rise from sitting or lying position gradually; to avoid hot tubs, hot showers, tub baths because hypotension may occur
• Instruct patient that in hot weather, heat stroke may occur; take extra precautions to stay cool

T

✦ Canada Only   Adverse effects: *italic* = common; **bold** = life-threatening

• Caution patient to avoid abrupt withdrawal of this drug, or extrapyramidal symptoms may result; drug should be withdrawn slowly

• Teach patient to avoid OTC preparations (cough, hay fever, cold) unless approved by prescriber—serious drug interactions may occur; avoid use with alcohol, CNS depressants—increased drowsiness may occur

• Advise patient to use a sunscreen and sunglasses to prevent burns

• Teach patient about extrapyramidal symptoms and necessity for meticulous oral hygiene because oral candidiasis may occur

• Advise patient to take antacids 2 hr before or after this drug

• Instruct patient to report sore throat, malaise, fever, bleeding, mouth sores; if these occur, CBC should be drawn and drug discontinued

Evaluation
Positive therapeutic outcome
• Decrease in emotional excitement, hallucinations, delusions, paranoia
• Reorganization of patterns of thought, speech

Treatment of overdose:
Lavage if orally ingested; provide airway; *do not induce vomiting or use epinephrine*

---

thiotepa (℞)
(thye-oh-tep′a)
Thioplex
Func. class.: Antineoplastic
Chem. class.: Alkylating agent
Pregnancy category   D

Action: Responsible for cross-linking DNA strands leading to cell death; activity is not cell–cycle-specific

➡ **Therapeutic Outcome:** Prevention of rapidly growing malignant cells

Uses: Hodgkin's disease, lymphomas; breast, ovarian, lung, bladder, cancer; neoplastic effusions

Dosage and routes
Adult: IV 0.3-0.4 mg/kg at 1-4 wk intervals

Neoplastic effusions
Adult: Intracavity 0.6-0.8 mg/kg

Bladder cancer
Adult: Instill 60 mg/30-60 ml water for inj instilled in bladder for 2 hr once weekly × 4 wk

Available forms: Powder for inj 15 mg

Adverse effects
CNS: Dizziness, headache
GI: Nausea, vomiting, anorexia
GU: Hyperuricemia, **hematuria, amenorrhea, azoospermia**
HEMA: **Thrombocytopenia, leukopenia, pancytopenia**
INTEG: Rash, pruritus

Contraindications: Hypersensitivity, pregnancy **D**

Precautions: Radiation therapy, bone marrow suppression, impaired renal or hepatic function

---

Pharmacokinetics

Absorption	Variably absorbed
Distribution	Unknown
Metabolism	Liver—extensively
Excretion	Kidneys
Half-life	Unknown

Pharmacodynamics

Unknown

Interactions
Individual drugs
Radiation: ↑ toxicity, bone marrow suppression
Succinylcholine: ↑ apnea
Drug classifications
Antineoplastics: ↑ toxicity, bone marrow suppression

NURSING CONSIDERATIONS
Assessment
◆• Assess symptoms indicating severe allergic reaction: rash, pruritus, urticaria, itching, flushing
• Monitor CBC, differential, platelet count weekly; withhold drug if WBC count is <4000/mm^3 or platelet count is <100,000/mm^3; notify prescriber of results if WBC <20,000/mm^3, platelets <150,000/mm^3
• Monitor renal function studies: BUN, creatinine, serum uric acid, urine CrCl before and during therapy; I&O ratio; report fall in urine output to <30 ml/hr
• Monitor temp q4h (may indicate beginning of infection)
• Monitor liver function tests before and during therapy [bilirubin, AST, ALT, LDH] as needed or monthly; jaundice, sclera, dark urine, clay-colored stools, itchy skin, abdominal pain, fever, diarrhea
• Assess for bleeding: hematuria, stool guaiac, bruising or petechiae, mucosa or orifices q8h; inflammation of mucosa, breaks in skin
• Identify dyspnea, rales, unproductive cough, chest pain, tachypnea
• Identify effects of alopecia on body image; discuss feelings about body changes

Nursing diagnoses
☑ Injury, risk for (adverse reactions)
☑ Body image disturbance (adverse reactions)
☑ Infection, risk for (adverse reactions)
☑ Knowledge deficit (teaching)

Implementation
• Give fluids **IV** or PO before chemotherapy to hydrate patient
• Give antacid before oral agent, give drug after evening meal, before bedtime; antiemetic 30-60 min before giving drug to prevent vomiting, and prn; antibiotics for prophylaxis of infection
• Give top or syst analgesics for pain
• Give liq diet: carbonated beverages; gelatin may be added if patient is not nauseated or vomiting
• Provide rinsing of mouth tid-qid with water, club soda; brushing of teeth bid-qid with soft brush or cotton-tipped applicators for stomatitis; use unwaxed dental floss
IV route
Direct route
• Give **IV** after diluting 15 mg/1.5 ml of sterile H_2O for inj; give over 1-3 min, use a 0.22 micron filter
Intermittent inf
• May be further diluted in 50-100 ml D_5W, 0.9% NaCl, Ringer's, LR

T

Syringe compatibilities:
Procaine HCl, (2%), epinephrine 1:1000

Y-site compatibilities:
Acyclovir, allopurinol, amifostine, amikacin, aminophylline, amphotericin B, ampicillin, ampicillin/sulbactam, aztreonam, bleomycin, bumetanide, buprenorphine, butorphanol, calcium gluconate, carboplatin, carmustine, cefazolin, cefepime, cefonicid, cefoperazone, cefotaxime, cefotetan, cefoxitin, ceftazidime, ceftizoxime, ceftriaxone, cefuroxime, chlorpromazine, cimetidine, ciprofloxacin, clindamycin, cyclophosphamide, cytarabine, dacarbazine, dactinomycin, daunorubicin, diphenhydramine, dobutamine, dopamine, doxorubicin, doxycycline, droperidol, enalaprilat, etoposide, famotidine, floxuridine, fluconazole, fludarabine, fluorouracil, furosemide, gallium, ganciclovir, gentamicin, granisetron, haloperidol, heparin, hydrocortisone, hydromorphone, hydroxyzine, idarubicin, ifosfamide, imipenemcilastatin, leucovorin, lorazepam, magnesium sulfate, mannitol, melphalan, meperidine, mesna, methotrexate, methylprednisolone, metoclopramide, metronidazole, mezlocillin, miconazole, mitomycin, mitoxantrone, morphine, nalbuphine, netilmicin, ofloxacin, ondansetron, paclitaxel, piperacillin, piperacillin/tazobactam, plicamycin, potassium chloride, prochlorperazine, promethazine, ranitidine, sodium bicarbonate, streptozocin, teniposide, ticarcillin, ticarcillin/clavulanate, tobramycin, trimethoprim-sulfamethoxazole, vancomycin, vinblastine, vincristine, zidovudine

Instill route
• Reconstitute solution, then mix 60 mg/30-60 ml sterile water; instill by Foley catheter; patient's position may be changed every few min; the patient must retain sol for 2 hr to provide for cell death

Intracavity route
• Reconstitute sol and administer by effusion tube as directed

Patient/family education
• Caution patient to avoid use of products containing aspirin or NSAIDs, razors, commercial mouthwash because bleeding may occur; to report symptoms of bleeding (hematuria, tarry stools)
• Advise patient to report signs of anemia, (fatigue, headache, irritability, faintness, shortness of breath)
• Advise patient to report any changes in breathing or coughing even several mo after treatment; to avoid crowds or persons with respiratory or other infections
• Inform patient that hair may be lost during treatment; a wig or hairpiece may make patient feel better; new hair may be different in color, texture
• Caution patient not to have any vaccinations without the advice of the prescriber because serious reactions can occur
• Advise patient that contraception is needed during treatment and for several mo after the completion of therapy

Evaluation
Positive therapeutic outcome
• Prevention of rapid division of malignant cells

☑ Herb/drug 🚫 Do Not Crush ◆ Alert ☞ Key Drug 🄶 Geriatric 🄿 Pediatric

thiothixene (℞)
(thye-oh-thix'een)
Navane, thiothixene
Func. class.:
Antipsychotic/neuroleptic
Chem. class.: Thioxan-
thene
Pregnancy category C

Action: Depresses cerebral
cortex, hypothalamus, limbic
system, which control activity,
aggression; blocks neurotransmission produced by dopamine
at synapse; exhibits strong
α-adrenergic blocking action;
mechanism for antipsychotic
effects is unclear

➡**Therapeutic Outcome:** Decreased signs and symptoms of
psychosis

Uses: Psychotic disorders,
schizophrenia, acute agitation

Dosage and routes
Adult: PO 2-5 mg bid-qid
depending on severity of condition; dose gradually increased
to 15-30 mg if needed; IM 4
mg bid-qid; max dose 30 mg
qd; administer PO dose as
soon as possible

G*Elderly:* PO 1-2 mg qd-bid,
increase by 1-2 mg q4-7 days
to desired dose

Available forms: Caps 1, 2, 5,
10, 20 mg; conc 5 mg/ml; inj
2 mg/ml; powder for inj 5
mg/ml

Adverse effects
*CNS: Extrapyramidal
symptoms: pseudoparkinsonism,
akathisia, dystonia, tardive
dyskinesia,* seizures, *headache*
CV: Orthostatic hypotension,
hypertension, **cardiac arrest,**
ECG changes, **tachycardia**

EENT: Blurred vision, glaucoma
*GI: Dry mouth, nausea, vomit-
ing, anorexia, constipation,*
diarrhea, jaundice, weight gain
GU: Urinary retention, urinary
frequency, enuresis, impotence,
amenorrhea, gynecomastia
HEMA: Anemia, **leukopenia,
leukocytosis, agranulocytosis**
INTEG: Rash, photosensitivity,
dermatitis
RESP: **Laryngospasm,** dyspnea, **respiratory depression**

Contraindications: Hypersen-
Psitivity, blood dyscrasias, child
<12 yr, bone marrow depres-
sion, circulatory collapse, CNS
depression, coma, alcoholism,
CV disease, hepatic disease,
Reye's syndrome, narrow-angle
glaucoma

Precautions: Pregnancy **C,**
lactation, seizure disorders,
hypertension, hepatic disease,
Gelderly

◆**Do Not Confuse:**
Navane/Norvasc

Pharmacokinetics	
Absorption	Well absorbed (PO, IM)
Distribution	Widely distributed, crosses placenta
Metabolism	Liver
Excretion	Kidneys, breast milk
Half-life	34 hr

Pharmacodynamics		
	PO	IM
Onset	Slow	15-30 min
Peak	2-8 hr	1-6 hr
Duration	Up to 12 hr	Up to 12 hr

Interactions
Individual drugs
Alcohol: ↑ effects of both
drugs, oversedation
Aluminum hydroxide: ↓ ab-
sorption

T

Adverse effects: *italic* = common; **bold** = life-threatening

Bromocriptine: ↓ antiparkinson activity

Disopyramide: ↑ anticholinergic effects

Guanethidine: ↓ antihypertensive response

Levodopa: ↓ antiparkinson activity

Lithium: ↓ chlorpromazine levels, ↑ extrapyramidal symptoms, masking of lithium toxicity

Magnesium hydroxide: ↓ absorption

Norepinephrine: ↓ vasoresponse, ↑ toxicity

Phenobarbital: ↓ effectiveness, ↑ metabolism

Drug classifications

Antacids: ↓ absorption

Anticholinergics: ↑ anticholinergic effects

Antidepressants: ↑ CNS depression

Antidiarrheals, adsorbent: ↓ absorption

Antihistamines: ↑ CNS depression

Antihypertensives: ↑ hypotension

Antithyroid agents: ↑ agranulocytosis

Barbiturate anesthetics: ↑ CNS depression

β-Adrenergic blockers: ↑ effects of both drugs

General anesthetics: ↑ CNS depression

MAOIs: ↑ CNS depression

Opiates: ↑ CNS depression

Sedative/hypnotics: ↑ CNS depression

Herb/drug

Kava: ↑ CNS depression

Lab test interferences

↑ Liver function tests, ↑ cardiac enzymes, ↑ cholesterol, ↑ blood glucose, ↑ prolactin, ↑ bilirubin, ↑ PBI, ↑ cholinesterase, ↑ ^{131}I, ↑ alk phosphatase, ↑ leukocytes, ↑ granulocytes, ↑ platelets

↓ Hormones (blood and urine)

False positive: Pregnancy tests, PKU, urine bilirubin

False negative: Urinary steroids, 17-OHCS

NURSING CONSIDERATIONS
Assessment

• Assess mental status: orientation, mood, behavior, presence of hallucinations (and type) before initial administration and monthly; this drug should significantly reduce psychotic behavior

• Check for swallowing of PO medication; check for hoarding or giving of medication to other patients

• Monitor I&O ratio, palpate bladder if low urinary output occurs, especially in elderly; urinalysis recommended before, during prolonged therapy

• Monitor bilirubin, CBC, liver function studies monthly

• Assess affect, orientation, LOC, reflexes, gait, coordination, sleep pattern disturbances

• Monitor B/P sitting, standing and lying, take pulse and respirations q4h during initial treatment; establish baseline before starting treatment; report drops of 30 mm Hg; obtain baseline ECG, Q-wave and T-wave changes

• Check for dizziness, faintness, palpitations, tachycardia on rising; severe orthostatic hypotension is common

• Identify for neuroleptic malignant syndrome: hyperpyrexia, muscle rigidity, increased CPK, altered mental status; drug should be discontinued

• Assess for extrapyramidal symptoms including akathisia (inability to sit still, no pattern

---

Herb/drug   Do Not Crush   ◆ Alert   Key Drug   G Geriatric   P Pediatric to movements), tardive dyskinesia (bizarre movements of the jaw, mouth, tongue, extremities), pseudoparkinsonism (ragged tremors, pill rolling, shuffling gait); an antiparkinson drug should be prescribed

• Assess for constipation, urinary retention daily; if these occur, increase bulk, water in diet

Nursing diagnoses
☑ Thought processes, altered (uses)
☑ Coping, ineffective individual (uses)
☑ Knowledge deficit (teaching)
☑ Noncompliance (teaching)

Implementation
PO route
• Give drug in liq form mixed in glass of juice or cola if hoarding is suspected; do not mix in caffeine drinks, tannics, pectins

G • Give decreased dose to elderly because metabolism is slowed in the elderly

• Give PO with full glass of water, milk; or give with food to decrease GI upset

• Store in tight, light-resistant container; store oral sol in amber bottle

IM route
• Dilute 10 mg vial/2.2 ml sterile water for inj to 5 mg/ml

• Inj in deep muscle mass, do not give SC; do not administer sol with a precipitate

Syringe compatibilities:
Benztropine, diphenhydramine, hydroxyzine

Patient/family education
• Teach patient to use good oral hygiene; frequent rinsing of mouth, sugarless gum for dry mouth

• Advise patient to avoid hazardous activities until drug response is determined; dizziness, blurred vision is common

• Inform patient that orthostatic hypotension occurs often and to rise from sitting or lying position gradually and to remain lying down after IM inj for at least 30 min; tell patient to avoid hot tubs, hot showers, tub baths because hypotension may occur; tell patient that in hot weather, heat stroke may occur, so to take extra precautions to stay cool

• Caution patient to avoid abrupt withdrawal of this drug, or extrapyramidal symptoms may result; drug should be withdrawn slowly

• Teach patient to avoid OTC preparations (cough, hayfever, cold) unless approved by prescriber, because serious drug interactions may occur; avoid use with alcohol, CNS depressants because increased drowsiness may occur

• Caution patient to use a sunscreen and sunglasses to prevent burns

• Teach patient about extrapyramidal symptoms and necessity of meticulous oral hygiene because oral candidiasis may occur

• Tell patient to take antacids 2 hr before or after this drug

• Advise patient to report sore throat, malaise, fever, bleeding, mouth sores; if these occur, CBC should be measured and drug discontinued

Evaluation
Positive therapeutic outcome
• Decrease in emotional excitement, hallucinations, delusions, paranoia

• Reorganization of patterns of thought, speech

Treatment of overdose:
Lavage if orally ingested; provide airway; *do not induce vomiting or use epinephrine*

thyroid USP (desiccated) (℞)
(thye′roid)
Armour Thyroid, Cholaxin ✦, S-P-T, Thyrar, Thyroid Strong, thyroid USP
Func. class.: Thyroid hormone
Chem. class.: Active thyroid hormone in natural state and ratio
Pregnancy category **A**

Action: Increases metabolic rates; controls protein synthesis; increases cardiac output, renal blood flow, O_2 consumption, body temp, blood volume, growth, development at cellular level

➡ **Therapeutic Outcome:** Correction of lack of thyroid hormone

Uses: Hypothyroidism, cretinism (juvenile hypothyroidism), myxedema

Dosage and routes
Hypothyroidism
Adult: PO 65 mg qd, increased by 65 mg q30d until desired response; maintenance dose 65-195 mg qd

G *Geriatric:* PO 7.5-15 mg qd, double dose q6-8w until desired response

Cretinism/juvenile hypothyroidism
P *Child over 1 yr:* PO up to 180 mg qd titrated to response
P *Child 4-12 mo:* PO 30-60 mg qd

P *Child 1-4 mo:* PO 15-30 mg qd; may increase q2w; titrated to response; maintenance dose 30-45 mg qd

Myxedema
Adult: PO 16 mg qd, double dose q2w, maintenance 65-195 mg/day

Available forms: Tabs 15, 30, 60, 90, 120 mg; enteric-coated tabs 30, 60, 120 mg; sugar-coated tabs 30, 60, 120, 180 mg; caps pork 60, 90, 120, 180 mg; tabs bovine 30, 60, 120 mg

Adverse effects
CNS: *Insomnia, tremors,* headache, thyroid storm
CV: *Tachycardia, palpitations, angina,* **dysrhythmias,** hypertension, **cardiac arrest**
GI: Nausea, diarrhea, increased or decreased appetite, cramps
MISC: Menstrual irregularities, weight loss, sweating, heat intolerance, fever

Contraindications: Adrenal insufficiency, MI, thyrotoxicosis

G **Precautions:** Elderly, angina pectoris, hypertension, ischemia, cardiac disease, pregnancy **A,** lactation

N **Do Not Confuse:**
Thyrar/Thyrolar

Pharmacokinetics	
Absorption	Well absorbed
Distribution	Widely distributed, does not cross placenta
Metabolism	Liver, tissues
Excretion	Feces via bile, breast milk
Half-life	T_3—2 days; T_4—1 wk

Pharmacodynamics	
Onset	1 hr
Peak	12-48 hr
Duration	Unknown

Interactions
Individual drugs
Cholestyramine: ↓ absorption of thyroid hormone

Colestipol: ↓ absorption of thyroid hormone

Digitalis: ↓ effect of digitalis

Insulin: ↑ requirement for insulin

Phenytoin (IV): ↑ release of thyroid hormone

Drug classifications
Amphetamines: ↑ CNS, cardiac stimulation

β-Adrenergic blockers: ↓ effect of beta blockers

Decongestants: ↑ CNS, cardiac stimulation

Oral anticoagulants: ↑ requirements for anticoagulants

Vasopressors: ↑ CNS, cardiac stimulation

Herb/drug
Bugleweed: Do not use together

Lab test interferences
↑ CPK, ↑ LDH, ↑ AST, ↑ PBI, ↑ blood glucose
↓ thyroid function tests

NURSING CONSIDERATIONS
Assessment
• Identify if the patient is taking anticoagulants, antidiabetic agents; document on chart

• Take B/P, pulse before each dose; monitor I&O ratio and weight every day in same clothing, using same scale, at same time of day

• Monitor height, weight, psychomotor development, and growth rate if given to a child

• Monitor T_3, T_4, FTIs, which are decreased; radioimmunoassay of TSH, which is increased; radio uptake, which is increased if patient is on too low a dose of medication

• Monitor pro-time—patient may require decreased dosage of anticoagulant; check for bleeding, bruising

• Assess for increased nervousness, excitability, irritability, which may indicate that dose of medication is too high, usually after 1-3 wk of treatment

• Assess cardiac status: angina, palpitation, chest pain, change in vital signs; the elderly patient may have undetected cardiac problems and baseline ECG should be completed before treatment

Nursing diagnoses
☑ Knowledge deficit (teaching)
☑ Noncompliance (teaching)

Implementation
• Give in AM if possible as a single dose to decrease sleeplessness; at same time each day to maintain drug level

• Give only for hormone imbalances; not to be used for obesity, male infertility, menstrual conditions, lethargy; give lowest dose that relieves symptoms; lower dose to the elderly and in cardiac diseases

• Store in tight, light-resistant container

• Wean patient off medication 4 wk before RAIU test

Patient/family education
• Teach patient that drug is not a cure but controls symptoms and that treatment is long-term

T

• Instruct patient to report excitability, irritability, anxiety, sweating, heat intolerance, chest pain, palpitations, which indicate overdose

• Advise patient not to switch brands unless approved by prescriber; bioavailability may differ; do not take with food; absorption will be decreased

• Teach patient that drug may be discontinued after giving birth; thyroid panel will be evaluated after 1-2 mo

P • Teach patient that hyperthyroid child will show almost immediate behavior/personality change; that hair loss will occur **P** in child and is temporary

• Caution patient that drug is not to be taken to reduce weight

• Caution patient to avoid OTC preparations containing iodine; read labels; other medications should not be used unless approved by health-care prescriber

• Teach patient to avoid iodine-containing food: iodized salt, soybeans, tofu, turnips, certain kinds of seafood and bread

Evaluation
Positive therapeutic outcome
• Absence of depression
• Weight loss, increased diuresis, pulse, appetite
• Absence of constipation, peripheral edema, cold intolerance, pale, cool dry skin, brittle nails, alopecia, coarse hair, menorrhagia, night blindness, paresthesias, syncope, stupor, coma, rosy cheeks
• Improved levels of T_3, T_4 by laboratory tests
P • Child: Age-appropriate weight, height, and psychomotor development

Treatment of overdose: Withhold dose for up to 1 wk, acute overdose—gastric lavage or induce emesis, then activated charcoal; provide supportive treatment to control symptoms

---

tiagabine (℞)
(tie-ah-ga′been)
Gabatril
Func. class.: Anticonvulsant

Pregnancy category   C

Action: Mechanism unknown; may increase seizure threshold

Uses: Adjunct treatment of partial seizures

Dosage and routes
Adult: PO 4 mg qd, may increase by 4-8 mg qwk until desired response, max 56 mg/day

P *Child 12-18 yr:* PO 4 mg qd, may increase by 4 mg at beginning of wk 2, may increase by 4-8 mg of wk until desired response, max 32 mg/day

Available forms: Tabs 4, 12, 16, 20 mg

Adverse effects
CNS: Dizziness, anxiety, somnolence, ataxia, amnesia, unsteady gait, depression
CV: Vasodilation
GI: Nausea, diarrhea, vomiting
INTEG: Pruritus, rash
RESP: Pharyngitis, coughing

Contraindications: Hypersensitivity to this drug

Precautions: Hepatic disease, **P** renal disease, pregnancy **C**, **G** lactation, child <12 yr, elderly

---

⬚ Herb/drug ⬔ Do Not Crush ◆ Alert ⚷ Key Drug **G** Geriatric **P** Pediatric

Pharmacokinetics

Absorption	>95%
Distribution	Unknown
Metabolism	Liver
Excretion	Kidneys
Half-life	7-9 hr

Pharmacodynamics

Unknown

Interactions: Unknown

NURSING CONSIDERATIONS
Assessment
• Monitor renal studies: urinalysis, BUN, urine creatinine q3mo
• Monitor hepatic studies: ALT, AST, bilirubin
• Assess description of seizures
• Assess mental status: mood, sensorium, affect, behavioral changes; if mental status changes, notify prescriber
• Assess eye problems, need for ophthalmic examinations before, during, after treatment (slit lamp, funduscopy, tonometry)
• Assess allergic reaction: purpura, red raised rash; if these occur, drug should be discontinued

Implementation
• Store at room temp away from heat and light
• Provide hard candy, frequent rinsing of mouth, gum for dry mouth
• Provide assistance with ambulation during early part of treatment; dizziness occurs
• Provide seizure precautions: padded side rails; move objects that may harm patient
• Provide increased fluids, bulk in diet for constipation

Patient/family education
• Advise patient to carry Medic Alert ID stating patient's name, drugs taken, condition, prescriber's name and phone number
• Advise patient to avoid driving, other activities that require alertness
• Teach patient not to discontinue medication quickly after long-term use

Evaluation
Positive therapeutic outcome
• Decreased seizure activity; document on patient's chart

Treatment of overdose: Lavage, VS

ticarcillin (℞)
(tye-kar-sill'in)
ticar
Func. class.: Broad-spectrum antiinfective
Chem. class.: Extended-spectrum penicillin
Pregnancy category B

Action: Interferes with cell wall replication of susceptible organisms; osmotically unstable cell wall swells, bursts from osmotic pressure

➡ **Therapeutic Outcome:** Decreased symptoms of infection

Uses: Respiratory, soft tissue, urinary tract infections, bacterial septicemia; effective for gram-positive cocci *(Staphylococcus aureus, Streptococcus faecalis, S. pneumoniae),* gram-negative cocci *(Neisseria gonorrhoeae),* gram-positive bacilli *(Clostridium perfringens, C. tetani),* gram-negative bacilli *(Bacteroides, F. nucleatum, E. coli, P. mirabilis, Salmonella, M. morganii, P. rettgeri, Enterobacter, P. aeruginosa, Serra-*

T

tia, Peptococcus, Peptostreptococcus, Eubacterium)

Dosage and routes
Adult: **IV**/IM 4-24 g/day in divided doses q4-6h; infuse over ½-2 hr

P *Child:* **IV**/IM 50-300 mg/kg/day in divided doses q4-8h

P *Neonate:* **IV** inf 75-100 mg/kg/8-12 hr

Renal dose
CrCl <30 ml/min reduce dose

Available forms: Inj 1, 3, 6, 20, 30 g

Adverse effects
CNS: Lethargy, hallucinations, anxiety, depression, twitching, **coma, convulsions**
GI: *Nausea, vomiting, diarrhea;* increased AST, ALT, abdominal pain, glossitis, colitis
GU: Oliguria, proteinuria, hematuria, *vaginitis, moniliasis,* **glomerulonephritis**
HEMA: Anemia, increased bleeding time, **bone marrow depression, granulocytopenia**
INTEG: Rash
META: Hypokalemia

Contraindications: Hypersensitivity to penicillins

Precautions: Hypersensitivity to cephalosporins, pregnancy **B**, lactation, renal disease

Pharmacokinetics

Absorption	Unknown
Distribution	Widely, breast milk
Metabolism	Liver, small amount
Excretion	Kidneys
Half-life	70 min

Pharmacodynamics

	IM	IV
Onset	Unknown	Unknown
Peak	1 hr	30-45 min
Duration	4-6 hr	4 hr

Interactions
Individual drugs
Aspirin: ↑ ticarcillin concentration
Heparin: ↑ effect of heparin
Probenecid: ↑ ticarcillin concentrations
Drug classifications
Aminoglycosides, IV: ↓ effect of ticarcillin
Erythromycins: ↓ effect of ticarcillin
Neuromuscular blockers: ↑ effect of neuromuscular blockers
Tetracyclines: ↓ effect of ticarcillin
☑ *Herb/drug*
Khat: ↓ absorption
Lab test interferences
False positive: Urine glucose, urine protein

NURSING CONSIDERATIONS
Assessment
• Monitor I&O ratio; report hematuria, oliguria, since penicillin in high doses is nephrotoxic
◆• Monitor any patient with compromised renal system, since drug is excreted slowly in poor renal system function; toxicity may occur rapidly
• Monitor liver studies: AST, ALT
• Monitor blood studies: WBC, RBC, Hgb, Hct, bleeding time
• Monitor renal studies: urinalysis, protein, blood, BUN, creatinine
• Monitor C&S before drug therapy; drug may be given as soon as culture is taken
• Assess bowel pattern before, during treatment
• Check for skin eruptions after administration of penicillin to 1 wk after discontinuing drug

- Assess respiratory status: rate, character, wheezing, tightness in chest
- Assess allergies before initiation of treatment, reaction of each medication; highlight allergies on chart

Implementation
- Give **IV** after diluting 1 g or less/4 ml sterile H_2O for inj; dilute further with 10-20 ml or more D_5W, NS, or sterile H_2O for inj sol; give 1 g or less/5 min or more or by intermittent inf over ½-2 hr or by continuous inf at prescribed rate

Y-site compatibilities: Acyclovir, allopurinol, amifostine, aztreonam, cyclophosphamide, diltiazem, famotidine, filgrastim, fludarabine, granisetron, hydromorphone, heparin, IL-2, regular insulin, magnesium sulfate, melphalan, meperidine, morphine, ondansetron, perphenazine, propofol, sargramostim, teniposide, theophylline, thiotepa, verapamil, vinorelbine

Additive compatibilities: Ranitidine, verapamil
- Give drug after C&S has been completed
- Have adrenalin, suction, tracheostomy set, endotracheal intubation equipment
- Provide adequate fluid intake (2 L) during diarrhea episodes
- Provide scratch test to assess allergy on order from prescriber; usually done when penicillin is only drug of choice
- Store at room temp, reconstituted sol 72 hr at room temp

Evaluation
Positive therapeutic outcome
- Absence of fever, purulent drainage, redness, inflammation

Patient/family education
- Advise that culture may be taken after completed course of medication
- Teach to report sore throat, fever, fatigue (may indicate superinfection)
- Teach to wear or carry Medic Alert ID if allergic to penicillins
- Advise to notify nurse of diarrhea

Treatment of overdose: Withdraw drug, maintain airway, administer epinephrine, aminophylline, O_2, **IV** corticosteroids for anaphylaxis

ticarcillin/ clavulanate (℞)
(tye-kar-sill'in)
Chem. class: Broad-spectrum antibiotic
Func. class.: Extended-spectrum penicillin
Pregnancy category B

Action: Interferes with cell wall replication of susceptible organisms; osmotically unstable cell wall swells, bursts from osmotic pressure

Therapeutic Outcome: Resolution of infection

Uses: Respiratory, soft tissue, urinary tract infections; bacterial septicemia; effective for gram-positive cocci (*Staphylococcus aureus, Streptococcus faecalis, S. pneumoniae*), gram-negative cocci (*Neisseria gonorrhoeae*), gram-positive bacilli (*Clostridium perfringens, C. tetani*), gram-negative bacilli (*Bacteroides, Fusobacterium nucleatum, Escherichia coli, Proteus mirabilis, Salmonella,*

Morganella morganii, Proteus rettgeri, Enterobacter, Pseudomonas aeruginosa, Serratia, Peptococcus, Peptostreptococcus, Eubacterium)

Dosage and routes
Adult: **IV** inf 1 vial containing ticarcillin 3 g, clavulanate K 0.1 g q4-6h, infuse over 30 min

P *Child <60 kg:* **IV** 200-300 mg ticarcillin/kg/day in divided doses q4-6h

Available forms: Inj IM, **IV** 3 g ticarcillin and 0.1 g clavulanate; **IV** inf 3 g ticarcillin and 0.1 g clavulanate; discs 75 µg ticarcillin, 10 µg clavulanate; powder for inj 3 g ticarcillin, 0.1 g clavulanate, 30 g ticarcillin, 1 g clavulanate

Adverse effects
CNS: Lethargy, hallucinations, anxiety, depression, twitching, **coma, convulsions**
GI: *Nausea, vomiting, diarrhea,* increased AST, ALT, abdominal pain, glossitis, colitis
GU: Oliguria, proteinuria, hematuria, *vaginitis, moniliasis,* **glomerulonephritis**
HEMA: Anemia, increased bleeding time, **bone marrow depression, granulocytopenia**
META: Hypokalemia, hypokalemia, alkalosis, hypernatremia

Contraindications: Hypersensitivity to penicillins

Precautions: Hypersensitivity to cephalosporins, pregnancy **B**

Pharmacokinetics
Absorption	Completely absorbed (**IV**)
Distribution	Widely distributed, crosses blood-brain barrier
Metabolism	Liver
Excretion	Kidneys
Half-life	64-68 min

Pharmacodynamics
	IV
Onset	Unknown
Peak	30-45 min
Duration	4 hr

Interactions
Individual drugs
Cholestyramine: ↓ absorption of thyroid hormone
Colestipol: ↓ absorption of thyroid hormone
Digitalis: ↓ effect of digitalis
Insulin: ↑ requirement for insulin
Phenytoin (IV): ↑ release of thyroid hormone
Drug classifications
Amphetamines: ↑ CNS, cardiac stimulation
β-Adrenergic blockers: ↓ effect of beta blockers
Decongestants: ↑ CNS, cardiac stimulation
Oral anticoagulants: ↑ requirements for anticoagulants
Vasopressors: ↑ CNS, cardiac stimulation
☑ *Herb/drug*
Khat: ↓ absorption
Lab test interferences
False positive: Urine glucose, urine protein Coombs' test

NURSING CONSIDERATIONS
Assessment
• Monitor I&O ratio; report hematuria, oliguria because penicillin in high doses is nephrotoxic
• Monitor any patient with compromised renal system

---

because drug is excreted slowly in poor renal system function; toxicity may occur rapidly
• Monitor liver studies: AST, ALT
• Monitor studies: WBC, RBC, H&H, bleeding time
• Monitor renal studies: urinalysis, protein, blood
• Obtain C&S test results before initiating drug therapy; drug may be given as soon as culture is taken
• Assess bowel pattern before, during treatment
• Assess skin eruptions after administration of penicillin to 1 wk after discontinuing drug
• Assess respiratory status: rate, character, wheezing, and tightness in chest
• Assess allergies before initiation of treatment, reaction of each medication; highlight allergies on chart, Kardex

Nursing diagnoses
☑ Infection, risk for (uses)
☑ Knowledge deficit (teaching)

Implementation
IV **IV route**
• Give **IV** after diluting 3.1 g or less/13 ml of sterile H_2O or NaCl (200 mg/ml), shake; may further dilute in 50-100 ml or more normal saline, D_5W, or LR sol and run over ½ hr

Y-site compatibilities:
Allopurinol, aztreonam, cefepime, cyclophosphamide, diltiazem, famotidine, filgrastim, fluconazole, fludarabine, foscarnet, heparin, regular insulin, melphalan, meperidine, morphine, ondansetron, perphenazine, sargramostim, teniposide, theophylline, vinorelbine
• Give drug after C&S has been completed

• Have adrenalin, suction, tracheostomy set, endotracheal intubation equipment available
• Give adequate fluid intake (2 L) during diarrhea episodes
• Obtain scratch test results to assess allergy after securing order from prescriber—usually done when penicillin is only drug of choice
• Store at room temp, reconstituted sol for 12-24 hr or 3-7 days refrigerated

Patient/family education
• Advise patient that culture may be taken after completed course of medication
• Instruct patient to report sore throat, fever, fatigue (may indicate super infection)
• Advise patient to wear or carry Medic Alert ID if allergic to penicillins

Evaluation
Positive therapeutic outcome
• Absence of fever, purulent drainage, redness, inflammation

Treatment of overdose:
Withdraw drug, maintain airway, administer epinephrine, aminophylline, O_2, **IV** corticosteroids for anaphylaxis

---

ticlopidine (Ⓡ)
(tye-cloe'pi-deen)
Ticlid
Func. class.: Platelet aggregation inhibitor
Pregnancy category   B

Action: Inhibits first and second phases of ADP-induced effects in platelet aggregation

➤**Therapeutic Outcome:** Decreased stroke by decreasing platelet aggregation

T

Uses: Reducing the risk of stroke in high-risk patients

Investigational uses: Intermittent claudication, chronic arterial occlusion, subarachnoid hemorrhage, uremic patients with AV shunts/fistulas, open heart surgery, coronary artery bypass grafts, primary glomerulonephritis

Dosage and routes
Adult: PO 250 mg bid with food

Available forms: Tab 250 mg

Adverse effects
CNS: Dizziness
GI: Nausea, vomiting, diarrhea, GI discomfort, **cholestatic jaundice, hepatitis,** increased cholesterol LDL, VLDL
HEMA: **Bleeding (epistaxis, hematuria, conjunctival hemorrhage, GI bleeding), agranulocytosis, neutropenia, thrombocytopenia**
INTEG: Rash, pruritus

Contraindications: Hypersensitivity, active liver disease, blood dyscrasias, active bleeding

Precautions: Past liver disease, G renal disease, elderly, pregnancy **B**, lactation, children, increased bleeding risk

Pharmacokinetics	
Absorption	Well absorbed
Distribution	Unknown
Metabolism	Liver—extensively
Excretion	Kidneys—unchanged drug
Half-life	Increased with repeat dosing; 4-5 days (multiple doses)

Pharmacodynamics	
Onset	Unknown
Peak	1-3 hr
Duration	Unknown

Interactions
Individual drugs
Aspirin: ↑ bleeding tendencies
Cimetidine: ↑ effects of ticlopidine
Digoxin: ↓ plasma levels of ticlopidine
Theophylline: ↑ effects of theophylline
Drug classifications
Antacids: ↓ plasma levels of ticlopidine
Anticoagulants: ↑ bleeding tendencies

NURSING CONSIDERATIONS
Assessment
• Monitor liver function studies: AST, ALT, bilirubin, creatinine if patient is on long-term therapy (4 mo or more)
• Monitor blood studies: CBC, Hct, Hgb, pro-time if patient is on long-term; CBC q2 wk × 3 mo therapy; thrombocytopenia, neutropenia may occur

Nursing diagnoses
☑ Injury, risk for (uses)
☑ Knowledge deficit (teaching)

Implementation
• Give with food to decrease gastric symptoms

Patient/family education
• Advise patient that blood work will be necessary during treatment
• Advise patient to report any unusual bleeding to prescriber
• Instruct patient to take with food or just after eating to minimize GI discomfort
• Caution patient to report side effects such as diarrhea, skin rashes, subcutaneous

---

bleeding, signs of cholestasis (yellow skin and sclera, dark urine, light-colored stools)

Evaluation
Positive therapeutic outcome
• Absence of stroke

---

tiludronate (℞)
(till-oo′droe-nate)
Skelid
Func. class.: Parathyroid agent (calcium regulator)
Chem. class.: Bisphos-phonate
Pregnancy category   C

Action: Decreases bone reabsorption and new bone development

▸**Therapeutic Outcome:** Decreased bone reabsorption and reduced calcium levels WNL

Uses: Paget's disease

Dosage and routes
Adult: PO 400 mg qd, with 8 oz water × 3 mo

Available forms: Tab 240 mg

Adverse effects
CNS: Headache, somnolence, dizziness, anxiety, vertigo, nervousness, involuntary movements
ENDO: Hyperparathyroidism
GI: Nausea, diarrhea, dry mouth, gastritis, vomiting, flatulence, gastric ulcers
GU: **Nephrotoxicity,** UTI
INTEG: Rash, epidermal necrosis, pruritus, sweating
MS: Bone pain, decreased mineralization of nonaffected bones, pathologic fractures
RESP: Rhinitis, rales, sinusitis, URI

Contraindications: Hypersensitivity to bisphosphonates, P pathologic fractures, children, colitis, severe renal disease with creatinine >5 mg/dl

Precautions: Pregnancy **C,** renal disease, lactation, restricted vit D/Ca, GI disease

Pharmacokinetics	
Absorption	Rapid
Distribution	Unknown, steady state 10 days
Metabolism	None
Excretion	Feces (unabsorbed), kidney (unchanged)
Half-life	150 hrs

Pharmacodynamics	
Onset	Unknown
Peak	Unknown
Duration	6 mo

Interactions
Individual drugs
Aspirin: ↓ effect of tiludronate
Indomethacin: ↑ effect of tiludronate
Drug classifications
Antacids: ↓ absorption of tiludronate
Mineral supplements with magnesium, calcium, or aluminum: ↓ absorption of tiludronate

NURSING CONSIDERATIONS
Assessment
• Assess for GI symptoms, polyuria, flushing, head swelling, tingling, headache—may indicate hypercalcemia; nervousness, irritability, twitching, seizures, spasm, paresthesia indicates hypocalcemia at start of treatment
• Identify nutritional status; evaluate diet for sources of vitamin D (milk, some seafood), calcium (dairy products,

T

dark green vegetables), phosphates
• Monitor BUN, creatinine, uric acid, chloride, electrolytes, urine pH, urinary calcium, magnesium, phosphate, urinalysis (calcium should be kept at 9-10 mg/dl), albumin, alk phosphatase baseline and q3-6 mo; check urine sediment for casts throughout treatment
• Assess for increased drug level—toxic reactions occur rapidly; have calcium chloride or gluconate on hand if calcium level drops too low; check for tetany

Nursing diagnoses
☑ Injury, risk for (adverse reactions)
☑ Pain, chronic (uses)
☑ Knowledge deficit (teaching)

Implementation
• Administer on empty stomach to improve absorption (2 hr ac), with 6-8 oz water

Patient/family education
• Caution patient to notify prescriber of hypercalcemic relapse: renal calculi, nausea, vomiting, thirst, lethargy, deep bone or flank pain
• Teach patient to follow a low-calcium diet as prescribed (Paget's disease, hypercalcemia)
• Advise patient to notify prescriber of diarrhea, nausea; dose may be divided to lessen these symptoms

Evaluation
Positive therapeutic outcome
• Calcium levels 9-10 mg/dl
• Decreasing symptoms of Paget's disease including pain

---

timolol (R)
(tye'moe-lole)
Apo-Timol ✦, Blocadren, timolol maleate, Timoptic
Func. class.: Antihypertensive; antiglaucoma
Chem. class.: Nonselective β-blocker
Pregnancy category C

Action: Competitively blocks stimulation of β-adrenergic receptor within vascular smooth muscle; (decreases rate of SA node discharge, increases recovery time), slows conduction of AV node, decreases heart rate, which decreases O_2 consumption in myocardium; also decreases renin-aldosterone-angiotensin system; at high doses inhibits β-2 receptors in bronchial system

▸**Therapeutic Outcome:** Decreased B/P, decreased arrhythmias, absence of death from MI, decreased aqueous humor in the eye, absence of migraine headaches

Uses: Mild to moderate hypertension, sinus tachycardia, persistent atrial extrasystoles, tachydysrhythmias, prophylaxis of angina pectoris, reduction of mortality after MI

Investigational uses: Mitral valve prolapse, hypertrophic cardiomyopathy, thyrotoxicosis, tremors, anxiety, pheochromocytoma, tachyarrhythmias, angina pectoris

Dosage and routes
Hypertension
Adult: PO 10 mg bid, or 20 mg qd, may increase by 10 mg q2-3d, not to exceed 60 mg/day

---

Myocardial infarction
Adult: 10 mg bid beginning
1-4 wk after MI

Glaucoma
Adult: Ophth i gtt qd or bid
P **Child:** Ophth i gtt qd or bid
(0.25% sol only)

*Migraine headache
prevention*
Adult: PO 10 mg bid, or 20
mg qd, may increase to 30
mg/day, 20 mg in AM, 10 mg
in PM

Available forms: Tabs 5, 10,
20 mg; ophth sol 0.25%, 0.5%

Adverse effects
CNS: Insomnia, dizziness,
hallucinations, anxiety
CV: Hypotension, bradycardia,
CHF, edema, chest pain,
bradycardia, claudication
EENT: Visual changes, sore
throat, *double vision,* dry burning eyes
GI: Nausea, vomiting, **ischemic colitis,** diarrhea, *abdominal pain,* **mesenteric arterial
thrombosis**
GU: Impotence, urinary frequency
HEMA: **Agranulocytosis,
thrombocytopenia, purpura**
INTEG: Rash, alopecia, pruritus, fever
META: Hypoglycemia
MUSC: Joint pain, muscle pain
RESP: **Bronchospasm,** dyspnea, cough, rales

Contraindications: Hypersensitivity to β-blockers, cardiogenic shock, heart block (2nd,
3rd degree), sinus bradycardia,
CHF, cardiac failure

Precautions: Major surgery,
pregnancy **C,** lactation, diabetes mellitus, renal disease,
thyroid disease, COPD, well-
compensated heart failure,
CAD, nonallergic broncho-
spasm

◼ **Do Not Confuse:**
Timoptic/Viroptic

Pharmacokinetics	
Absorption	Well absorbed (PO), ophth (minimal)
Distribution	Not known
Metabolism	Liver—extensively
Excretion	Breast milk
Half-life	3-4 hr

Pharmacodynamics	
	PO
Onset	Unknown
Peak	2-4 hr
Duration	12-24 hr

Interactions
Individual drugs
Alcohol: ↑ hypotension (large
amounts)
Epinephrine: α-Adrenergic
stimulation
Hydralazine: ↑ hypotension,
bradycardia
Indomethacin: ↓ antihyper-
tensive effect
Insulin: ↑ hypoglycemia
Methyldopa: ↑ hypotension,
bradycardia
Prazosin: ↑ hypotension,
bradycardia
Reserpine: ↑ hypotension,
bradycardia
Thyroid: ↓ effect of timolol
Verapamil: ↑ myocardial de-
pression
Drug classifications
Antihypertensives: ↑ hypo-
tension
β₂-Agonists: ↓ bronchodilata-
tion
Cardiac glycosides: ↑ brady-
cardia
Nitrates: ↑ hypotension
Sulfonylureas: ↓ hypoglyce-
mic effect
Theophyllines: ↓ bronchodila-
tation

T

✤ Canada Only   Adverse effects: *italic* = common; **bold** = life-threatening

Lab test interferences
False: ↑ Urinary catechol-amines

NURSING CONSIDERATIONS
Assessment
• Monitor B/P during beginning treatment, periodically thereafter; pulse q4h; note rate, rhythm, quality: apical/radial pulse before administration; notify prescriber of any significant changes (pulse <50 bpm)
• Check for baselines in renal, liver function tests before therapy begins
• Assess for edema in feet, legs daily, monitor I&O, daily weight; check for jugular vein distention, rales, bilaterally, dyspnea (CHF)
• Monitor skin turgor, dryness of mucous membranes for hydration status, especially
G elderly

Nursing diagnoses
☑ Cardiac output, decreased (uses)
☑ Injury, risk for physical (side effects)
☑ Knowledge deficit (teaching)
☑ Noncompliance (teaching)

Implementation
PO route
• Given ac, hs, tab may be crushed or swallowed whole; give with food to prevent GI upset; reduced dosage in renal dysfunction
• Store protected from light, moisture; place in cool environment

Patient/family education
• Teach patient not to discontinue drug abruptly; taper over 2 wk; may cause precipitate angina if stopped abruptly
• Advise patient not to use OTC products containing α-adrenergic stimulants (such as nasal decongestants, cold preparations); to avoid alcohol, smoking and to limit sodium intake as prescribed
• Teach patient how to take pulse and B/P at home—advise patient when to notify prescriber
• Instruct patient to comply with weight control, dietary adjustments, modified exercise program
• Advise patient to carry/wear Medic Alert ID to identify drug being taken, any allergies; tell patient drug controls symptoms but does not cure
• Caution patient to avoid hazardous activities if dizziness, drowsiness is present
• Teach patient to report symptoms of CHF; difficult breathing, especially on exertion or when lying down; night cough; swelling of extremities or bradycardia; dizziness; confusion; depression; fever
• Teach patient to take drug as prescribed, not to double doses, skip doses; take any missed doses as soon as remembered if at least 4 hr until next dose

Evaluation
Positive therapeutic outcome
• Decreased B/P in hypertension (after 1-2 wk)
• Absence of dysrhythmias

Treatment of overdose: Lavage, **IV** atropine for bradycardia, **IV** theophylline for bronchospasm, digitalis, O_2, diuretic for cardiac failure, hemodialysis, **IV** glucose for hyperglycemia, **IV** diazepam (or phenytoin) for seizures

---

tirofiban (℞)

(tie-roh-fee'ban)

Aggrastat

Func. class.: Antiplatelet

Chem. class.: Nonpeptide antagonist

Pregnancy category B

Action: Activation of platelet glycoprotein (GP) IIb/IIIa receptor that leads to binding of fibrongen and von Willebrand's factor, which causes platelet aggregation

➡ **Therapeutic Outcome:** Increased platelet count

Uses: Acute coronary syndrome

Dosage and routes

Adult: **IV** 0.4 μg/kg/min × 30 min, then 0.1 μg/kg/min; give ½ dose in renal disease

Available forms: Inj for sol 250 μg/ml, inj 50 μg/ml

Adverse effects

CNS: Dizziness

CV: Bradycardia

HEMA: Bleeding

INTEG: Rash

OTHER: Dissection, coronary artery edema, pain in legs/pelvis, sweating

Contraindications: Hypersensitivity, active internal bleeding, stroke, major surgery, severe trauma, intracranial neoplasm, aneurysm, hemorrhage

Precautions: Pregnancy **B**, ◨ lactation, elderly, renal disease, bleeding tendencies

Pharmacokinetics

Absorption	Unknown
Distribution	Plasma clearance 20%-25%
Metabolism	Liver
Excretion	Urine/feces
Half-life	2 hr

Pharmacodynamics

Onset	Unknown
Peak	Unknown
Duration	Unknown

Interactions

Individual drugs

Aspirin: ↑ bleeding

Heparin: ↑ bleeding

Levothyroxine: ↑ clearance of tirofiban

Omeprazole: ↑ clearance of tirofiban

NURSING CONSIDERATIONS

Assessment

• Monitor B/P pulse during treatment until stable; take B/P lying, standing; orthostatic hypotension is common

• Monitor platelet counts, Hct, Hgb, prior to treatment, within 6 hr of loading dose and at least qd thereafter

Nursing diagnoses

✓ Tissue perfusion, altered (uses)

Implementation

• **IV:** Give ½ dose in renal disease

• Dilute inj: withdraw and discard 100 ml from a 500 ml bag of sterile 0.9% NaCl or D₅ and replace this vol with 50 ml of tirofiban inj from one vial

• Tirofiban inj for sol is premixed in containers of 500 ml 0.9% NaCl (50 mg/ml)

• Minimize other arterial/venous punctures IM inj, catheter use, intubation, to reduce bleeding risks

Patient/family education

• Advise patient that it is necessary to quit smoking to prevent excessive vasoconstriction

• Teach patient to avoid hazardous activities; dizziness may occur

T

♣ Canada Only   Adverse effects: *italic* = common; **bold** = life-threatening

Evaluation
Positive therapeutic outcome
• Decreased platelet count

---

tizanidine (℞)
(tye-za′na-deen)
Zanaflex
Func. class.: Skeletal muscle relaxant, central acting
Chem. class.: Imidazole
Pregnancy category   C

Action: Unknown; possesses central α_2-adrenergic agonist properties; reduces excitation of spinal cord interneurons; also acts on the basal ganglia, producing muscle relaxation

➔Therapeutic Outcome: Decreased spasticity of muscles

Uses: Spinal cord injury, spasticity in multiple sclerosis, tension headache

Dosage and routes
Adult: Reduce dose in renal failure; 4-36 mg qd in 3 divided doses

Spasticity:
Adult: PO 8 mg as a single dose; may increase in 2-4 mg increments until desired response, may repeat q6-8h up to 3 doses/24 hr, max 36 mg/day

Tension headache:
Adult: PO 2 mg tid, may increase by 4-6 mg tid after 2 wk interval

Available forms: Tabs 4 mg

Adverse effects
CNS: Dizziness, asthenia, somnolence, *fatigue, insomnia,* severe sedation
CV: Hypotension
GI: Nausea, constipation, *vomiting,* diarrhea, **hepatotoxicity,** *dry mouth,* anorexia
GU: Urinary frequency, UTI
INTEG: Rash, pruritus, sweating, skin ulcer

Contraindications: Hypersensitivity

Precautions: Renal disease, hepatic disease, stroke, cardiac **G** disease, pregnancy **C,** elderly

Pharmacokinetics	
Absorption	Complete
Distribution	Widely
Metabolism	Liver, extensively
Excretion	Kidneys, feces
Half-life	2½ hr

Pharmacodynamics	
Onset	Unknown
Peak	1-2 hr
Duration	3-6 hr

Interactions
Individual drugs
Alcohol: CNS depression
Drug classifications
Antidepressants, tricyclic: ↑ CNS depression
Barbiturates: ↑ CNS depression
Diuretics: ↑ hypotensive effects
Opiates: ↑ CNS depression
Oral contraceptives: ↑ adverse reactions of tizanidine
Sedative/hypnotics: ↑ CNS depression

Lab test interferences
↑ AST, ↑ alkaline phosphatase

NURSING CONSIDERATIONS
Assessment
• Monitor B/P, heart rate
• Perform neuroexam in spasticity: deep tendon reflexes, muscle tone, clonus, sensory function
• Monitor liver, renal function

---

tests, electrolytes, CBC with diff during long-term treatment
• Assess for allergic reactions: rash, fever, respiratory distress; severe weakness, numbness in extremities
• Assess CNS depression: dizziness, drowsiness, psychiatric symptoms
• Check dosage, as individual titration is required

Nursing diagnoses
☑ Mobility, impaired uses
☑ Injury, risk for (adverse reactions)
☑ Knowledge deficit (teaching)

Implementation
• Give with meals for GI symptoms; gum, frequent sips of water for dry mouth
• Store in airtight container at room temperature

Patient/family education
• Advise patient not to discontinue medication quickly; spasticity, will occur; drug should be tapered off over 1-2 wk
• Advise patient not to take with alcohol, other CNS depressants, take as directed, if dose is missed, take as soon as remembered, unless it is almost time for next dose
• Caution patient to avoid altering activities while taking this drug; to avoid hazardous activities if drowsiness or dizziness occurs; to rise from sitting or lying slowly to prevent fainting
• Advise patient to avoid using OTC medication: cough preparations, antihistamines unless directed by prescriber
• Notify prescriber if fainting, hallucinations, dark urine, stomach pain, yellowing of skin/eyes occur

Evaluation
Positive therapeutic outcome
• Decreased pain, spasticity

---

tobramycin (℞)
(toe-bra-mye'sin)
Nebcin, tobramycin sulfate, Tobrex, Tobi
Func. class.: Antiinfective
Chem. class.: Aminoglycoside
Pregnancy category C

Action: Interferes with protein synthesis in bacterial cell by binding to ribosomal subunit, causing inaccurate peptide sequence to form in protein chain, causing bacterial death

Therapeutic Outcome: Bactericidal effects for the following organisms: *Pseudomonas aeruginosa, Enterobacter, Escherichia coli, Providencia, Citrobacter, Staphylococcus, Proteus, Klebsiella, Serratia*

Uses: Severe systemic infections of CNS, respiratory, GI, urinary tract, bone, skin, soft tissues, eye, cystic fibrosis (nebulizer) for *Pseudomonas aeruginosa*

Dosage and routes
Adult: IM/**IV** 3 mg/kg/day in divided doses q8h; may give up to 5 mg/kg/day in divided doses q6-8h; once qd dosing is an option

P *Child:* IM/**IV** 6-7.5 mg/kg/day in 3-4 equal divided doses

P *Child ≥6 yr:* Neb 300 mg bid in repeating cycles of 28 days on/28 days off; give inh over 10-15 mins using a hand-held PARI LC PLUS reusable nebulizer with a DeVilbiss Pulmo-Aid compressor

---

P *Neonates <1 wk:* IM up to 4 mg/kg/day in divided doses q12h; **IV** up to 4 mg/kg/day in divided doses q12h diluted in 50-100 mg NS or D_5W; give over 30-60 min

Available forms: Inj 10, 40 mg/ml; powder for inj 1.2 g; inj 20 mg/2 ml; 0.3% ophth, neb sol 300 mg/5 ml

Adverse effects

CNS: Confusion, depression, numbness, tremors, **convulsions,** muscle twitching, **neurotoxicity,** dizziness, vertigo
CV: Hypotension, hypertension, palpitations
EENT: Ototoxicity, deafness, visual disturbances, tinnitus
GI: Nausea, vomiting, anorexia, increased ALT, AST, bilirubin, hepatomegaly, **hepatic necrosis,** splenomegaly
GU: **Oliguria, hematuria, renal damage, azotemia, renal failure, nephrotoxicity**
HEMA: **Agranulocytosis, thrombocytopenia, leukopenia, eosinophilia,** anemia
INTEG: Rash, burning, urticaria, dermatitis, alopecia

Contraindications: Severe renal disease, hypersensitivity to aminoglycosides

P **Precautions:** Neonates, mild renal disease, pregnancy **C,** myasthenia gravis, lactation, hearing deficits, Parkinson's disease

N **Do Not Confuse:**
Tobrex/Tobra Dex

Pharmacokinetics

Absorption	Well absorbed (IM), completely absorbed (**IV**)
Distribution	Widely distributed in extracellular fluids
Metabolism	Minimal—liver
Excretion	Mostly unchanged (>90%) kidneys
P **Half-life**	2-3 hr, increased in renal disease, neonates

Pharmacodynamics

	IM	IV	OPHTH
Onset	Rapid	Rapid	Rapid
Peak	1 hr	Inf end	Unknown

Interactions
Individual drugs
Amphotericin B: ↑ ototoxicity, neurotoxicity, nephrotoxicity
Cisplatin: ↑ ototoxicity, neurotoxicity, nephrotoxicity
Ethacrynic acid: ↑ ototoxicity, neurotoxicity, nephrotoxicity
Furosemide: ↑ ototoxicity, neurotoxicity, nephrotoxicity
Mannitol: ↑ ototoxicity, neurotoxicity, nephrotoxicity
Methoxyflurane: ↑ ototoxicity, neurotoxicity, nephrotoxicity
Polymyxin: ↑ ototoxicity, neurotoxicity, nephrotoxicity
Succinylcholine: ↑ neuromuscular blockade, respiratory depression
Vancomycin: ↑ ototoxicity, neurotoxicity, nephrotoxicity
Drug classifications
Aminoglycosides: ↑ otoxicity, neurotoxicity, nephrotoxicity
Anesthetics: ↑ neuromuscular blockade, respiratory depression
Nondepolarizing neuromuscular blockers: ↑ neuromuscular blockade, respiratory depression

---

Penicillins: ↑ ototoxicity, neurotoxicity, nephrotoxicity

NURSING CONSIDERATIONS
Assessment
• Assess patient for previous sensitivity reaction

Syst route
• Assess patient for signs and symptoms of infection including characteristics of wounds, sputum, urine, stool WBC >10,000, temp; obtain baseline information before and during treatment
• Complete C&S testing before beginning drug therapy to identify if correct treatment has been initiated
• Assess for allergic reactions: rash, urticaria, pruritus, chills, fever, joint pain
• Identify urine output; if decreasing, notify prescriber (may indicate nephrotoxicity); also, obtain BUN, creatinine, urine CrCl (<80 ml/min) values
• Monitor blood studies: AST, ALT, CBC, Hct, bilirubin, LDH, alk phosphatase, Coombs' test monthly if patient is on long-term therapy
• Monitor electrolytes: potassium, sodium, chloride, magnesium monthly if patient is on long-term therapy
• Monitor for bleeding: ecchymosis, bleeding gums, hematuria, stool guaiac daily if patient is on long-term therapy
• Assess for overgrowth of infection: perineal itching, fever, malaise, redness, pain, swelling, drainage, rash, diarrhea, change in cough, sputum
• Obtain weight before treatment; calculation of dosage is usually based on ideal body weight, but may be calculated on actual body weight

• Monitor I&O ratio; urinalysis daily for proteinuria, cells, casts; report sudden change in urine output
• Monitor VS during inf, watch for hypotension, change in pulse
• Assess **IV** site for thrombophlebitis including pain, redness, swelling q30 min, change site if needed; apply warm compresses to discontinued site
• Obtain serum peak, drawn at 30-60 min after **IV** inf or 60 min after IM inj, trough level drawn just before next dose; peak 4-12 µg/ml, trough 1-2 µg/ml
• Monitor for deafness by audiometric testing, ringing, roaring in ears, vertigo; assess hearing before, during, after treatment
• Monitor for dehydration: high sp gr, decrease in skin turgor, dry mucous membranes, dark urine
• Monitor for overgrowth of infection including increased temp, malaise, redness, pain, swelling, perineal itching, diarrhea, stomatitis, change in cough, sputum

Nursing diagnoses
☑ Infection, risk for (uses)
☑ Diarrhea (adverse reactions)
☑ Injury, risk for (adverse reactions)
☑ Knowledge deficit (teaching)
☑ Noncompliance (teaching)

Implementation
IM route
• Give deeply in large muscle mass

IV route
• Give **IV** diluted in 50-100 ml NS $D_{10}W$, D_5/0.9% NaCl, 0.9% NaCl, Ringers, LR, D_5W (adult), infuse over 20-60 min

---

• Flush after inf with D$_5$W, 0.9% NaCl
• Separate aminoglycosides and penicillins by ≥1 hr

Syringe compatibilities:
Doxapram

Syringe incompatibilities:
Cefamandole, clindamycin, heparin, sargramostim

Y-site compatibilities:
Acyclovir, amifostine, amiodarone, amsacrine, aztreonam, ciprofloxacin, cyclophosphamide, diltiazem, enalaprilat, esmolol, filgrastim, fluconazole, fludarabine, foscarnet, furosemide, granisetron, hydromorphone, IL-2, regular insulin, labetalol, magnesium sulfate, melphalan, meperidine, midazolam, morphine, perphenazine, tacrolimus, teniposide, theophylline, thiotepa, tolazoline, vinorelbine, zidovudine

Additive compatibilities:
Aztreonam, bleomycin, calcium gluconate, cefoxitin, ciprofloxacin, clindamycin, furosemide, metronidazole, ofloxacin, ranitidine, verapamil

Additive incompatibilities:
Cefamandole, floxacillin

Nebulizer route
• Give as close to q12h apart as possible; do not use <6 hr apart
• Do not mix with dornase alfa in the nebulizer

Patient/family education
Nebulizer
• Have patient inhale sitting or standing, breathe normally through the mouthpiece, may use nose clips
• Advise to use multiple therapies first, then tobramycin

Syst route
• Teach patient to report sore throat, bruising, bleeding, joint pain—may indicate blood dyscrasias (rare)
• Advise patient to contact prescriber if vaginal itching, loose, foul-smelling stools, furry tongue occur—may indicate superimposed infection
• Advise patient to notify prescriber of diarrhea with blood or pus, which may indicate pseudomembranous colitis

Evaluation
Positive therapeutic outcome
• Absence of signs/symptoms of infection (WBC <10,000, temp WNL, absence of red, draining wounds)
• Reported improvement in symptoms of infection

Treatment of overdose:
Withdraw drug, hemodialysis, exchange transfusion in the newborn, monitor serum levels of drug, may give ticarcillin or carbenicillin

---

tocainide (℞)
(toe-kay′nide)
Tonocard
Func. class.: Antidysrhythmic (Class IB)
Chem. class.: Lidocaine analog
Pregnancy category   C

Action: Increases electrical stimulation threshold of ventricle, His-Purkinje system, which stabilizes cardiac membrane and decreases automaticity

▷**Therapeutic Outcome:** Decreased ventricular dysrhythmia

Uses: Life-threatening ventricular dysrhythmias (multi-focal/unifocal PVCs), ventricular tachycardia

---

☑ Herb/drug   🚫 Do Not Crush   ◆ Alert   ⚮ Key Drug   🅖 Geriatric   🅟 Pediatric

Dosage and routes
Adult: PO 400 mg q8h

Available forms: Tabs 400, 600 mg

Adverse effects
CNS: Headache, dizziness, involuntary movement, confusion, psychosis, restlessness, irritability, paresthesias, tremors, **seizures**
CV: Hypotension, bradycardia, angina, PVCs, **heart block, cardiovascular collapse, arrest, CHF,** chest pain, tachycardia, prodysrhythmias
EENT: Tinnitus, blurred vision, hearing loss
GI: Nausea, vomiting, anorexia, diarrhea, hepatitis
HEMA: **Blood dyscrasias: leukopenia, agranulocytosis, hypoplastic anemia, thrombocytopenia**
INTEG: Rash, urticaria, edema, swelling
RESP: Dyspnea, **respiratory depression, pulmonary fibrosis**

Contraindications: Hypersensitivity to amides, severe heart block

Precautions: Pregnancy **C,** lactation, children, renal disease, liver disease, CHF, respiratory depression, myasthenia gravis, blood dyscrasias

Pharmacokinetics	
Absorption	Well absorbed
Distribution	Widely distributed, crossed blood-brain barrier
Metabolism	Liver
Excretion	Kidney (up to 50% unchanged)
Half-life	10-17 hr

Pharmacodynamics	
Onset	1 hr
Peak	½-2 hr
Duration	8-12 hr

Interactions
Individual drugs
Cimetidine: ↓ levels of tocainide
Digoxin: ↑ blood levels, ↑ toxicity
Disopyramide: ↑ levels, ↑ toxicity
Flecainide: ↑ levels, ↑ toxicity
Lidocaine: ↑ effect
Mexiletine: ↑ levels, ↑ toxicity
Phenytoin: ↑ blood levels
Procainamide: ↑ levels, ↑ toxicity
Quinidine: ↑ levels, ↑ toxicity
Rifampin: ↓ tocainide levels
Warfarin: ↑ levels, ↑ bleeding
Drug classifications
β-Adrenergic blockers: ↑ dysrhythmias, arrest
Calcium channel blockers: ↑ dysrhythmias, arrest
Herb/drug
Aloe: ↑ hypokalemia
Buckthorn: ↑ hypokalemia
Cascara sagrada: ↑ hypokalemia
Senna: ↑ hypokalemia
Lab test interferences
↑ CPK

NURSING CONSIDERATIONS
Assessment
• Assess for oxygenation or perfusion deficit: decreased B/P, chest pain, dizziness, loss of consciousness
• Assess respiratory status: auscultate lung fields for bibasilar crackles in patients with advanced CHF
• Assess for urinary retention: check for pain, abdominal absorption, palpate bladder; check males with benign prostatic hypertrophy—

T

anticholinergic reaction may cause retention
• Monitor I&O ratio; electrolytes: (potassium, sodium, chloride); watch for decreasing urinary output, possible retention
• Monitor liver function studies: AST, ALT, bilirubin, alk phosphatase
• Monitor ECG to determine drug effectiveness; measure PR, QRS, QT intervals; check for PVCs, other dysrhythmias; monitor B/P for hypotension, hypertension; for rebound hypertension after 1-2 hr
• Monitor patient for CNS symptoms: confusion, psychosis, numbness, depression, involuntary movements; if these occur, drug should be discontinued
• Assess pulmonary toxicity: dyspnea, fatigue, cough, fever, chest pain; drug should be discontinued if these occur
• Assess cardiac rate, respiration: rate, rhythm, character, chest pain, ventricular tachycardia, supraventricular tachycardia or fibrillation

Nursing diagnoses
☑ Cardiac output, decreased (uses)
☑ Impaired gas exchange (adverse reactions)
☑ Knowledge deficit (teaching)

Implementation
• Give with meals for GI upset occurrences

Patient/family education
• Inform patient or family of reason for use of medication and expected results
• Teach patient method for taking pulse at home and what to report to prescriber
• Advise patient to avoid hazardous activities until drug

response is known; dizziness, confusion, sedation may occur
• Advise patient to use a Medic Alert bracelet or other ID indicating medications taken, condition, and prescriber's name and phone number
• Instruct patient to report bleeding, bruising, respiratory symptoms, chills, fever, sore throat to prescriber

Evaluation
Positive therapeutic outcome
• Decreased dysrhythmias

Treatment of overdose: Defibrillation, vasopressor for hypotension

---

tolazoline (℞)
(toe-laz′a-leen)
Priscoline
Func. class.: Peripheral vasodilator
Chem. class.: Imidazoline derivative
Pregnancy category   C

Action: Peripheral vasodilation occurs by direct relaxation on vascular smooth muscle; also has weak α- and β-adrenergic properties

➥**Therapeutic Outcome:** Decreased pulmonary hypertension

Uses: Persistent pulmonary hypertension of newborn; also hypoxic pulmonary hypertension

Dosage and routes
℗ *Newborn:* IV 1-2 mg/kg via scalp vein; **IV** inf 1-2 mg/kg/hr

Available forms: Inj 25 mg/ml

Adverse effects
CV: Orthostatic hypotension, **tachycardia,** dysrhythmias, hypertension, **cardiovascular collapse**
GI: Nausea, vomiting, diarrhea, peptic ulcer, **GI hemorrhage, hepatitis**
GU: Edema, oliguria, hematuria
HEMA: **Thrombocytopenia, leukopenia**
INTEG: Flushing, tingling, rash, chills, sweating, increased pilomotor activity
RESP: **Pulmonary hemorrhage**

Contraindications: Hypersensitivity, CVA, CAD

Precautions: Pregnancy **C,** active peptic ulcer, lactation, mitral stenosis

Pharmacokinetics	
Absorption	Complete
Distribution	Unknown
Metabolism	Liver
Excretion	Kidneys
Half-life	3-10 hr

Pharmacodynamics	
Onset	½ hr
Peak	½-1 hr
Duration	3-4 hr

Interactions
Individual drugs
Alcohol: ↑ effects
Epinephrine: ↓ B/P, rebound hypertension
Drug classifications
Antihypertensives: ↑ effects
β-Adrenergic blockers: ↑ effects

NURSING CONSIDERATIONS
Assessment
• Monitor ABGs, electrolytes, VS in newborn
• Monitor B/P, pulse during treatment until stable; take B/P with patient in lying and standing position; orthostatic hypotension is common
• Monitor hepatic tests: AST, ALT, bilirubin; liver enzymes may increase
• Monitor blood studies: CBC, platelets; watch for thrombocytopenia, agranulocytosis
• Monitor hepatic involvement: nausea, vomiting, jaundice; drug should be discontinued if this occurs
• Monitor for bleeding from GI tract: coffee grounds vomitus, increased pulse, pain in upper gastric area
• Assess affected areas for changes in temp, color

Nursing diagnoses
☑ Tissue, perfusion, altered (uses)
☑ Knowledge deficit (teaching)

Implementation
• Give **IV** undiluted; give 10 mg or less over 1 min; in scalp vein may be diluted in D₅, D₅NS, LR, NS, ½NS, Ringer's sol; run over 1 hr
• Give decreased dose for patients with low urine output (<1 cc/kg/h)
• Give ordered analgesic if headache develops
• Give intraarterially to patient in supine position
• Give to patient who is sitting or lying down during treatment
• Store at room temp, protect from light

Y-site compatibilities:
Aminophylline, ampicillin, calcium gluconate, cefotaxime, cimetidine, dobutamine, dopamine, furosemide, gentamicin, phytonadione, sodium bicarbonate, tobramycin, vancomycin

T

Additive compatibilities: Verapamil

Patient/family education
• Advise patient to report jaundice, dark urine, joint pain, fatigue, malaise, bruising, easy bleeding, which may indicate blood dyscrasias
• Instruct patient that it is necessary to quit smoking to prevent excessive vasoconstriction if prescribed for PVD
• Caution to avoid hazardous activities until stabilized on medication; dizziness may occur

Evaluation
Positive therapeutic outcome
• Decrease in pulmonary hypertension or pulse volume, increased temperature in extremities, ability to walk without pain

Treatment of overdose: Administer **IV** fluids, position patient's head in low position

---

tolcapone (℞)
(toll'cah-pone)
Tasmar
Func. class.: Antiparkinson agent
Chem. class.: Catecholamine inhibitor

Pregnancy category C

Action: Selective, reversible inhibitor of catecholamine; used as adjunct to levodopa/carbidopa therapy

➡ Therapeutic Outcome: Increased ability to move and speak

Uses: Parkinsonism

Dosage and routes
Adult: PO 100-200 mg tid, with levodopa/carbidopa therapy; max 600 mg/day

Available forms: Tabs 100, 200 mg

Adverse effects
CNS: Dystonia, dyskinesia, dreaming, *fatigue, headache, confusion,* psychosis, hallucination, dizziness
CV: Orthostatic hypotension, chest pain, hypotension
EENT: Cataract, eye inflammation
GI: Nausea, vomiting, abdominal distress, diarrhea, constipation, **fatal liver failure**
GU: UTI, urine discoloration, uterine tumor, micturition disorder
HEMA: **Hemolytic anemia, leukopenia, agranulocytosis**
INTEG: Sweating, alopecia

Contraindications: Hypersensitivity

Precautions: Renal disease, cardiac disease, hepatic disease, hypertension, pregnancy **C,** asthma, lactation

Pharmacokinetics	
Absorption	Rapidly
Distribution	Protein binding 99%
Metabolism	Liver (extensively)
Excretion	Urine (60%), feces (40%)
Half-life	2-3 hr

Pharmacodynamics	
Onset	Unknown
Peak	2 hr
Duration	Unknown

Interactions
Individual drugs
α-Methyldopa: May influence pharmacokinetics
Apomorphine: May influence pharmacokinetics
Dobutamine: May influence pharmacokinetics

Isoproterenol: May influence pharmacokinetics

Drug classifications
MAOIs: ↓ normal catecholamine metabolism; MAO-B inhibitor may be used

NURSING CONSIDERATIONS
Assessment
• Monitor liver function enzymes: AST, ALT, alk phosphatase, LDH, bilirubin, CBC
• Assess involuntary movements in parkinsonism: akinesia, tremors, staggering gait, muscle rigidity, drooling
• Monitor B/P, respiration during initial treatment; hypo/hypertension should be reported
• Monitor mental status: affect, mood, behavioral changes

Nursing diagnoses
☑Physical mobility, impaired (uses)
☑Injury, risk for (uses)
☑Knowledge deficit (teaching)

Implementation
PO route
• Administer tid with levodopa/carbidopa therapy
• Provide assistance with ambulation during beginning therapy

Patient/family education
• Advise patient to change positions slowly to prevent orthostatic hypotension
• Advise patient that urine, sweat may change color
• Teach patient that food taken within 1 hr ac or 2 hr pc increases action of drug by 20%
• Teach patient to report nausea, vomiting, anorexia

Evaluation
Positive therapeutic outcome
• Decrease in akathisia, increased mood

---

tolmetin (℞)
(tole′met-in)
Tolectin DS, Tolectin 200, Tolectin 600, tolmetin sodium
Func. class.: Nonsteroidal antiinflammatory
Chem. class.: Pyrrole acetic acid derivative

Pregnancy category B

Action: Inhibits prostaglandin synthesis by decreasing an enzyme needed for biosynthesis; analgesic, antiinflammatory, antipyretic

Therapeutic Outcome: Decreased pain, inflammatory

Uses: Mild to moderate pain, osteoarthritis, rheumatoid arthritis

Dosage and routes
Adult: PO 400 mg tid-qid, not to exceed 2 g/day
Child >2 yr: PO 15-30 mg/kg/day in 3 or 4 divided doses

Available forms: Cap 400 mg; tabs 200, 600 mg

Adverse effects
CNS: Dizziness, drowsiness, fatigue, tremors, confusion, insomnia, anxiety, depression, headache
CV: Tachycardia, peripheral edema, palpitations, dysrhythmias, hypertension
EENT: Tinnitus, hearing loss, blurred vision
GI: Nausea, anorexia, vomiting, diarrhea, jaundice, **cholestatic hepatitis,** constipation, flatulence, cramps, dry mouth, peptic ulcer, ulceration, bleeding, perforation
GU: **Nephrotoxicity: dysuria, hematuria, oliguria, azotemia, pseudoproteinuria**

HEMA: Blood dyscrasias
INTEG: Purpura, rash, pruritus, sweating

Contraindications: Hypersensitivity, asthma, severe renal disease, severe hepatic disease, ulcer disease

Precautions: Pregnancy **B**, **P** lactation, children, bleeding disorders, GI disorders, cardiac disorders, hypersensitivity to other antiinflammatory agents, peptic ulcer disease

Pharmacokinetics	
Absorption	Well absorbed
Distribution	Not known
Metabolism	Extensively
Excretion	Unchanged kidneys—20%
Half-life	3-3½ hr

Pharmacodynamics	
Onset	Unknown
Peak	2 hr
Duration	Unknown

Interactions
Individual drugs
Acetaminophen (long-term use): ↑ renal reactions
Alcohol: ↑ adverse reactions
Aspirin: ↓ effectiveness, ↑ adverse reactions
Digoxin: ↑ toxicity, ↑ levels
Insulin: ↓ insulin effect
Lithium: ↑ toxicity
Methotrexate: ↑ toxicity
Phenytoin: ↑ toxicity
Probenecid: ↑ toxicity
Radiation: ↑ risk of hematologic toxicity
Sulfonylurea: ↑ toxicity
Drug classifications
Anticoagulants: ↑ risk of bleeding
Antihypertensives: ↓ effect of antihypertensives
Antineoplastics: ↑ risk of hematologic toxicity

β-Adrenergic blockers: ↑ antihypertension
Cephalosporins: ↑ risk of bleeding
Diuretics: ↓ effectiveness of diuretics
Glucocorticoids: ↑ adverse reactions
Hypoglycemics: ↓ hypoglycemic effect
NSAIDs: ↑ adverse reactions
Potassium supplements: ↑ adverse reactions
Sulfonamides: ↑ toxicity
Lab test interferences
↑ Serum potassium, ↑ liver function studies, ↑ BUN
False positive: Urine protein

NURSING CONSIDERATIONS
Assessment
• Monitor blood counts during therapy; watch for decreasing platelets; if low, therapy may need to be discontinued, restarted after hematologic recovery; and for blood dyscrasia (thrombocytopenia): bruising, fatigue, bleeding, poor healing

Nursing diagnoses
☑ Pain (uses)
☑ Mobility, impaired physical (uses)
☑ Injury, risk for (adverse reactions)
☑ Knowledge deficit (teaching)

Implementation
• Administer with food or milk to decrease gastric symptoms—food will slow absorption slightly, but will not decrease absorption

Patient/family education
• Inform patient that drug must be continued for prescribed time to be effective; to avoid aspirin, alcoholic beverages
• Caution patient to report

☑ Herb/drug 🚫 Do Not Crush ◆ Alert ⊶ Key Drug **G** Geriatric **P** Pediatric

bleeding, bruising, fatigue, malaise because blood dyscrasias do occur
• Instruct patient to use caution when driving; drowsiness, dizziness may occur
• Teach patient to take with a full glass of water to enhance absorption; do not crush, break or chew

Evaluation
Positive therapeutic outcome
• Decreased pain
• Decreased inflammation
• Increased mobility

tolterodine (℞)
(tol-tehr'oh-deen)
Detrol
Func. class.: Overactive bladder product
Chem. class.: Muscarinic receptor antagonist
Pregnancy category C

Action: Relaxes smooth muscles in urinary tract by inhibiting acetylcholine at postganglionic sites

Therapeutic Outcome: Decreased symptoms of overactive bladder

Uses: Overactive bladder, (frequency, urgency)

Dosage and routes
Adult: PO 2 mg bid, hepatic disease 1 mg bid

Available forms: Tabs 1, 2 mg

Adverse effects
CNS: Anxiety, paresthesia, fatigue, *dizziness,* headache
CV: Chest pain, hypertension
EENT: Vision abnormalities, xerophthalmia
GI: Nausea, vomiting, an-

orexia, abdominal pain constipation, dry mouth, dyspepsia
GU: Dysuria, retention, frequency, UTI
INTEG: Rash, pruritis
RESP: Bronchitis, cough, pharyngitis, URI

Contraindications: Hypersensitivity, uncontrolled narrow-angle glaucoma, urinary retention, gastric retention

Precautions: Pregnancy C, lactation, children, renal/hepatic disease, controlled narrow-angle glaucoma

Pharmacokinetics

Absorption	Rapidly
Distribution	Highly protein bound
Metabolism	Liver (extensively)
Excretion	Urine/feces
Half-life	Unknown

Pharmacodynamics

Onset	Unknown
Peak	Unknown
Duration	Unknown

Interactions
Drug classifications
Antibiotics, macrolide: ↑ action of tolterodine
Antifungals: ↑ action of tolterodine
Food/drug
↑ bioavailability of tolterodine

NURSING CONSIDERATIONS
Assessment
• Assess urinary patterns: distension, nocturia, frequency, urgency, incontinence
• Assess allergic reactions: rash; if this occurs, drug should be discontinued
Nursing diagnoses
✓ Urinary elimination, altered (uses)
✓ Incontinence, functional (uses)

✓ Knowledge deficit (teaching)
✓ Activity intolerance (uses)
Patient/family education
• Advise patient to avoid hazardous activities; dizziness may occur

Evaluation
Positive therapeutic outcome
• Decreased urinary frequency, urgency

topiramate (℞)
(to-pi-ra′mate)
Topamax
Func. class.: Anticonvulsant, misc
Chem. class.: Carbamate derivative

Pregnancy category   C

Action: Mechanism of action unknown; may prevent seizure spread as opposed to an elevation of seizure threshold

➡**Therapeutic Outcome:** Absence of seizures

Uses: Partial seizures, with or without generalization in adults

Dosage and routes
Adjunctive therapy
Adult: PO add 400 mg in 2 divided doses

Renal dose
CrCl <70 ml/min give ½ dose
Available forms: Tabs 25, 100, 200 mg; sprinkle cap 15, 25, 50 mg

Adverse effects
CNS: Dizziness, fatigue, cognitive disorder, *insomnia,* anxiety, depression, paresthesia
EENT: Diplopia, vision abnormality
ENDO: Weight loss

GI: Diarrhea, anorexia, nausea, dyspepsia, abdominal pain, constipation, dry mouth
GU: Breast pain, dysmenorrhea, menstrual disorder
INTEG: Rash
MISC: Weight loss, leukopenia
RESP: URI, pharyngitis, sinusitis

Contraindications: Hypersensitivity

Precautions: Hepatic disease, renal disease, cardiac disease,
G elderly, lactation, children,
P pregnancy **C**

Pharmacokinetics

Absorption	Well absorbed
Distribution	Crosses placenta, plasma protein binding (9%-17%); steady state 4 days
Metabolism	Unknown
Excretion	Kidneys unchanged 55%-97%
Half-life	21 hr

Pharmacodynamics

Onset	Unknown
Peak	2-4 hr
Duration	Unknown

Interactions
Individual drugs
Alcohol: ↑ levels of alcohol
Carbamazepine: ↓ levels of topiramate
Digoxin: ↓ levels of digoxin
Phenytoin: ↓ levels of topiramate
Valproic acid: ↓ levels of topiramate
Drug classifications
Carbonic anhydrase inhibitors: ↑ levels of carbonic anhydrase inhibitors
CNS depressants: ↑ CNS depression
Contraceptives, oral: ↓ level of oral contraceptives

Food/drug
↓ levels of topiramate

NURSING CONSIDERATIONS
Assessment
• Assess mental status: mood, sensorium, affect, memory (long, short), especially in G elderly
• Assess for blood dyscrasias: fever, sore throat, bruising, rash, jaundice, epistaxis (long-term treatment only)
• Assess seizure activity including type, location, duration, and character; provide seizure precaution
• Monitor CBC during long-term therapy
• Assess body weight and evidence of cognitive disorder

Nursing diagnoses
☑ Injury, risk for (side effects)
☑ Knowledge deficit (teaching)

Implementation
• May take with food
🚫• Do not crush, or break tabs; very bitter

Patient/family education
• Teach patient to carry Medic Alert ID stating name, drugs taken, condition, prescriber's name, phone number
• Advise patient to avoid driving, other activities that require alertness
• Teach patient not to discontinue medication abruptly after long-term use

Evaluation
Positive therapeutic outcome
• Decreased seizure activity

Treatment of overdose:
Lavage, vital signs

---

topotecan (℞)
(to-poe′ti-kan)
Hycamtin
Func. class: Antineoplastic hormone
Chem. class: Semi-synthetic derivative of camptothecin (topoisomerase inhibitor)
Pregnancy category   C

Action: Antitumor drug with topoisomerase I-inhibitory activity; topoisomerase I relieves torsional strain in DNA by causing single-strand breaks; causes double-strand DNA damage

⮕**Therapeutic Outcome:** Decreased tumor size

Uses: Metastatic carcinoma of the ovary after failure of traditional chemotherapy

Dosage and routes
Adult: **IV** inf 1.5 mg/m² over 30 min qd × 5 days starting on day 1 of a 2-day course × 4 courses; may be reduced to 0.25 mg/m² for subsequent courses if severe neutropenia occurs

Available forms: Lyophilized powder for inj 4 mg (free base)

Adverse effects
CNS: Arthralgia, asthenia, headache, myalgia, pain
GI: Abdominal pain, constipation, diarrhea, obstruction, nausea, stomatitis, vomiting, increased ALT, AST; anorexia
HEMA: **Neutropenia, leukopenia, thrombocytopenia, anemia, sepsis**
INTEG: Total alopecia
RESP: Dyspnea

T

Contraindications: Hypersensitivity, lactation, severe bone marrow depression

P **Precautions:** Children, pregnancy **C**

Pharmacokinetics	
Absorption	Rapidly/completely
Distribution	Unknown
Metabolism	Liver
Excretion	Urine, feces to metabolites
Half-life	8 hr

Pharmacodynamics
Unknown

Interactions
Individual drugs
Cisplatin: ↑ myelosuppression
G-CSF: ↑ duration of neutropenia

NURSING CONSIDERATIONS
Assessment
• Monitor liver function studies: AST, ALT, alk phosphatase, which may be elevated
• Monitor for CNS symptoms: drowsiness, confusion, depression, anxiety
• Monitor CBC, differential, platelet count weekly; withhold drug if WBC is <3500/mm^3 or platelet count is <100,000/mm^3; notify prescriber of these results; drug should be discontinued
• Assess buccal cavity q8h for dryness, sores or ulceration, white patches, oral pain, bleeding, dysphagia
• Assess GI symptoms: frequency of stools, cramping
• Assess signs of dehydration: rapid respiration, poor skin turgor, decreased urine output, dry skin, restlessness, weakness

Nursing diagnoses
☑ Infection, risk for (adverse reactions)
☑ Knowledge deficit (teaching)

Implementation
• Provide increased fluid intake to 2-3 L/day to prevent dehydration, unless contraindicated
• Change **IV** site q48h
• Rinse mouth tid-qid with water, club soda; brush teeth bid-tid with soft brush or cotton-tipped applicator for stomatitis; use unwaxed dental floss
• Provide nutritious diet with iron, vit K supplements, low fiber, few dairy products

Patient/family education
• Advise to avoid foods with citric acid or hot or rough texture if stomatitis is present; to drink adequate fluids
• Advise to report stomatitis; any bleeding, white spots, ulcerations in mouth; tell patient to examine mouth qd; report symptoms
• Assess to report signs of anemia; fatigue, headache, faintness, shortness of breath, irritability
• Teach to use contraception during therapy

Evaluation
Positive therapeutic outcome
• Decreased tumor size, spread of malignancy

toremifene (℞)
(tore'me-feen)
Fareston
Func. class.: Antineoplastic
Chem. class.: Antiestrogen hormone
Pregnancy category   D

Action: Inhibits cell division by binding to cytoplasmic estrogen receptors; resembles normal cell complex but inhibits DNA synthesis and estrogen response of target tissue

⇒**Therapeutic Outcome:** Prevention of rapidly growing malignant cells

Uses: Advanced breast carcinoma that has not responded to other therapy in estrogen-receptor-positive patients (usually postmenopausal)

Dosage and routes
Adult: PO 60 mg qd

Available forms: Tabs 60 mg

Adverse effects
CNS: Hot flashes, headache, lightheadedness, depression
CV: Chest pain
EENT: Ocular lesions, retinopathy, corneal opacity, blurred vision (high doses)
GI: Nausea, vomiting, altered taste (anorexia)
GU: Vaginal bleeding, pruritus vulvae
HEMA: **Thrombocytopenia, leukopenia**
INTEG: Rash, alopecia
META: Hypercalcemia

Contraindications: Hypersensitivity, pregnancy **D**

Precautions: Leukopenia, thrombocytopenia, lactation, cataracts

Pharmacokinetics	
Absorption	Adequately absorbed
Distribution	Unknown
Metabolism	Liver, extensively
Excretion	Feces, slowly, small amounts (kidneys)
Half-life	Unknown

Pharmacodynamics	
Onset	Unknown
Peak	3 hr
Duration	Unknown

Interactions
Lab test interferences
↑ Serum Ca

NURSING CONSIDERATIONS
Assessment
• Monitor CBC, differential, platelet count weekly; withhold drug if WBC is <4000 or platelet count is <75,000; notify prescriber of results; monitor calcium levels (hypercalcemia is common)
• Assess for tumor flare: increase in bone, tumor pain during beginning treatment; give analgesics as ordered to decrease pain
• Assess for bleeding: hematuria, guaiac, bruising or petechiae, mucosa or orifices q8h, no rec temp

Nursing diagnoses
☑ Injury, risk for (adverse reactions)
☑ Knowledge deficit (teaching)

Implementation
• Give with food or fluids for GI upset; do not break, crush, or chew enteric products; repeat dose may be needed if vomiting occurs
• Store in light-resistant container at room temp

Patient/family education
• Instruct patient to report any complaints, side effects to health care prescriber; if dose is missed, do not double next dose
• Advise patient that vaginal bleeding, pruritus, hot flashes, can occur, and are reversible after discontinuing treatment
• Instruct patient to report immediately decreased visual acuity, which may be irreversible; stress need for routine eye exams

- Inform patient about who should be told about toremifene therapy
- Advise patient to report vaginal bleeding immediately; that tumor flare—increase in size or tumor, increased bone pain—may occur and will subside rapidly; may take analgesics for pain; that premenopausal women must use mechanical birth control method because ovulation may be induced (teratogenic drug)
- Caution patient to use sunscreen and protective clothing to prevent burns because photosensitivity is common
- Teach patient that hair loss may occur during treatment; a wig or hairpiece may make patient feel better; new hair may be different in color, texture
- Inform patient rash or lesions are temporary and may become large during beginning therapy

Evaluation

Positive therapeutic outcome
- Decreased spread of malignant cells in breast cancer

---

trace elements (chromium, copper, iodide, manganese, selenium, zinc) (℞)

Concentrated Multiple Trace Elements, ConTE-PAK-4, M.T.E.-4 Concentrated, M.T.E.-5, M.T.E.-5 Concentrated, M.T.E.-6, M.T.E.-6 Concentrated, M.T.E.-7, MulTE-PAK-4, MulTE-PAK-5, Multiple Trace Element, Multiple Trace Element Neonatal, Multiple Trace Element Pediatric, Neotrace 4, Ped TE-PAK-4, Pedtrice-4, P.T.E.-4, P.T.E.-5

Func. class.: Mineral supplement

Pregnancy category **C**

Action: Needed for adequate absorption and synthesis of amino acids

Therapeutic Outcome: Replacement for mineral deficiencies

Uses: Prevention of trace element deficiency, a component of TPN

Dosage and routes

Usual dosage may be given in TPN sol

Chromium
Adult: **IV** 10-15 µg qd

P *Child:* **IV** 0.14-0.20 µg/kg/day

Copper
Adult: **IV** 0.5-1.5 mg/day

P *Child:* **IV** .05-0.2 mg/kg/day

Iodide
Adult: **IV** 1 µg/kg/day

Manganese
Adult: **IV** 1-3 mg/day

Selenium
Adult: 40-120 µg/day
P *Child:* 3 µg/kg/day
Zinc
Adult: **IV** 2-4 mg/day
P *Child:* **IV** 0.05 mg/kg/day
Available forms: Many forms available—see particular elements

Adverse effects
CHROMIUM: **Seizures, coma,** nausea, vomiting, ulcers, **renal/hepatic toxicity**
COPPER: Personality changes, diarrhea, weakness, photophobia, muscle weakness
IODINE: Headache, edema of eyelids, acne, metallic taste, sore mouth, running nose
MANGANESE: Incoordination, headache, irritability, lability, slurred speech, impotence
SELENIUM: Alopecia, depression, vomiting, GI cramping, nervousness, garlic smell
ZINC: Vomiting, oliguria, **hypothermia,** vision changes, **tachycardia,** jaundice, **coma**
Precautions: Liver, biliary disease, pregnancy **C,** lactation, severe vomiting or diarrhea

Pharmacokinetics	
Absorption	Completely absorbed
Distribution	Widely distributed
Metabolism	Unknown
Excretion	Depends on element
Half-life	Unknown

Pharmacodynamics
Unknown

Interactions: None

NURSING CONSIDERATIONS
Assessment
• Assess trace element levels; notify prescriber if low copper

0.07-0.15 mg/ml, zinc 0.05-0.15 mg/100 ml, manganese 4-20 µg/100 ml, selenium 0.1-0.19 µg/ml
• Assess trace element deficiency if patient is receiving TPN for extended period
• Obtain calorie count to identify nutritional deficiencies
• Assess for toxicity to individual element (see side effects/adverse reactions)

Nursing diagnoses
☑ Nutrition: less than body requirements (uses)
☑ Knowledge deficit (teaching)

Implementation
• Give by **IV** inf, often mixed with TPN sol
• Discard unused portions
• Give by continuous inf diluted in 1 L or more **IV** sol; give at prescribed rate

Patient/family education
• Explain reason for and expected results of medication

Evaluation
Positive therapeutic outcome
• Absence of element deficiency

---

tramadol (℞)
(trah'mah-dol)
Ultram
Func. class.: Central analgesic
Pregnancy category   C

Action: Not completely understood, binds to opioid receptors and inhibits reuptake of norepinephrine, serotonin; does not cause histamine release or affect heart rate
➡ **Therapeutic Outcome:** Relief of pain

T

Uses: Management of moderate to severe pain

Dosage and routes

Adult: PO 50-100 mg prn q4-6h, max 400 mg/day

G *Elderly >75 yrs:* PO <300 mg/day in divided dose

Hepatic dose

PO 50 mg q12h

Renal dose

CrCl <30 ml/min give q12h, max 200 mg/day

Available forms: Tab 50 mg

Adverse effects

CNS: Dizziness, CNS stimulation, somnolence, headache, anxiety, confusion, euphoria, **seizure,** hallucinations

CV: Vasodilation, orthostatic hypotension, tachycardia, hypertension, abnormal ECG

GI: Nausea, constipation, vomiting, dry mouth, diarrhea, abdominal pain, anorexia, flatulence, GI bleeding

GU: Urinary retention/ frequency, menopausal symptoms, dysuria, menstrual disorder

INTEG: Pruritus, rash, urticaria, vesicles

Contraindications: Hypersensitivity, acute intoxication with any CNS depressant

Precautions: Seizure disorder, P pregnancy **C,** lactation, chil- G dren, elderly, renal, hepatic disease, respiratory depression, head trauma, increased intracranial pressure, acute abdominal condition, drug abuse

N **Do Not Confuse:**

tramadol/Toradol

Pharmacokinetics

Absorption	Rapidly, almost completely absorbed
Distribution	Steady state 2 days
Metabolism	Extensively in liver, may cross bloodbrain barrier
Excretion	Unchanged drug 30% in urine
Half-life	Unknown

Pharmacodynamics

Unknown

Interactions

Individual drugs

Carbamazepine: ↓ of tramadol

Drug classifications

MAOIs: Inhibition of norepinephrine and serotonin reuptake; use together with caution

Sedatives/hypnotics: ↑ CNS depression

Herb/drug

Kava: ↑ CNS depression

Lab test interferences

↑ Creatinine, ↑ liver enzymes ↓ Hgb

NURSING CONSIDERATIONS

Assessment

• Assess pain: location, type, character; give before pain becomes extreme

• Monitor I&O ratio: check for decreasing output; may indicate urinary retention

• Assess need for drug

• Assess for constipation; increase fluids, bulk in diet

• Monitor CNS changes: dizziness, drowsiness, hallucinations, euphoria, LOC, pupil reaction

• Determine allergic reactions: rash, urticaria

Nursing diagnoses

☑ Pain (uses)

☑ Sensory, perceptual alteration: visual, auditory (adverse reactions)

☑ Injury, risk for (adverse reactions)
☑ Knowledge deficit (teaching)

Implementation
- Give with antiemetic for nausea, vomiting
- Administer when pain is beginning to return; determine dosage interval by patient response
- Store in cool environment, protect from sunlight

Patient/family education
- Teach patient to report any symptoms of CNS changes, allergic reactions
- Teach patient that drowsiness, dizziness, and confusion may occur; to call for assistance
- Instruct patient to make position changes slowly, orthostatic hypotension may occur
- Tell patient to avoid OTC medication and alcohol unless approved by prescriber

Evaluation
Positive therapeutic outcome
- Decreased pain

---

trandolapril (℞)
(tran-doe′la-prill)
Mavik
Func. class.: Antihypertensive
Chem. class.: Angiotensin-converting enzyme inhibitor

Pregnancy category **D** (2nd/3rd trimesters); **C** (1st trimester)

Action: Selectively suppresses renin-angiotensin-aldosterone system; inhibits ACE; prevents conversion of angiotensin I to angiotensin II, resulting in dilatation of arterial and venous vessels and lowered B/P

➡ **Therapeutic Outcome:** Decreased B/P in hypertension

Uses: Hypertension alone or in combination, heart failure, post MI/left ventricular dysfunction post MI

Dosage and routes
Hypertension
Adult: PO 1 mg/day, 2 mg/day in African Americans, make dosage adjustment ≥wk; up to 8 mg/day

Heart failure (post MI/left ventricular dysfunction)
Adult: PO 1 mg/day, titrate upward to 4 mg/day if tolerated

Renal dose
CrCl <30 ml/min give 0.5 mg/day may increase gradually up to 4 mg/day

Available forms: Tabs 1, 2, 4 mg

Adverse effects
CNS: Dizziness, paresthesias, headache, fatigue, drowsiness, depression, sleep disturbances
CV: Hypotension, MI, palpitations, angina, TIAs, stroke, bradycardia, dysrhythmias
GI: Nausea, vomiting, cramps, diarrhea, constipation, ileus, pancreatitis, hepatitis, *dyspepsia*
GU: **Proteinuria, renal failure**
HEMA: **Agranulocytosis, neutropenia, leukopenia,** anemia
INTEG: Rash, purpura
MISC: Hyperkalemia, hyponatremia, impotence, *myalgia*
RESP: Dyspnea, cough

Contraindications: Hypersensitivity, history of angio-

T

---

edema, pregnancy **D** (2nd/3rd trimesters)

Precautions: Renal disease, hyperkalemia, hepatic disease, bilateral renal stenosis, post kidney transplant, aortal/mitral valve stenosis, cirrhosis, severe renal disease, untreated CHF, autoimmune diseases, severe hypertension, pregnancy **C** (1st trimester)

Pharmacokinetics

Absorption	40-60%
Distribution	Unknown
Metabolism	Liver
Excretion	Kidneys, feces
Half-life	0.6-1.1 hr, 16-24 hr

Pharmacodynamics

Onset	½ hr
Peak	4-10 hr
Duration	>8 days

Interactions
Individual drugs
Alcohol: ↑ hypotension (large amounts)
Allopurinol: ↑ hypersensitivity
Capsaicin: ↑ coughing
Digoxin: ↑ serum levels of digoxin
Hydralazine: ↑ toxicity
Indomethacin: ↓ antihypertensive effect
Lithium: ↑ serum levels of lithium
Prazosin: ↑ toxicity
Drug classifications
Adrenergic blockers: ↑ hypotension
Antacids: ↓ absorption
Antihypertensives: ↑ hypotension
Diuretics: ↑ hypotension
Diuretics, potassium-sparing: ↑ toxicity
Ganglionic blockers: ↑ hypotension
Phenothiazines: ↑ antihypertensive effects

Potassium supplements: ↑ toxicity of potassium
Sympathomimetics: ↑ toxicity

NURSING CONSIDERATIONS
Assessment
• Monitor blood studies: neutrophils, decreased platelets
• Monitor B/P, orthostatic hypotension, syncope; if changes occur dosage change may be required
• Monitor renal studies: protein, BUN, creatinine; increased levels may indicate nephrotic syndrome and renal failure
• Monitor renal symptoms: polyuria, oliguria, frequency, dysuria
• Establish baselines in renal, liver function tests before therapy begins
• Check potassium levels throughout treatment, although hyperkalemia rarely occurs
• Check for edema in feet, legs daily
• Assess for allergic reactions: rash, fever, pruritus, urticaria; drug should be discontinued if antihistamines fail to help

Nursing diagnoses
☑ Cardiac output, decreased (uses)
☑ Injury, potential for (adverse reactions)
☑ Knowledge deficit (teaching)
☑ Noncompliance (teaching)

Implementation
• Store in air-tight container at 86° F (36° C) or less

Patient/family education
• Advise patient not to discontinue drug abruptly; advise patient to tell all persons associated with health care
• Teach patient not to use OTC products (cough, cold,

☑ Herb/drug ⓢ Do Not Crush ◆ Alert ✆ Key Drug ⒼGeriatric ⓅPediatric allergy medications) unless directed by physician; serious side effects can occur; xanthines, such as coffee, tea, chocolate, cola can prevent action of drug

• Instruct patient on the importance of complying with dosage schedule, even if feeling better; to continue with medical regimen to decrease B/P: exercise, cessation of smoking, decreasing stress, diet modifications

• Emphasize the need to rise slowly to sitting or standing position to minimize orthostatic hypotension; not to exercise in hot weather, which can cause increased hypotension

• Advise patient to notify prescriber of mouth sores, sore throat, fever, swelling of hands or feet, irregular heartbeat, chest pain, coughing, shortness of breath

• Caution patient to report excessive perspiration, dehydration, vomiting, diarrhea; may lead to fall in B/P

• Caution patient that drug may cause dizziness, fainting, lightheadedness; may occur during 1st few days of therapy; to avoid activities that may be hazardous

• Teach patient how to take B/P, and normal readings for age group

Evaluation
Positive therapeutic outcome
• Decreased B/P in hypertension

Treatment of overdose: Lavage, **IV** atropine for bradycardia, **IV** theophylline for bronchospasm, digitalis, O_2, diuretic for cardiac failure, hemodialysis

tranylcypromine (R)
(tran-ill-sip'roe-meen)
Parnate
Func. class: Antidepressant—MAOI
Chem. class: Nonhydrazine
Pregnancy category   C

Action: Increases concentrations of endogenous epinephrine, norepinephrine, serotonin, dopamine in storage sites in CNS by inhibition of MAO; increased concentration reduces depression

▶**Therapeutic Outcome:** Decreased symptoms of depression after 2-3 wk

Uses: Depression, when uncontrolled by other means

Investigational uses: Bulimia, cocaine addiction, migraines, seasonal affective disorder, panic disorder

Dosages and routes
Adult: PO 10 mg bid; may increase to 30 mg/day after 2 wk

Available forms: Tab 10 mg

Adverse effects
CNS: Dizziness, drowsiness, confusion, headache, anxiety, tremors, stimulation, weakness, hyperreflexia, mania, insomnia, fatigue, weight gain
CV: Orthostatic hypotension, hypertension, **dysrhythmias, hypertensive crisis**
EENT: Blurred vision
ENDO: **SIADH-like syndrome**
GI: Constipation, dry mouth, nausea, vomiting, *anorexia,* diarrhea, weight gain
GU: Change in libido, frequency
HEMA: Anemia
INTEG: Rash, flushing, increased perspiration

T

Contraindications: Hypersensitivity to MAOIs, elderly, hypertension, CHF, severe hepatic disease, pheochromocytoma, severe renal disease, severe cardiac disease

Precautions: Suicidal patients, convulsive disorders, severe depression, schizophrenia, hyperactivity, diabetes mellitus, pregnancy **C**

Pharmacokinetics

Absorption	Well absorbed
Distribution	Crosses placenta
Metabolism	Liver, extensively
Excretion	Kidneys, breast milk
Half-life	Unknown

Pharmacodynamics

Unknown

Interactions
Individual drugs
Alcohol: ↑ CNS depression
Buspirone: ↑ pressor effect
Dextromethorphan: ↑ hypertensive crisis
Fluoxetine: Serotonin syndrome, do not use together
Fluvoxame: Serotonin syndrome, do not use together
Guanethidine: ↓ hypertensive crisis
Methylphenidate: ↑ hypertensive crisis
Paroxetine: Serotonin syndrome, do not use together
Sertraline: Serotonin syndrome, do not use together
Sumatriptan: ↑ effects
Drug classifications
Antidepressants, tricyclic: ↑ hypertensive crisis
Antidiabetics: ↑ effects
Antihypertensives: ↑ hypotension
β-Adrenergic blockers: ↑ effects
Diuretics, thiazide: ↑ effects

Opiates: ↑ CNS depression
Rauwolfia alkaloids: ↑ effects
Sulfonamides: ↑ effects
Food/drug
Foods containing tyramine: ↑ hypertensive crisis
Herb/drug
Ephedra: ↑ sympathomimetic action
L-**Tryptophan:** ↑ effects

NURSING CONSIDERATIONS
Assessment
• Monitor B/P (lying, standing), pulse q4h; if systolic B/P drops 20 mm hg hold drug, notify prescriber; take vital signs q4h in patients with cardiovascular disease
• Monitor hepatic studies: AST, ALT, bilirubin
• Check weight qwk; appetite may increase with drug
• Assess mental status: mood, sensorium, affect, suicidal tendencies; increase in psychiatric symptoms: depression, panic
• Monitor urinary retention, constipation; constipation is more likely to occur in children or elderly
• Assess for withdrawal symptoms: headache, nausea, vomiting, muscle pain, weakness; do not usually occur unless drug was discontinued abruptly
• Identify alcohol consumption; if alcohol is consumed, hold dose until morning

Nursing diagnoses
✓ Coping, ineffective individual (uses)
✓ Injury, risk for (side effects)
✓ Knowledge deficit (teaching)
✓ Noncompliance (teaching)

Implementation
• Give with food or milk for GI symptoms; crush if patient

---

is unable to swallow medication whole
• Store at room temp; do not freeze

Patient/family education
• Advise patient that therapeutic effects may take 48 hr-3 wk
• Teach patient to use caution in driving or other activities requiring alertness because of drowsiness, dizziness, blurred vision; to avoid rising quickly from sitting to standing, especially elderly G
• Caution patient to avoid alcohol ingestion, other CNS depressants
• Advise patient not to discontinue medication quickly after long-term use: may cause nausea, headache, malaise
• Advise patient to increase fluids, bulk in diet if constipation, urinary retention occur, especially elderly G
• Teach patient to take gum, hard sugarless candy, or frequent sips of water for dry mouth
• Teach patient to avoid high-tyramine foods; cheese (aged), sour cream, beer, wine, pickled products, liver, raisins, bananas, figs, avocados, meat tenderizers, chocolate, yogurt; increased caffeine, ginseng
• Teach patient to report headache, palpitation, neck stiffness
• Instruct patient to wear or carry Medic Alert Bracelet or ID with medications taken, condition treated, and prescriber's name and phone number

Evaluation
Positive therapeutic outcome
• Decrease in depression
• Absence of suicidal thoughts

Treatment of overdose: Lavage, activated charcoal, monitor electrolytes, vital signs, diazepam **IV**, NaHCO$_3$

trastuzumab (℞)
(tras-tuz'uh-mab)
Herceptin
Func. class.: Miscellaneous antineoplastic
Chem. class.: Humanized monoclonal antibody
Pregnancy category   B

Action: DNA-derived monoclonal antibody selectively binds to extracellular portion of human epidermal growth factor receptor 2; it inhibits proliferation of cancer cells

Therapeutic Outcome: Decreasing symptoms of breast cancer

Uses: Breast cancer; metastatic with overexpression of HER2

Dosage and routes
Adult: **IV** 4 mg/kg given over 90 min, then maintenance 2 mg/kg given over 30 min; do not give as **IV** push or bol

Available forms: Lyophilized powder 440 mg

Adverse effects
CNS: Dizziness, numbness, paresthesias, depression, insomnia, neuropathy, peripheral neuritis
CV: **Tachycardia, CHF**
GI: Nausea, vomiting, anorexia, diarrhea
HEMA: Anemia, **leukopenia**
INTEG: Rash, acne, herpes simplex
META: Edema, peripheral edema
MISC: Flulike syndrome; fever, headache, chills

T

MS: Arthralgia, bone pain
RESP: Cough, dyspnea, pharyngitis, rhinitis, sinusitis
Contraindications: Hypersensitivity to this drug, Chinese hamster ovary cell protein
P **Precautions:** Pregnancy **B**,
G lactation, children, elderly, cardiac disease, anemia, leukopenia

Pharmacokinetics

Absorption	Unknown
Distribution	Unknown
Metabolism	Unknown
Excretion	Unknown
Half-life	1.7-12 days

Pharmacodynamics

Onset	Unknown
Peak	Unknown
Duration	Unknown

Interactions
Unknown

NURSING CONSIDERATIONS
Assessment

• Assess for symptoms of infection; may be masked by drug
• Assess CNS reaction: LOC, mental status, dizziness, confusion

Nursing diagnoses

☑ Infection, risk for (side effects)
☑ Nutrition, altered, less than body requirements (side effects)
☑ Knowledge deficit (teaching)

Implementation

• Give acetaminophen as ordered to alleviate fever and headache
• Increase fluid intake to 2-3 L/day

IV route

• Administer after reconstituting vial with 20 ml bacteriostatic water for inj, 1.1% benzyl alcohol preserved (supplied) to yield 21 mg/ml, mark date on vial 28 days from reconstitution date, if pt is allergic to benzyl alcohol, reconstitute with sterile water for inj—use immediately
• Do not mix or dilute with other drugs or dextrose sol

Patient/family education

• Advise patient to take acetaminophen for fever
• Teach patient to avoid hazardous tasks, since confusion, dizziness may occur
• Teach patient to report signs of infection: sore throat, fever, diarrhea, vomiting
• Inform patient that emotional lability is common; instruct patient to notify prescriber if severe or incapacitating

Evaluation

Positive therapeutic outcome
• Decrease in size of tumors

---

trazodone (℞)
(tray'zoe-done)
Desyrel, Desyrel Dividose, trazodone HCl
Func. class.: Antidepressant, miscellaneous
Chem. class.: Triazolopyridine
Pregnancy category **C**

Action: Selectively inhibits serotonin uptake by brain, potentiates behavioral changes
➡ **Therapeutic Outcome:** Decreased symptoms of depression after 2-3 wk
Uses: Depression
Investigational uses:
Chronic pain syndromes

Dosage and routes:
Adult: PO 150 mg/day in divided doses; may increase by 50 mg/day q3-4d, not to exceed 600 mg/day

G *Elderly:* PO 25-50 hs, ↑ by 25-50 mg q3-7 days, to desired dose

Available forms: Tabs 50, 100, 150, 300 mg

Adverse effects

CNS: Dizziness, drowsiness, confusion, headache, anxiety, tremors, stimulation, weakness, insomnia, nightmares, EPS
G (elderly), increase in psychiatric symptoms

CV: Orthostatic hypotension, ECG changes, tachycardia, **hypertension,** palpitations

EENT: Blurred vision, tinnitus, mydriasis

GI: Diarrhea, dry mouth, nausea, vomiting, **paralytic ileus,** increased appetite, cramps, epigastric distress, jaundice, **hepatitis,** stomatitis

GU: Retention, **acute renal failure, priapism**

HEMA: **Agranulocytosis, thrombocytopenia, eosinophilia, leukopenia**

INTEG: Rash, urticaria, sweating, pruritus, photosensitivity

Contraindications: Hypersensitivity to tricyclic antidepressants, recovery phase of MI, convulsive disorders, prostatic hypertrophy

Precautions: Suicidal patients, severe depression, increased intraocular pressure, narrow-angle glaucoma, urinary retention, cardiac disease, hepatic disease, hyperthyroidism, electroshock therapy, elective surgery, pregnancy **C**

Pharmacokinetics

Absorption	Well absorbed
Distribution	Widely distributed
Metabolism	Liver, extensively
Excretion	Kidneys—unchanged minimally
Half-life	4½-7½ hr

Pharmacodynamics

Unknown

Interactions
Individual drugs

Alcohol: ↑ CNS depression
Cimetidine: ↑ levels, ↑ toxicity
Clonidine: Severe hypotension, avoid use
Disulfiram: Organic brain syndrome
Fluoxetine: ↑ levels, ↑ toxicity
Guanethidine: ↓ effects

Drug classifications

Analgesics: ↑ CNS depression
Anticholinergics: ↑ side effects
Antihistamines: ↑ CNS depression
Antihypertensives: may block antihypertensive effect
Barbiturates: ↑ effects
Benzodiazepines: ↑ effects
CNS depressants: ↑ effects
MAOIs: ↑ hypertensive crisis, convulsions
Oral contraceptives: effects, toxicity
Phenothiazines: ↑ toxicity
Sedative/hypnotics: ↑ CNS depression
Sympathomimetics, indirect-acting: ↓ effects

Smoking

↑ metabolism, ↓ effects

Herb/drug

Kava: ↑ CNS depression

Lab test interferences

↑ Serum bilirubin, ↑ blood glucose, ↑ alk phosphatase ↓ VMA, ↓ 5-HIAA, ↓ blood glucose

T

False increase: Urinary cat-echolamines

NURSING CONSIDERATIONS
Assessment

• Monitor B/P (lying, stand-ing), pulse q4h; if systolic B/P drops 20 mm hg hold drug, notify prescriber; take vital signs q4h in patients with cardiovascular disease
• Monitor blood studies: CBC, leukocytes, differential, cardiac enzymes if patient is receiving long-term therapy
• Monitor hepatic studies: AST, ALT, bilirubin
• Check weight qwk; appetite may increase with drug
• Assess ECG for flattening of T wave, bundle branch block, AV block, dysrhythmias in cardiac patients
G • Assess for EPS primarily in elderly; rigidity, dystonia, akathisia
• Assess mental status: mood, sensorium, affect, suicidal tendencies; increase in psychi-atric symptoms: depression, panic
P • Monitor urinary retention, constipation; constipation is more likely to occur in children
G or elderly
• Assess for withdrawal symptoms: headache, nausea, vomiting, muscle pain, weak-ness; do not usually occur unless drug was discontinued abruptly
• Identify alcohol consump-tion; if alcohol is consumed, hold dose until AM

Nursing diagnoses

☑ Coping, ineffective individual (uses)
☑ Injury, risk for (adverse reac-tions)
☑ Knowledge deficit (teaching)
☑ Noncompliance (teaching)

Implementation

• Give with food or milk for GI symptoms; crush if patient is unable to swallow medica-tion whole
G • Give dosage hs if overseda-tion occurs during day; may take entire dose hs; elderly may not tolerate once/day dosing
• Store at room temp; do not freeze

Patient/family education

• Teach patient that therapeu-tic effects may take 2-3 wk
G • Teach patient to use caution in driving or other activities requiring alertness because of drowsiness, dizziness, blurred vision; to avoid rising quickly from sitting to standing, especially elderly
• Caution patient to avoid alcohol ingestion, other CNS depressants
• Teach patient not to discon-tinue medication quickly after long-term use: may cause nausea, headache, malaise
• Advise patient to wear sun-screen or large hat because photosensitivity occurs
G • Teach patient to increase fluids, bulk in diet if constipa-tion, urinary retention occur, especially elderly
• Advise patient to take gum, hard sugarless candy, or fre-quent sips of water for dry mouth

Evaluation
Positive therapeutic outcome
• Decrease in depression
• Absence of suicidal thoughts

Treatment of overdose:
ECG monitoring, induce eme-sis, lavage, activated charcoal, administer anticonvulsant

---

☑ Herb/drug 🚫 Do Not Crush ◆ Alert ☛ Key Drug **G** Geriatric **P** Pediatric

tretinoin (vitamin A acid, retinoic acid) (℞)
(tret′i-noyn)
Retin-A, Stievaa ♣,
Tretinoin LF IV, Vesanoid
Func. class.: Vitamin A acid/acne product, antineoplastic-misc.
Chem. class.: Tretinoin derivative

Pregnancy category C (top), D (PO)

Action: Decreases cohesiveness of follicular epithelium, decreases microcomedone formation (top); induces maturation of acute promyelocytic leukemia, exact action is unknown (PO)

▶**Therapeutic Outcome:** Decreased signs/symptoms of leukemia

Uses: Acne vulgaris (grades 1-3) (top); acute promyelocytic leukemia (PO)

Investigational uses: Skin cancer

Dosage and routes
▣*Adult and child:* Top cleanse area, apply hs; cover lightly

Promyelocytic leukemia
Adult: PO 45 mg/m^2/day given as 2 evenly divided doses until remission, discontinue treatment 30 days after remission or 90 days of treatment, whichever is first

Available forms: Top cream 0.05%, 0.01%; top gel 0.025%, 0.01%; top liq 0.05%; cap 10 mg

Adverse effects
Top
INTEG: Rash, stinging, warmth, redness, erythema, blistering, crusting, peeling, contact dermatitis, hypopigmentation, hyperpigmentation

PO
CNS: Headache, fever, sweating
GI: Nausea, vomiting, **hemorrhage,** abdominal pain, diarrhea, constipation, dyspepsia, distention, **hepatitis**

Contraindications: Hypersensitivity to retinoids or sensitive to parabens, pregnancy **D** (PO)

Precautions: Pregnancy **C** (top), lactation, eczema, sunburn

Pharmacokinetics

Absorption	Small amounts
Distribution	Unknown
Metabolism	Unknown
Excretion	Kidneys
Half-life	Unknown

Pharmacodynamics

Unknown

Interactions
Individual drugs
Benzoyl peroxide: ↑ peeling
Resorcinol: ↑ peeling
Salicylic acid: ↑ peeling
Sulfur: ↑ peeling
Drug classifications
Abrasive soaps: ↑ peeling
Alcohol astringents: ↑ peeling

NURSING CONSIDERATIONS T
Assessment

Top
• Assess part of body involved, including time involved, what helps or aggravates condition, cysts, dryness, itching; lesions may become worse at beginning of treatment
Nursing diagnoses
☑ Skin integrity, impaired (uses)

☑ Body image disturbances (uses)
☑ Knowledge deficit (teaching)

Implementation
Top route
• Apply using gloves, once daily before hs; cover area lightly using gauze
• Store at room temp
• Wash hands after application
Liq
• Apply with gloves or cotton; apply only to affected areas

Patient/family education
Top
• Instruct patient to avoid application on normal skin, and to avoid getting cream in eyes, nose, other mucous membranes
• Advise patient to avoid sunlight, sunlamps or to use protective clothing or sunscreen to prevent burns
• Advise patient that treatment may cause warmth, stinging; dryness; peeling will occur
• Inform patient that cosmetics may be used over drug; not to use shaving lotions
• Inform patient that rash may occur during first 1-3 wk of therapy
• Caution patient that drug does not cure condition; only relieves symptoms; that therapeutic results may be seen in 2-3 wk but may not be optimal until after 6 wk

Evaluation
Positive therapeutic outcome
• Decrease in size and number of lesions

triamcinolone (℞)
(trye-am-sin'oh-lone)
Amcort, Aristocort, Aristocort Forte, Aristocort Intralesional, Aristospan Intra-Articular, Aristospan Intralesional, Articulose L.A., Atolone, Azmacort, Cenocort A-40, Cenocort Forte, Kenacort, Kenaject-40, Kenalog, Kenalog-10, Kenalog-40, Tac-3, Tac-40, Triam-A, triamcinolone, triamcinolone acetonide, Triam Forte, Triamolone 40, Triamonide 40, Tri-Kort, Trilog, Trilone, Trisoject
Func. class.: Corticosteroid; antiinflammatory
Chem. class.: Glucocorticoid, intermediate-acting
Pregnancy category   C

Action: Decreases inflammation by suppression of migration of polymorphonuclear leukocytes, fibroblasts, reversal to increase capillary permeability and lysosomal stabilization

▶**Therapeutic Outcome:** Decreased inflammation, normal immune response

Uses: Severe inflammation, immunosuppression, neoplasms, asthma (steroid dependent), collagen, respiratory, dermatologic disorders

Dosage and routes
Adult: PO 4-12 mg/day in divided doses qd-qid; IM 40 mg qwk (acetonide, or diacetate), 5-48 mg into neoplasms (diacetate, acetonide), 2-40 mg into joint or soft tissue (diac-

---

☑ Herb/drug   Ⓢ Do Not Crush   ◆ Alert   ☞ Key Drug   Ⓖ Geriatric   Ⓟ Pediatric

etate, acetonide), 0.5 mg/sq in of affected intralesional skin (hexacetonide), 2-20 mg into joint or soft tissue (hexacetonide)

P *Child:* PO 117 µg/kg/day as a single dose or divided doses

Asthma
Adult: Inh 2 tid-qid, not to exceed 16 inh/day

P *Child 6-12 yr:* Inh 1-2 tid-qid, not to exceed 12 inh/day

Available forms: Tabs 1, 2, 4, 8 mg; syr 2 mg/5 ml, 4.85 mg/5 ml; inj 25, 40 mg/ml diacetate; inj 3, 10, 40 mg/ml acetonide; inj 5, 20 mg/ml hexacetonide; inh 100 µg/spray; intranasal 55 µg/spray

Adverse effects
CNS: Depression, flushing, sweating, headache, mood changes
CV: Hypertension, **circulatory collapse, thrombophlebitis, embolism,** tachycardia, edema
EENT: Fungal infections, increased intraocular pressure, blurred vision
GI: Diarrhea, nausea, abdominal distention, **GI hemorrhage,** *increased appetite,* **pancreatitis**
HEMA: **Thrombocytopenia**
INTEG: Acne, poor wound healing, ecchymosis, petechiae
MS: Fractures, osteoporosis, weakness

Contraindications: Psychosis, hypersensitivity, idiopathic thrombocytopenia, acute glomerulonephritis, amebiasis, fungal infections, nonasthmatic P bronchial disease, child <2 yr, AIDS, TB

Precautions: Pregnancy **C,** diabetes mellitus, glaucoma, osteoporosis, seizure disorders, ulcerative colitis, CHF, myasthenia gravis, renal disease, esophagitis, peptic ulcer

Interactions
Individual drugs
Amphotericin B: ↑ hypokalemia
Azlocillin: ↑ hypokalemia
Insulin: ↑ need for insulin
Mezlocillin: ↑ hypokalemia
Phenytoin: ↓ action, ↑ metabolism
Piperacillin: ↑ hypokalemia
Rifampin: ↓ action, ↑ metabolism
Ticarcillin: ↑ hypokalemia
Drug classifications
Barbiturates: ↓ action, ↑ metabolism
Diuretics: ↑ hypokalemia
Hypoglycemic agents: ↑ need for hypoglycemic agents
Herb/drug
Aloe: ↑ hypokalemia
Buckthorn: ↑ hypokalemia
Rhubarb: ↑ hypokalemia
Senna: ↑ hypokalemia
Lab test interferences
↑ Cholesterol, ↑ sodium, ↑ blood glucose, ↑ uric acid, ↑ calcium, ↑ urine glucose
↓ Calcium, ↓ potassium, ↓ T_4, ↓ T_3, ↓ thyroid ^{131}I uptake test, ↓ urine 17-OHCS, ↓ 17-KS, ↓ PBI
False negative: Skin allergy tests

Pharmacokinetics		T
Absorption	Well absorbed (PO, IM)	
Distribution	Crosses placenta, widely distributed	
Metabolism	Liver—extensively	
Excretion	Kidney, breast milk	
Half-life	2-5 hr, adrenal suppression 3-4 days	

Pharmacodynamics					
	PO	IM	TOP	INH	INTRANASAL
Onset	Unknown	Unknown	Min to hr	1-2 wk	Unknown
Peak	1-2 hr	1-2 hr	Hr to days	Unknown	2-3 wk
Duration	3 days	Unknown	Hr to days	Unknown	Unknown

NURSING CONSIDERATIONS
Assessment
• Monitor potassium, blood sugar, urine glucose while on long-term therapy; hypokalemia and hyperglycemia
• Monitor weight daily; notify prescriber of weekly gain >5 lb; I&O ratio; be alert for decreasing urinary output and increasing edema
• Monitor B/P q4h, pulse; notify prescriber if chest pain occurs
• Monitor plasma cortisol levels during long-term therapy (normal level; 138-635 nmol/L SI units when drawn at 8 AM); adrenal function periodically for HPA axis suppression
• Assess for infection: increase temp, WBC even after withdrawal of medication; drug masks infection symptoms
• Assess for potassium depletion: paresthesias, fatigue, nausea, vomiting, depression, polyuria, dysrhythmias, weakness
• Assess mental status: affect, mood, behavioral changes, aggression
• Assess nasal passages during long-term treatment for changes in mucus (nasal)
• Monitor temp; if fever develops, drug should be discontinued
• Assess for systemic absorption: increased temp, inflammation, irritation (top)
Nursing diagnoses
☑ Infection, risk for (adverse reactions)

☑ Knowledge deficit (teaching)
☑ Noncompliance (teaching)

Implementation
IM route
• Give IM inj deeply in large muscle mass, rotate sites, avoid deltoid, use 21-gauge needle
• Give in one dose in AM to prevent adrenal suppression; avoid SC administration—may damage tissue
PO route
• Give with food or milk to decrease GI symptoms
Inh route
G • Use spacer device for elderly
• Give inh with water to decrease possibility of fungal infections; titrated dose, use lowest effective dose
• Give after cleaning aerosol top daily with warm water, dry thoroughly
• Store in cool environment; do not puncture or incinerate container
Top route
• Apply only to affected areas; do not get in eyes
• Apply medication, then cover with occlusive dressing (only if prescribed), seal to normal skin, change q12h; systemic absorption may occur
• Apply only to dermatoses; do not use on weeping, denuded, or infected areas
• Cleanse skin before applying drug
• Continue treatment for a few days after area has cleared
• Store at room temp

Nasal route

• Have patient clear nasal passages before administration; use decongestant if needed; shake inhaler, invert, tilt head backward, insert nozzle into nostril, away from septum; hold other nostril closed and depress activator, inhale through nose, exhale through mouth

Patient/family education

• Advise patient that ID as steroid user should be carried

• Instruct patient to notify patient if therapeutic response decreases; dosage adjustment may be needed; not to discontinue abruptly; adrenal crisis can result

• Caution patient to avoid OTC products: salicylates, alcohol in cough products, cold preparations unless directed by prescriber

• Advise patient on all aspects of drug usage including cushingoid symptoms

• Teach patient symptoms of adrenal insufficiency: nausea, anorexia, fatigue, dizziness, dyspnea, weakness, joint pain

• Teach patient that long-term therapy may be needed to clear infection (1-2 mo depending on type of infection)

Nasal route

• Instruct patient to clear nasal passages if sneezing attack occurs, repeat dose

• Advise patient to continue using product even if mild nasal bleeding occurs; is usually transient

• Teach patient method of instill after providing written instruction from manufacturer

Inh route

• Teach patient proper administration technique; to wash inhaler with warm water and dry after each use

• Teach patient all aspects of drug usage including cushingoid symptoms

Top route

• Instruct patient to avoid sunlight on affected area; burns may occur

Evaluation

Positive therapeutic outcome

• Decrease in runny nose (nasal)

• Decreased dyspnea, wheezing, dry rales on auscultation (inh)

• Ease of respirations, decreased inflammation

• Absence of severe itching, patches on skin, flaking (top)

---

triamterene (℞)

(try-am′ter-een)

Dyrenium

Func. class.: Potassium-sparing diuretic

Chem. class.: Pteridine derivative

Pregnancy category   B

Action: Acts primarily on distal tubule to inhibit reabsorption of sodium, chloride; increase potassium retention and conserve hydrogen ions

▶ **Therapeutic Outcome:** Diuretic and antihypertensive effect while retaining potassium

Uses: Edema, hypertension, diuretic-induced hypokalemia

Dosage and routes

Adult: PO 100 mg bid pc, not to exceed 300 mg/day

G *Elderly:* PO 50 mg qd, max 100 mg/day

Available forms: Caps 50, 100 mg

Adverse effects
CNS: Weakness, headache, dizziness, fatigue
ELECT: Hyperkalemia, hyponatremia, hypochloremia
GI: Nausea, diarrhea, vomiting, dry mouth, jaundice, liver disease
GU: **Azotemia, interstitial nephritis,** increased BUN, creatinine, renal stones, bluish discoloration of urine
HEMA: **Thrombocytopenia, megaloblastic anemia,** low folic acid levels
INTEG: Photosensitivity, rash

Contraindications: Hypersensitivity, anuria, severe renal, hepatic disease; hyperkalemia

Precautions: Dehydration, hepatic disease, lactation, CHF, renal disease, cirrhosis, pregnancy **B,** lactation

Pharmacokinetics	
Absorption	GI tract; well absorbed
Distribution	Crosses placenta
Metabolism	Liver
Excretion	Renal; breast milk
Half-life	3 hr

Pharmacodynamics	
Onset	2 hr
Peak	6-8 hr
Duration	12-16 hr

Interactions
Individual drugs
Amantadine: ↑ toxicity of amantadine
Cimetidine: ↓ renal clearance of triamterene
Indomethacin: ↑ nephrotoxicity

Drug classifications
ACE inhibitors: ↑ hyperkalemia

Antihypertensives: ↑ action
Diuretics, potassium-sparing: ↑ hyperkalemia
NSAIDs: ↓ nephrotoxicity
Potassium products: ↑ hyperkalemia
Salt substitutes: ↑ hyperkalemia

Food/drug
Potassium foods: ↑ hyperkalemia

Lab test interferences
Interference: Quinidine serum levels, LDH

NURSING CONSIDERATIONS
Assessment
• Monitor for manifestations of hyperkalemia: *Renal:* acidic urine, reduced urine osmolality, nocturia, polyuria, polydipsia; *Cardiac:* hypotension, broad T wave, U wave, ectopy, tachycardia, weak pulse; *Neuro:* muscle weakness, altered LOC, drowsiness, apathy, lethargy, confusion, depression, anorexia, nausea, cramps, constipation, distension, paralytic ileus, hypoventilation, respiratory muscle weakness
• Monitor for manifestations of hyponatremia: *CV:* ↑ B/P, cold, clammy skin, hypo- or hypervolemia; *GI:* anorexia, nausea, vomiting, diarrhea, abdominal cramps; *Neuro:* lethargy, increased ICP, confusion, headache, seizures, coma, fatigue, tremors, hyperreflexia
• Monitor for manifestations of hyperchloremia: *Neuro:* weakness, lethargy, coma; *Resp:* deep rapid breathing
• Assess fluid volume status: I&O ratios and record, weight, distended red veins, crackles in lung, color, quality and sp gr of urine, skin turgor, adequacy of pulses, moist mucous membranes, bilateral lung sounds,

peripheral pitting edema; dehydration symptoms of decreasing output, thirst, hypotension, dry mouth and mucous membranes should be reported
• Monitor electrolytes: potassium, sodium, calcium, magnesium; also include BUN, ABGs, uric acid, CBC, blood sugar

Nursing diagnoses
☑ Urinary elimination, altered (adverse reactions)
☑ Fluid volume deficit (adverse reactions)
☑ Fluid volume excess (uses)
☑ Knowledge deficit (teaching)

Implementation
• Give in AM to avoid interference with sleep
• With food, if nausea occurs

Patient/family education
• Teach patient to take medication early in the day to prevent nocturia
• Instruct the patient to take with food or milk if GI symptoms of nausea and anorexia occur
• Teach patient to maintain a record of weight on a weekly basis and notify prescriber of weight loss of 5 lb
• Caution the patient that this drug causes an increase in potassium levels, that foods high in potassium should be avoided; refer to dietician for assistance planning
• Caution the patient not to exercise in hot weather, and stand for prolonged periods of time because orthostatic hypotension will be enhanced
• Advise patient to wear protective clothing and sunscreen in the sun to prevent photosensitivity
• Teach patient not to use alcohol, or any OTC medications without prescriber's approval because serious drug reactions may occur
• Emphasize the need to contact prescriber immediately if muscle cramps, weakness, nausea, dizziness, or numbness occur
• Teach patient to take own B/P and pulse and record
• Advise patient that dizziness and confusion may occur; avoid driving or other hazardous activities if alertness is decreased
• Teach patient to continue taking medication even if feeling better; this drug controls symptoms but does not cure the condition
• Advise the patient with hypertension to continue other medical treatment (exercise, weight loss, relaxation techniques, cessation of smoking)

Evaluation
Positive therapeutic outcome
• Prevention of hypokalemia (diuretic use)
• Decreased edema
• Decreased B/P
• Increased diuresis

Treatment of overdose:
Lavage if taken orally; monitor electrolytes; administer sodium bicarbonate for K 6.5 mEq/L; monitor hydration, CV, renal status

T

triazolam (℞)
(trye-az'oh-lam)
Apo-Triazo ✦, Halcion,
Novotriolam ✦, Nu-
Triazol ✦
Func. class.: Sedative-
hypnotic
Chem. class.: Benzodiaze-
pine

Pregnancy category **X**
**Controlled substance
schedule** **IV** (USA),
schedule **F** (Canada)

Action: Produces CNS depression at limbic, thalamic, hypothalamic levels of CNS; may be
mediated by neurotransmitter;
γ-aminobutyric acid (GABA);
results are sedation, hypnosis,
skeletal muscle relaxation,
anticonvulsant activity, anxiolytic action

➡ **Therapeutic Outcome:** Decreased anxiety, insomnia

Uses: Insomnia (short-term),
sedative/hypnotic

Dosage and routes
Adult: PO 0.125-0.5 mg hs

G *Elderly:* PO 0.625-0.125
mg hs

Available forms: Tabs 0.125,
0.25 mg

Adverse effects
*CNS: Headache, lethargy,
drowsiness, daytime sedation,*
dizziness, confusion, light-
headedness, anxiety, irritability,
amnesia, poor coordination
CV: Chest pain, pulse changes
GI: Nausea, vomiting, diarrhea, heartburn, abdominal
pain, constipation
HEMA: **Leukopenia, granulocytopenia** (rare)

Contraindications: Hypersensitivity to benzodiazepines,

pregnancy **X,** lactation, intermittent porphyria

Precautions: Anemia, hepatic
disease, renal disease, suicidal
G individuals, drug abuse, elderly,
P psychosis, child <15 yr, acute
narrow-angle glaucoma, seizure disorders

Pharmacokinetics	
Absorption	Well absorbed
Distribution	Widely distributed, crosses placenta, crosses blood-brain barrier
Metabolism	Liver
Excretion	Kidneys, breast milk
Half-life	2-3 hr

Pharmacodynamics	
Onset	½ hr
Peak	Unknown
Duration	6-8 hr

Interactions
Individual drugs
Alcohol: ↑ CNS depression
Cimetidine: ↑ action
Disulfiram: ↑ action
Fluoxetine: ↑ action
Isoniazid: ↑ action
Ketoconazole: ↑ action
Levodopa: ↓ action of levo-
dopa
Metoprolol: ↑ action
Propoxyphene: ↑ action
Propranolol: ↑ action
Rifampin: ↓ action of tria-
zolam
Theophylline: ↓ sedative
effects
Valproic acid: ↑ action
Drug classifications
Antidepressants: ↑ CNS
depression
Antihistamines: ↑ CNS de-
pression
Barbiturates: ↓ effect of tria-
zolam
Contraceptives: ↑ effect
Opiates: ↑ CNS depression

☑ Herb/drug   ⑤ Do Not Crush   ◆ Alert   ⬩ᴛ Key Drug   G Geriatric   P Pediatric

Herb/drug
Kava: ↑ CNS depression
Lab test interferences
↑ AST/ALT, ↑ serum bilirubin
False: ↑ 17-OHCS
↓ RAIU

NURSING CONSIDERATIONS
Assessment
• Assess patient's mental
status: mood, sensorium, anxiety, affect, sleeping pattern,
drowsiness, dizziness, especially
🄶 elderly; physical dependency,
withdrawal symptoms: anxiety,
panic attacks, agitation, convulsions, headache, nausea,
vomiting, muscle pain,
weakness; suicidal tendencies;
for indications of increasing
tolerance and abuse
• Monitor patient's B/P (lying, standing), pulse; if systolic
B/P drops 20 mm Hg, hold
drug, notify prescriber
• Monitor blood studies: CBC
during long-term therapy;
blood dycrasias have occurred
rarely; decreased hematocrit,
neutropenia may occur
• Monitor hepatic studies:
AST, ALT, bilirubin, creatinine
LDH, alk phosphatase
• Monitor I&O; indicate renal
dysfunction

Nursing diagnoses
☑ Anxiety (uses)
☑ Depression (uses)
☑ Injury, risk for (adverse reac-
tions)
☑ Knowledge deficit (teaching)

Implementation
• Give with food or milk for
GI symptoms; if patient is
unable to swallow medication
whole, tab may be crushed and
mixed with foods or fluids
• Give sugarless gum, hard
candy, frequent sips of water
for dry mouth

Patient/family education
• Advise patient that drug may
be taken with food or fluids,
and tab may be crushed or
swallowed whole
• Caution patient not to use
for everyday stress or longer
than 3 mo unless directed by
prescriber; not to take more
than prescribed amount; may
be habit forming; not to
double doses or skip doses
• Instruct patient to avoid
OTC preparations unless approved by health care
prescriber; alcohol and CNS
depressants will increase CNS
depression
• Caution patient to avoid
driving, activities that require
alertness because drowsiness
may occur; to avoid alcohol
ingestion or other psychotropic
medications; to rise slowly or
fainting may occur, especially
🄶 elderly; that drowsiness may
worsen at beginning of treatment
• Advise patient not to discontinue medication abruptly after
long-term use; withdrawal
symptoms include vomiting,
cramping, tremors, seizures

Evaluation
Positive therapeutic outcome
• Decreased anxiety, restlessness, sleeplessness (short-term
treatment only)

Treatment of overdose:
Lavage, VS, supportive care

T

---

trifluoperazine (℞)
(trye-floo-oh-per'a-zeen)
Novoflurazine ♣,
Solazine ♣, Stelazine,
Suprazine, Terfluzine,
trifluoperazine HCl, Triflurin
Func. class.:
Antipsychotic/neuroleptic
Chem. class.: Phenothi-
azine, piperazine
Pregnancy category   C

Action: Depresses cerebral
cortex, hypothalamus, limbic
system, which control activity,
aggression; blocks neurotransmission produced by dopamine
at synapse; exhibits strong
α-adrenergic, anticholinergic
blocking action; mechanism for
antipsychotic effects is unclear

➡Therapeutic Outcome: Decreased signs and symptoms of
psychosis

Uses: Psychotic disorders,
nonpsychotic anxiety, schizophrenia

Dosage and routes
Adult: PO 2-5 mg bid, usual
range 15-20 mg/day, may
require 40 mg/day or more;
IM 1-2 mg q4-6h

G*Elderly:* PO 0.5-1 mg qd-bid,
q4-7 days by 0.5-1 mg/day to
desired dose

P*Child >6 yr:* PO 1 mg qd or
bid; IM *not recommended for
children,* but 1 mg may be
given qd or bid

Nonpsychotic anxiety
Adult: PO 1-2 mg bid, not to
exceed 5 mg/day; do not give
longer than 12 wk

Available forms: Tabs 1, 2, 5,
10 mg; conc 10 mg/ml; inj 2
mg/ml

Adverse effects
*CNS: Extrapyramidal
symptoms: pseudoparkinsonism,
akathisia, dystonia, tardive
dyskinesia,* **seizures,** *headache,*
**neuroleptic malignant syn-
drome**
CV: Orthostatic hypotension,
hypertension, **cardiac arrest,**
ECG changes, **tachycardia**
EENT: Blurred vision, glaucoma, dry eyes
*GI: Dry mouth, nausea, vomit-
ing, anorexia, constipation,*
diarrhea, jaundice, weight gain
GU: Urinary retention, urinary
frequency, enuresis, impotence,
amenorrhea, gynecomastia
HEMA: Anemia, **leukopenia,
leukocytosis, agranulocytosis**
INTEG: **Rash,** photosensitivity,
dermatitis
RESP: **Laryngospasm,** dyspnea, **respiratory depression**

Contraindications: Hypersensitivity, cardiovascular disease,
coma, blood dyscrasias, severe
Phepatic disease, child <6 yr,
glaucoma

Precautions: Breast cancer,
seizure disorders, pregnancy C,
lactation, diabetes mellitus,
respiratory conditions, pros-
Gtatic hypertrophy, elderly

◨Do Not Confuse:
trifluoperazine/trihexyphenidyl

Pharmacokinetics	
Absorption	Variably absorbed (tab), well absorbed (IM)
Distribution	Widely distributed, high concentrations in CNS, crosses placenta
Metabolism	Liver—extensively
Excretion	Kidneys, breast milk
Half-life	Unknown

☑ Herb/drug 🚫 Do Not Crush ◆ Alert ✺☌ Key Drug **G** Geriatric **P** Pediatric

Pharmacodynamics		
	PO	IM
Onset	Rapid	Immediate
Peak	2-3 hr	1 hr
Duration	12 hr	12 hr

Interactions
Individual drugs
Alcohol: ↑ effects of both drugs, oversedation
Aluminum hydroxide: ↓ absorption
Bromocriptine: ↓ antiparkinson activity
Disopyramide: ↑ anticholinergic effects
Epinephrine: ↑ toxicity
Guanethidine: ↓ antihypertensive response
Levodopa: ↓ antiparkinson activity
Lithium: ↓ chlorpromazine levels, ↑ extrapyramidal symptoms, masking of lithium toxicity
Magnesium hydroxide: ↓ absorption
Norepinephrine: ↓ vasoresponse, ↑ toxicity
Phenobarbital: ↓ effectiveness, ↑ metabolism
Drug classifications
Antacids: ↓ absorption
Anticholinergics: ↑ anticholinergic effects
Antidepressants: ↑ CNS depression
Antidiarrheals, adsorbent: ↓ absorption
Antihistamines: ↑ CNS depression
Antihypertensives: ↑ hypotension
Antithyroid agents: ↑ agranulocytosis
Barbiturate anesthetics: ↑ CNS depression
β-Adrenergic blockers: ↑ effects of both drugs

General anesthetics: ↑ CNS depression
MAOIs: ↑ CNS depression
Opiates: ↑ CNS depression
Sedative/hypnotics: ↑ CNS depression
Herb/drug
Kava: ↑ CNS depression
Lab test interferences
↑ Liver function tests, ↑ cardiac enzymes, ↑ cholesterol, ↑ blood glucose, ↑ prolactin, ↑ bilirubin, ↑ PBI, ↑ cholinesterase, ↑ alk phosphatase, ↑ leukocytes, ↑ granulocytes, ↑ platelets
↓ Hormones (blood and urine)
False positive: Pregnancy tests, PKU, urine bilirubin
False negative: Urinary steroids, 17-OHCS

NURSING CONSIDERATIONS
Assessment
• Assess mental status: orientation, mood, behavior, presence of hallucinations, and type before initial administration and monthly; drug should significantly reduce psychotic behavior
• Check for swallowing of PO medication; check for hoarding or giving of medication to other patients
• Monitor I&O ratio, palpate bladder if low urinary output occurs, especially in elderly; urinalysis recommended before, during prolonged therapy
• Monitor bilirubin, CBC, liver function studies monthly
• Assess affect, orientation, LOC, reflexes, gait, coordination, sleep pattern disturbances
• Monitor B/P sitting, standing and lying, take pulse and respirations q4h during initial treatment; establish baseline before starting treatment; report drops of 30 mm Hg;

obtain baseline ECG, Q-wave and T-wave changes
• Check for dizziness, faintness, palpitations, tachycardia on rising; severe orthostatic hypotension is common
◆• Identify for neuroleptic malignant syndrome: hyperpyrexia, muscle rigidity, increased CPK, altered mental status; drug should be discontinued
• Assess for extrapyramidal symptoms including akathisia (inability to sit still, no pattern to movements), tardive dyskinesia (bizarre movements of the jaw, mouth, tongue, extremities), pseudoparkinsonism (ragged tremors, pill rolling, shuffling gait); an antiparkinson drug should be prescribed
• Assess for constipation, urinary retention daily; if these occur, increase bulk, water in diet
• Assess for hypo-/hyperglycemia; appetite patterns

Nursing diagnoses
☑ Thought processes, altered (uses)
☑ Coping, ineffective individual (uses)
☑ Knowledge deficit (teaching)
☑ Noncompliance (teaching)

Implementation
PO route
• Drug in liq form mixed in glass of juice or cola if hoarding is suspected; do not mix in caffeine drinks, tannics, pectins
G • Decreased dose in elderly; metabolism is slowed in the elderly
• PO with full glass of water, milk; or give with food to decrease GI upset
• Storage in tight, light-resistant container, oral sol in amber bottle

IM route
• Inj in deep muscle mass, do not give SC; do not administer sol with a precipitate
IV route
• Give **IV** after diluting 10 mg/9 ml of NS; give 1 mg or less/2 min

Syringe compatibilities:
Glycopyrrolate

Additive compatibilities:
Meperidine, netilmicin

Patient/family education
• Teach patient to use good oral hygiene; frequent rinsing of mouth, sugarless gum for dry mouth
• Caution patient to avoid hazardous activities until drug response is determined; dizziness, blurred vision is common
• Inform patient that orthostatic hypotension occurs often and to rise from sitting or lying position gradually and to remain lying down after IM inj for at least 30 min
• Caution patient to avoid tubs, hot showers, tub baths because hypotension may occur
• Instruct patient that heat stroke may occur in hot weather, so take extra precautions to stay cool
• Advise patient to avoid abrupt withdrawal of this drug, or extrapyramidal symptoms may result; drug should be withdrawn slowly
• Teach patient to avoid OTC preparations (cough, hay fever, cold) unless approved by prescriber because serious drug interactions may occur; avoid use with alcohol, CNS depressants because increased drowsiness may occur
• Advise patient to use a sun-

☑ Herb/drug ⓢ Do Not Crush ◆ Alert ⊶ Key Drug **G** Geriatric **P** Pediatric

screen and sunglasses to prevent burns
- Teach patient about extrapyramidal symptoms and necessity of meticulous oral hygiene because oral candidiasis may occur
- Advise patient to take antacids 2 hr before or after this drug
- Instruct patient to report sore throat, malaise, fever, bleeding, mouth sores; if these occur, CBC should be drawn and drug discontinued

Evaluation
Positive therapeutic outcome
- Decrease in emotional excitement, hallucinations, delusions, paranoia
- Reorganization of patterns of thought, speech

Treatment of overdose: Lavage if orally ingested; provide airway; *do not induce vomiting or use epinephrine*

---

trihexyphenidyl (℞)
(trye-hex-ee-fen′i-dill)
Artane, Artane Sequels, Novohexidyl ✣, Trihexy-2, Trihexy-5, trihexyphenidyl HCl, Trihexane
Func. class.: Cholinergic blocker; antiparkinson
Chem. class.: Synthetic tertiary amine

Pregnancy category C

Action: Blocks central muscarinic receptors, which decreases involuntary movements, sweating, salivation

▶**Therapeutic Outcome:** Decreased involuntary movements

Uses: Parkinson symptoms, drug-induced extrapyramidal symptoms

Dosage and routes
Parkinson symptoms
Adult: PO 1 mg, increased by 2 mg q3-5d to a total of 6-10 mg/day

Drug-induced extrapyramidal symptoms
Adult: PO 1 mg/day; usual dose 5-15 mg/day

Available forms: Tabs 2, 5 mg; caps sus-rel 5 mg; elix 2 mg/5 ml

Adverse effects
CNS: Confusion, anxiety, restlessness, irritability, delusions, hallucinations, headache, sedation, depression, incoherence, dizziness, flushing, weakness
CV: Palpitations, tachycardia, postural hypotension
EENT: Blurred vision, photophobia, dilated pupils, difficulty swallowing, dry eyes, increased intraocular tension, angle-closure glaucoma
GI: Dryness of mouth, constipation, nausea, vomiting, abdominal distress, **paralytic ileus**
GU: Urinary hesitancy, urinary retention, dysuria
INTEG: Urticaria, rash
MISC: Suppression of lactation, nasal congestion, decreased sweating, increased temp, hyperthermia, heat stroke, numbness of fingers
MS: Weakness, cramping

Contraindications: Hypersensitivity, narrow-angle glaucoma, myasthenia gravis, GI/GU obstruction, tachycardia, myocardial ischemia, unstable CV disease, prostatic hypertrophy

T

Precautions: Pregnancy **C,**
[G] elderly, lactation, tachycardia,
abdominal obstruction, infec-
[P] tion, children, gastric ulcer

Do Not Confuse:
trihexyphenidyl/trifluoperazine,
Artane/Altace

Pharmacokinetics

Absorption	Well absorbed
Distribution	Unknown
Metabolism	Unknown
Excretion	Unknown
Half-life	5-10 hr

Pharmacodynamics

	PO	PO-ER
Onset	1 hr	Unknown
Peak	2-3 hr	Unknown
Duration	6-12 hr	Up to 24 hr

Interactions
Individual drugs
Alcohol: ↑ CNS depression
Disopyramide: ↑ anticholiner-
gic effects
Quinidine: ↑ anticholinergic
effects
Drug classifications
Analgesics: ↑ CNS depression
Antacids: ↓ absorption
Antidepressants, tricyclic:
↑ anticholinergic effects
Antihistamines: ↑ anticholin-
ergic effects
Phenothiazines: ↑ anticholin-
ergic effects
Sedatives/hypnotics: ↑ CNS
depression

NURSING CONSIDERATIONS
Assessment
• Monitor I&O ratio; retention commonly causes de-
creased urinary output, distention, frequency, incontinence
• Assess for parkinsonism,
extrapyramidal symptoms:
shuffling gait, muscle rigidity,
involuntary movements, pill
rolling, muscle spasms, drool-

ing before and during treatment
• Monitor for urinary hesitancy, retention; palpate bladder if retention occurs
• Monitor for constipation,
cramping, pain in abdomen,
abdominal distention; increase
fluids, bulk, exercise if this
occurs
• Assess for tolerance over
long-term therapy; dose may
have to be increased or
changed
• Assess for mental status:
affect, mood, CNS depression,
worsening of mental symptoms
during early therapy
Nursing diagnoses
☑ Physical mobility, impaired
(uses)
☑ Knowledge deficit (teaching)
Implementation
• Give with or pc to prevent
GI upset; may give with fluids
other than water; offer hard
candy, frequent drinks, gum to
relieve dry mouth
• Give at hs to avoid daytime
drowsiness in patient with
parkinsonism
• Store at room temp
Patient/family education
• Teach patient to use caution
in hot weather; drug may
increase susceptibility to stroke
because perspiration is decreased; patient should remain
indoors
• Teach patient not to discontinue this drug abruptly; to
taper off over 1 wk to prevent
withdrawal symptoms (insomnia, involuntary movements,
anxiety, tachycardias)
• Caution patient to avoid
driving or other hazardous
activities; drowsiness, dizziness
may occur

• Advise patient to avoid OTC medications: cough, cold preparations with alcohol, antihistamines unless directed by prescriber; increased CNS depression may occur
• Instruct patient to rise from sitting or recumbent position slowly to minimize orthostatic hypotension
• Advise patient to use gum, hard candy, frequent sips of water to decrease dry mouth; if dry mouth continues, saliva substitutes may be prescribed
• Instruct patient that doses should not be doubled, but missed dose may be taken up to 2 hr before next dose

Evaluation
Positive therapeutic outcome
• Absence of involuntary movements (pill rolling, tremors, muscle spasms)

---

trimethobenzamide (R)
(trye-meth-oh-ben'za-mide)
Arrestin, Benzacot, Brogan, Stemetic, T-Gen, Tebamide, Ticon, Tigan, Tijet-20, Tribun, Trimazide, trimethobenzamide, trimethobenzamide HCl
Func. class.: Antiemetic, anticholinergic
Chem. class.: Ethanolamine derivative
Pregnancy category C

Action: Acts centrally by blocking chemoreceptor trigger zone, which in turn acts on vomiting center

➡ **Therapeutic Outcome:** Absence of nausea and vomiting

Uses: Nausea, vomiting, prevention of postoperative vomiting

Dosage and routes
Postoperative vomiting
Adult: IM/rec 200 mg before or during surgery; may repeat 3 hr after

Discontinuing anesthesia
P *Child 13-40 kg:* PO/rec 100-200 mg tid-qid
P *Child <13 kg:* PO/rec 100 mg tid-qid

Nausea/vomiting
Adult: PO 250 mg tid-qid; IM/rec 200 mg tid-qid

Available forms: Caps 100, 250, mg; supp 100, 200 mg; inj 100 mg/ml

Adverse effects
CNS: Drowsiness, restlessness, headache, dizziness, insomnia, confusion, nervousness, tingling, *vertigo,* extrapyramidal symptoms
CV: Hypertension, hypotension, palpitations
EENT: Dry mouth, blurred vision, diplopia, nasal congestion, photosensitivity
GI: Nausea, anorexia, diarrhea, vomiting, constipation
INTEG: Rash, urticaria, fever, chills, flushing

Contraindications: Hypersensitivity to narcotics, shock, P children (parenterally)

P **Precautions:** Children, cardiac
G dysrhythmias, elderly, asthma, pregnancy **C**, prostatic hypertrophy, bladder-neck obstruction, narrow-angle glaucoma, stenosing peptic ulcer, pyloroduodenal obstruction

T

Pharmacokinetics

Absorption	Unknown
Distribution	Unknown
Metabolism	Liver, extensively
Excretion	Kidneys
Half-life	Unknown

Pharmacodynamics

	PO	IM	REC
Onset	20-40 min	15 min	10-40 min
Peak	Un-known	Un-known	Un-known
Duration	3-4 hr	2-3 hr	3-4 hr

Interactions
Individual drugs
Alcohol: ↑ CNS depression
Drug classifications
Analgesics: ↑ CNS effect
Antidepressants: ↑ CNS effect
Antihistamines: ↑ CNS effect
CNS depressants: ↑ CNS effect
Sedative/hypnotics: ↑ CNS effect

NURSING CONSIDERATIONS
Assessment
• Monitor VS, B/P; check patients with cardiac disease more often
• Assess for signs of toxicity of other drugs or masking of symptoms of disease: brain tumor, intestinal obstructions
• Observe for drowsiness, dizziness
• Assess for nausea, vomiting before and after treatment

Nursing diagnoses
☑ Knowledge deficit (teaching)

Implementation
IM route
• Administer IM inj in large muscle mass; aspirate to avoid **IV** administration

Syringe compatibilities:
Glycopyrrolate, hydromorphone, midazolam, nalbuphine

Y-site compatibilities:
Heparin, hydrocortisone, potassium chloride, vit B/C
PO route
• Cap may be swallowed whole or opened and mixed with food or fluids

Patient/family education
• Teach patient to use good oral hygiene; frequent rinsing of mouth, sugarless gum for dry mouth
• Caution patient to avoid hazardous activities until drug response is determined, drowsiness may occur
• Inform patient that orthostatic hypotension occurs often and to rise from sitting or lying position gradually and to remain lying down after IM inj for at least 30 min
• Advise patient to avoid hot tubs, hot showers, tub baths because hypotension may occur
• Inform patient that in hot weather, heat stroke may occur; take extra precautions to stay cool
• Teach patient to avoid OTC preparations (cough, hayfever, cold) unless approved by prescriber because serious drug interactions may occur; avoid use with alcohol, CNS depressants because increased drowsiness may occur
• Teach patient about extrapyramidal symptoms
• Instruct patient to report sore throat, malaise, fever, bleeding, mouth sores; if these occur, CBC should be drawn and drug discontinued

Evaluation
Positive therapeutic outcome
• Decreased nausea, vomiting

**trimethoprim/
sulfamethoxazole (co-
trimoxazole) (R)**
(trye-meth'oh-prim/sul-fa-
meth-ox'a-zole [ko-trye-
mox'a-zole])
Apo-Sulfatrim*, Bactrim,
Bactrim IV, Bethaprim,
Comoxol, Cotrim, Septra,
Sulfatrim
Func. class.: Antiinfective
Chem. class.: Miscella-
neous sulfonamide
Pregnancy category   **C**

Action: Sulfamethoxazole
(SMZ) interferes with bacterial
biosynthesis of proteins by
competitive antagonism of
PABA when adequate levels are
maintained; trimethoprim
(TMP) blocks synthesis of
tetrahydrofolic acid; combination blocks 2 consecutive steps
in bacterial synthesis of essential nucleic acids, protein

⮞Therapeutic Outcome: Ab-
sence of infection, based on
C&S

Uses: UTI, otitis media, acute
and chronic prostatitis, shigel-
losis, *Pneumocystis carinii*
pneumonitis, chronic bronchitis, chancroid, traveler's diarrhea

Dosage and routes
UTI
Adult: PO 160 mg TMP/800
mg SMZ q12h × 10-14 days
🅿 *Child:* PO 8 mg/kg TMP/40
mg/kg SMZ qd in 2 divided
doses q12h
Otitis media
🅿 *Child:* PO 8 mg/kg TMP/40
mg/kg SMZ qd in 2 divided
doses q12h × 10 days

Bacterial infections
🅿 *Adult and child ≥40 kg:* 160
mg TMP/800 mg SMZ q12h
🅿 *Adult and child >2 mo:*
4-6 mg/kg TMP/20-30
mg/kg SMZ q12h; **IV** 2-2.5
mg/kg TMP/10-12.5 mg/kg
SMZ q6h or 4-5 mg/kg
TMP/20-25 mg/kg SMZ
q12h
Chronic bronchitis
Adult: PO 160 mg TMP/800
mg SMZ q12h × 14 days
*Pneumocystis carinii
pneumonitis*
🅿 *Adult and child >2 mo:* PO
3.75-5 mg/kg TMP/18.75-25
mg SMZ q6h × 14 days; **IV**
3.75-5 mg/kg TMP/18.5-25
mg SMZ q6h or 5-6.7 mg/kg
TMP/25-33.3 mg SMZ q8h
divided doses for up to 14 days
• Dosage reduction necessary
in moderate to severe renal
impairment (CrCl <30 ml/
min)

Available forms: Tabs 80 mg
TMP/400 mg SMZ, 160 mg
TMP/800 mg SMZ; susp 40
mg/200 mg/5 ml; **IV** 16
mg/80 mg/ml

Adverse effects
CNS: Headache, insomnia,
hallucinations, depression,
vertigo, fatigue, anxiety, convulsions, drug fever, chills,
aseptic meningitis
CV: **Allergic myocarditis**
GI: *Nausea, vomiting, abdominal pain,* stomatitis, **hepatitis,**
glossitis, pancreatitis, diarrhea,
enterocolitis, anorexia
GU: **Renal failure, toxic
nephrosis;** increased BUN,
creatinine; crystalluria
HEMA: **Leukopenia, neutropenia, thrombocytopenia,
agranulocytosis, hemolytic
anemia, hypoprothrombin-**

T

emia, Henoch-Schönlein purpura, methemoglobinemia, eosinophilia I
INTEG: Rash, dermatitis, urticaria, ***Stevens-Johnson syndrome,*** erythema, photosensitivity, pain, inflammation at injection site
RESP: Cough, shortness of breath
SYST: **Anaphylaxis, SLE**

Contraindications: Hypersensitivity to trimethoprim or sulfonamides, pregnancy at term, megaloblastic anemia, **P** infants <2 mo, CrCl <15 ml/min, lactation, porphyria

Precautions: Pregnancy **C**, **G** renal disease, elderly, G6PD deficiency, impaired hepatic/renal function, possible folate deficiency, severe allergy, bronchial asthma

Pharmacokinetics	
Absorption	Rapid
Distribution	Breast milk, crosses placenta, 68% protein bound
Metabolism	Liver
Excretion	Kidneys
Half-life	8-13 hr

Pharmacodynamics	
Onset	Unknown
Peak	1-4 hr
Duration	Unknown

Interactions
Individual drugs
Cyclosporine: ↓ response
Methotrexate: ↑ bone marrow depression
Phenytoin: ↓ hepatic clearance of phenytoin
Drug classifications
Anticoagulants, oral: ↑ anticoagulant effect
Diuretics, thiazide: ↑ thrombocytopenia

Sulfonylureas: ↑ hypoglycemic response
Lab test interferences
↑ Alk phosphatase, ↑ creatinine, ↑ bilirubin
False positive: Urinary glucose test

NURSING CONSIDERATIONS
Assessment
• Assess allergic reactions: rash, fever (AIDS patients more susceptible)
• Monitor I&O ratio; note color, character, pH of urine if drug administered for UTI; output should be 800 ml less than intake; if urine is highly acidic, alkalization may be needed
• Monitor kidney function studies: BUN, creatinine, urinalysis (long-term therapy)
• Assess type of infection; obtain C&S before starting therapy
• Assess blood dyscrasias, skin rash, fever, sore throat, bruising, bleeding, fatigue, joint pain
• Assess allergic reaction: rash, dermatitis, urticaria, pruritus, dyspnea, bronchospasm

Nursing diagnoses
☑ Infection, risk for (uses)
☑ Knowledge deficit (teaching)
☑ Noncompliance (teaching)

Implementation
• Give with full glass of water to maintain adequate hydration; increase fluids to 2 L/day to decrease crystallization in kidneys
• Give medication after C&S; repeat C&S after full course of medication
• Store in tight, light-resistant container at room temp
• Dilute 5 ml ampule/100-125 ml D₅W, stable for 6 hr,

---

give over 1-½ hr, do not refrigerate

IV route

Syringe compatibilities:
Heparin

Y-site compatibilities:
Acyclovir, aldesleukin, allopurinol, amifostine, atracurium, aztreonam, cefepime, cyclophosphamide, diltiazem, enalaprilat, esmolol, filgrastim, fludarabine, gallium, granisetron, hydromorphone, labetalol, lorazepam, magnesium sulfate, melphalan, meperidine, morphine, pancuronium, perphenazine, piperacillin/tazobactam, sargramostim, tacrolimus, teniposide, thiotepa, vecuronium, zidovudine

Patient family education
• Teach patient to take each oral dose with full glass of water to prevent crystalluria; drink 8-10 glasses of water/day
• Teach patient to complete course of full treatment to prevent superinfection
• Teach patient to avoid sunlight or use sunscreen to prevent burns
• Teach patient to avoid OTC medications (aspirin, vit C) unless directed by prescriber
• If diabetic, teach patient to use Clinistix or Tes-Tape
• Teach patient to use alternative contraceptive measures; decreased effectiveness of oral contraceptives may result
• Teach patient to notify prescriber if skin rash, sore throat, fever, mouth sores, unusual bruising, bleeding occur

Evaluation
Positive therapeutic outcome
Absence of pain, fever, C&S negative

triprolidine (℞)
(trye-proe′li-deen)
Actidil, Alleract, Myidil, triprolidine HCl
Func. class.: Antihistamine
Chem. class.: Alkylamine, H_1-receptor antagonist
Pregnancy category   C

Action: Acts on blood vessels, GI, respiratory systems by competing with histamine for H_1-receptor site; decreases allergic response by blocking histamine

Therapeutic Outcome: Absence of allergy symptoms and rhinitis

Uses: Rhinitis, allergy symptoms

Dosage and routes
Adult: PO 2.5 mg tid-qid
Child >6 yr: PO 1.25 mg tid-qid
Child 4-6 yr: PO 0.9 mg tid-qid
Child 2-4 yr: PO 0.6 mg tid-qid
Child 4 mo-2 yr: PO 0.3 mg tid-qid

Available forms: Tab 2.5 mg; syr 1.25 mg/5 ml

Adverse effects
CNS: Dizziness, drowsiness, poor coordination, fatigue, anxiety, euphoria, confusion, paresthesia, neuritis
CV: Hypotension, palpitations, tachycardia
EENT: Blurred vision, dilated pupils, tinnitus, nasal stuffiness, dry nose, throat, mouth
GI: Constipation, dry mouth, nausea, vomiting, anorexia, diarrhea
GU: Retention, dysuria, frequency

HEMA: **Thrombocytopenia, agranulocytosis, hemolytic anemia**
INTEG: Rash, urticaria, photosensitivity
RESP: Increased thick secretions, wheezing, chest tightness

Contraindications: Hypersensitivity to H_1-receptor antagonist, acute asthma attack, lower respiratory tract disease

Precautions: Increased IOP, renal disease, cardiac disease, hypertension, bronchial asthma, seizure disorder, stenosed peptic ulcers, hyperthyroidism, prostatic hypertrophy, bladder neck obstruction, pregnancy **C**

Pharmacokinetics	
Absorption	Well absorbed
Distribution	Widely distributed, crosses blood-brain barrier
Metabolism	Liver—extensively
Excretion	Kidneys
Half-life	5 hr

Pharmacodynamics	
Onset	15-60 min
Peak	1-2 hr
Duration	6-8 hr

Interactions
Individual drugs
Alcohol: ↑ CNS depression
Atropine: ↑ anticholinergic reactions
Disopyramide: ↑ anticholinergic reactions
Haloperidol: ↑ anticholinergic reactions
Quinidine: ↑ anticholinergic reactions
Drug classifications
Antidepressants: ↑ anticholinergic reactions
Antihistamines: ↑ anticholinergic reactions

CNS depressants: ↑ CNS depression
MAOIs: ↑ anticholinergic effect
Opiates: ↑ CNS depression
Phenothiazines: ↑ anticholinergic reactions
Sedative/hypnotics: ↑ CNS depression
☑ *Herb/drug*
Henbane: ↑ anticholinergic effect
Lab test interferences
False negative: Skin allergy tests (discontinue antihistamines 3 days before testing)

NURSING CONSIDERATIONS
Assessment
• Assess respiratory status: rate, rhythm, increase in bronchial secretions, wheezing, chest tightness; provide fluids to 2 L/day to decrease thickness of secretions
• Monitor I&O ratio: be alert for urinary retention, frequency, dysuria, especially in **G** elderly; drug should be discontinued if these occur
• Monitor CBC during long-term therapy; blood dyscrasias may occur but are rare

Nursing diagnoses
✓ Airway clearance, ineffective (uses)
✓ Injury, risk for (adverse reactions)
✓ Knowledge deficit (teaching)
✓ Noncompliance (teaching—overuse)

Implementation
• Give on an empty stomach, 1 hr ac or 2 hr pc after meals to facilitate absorption
• Store in tight, light-resistant container

Patient/family education
• Teach patient all aspects of drug uses; to notify prescriber

if confusion, sedation, hypotension occur; to avoid driving or other hazardous activity if drowsiness occurs; to avoid alcohol or other CNS depressants that may potentiate effect
• Advise patient to take medication 1 hr ac or 2 hr pc to facilitate absorption
• Caution patient not to exceed recommended dose because dysrhythmias may occur
• Inform patient that hard candy, gum, frequent rinsing of mouth may be used for dryness

Evaluation
Positive therapeutic outcome
• Absence of running or congested nose, rashes

Treatment of overdose: Administer ipecac syrup or lavage, diazepam, vasopressors, barbiturates (short-acting)

tubocurarine ⊶ (℞)
(too-boh-cure'a-reen)
Tubarine ✦, Tubocuraine
Func. class.: Neuromuscular blocker
Chem. class.: Synthetic curariform
Pregnancy category   C

Action: Inhibits transmission of nerve impulses by binding with cholinergic receptor sites, antagonizing action of acetylcholine; no analgesic response

Therapeutic Outcome: Skeletal muscle paralysis during anesthesia

Uses: Facilitation of endotracheal intubation, skeletal muscle relaxation during mechanical ventilation, surgery, or general anesthesia

Dosage and routes
Adult: **IV** bol 0.4-0.5 mg/kg, then 0.08-0.10 mg/kg 20-45 min after 1st dose if needed for prolonged procedures

Available forms: Inj 3 mg/ml, (20 U/ml)

Adverse effects
CV: Bradycardia, tachycardia, increased, decreased B/P
EENT: Increased secretions
INTEG: Rash, flushing, pruritus, urticaria
RESP: Prolonged apnea, bronchospasm, cyanosis, respiratory depression

Contraindications: Hypersensitivity

Precautions: Pregnancy **C**, cardiac disease, lactation, children <2 yr, electrolyte imbalances, dehydration, neuromuscular disease, respiratory disease

Pharmacokinetics
Absorption	Complete bioavailability
Distribution	Extensive, crosses placenta
Metabolism	Liver, small amount
Excretion	Kidneys—unchanged (30%-75%), bile (11%)
Half-life	2 hr

Pharmacodynamics
	IV	IM
Onset	1 min	15-30 min
Peak	5 min	Unknown
Duration	½-1½ hr	Unknown

Interactions
Individual drugs
Clindamycin: ↑ paralysis, length and intensity
Colistin: ↑ paralysis, length and intensity
Lidocaine: ↑ paralysis, length and intensity

Lithium: ↑ paralysis, length and intensity
Magnesium: ↑ paralysis, length and intensity
Polymyxin B: ↑ paralysis, length and intensity
Procainamide: ↑ paralysis, length and intensity
Quinidine: ↑ paralysis, length and intensity
Succinylcholine: ↑ paralysis, length and intensity
Drug classifications
Aminoglycosides: ↑ paralysis, length and intensity
β-Adrenergic blockers: ↑ paralysis, length and intensity
Diuretics, potassium-losing: ↑ paralysis, length and intensity
General anesthesia: ↑ paralysis, length and intensity

NURSING CONSIDERATIONS
Assessment
• Monitor for electrolyte imbalances (potassium, magnesium), before drug is used; electrolyte imbalances may lead to increased action of this drug
• Monitor vital signs (B/P, pulse, respirations, airway) until fully recovered; rate, depth, pattern of respirations, strength of hand grip; patient should be intubated before use
• Monitor recovery: decreased paralysis of face, diaphragm, leg, arm, rest of body; residual weakness and respiratory problems may occur during recovery period
• Monitor allergic reactions: rash, fever, respiratory distress, pruritus; drug should be discontinued

Nursing diagnoses
☑ Breathing pattern, ineffective (uses)
☑ Communication, impaired verbal (adverse reactions)
☑ Fear (adverse reactions)
☑ Knowledge deficit (teaching)

Implementation
• Use peripheral nerve stimulator by anesthesiologist to determine neuromuscular blockade; deep tendon reflexes should be monitored during extended periods
• Give **IV** undiluted by direct **IV** over 1-1½ min, (only by qualified person, usually an anesthesiologist)

Syringe compatibilities:
Pentobarbital, thiopental

Additive incompatibilities:
Barbiturates, sodium bicarbonate

Solution compatibilities:
D_5, $D_{10}W$, 0.9% NaCl, 0.45% NaCl, Ringer's, LR, dextrose/Ringer's or dextrose/LR combinations

Patient/family education
• Provide reassurance if communication is difficult during recovery from neuromuscular blockade
• Provide explanation to patients regarding all procedures or treatments; patient will remain conscious if anesthesia is not given also

Evaluation
Positive therapeutic outcome
• Paralysis of jaw, eyelid, head, neck, rest of body as evaluated by peripheral nerve stimulator

Treatment of overdose:
Edrophonium or neostigmine, atropine, monitor VS; patient may require mechanical ventilation

---

urokinase (℞)
(yoor-oh-kin'ase)
Abbokinase, Abbokinase
Open-Cath
Func. class.: Thrombolytic
enzyme
Chem. class.: β-hemolytic
streptococcus filtrate
(purified)
Pregnancy category   B

Action: Promotes thrombolysis by directly converting plasminogen to plasmin

Therapeutic Outcome: Lysis of emboli, or thrombosis in various parts of the body

Uses: Venous thrombosis, pulmonary embolism, arterial thrombosis, arterial embolism, arteriovenous cannula occlusion, lysis of coronary artery thrombi after MI

Dosage and routes
Lysis of pulmonary emboli
Adult and child: **IV** 4400 IU/kg/hr × 12-24 hr, not to exceed 200 ml; then **IV** heparin, then anticoagulants

Coronary artery thrombosis
Adult: Instill 6000 IU/min into occluded artery for 1-2 hr after giving **IV** bol of heparin 2500-10,000 U; may also give as **IV** inf of 2-3 million U over 45-90 min

Venous catheter occlusion
Adult and child: Instill 5000 IU into line, wait 5 min, then aspirate; repeat aspiration attempts q5min × ½ hr; if occlusion has not been removed, then cap line and wait ½-1 hr, then aspirate; may need 2nd dose if still occluded

Available forms: Powder for inj, 250,000 IU/vial; powder for catheter clearance

Adverse effects
CNS: Headache, fever
CV: Hypertension, dysrhythmias, hypertension
EENT: Periorbital edema
GI: Nausea, vomiting
HEMA: Decreased Hct,
bleeding
INTEG: Rash, urticaria, phlebitis at **IV** inf site, itching, flushing
MS: Low back pain
RESP: Altered respirations, cyanosis, SOB, **bronchospasm**
SYST: **GI, GU, intracranial, retroperitoneal bleeding;** surface bleeding; **anaphylaxis** (rare)

Contraindications: Hypersensitivity, active bleeding, intraspinal surgery, neoplasms of CNS, ulcerative colitis/enteritis, severe hypertension, renal disease, hepatic disease, hypocoagulation, COPD, subacute bacterial endocarditis, rheumatic valvular disease, cerebral embolism/thrombosis/hemorrhage, intraarterial diagnostic procedure or surgery (10 days), recent major surgery

Precautions: Arterial emboli from left side of heart, pregnancy **B**

Pharmacokinetics	
Absorption	Completely
Distribution	Unknown
Metabolism	Liver
Excretion	Kidneys
Half-life	10-20 min

Pharmacodynamics	
Onset	Rapid
Peak	Rapid
Duration	12 hr

U

Interactions
Individual drugs
Aspirin: ↑ bleeding
Dipyridamole: ↑ bleeding
Heparin: ↑ bleeding
Plicamycin: ↑ bleeding
Valproic acid: ↑ bleeding
Drug classifications
Cephalosporins: ↑ bleeding
Anticoagulants, oral:
↑ bleeding
NSAIDs: ↑ bleeding
Lab test interferences
↑ PT, ↑ APTT, ↑ TT

NURSING CONSIDERATIONS
Assessment
• Monitor VS, B/P, pulse, respirations (including peripheral), neurologic signs, temp at least q4hr; temp >104° F (40° C) indicates internal bleeding; monitor rhythm closely; ventricular dysrhythmias may occur with hyperfusion; monitor heart, breath sounds, neuro status, peripheral pulses
• Assess for bleeding during first hr of treatment: hematuria, hematemesis, bleeding from mucous membranes, epistaxis, ecchymosis; guaiac all body fluids, stools; blood studies (Hct, platelets, PTT, PT, TT, APTT) before starting therapy; PT or APTT must be less than 2 × control before starting therapy TT or PT q3-4h during treatment
• Assess allergy: fever, rash, itching, chills; mild reaction may be treated with antihistamines; report to health care prescriber
• Monitor ECG on monitor, watch for segment changes, changes in rhythm; sinus bradycardia, ventricular tachycardia, accelerated idioventricular rhythm may occur because of reperfusion

Nursing diagnoses
☑ Tissue perfusion, altered (uses)
☑ Injury, high risk for (adverse reactions)
☑ Impaired gas exchange (uses)

Implementation
IV Int IV
• Give **IV** loading dose over 30 min to avoid hypotension
• **IV** after dilution with 4-5 g/250 ml NS, D_5W, LR, give over 1 hr; may give by continuous inf after loading dose(s) of 1 g/hr diluted in 50-100 ml of compatible sol; use inf pump; do not give by direct **IV**
• Give heparin therapy after thrombolytic therapy is discontinued, TT, ACT, or APTT less than 2 × control (about 3-4 hr)
• Avoid invasive procedures, inj, rec temp
• Apply pressure for 30 sec to minor bleeding sites; 30 min to sites of atrial puncture, followed by pressure dressing; inform prescriber if this does not attain hemostasis; apply pressure dressing
• Store powder at room temp or refrigerate; protect from excessive light

Additive incompatibilities:
Do not mix with other medications

Patient/family education
• Teach patient reason for medication, signs and symptoms of bleeding, allergic reactions, when to notify health care prescriber

Evaluation
Positive therapeutic outcome
• Lysis of thrombi or emboli

valacyclovir (℞)
(val-a-sye′kloh-vir)
Valtrex
Func. class.: Antiviral
Chem. class.: Acyclic
purine nucleoside analog
Pregnancy category **B**

Action: Interferes with DNA
synthesis by conversion to
acyclovir, causing decreased
viral replication, time of
lesional healing

➤**Therapeutic Outcome:** Absence of itching, painful
lesions; crusting and healing of
lesions

Uses: Herpes zoster (not
immunosuppressed), recurrent
genital herpes (not immunosuppressed)

Dosage and routes
Genital herpes
Adult: PO 1 g bid × 10 days
initially; 1 g qd or 500 mg
bid in those with <10 recur-
rences/yr

Herpes zoster
Adult: PO 1 g tid × 1 wk

Available forms: Tabs 500,
1000 mg

Adverse effects
CNS: Tremors, lethargy, *dizziness, headache, weakness*
*GI: Nausea, vomiting, diar-
rhea, abdominal pain, constipation*
INTEG: Rash

Contraindications: Hypersensitivity to this drug or acyclovir

Precautions: Lactation, hepatic disease, renal disease,
electrolyte imbalance, dehydration, pregnancy **B**

Pharmacokinetics

Absorption	Unknown
Distribution	Crosses placenta, enters breast milk
Metabolism	Converts to acyclovir
Excretion	Unknown
Half-life	2½-3½ hr

Pharmacodynamics

Onset	Unknown
Peak	Unknown
Duration	Unknown

Interactions
Individual drugs
Cimetidine: Increased blood
levels of valacyclovir
Probenecid: Increased blood
levels of valacyclovir

NURSING CONSIDERATIONS
Assessment
• Assess for signs of infection;
characteristics of lesions
• Assess C&S before drug
therapy; drug may be taken as
soon as culture is taken; repeat
C&S after treatment; determine the presence of other
sexually transmitted diseases
• Assess bowel pattern before,
during treatment
• Assess for skin eruptions:
rash
• Assess allergies before treatment, reaction of each
medication; place allergies on
chart in bright red letters

Nursing diagnoses
✔ Potential infection (uses)

Patient/family education
• Advise patient to take as
prescribed; if dose is missed,
take as soon as remembered up
to 1 hr before next dose; do
not double dose
• Instruct patient to take drug
orally before infection occurs;
drug should be taken when
itching or pain occurs, usually
before eruptions

V

• Inform patient that partners need to be told that patient has herpes; they can become infected; condoms must be worn to prevent reinfections

• Tell patient that drug does not cure infection, just controls symptoms and does not prevent infection to others

Evaluation
Positive therapeutic outcome
• Absence of itching, painful lesions; crusting and healed lesions

Treatment of overdose:
• Discontinue drug
• Provide hemodialysis, resuscitation if needed

---

valproate (℞)
(val-proh′ate)
Depacon
valproic acid (℞)
Depakene, Myproic acid
divalproex sodium (℞)
Depakote, Epival
Func. class.: Anticonvulsant
Chem. class.: Carboxylic acid derivative
Pregnancy category **D**

Action: Increases levels of γ-aminobutyric acid (GABA) in brain, which decreases seizure activity

Therapeutic Outcome: Decreased symptoms of epilepsy, bipolar disorder

Uses: Simple (petit mal), complex (petit mal) absence, mixed, manic episode associated with bipolar disorder

Investigational uses: Tonic-clonic (grand mal), myoclonic seizures, migraines

Dosage and routes
P *Adult and child:* PO 15 mg/kg/day divided in 2-3 doses, may increase by 5-10 mg/kg/day qwk, not to exceed 60 mg/kg/day in 2-3 divided doses

Available forms: Valproic acid caps 250 mg; divalproex delayed rel tabs 125, 250, 500 mg; 125 mg sprinkle cap; valproate sodium syr 250 mg/5 ml

Adverse effects
CNS: Sedation, drowsiness, dizziness, headache, incoordination, paresthesia, depression, hallucinations, behavioral changes, tremors, aggression, weakness
EENT: Visual disturbances
GI: Nausea, vomiting, constipation, diarrhea, heartburn, anorexia, cramps, **hepatic failure, pancreatitis, toxic hepatitis,** stomatitis
GU: Enuresis, irregular menses
HEMA: **Thrombocytopenia, leukopenia, lymphocytosis,** increased pro-time
INTEG: Rash, alopecia, bruising

Contraindications: Hypersensitivity, pregnancy **D**, hepatic disease

P **Precautions:** Lactation, child <2 yr

Pharmacokinetics

Absorption	Unknown
Distribution	Breast milk, crosses placenta, widely distributed
Metabolism	Liver
Excretion	Kidneys
Half-life	9-16 hr

Pharmacodynamics	
Onset	15-30 min
Peak	1-4 hr
Duration	4-6 hr

Interactions
Individual drugs
Cimetidine: ↑ metabolism of valproic acid
Phenobarbital: ↑ CNS depressants
Phenytoin: ↑ action of phenytoin
Primidone: ↑ CNS depressants
Warfarin: ↑ toxicity of warfarin
Drug classifications
Benzodiazepines: ↑ sedation
Salicylates: ↑ toxicity of valproic acid
Lab test interferences
False positive: Ketones

NURSING CONSIDERATIONS
Assessment
• Monitor blood studies: Hct, Hgb, RBC, serum folate, platelets, pro-time, vit D if on long-term therapy
• Monitor hepatic studies: AST, ALT, bilirubin, creatinine, failure
• Monitor blood levels: therapeutic level 50-100 μg/ml
• Assess mental status: mood, sensorium, affect, memory (long, short)
• Assess respiratory dysfunction: respiratory depression, character, rate, rhythm; hold drug if respirations are <12/min or if pupils are dilated

Implementation
🚫 • Give tablets or capsules whole
• Give elixir alone; do not dilute with carbonated beverage; do not give syrup

to patients on sodium restriction
• Give with food or milk to decrease GI symptoms

Patient/family education
• Teach patient that physical dependency may result from extended use
• Instruct patient to avoid driving, other activities that require alertness
• Advise patient not to discontinue medication quickly after long-term use; convulsions may result
• Advise patient to report visual disturbances, rash, diarrhea, light-colored stools, jaundice, protracted vomiting to prescriber

Evaluation
Positive therapeutic outcome
• Decreased seizures

---

valrubicin (℞)
(val-roo'bih-sin)
Valstar
Func. class.: Antineoplastic, antibiotic
Chem. class.: Anthracycline glycoside
Pregnancy category   C

Action: A semisynthetic analog of doxorubicin that inhibits DNA synthesis primarily; replication is decreased by binding to DNA, which causes strand splitting; active throughout entire cell cycle; a vesicant

⮕**Therapeutic Outcome:** Decreased symptoms of breast cancer

Uses: Bladder cancer

Dosage and routes
Adult: **INTRAVESICALLY** 800 mg qwk × 6 wk, delay adminis-

V

tration ≥2 wks after transurethral resection of fulguration

Available forms: Sol for intravesical instillation: 40 mg/ml

Adverse effects

CV: Chest pain
GI: Nausea, vomiting, anorexia, diarrhea
GU: UTI, urinary retention, hematuria
HEMA: Thrombocytopenia, leukopenia, *anemia*
INTEG: Rash

Contraindications: Hypersensitivity to anthracyclines or Cremophor El, urinary tract infection, small bladder

Precautions: Pregnancy C, **P** lactation, children

Pharmacokinetics	
Absorption	Unknown
Distribution	Penetrates bladder wall
Metabolism	Unknown
Excretion	Unknown
Half-life	Unknown

Pharmacodynamics	
Onset	Unknown
Peak	Unknown
Duration	Unknown

Interactions
Unknown

NURSING CONSIDERATIONS
Assessment
• Monitor I&O ratio; report fall in urine output of <30 ml/hr
• Monitor temperature q4h; fever may indicate beginning infection
• Monitor local irritation, pain, burning at injection site

Nursing diagnoses
☑ Infection, risk for (side effects)
☑ Nutrition, altered, less than body requirements (side effects)
☑ Knowledge deficit (teaching)

Implementation
• Administer after urinary catheter is inserted under aseptic conditions, drain bladder and instill the diluted 75 ml valrubicin by gravity for several min, withdraw catheter; drug should be retained for 2 hr, then void
• Use procedure for handling and disposal of cytotoxic agents
• Do not use polyvinyl chloride (PVC) or IV tubing
• Prepare/store valrubicin sol in glass, polypropylene, or polyolefin tubing/containers
• For instillation, 5 ml vials (200 mg valrubicin/5 ml/vial) should be warmed to room temp, withdraw 20 ml from the 4 vials and dilute with 55 ml 0.9% NaCl inj to 75 ml of diluted valrubicin sol
• Valrubicin sol is clear red, at lower temps a waxy precipitate may form, warm in hand until sol is clear
• Perform strict hand-washing technique, gloves, protective clothing
• Provide increased fluid intake to 2-3L/day to prevent urate, calculi formation
• Store at room temperature for 12 hr after reconstituting

Patient/family education
• Advise patient to report any complaints, side effects to nurse or prescriber
• Teach patient that urine and other body fluids may be red-orange for 48 hr
• Teach patient that contraceptive measures are recommended during therapy

Evaluation
Positive therapeutic outcome
• Decreased tumor size, spread of malignancy

valsartan (R̸)
(val-zar'tan)
Diovan
Func. class.: Antihypertensive
Chem. class.: Angiotensin II receptor (Type AT_1)
Pregnancy category **UK**

Action: Blocks the vasoconstrictor and aldosterone-secreting effects of angiotensin II; selectively blocks the binding of angiotensin II to the AT_1 receptor found in tissues

➡ **Therapeutic Outcome:** Decreased B/P

Uses: Hypertension, alone or in combination

Dosage and routes
Adult: PO 80-160 mg qd alone or when used in combination

Available forms: Tabs 80, 160 mg

Adverse effects
CNS: Dizziness, insomnia, depression, drowsiness, vertigo
CV: Angina pectoris, 2nd-degree AV block, **cerebrovascular accident,** hypotension, **myocardial infarction, dysrhythmias**
EENT: Conjunctivitis
GI: Diarrhea, abdominal pain, nausea, **hepatotoxicity**
GU: Impotence, nephrotoxicity
HEMA: Anemia, neutropenia
MS: Cramps, myalgia, pain, stiffness
RESP: Cough

Contraindications: Hypersensitivity, pregnancy **UK,** severe hepatic disease, bilateral renal artery stenosis

Precautions: Hypersensitivity to ACE inhibitors, congestive heart failure, hypertrophic cardiomyopathy, aortic/mitral valve stenosis, CAD; lactation, children, elderly

Pharmacokinetics	
Absorption	Well
Distribution	Bound to plasma proteins
Metabolism	Extensive
Excretion	Feces, urine, breast milk
Half-life	9 hr

Pharmacodynamics	
Onset	Unknown
Peak	2 hr
Duration	24 hr

Interactions: None significant

NURSING CONSIDERATIONS
Assessment
• Assess B/P, pulse q4h; note rate, rhythm, quality
• Monitor electrolytes: potassium, sodium, chloride; total CO_2
• Obtain baselines in renal, liver function tests before therapy begins
• Assess blood studies: BUN, creatinine, LFTs before treatment
• Monitor for edema in feet, legs daily
• Assess for skin turgor, dryness of mucous membranes for hydration status

Nursing diagnoses
✓ Fluid volume deficit (side effects)
✓ Noncompliance (teaching)
✓ Knowledge deficit (teaching)

V

Implementation
• Administer without regard to meals

Patient/family education
• Teach patient not to take this drug if breastfeeding or pregnant, or have had an allergic reaction to this drug
• If a dose is missed, instruct patient to take as soon as possible, unless it is within an hour before next dose
• Advise patient to comply with dosage schedule, even if feeling better
• Teach patient to notify prescriber of fever, swelling of hands or feet, irregular heartbeat, chest pain
• Advise patient excessive perspiration, dehydration, diarrhea may lead to fall in blood pressure—consult prescriber if these occur
• Inform patient that drug may cause dizziness, fainting; lightheadedness may occur
• Caution patient to rise slowly to sitting or standing position to minimize orthostatic hypotension

Evaluation
Positive therapeutic outcome
• Decreased B/P

---

vancomycin
(van-koe-mye′sin)
Vancocin, vancomycin HCl
Func. clas.: Antiinfective, misc.
Chem. class.: Tricyclic glycopeptide
Pregnancy category   C

Action: Inhibits bacterial cell wall synthesis

➡**Therapeutic Outcome:** Bactericidal for the following

organisms: Staphylococci, Streptococci, Corynebacterium, Clostridium

Uses: Resistant staphylococcal infections, pseudomembranous colitis, staphylococcal enterocolitis, group A β-hemolytic streptococci, endocarditis prophylaxis for dental procedures, diphtheroid endocarditis

Dosage and routes
Serious staphylococcal infections
Adult: **IV** 500 mg (7.5 mg/kg) q6-8h or 1 g (15 mg/kg) q12h max 4 g/day
P *Child:* **IV** 40 mg/kg/day divided q6-12h
P *Neonates:* **IV** 15 mg/kg initially followed by 10 mg/kg q8-24h

Pseudomembranous/staphylococcal enterocolitis
Adult: PO 500 mg-2 g/day in 3-4 divided doses for 7-10 days
P *Child:* PO 40 mg/kg/day divided q6h, not to exceed 2 g/day
P *Neonates:* PO 10 mg/kg/day in divided doses

Endocarditis prophylaxis
Adult: **IV** 1 g over 1 hr, 1 hr before dental procedure
P *Child:* 20 mg/kg over 1 hr, 1 hr before procedure

Available forms: Pulvules 125, 250 mg; powder for oral sol 1, 10 g; powder for inj **IV** 500 mg; vials 1, 5, 10 g

Adverse effects
CV: **Cardiac arrest, vascular collapse** (rare)
EENT: Ototoxicity, permanent deafness, tinnitus
GI: Nausea, **pseudomembranous colitis**

GU: **Nephrotoxicity, increased BUN, creatinine, albumin, fatal uremia**
HEMA: **Leukopenia, eosinophilia, neutropenia**
INTEG: Chills, fever, rash, thrombophlebitis at inj site, urticaria, pruritus, necrosis (Redman's syndrome)
RESP: Wheezing, dyspnea
SYST: **Anaphylaxis**

Contraindications: Hypersensitivity, previous hearing loss

Precautions: Renal disease,
G pregnancy **C,** lactation, elderly,
P neonates

Pharmacokinetics
Absorption	Poorly absorbed (PO), completely absorbed (**IV**)
Distribution	Widely distributed, crosses placenta
Metabolism	Liver
Excretion	PO—feces, IV—kidneys
Half-life	4-8 hr

Pharmacodynamics
	IV
Onset	Immediate
Peak	Inf end

Interactions
Individual drugs
Amphotericin B: ↑ toxicity
Bacitracin: ↑ toxicity
Cisplatin: ↑ toxicity
Polymyxin B: ↑ toxicity
Drug classifications
Aminoglycosides: ↑ toxicity
Cephalosporins: ↑ toxicity
Nondepolarizing muscle relaxants: ↑ toxicity

NURSING CONSIDERATIONS
Assessment
• Monitor I&O ratio; report hematuria, oliguria because nephrotoxicity may occur
• Monitor any patient with compromised renal system; drug is excreted slowly in poor renal system function; toxicity may occur rapidly; BUN, creatinine
• Monitor blood studies: WBC; serum levels; peak 1 hr after 1-hr inf 25-40 mg/ml; trough prior to next dose 5-10 mg/ml
• Obtain C&S before drug therapy; drug may be given as soon as culture is taken
• Assess auditory function during, after treatment; hearing loss, ringing, roaring in ears; drug should be discontinued
• Monitor B/P during administration; sudden drop may indicate Red Man's syndrome
• Assess for signs of infection
• Assess respiratory status: rate, character, wheezing, tightness in chest
• Identify allergies before treatment, reaction of each medication; place allergies on chart in bright letters; notify all people giving drugs

Nursing diagnoses
☑ Infection, risk for (uses)
☑ Knowledge deficit (teaching)

Implementation
IV **IV route**
• Give after reconstitution with 10 ml sterile water for inj (500 mg/10 ml); further dilution is needed for **IV,** 500 mg/ 100 ml NS, D$_5$W given as int inf over 1 hr; decrease rate of infusion if Red Man's syndrome occurs

Y-site compatibilities: Acyclovir, allopurinol, amiodarone, amsacrine, atracurium, cyclophosphamide, diltiazem, enalaprilat, esmolol, filgrastim, fluconazole, fludarabine, gal-

V

lium, granisetron, hydromorphone, regular insulin, labetalol, lorazepam, magnesium sulfate, melphalan, meperidine, meropenem, midazolam, morphine, ondansetron, paclitaxel, pancuronium, perphenazine, propofol, sodium bicarbonate, tacrolimus, teniposide, theophylline, thiotepa, tolazoline, vecuronium, vinorelbine, warfarin, zidovudine

Additive compatibilities:
Amikacin, atracurium, calcium gluconate, cefepime, cimetidine, corticotropin, dimenhydrinate, hydrocortisone, meropenem, ofloxacin, potassium chloride, ranitidine, verapamil, vit B/C
• Give antihistamine if Red Man's syndrome occurs: decreased B/P, flushing of neck, face
• Give dose based on serum concentration
• Store at room temp for up to 2 wk after reconstitution
• Have adrenalin, suction, tracheostomy set, endotracheal intubation equipment on unit; anaphylaxis may occur
• Provide adequate intake of fuids (2 L) to prevent nephrotoxicity

Patient/family education
• Teach patient aspects of drug therapy: need to complete entire course of medication to ensure organism death (7-10 days); culture may be taken after completed course of medication
• Advise patient to report sore throat, fever, fatigue; could indicate superinfection
• Instruct patient that drug must be taken in equal intervals around clock to maintain blood levels

Evaluation
Positive therapeutic outcome
• Absence of fever, sore throat
• Negative culture after treatment

vecuronium (℞)
(ve-kure-oh′nee-yum)
Norcuron
Func. class.: Neuromuscular blocker
Chem. class.: Synthetic curariform
Pregnancy category   C

Action: Inhibits transmission of nerve impulses by binding with cholinergic receptor sites, antagonizing action of acetylcholine; no analgesic response

➡ **Therapeutic Outcome:** Skeletal muscle paralysis during anesthesia

Uses: Facilitation of endotracheal intubation; skeletal muscle relaxation during mechanical ventilation, surgery, or general anesthesia

Dosage and routes
🅟 *Adult and child >9 yr:* **IV** bol 0.08-0.10 mg/kg, then 0.010-0.015 mg/kg for prolonged procedures

Available forms: 10 mg/5 ml vial

Adverse effects
CNS: Skeletal muscle weakness or paralysis (rarely)
RESP: **Prolonged apnea, possible respiratory paralysis**

Contraindications: Hypersensitivity

Precautions: Pregnancy **C**, cardiac disease, lactation, 🅟 children <2 yr, electrolyte imbalances, dehydration, neuromuscular disease, respiratory, hepatic disease

◼ **Do Not Confuse:**
Nocuron/Narcan

Pharmacokinetics	
Absorption	Completely absorbed
Distribution	Rapid—to extracellular fluids
Metabolism	Liver (20%)
Excretion	Kidneys—unchanged (35%)
Half-life	1½ hr, increased in liver disease

Pharmacodynamics	
Onset	1 min
Peak	5 min
Duration	15-25 min

Interactions
Individual drugs
Clindamycin: ↑ paralysis, length and intensity
Colistin: ↑ paralysis, length and intensity
Lidocaine: ↑ paralysis, length and intensity
Lithium: ↑ paralysis, length and intensity
Magnesium: ↑ paralysis, length and intensity
Polymyxin B: ↑ paralysis, length and intensity
Procainamide: ↑ paralysis, length and intensity
Quinidine: ↑ paralysis, length and intensity
Succinylcholine: ↑ paralysis, length and intensity
Drug classifications
Aminoglycosides: ↑ paralysis, length and intensity
β-Adrenergic blockers: ↑ paralysis, length and intensity
Diuretics, potassium-losing: ↑ paralysis, length and intensity
General anesthesia: ↑ paralysis, length and intensity

NURSING CONSIDERATIONS
Assessment
• Monitor for electrolyte imbalances (potassium, magnesium), before drug is used; electrolyte imbalances may lead to increased action of this drug
• Monitor patient's vital signs (B/P, pulse, respirations, airway) until fully recovered; rate, depth, pattern of respirations, strength of hand grip; patient should be intubated before use
• Monitor patient's recovery: decreased paralysis of face, diaphragm, leg, arm, rest of body; residual weakness and respiratory problems may occur during recovery period
• Monitor allergic reactions: rash, fever, respiratory distress, pruritus; drug should be discontinued

Nursing diagnoses
☑ Breathing pattern, ineffective (uses)
☑ Communication, impaired verbal (adverse reactions)
☑ Fear (adverse reactions)
☑ Knowledge deficit (teaching)

Implementation
• Use peripheral nerve stimulator by anesthesiologist to determine neuromuscular blockade; deep tendon reflexes should be monitored during extended periods
• Give by direct **IV** after reconstituting with bacteriostatic water, over 5 min, D₅W, 0.9% NaCl or LR
• Give by direct **IV** after reconstituting dose in 5-10 ml; give by titrating to patient response
• Give by continuous inf after diluting to 10-20 mg/100 ml and by titrating to patient response (only by qualified

V

person, usually an anesthesiologist); do not administer IM
• Store in light-resistant area

Syringe incompatibilities:
Barbiturates

Y-site compatibilities:
Aminophylline, cefazolin, cefuroxime, cimetidine, diltiazem, dobutamine, dopamine, epinephrine, esmolol, fentanyl, fluconazole, gentamicin, heparin, hydrocortisone, hydromorphone, isoproterenol, labetalol, lorazepam, midazolam, milrinone, morphine, nicardipine, nitroglycerin, nitroprusside, norepinephrine, propofol, ranitidine, trimethoprim/sulfamethoxazole, vancomycin

Y-site incompatibilities:
Barbiturates

Patient/family education
• Provide reassurance if communication is difficult during recovery from neuromuscular blockade
• Provide explanation to patients regarding all procedures or treatments; patient will remain conscious if anesthesia is not given also

Evaluation
Positive therapeutic outcome
• Paralysis of jaw, eyelid, head, neck, rest of body as evaluated by peripheral nerve stimulator

Treatment of overdose:
Edrophonium or neostigmine, atropine, monitor VS; may require mechanical ventilation

---

venlafaxine (℞)
(ven-la-fax′een)
Effexor
Func. class.: Second-generation antidepressant-misc

Pregnancy category C

Action: Potent inhibitor of neuronal serotinin and norepinephrine uptake, weak inhibitor of dopamine; no muscarinic, histaminergic, or α-adrenergic receptors in vitro

▧**Therapeutic Outcome:** Relief of depression

Uses: Depression

Dosage and routes
Depression
Adult: PO 75 mg/day in 2 or 3 divided doses; taken with food, may be increased to 150 mg/day; if needed may be further increased to 225 mg/day; increments of 75 mg/day should be made at intervals of no less than 4 days; some hospitalized patients may require up to 375 mg/day in 3 divided doses; ext rel 37.5-75 mg PO qd, max 225 mg/day

Hepatic dose
Moderate impairment 50% of dose

Renal dose
Mild to moderate impairment 75% of dose

Available forms: Tabs scored 25, 37.5, 50, 75, 100 mg; cap ext rel 37.5, 75, 150 mg

Adverse effects
CNS: Emotional lability, vertigo, apathy, ataxia, CNS stimulation, euphoria, hallucinations, hostility, increased libido, hypertonia, hypotonia, psychosis

---

CV: Migraine, angina pectoris, extrasystoles, postural hypotension, syncope, thrombophlebitis, hypertension
EENT: Abnormal vision, ear pain, cataract, conjunctivitis, corneal lesions, dry eyes, otitis media, photophobia
GI: Dysphagia, eructation, colitis, gastritis, gingivitis, **rectal hemorrhage,** stomatitis, stomach and mouth ulceration
GU: Anorgasmia, dysuria, hematuria, metrorrhagia, vaginitis, impaired urination, albuminaria, amenorrhea, kidney calculus, cystitis, nocturia, breast and bladder pain, polyuria, **uterine hemorrhage, vaginal hemorrhage,** moniliasis
INTEG: Ecchymosis, acne, alopecia, brittle nails, dry skin, photosensitivity
META: Peripheral edema, weight loss or gain, diabetes mellitus, edema, glycosuria, hyperlipemia, hypokalemia
MS: Arthritis, bone pain, bursitis, myasthenia tenosynovitis
RESP: Bronchitis, dyspnea, asthma, chest congestion, epistaxis, hyperventilation, laryngitis
SYST: Accidental injury, malaise, neck pain, enlarged abdomen, cyst, facial edema, hangover effect, hernia

Contraindications: Hypersensitivity

Precautions: Mania, pregnancy **C,** lactation, children, elderly

Pharmacokinetics

Absorption	Well absorbed
Distribution	Widely distributed, 27% protein binding
Metabolism	Liver—extensively
Excretion	Kidneys, 87%
Half-life	5-7 hr, 11-13 hr (active metabolite)

Pharmacodynamics

Unknown

Interactions
Drug classifications
MAOIs: Hypertensive crisis, convulsions
Lab test interferences
↑ Serum bilirubin, ↑ blood glucose, ↑ alk phosphatase
↓ VMA, ↓ 5-HIAA
False: ↑ Urinary catecholamines

NURSING CONSIDERATIONS
Assessment
• Monitor B/P (lying, standing), pulse q4h; if systolic B/P drops 20 mm hg hold drug, notify prescriber; take vital signs q4h in patients with cardiovascular disease
• Monitor blood studies: CBC, leukocytes, differential, cardiac enzymes if patient is receiving long-term therapy
• Monitor hepatic studies: AST, ALT, bilirubin
• Check weight qwk; weight loss or gain; appetite may increase
• Assess mental status: mood, sensorium, affect, suicidal tendencies; increase in psychiatric symptoms: depression, panic
• Monitor urinary retention, constipation; constipation is more likely to occur in children or elderly
• Assess for withdrawal symptoms: headache, nausea, vomiting, muscle pain, weak-

ness; do not usually occur unless drug was discontinued abruptly
• Identify alcohol consumption; if alcohol is consumed, hold dose

Nursing diagnoses
☑ Coping, ineffective individual (uses)
☑ Injury, risk for physical (side effects)
☑ Knowledge deficit (teaching)
☑ Noncompliance (teaching)

Implementation
• Give with food or milk for GI symptoms
• Crush if patient is unable to swallow medication whole
• Store at room temp; do not freeze

Patient/family education
• Teach patient that therapeutic effects may take 2-3 wk
• Teach patient to use caution in driving or other activities requiring alertness because of drowsiness, dizziness, blurred vision; to avoid rising quickly from sitting to standing, especially elderly
• Teach patient to avoid alcohol ingestion, other CNS depressants

Evaluation
Positive therapeutic outcome
• Decreased depression
• Absence of suicidal thoughts

Treatment of overdose:
ECG monitoring, induce emesis, lavage, activated charcoal, administer anticonvulsant

verapamil ⚷ (℞)
(ver-ap'a-mil)
Calan, Calan SR, Isoptin, Isoptin SR, verapamil HCl, verapamil HCl SR, Verelan
Func. class.: Calcium-channel blocker; antihypertensive; antianginal
Chem. class.: Phenylalkylamine

Pregnancy category　C

Action: Inhibits calcium ion influx across cell membrane during cardiac depolarization; produces relaxation of coronary vascular smooth muscle; peripheral vascular smooth muscle; dilates coronary vascular arteries; increases myocardial oxygen delivery in patients with vasospastic angina

▷**Therapeutic Outcome:** Decreased angina pectoris, dysrhythmias, B/P

Uses: Chronic stable angina pectoris, vasospastic angina, dysrhythmias, hypertension

Investigational uses: Prevention of migraine headaches, ventricular outflow obstruction in hypertrophic cardiomyopathy

Dosage and routes
Adult: PO 80 mg tid or qid, increase qwk; **IV** bol 5-10 mg >2 min, repeat if necessary in 30 min

🅿 *Child 1-15 yr:* **IV** bol 0.1-0.3 mg/kg over >2 min, repeat in 30 min, not to exceed 10 mg in a single dose

Available forms: Tabs 40, 80, 120 mg; sus-rel tabs, 120, 180, 240 mg; inj 5 mg/ml; sus-rel caps 120, 180, 240, 360 mg

---

☑ Herb/drug　🚫 Do Not Crush　◆ Alert　⚷ Key Drug　🅖 Geriatric　🅿 Pediatric

Adverse effects
CNS: Headache, drowsiness, dizziness, anxiety, depression, weakness, insomnia, confusion, lightheadedness
CV: Edema, CHF, bradycardia, hypotension, palpitations, AV block
GI: Nausea, diarrhea, gastric upset, *constipation,* increased liver function studies
GU: Nocturia, polyuria

Contraindications: Sick sinus syndrome, 2nd- or 3rd-degree heart block, hypotension less than 90 mm Hg systolic, cardiogenic shock, severe CHF

Precautions: CHF, hypotension, hepatic injury, pregnancy **P** C, lactation, children, renal disease, concomitant β-blocker therapy

Pharmacokinetics

Absorption	Well absorbed (PO)
Distribution	Not known
Metabolism	Liver—extensively
Excretion	Kidneys
Half-life	Biphasic 4 min, 3-7 hr

Pharmacodynamics

	PO	PO-ER	IV
Onset	1-2 hr	Unknown	1-5 min
Peak	½-1½ hr	5-7 hr	3-5 min
Duration	3-7 hr	24 hr	2 hr

Interactions
Individual drugs
Alcohol: ↑ hypotension
Carbamazepine: ↑ toxicity
Digoxin: ↑ digoxin levels, ↑ bradycardia, CHF
Phenobarbital: ↓ effectiveness
Phenytoin: ↓ effectiveness
Propranolol: ↑ toxicity
Drug classifications
Antihypertensives: ↑ hypotension

β-Adrenergic blockers: ↑ bradycardia, CHF
Nitrates: ↑ nitrates
Food/drug
Grapefruit: ↑ hypotension

NURSING CONSIDERATIONS
Assessment
• Assess fluid volume status: I&O ratio and record; weight; distended red veins; crackles in lung; color; quality, and specific gravity of urine; skin turgor; adequacy of pulses; moist mucous membranes; bilateral lung sounds; peripheral pitting edema—dehydration symptoms of decreasing output, thirst, hypotension, dry mouth, and mucous membranes should be reported
• Monitor B/P and pulse, pulmonary capillary wedge pressure (PCWP), central venous pressure, index, often during inf; if B/P drops 30 mm Hg, stop inf and call prescriber
• Monitor ALT, AST, bilirubin daily; if these are elevated, hepatotoxicity is suspected
• Monitor if platelets are <150,000/mm³—if so, drug is usually discontinued and another drug started
• Assess for extravasation; change site q48h
• Monitor cardiac status: B/P, pulse, respiration, ECG

Nursing diagnoses
☑ Cardiac output, decreased (uses)
☑ Knowledge deficit (teaching)

Implementation
PO route
• Give once a day, with food for GI symptoms
IV route
• Give by direct **IV** undiluted (Y-site, 3-way stopcock) over

V

---

at least 2 min; to prevent serious hypotension, patient should be recumbent for 1 hr or more

Syringe compatibilities:
Amrinone, heparin, milrinone

Y-site compatibilities:
Amrinone, aprofloxacin, dobutamine, dopamine, famotidine, hydralazine, meperidine, methicillin, milrinone, penicillin G potassium, piperacillin, propofol, ticarcillin

Y-site incompatibilities:
Albumin, ampicillin, mezlocillin, nafcillin, oxacillin, sodium bicarbonate

Additive compatibilities:
Amikacin, amiodarone, ascorbic acid, atropine, bretylium, calcium chloride, calcium gluconate, cefamandole, cefazolin, cefotaxime, cefoxitin, cephapirin, chloramphenicol, cimetidine, clindamycin, dexamethasone, diazepam, digoxin, dopamine, epinephrine, erythromycin, gentamicin, heparin, hydrocortisone hydromorphone, hydrocortisone sodium phosphate, insulin (regular), isoproterenol, lidocaine, magnesium sulfate, mannitol, meperidine, metaraminol, methicillin, methyldopate, methylprednisolone, metoclopramide, mezlocillin, morphine, moxalactam, multivitamins, naloxone, nitroglycerin, norepinephrine, oxytocin, pancuronium, penicillin G potassium, penicillin G sodium, pentobarbital, phenobarbital, phentolamine, phenytoin, piperacillin, potassium chloride, potassium phosphates, procainamide, propranolol, protamine, quinidine, sodium bicarbonate, sodium nitroprusside, theophylline, ticarcillin, tobramycin, tolazoline, vancomycin, vasopressin, vit B/C

Patient/family education
• Advise patient to increase fluids/fiber to counteract constipation
• Caution patient to avoid hazardous activities until stabilized on drug, dizziness is no longer a problem
• Instruct patient to limit caffeine consumption; to avoid alcohol and OTC drugs unless directed by prescriber
• Advise patient to comply with medical regimen: diet, exercise, stress reduction, drug therapy; to notify prescriber of irregular heart beat, shortness of breath, swelling of feet and hands, pronounced dizziness, constipation, nausea, hypotension
• Teach patient to use as directed even if feeling better; may be taken with other cardiovascular drugs (nitrates, β blockers)

Evaluation
Positive therapeutic outcome
• Decreased anginal pain
• Decreased dysrhythmias
• Decreased B/P

Treatment of overdose:
Defibrillation, atropine for AV block, vasopressor for hypotension

---

 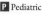

vinblastine (VLB) (℞)
(vin-blast′een)
Alkaban-AQ, Velban,
Velbe ✤, Velsar, vinblastine
sulfate
Func. class.: Antineoplastic
Chem. class.: Vinca rosea
alkaloid
Pregnancy category   D

Action: Inhibits mitotic activity, arrests cell cycle at metaphase; inhibits RNA synthesis, blocks cellular use of glutamic acid needed for purine synthesis; a vesicant

➡ **Therapeutic Outcome:** Prevention of rapid growth of malignant cells, immunosuppressive

Uses: Breast, testicular cancer; lymphomas; neuroblastoma; Hodgkin's, non-Hodgkin's lymphomas; mycosis fungoides; histiocytosis; Kaposi's sarcoma

Dosage and routes
Adult: **IV** 0.1 mg/kg or 3.7 mg/m² q wk or q2 wk, not to exceed 0.5 mg/kg or 18.5 mg/m² q wk

P *Child:* 2.5 mg/m² then dose of 3.75, 5.0, 6.25, and 7.5 at 7-day intervals

Available forms: Inj powder 10 mg for 10 ml **IV** inj

Adverse effects
CNS: Paresthesias, peripheral neuropathy, depression, headache, **convulsions**
CV: Tachycardia, orthostatic hypotension
GI: Nausea, vomiting, ileus, *anorexia, stomatitis,* constipation, abdominal pain, GI and rectal bleeding, **hepatotoxicity,** pharyngitis

GU: Urinary retention, **renal failure**
HEMA: **Thrombocytopenia, leukopenia, myelosuppression**
INTEG: Rash, alopecia, photosensitivity
META: SIADH
RESP: **Fibrosis, pulmonary infiltrate**

Contraindications: Hypersensitivity, infants, pregnancy **D**

Precautions: Renal disease, hepatic disease

⊠ **Do Not Confuse:**
vinblastine/vincristine

Pharmacokinetics	
Absorption	Complete bioavailability
Distribution	Crosses blood-brain barrier slightly
Metabolism	Liver—active antineoplastic
Excretion	Biliary, kidneys
Half-life	Triphasic—35 min, 53 min, 19 hr

Pharmacodynamics
Unknown

Interactions
Individual drugs
Mitomycin: ↑ bronchospasm
Radiation: ↑ toxicity, bone marrow suppression
Drug classifications
Antineoplastics: ↑ toxicity, bone marrow suppression
Live virus vaccines: ↑ adverse reactions

NURSING CONSIDERATIONS
Assessment
• Monitor B/P, (baseline and q15 min) during administration
• Monitor CBC, differential, platelet count weekly; withhold drug if WBC is <4000 or platelet count is <75,000; notify

V

prescriber of results, recovery will take 3 wk
• Assess for dyspnea, rales, unproductive cough, chest pain, tachypnea
• Monitor renal function studies: BUN, serum uric acid, urine CrCl before, during therapy; I&O ratio; report fall in urine output of 30 ml/hr; for decreased hyperuricemia
• Monitor for cold, fever, sore throat (may indicate beginning infection); notify health care prescriber if these occur
• Assess for bleeding: hematuria, guaiac, bruising or petechiae, mucosa or orifices q8h, no rectal temp; avoid IM inj; use pressure to venipuncture sites
• Identify nutritional status: an antiemetic may need to be prescribed
• Assess for symptoms indicating severe allergic reactions: rash, pruritus, urticaria, itching, flushing, bronchospasm, hypotension; epinephrine and crash cart should be nearby

Nursing diagnoses
☑ Injury, risk for (adverse reactions)
☑ Body image disturbance (adverse reactions)
☑ Infection, risk for (adverse reactions)
☑ Knowledge deficit (teaching)

Implementation
• Give by intermittent inf
• Sol should be prepared by qualified personnel only under controlled conditions
• Use Luer-Loc tubing to prevent leakage; do not let sol come in contact with skin; if contact occurs, wash well with soap and water
• Administer **IV** after diluting 10 mg/10 ml NaCl; give

through Y-tube or 3-way stopcock or directly over 1 min
• Give hyaluronidase 150 U/ml in 1 ml NaCl, warm compress for extravasation for vesicant activity treatment

Syringe compatibilities:
Bleomycin, cisplatin, cyclophosphamide, droperidol, fluorouracil, leucovorin, methotrexate, metoclopramide, mitomycin, vincristine

Y-*site compatibilities:*
Allopurinol, amifostine, aztreonam, bleomycin, cisplatin, cyclophosphamide, doxorubicin, droperidol, filgrastim, fludarabine, fluorouracil, granisetron, heparin, leucovorin, melphalan, methotrexate, metoclopramide, mitomycin, ondansetron, paclitaxel, piperacillin/tazobactam, sargramostim, teniposide, thiotepa, vincristine, vinorelbine

Y-*site incompatibilities:*
Furosemide

Additive compatibilities:
Bleomycin

Patient/family education
• Teach patient to avoid use of products containing aspirin or NSAIDs, razors, commercial mouthwash because bleeding may occur; to report symptoms of bleeding (hematuria, tarry stools)
• Instruct patient to report signs of anemia, (fatigue, headache, irritability, faintness, shortness of breath)
• Caution patient to report any changes in breathing or coughing even several mo after treatment
• Advise patient that contraception will be necessary during treatment; teratogenesis may occur

---

• Inform patient that hair may be lost during treatment; a wig or hairpiece may make patient feel better; new hair will be different in color, texture
• Advise patient to avoid vaccinations during treatment; serious reactions may occur
• Teach patient to report signs/symptoms of infection: fever, chills, sore throat; patient should avoid crowds and persons with known infections

Evaluation
Positive therapeutic outcome
• Decreased spread of malignant cells

---

vincristine (VCR)
Oₙ (℞)
(vin-kris'teen)
Oncovin, Vincasar PFS, vincristine sulfate
Func. class.: Antineoplastic-misc
Chem. class.: Vinca alkaloid
Pregnancy category   D

Action: Inhibits mitotic activity, arrests cell cycle at metaphase; inhibits RNA synthesis, blocks cellular use of glutamic acid needed for purine synthesis; a vesicant

Therapeutic Outcome: Prevention of rapid growth of malignant cells, immunosuppression

Uses: Breast, lung cancer; lymphomas; neuroblastomas; Hodgkin's disease; acute lymphoblastic and other leukemias; rhabdomyosarcoma, Wilms' tumor; osteogenic and other sarcomas

Dosage and routes
Adult: **IV** 1-2 mg/m²/wk, not to exceed 2 mg
P *Child:* **IV** 1.5-2 mg/m²/wk, not to exceed 2 mg

Available forms: Inj 1 mg/ml

Adverse effects
CNS: Decreased reflexes, numbness, weakness, motor difficulties, CNS depression, cranial nerve paralysis, **seizures**
CV: Orthostatic hypotension
GI: Nausea, vomiting, anorexia, stomatitis, constipation, **paralytic ileus, abdominal pain, hepatotoxicity**
HEMA: **Thrombocytopenia, leukopenia, myelosuppression, anemia**
INTEG: Alopecia

Contraindications: Hypersensitivity, infants, pregnancy **D**

Precautions: Renal disease, hepatic disease, hypertension, neuromuscular disease

Do Not Confuse:
vincristine/vinblastine

Pharmacokinetics	
Absorption	Complete bioavailability
Distribution	Rapidly, widely distributed; blood-brain barrier
Metabolism	Liver
Excretion	Biliary, in feces, crosses placenta
Half-life	Triphasic 0.85 min, 7.4 min, 1.64 min

Pharmacodynamics	
Onset	Unknown
Peak	Unknown
Duration	1 wk

Interactions
Individual drugs
L-asparaginase: ↓ metabolism of vincristine

V

Mitomycin: ↑ bronchospasm
Radiation: ↑ toxicity, bone marrow suppression
Drug classifications
Antineoplastics: ↑ toxicity, bone marrow suppression
Live virus vaccines: ↓ antibody response

NURSING CONSIDERATIONS
Assessment
• Monitor CBC, differential, platelet count weekly; withhold drug if WBC is <4000 or platelet count is <75,000; notify prescriber of results; platelets may increase or decrease
• Assess neurologic status: paresthesia, weakness, cranial nerve palsies, orthostatic hypotension, lethargy, agitation, psychosis; notify health care prescriber
• Monitor renal function studies: BUN, serum uric acid, urine CrCl before, during therapy; I&O ratio; report fall in urine output of 30 ml/hr; for decreased hyperuricemia, hyponatremia, and increased fluid retention (SIADH)
• Monitor for cold, fever, sore throat (may indicate beginning infection)
• Identify for increased uric acid levels, joint pain in extremities; increase fluid intake to 2-3 L/day unless contraindicated

Nursing diagnoses
☑ Injury, risk for (adverse reactions)
☑ Body image disturbance (adverse reactions)
☑ Infection, risk for (adverse reactions)
☑ Knowledge deficit (teaching)

Implementation
• Administer **IV** after diluting with diluent provided or 1

mg/10 ml of sterile H_2O or NaCl; give through Y-tube or 3-way stopcock or directly over 1 min
• Hyaluronidase 150 U/ml in 1 ml NaCl; apply warm compress for extravasation

Syringe compatibilities:
Bleomycin, cisplatin, cyclophosphamide, doxapram, doxorubicin, droperidol, fluorouracil, heparin, leucovorin, methotrexate, metoclopramide, mitomycin, ondansetron, vincristine

Syringe incompatibilities:
Furosemide

Y-site compatibilities:
Allopurinol, amifostine, aztreonam, bleomycin, cisplatin, cladribine, cyclophosphamide, doxorubicin, droperidol, filgrastim, fludarabine, fluorouracil, granisetron, heparin, leucovorin, methotrexate, metoclopramide, mitomycin, ondansetron, paclitaxel, sargramostim, teniposide, thiotepa, vincristine, vinorelbine

Y-site incompatibilities:
Furosemide

Patient/family education
• Teach patient to avoid use of products containing aspirin or NSAIDs, razors, commercial mouthwash because bleeding may occur; to report symptoms of bleeding (hematuria, tarry stools)
• Instruct patient to report signs of anemia, (fatigue, headache, irritability, faintness, shortness of breath)
• Caution patient to report any changes in breathing or coughing, even several mo after treatment
• Advise patient that contraception will be necessary dur-

---

ing treatment; teratogenesis
may occur
• Inform patient that hair may
be lost during treatment; a wig
or hairpiece may make patient
feel better; new hair will be
different in color, texture
• Advise patient to avoid vaccinations during treatment;
serious reactions may occur
• Teach patient to report
signs/symptoms of infection:
fever, chills, sore throat; patient
should avoid crowds, or persons with known infections

Evaluation
Positive therapeutic outcome
• Decreased spread of malig-
nancies

---

vinorelbine (R)
(vi-nor'el-bine)
Navelbine
Func. class.: Antineo-
plastic-misc
Chem. class.: Semi
synthetic Vinca alkaloid
Pregnancy category   D

Action: Inhibits mitotic activity, arrests cell cycle at
metaphase; inhibits RNA synthesis, blocks cellular use of
glutamic acid needed for purine synthesis; a vesicant

Therapeutic Outcome: Decreased spread of malignancy

Uses: Breast cancer; unresectable, advanced non–small-cell
lung cancer (NSCLC) stage
IV; may be used alone or in
combination with cisplatin for
stage III or IV NSCLC

Dosage and routes
Adult: **IV** 30 mg/m² qwk

Breast cancer
Adult: **IV** 30 mg/m² qwk

Available forms: Inj **IV**,
powder 10 mg for 10 ml **IV** inj
Adverse effects
CNS: Paresthesias, peripheral
neuropathy, depression, headache, **convulsions,** weakness,
jaw pain
GI: Nausea, vomiting, ileus,
anorexia, stomatitis, constipation, abdominal pain, GI,
diarrhea, **hepatotoxicity**
HEMA: **Neutropenia, anemia, thrombocytopenia**
INTEG: Rash, alopecia, photosensitivity
META: SIADH
MS: Myalgia

Contraindications: Hypersensitivity, infants, pregnancy **D**

Precautions: Renal disease,
hepatic disease

Pharmacokinetics

Absorption	Poor bioavailability (<50%)
Distribution	Unknown
Metabolism	Liver—to metabolite
Excretion	Bile
Half-life	43 hr

Pharmacodynamics

Onset	Unknown
Peak	1-2 hr
Duration	Unknown

Interactions
Individual drugs
Fluorouracil: ↑ toxicity a
possibility

NURSING CONSIDERATIONS
Assessment
• Monitor B/P, (baseline and
q15 min) during administration
• Monitor CBC, differential,
platelet count weekly; withhold
drug if WBC is <4000 or platelet count is <75,000; notify

V

---

prescriber of results, recovery will take 3 wk
• Assess for dyspnea, rales, unproductive cough, chest pain, tachypnea
• Monitor renal function studies: BUN, serum uric acid, urine CrCl before, during therapy, I&O ratio; report fall in urine output of 30 ml/hr; for decreased hyperuricemia
• Monitor for cold, fever, sore throat (may indicate beginning infection); notify health care prescriber if these occur
• Assess for bleeding: hematuria, guaiac, bruising or petechiae, mucosa or orifices q8h: no rectal temp; avoid IM inj; use pressure on venipuncture sites
• Identify nutritional status: an antiemetic may need to be prescribed
• Assess for symptoms indicating severe allergic reactions: rash, pruritus, urticaria, itching, flushing, bronchospasm, hypotension; epinephrine and crash cart should be nearby

Nursing diagnoses
☑ Injury, risk for (adverse reactions)
☑ Body image disturbance (adverse reactions)
☑ Infection, risk for (adverse reactions)
☑ Knowledge deficit (teaching)

Implementation
• Hyaluronidase 150 U/ml in 1 ml NaCl, warm compress for extravasation for vesicant activity treatment
• Antacid before oral agent; give drug after evening meal before bedtime
• Antiemetic 30-60 min before giving drug and prn to prevent vomiting

Cont inf
• Give 40 mg/m^2 q 3 wk after **IV** bol of 8 mg/m^2; may be given in combination with doxorubicin, fluorouracil, cisplatin

Y-site compatibilities:
Amikacin, aztreonam, bleomycin, buprenorphine, butorphanol, calcium gluconate, carboplatin, cefotaxime, cisplatin, cimetidine, clindamycin, dexamethasone, enalaprilat, etoposide, famotidine, filgrastim, fluconazole, fludarabine, gentamicin, hydrocortisone, lorazepam, meperidine, morphine, netilmicin, ondansetron, plicamycin, streptozocin, teniposide, ticarcillin, tobramycin, vancomycin, vinblastine, vincristine, zidovudine

Patient/family education
• Teach patient to use liq diet: cola, Jell-O; dry toast or crackers may be added if patient is not nauseated or vomiting
• Advise patient to rinse mouth 3-4 × day with water and brush teeth 2-3 × day with soft brush or cotton-tipped applicators for stomatitis; use unwaxed dental floss
• Inform patient that a nutritious diet with iron, vitamin supplements is necessary

Evaluation
Positive therapeutic outcome
• Decreased spread of malignant cells

☑ Herb/drug Ⓢ Do Not Crush ◆ Alert ☛ Key Drug Ⓖ Geriatric Ⓟ Pediatric

vitamin A (PO, OTC; IM, ℞)
Aquasol A, Del-Vi-A, Vitamin A
Func. class.: Vitamin, fat-soluble
Chem. class.: Retinol
Pregnancy category **C**

Action: Needed for normal bone and tooth development, visual dark adaptation, skin disease, mucosa tissue repair, assists in production of adrenal steroids, cholesterol, RNA

⇒ **Therapeutic Outcome:** Prevention, absence of vitamin A deficiency

Uses: Vitamin A deficiency

Dosage and routes
🅟 *Adult and child >8 yr:* PO 100,000-500,000 IU qd 3 days, then 50,000 qd × 2 wk; dose based on severity of deficiency; maintenance 10,000-20,000 IU for 2 mo

🅟 *Child 1-8 yr:* IM 5,000-15,000 IU qd × 10 days

🅟 *Infants <1 yr:* IM 5,000-15,000 IU × 10 days

Maintenance
🅟 *Child 4-8 yr:* IM 15,000 IU qd × 2 mo

🅟 *Child <4 yr:* IM 10,000 IU qd × 2 mo

Available forms: Caps 10,000, 25,000, 50,000 IU; drops 5000 IU; inj 50,000 IU/ml; tabs 10,000, 25,000, 50,000 IU

Adverse effects
CNS: Headache, increased intracranial pressure, intracranial hypertension, lethargy, malaise
EENT: Gingivitis, papilledema, exophthalmos, inflammation of tongue and lips
GI: Nausea, vomiting, anorexia, abdominal pain, *jaundice*
INTEG: Drying of skin, pruritus, increased pigmentation, night sweats, alopecia
MS: Arthralgia, retarded growth, hard areas on bone
META: Hypomenorrhea, hypercalcemia

Contraindications: Hypersensitivity to vit A, malabsorption syndrome (PO)

Precautions: Lactation, impaired renal function, pregnancy **C**

Pharmacokinetics	
Absorption	Rapidly absorbed
Distribution	Stored in liver, kidneys, lungs
Metabolism	Liver
Excretion	Breast milk
Half-life	Unknown

Pharmacodynamics
Unknown

Interactions
Individual drugs
Cholestyramine: ↓ absorption of vitamin A
Colestipol: ↓ absorption of vitamin A
Mineral oil: ↓ absorption of vitamin A
Drug classifications
Corticosteroids: ↑ levels of vitamin A
Oral contraceptives: ↑ level of vitamin A
Lab test interferences
False: ↑ Bilirubin, ↑ serum cholesterol

NURSING CONSIDERATIONS
Assessment
• Assess nutritional status: increase intake of yellow and dark

V

---

green vegetables, yellow/ orange fruits, vitamin A-fortified foods, liver, egg yolks

• Assess vitamin A deficiency: decreased growth; night blindness; dry, brittle nails; hair loss; urinary stones; increased infection; hyperkeratosis of skin; drying of cornea

• Identify vitamin A deficiency by plasma vitamin A, carotene level

• Assess for chronic vitamin A toxicity: increased calcium, BUN, glucose, cholesterol, triglyceride level

Nursing diagnoses

☑ Nutrition: less than body requirements (uses)

☑ Knowledge deficit (teaching)

Implementation

PO route

• Give with food (PO) for better absorption; do not give **IV** because anaphylaxis may occur

• Store in tight, light-resistant container

Patient/family education

• Instruct patient that if dose is missed, it should be omitted

• Inform patient that ophth exams may be required periodically throughout therapy

• Instruct patient not to use mineral oil while taking this drug because absorption will be decreased

• Advise patient to notify a prescriber of nausea, vomiting, lip cracking, loss of hair, headache

• Caution patient not to take more than the prescribed amount

Evaluation

Positive therapeutic outcome

• Increase in growth rate, weight

• Absence of dry skin and mucous membranes, night blindness

Treatment of overdose: Discontinue drug

(vitamin B₁₂) cyanocobalamin/ (vitamin B₁₂a) hydroxocobalamin
(PO, OTC; IM/SC, ℞)
(sye-an-oh-koe-bal'a-min)

Acti-B₁₂ ✦, Alphamine, Anacobin ✦, Bedoz ✦, B₁₂, Resin, Cobex, Crystamine, Crysti-12, Cyanoject, Cyomin, Hydrobexan, Hydro Cobex, Rubesol-1000, Rubion ✦, Rubramin PC, Vitamin B₁₂

Func. class.: Vitamin B₁₂, water-soluble vitamin

Pregnancy category   A

Action: Needed for adequate nerve functioning, protein and carbohydrate metabolism, normal growth, RBC development and cell reproduction

➡ **Therapeutic Outcome:** Prevention, correction of vitamin B₁₂ deficiency

Uses: Vitamin B₁₂ deficiency; pernicious anemia; vitamin B₁₂ malabsorption syndrome; Schilling test; increased requirements with pregnancy, thyrotoxicosis, hemolytic anemia, hemorrhage, renal and hepatic disease

Dosage and routes

Adult: PO 25 µg qd × 5-10 days, maintenance 100-200 mg IM qmo; IM/SC 30-100 µg qd × 5-10 days, maintenance 100-200 µg IM qmo

🅿 *Child:* PO 1 µg qd × 5-10 days, maintenance 60 µg IM

---

qmo or more; IM/SC 1-30 µg
qd × 5-10 days, maintenance
60 µg IM qmo or more

*Pernicious anemia/
malabsorption syndrome*
Adult: IM 100-1000 µg
qd × 2 wk, then 100-1000 µg
IM qmo

P *Child:* IM 100-500 µg over 2
wk or more given in 100-500
µg doses, then 60 µg IM/SC
monthly

Schilling test
P *Adult and child:* IM 1000 µg
in one dose

Available forms: Tabs 25, 50,
100, 250, 500, 1000 µg; inj
100, 120, 1000 µg/ml

Adverse effects
CNS: Flushing, optic nerve
atrophy
CV: **CHF,** peripheral vascular
thrombosis, **pulmonary edema**
GI: Diarrhea
INTEG: Itching, rash, pain at
site
META: Hypokalemia
SYST: **Anaphylactic shock**

Contraindications: Hypersensitivity, optic nerve atrophy

Precautions: Pregnancy **A,**
P lactation, children, cardiac
disease, uremia, iron deficiency,
folic acid deficiency

Pharmacokinetics	
Absorption	Well absorbed (IM, SC)
Distribution	Crosses placenta
Metabolism	Stored in liver, kidney, stomach
Excretion	50%-90% (urine), breast milk
Half-life	Unknown

Pharmacodynamics
Unknown

Interactions
Individual drugs
Alcohol: ↓ absorption
Aminosalicylic acid: ↓ absorp-
tion
Chloramphenicol: ↓ absorp-
tion
Cimetidine: ↓ absorption
Colchicine: ↓ absorption
Drug classifications
Aminoglycosides: ↓ absorp-
tion
Anticonvulsants: ↓ absorption
Potassium products: ↓ ab-
sorption
Lab test interferences
False positive: Intrinsic factor

NURSING CONSIDERATIONS
Assessment
• Assess for deficiency: anorexia, dyspepsia or exertion,
palpitations, paresthesias, psychosis, visual disturbances,
pallor, red inflamed tongue,
neuropathy, edema of legs
• Monitor potassium levels
during beginning treatment in
patients with megaloblastic
anemia
• Monitor CBC for increase in
reticulocyte count during 1st
wk of therapy, then increase in
RBC and hemoglobin; folic
acid levels, vitamin B$_{12}$ levels
• Assess nutritional status: egg
yolks, fish, organ meats, dairy
products, clams, oysters, which
are good sources for vit B$_{12}$
• Monitor for pulmonary
edema or worsening of CHF
in cardiac patients

Nursing diagnoses
☑ Nutrition; less than body re-
quirements (uses)
☑ Knowledge deficit (teaching)
☑ Noncompliance (teaching)
(overuse)

V

Implementation
PO route
• Give with fruit juice to disguise taste; administer immediately after mixing
• Give with meals if possible for better absorption
IM route
• Give by IM inj for pernicious anemia for life unless contraindicated
🔳 IV route
• May be mixed with TPN sol, but **IV** route is not recommended

Y-site compatibilities:
Heparin, hydrocortisone sodium succinate, potassium chloride

Solution compatibilities:
Dextrose/Ringer's or lactated Ringer's combinations, dextrose/saline combinations, D_5W, $D_{10}W$, 0.45% NaCl, Ringer's or lactated Ringer's sol, ascorbic acid

Patient/family education
• Instruct patient that treatment must continue for life if diagnosed as having pernicious anemia
• Advise patient to eat well-balanced diet from the food pyramid and comply with dietary recommendation
• Caution patient not to exceed the RDA of vitamin B_{12} because adverse reactions may occur
Evaluation
Positive therapeutic outcome
• Decreased anorexia, dyspnea on exertion, palpitations, paresthesias, psychosis, visual disturbances, edema of legs
• Prevention or correction of vitamin B_{12} deficiency
Treatment of overdose:
Discontinue drug

**vitamin D
(cholecalciferol,
vitamin D_3 or
ergocalciferol,
vitamin D_2)** (℞, OTC)
Calciferol, Drisdol, Radiostol ✦, Radiostol Forte ✦, Delta-D, Vitamin D, Vitamin D_3
Func. class.: Vitamin D
Chem. class: Fat soluble
Pregnancy category   C

Action: Needed for regulation of calcium, phosphate levels; normal bone development; parathyroid activity; neuromuscular functioning

▷**Therapeutic Outcome:** Prevention of rickets, osteomalacia, normal calcium/phosphate levels

Uses: Vitamin D deficiency, rickets, renal osteodystrophy, hypoparathyroidism, hypophosphatemia, psoriasis, rheumatoid arthritis

Dosage and routes
Deficiency
Adult: PO/IM 12,000 IU qd, then increased to 500,000 IU/day

🔳 **Child:** PO/IM 1500/5000 IU qd × 2-4 wk, may repeat after 2 wk or 600,000 IU as single dose

Hypoparathyroidism
🔳 **Adult and child:** PO/IM 200,000 IU given with 4 g calcium tab

Available forms: Tabs 400, 1000, 50,000 IU; caps 25,000, 50,000; oral sol 8000 IU/ml; inj 500,000 IU/ml, 500,000 IU/5 ml

Adverse effects
CNS: Fatigue, weakness,

---

drowsiness, **convulsions,** headache, psychosis
CV: Hypertension, dysrhythmias
GI: Nausea, vomiting, anorexia, cramps, diarrhea, constipation, metallic taste, dry mouth, decreased libido
GU: Polyuria, nocturia, **hematuria, albuminuria, renal failure**
INTEG: Pruritus, photophobia
MS: Decreased bone growth, early joint pain, early muscle pain

Contraindications: Hypersensitivity, hypercalcemia, renal dysfunction, hyperphosphatemia

Precautions: Cardiovascular disease, renal calculi, pregnancy **C**

▧ **Do Not Confuse:**
Calciferol/calcitriol

Pharmacokinetics	
Absorption	Well absorbed
Distribution	Stored in liver
Metabolism	Liver, sun
Excretion	Bile, kidney
Half-life	12-22 hr

Pharmacodynamics		
	PO	IM
Onset	Unknown	Unknown
Peak	4 hr	Unknown
Duration	15-20 days	Unknown

Interactions
Individual drugs
Cholestyramine: ↓ absorption of vitamin D
Colestipol: ↓ absorption of vitamin D
Mineral oil: ↓ absorption of vitamin D
Drug classifications
Cardiac glycosides: ↑ dysrhythmias
Corticosteroids: ↓ effects

Diuretics, thiazide: ↑ hypercalciuria
Lab test interferences
False: ↑ Cholesterol

NURSING CONSIDERATIONS
Assessment
• Monitor BUN, urinary calcium, AST, ALT, cholesterol, creatinine, uric acid, chloride, magnesium, electrolytes, urine pH, phosphate—may increase; calcium should be kept at 9-10 mg/dl; vitamin D 50-135 IU/dl, phosphate 70 mg/dl; ALK phosphatase—may be decreased
• Monitor for increased blood level—toxic reactions may occur rapidly
• Assess for dry mouth, metallic taste, polyuria, bone pain, muscle weakness, headache, fatigue, tinnitus, change in LOC, irregular pulse, dysrhythmias, increased respirations, anorexia, nausea, vomiting, cramps, diarrhea, constipation—may indicate hypercalcemia
• Assess renal status: decreased urinary output (oliguria, anuria), edema in extremities, weight gain 5 lb, periorbital edema
• Assess nutritional status, diet for sources of vitamin D (milk, cod, halibut, salmon, sardines, egg yolk) calcium (dairy products, dark green vegetables), phosphates (dairy products)
Nursing diagnoses
☑ Nutrition, less than body requirements (uses)
☑ Knowledge deficit (teaching)
Implementation
PO route
• PO may be increased q4wk depending on blood level

- Store in airtight, light-resistant container at room temp

IM route
- Give deeply in large muscle mass, administer slowly, aspirate to avoid **IV** administration, rotate inj site

Patient/family education
- Advise patient to omit dose if missed; to avoid vitamin supplements unless directed by prescriber
- Inform patient of necessary foods to be included in diet
- Advise patient to keep appointments for evaluation because therapeutic and toxic levels are narrow
- Instruct patient to report weakness, lethargy, headache, anorexia, loss of weight; to report nausea, vomiting, abdominal cramps, diarrhea, constipation, excessive thirst, polyuria, muscle and bone pain
- Caution patient to decrease intake of antacids and laxatives containing magnesium

Evaluation
Positive therapeutic outcome
- Calcium levels 9-10 ml/dl
- Decreasing symptoms of bone disease

---

vitamin E (OTC)

Amino-Opti-E, Aquasol E, Daltose ✤, E-Complex-600, E-Ferol, E-Vitamin Succinate, E-200 I.U. Softgels, Gordo-Vite E, Tocopherol, vitamin E, Vita-Plus E Softgells, Vitec
Func. class.: Vitamin E
Chem. class.: Fat soluble

Pregnancy category   A

Action: Needed for digestion and metabolism of polyunsaturated fats, decreases platelet aggregation, decreases blood clot formation, promotes normal growth and development of muscle tissue, prostaglandin synthesis

Therapeutic Outcome: Prevention and treatment of vitamin E deficiency

Uses: Vitamin E deficiency, impaired fat absorption, hemolytic anemia in premature neonates, prevention of retrolental fibroplasia, sickle cell anemia, supplement in malabsorption syndrome

Dosage and routes
Deficiency
Adult: PO 60-75 IU qd
P *Child:* PO 1 mg/0.6 g of dietary fat

Prevention of deficiency
Adult: PO 30 U/day
P *Infant:* PO 5 IU/day

Top
P *Adult and child:* Top apply to affected areas as needed

Available forms: Caps 100, 200, 400, 500, 600, 800 ✤, 1000 IU; tabs 100, 200, 400 IU; drops 50 mg/ml; chew tab 400 U; ointment, cream, lotion, oil

Adverse effects
CNS: Headache, fatigue
CV: Increased risk of thrombophlebitis
EENT: Blurred vision
GI: Nausea, cramps, diarrhea
GU: Gonadal dysfunction
INTEG: Sterile abscess, contact dermatitis
META: Altered metabolism of hormones, thyroid, pituitary, adrenal, altered immunity
MS: Weakness

Contraindications: None significant

Precautions: Pregnancy **A**

Pharmacokinetics

Absorption	20%-80% (PO)
Distribution	Widely distributed, stored in fat
Metabolism	Liver
Excretion	Bile
Half-life	Unknown

Pharmacodynamics

Unknown

Interactions
Individual drugs
Cholestyramine: ↓ absorption
Colestipol: ↓ absorption
Mineral oil: ↓ absorption
Sucralfate: ↓ absorption
Drug classification
Oral anticoagulants: ↑ action of anticoagulants

NURSING CONSIDERATIONS
Assessment
• Monitor vitamin E levels during treatment
• Assess nutritional status: intake of wheat germ, dark green leafy vegetables, nuts, eggs, liver, vegetable oils, dairy products, cereals
• Assess for vitamin E deficiency (usually in neonates): irritability, restlessness, hemolytic anemia
Nursing diagnoses
✓ Nutrition: less than body requirements (uses)
✓ Knowledge deficit (teaching)
Implementation
PO route
• Chewable tab: chew well
• Sol: may be dropped in mouth or mixed with food
• Store in tight, light-resistant container

Top route
• Apply top to moisturize dry skin
Patient/family education
• Inform patient necessary foods to be included in diet high in vitamin E
• Instruct patient to omit if dose missed
• Instruct patient to avoid vitamin supplements unless directed by prescriber because overdose may occur
Evaluation
Positive therapeutic outcome
• Absence of hemolytic anemia
• Adequate vitamin E levels
• Improvement in skin lesions
• Decrease in edema

warfarin ⚬━ (℞)
(war′far-in)
Coumadin, Sofarin, warfarin sodium, Warfilone
Sodium ♣
Func. class.: Anticoagulant
Pregnancy category **D**

Action: Interferes with blood clotting by indirect means; depresses hepatic synthesis of vitamin K-dependent coagulation factors (II, VII, IX, X)

→**Therapeutic Outcome:** Prevention of clotting

Uses: Pulmonary emboli, deep vein thrombosis, MI, atrial dysrhythmias, postcardiac valve replacement

Dosage and routes
Adult: PO 10-15 mg/day × 3 days, then titrated to prothrombin time qd
🅿 *Child:* 0.1 mg/kg/day titrated to INR

W

Available forms: Tabs 1, 2, 2.5, 5, 7.5, 10 mg; inj 50 mg/2 ml

Adverse effects
CNS: Fever
GI: Diarrhea, nausea, vomiting, anorexia, stomatitis, cramps, **hepatitis**
GU: **Hematuria**
HEMA: **Hemorrhage, agranulocytosis, leukopenia, eosinophilia**
INTEG: Rash, dermatitis, urticaria, alopecia, pruritus

Contraindications: Hypersensitivity, hemophilia, leukemia with bleeding, peptic ulcer disease, thrombocytopenic purpura, hepatic disease (severe), severe hypertension, subacute bacterial endocarditis, acute nephritis, blood dyscrasias, pregnancy **D**, eclampsia, preeclampsia, lactation

Precautions: Alcoholism, G elderly

Do Not Confuse:
Coumadin/Cardura,
Coumadin/Compazine

Pharmacokinetics	
Absorption	Well absorbed (PO), completely absorbed
Distribution	Crosses placenta, 99% plasma protein binding
Metabolism	Liver
Excretion	Kidney, feces (active, inactive metabolites)
Half-life	½-2½ days

Pharmacodynamics	
	PO
Onset	12-24 hr
Peak	½-3 days
Duration	3-5 days

Interactions
Individual drugs
Allopurinol: ↑ warfarin action
Amiodarone: ↑ warfarin action
Carbamazepine: ↓ warfarin action
Cefamandole: ↑ warfarin action
Chloramphenicol: ↑ warfarin action
Cimetidine: ↑ warfarin action
Clofibrate: ↑ warfarin action
Cotrimoxazole: ↑ warfarin action
Diflunisal: ↑ warfarin action
Erythromycin: ↑ warfarin action
Heparin: ↑ warfarin action
Isoniazid: ↑ warfarin action
Phenytoin: ↓ warfarin action
Rifampin: ↓ warfarin action
Sucralfate: ↓ warfarin action
Drug classifications
Barbiturates: ↓ warfarin action
Corticosteroids: ↓ warfarin action
Estrogens: ↓ warfarin action
NSAIDs: ↑ warfarin action
Oral contraceptives: ↓ warfarin action
Quinolones: ↑ warfarin action
Salicylates: ↑ warfarin action
Thrombolytics: ↑ warfarin action
Tricyclic antidepressants: ↑ warfarin action
Herb/drug
Alfalfa: ↓ anticoagulation
Bromelain: ↑ risk of bleeding
Cayenne: ↑ risk of bleeding
Cinchona: ↑ risk of bleeding
Danshen: ↑ risk of bleeding
Feverfew: ↑ risk of bleeding
Garlic: ↑ risk of bleeding
Ginger: ↑ risk of bleeding
Ginkgo biloba: ↑ risk of bleeding
Ginseng: ↓ anticoagulation
Quinine: ↑ risk of bleeding

Lab test interferences
↑ T_3 uptake
↓ Uric acid

NURSING CONSIDERATIONS
Assessment
• Monitor blood studies (Hct, occult blood in stools) q3mo; partial prothrombin time, which should be 1½-2 × control, PTT; often done qd, APTT, ACT; platelet count q2-3 days; thrombocytopenia may occur
• Monitor B/P, watch for increasing signs of hypertension
• Assess for bleeding: bleeding gums, petechiae, ecchymosis, black tarry stools, hematuria, epistaxis; decreased B/P may indicate bleeding and possible hemorrhage
• Assess for fever, skin rash, urticaria
• Assess for needed dosage change q1-2 wk
◆ Assess patients carefully for symptoms of Churg-Strauss syndrome (rare): eosinophilia, vasculitis, rash, worsening pulmonary symptoms, cardiac complications, neuropathy

Nursing diagnoses
✓ Injury, risk for (uses, adverse reactions)
✓ Tissue perfusion, altered (uses)
✓ Knowledge deficit (teaching)

Implementation
PO route
• Warfarin is usually given with **IV** heparin for 3 or more days, warfarin blood level may take several days
IV IV route
• Protect from light, **IV** form is in short supply

Additive compatibilities:
Cephapirin

Patient/family education
• Caution patient to avoid OTC preparations unless directed by prescriber—may cause serious drug interactions
• Advise patient that drug may be withheld during active bleeding (menstruation), depending on condition
• Advise patient to use soft-bristle toothbrush to avoid bleeding gums, avoid contact sports, use electric razor, avoid IM inj
• Instruct patient to carry a Medic Alert ID identifying drug taken
• Advise patient to report any signs of bleeding: gums, under skin, urine, stools
• Teach patient to read food labels—limited intake of vitamin K foods is necessary to maintain consistent prothrombin levels

Evaluation
Positive therapeutic outcome
• Decrease of deep vein thrombosis
• Prothrombin time (1.3-2.0 × control)

---

zafirlukast (℞)
(za-feer'loo-cast)
Accolate
Func. class.: Bronchodilator
Chem. class: Leukotriene receptor antagonist
Pregnancy category   UK

Action: Antagonizes the contractile action of leukotrienes (LTC_4, LTD_4, LTE_4) in airway smooth muscle; inhibits bronchoconstriction caused by antigens

➡️**Therapeutic Outcome:** Ability to breathe more easily

P **Uses:** Prophylaxis and chronic treatment of asthma in adults/children >12 yr

Dosage and routes
Adult: PO 20 mg bid, take 1 hr ac or 2 hr pc

Available forms: Tab 20 mg

Adverse effects
CNS: Headache, dizziness
GI: Nausea, diarrhea, abdominal pain, vomiting
OTHER: Infections, pain, asthenia, myalgia, fever, dyspepsia, increased ALT

Contraindications: Hypersensitivity

Precautions: Pregnancy **UK**,
G elderly, lactation, children,
P hepatic disease

Pharmacokinetics

Unknown

Pharmacodynamics

Unknown

Interactions
Individual drugs
Aspirin: ↑ plasma levels of zafirlukast
Erythromycin: ↓ plasma levels of zafirlukast
Theophylline: ↓ plasma levels of zafirlukast
Warfarin: ↑ pro-time
Food/drug
↓ Bioavailability of zafirlukast

NURSING CONSIDERATIONS
Assessment

• Assess respiratory rate, rhythm, depth; auscultate lung fields bilaterally; notify prescriber of abnormalities

Nursing diagnoses
☑ Breathing pattern, ineffective (uses)
☑ Knowledge deficit (teaching)
☑ Noncompliance (teaching)

Implementation
• Give after meals for GI symptoms; absorption may be affected

Patient/family education
• Advise patient to check OTC medications, current prescription medications, which will increase stimulation
• Advise patient to avoid hazardous activities; dizziness may occur
• Advise patient that if GI upset occurs, to take drug with 8 oz water; avoid food if possible, absorption may be decreased
• Advise patient to notify prescriber of nausea, vomiting, diarrhea, abdominal pain

Evaluation
Positive therapeutic outcome
• Ability to breathe more easily

zalcitabine (℞)
(zal-sit'a-bin)
HIVID, ddC, Dideoxycitidine
Func. class.: Antiviral
Chem. class.: Synthetic pyrimidine nucleoside analog of 2'-deoxycytidine
Pregnancy category **C**

Action: Inhibits HIV replication by the conversion of this drug by cellular enzymes to an active antiviral metabolite

➡️**Therapeutic Outcome:** Improved symptoms of HIV infection

P **Uses:** Advanced HIV infections in adults and children >13 yrs who have been unable to use zidovudine or who have not responded to treatment

Dosage and routes
Adult: PO combined with zidovudine in advanced HIV infection: 0.75 mg administered concomitantly with 200 mg zidovudine q8h; dosage reduction not necessary for patients weighing >30 kg; in presence of peripheral neuropathy initiate dose at 0.375 mg q8h of zalcitabine

Available forms: Tabs 0.375, 0.75 mg

Adverse effects
CNS: Headache, peripheral neuropathy, **seizures,** confusion, anxiety, hypertonia, abnormal thinking, asthenia, insomnia, CNS depression, pain, *dizziness,* chills, *fever*
CV: Hypertension, vasodilation, dysrhythmia, syncope, palpitation, tachycardia
EENT: Ear pain, otitis, photophobia, visual impairment
ENDO: Hypoglycemia, hyponatremia, hyperbilirubinemia, hyperglycemia
GI: Pancreatitis, diarrhea, nausea, vomiting, abdominal pain, constipation, stomatitis, dysplasia, liver abnormalities, *oral ulcers,* flatulence, taste perversion, dry mouth, oral thrush, melena, *increased ALT, AST, alk phosphatase, amylase,* increased bilirubin
GU: Uric acid, **toxic nephropathy,** polyuria
HEMA: **Leukopenia, granulocytopenia, thrombocytopenia,** anemia
INTEG: Rash, pruritus, alopecia, sweating, acne
MS: Myalgia, arthritis, myopathy, muscular atrophy
RESP: Cough, pneumonia, dyspnea, asthma, hypoventilation

Contraindications: Hypersensitivity

Precautions: Renal, hepatic, cardiac disease, pregnancy **C,** lactation, children (<13 yr), patients with peripheral neuropathy

Pharmacokinetics
Absorption	Minimally absorbed
Distribution	Unknown
Metabolism	Liver
Excretion	Unknown
Half-life	1.62 hr, increased in renal disease

Pharmacodynamics
Onset	Unknown
Peak	1½-2½
Duration	Unknown

Interactions
Individual drugs
Amphotericin B: ↑ neurotoxicity, nephrotoxicity
Cimetidine: ↑ neurotoxicity, nephrotoxicity
Foscarnet: ↑ neurotoxicity, nephrotoxicity
Interferon: ↑ neurotoxicity, nephrotoxicity
Methotrexate: ↑ neurotoxicity, nephrotoxicity
Probenecid: ↑ neurotoxicity, nephrotoxicity
Drug classifications
Aminoglycosides: ↑ neurotoxicity, nephrotoxicity
Antacids: ↓ absorption

NURSING CONSIDERATIONS
Assessment
• Assess for peripheral neuropathy: tingling or pain in hands and feet, distal numbness; if these occur during therapy, drug may be decreased or discontinued

• Assess for pancreatitis: abdominal pain, nausea, vomiting, elevated liver enzymes; drug should be discontinued because condition can be fatal

[P] • Assess children by dilated retinal examination q6mo to rule out retinal depigmentation

• Monitor CBC, differential, platelet count qmo; withhold drug if WBC is <4000 or platelet count is <75,000; notify prescriber of results

• Monitor renal function studies; BUN, serum uric acid, urine CrCl before, during therapy; these may be elevated throughout treatment

• Monitor temp q4h, may indicate beginning infection

• Monitor liver function tests before, during therapy (bilirubin, AST, ALT, amylase, alk phosphatase, triglycerides as needed or qmo

Nursing diagnoses

☑ Infection, risk for (uses)
☑ Injury, risk for (adverse reactions)
☑ Knowledge deficit (teaching)

Implementation

• Give on empty stomach, q8h around the clock

Patient/family education

• Advise patient to take on empty stomach; not to take dapsone at same time as ddC; to use exactly as prescribed

• Instruct patient to report signs of infection: increased temp, sore throat, flu symptoms; to avoid crowds and those with known infections

• Caution patient to report signs of anemia; fatigue, headache, faintness, shortness of breath, irritability

• Advise patient to report bleeding; avoid use of razors or commercial mouthwash

• Inform patient that hair may be lost during therapy (rare); a wig or hairpiece may make patient feel better

• Caution patient to avoid OTC products or other medications without approval of prescriber

• Caution patient not to have any sexual contact without use of a condom, that needles should not be shared, that blood from infected individual should not come in contact with another's mucus membranes

Evaluation

Positive therapeutic outcome

• Absence of infection; symptoms of HIV

---

zaleplon
See Appendix A,
Selected New Drugs

---

zanamivir
See Appendix A,
Selected New Drugs

---

zidovudine ⚷π (℞)
(zye-doe'vue-deen)
Apo-Zidovudine ✦,
Azidothymidine, AZT,
Novo-AZT ✦, Retrovir
Func. class.: Antiviral
Chem. class.: Thymidine analog

Pregnancy category   C

Action: Inhibits replication of HIV by incorporating into cellular DNA by viral reverse transcriptase, thereby terminating the cellular DNA chain

---

☑ Herb/drug 🚫 Do Not Crush ⬧ Alert ⚷π Key Drug [G] Geriatric [P] Pediatric

➔**Therapeutic Outcome:** Decreased symptoms of HIV

Uses: Symptomatic/asymptomatic HIV infections (AIDS, ARC), confirmed *P. carinii* pneumonia, or absolute CD4 lymphocytes <200/mm³, prevention of maternal-fetal HIV transmission

Dosage and routes
Adult: PO 200 mg q4h; may have to stop treatment if severe bone marrow depression occurs, and restart after bone marrow recovery; **IV** 1-2 mg/kg q4h, initiate PO as soon as possible

🄿 *Child:* PO 90-180 mg/m²/dose q6h; **IV** same as adult

🄿 *Neonates:* PO 2-3 mg/kg/dose q6h; **IV** same as adult

Prevention of maternal-fetal HIV transmission
🄿 *Neonatal:* PO 2 mg/kg/dose q6h × 6 wk beginning 8-12 hr after birth; **IV** 1.5 mg/kg/dose over 30 min q6h until able to take PO

Maternal (>14 wk gestation): PO 100 mg 5×/day until start of labor, then **IV** 2 mg/kg over 1 hr followed by **IV** inf 1 mg/kg/hr until umbilical cord clamped

Asymptomatic HIV infection
🄿 *Child 3 mo to 12 yr:* PO 90-180 mg/m² q6h (max 200 mg q6h); **IV** 1-2 mg/kg over 1 hr q4h

Adult: PO 100 mg q4h while awake (5×/day)

Symptomatic HIV infection
🄿 *Child 3 mo to 12 yr:* PO 90-180 mg/m² q6h (max 200 ng q6h); **IV** 1-2 mg/kg over 1 hr q4h

Adult: PO 100 mg q4h; **IV** 1-2 mg/kg over 1 hr q4h

Prevention of HIV following needlestick
Adult: PO 200 mg tid plus lamivudine 150 mg bid, plus a protease inhibitor for high-risk exposure; begin within 2 hrs of exposure

Available forms: Cap 100 mg; inj 200 mg/20 ml; oral syr 50 mg/5 ml

Adverse effects
CNS: Fever, headache, malaise, diaphoresis, *dizziness, insomnia,* paresthesia, somnolence, chills, tremor, twitching, anxiety, confusion, depression, lability, vertigo, loss of mental acuity
EENT: Taste change, hearing loss, photophobia
GI: Nausea, vomiting, diarrhea, anorexia, cramps, *dyspepsia,* constipation, dysphagia, *flatulence,* rec bleeding, mouth ulcer
GU: Dysuria, polyuria, frequency, hesitancy
HEMA: **Granulocytopenia, anemia**
INTEG: Rash, acne, pruritus, urticaria
MS: Myalgia, arthralgia, muscle spasm
RESP: Dyspnea

Contraindications: Hypersensitivity

Precautions: Granulocyte count <1000/mm³ or Hgb <9.5 g/dl, pregnancy **C**, lactation, 🄿 children, severe renal disease, severe hepatic function

Pharmacokinetics

Absorption	Well absorbed (PO), completely absorbed (**IV**)
Distribution	Widely distributed—crosses placenta, CSF
Metabolism	Liver—mostly
Excretion	Kidneys
Half-life	1 hr

Pharmacodynamics

	PO	IV
Onset	Unknown	Rapid
Peak	½-1½ hr	Inf end
Duration	Unknown	Unknown

Interactions
Individual drugs
Amphotericin B: ↑ neurotoxicity, nephrotoxicity
Interferon: ↑ neurotoxicity, nephrotoxicity
Methotrexate: ↑ neurotoxicity, nephrotoxicity
Probenecid: ↑ neurotoxicity, nephrotoxicity
Drug classifications
Aminoglycosides: ↑ neurotoxicity, nephrotoxicity

NURSING CONSIDERATIONS
Assessment
• Assess for peripheral neuropathy: tingling or pain in hands and feet, distal numbness; if these occur, drug may be decreased or discontinued
• Assess for pancreatitis: abdominal pain, nausea, vomiting, elevated liver enzymes; drug should be discontinued because condition can be fatal
P • Assess children by dilated retinal examination q6mo to rule out retinal depigmentation
• Monitor CBC, differential, platelet count qmo; withhold drug if WBC is <4000 or platelet count is <75,000; notify prescriber of results
• Monitor renal function studies; BUN, serum uric acid, urine CrCl before, during therapy; these may be elevated throughout treatment
• Monitor temp q4h, may indicate beginning infection
• Monitor liver function tests before, during therapy (bilirubin, AST, ALT amylase, alkaline phosphatase prn or qmo

Nursing diagnoses
☑ Infection, risk for (uses)
☑ Injury, risk for physical injury (adverse reactions)
☑ Knowledge deficit (teaching)

Implementation
PO route
• Give on empty stomach, q4h around the clock
IV IV route
• Give by intermittent inf after diluting with D_5W; give over 1 hr (<4 mg/ml), do not give by direct **IV**

Y-site compatibilities:
Acyclovir, allopurinol, amikacin, amphotericin B, aztreonam, ceftazidime, ceftriaxone, cimetidine, clindamycin, dexamethasone, dobutamine, dopamine, erythromycin, fluconazole, fludarabine, gentamicin, heparin, imipenem/cilastatin, lorazepam, metoclopramide, morphine, nafcillin, ondansetron, oxacillin, pentamidine, phenylephrine, piperacillin, potassium chloride, ranitidine, sargramostim, tobramycin, trimethoprim-sulfamethoxazole, vancomycin

Additive incompatibilities:
Blood products or protein solutions

Patient/family education
• Caution patient to take on empty stomach; not to take

---

dapsone at same time as ddl; to use exactly as prescribed
• Advise patient to report signs of infection: increased temp, sore throat, flu symptoms; to avoid crowds and those with known infections
• Instruct patient to report signs of anemia: fatigue, headache, faintness, shortness of breath, irritability
• Advise patient to report bleeding; avoid use of razors or commercial mouthwash
• Inform patient that hair may be lost during therapy (rare); a wig or hairpiece may make patient feel better
• Caution patient to avoid OTC products or other medications without approval of prescriber
• Caution patient not to have any sexual contact without use of a condom, needles should not be shared, blood from infected individual should not come in contact with another's mucus membranes

Evaluation
Positive therapeutic outcome
• Decreased infection; symptoms of HIV

---

zileuton (℞)
(zye-loo'tahn)
Zyflo
Func. class.: Bronchodilator
Chem. class.: 5-1 poxygenase inhibitor, leukotriene pathway inhibitor
Pregnancy category C

Action: Inhibits leukotriene (LT) formation; leukotrienes exert their effects by increasing neutrophil, eosinophil migration; aggregation of neutrophils, monocytes; smooth muscle contraction, capillary permeability; these actions further lead to bronchoconstriction, inflammation, edema

➤**Therapeutic Outcome:** Ability to breathe more easily

Uses: Allergic rhinitis, asthma

Investigational uses: Ulcerative colitis, rheumatoid arthritis

Dosage and routes
Asthma
🅟 *Adult and child >12 yr:* PO 600 mg qid, may be given with meal and hs
Ulcerative colitis
Adult: PO 600 mg bid

Available forms: Tab 600 mg

Adverse effects
CNS: Dizziness, insomnia, fatigue, paresthesias, headache
GI: Nausea, abdominal pain, dyspepsia, diarrhea, LFTs abnormalities
INTEG: Hives
MS: Myalgia, asthenia

Contraindications: Hepatic disease, elevations in LFTs 3× upper limits, hypersensitivity

Precautions: Acute attacks of asthma, alcohol consumption, pregnancy **C**

Pharmacokinetics	
Absorption	Rapid
Distribution	Protein-binding 93%
Metabolism	Liver
Excretion	Urine
Half-life	2.1-2.5 hr

Pharmacodynamics	
Onset	Unknown
Peak	1-3 hr
Duration	Unknown

Interactions
Individual drugs
Propranolol: ↑ action of zilenton
Theophylline: ↑ action of zilenton
Drug classifications
Anticoagulants: ↑ effects

NURSING CONSIDERATIONS
Assessment
• Assess CBC, blood chemistry, during treatment
• Assess LFTs before and qmo × 3 mo, their q2-3mo during treatment
• Assess respiratory rate, rhythm, depth; auscultate lung fields bilaterally; notify prescriber of abnormalities
• Assess allergic reactions: rash, urticaria; drug should be discontinued

Nursing diagnoses
✓ Breathing pattern, ineffective (uses)
✓ Knowledge deficit (teaching)
✓ Noncompliance (teaching)

Implementation
• Give PO after meals for GI symptoms; absorption may be affected

Patient/family education
• Advise patient to check OTC medications, current prescription medications for ephedrine, which will increase stimulation; to avoid alcohol
• Advise patient to avoid hazardous activities; dizziness may occur
• Advise patient that if GI upset occurs, to take drug with 8 oz water or food; absorption may be decreased slightly
• Advise patient to notify prescriber of nausea, vomiting, anxiety, insomnia

Evaluation
Positive therapeutic outcome
• Ability to breathe more easily

---

zinc sulfate
(PO, OTC; IV, ℞)
(zink sul'fate)
Orazinc, PMS Egozine ✽, Verazinc, Zinca-Pak, Zincate, Zinc 15, Zinc-220, zinc sulfate
Func. class.: Trace element; nutritional supplement
Pregnancy category A

Action: Needed for adequate healing, bone and joint development, taste and smell (23% zinc)

⇒ **Therapeutic Outcome:** Replacement of zinc

Uses: Prevention of zinc deficiency, adjunct to vitamin A therapy

Investigational uses: Wound healing

Dosage and routes
Dietary supplement
Adult: PO 25-50 mg/day

Nutritional supplement **(IV)**
Adult: 2.5-4 mg/day, may increase by 2 mg/day if needed

P *Child to 5 yr:* **IV** 100 µg/kg/day

P *Infants: <1500 gm to 3 kg;* **IV** 300 µg/kg/day

Available forms: Tabs 66, 110 mg; cap 220 mg; inj 1 mg, 5 mg/ml

Adverse effects
GI: Nausea, vomiting, cramps, heartburn, ulcer formation

☑ Herb/drug 🚫 Do Not Crush ◆ Alert ⚷ Key Drug **G** Geriatric **P** Pediatric

OVERDOSE: Diarrhea, rash, dehydration, restlessness

Precautions: Pregnancy **A**

Pharmacokinetics

Absorption	Poorly absorbed (PO), completely absorbed (**IV**)
Distribution	Widely distributed
Metabolism	Liver
Excretion	90%—feces, 10%—kidneys
Half-life	Unknown

Pharmacodynamics

Unknown

Interactions
Individual drugs
Tetracycline: ↓ absorption of tetracycline

NURSING CONSIDERATIONS
Assessment
• Monitor zinc levels during treatment

Nursing diagnoses
☑ Nutrition: less than body requirements (uses)
☑ Knowledge deficit (teaching)

Implementation
PO route
• Give with meals to decrease gastric upset; restrict dairy products, caffeine, which decrease absorption

IV **IV route**
• Part of total parenteral nutrition (TPN)

Patient/family education
• Inform patient that element must be taken for 2 mo to be effective
• Advise patient to report immediately nausea, diarrhea, rash, severe vomiting, restlessness, abdominal pain, tarry stools

Evaluation
Positive therapeutic outcome
• Absence of zinc deficiency
• Improved wound healing

---

zolmitriptan (Ŗ)
(zole-mih-trip′tan)
Zomig
Func. class.: Migraine agent
Chem. class.: 5-HT₁ receptor agonist
Pregnancy category C

Action: Binds selectively to the vascular 5-HT₁ receptor subtype, exerts antimigraine effect; causes vasoconstriction in cranial arteries

➙**Therapeutic Outcome:** Decreased severity, frequency of headache

Uses: Acute treatment of migraine with or without aura

Dosage and routes:
Adult: PO ≤2.5 mg (tab may be broken), may repeat after 2 hr, max 10 mg/24 hr

Available forms: Tabs 2.5, 5 mg

Adverse effects:
CV: Palpitations
GI: Abdominal discomfort
MS: Weakness, neck stiffness, myalgia
NEURO: Tingling, hot sensation, burning, feeling of pressure, tightness, numbness, dizziness, sedation
RESP: Chest tightness, pressure

Contraindications: Angina pectoris, history of MI, documented silent ischemia, ischemic heart disease, concurrent ergotamine-containing preparations, uncontrolled hypertension, hypersensitivity, basilar or hemiplegic migraine

Precautions: Postmenopausal women, men >40 yr, risk factors for CAD, hypercholesterolemia, obesity, diabetes, impaired hepatic or renal **P** function, pregnancy **C,** lacta-**G** tion, children, elderly

Pharmacokinetics

Absorption	Unknown
Distribution	25% protein binding
Metabolism	Unknown
Excretion	Unknown
Half-life	3-3½ hr

Pharmacodynamics

Onset	Unknown
Peak	Unknown
Duration	2-3½ hr

Interactions
Individual drugs
Cimetidine: ↑ half-life of zolmitriptan
Ergot: ↑ vasospastic effects
Drug classifications
Ergot derivatives: ↑ vasospastic effects
MAOIs: Do not use within 2 wk
SSRIs: ↑ weakness, hyperreflexia, incoordination

NURSING CONSIDERATIONS
Assessment
• Assess tingling, hot sensation, burning, feeling of pressure, numbness, flushing
• Assess for stress level, activity, recreation, coping mechanisms
• Assess neurologic status: LOC, blurring vision, nausea, vomiting, tingling in extremities preceding headache
• Monitor ingestion of tyramine foods (pickled products, beer, wine, aged cheese), food additives, preservatives, color-

ings, artifical sweeteners, chocolate, caffeine, which may precipitate these types of headaches
• Assess for serotonin syndrome, if also taking an SSRI

Nursing diagnoses
✓ Pain (uses)
✓ Noncompliance (teaching)
✓ Knowledge deficit (teaching)

Implementation
• Give with fluids as soon as symptoms of migraine occur
• Provide quiet, calm environment with decreased stimulation for noise, bright light, excessive talking

Patient/family education
• Teach patient to report any side effects to prescriber
• Advise patient to use contraception while taking drug

Evaluation
Positive therapeutic outcome
• Decrease in frequency, severity of headache

---

zolpidem (℞)
(zole-pi′dem)
Ambien
Func. class.: Sedative-hypnotic
Chem. class.: Nonbenzodiazepine of imidazopyridine class

Pregnancy category B
Controlled substance schedule IV

Action: Produces CNS depression at limbic, thalamic, hypothalamic levels of CNS; may be mediated by neurotransmitter γ-aminobutyric acid (GABA); results are sedation, hypnosis, skeletal muscle relaxation, anticonvulsant activity, anxiolytic action

Therapeutic Outcome: Ability to sleep, sedation

Uses: Insomnia, short-term treatment

Dosage and routes
Adult: PO 10 mg hs × 7-10 days only; total dose should not exceed 10 mg

Elderly: PO 5 mg hs

Available forms: Tabs 5, 10 mg

Adverse effects
CNS: Headache, lethargy, drowsiness, daytime sedation, dizziness, confusion, lightheadedness, anxiety, irritability, amnesia, poor coordination
CV: Chest pain, palpitation
GI: Nausea, vomiting, diarrhea, heartburn, abdominal pain, constipation

Contraindications: Hypersensitivity to benzodiazepines

Precautions: Anemia, hepatic disease, renal disease, suicidal individuals, drug abuse, elderly, psychosis, child <18 yr, seizure disorders, pregnancy **B**, lactation

Pharmacokinetics

Absorption	Rapidly absorbed
Distribution	Unknown
Metabolism	Liver—inactive metabolite
Excretion	Kidneys, breast milk
Half-life	2½ hr, increased in elderly

Pharmacodynamics

Unknown

Interactions
Individual drugs
Alcohol: ↑ CNS depression
Fluoxetine: ↑ action
Propoxyphene: ↑ action

Drug classifications
Antidepressants: ↑ CNS depression
Antihistamines: ↑ CNS depression
Opiates: ↑ CNS depression
Sedative/hypnotics: ↑ CNS depression
Food/drug
↓ absorption
Herb/drug
Kava: ↑ CNS depression
Lab test interferences
↑ ALT, ↑ AST, ↑ serum bilirubin
↓ RAI uptake
False: ↑ Urinary 17-OHCS

NURSING CONSIDERATIONS
Assessment
• Assess mental status: mood, sensorium, anxiety, affect, sleeping pattern, drowsiness, dizziness, especially elderly; physical dependency, withdrawal symptoms: anxiety, panic attacks, agitation, convulsions, headache, nausea, vomiting, muscle pain, weakness; suicidal tendencies; for indications of increasing tolerance and abuse
• Monitor B/P (lying, standing), pulse; if systolic B/P drops 20 mm Hg, hold drug, notify prescriber
• Monitor blood studies: CBC during long-term therapy; blood dycrasias have occurred rarely; decreased hematocrit, neutropenia may occur
• Monitor hepatic studies: AST, ALT, bilirubin, creatinine LDH, alk phosphatase
• Monitor I&O for renal dysfunction
Nursing diagnoses
☑ Anxiety (uses)
☑ Depression (uses)

☑ Injury, risk for (adverse reactions)

☑ Knowledge deficit (teaching)

Implementation

• Give ½-1 hr before hs for sleeplessness; give several hr before patient is to arise (to avoid hangover)

• Store in tight container in cool environment

Patient/family education

• Instruct patient that drug may be taken with food, or fluids and tab may be crushed or swallowed whole

• Caution patient not to use for everyday stress or longer than 3 mo unless directed by prescriber; not to take more than prescribed amount; may be habit forming; not to double or skip doses

• Caution patient to avoid OTC preparations unless approved by health care prescriber; alcohol and CNS depressants will increase CNS depression

• Advise patient to avoid driving, activities that require alertness, because drowsiness may occur; to avoid alcohol ingestion or other psychotropic medications; to rise slowly or fainting may occur, especially G elderly; that drowsiness may worsen at beginning of treatment

• Instruct patient not to discontinue medication abruptly after long-term use; withdrawal symptoms include vomiting, cramping, tremors, seizures

Evaluation

Positive therapeutic outcome

• Ability to sleep at night

• Decreased amount of early morning awakening if taking drug for insomnia

Treatment of overdose: Lavage, VS, supportive care

☒ Herb/drug ◎ Do Not Crush ◆ Alert ☞ Key Drug G Geriatric P Pediatric

ALPHA-ADRENERGIC BLOCKERS

Action: Binds to α-adrenergic receptors, causing dilatation of peripheral blood vessels; lowers peripheral resistance, resulting in decreased blood pressure.

Uses: Used for pheochromocytoma, prevention of tissue necrosis, and sloughing associated with extravasation of IV vasopressors.

Adverse effects: The most common side effects are hypotension, tachycardia, nasal stuffiness, nausea, vomiting, and diarrhea.

Contraindications: Hypersensitive reactions may occur, and allergies should be identified before these products are given. Patients with myocardial infarction, coronary insufficiency, angina, or other evidence of coronary artery disease should not use these products.

Pharmacokinetics: Onset, peak, and duration vary among products.

Interactions: Vasoconstrictive and hypertensive effects of epinephrine are antagonized by α-adrenergic blockers.

NURSING CONSIDERATIONS
Assessment
- Monitor electrolytes: potassium, sodium chloride, carbon dioxide
- Monitor weight daily, I&O
- Monitor B/P with patient lying, standing before starting treatment, q4h thereafter
- Assess for nausea, vomiting, diarrhea
- Assess for skin turgor, dryness of mucous membranes for hydration status

Nursing diagnoses
☑ Altered tissue perfusion (uses)
☑ Risk for injury (adverse reactions)
☑ Sleep pattern disturbance (adverse reactions)

Implementation
PO Route
- Start with low dose, gradually increasing to prevent side effects
- Give with food or milk for GI symptoms

Evaluation
- Therapeutic response: decreased B/P, increased peripheral pulses

Patient/family education
- Caution patient to avoid alcoholic beverages
- Advise patient to report dizziness, palpitations, fainting
- Instruct patient to change position slowly or fainting may occur

• Teach patient to take drug exactly as prescribed; to avoid all OTC products (cough, cold, allergy) unless directed by prescriber

---

Generic Names

phenoxybenzamine

phentolamine

ANESTHETICS—GENERAL/LOCAL

Action: Anesthetics (general) act on the CNS to produce tranquilization and sleep before invasive procedures. Anesthetics (local) inhibit conduction of nerve impulses from sensory nerves.

Uses: General anesthetics are used to premedicate for surgery, and for induction and maintenance in general anesthesia. For local anesthetics, refer to individual product listing for indications.

Adverse effects: The most common side effects are dystonia, akathisia, flexion of arms, fine tremors, drowsiness, restlessness, and hypotension. Also common are chills, respiratory depression, and laryngospasm.

Contraindications: Persons with CVA, increased intracranial pressure, severe hypertension, cardiac decompensation should not use these products, since severe adverse reactions can occur.

Precautions: Anesthetics (general) should be used with caution in the **G** elderly, cardiovascular disease (hypotension, bradydysrhythmias), renal **P** disease, liver disease, Parkinson's disease, children <2 yr. The precaution for anesthetics (local) is pregnancy.

Pharmacokinetics: Onset, peak, and duration vary widely among products. Most products are metabolized in the liver and excreted in urine.

Interactions: MAOIs, tricyclics, phenothiazines may cause severe hypotension or hypertension when used with local anesthetics. CNS depressants will potentiate general and local anesthetics.

NURSING CONSIDERATIONS
Assessment
• Monitor VS q10 min during **IV** administration, q30 min after IM dose

Nursing diagnoses
General
✓ Risk for injury (adverse reactions)
✓ Knowledge deficit (teaching)

Local

✓ Pain (uses)
✓ Knowledge deficit (teaching)

Implementation

- Give anticholinergic preoperatively to decrease secretions
- Administer only with crash cart, resuscitative equipment nearby
- Provide quiet environment for recovery to decrease psychotic symptoms

Evaluation

- Therapeutic response: maintenance of anesthesia, decreased pain

---

Generic Names

General anesthetics:
droperidol
etomidate
fentanyl citrate
   fentanyl citrate/droperidol
ketamine
methohexital
midazolam
procaine
thiopental

Local anesthetics:
🔑 lidocaine HCl
propofol
ropivacaine
tetracaine

ANTACIDS

Action: Antacids are basic compounds that neutralize gastric acidity and decrease the rate of gastric emptying. Products are divided into those containing aluminum, magnesium, calcium, or a combination of these.

Uses: Hyperacidity is decreased by antacids in conditions such as peptic ulcer disease, reflux esophagitis, gastritis, or hiatal hernia.

Adverse effects: The most common side effect caused by aluminum-containing antacids is constipation, which may lead to fecal impaction and bowel obstruction. Diarrhea occurs often when magnesium products are given. Alkalosis may occur when systemic products are used. Constipation occurs more frequently than laxation with calcium carbonate. The release of CO_2 from carbonate-containing antacids causes belching, abdominal distention, and flatulence. Sodium bicarbonate may act as a systemic antacid and produce systemic electrolyte disturbances and alkalosis. Calcium carbonate and sodium bicarbonate may cause rebound hyperacidity and milk-alkali syndrome. Alkaluria may occur when products are used on a long-term basis, particularly in persons with abnormal renal function.

Contraindications: Sensitivity to aluminum or magnesium products may cause hypersensitive reactions. Aluminum products should not be used by persons sensitive to aluminum; magnesium products should not be used by persons sensitive to magnesium. Check for sensitivity before administering.

Precautions: Magnesium products should be given cautiously to patients with renal insufficiency, during pregnancy, or lactation. Sodium content of antacids may be significant; use with caution for patients with hypertension, CHF, or those on a low-sodium diet.

Pharmacokinetics: Duration is 20-40 min. If ingested 1 hr pc, acidity is reduced for at least 3 hr.

Interactions: Drugs whose effects may be increased by some antacids: quinidine, amphetamines, pseudoephedrine, levodopa, valproic acid, dicumarol. Drugs whose effects may be decreased by some antacids: cimetidine, corticosteroids, ranitidine, iron salts, phenothiazines, phenytoin, digoxin, tetracyclines, ketoconazole, salicylates, isoniazid.

NURSING CONSIDERATIONS
Assessment
- Assess for aggravating and alleviating factors of epigastric pain or hyperacidity; identify the location, duration, and characteristics of epigastric pain
- Assess GI symptoms, including constipation, diarrhea, abdominal pain; if severe abdominal pain with fever occurs, these drugs should not be given
- Assess renal symptoms, including increasing urinary pH, electrolytes

Nursing diagnoses
☑ Pain (uses)
☑ Constipation (adverse reactions)
☑ Diarrhea (adverse reactions)

Implementation
- Give all products with an 8-oz glass of water to ensure absorption in the stomach
- Give another antacid if constipation occurs with aluminum products

Evaluation
- Therapeutic response: absence of epigastric pain, decreased acidity

Patient/family education

- Advise patient not to take other drugs within 1-2 hr of antacid administration, since antacids may impair absorption of other drugs

---

Generic Names

aluminum hydroxide
bismuth subsalicylate
calcium carbonate

magaldrate
magnesium oxide
sodium bicarbonate

ANTIANGINALS

Action: The antianginals are divided into the nitrates, calcium channel blockers, and β-adrenergic blockers. The nitrates dilate coronary arteries, causing decreased preload, and dilate systemic arteries, causing decreased afterload. Calcium channel blockers dilate coronary arteries, decrease SA/AV node conduction. β-Adrenergic blockers decrease heart rate so that myocardial O_2 use is decreased. Dipyridamole selectively dilates coronary arteries to increase coronary blood flow.

Uses: Antianginals are used in chronic stable angina pectoris, unstable angina, vasospastic angina. Some (i.e., calcium channel blockers and β-blockers) may be used as dysrhythmias and in hypertension.

Adverse effects: The most common side effects are postural hypotension, headache, flushing, dizziness, nausea, edema, and drowsiness. Also common are rash, dysrhythmias, and fatigue.

Contraindications: Persons with known hypersensitivity, increased intracranial pressure, or cerebral hemorrhage should not use some of these products.

Precautions: Antianginals should be used with caution in postural [P] hypotension, pregnancy, lactation, children, renal disease, and hepatic injury.

Pharmacokinetics: Onset, peak, and duration vary widely among coronary products. Most products are metabolized in the liver and excreted in urine.

Interactions: Please check individual monographs, since interactions vary widely among products.

NURSING CONSIDERATIONS
Assessment

- Orthostatic B/P, pulse
- Assess for pain: duration, time started, activity being performed, character

- Assess for tolerance if taken over long period
- Assess for headache, lightheadedness, decreased B/P; may indicate a need for decreased dosage

Nursing diagnoses
☑ Altered tissue perfusion: cardiopulmonary (uses)
☑ Pain (uses)
☑ Risk for injury (uses)
☑ Knowledge deficit (teaching)
☑ Decreased cardiac output (adverse reactions)

Implementation
- Store protected from light, moisture; place in cool environment

Evaluation
- Therapeutic response: decreased, prevention of anginal pain

Patient/family education
- Instruct patient to keep tabs in original container
- Instruct patient not to use OTC products unless directed by prescriber
- Advise patient to report bradycardia, dizziness, confusion, depression, fever
- Teach patient to take pulse at home; advise when to notify prescriber
- Advise patient to avoid alcohol, smoking, sodium intake
- Advise patient to comply with weight control, dietary adjustments, modified exercise program
- Teach patient to carry Medic Alert ID to identify drug being taken, allergies
- Caution patient to make position changes slowly to prevent fainting

---

Generic Names

Nitrates:
amyl nitrite
isosorbide
� nitroglycerin

β-adrenergic blockers:
atenolol
metoprolol
nadolol
propranolol

Calcium channel blockers:
amlodipine
bepridil
diltiazem
nicardipine
nifedipine
� verapamil

ANTICHOLINERGICS

Action: Anticholinergics inhibit the muscarinic actions of acetylcholine at receptor sites in the autonomic nervous system; anticholinergics are also known as antimuscarinic drugs.

Uses: Anticholinergics are used for a variety of conditions: gastrointestinal anticholinergics are used to decrease motility (smooth muscle tone) in the GI, biliary, and urinary tracts and for their ability to decrease gastric secretions (propantheline, glycopyrrolate); decreasing involuntary movements in parkinsonism (benztropine, trihexyphenidyl); bradydysrhythmias (atropine); nausea and vomiting (scopolamine); and as cycloplegic mydriatics (atropine, hematropine, scopalamine, cyclopentolate, tropicamide).

Adverse effects: The most common side effects are dry mouth, constipation, urinary retention, urinary hesitancy, headache, and dizziness. Also common is paralytic ileus.

Contraindications: Persons with narrow-angle glaucoma, myasthenia gravis, or GI/GU obstruction should not use some of these products.

Precautions: Anticholinergics should be used with caution in patients who are elderly, pregnant, or lactating or in those with prostatic hypertrophy, CHF, or hypertension; use with caution in presence of high environmental temp.

Pharmacokinetics: Onset, peak, and duration vary widely among products. Most products are metabolized in the liver and excreted in urine.

Interactions: Increased anticholinergic effects may occur when used with MAOIs and tricyclic antidepressants and amantadine. Anticholinergics may cause a decreased effect of phenothiazines and levodopa.

NURSING CONSIDERATIONS
Assessment
- Assess I&O ratio; retention commonly causes decreased urinary output
- Assess for urinary hesitancy, retention; palpate bladder if retention occurs
- Assess for constipation; increase fluids, bulk, exercise if this occurs
- Identify tolerance over long-term therapy; dosage may need to be increased or changed
- Assess mental status: affect, mood, CNS depression, worsening of mental symptoms during early therapy

Nursing diagnoses
☑ Decreased cardiac output (uses)
☑ Constipation (adverse reactions)
☑ Knowledge deficit (teaching)

Implementation
ⅣV IM/IV Routes
- Give parenteral dose with patient recumbent to prevent postural hypotension
- Give parenteral dose slowly; keep in bed for at least 1 hr after dose; monitor VS
- Give after checking dose carefully; even slight overdose could lead to toxicity

PO Route
- Give with or after meals to prevent GI upset; may give with fluids other than water
- Store at room temp
- Give hard candy, frequent drinks, sugarless gum to relieve dry mouth

Evaluation
- Therapeutic response: decreased secretions, absence of nausea and vomiting

Patient/family education
- Caution patient to avoid driving and other hazardous activities; drowsiness may occur
- Advise patient to avoid OTC medication: cough, cold preparations with alcohol, antihistamines unless directed by prescriber

---

Generic Names

⌀π atropine	propantheline
⌀π benztropine	scopolamine
biperiden	scopolamine (transdermal)
cyclopentolate (Appx C)	trihexyphenidyl
glycopyrrolate	tropicamide (Appx C)
homatropine (Appx C)	

ANTICOAGULANTS

Action: Anticoagulants interfere with blood clotting by preventing clot formation.

Uses: Anticoagulants are used for deep vein thrombosis, pulmonary emboli, myocardial infarction, open heart surgery, disseminated intravascular clotting syndrome, atrial fibrillation with embolization, and in transfusion and dialysis.

Adverse effects: The most serious adverse reactions are hemorrhage, agranulocytosis, leukopenia, eosinophilia, and thrombocytopenia, depending on the specific product. The most common side effects are diarrhea, rash, and fever.

Contraindications: Persons with hemophilia, leukemia with bleeding, peptic ulcer disease, thrombocytopenic purpura, blood dyscrasias, acute nephritis, and subacute bacterial endocarditis should not use these products.

Precautions: Anticoagulants should be used with caution in alcoholism, elderly, and pregnancy.

Pharmacokinetics: Onset, peak, and duration vary widely among products. Most products are metabolized in the liver and excreted in urine.

Interactions: Salicylates, steroids, and nonsteroidal antiinflammatories will potentiate the action of anticoagulants. Anticoagulants may cause serious effects; please check individual monographs.

NURSING CONSIDERATIONS
Assessment
- Monitor blood studies (Hct, platelets, occult blood in stools) q3 mo
- Monitor partial prothrombin time, which should be 1½-2 × control, PPT; often qd, APTT, ACT, INR
- Monitor B/P; watch for increasing signs of hypertension
- Monitor for bleeding gums, petechiae, ecchymosis, black tarry stools, hematuria
- Monitor for fever, skin rash, urticaria
- Monitor for needed dosage change q1-2wk

Nursing diagnoses
- ✓ Altered tissue perfusion (uses)
- ✓ Risk for injury (side effects)
- ✓ Knowledge deficit (teaching)

Implementation
SC Route
- Give at same time each day to maintain steady blood levels
- Do not massage area or aspirate when giving SC inj; give in abdomen between pelvic bones; rotate sites; do not pull back on plunger, leave in for 10 sec; apply gentle pressure for 1 min
- Do not change needles
- Avoid all IM inj that may cause bleeding
- Store in tight container (PO dose)

Evaluation
• Therapeutic response: decrease of deep vein thrombosis

Patient/family education
• Advise patient to avoid OTC preparations that may cause serious drug interactions unless directed by prescriber
• Inform patient that drug may be held during active bleeding (menstruation), depending on condition
• Caution patient to use soft-bristle toothbrush to avoid bleeding gums; avoid contact sports; use electric razor
• Instruct patient to carry a Medic-Alert ID identifying drug taken
• Instruct patient to report any signs of bleeding: gums, under skin, urine, stools

---

Generic Names

ardeparin (Appx E)
dalteparin
danaparoid
enoxaparin

🔑 heparin
lepirudin
🔑 warfarin

ANTICONVULSANTS

Action: Anticonvulsants are divided into the barbiturates (p. 1298), benzodiazepines (p. 1299), hydantoins, succinimides, and miscellaneous products. Barbiturates and benzodiazepines are discussed in separate sections. Hydantoins act by inhibiting the spread of seizure activity in the motor cortex. Succinimides act by inhibiting spike and wave formation; they also decrease amplitude, frequency, duration, and spread of discharge in seizures.

Uses: Hydantoins are used in generalized tonic-clonic seizures, status epilepticus, and psychomotor seizures. Succinimides are used for absence of (petit mal) seizures. Barbiturates are used in generalized tonic-clonic and cortical focal seizures.

Adverse effects: Bone marrow depression is the most life-threatening adverse reaction associated with hydantoins or succinimides. The most common side effects are GI symptoms. Other common side effects for hydantoins are gingival hyperplasia and CNS effects such as nystagmus, ataxia, slurred speech, and confusion.

Contraindications: Hypersensitive reactions may occur, and allergies should be identified before these products are given.

Precautions: Persons with renal or hepatic disease should be watched closely.

Pharmacokinetics: Onset, peak, and duration vary widely among products. Most products are metabolized in the liver and excreted in urine, bile, and feces.

Interactions: Decreased effects of estrogens, oral contraceptives (hydantoins).

NURSING CONSIDERATIONS
Assessment
- Monitor renal function studies, including BUN, creatinine, serum uric acid, urine creatinine clearance before and during therapy
- Monitor blood studies: RBC, Hct, Hgb, reticulocyte counts weekly for 4 wk then monthly
- Monitor hepatic studies: AST, ALT, bilirubin, creatinine
- Assess mental status, including mood, sensorium, affect, behavioral changes; if mental status changes, notify prescriber
- Assess for eye problems, including need for ophth examinations before, during, and after treatment (slit lamp, fundoscopy, tonometry)
- Assess for allergic reaction, including red raised rash; if this occurs, drug should be discontinued
- Assess for blood dyscrasias, including fever, sore throat, bruising, rash, jaundice
- Monitor toxicity, including bone marrow depression, nausea, vomiting, ataxia, diplopia, cardiovascular collapse, Stevens-Johnson syndrome

Nursing diagnoses
☑Risk for injury (uses)
☑Noncompliance (teaching)
☑Sleep pattern disturbance (adverse reactions)

Implementation
PO Route
- Give with food, milk to decrease GI symptoms
- Good oral hygiene is important for patients taking hydantoins

Evaluation
- Therapeutic response, including decreased seizure activity; document on patient's chart

Patient/family education
- Advise patient to carry ID card or Medic Alert bracelet stating drugs taken, condition, prescriber's name, phone number
- Advise patient to avoid driving, other activities that require alertness

Generic Names

Hydantoins:
fosphenytoin
⊙ᴨ phenytoin

Succinimides:
ethosuximide

Miscellaneous:
acetazolamide
carbamazepine
clonazepam
⊙ᴨ diazepam
felbamate
gabapentin

lamotrigine
magnesium sulfate
tiagabine
topiramate
valproate/valproic acid/
　　divalproex sodium

Barbiturates:
amobarbital
⊙ᴨ phenobarbital
primidone
thiopental

ANTIDEPRESSANTS

Action: Antidepressants are divided into the tricyclics, MAOIs, and miscellaneous antidepressants. The tricyclics work by blocking re-uptake of norepinephrine and serotonin into nerve endings and increasing action of norepinephrine and serotonin in nerve cells. MAOIs act by increasing concentrations of endogenous epinephrine, norepinephrine, serotonin, dopamine in storage sites in CNS by inhibition of MAO; increased concentration reduces depression.

Uses: Antidepressants are used for depression and in some cases 🅿 enuresis in children.

Adverse effects: The most serious adverse reactions are paralytic ileus, acute renal failure, hypertension, and hypertensive crisis, depending on the specific product. Common side effects are dizziness, drowsiness, diarrhea, dry mouth, urinary retention, and orthostatic hypotension.

Contraindications: The contraindications for antidepressants are convulsive disorders, prostatic hypertrophy, severe renal, hepatic, cardiac disease depending on the type of medication.

Precautions: Antidepressants should be used cautiously in suicidal patients, severe depression, schizophrenia, hyperactivity, diabetes mel-🅖 litus, pregnancy, and the elderly.

Pharmacokinetics: Onset, peak, and duration vary widely among products. Most products are metabolized in the liver and excreted in urine.

Interactions: Please check individual monographs, since interactions vary widely among products.

NURSING CONSIDERATIONS
Assessment

- Monitor B/P (lying, standing), pulse q4h; if systolic B/P drops 20 mm Hg, hold drug, notify prescriber; take VS q4h in patients with cardiovascular disease
- Monitor blood studies: CBC, leukocytes, differential, cardiac enzymes if patient is receiving long-term therapy
- Monitor hepatic studies: AST, ALT, bilirubin, creatinine
- Monitor weight weekly; appetite may increase with drug
- **G** Monitor for EPS primarily in elderly: rigidity, dystonia, akathisia
- Assess mental status: mood, sensorium, affect, suicidal tendencies, increase in psychiatric symptoms (depression, panic)
- **P** Check for urinary retention, constipation; constipation is more
- **G** likely to occur in children, elderly
- Assess for withdrawal symptoms: headache, nausea, vomiting, muscle pain, weakness; do not usually occur unless drug was discontinued abruptly
- Identify alcohol consumption; if alcohol is consumed, hold dose until AM

Nursing diagnoses
- ✓ Ineffective individual coping (uses)
- ✓ Risk for injury (uses/adverse reactions)
- ✓ Knowledge deficit (teaching)

Implementation
PO Route
- Give increased fluids, bulk in diet if constipation, urinary retention occur
- Give with food or milk for GI symptoms
- Give gum, hard candy, or frequent sips of water for dry mouth
- Store in tight container at room temp; do not refreeze
- Provide assistance with ambulation during beginning therapy, since drowsiness/dizziness occurs

Evaluation
- Therapeutic response: decreased depression

Patient/family education
- Teach patient that therapeutic effects may take 2-3 wk
- Advise patient to use caution in driving or other activities requiring alertness because of drowsiness, dizziness, blurred vision
- Caution patient to avoid alcohol ingestion, other CNS depressants
- Instruct patient not to discontinue medication quickly after long-term use; may cause nausea, headache, malaise

• Instruct patient to wear sunscreen or large hat, since photosensitivity may occur

---

Generic Names

Tetracyclic:
mirtazapine

Tricyclics:
amitriptyline
amoxapine
clomipramine
desipramine
doxepin
⚷ imipramine
nortriptyline
protriptyline
trimipramine

Miscellaneous:
bupropion

maprotiline
nefazodone
trazodone
venlafaxine

MAOIs:
phenelzine
tranylcypromine

SSRIs
citalopram
fluoxetine
paroxetine
sertraline

ANTIDIABETICS

Action: Antidiabetics are divided into the insulins that decrease blood sugar, phosphate, and potassium and increase blood pyruvate and lactate; and oral antidiabetics that cause functioning β-cells in the pancreas to release insulin, improves the effect of endogenous and exogenous insulin.

Uses: Insulins are used for ketoacidosis and diabetes mellitus types I (IDDM) and II (NIDDM); oral antidiabetics are used for stable adult-onset diabetes mellitus type II (NIDDM).

Adverse effects: The most common side effect of insulin and oral antidiabetics is hypoglycemia. Other adverse reactions for oral antidiabetics include blood dyscrasias, hepatotoxicity, and, rarely, cholestatic jaundice. Adverse reactions for insulin products include allergic responses and, more rarely, anaphylaxis.

Contraindications: Hypersensitive reactions may occur, and allergies should be identified before these products are given. Oral antidiabetics should not be used in juvenile or brittle diabetes, diabetic ketoacidosis, severe renal disease, or severe hepatic disease.

Precautions: Oral antidiabetics should be used with caution in the
G elderly, in cardiac disease, pregnancy, lactation, and in the presence of
alcohol.

Pharmacokinetics: Onset, peak, and duration vary widely among
products. Oral antidiabetics are metabolized in the liver, with metabolites excreted in urine, bile, and feces.

Interactions: Interactions vary widely among products. Check individual monograph for specific information.

NURSING CONSIDERATIONS
Assessment
- Monitor blood, urine glucose levels during treatment to determine
  diabetes control (oral products)
- Monitor fasting blood glucose, 2 hr PP (60-100 mg/dl normal
  fasting level) (70-130 mg/dl—normal 2-hr level)
- Assess for hypoglycemic reaction that can occur during peak time

Nursing diagnoses
☑ Altered nutrition: more than body requirements (uses)

Implementation
SC Route
- Give insulin after warming to room temp by rotating in palms to
  prevent lipodystrophy from injecting cold insulin
- Give human insulin to those allergic to beef or pork
- Rotate inj sites when giving insulin; use abdomen, upper back,
  thighs, upper arm, buttocks; keep a record of sites
PO Route
- Give oral antidiabetic 30 min ac

Evaluation
- Therapeutic response, including decrease in polyuria, polydipsia,
  polyphagia, clear sensorium, absence of dizziness, stable gait

Patient/family education
- Advise patient to avoid alcohol and salicylates except on advice of
  prescriber
- Teach patient symptoms of ketoacidosis: nausea, thirst, polyuria,
  dry mouth, decreased B/P, dry, flushed skin, acetone breath,
  drowsiness, Kussmaul respirations
- Teach patient symptoms of hypoglycemia: headache, tremors,
  fatigue, weakness; and that candy or sugar should be carried to
  treat hypoglycemia
- Advise patient to test urine for glucose/ketones tid if this drug is
  replacing insulin

• Advise patient to continue weight control, dietary restrictions, exercise, hygiene

---

Generic Names

acetohexamide	insulin, zinc suspension (Lente)
chlorpropamide	metformin
glipizide	miglitol
glyburide	pioglitazone
Oπ insulin, isophane suspension	repaglinide
insulin, lispro	rosiglitazone
Oπ insulin, regular	tolazamide
Oπ insulin, regular concentrated	tolbutamide
insulin, zinc suspension (Ultralente)	

ANTIDIARRHEALS

Action: Antidiarrheals work by various actions including direct action on intestinal muscles to decrease GI peristalsis; or by inhibiting prostaglandin synthesis responsible for GI hypermotility; acting on mucosal receptors responsible for peristalsis; or decreasing water content of stools.

Uses: Antidiarrheals are used for diarrhea of undetermined causes.

Adverse effects: The most serious adverse reactions of some products are paralytic ileus, toxic megacolon, and angioneurotic edema. The most common side effects are constipation, nausea, dry mouth, and abdominal pain.

Contraindications: Persons with severe ulcerative colitis, pseudo-membranous colitis with some products.

G
P **Precautions:** Antidiarrheal should be used with caution in the elderly, pregnancy, lactation, children, dehydration.

Pharmacokinetics: Onset, peak, and duration vary widely among products. Most products are metabolized in the liver and excreted in urine.

Interactions: Please check individual monographs, since interactions vary widely among products.

NURSING CONSIDERATIONS
Assessment

• Monitor electrolytes (potassium, sodium, chloride) if on long-term therapy

- Monitor bowel pattern before; for rebound constipation after termination of medication
- Assess response after 48 hr; if no response, drug should be discontinued
P• Identify dehydration in children

Nursing diagnoses
✓Diarrhea (uses)
✓Constipation (adverse reactions)
✓Fluid volume deficit (adverse reactions)
✓Knowledge deficit (teaching)

Implementation
PO Route
- Give for 48 hr only

Evaluation
- Therapeutic response: decreased diarrhea

Patient/family education
- Advise patient to avoid OTC products
- Caution patient not to exceed recommended dose

Generic Names
bismuth subsalicylate
difenoxin

kaolin/pectin
loperamide

ANTIDYSRHYTHMICS

Action: Antidysrhythmics are divided into four classes and miscellaneous antidysrhythmics:
- Class I increases the action potential duration and the effective refractory period and reduces disparity in the refractory period between a normal and infarcted myocardium; further subclasses include Ia, Ib, Ic
- Class II decreases the rate of SA node discharge, increases recovery time, slows conduction through the AV node, and decreases heart rate, which decreases O_2 consumption in the myocardium
- Class III increases the action potential duration and the effective refractory period
- Class IV inhibits calcium ion influx across the cell membrane during cardiac depolarization; decreases SA node discharge, decreases conduction velocity through the AV node

- Miscellaneous antidysrhythmics include those such as adenosine, which slows conduction through the AV node, and digoxin, which decreases conduction velocity and prolongs the effective refractory period in the AV node

Uses: These products are used for PVCs, tachycardia, hypertension, atrial fibrillation, angina pectoris.

Adverse effects: Side effects and adverse reactions vary widely among products.

Contraindications: Contraindications vary widely among products.

Precautions: Precautions vary widely among products.

Pharmacokinetics: Onset, peak, and duration vary widely among products.

Interactions: Interactions vary widely among products; check individual monograph for specific information.

NURSING CONSIDERATIONS
Assessment
- Monitor ECG continuously to determine drug effectiveness, PVCs, or other dysrhythmias
- Assess for dehydration or hypovolemia
- Monitor B/P continuously for hypotension, hypertension
- Monitor I&O ratio
- Monitor serum potassium
- Assess for edema in feet and legs daily

Nursing diagnoses
- ☑ Altered tissue perfusion: cardiopulmonary (uses)
- ☑ Decreased cardiac output (uses)
- ☑ Diarrhea (adverse reactions)
- ☑ Impaired gas exchange (adverse reactions)

Evaluation
- Therapeutic response, including decrease in B/P in hypertension, decreased B/P, edema, moist rales in CHF

Patient/family education
- Advise patient to comply with dosage schedule, even if patient is feeling better
- Instruct patient to report bradycardia, dizziness, confusion, depression, fever

Generic Names

Class I:
moricizine

Class Ia:
disopyramide
Ⓞ▣ procainamide
Ⓞ▣ quinidine

Class Ib:
lidocaine
mexiletine
Ⓞ▣ phenytoin
tocainide

Class Ic:
flecainide
indecainide

Class II:
acebutolol
esmolol
Ⓞ▣ propranolol
sotalol

Class III:
amiodarone
Ⓞ▣ bretylium
ibutilide

Class IV:
Ⓞ▣ verapamil

Miscellaneous:
adenosine
atropine
Ⓞ▣ digoxin

ANTIFUNGALS (SYSTEMIC)

Action: Antifungals act by increasing cell membrane permeability in susceptible organisms by binding sterols and decreasing potassium, sodium, and nutrients in the cell.

Uses: Antifungals are used for infections of histoplasmosis, blastomycosis, coccidioidomycosis, cryptococcosis, aspergillosis, phycomycosis, candidiasis, sporotrichosis causing severe meningitis, septicemia, and skin infections.

Adverse effects: The most serious adverse reactions include renal tubular acidosis, permanent renal impairment, anuria, oliguria, hemorrhagic gastroenteritis, acute liver failure, and blood dyscrasias. Some common side effects include hypokalemia, nausea, vomiting, anorexia, headache, fever, and chills.

Contraindications: Persons with severe bone depression or hypersensitivity should not use these products.

Precautions: Antifungals should be used with caution in renal disease, pregnancy, and hepatic disease.

Pharmacokinetics: Onset, peak, and duration vary widely among products. Most products are metabolized in the liver and excreted in urine.

Interactions: Please check individual monographs, since interactions vary widely among products.

NURSING CONSIDERATIONS
Assessment
- Monitor VS q15-30 min during first inf; note changes in pulse, B/P
- Monitor I&O ratio; watch for decreasing urinary output, change in sp gr; discontinue drug to prevent permanent damage to renal tubules
- Monitor blood studies; CBC, potassium, sodium, calcium, magnesium q2 wk
- Monitor weight weekly; if weight increases over 2 lb/wk, edema is present; renal damage should be considered
- Assess for renal toxicity: increasing BUN, is >40 mg/dl or if serum creatinine >3 mg/dl; drug may be discontinued or dosage reduced
- Assess for hepatotoxicity: increasing AST, ALT, alkaline phosphatase, bilirubin
- Assess for allergic reaction: dermatitis, rash; drug should be discontinued; antihistamines (mild reaction) or epinephrine (severe reaction) administered
- Assess for hypokalemia: anorexia, drowsiness, weakness, decreased reflexes, dizziness, increased urinary output, increased thirst, paresthesias
- Assess for ototoxicity: tinnitus (ringing, roaring in ears), vertigo, loss of hearing (rare)

Nursing diagnoses
☑Risk for infection (uses)
☑Risk for injury (adverse reactions)
☑Knowledge deficit (teaching)

Implementation
IV **IV Route**
- Give by **IV** using in-line filter (mean pore diameter >1 μm) using distal veins; check for extravasation, necrosis q8h
- Give drug only after C&S confirms organism, drug needed to treat condition; make sure drug is used in life-threatening infections
- Provide protection from light during inf; cover with foil
- Give symptomatic treatment as ordered for adverse reactions: aspirin, antihistamines, antiemetics, antispasmodics
- Store protected from moisture and light; diluted sol is stable for 24 hr

Evaluation
- Therapeutic response: decreased fever, malaise, rash, negative C&S for infecting organism

Patient/family education
- Teach patient that long-term therapy may be needed to clear infection (2 wk-3 mo depending on type of infection)

Generic Names

Om amphotericin B
fluconazole
flucytosine
griseofulvin

itraconazole
ketoconazole
Om miconazole
nystatin

ANTIHISTAMINES

Action: Antihistamines compete with histamines for H_1 receptor sites. They antagonize in varying degrees most of the pharmacologic effects of histamines.

Uses: Products are used to control the symptoms of allergies, rhinitis, and pruritus.

Adverse effects: Most products cause drowsiness; however, two of the newer products, loratadine and fexofenadine, produce little, if any, drowsiness. Other common side effects are headache and thickening of bronchial secretions. Serious blood dyscrasias may occur, but are rare. Urinary retention, GI effects occur with many of these products.

Contraindications: Hypersensitivity to H_1-receptor antagonists occurs rarely. Patients with acute asthma and lower respiratory tract disease should not use these products, since thick secretions may result. Other contraindications include narrow-angle glaucoma, bladder neck obstruction, stenosing peptic ulcer, symptomatic prostatic hypertrophy, newborn, lactation.

Precautions: These products must be used cautiously in conjunction with intraocular pressure, since they increase intraocular pressure. Caution should also be used in patients with renal and cardiac disease, hypertension, and seizure disorders, pregnancy, lactation and in the elderly.

Pharmacokinetics: Onset varies from 20-60 min, with duration lasting 4-12 hr. In general, pharmacokinetics vary widely among products.

Interactions: Barbiturates, narcotics, hypnotics, tricyclic antidepressants, and alcohol can increase CNS depression when taken with antihistamines.

NURSING CONSIDERATIONS
Assessment
- Check I&O ratio; be alert for urinary retention, frequency, dysuria; drug should be discontinued if these occur
- Assess for blood dyscrasias: thrombocytopenia, agranulocytosis (rare)
- Assess for respiratory status, including rate rhythm, increase in bronchial secretions, wheezing, chest tightness
- Assess for cardiac status, including palpitations, increased pulse, hypotension
- Assess CBC during long-term therapy, since hemolytic anemia, although rare, may occur
- Administer with food or milk to decrease GI symptoms; absorption may be decreased slightly
- ⊘ Administer whole (sustained-release tab)
- Provide hard candy, gum, frequent rinsing of mouth for dryness

Nursing diagnoses
✓ Ineffective airway clearance (uses)

Evaluation
- Therapeutic response: absence of allergy symptoms, itching

Patient/family education
- Advise patient to notify prescriber if confusion, sedation, hypotension occur
- Caution patient to avoid driving and other hazardous activity if drowsiness occurs
- Instruct patient to avoid concurrent use of alcohol and other CNS depressants
- Inform patient to discontinue a few days before skin testing

---

Generic Names

azatadine
brompheniramine
cetirizine
chlorpheniramine
clemastine
cyproheptadine

🔑 diphenhydramine
fexofenadine
loratadine
promethazine
triprolidine

ANTIHYPERTENSIVES

Action: Antihypertensives are divided into angiotensin converting enzyme (ACE) inhibitors, β-adrenergic blockers, calcium channel blockers, centrally acting adrenergics, diuretics, peripherally acting antiadrenergics, and vasodilators. β-Blockers, calcium channel blockers, and diuretics are discussed in separate sections. ACE inhibitors selectively suppress conversion of renin-angiotensin I to angiotensin II; dilatation of arterial and venous vessels occurs. Centrally acting adrenergics act by inhibiting the sympathetic vasomotor center in the CNS, which reduces impulses in the sympathetic nervous system; blood pressure, pulse rate, and cardiac output decrease. Peripherally acting antiadrenergics inhibit sympathetic vasoconstriction by inhibiting release of norepinephrine and/or depleting norepinephrine stores in adrenergic nerve endings. Vasodilators act on arteriolar smooth muscle by producing direct relaxation or vasodilatation; a reduction in blood pressure, with concomitant increases in heart rate and cardiac output, occurs.

Uses: Used for hypertension and for heart failure not responsive to conventional therapy. Some products are used in hypertensive crisis, angina, and for some cardiac dysrhythmias.

Adverse effects: The most common side effects are marked hypotension, bradycardia, tachycardia, headache, nausea, and vomiting. Side effects and adverse reactions may vary widely between classes and specific products.

Contraindications: Hypersensitive reactions may occur, and allergies should be identified before these products are given. Antihypertensives **P** should not be used in patients with heart block or in children.

Precautions: Antihypertensives should be used with caution in the **G** elderly, in dialysis patients, and in the presence of hypovolemia, leukemia, and electrolyte imbalances.

Pharmacokinetics: Onset, peak, and duration vary widely among products. Most products are metabolized in the liver, with metabolites excreted in urine, bile, and feces.

Interactions: Interactions vary widely among products; check individual monograph for specific information.

NURSING CONSIDERATIONS
Assessment
- Monitor blood studies: neutrophil; decreased platelets occur with many of the products
- Monitor renal studies: protein, BUN, creatinine; watch for increased levels, which may indicate nephrotic syndrome; obtain baselines in renal and liver function studies before beginning treatment
- Assess for edema in feet and legs daily
- Identify allergic reaction, including rash, fever, pruritus, urticaria: drug should be discontinued if antihistamines fail to help
- Identify symptoms of CHF: edema, dyspnea, wet rales, B/P
- Assess for renal symptoms: polyuria, oliguria, frequency

Nursing diagnoses
☑ Altered tissue perfusion (uses)
☑ Decreased cardiac output (uses)
☑ Diarrhea (adverse reactions)
☑ Impaired gas exchange (adverse reactions)

Implementation
- Place patient in supine or Trendelenburg position for severe hypotension

Evaluation
- Therapeutic response: decrease in B/P in hypotension; decreased B/P, edema, moist rales in CHF

Patient/family education
- Instruct patient to comply with dosage schedule, even if feeling better
- Advise patient to rise slowly to sitting or standing position to minimize orthostatic hypotension

---

Generic Names

ACE inhibitors:
benazepril
captopril
enalapril
esoprostenol
fosinopril
lisinopril
quinapril
ramipril
spirapril
trandolapril

Angiotension II receptors
candesartan
irbesartan
losartan
telmisartan
valsartan

Centrally acting adrenergics:
⚷ clonidine
guanabenz

guanfacine
methyldopa

Peripherally acting antiadrenergics:
doxazosin
guanadrel
guanethidine
⚷ prazosin
reserpine
terazosin

Vasodilators:
diazoxide
fenoldopam
hydralazine
minoxidil
nitroprusside

Antidrenergic:
Combined α-/β-blocker:
    labetalol

ANTIINFECTIVES

Action: Antiinfectives are divided into several groups, which include but are not limited to penicillins, cephalosporins, aminoglycosides, sulfonamides, tetracyclines, monobactam, erythromycins, and quinolones. These drugs inhibit the growth and replication of susceptible bacterial organisms.

Uses: Used for infections of susceptible organisms. These products are effective against bacterial, rickettsial, and spirochete infections.

Adverse effects: The most common side effects are nausea, vomiting, and diarrhea. Adverse reactions include bone marrow depression and anaphylaxis.

Contraindications: Hypersensitive reactions may occur, and allergies should be identified before these products are given. Cross-sensitivity can occur between products of different classes (penicillins or cephalosporins). Often persons allergic to penicillins are also allergic to cephalosporins.

Precautions: Antiinfectives should be used with caution in persons with renal and liver disease.

Pharmacokinetics: Onset, peak, and duration vary widely among products. Most products are metabolized in the liver, and metabolites are excreted in urine, bile, and feces.

Interactions: Interactions vary widely among products; check individual monograph for specific information.

NURSING CONSIDERATIONS
Assessment
- Assess for nephrotoxicity, including increased BUN, creatinine
- Monitor blood studies: AST, ALT, CBC, Hct, bilirubin; test monthly if patient is on long-term therapy
- Monitor bowel pattern qd; if severe diarrhea occurs, drug should be discontinued
- Monitor urine output; if decreasing, notify prescriber; may indicate nephrotoxicity
- Assess for allergic reaction, including rash, fever, pruritus, urticaria; drug should be discontinued
- Assess for bleeding: ecchymosis, bleeding gums, hematuria, stool guaiac daily
- Assess for overgrowth of infection: perineal itching, fever, malaise, redness, pain, swelling, drainage, rash, diarrhea, change in cough, sputum

Nursing diagnoses

✓ Risk for infection (uses)
✓ Diarrhea (adverse reactions)

Implementation

* Give for 10-14 days to ensure organism death, prevention of superinfection
* Give after C&S completed; drug may be taken as soon as culture is obtained

Evaluation

* Therapeutic response: absence of fever, fatigue, malaise, draining wounds

Patient/family education

* Teach patient to comply with dosage schedule, even if feeling better
* Advise patient to report sore throat, bruising, bleeding, joint pain; may indicate blood dyscrasias (rare)

Generic Names

Aminoglycosides:
amikacin
gentamicin
kanamycin
neomycin
netilmicin
streptomycin
tobramycin

Cephalosporins:
cefaclor
cefadroxil
cefamandole
cefazolin
cefdinir
cefepime
cefixime
cefmetazole
cefonicid
cefoperazone
ceforanide
cefotaxime

cefprozil
ceftibuten
cefuroximine ·
⚿ cephalexin
cephalothin
cephapirin
cephradine
moxalactam

Fluoroquinolones:
alatrofloxacin
ciprofloxacin
levofloxacin
lomefloxacin
norfloxacin
ofloxacin
sparfloxacin
trovafloxacin

Macrolides:
azithromycin
clarithromycin
erythromycin

Misc:
meropenem

Penicillins:
amoxicillin/clavulanate
ampicillin/sulbactam
cloxacillin
dicloxacillin
imipenem/cilastatin
methicillin
mezlocillin
nafcillin
oxacillin
penicillin G benzathine

penicillin G potassium
penicillin G procaine
⚷π penicillin G sodium
penicillin V
piperacillin
ticarcillin/clavulanate

Sulfonamides:
sulfasalazine
sulfisoxazole

Tetracyclines:
doxycycline
minocycline
tetracycline

ANTINEOPLASTICS

Action: Antineoplastics are divided into alkylating agents, antimetabolites, antibiotic agents, hormonal agents, and miscellaneous agents. Alkylating agents act by cross-linking strands of DNA. Antimetabolites act by inhibiting DNA synthesis. Antibiotic agents act by inhibiting RNA synthesis and by delaying or inhibiting mitosis. Hormones alter the effect of androgens, luteinizing hormone, follicle-stimulating hormone, or estrogen by changing the hormonal environment.

Uses: Uses vary widely among products and classes of drugs. They are used to treat leukemia, Hodgkin's disease, lymphomas, and other tumors throughout the body.

Adverse effects: Most products cause thrombocytopenia, leukopenia, and anemia, and, if these reactions occur, the drug may need to be stopped until the problem is corrected. Other side effects include nausea, vomiting, glossitis, and hair loss. Some products also cause hepatotoxicity, nephrotoxicity, and cardiotoxicity.

Contraindications: Hypersensitive reactions may occur, and allergies should be identified before these products are given. Also, persons with severe liver and kidney disease should not use these products unless the benefits outweigh the risks.

Precautions: Persons with bleeding, severe bone marrow depression, or renal or hepatic disease should be watched closely.

Pharmacokinetics: Onset, peak, and duration vary widely among products. Most products cross the placenta and are excreted in breast milk and in urine.

Interactions: Toxicity may occur when used with other antineoplastics or radiation.

NURSING CONSIDERATIONS
Assessment
- Monitor CBC, differential, platelet count weekly; withhold drug if WBC is <4000 or platelet count is <75,000; notify prescriber of results
- Monitor renal function studies, including BUN, creatinine, serum uric acid, and urine creatinine clearance before and during therapy
- Monitor I&O ratio; report fall in urine output of 30 ml/hr
- Monitor temp q4h (may indicate beginning infection)
- Monitor liver function tests before and during therapy (bilirubin, AST, ALT, LDH) prn or monthly
- Assess for bleeding, including hematuria, guaiac, bruising or petechiae, mucosa, or orifices q8h; obtain prescription for viscous lidocaine (Xylocaine)
- Identify jaundice of skin, sclera, dark urine, clay-colored stools, itchy skin, abdominal pain, fever, diarrhea
- Assess for edema in feet, joint pain, stomach pain, shaking
- Assess for inflammation of mucosa, breaks in skin

Nursing diagnoses
- ✓Risk for infection (adverse reactions)
- ✓Altered nutrition: less than body requirements (adverse reactions)
- ✓Altered oral mucous membrane (adverse reactions)

Implementation
- Check **IV** site for irritation; phlebitis
- Have epinephrine available for hypersensitivity reaction
- Give antibiotics for prophylaxis of infection
- Provide strict medical asepsis, protective isolation if WBC levels are low
- Provide comprehensive oral hygiene, using careful technique and soft-bristle brush

Evaluation
- Therapeutic response: decreased tumor size

Patient/family education
- Advise patient to report signs of infection, including increased temp, sore throat, malaise
- Instruct patient to report signs of anemia, including fatigue, headache, faintness, shortness of breath, irritability
- Instruct patient to report bleeding and to avoid use of razors and commercial mouthwash

Generic Names

Alkylating agents:
busulfan
carboplatin
carmustine
chlorambucil
cisplatin
⚷ cyclophosphamide
dacarbazine
lomustine
mechlorethamine
melphalan
streptozocin
thiotepa

Antimetabolites:
capecitabine
cytarabine
⚷ doxorubicin
etoposide
fludarabine
fluorouracil
mercaptopurine
thioguanine (6-TG)

Antibiotic agents:
⚷ bleomycin
dactinomycin
daunorubicin
epirubicin
⚷ methotrexate
mitomycin
mitoxantrone
plicamycin

Hormonal agents:
aminoglutethimide
estramustine
flutamide
goserelin acetate
irinotecan
leuprolide
megestrol
mitotane
nilutamide
tamoxifen
testolactone
topotecan

Miscellaneous agents:
altretamine
anastrozole
asparaginase
cladribine
gemcitabine
interferon alfa-2A,
    interferon alfa-2B
irinotecan
pentostatin
porfimer
procarbazine
rituximab
vinblastine
⚷ vincristine

ANTIPARKINSONIAN AGENTS

Action: Antiparkinsonian agents are divided into cholinergics and dopamine agonists. Cholinergics work by the blocking or competing at central acetylcholine receptors; dopamine agonists work by decarboxylation to dopamine or by activation of dopamine receptors; monoamine oxidase type B inhibitors increase dopamine activity by inhibiting MAO type B activity.

Uses: These agents are used alone or in combination for patients with Parkinson's disease.

Adverse effects: Side effects and adverse reactions vary widely among products. The most common side effects include involuntary movements, headache, numbness, insomnia, nightmares, nausea, vomiting, dry mouth, and orthostatic hypotension.

Contraindications: Persons with hypersensitivity, narrow-angle laucoma, and undiagnosed skin lesions should not use these products.

Precautions: Antiparkinsonian agents should be used with caution in pregnancy, lactation, children, renal, cardiac, hepatic disease, and affective disorder.

Pharmacokinetics: Onset, peak, and duration vary widely among products. Most products are metabolized in the liver and excreted in urine.

Interactions: Please check individual monographs, since interactions vary widely among products.

NURSING CONSIDERATIONS
Assessment
- Monitor B/P, respiration
- Assess mental status: affect, behavioral changes, depression, complete suicide assessment

Nursing diagnoses
- Risk for injury (uses)
- Risk for impaired mobility (uses)
- Knowledge deficit (teaching)

Implementation
- Give drug up until NPO before surgery
- Adjust dosage depending on patient response
- Give with meals; limit protein taken with drug
- Give only after MAOIs have been discontinued for 2 wk
- Assist with ambulation, during beginning therapy if needed
- Test for diabetes mellitus and acromegaly if on long-term therapy

Evaluation
- Therapeutic response: decrease in akathisia, improvement in mood

Patient/family education
- Advise patient to change positions slowly to prevent orthostatic hypotension

- Instruct patient to report side effects: twitching, eye spasm; indicate overdose
- Advise patient to use drug exactly as prescribed; if drug is discontinued abruptly, parkinsonian crisis may occur

---

Generic Names

amantadine
🗝 benztropine
biperiden
bromocriptine
cabergoline
carbidopa-levodopa

🗝 levodopa
pramipexole
procyclidine
selegiline
tolcapone
trihexyphenidyl

ANTIPSYCHOTICS

Action: Antipsychotics/neuroleptics are divided into several subgroups: phenothiazines, thioxanthenes, butyrophenones, dibenzoxazepines, dibenzodiazepines, and indolones and other heterocyclic compounds. Although chemically different, these subgroups share many pharmacologic and clinical properties. All antipsychotics work to block postsynaptic dopamine receptors in the brain that are responsible for psychotic behavior, including hallucinations, delusions, and paranoia.

Uses: Antipsychotic behavior is decreased in conditions such as schizophrenia, paranoia, and mania. These agents are also effective for severe anxiety, intractable hiccups, nausea, vomiting, behavioral problems in children, and before surgery for relaxation.

Adverse effects: The most common side effects include extrapyramidal symptoms such as pseudoparkinsonism, akathisia, dystonia, and tardive dyskinesia, which may be controlled by use of antiparkinsonian agents. Serious adverse reactions such as hypotension, agranulocytosis, cardiac arrest, and laryngospasm have occurred. Other common side effects include dry mouth and photosensitivity.

Contraindications: Persons with liver damage, severe hypertension or coronary disease, cerebral arteriosclerosis, blood dyscrasias, bone marrow depression, parkinsonism, severe depression, or narrow angle glaucoma, children <12 yr, or persons withdrawing from alcohol or barbiturates should not use antipsychotics until these conditions are corrected.

Precautions: Caution must be used when antipsychotics are given to the elderly, since metabolism is slowed and adverse reactions can occur rapidly. Hepatic and renal disease may cause poor metabolism and excretion of the drug. Seizure threshold is decreased with these products; increases in the dose of anticonvulsants may be required. Persons with diabetes mellitus, prostatic hypertrophy, chronic respiratory disease, and peptic ulcer disease should be monitored closely.

Pharmacokinetics: Onset, peak, and duration vary widely with different products and routes. Products are metabolized by the liver, are excreted in urine as metabolites, are highly bound to plasma proteins, cross the placenta, and enter breast milk. Half-life can be extended over 3 days.

Interactions: Because other CNS depressants can cause oversedation, these combinations should be used carefully. Anticholinergics may decrease the therapeutic actions of phenothiazines and also cause increased anticholinergic effects.

NURSING CONSIDERATIONS
Assessment
- Monitor bilirubin, CBC, liver function studies monthly, since these drugs are metabolized in the liver and excreted in urine
- Monitor I&O ratio: palpate bladder if low urinary output occurs, since urinary retention occurs with many of these products
- Assess affect, orientation, LOC, reflexes, gait, coordination, sleep pattern disturbances
- Assess dizziness, faintness, palpitations, tachycardia on rising
- Check B/P with patient lying and standing; wide fluctuations between lying and standing B/P may require dosage or product change, since orthostatic hypotension is occurring
- Assess for EPS, including akathisia, tardive dyskinesia, pseudoparkinsonism

Nursing diagnoses
☑ Altered thought processes (uses)
☑ Sensory-perceptual alterations(uses)

Implementation
- Give antiparkinsonian agent if EPS occur
- Administer liq concentrates mixed in glass of juice or cola, since taste is unpleasant; avoid contact with skin when preparing liq concentrate or parenteral medications
- Supervise ambulation until stabilized on medication; do not involve in strenuous exercise program, since fainting is possible; patient should not stand still for long periods
- Increase fluids to prevent constipation
- Give sips of water, candy, gum for dry mouth

Evaluation
- Therapeutic response: decrease in excitement, hallucinations, delusions, paranoia, reorganization of thought patterns, speech

Patient/family education
- Advise patient to rise from sitting or lying position gradually, since fainting may occur
- Instruct patient to remain lying down for at least 30 min after IM inj
- Caution patient to avoid hot tubs, hot showers, or tub baths, since hypotension may occur
- Advise patient to wear a sunscreen or protective clothing to prevent burns
- Advise patient to take extra precautions during hot weather to stay cool; heat stroke can occur
- Caution patient to avoid driving and other activities requiring alertness until response to medication is known
- Inform patient that drowsiness or impaired mental/motor activity is evident the first 2 wk, but tends to decrease over time

---

Generic Names

Phenothiazines:
⚷ chlorpromazine
fluphenazine
mesoridazine
perphenazine
prochlorperazine
promazine
thioridazine
thiothixene
trifluoperazine

Butyrophenone:
⚷ haloperidol

Miscellaneous:
loxapine
molindone
olanzapine
quetiapine
risperidone

ANTITUBERCULARS

Action: Antituberculars act by inhibiting RNA or DNA, or interfering with lipid and protein synthesis, thereby decreasing tubercle bacilli replication.

Uses: Antituberculars are used for pulmonary tuberculosis.

Adverse effects: They vary widely among products. Most products can cause nausea, vomiting, anorexia, and rash. Serious adverse reactions include renal failure, nephrotoxicity, ototoxicity, and hepatic necrosis.

Contraindications: Persons with severe renal disease or hypersensitivity should not use these products.

Precautions: Antituberculars should be used with caution in pregnancy, lactation, and hepatic disease.

Pharmacokinetics: Onset, peak, and duration vary widely among products. Most products are metabolized in the liver and excreted in urine.

Interactions: Please check individual monographs, since interactions vary widely among products.

NURSING CONSIDERATIONS
Assessment
- Assess for signs of anemia: Hct, Hgb, fatigue
- Monitor liver studies weekly: ALT, AST, bilirubin
- Monitor renal status before treatment and monthly thereafter: BUN, creatinine, output, sp gr, urinalysis
- Monitor hepatic status: decreased appetite, jaundice, dark urine, fatigue

Nursing diagnoses
- ✓ Risk for infection (uses)
- ✓ Risk for injury (adverse reactions)
- ✓ Knowledge deficit (teaching)
- ✓ Noncompliance (teaching)

Implementation
- Give some of these agents on empty stomach, 1 hr ac (only for isoniazid and rifampin) or 2 hr pc
- Give antiemetic if vomiting occurs
- Give after C&S is completed; monthly to detect resistance

Evaluation
- Therapeutic response: decreased symptoms of TB, culture negative

Patient/family education
- Teach patient that compliance with dosage schedule, duration is necessary
- Teach patient that scheduled appointments must be kept; relapse may occur
- Advise patient to avoid alcohol while taking drug

- Advise patient to report flulike symptoms: excessive fatigue, anorexia, vomiting, sore throat; unusual bleeding, yellowish discoloration of skin/eyes

---

Generic Names

ethambutol
⦿π isoniazid
pyrazinamide

rifabutin
rifampin
streptomycin

ANTITUSSIVES/EXPECTORANTS

Action: Antitussives suppress the cough reflex by direct action on the cough center in the medulla. Expectorants act by liquefying and reducing the viscosity of thick, tenacious secretions.

Uses: Antitussives/expectorants are used to treat cough occurring in pneumonia, bronchitis, TB, cystic fibrosis, and emphysema; as an adjunct in atelectasis (expectorants); and for nonproductive cough (antitussives).

Adverse effects: The most common side effects are drowsiness, dizziness, and nausea.

Contraindications: Some products are contraindicated in hypothyroidism, iodine sensitivity, pregnancy, and lactation.

Precautions: Some products should be used cautiously in asthma, **G** elderly, and debilitated patients.

Pharmacokinetics: Onset, peak, and duration vary widely among products. Some products are metabolized in the liver and excreted in urine.

Interactions: Please check individual monographs, since interactions vary widely among products.

NURSING CONSIDERATIONS
Assessment
- Assess cough: type, frequency, character including sputum

Nursing diagnoses:
☑ Ineffective breathing pattern (uses)
☑ Ineffective airway clearance (uses)
☑ Knowledge deficit (teaching)

Implementation

G• Give decreased dosage to elderly patients; their metabolism may be slowed
• Increase fluids to liquefy secretions
• Humidify patient's room

Evaluation

• Therapeutic response: absence of cough

Patient/family education

• Advise patient to avoid driving and other hazardous activities until stabilized on this medication
• Caution patient to avoid smoking, smoke-filled rooms, perfumes, dust, environmental pollutants, cleaners that increase cough

---

Generic Names

○ϖ acetylcysteine
○ϖ codeine
dextromethorphan
○ϖ diphenhydramine

guaifenesin
hydrocodone
potassium iodide

ANTIVIRALS

Action: Antivirals act by interfering with DNA synthesis that is needed for viral replication.

Uses: Antivirals are used for mucocutaneous herpes simplex virus, herpes genitalis (HSV_1, HSV_2), advanced HIV infections, herpes simplex virus encephalitis, varicella-zoster encephalomyelitis.

Adverse effects: Serious adverse reactions are fatal metabolic encephalopathy, blood dyscrasias, and acute renal failure. Common side effects are nausea, vomiting, anorexia, diarrhea, headache, vaginitis, and moniliasis.

Contraindications: Persons with hypersensitivity and immunosuppressed individuals with herpes zoster should not use these products.

Precautions: Antivirals should be used with caution in renal disease, liver disease, lactation, pregnancy, and dehydration.

Pharmacokinetics: Onset, peak, and duration vary widely among products. Most products are metabolized in the liver and excreted in urine.

Interactions: Please check individual monographs, since interactions vary widely among products.

NURSING CONSIDERATIONS
Assessment

- Assess for signs of infection, anemia
- Monitor I&O ratio; report hematuria, oliguria, fatigue, weakness; may indicate nephrotoxicity; check for protein in urine during treatment
- Monitor any patient with compromised renal system, since drug is excreted slowly in poor renal system function; toxicity may occur rapidly
- Check liver studies: AST, ALT
- Check blood studies: WBC, RBC, Hct, Hgb, bleeding time; blood dyscrasias may occur; drug should be discontinued
- Check renal studies: urinalysis, protein, BUN, creatinine, Cr Cl
- Obtain C&S before drug therapy; drug may be taken as soon as culture is obtained; repeat C&S after treatment
- Assess bowel pattern before, during treatment; if severe abdominal pain with bleeding occurs, drug should be discontinued
- Identify skin eruptions: rash, urticaria, itching
- Assess for allergies before treatment, reaction of each medication; place allergies on chart, Kardex in bright red letters

Nursing diagnoses

✓ Risk for infection (uses)
✓ Risk for injury (adverse reactions)
✓ Knowledge deficit (teaching)

Implementation

- Give increased fluids to 3 L/day to decrease crystalluria when given IB
- Store at room temp for up to 12 hr after reconstitution
- Give adequate intake of fluids (2000 ml) to prevent deposit in kidneys

Evaluation

- Therapeutic response: absence of or control of infection

Patient/family education

- Inform patient that drug does not cure infection, just controls symptoms
- Instruct patient to report sore throat, fever, fatigue; could indicate superinfection
- Advise patient that drug must be taken in equal intervals around the clock to maintain blood levels for duration of therapy
- Advise patient to notify prescriber of side effects of bruising, bleeding, fatigue, malaise; may indicate blood dyscrasias

Generic Names

abacavir	indinavir
⊶ acyclovir	nelfinavir
amantadine	nevirapine
cidofovir	rimantadine
delavirdine	ritonavir
didanosine	saquinavir
famciclovir	stavudine
foscarnet	vidarabine
ganciclovir	zalcitabine
idoxuridine	⊶ zidovudine

BARBITURATES

Action: Barbiturates act by decreasing impulse transmission to the cerebral cortex.

Uses: All forms of epilepsy can be controlled, since the seizure threshold is increased. Uses also include febrile seizures in children, sedation, insomnia, hyperbilirubinemia, chronic cholestasis with some of these products. Ultra-short acting barbiturates are used as anesthetics.

Adverse effects: The most common side effects are drowsiness and nausea. Serious adverse reactions such as Stevens-Johnson syndrome and blood dyscrasias may occur with high doses and long-term treatment.

Contraindications: Hypersensitivity may occur, and allergies should be identified before administering. Barbiturates are identified as pregnancy category **D** and should not be used in pregnancy. Other contraindications include porphyria and marked impairment of liver function.

Precautions: Caution must be used when these products are given to the elderly or debilitated; usually smaller doses are needed, since metabolism is slowed. Persons with renal and hepatic disease may show delayed excretion. Barbiturates may produce excitability in children.

Pharmacokinetics: Onset of action can be slow, up to 1 hr, with a peak of 8 hr and a duration of 3-10 hr. These drugs are metabolized by the liver, excreted by the kidneys, cross the placenta, and enter breast milk.

Interactions: Increased CNS depressant effect may occur with alcohol, MAOIs, sedatives, or narcotics. These products should be used together cautiously. Oral anticoagulants, corticosteroids, griseofulvin, quinidine, oral contraceptives, and theophylline may show a decreased effect when used with barbiturates.

NURSING CONSIDERATIONS
Assessment
- Monitor hepatic and renal studies: AST, ALT, bilirubin, creatinine, LDH, alkaline phosphatase, BUN if patient is on long-term therapy, since these products are metabolized and excreted by the liver and kidney
- Monitor blood studies: CBC, hematocrit, hemoglobin, and prothrombin time if patient is on long-term therapy, since these products increase the possibility of bleeding and blood dyscrasias
- Identify barbiturate toxicity: hypotension, pulmonary constriction, cold, clammy skin, cyanosis of lips, insomnia, nausea, vomiting, hallucinations, delirium, weakness

Nursing diagnoses
☑ Sleep pattern disturbance (uses)
☑ Risk for injury (adverse reactions)

Evaluation
- Therapeutic response: appropriate sedation or seizure control

Patient/family education
- Inform patient that physical dependency may result when used for extended periods (45-90 days, depending on dosage)
- Advise patient to avoid driving and activities that require alertness, since drowsiness and dizziness may occur
- Caution patient to abstain from alcohol and other psychotropic medications unless prescribed by prescriber
- Instruct patient not to discontinue medication abruptly after long-term use; withdrawal symptoms will occur

---

Generic Names
amobarbital
pentobarbital
⚷ phenobarbital

secobarbital
thiopental

BENZODIAZEPINES

Action: Benzodiazepines potentiate the effects of GABA, including any other inhibitory transmitters in the CNS, resulting in decreased anxiety.
Uses: Anxiety is relieved in conditions such as phobic disorders.

Benzodiazepines are also used for acute alcohol withdrawal to relieve the possibility of delirium tremens, and some products are used before surgery for relaxation.

Adverse effects: The most common side effects are dizziness, drowsiness, blurred vision, and orthostatic hypotension. Most adverse effects are mediated through the CNS. There is a risk for physical dependence and abuse.

Contraindications: Hypersensitivity, acute narrow-angle glaucoma, **P** children <6 months, liver disease (clonazepam), lactation (diazepam).

Precautions: Caution must be used when these products are given **G** to the elderly or debilitated; usually smaller dosages are needed, since metabolism is slowed. Persons with renal and hepatic disease may show delayed excretion. Clonazepam may increase incidence of seizures.

Pharmacokinetics: Onset of action is ½-1 hr, with a peak of 1-2 hr and a duration of 4-6 hr. These drugs are metabolized by the liver, excreted by the kidneys, cross the placenta, and enter breast milk.

Interactions: Increased CNS depressant effect may occur with other CNS depressants. These products should be used together cautiously. Alcohol should not be used; fatal reactions can occur. The serum concentration and toxicity of digoxin may be increased.

NURSING CONSIDERATIONS
Assessment
- Monitor B/P (with patient lying, standing), pulse; if systolic B/P drops 20 mm Hg, hold drug, notify prescriber; orthostatic hypotension is severe
- Monitor hepatic and renal studies: AST, ALT, bilirubin, creatinine, LDH, alkaline phosphatase
- Assess for physical dependency, withdrawal symptoms, including headache, nausea, vomiting, muscle pain, weakness after long-term use

Nursing diagnoses
✓Anxiety (uses)
✓Risk for injury (adverse reactions)

Implementation
- Give with food or milk for GI symptoms; may give crushed if patient is unable to swallow medication whole

Evaluation
- Therapeutic response: relaxation or decreased anxiety

Patient/family education

- Teach patient that drug should not be used for everyday stress or long term; not to take more than prescribed amount, since drug is habit forming
- Caution patient to avoid driving and activities that require alertness, since drowsiness and dizziness occur
- Caution patient to abstain from alcohol and other psychotropic medications unless prescribed by prescriber
- Advise patient not to discontinue medication abruptly after long-term use; withdrawal symptoms will occur

---

Generic Names

alprazolam

chlordiazepoxide

clonazepam

✳ diazepam

flurazepam

halazepam

lorazepam

midazolam

oxazepam

prazepam

quazepam

temazepam

triazolam

β-ADRENERGIC BLOCKERS

Action: β-Blockers are divided into selective and nonselective blockers. Nonselective blockers produce a fall in blood pressure without reflex tachycardia or reduction in heart rate through a mixture of β-blocking effects; elevated plasma renins are reduced. Selective β-blockers competitively block stimulation of β_1-receptors in cardiac smooth muscle; these drugs produce chronotropic and inotropic effects.

Uses: β-Blockers are used for hypertension, ventricular dysrhythmias, and prophylaxis of angina pectoris.

Adverse effects: The most common side effects are orthostatic hypotension, bradycardia, diarrhea, nausea, vomiting. Serious adverse reactions include blood dyscrasias, bronchospasm, and CHF.

Contraindications: Hypersensitive reactions may occur, and allergies should be identified before these products are given. β-Adrenergic blockers should not be used in heart block, CHF, or cardiogenic shock.

G Precautions: β-Blockers should be used with caution in the elderly or in renal and thyroid disease, COPD, CAD, diabetes mellitus, pregnancy, or asthma.

Pharmacokinetics: Onset, peak, and duration vary widely among products. Most products are metabolized in the liver, with metabolites excreted in urine, bile, and feces.

Interactions: Interactions vary widely among products; check individual monograph for specific information.

NURSING CONSIDERATIONS
Assessment
- Monitor renal studies, including protein, BUN, creatinine; watch for increased levels that may indicate nephrotic syndrome; obtain baselines in renal and liver function studies before beginning treatment
- Monitor I&O, weight daily
- Monitor B/P during beginning treatment and periodically thereafter, pulse q4h; note rate, rhythm, quality
- Monitor apical/radial pulse before administration; notify prescriber of significant changes
- Check for edema in feet and legs daily

Nursing diagnoses
- ✓ Altered tissue perfusion (uses)
- ✓ Decreased cardiac output (uses)
- ✓ Diarrhea (adverse reactions)
- ✓ Impaired gas exchange (adverse reactions)

Implementation
- Give PO ac, hs; tab may be crushed or swallowed whole
- Give reduced dosage in renal dysfunction

Evaluation
- Therapeutic response: decrease in B/P in hypertension; decreased B/P, edema, moist rales in CHF

Patient/family education
- Instruct patient to comply with dosage schedule, even if feeling better
- Caution patient to rise slowly to sitting or standing position to minimize orthostatic hypotension
- Advise patient to report bradycardia, dizziness, confusion, depression, fever
- Teach patient to take pulse at home; advise when to notify prescriber
- Instruct patient to comply with weight control, dietary adjustment, modified exercise program
- Advise patient to wear support hose to minimize effects of orthostatic hypotension

- Advise patient not to discontinue drug abruptly; taper over 2 wk; may precipitate angina

---

Generic Names

Selective β₁-receptor blockers:
acebutolol
atenolol
esmolol
metoprolol

Nonselective β₁ and β₂-blockers:
carteolol

nadolol
pindolol
⚷ propranolol
timolol

Combined α₁, β₁, and β₂-receptor blocker:
labetalol

BRONCHODILATORS

Action: Bronchodilators are divided into anticholinergics, α/β-adrenergics agonists, β-adrenergic agonists, and phosphodiesterase inhibitors. Anticholinergics act by inhibiting interaction of acetylcholine at receptor sites on bronchial smooth muscle; α/β-adrenergic agonists by relaxing bronchial smooth muscle and increasing diameter of nasal passages; β-adrenergic agonists by action on β₂-receptors, which relaxes bronchial smooth muscle; phosphodiesterase inhibitors by blocking phosphodiesterase and increasing cAMP, which mediates smooth muscle relaxation in the respiratory system.

Uses: Bronchodilators are used for bronchial asthma, bronchospasm associated with bronchitis, emphysema, other obstructive pulmonary diseases, and Cheyne-Stokes respirations, as well as prevention of exercise-induced asthma.

Adverse effects: The most common side effects are tremors, anxiety, nausea, vomiting, and irritation in the throat. The most serious adverse reactions include bronchospasm and dyspnea.

Contraindications: Persons with hypersensitivity, narrow-angle glaucoma, tachydysrhythmias, and severe cardiac disease should not use some of these products.

Precautions: Bronchodilators should be used with caution in lactation, pregnancy, hyperthyroidism, hypertension, prostatic hypertrophy, and seizure disorders.

Pharmacokinetics: Onset, peak, and duration vary widely among products. Most products are metabolized in the liver and excreted in urine.

Interactions: Please check individual monographs, since interactions vary widely among products.

NURSING CONSIDERATIONS
Assessment
- Monitor respiratory function: vital capacity, FEV, ABGs, lung sounds, heart rate and rhythm

Nursing diagnoses
☑ Ineffective airway clearance (uses)
☑ Activity intolerance (uses)
☑ Risk for injury (adverse reactions)
☑ Knowledge deficit (teaching)

Implementation
- Give after shaking; exhale, place mouthpiece in mouth, inhale slowly, hold breath, remove, exhale slowly
- Give gum, sips of water for dry mouth
- Give PO with meals to decrease gastric irritation
- Store in light-resistant container; do not expose to temp over 86° F

Evaluation
- Therapeutic response: absence of dyspnea, wheezing

Patient/family education
- Advise patient not to use OTC medications; extra stimulation may occur
- Teach patient use of inhaler; review package insert with patient; to wash inhaler in warm water qd and dry
- Advise patient to avoid getting aerosol in eyes
- Caution patient to avoid smoking, smoke-filled rooms, persons with respiratory tract infections

Generic Names
⚷ albuterol
aminophylline
⚷ atropine
bitolterol
dyphylline
ephedrine
⚷ epinephrine
ipratropium

isoproterenol
levalbuterol
metaproterenol
mibefradil
oxtriphylline
pirbuterol
terbutaline
⚷ theophylline

CALCIUM CHANNEL BLOCKERS

Action: These products inhibit calcium ion influx across the cell membrane in cardiac and vascular smooth muscle. This action produces relaxation of coronary vascular smooth muscle, dilates coronary arteries, slows SA/AV node conduction, and dilates peripheral arteries.

Uses: These products are used for chronic stable angina pectoris, vasospastic angina, dysrhythmias, hypertension, and unstable angina.

Adverse effects: The most common side effects are dysrhythmias and edema. Also common are headache, fatigue, drowsiness, and flushing.

Contraindications: Persons with 2nd- or 3rd-degree heart block, sick sinus syndrome, hypotension of <90 mm Hg systolic, Wolff-Parkinson-White syndrome, or cardiogenic shock should not use these products, since worsening of those conditions may occur.

Precautions: CHF may worsen, since edema may be increased. Hypotension may worsen, since B/P is decreased. Patients with renal and liver disease should use these products cautiously, since they are metabolized in the liver and excreted by the kidneys.

Pharmacokinetics: Onset, peak, and duration vary widely with route of administration. Drugs are metabolized by the liver and excreted in the urine primarily as metabolites.

Interactions: Increased levels of digoxin and theophylline may occur when used with these products. Increased effects of β-blockers and antihypertensives may occur with calcium channel blockers.

NURSING CONSIDERATIONS
Assessment
- Monitor cardiac system, including B/P, pulse, respirations, ECG intervals (PR, QRS, QT)

Nursing diagnoses
☑Altered tissue perfusion: cardiopulmonary (uses)
☑Decreased cardiac output (adverse reactions)

Implementation
- Give PO ac and hs

Evaluation
- Therapeutic response: decreased anginal pain, decreased B/P, dysrhythmias

Patient/family education
- Teach patient how to take pulse before taking drug; patient should record or graph pulses to identify changes

- Advise patient to avoid hazardous activities until stabilized on this drug, since dizziness occurs frequently
- Inform patient of need for compliance to all areas of medical regimen, including diet, exercise, stress reduction, drug therapy

---

Generic Names

amlodipine

bepridil

diltiazem

felodipine

isradipine

nicardipine

nifedipine

⊙π verapamil

CARDIAC GLYCOSIDES

Action: Products act by inhibiting sodium and potassium ATPase and then making more calcium available to activate contracted proteins. Cardiac contractility and cardiac output are increased.

Uses: These products are used for CHF, atrial fibrillation, atrial flutter, atrial tachycardia, and rapid digitalization in these disorders.

Adverse effects: The most common side effects are cardiac disturbances, headache, hypotension, GI symptoms. Also common are blurred vision and yellow-green halos.

Contraindications: Hypersensitive reactions may occur, and allergies should be identified before these products are given. Also, persons with ventricular tachycardia, ventricular fibrillation, and carotid sinus syndrome should not use these products.

Precautions: Persons with acute MI and those who have or may develop serum potassium, calcium, or magnesium imbalances should use these products cautiously. Also, persons with AV block, severe respiratory disease, hypothyroidism, renal and liver disease, and the ⓖ elderly should exercise caution when these drugs are prescribed.

Pharmacokinetics: Onset, peak, and duration vary widely with the route of administration. Digitoxin is inactivated by the liver, and inactive metabolites are excreted in urine. Digoxin is excreted in urine mainly as the parent drug and metabolites.

Interactions: Toxicity may occur when used with diuretics, succinylcholine, quinidine, and thioamines. Increased blood levels may occur with propantheline bromide, spironolactone, quinidine, verapamil, aminoglycosides (PO), amiodarone, anticholinergics, and quinine. Diuretics may increase toxicity.

NURSING CONSIDERATIONS
Assessment
- Montior cardiac system, including B/P, pulse, respirations, and increased urine output
- Monitor apical pulse for 1 min before giving drug; if pulse <60, take again in 1 hr; if <60 notify prescriber
- Monitor electrolytes, including potassium, sodium, chloride, calcium, magnesium; renal function studies, including BUN and creatinine; and blood studies, including AST, ALT, bilirubin
- Monitor I&O ratio, daily weights
- Monitor therapeutic drug levels

Nursing diagnoses
☑ Altered tissue perfusion: cardiopulmonary (uses)
☑ Decreased cardiac output (adverse reactions)

Implementation
- Give potassium supplements if ordered for potassium levels <3

Evaluation
- Therapeutic response: decreased weight, edema, pulse, respiration, and increased urine output

Patient/family education
- Teach patient how to take pulse before taking drug; patient should record or graph pulse to identify changes
- Advise patient to avoid hazardous activities until stabilized on this drug, since dizziness occurs frequently
- Inform patient of need for compliance to all areas of medical regimen, including diet, exercise, stress reduction, drug therapy

---

Generic Names
digitoxin   ⚷ digoxin

CHOLINERGICS

Action: Cholinergics act by preventing destruction of acetylcholine, which increases concentration at sites where acetylcholine is released; this exaggerates the effects of acetylcholine and facilitates transmission of impulses across myoneural junction. Cholinergics may also act by stimulating receptors for acetylcholine.

Uses: Cholinergics are used for myasthenia gravis, as antagonists of nondepolarizing neuromuscular blockade, postoperative bladder distention and urinary distention, postoperative ileus.

Adverse effects: The most serious adverse reactions are respiratory depression, bronchospasm, constriction, laryngospasm, respiratory arrest, convulsions, and paralysis. The most common side effects are nausea, diarrhea, and vomiting.

Contraindications: Persons with obstruction of the intestine or renal system should not use these products.

Precautions: Caution should be used in patients with bradycardia, hypotension, seizure disorders, bronchial asthma, coronary occlusion, hyperthyroidism, and in lactation and children.

Pharmacokinetics: Onset, peak, and duration vary widely among products. Most products are metabolized in the liver and excreted in urine.

Interactions: Please check individual monographs since interactions vary widely among products.

NURSING CONSIDERATIONS
Assessment
- Monitor VS, respiration q8h
- Monitor I&O ratio; check for urinary retention of incontinence
- Assess for bradycardia, hypotension, bronchospasm, headache, dizziness, convulsions, respiratory depression; drug should be discontinued if toxicity occurs

Nursing diagnoses
- ☑ Altered urinary elimination (uses)
- ☑ Ineffective breathing pattern (uses)
- ☑ Knowledge deficit (teaching)
- ☑ Noncompliance (teaching)

Implementation
- Give only with atropine sulfate available for cholinergic crisis
- Give only after all other cholinergics have been discontinued
- Give increased dosages if tolerance occurs
- Give larger doses after exercise or fatigue
- Give on empty stomach for better absorption
- Store at room temp

Evaluation
- Therapeutic response: increased muscle strength, hand grasp, improved muscle gait, absence of labored breathing (if severe)

Patient/family education
- Inform patient that drug is not a cure; it only relieves symptoms (myasthenia gravis)
- Advise patient to wear Medic Alert ID specifying myasthenia gravis, drugs taken

Generic Names

bethanechol
edrophonium
neostigmine

physostigmine
pyridostigmine

CHOLINERGIC BLOCKERS

Action: Cholinergic blockers inhibit or block acetylcholine at receptor sites in the autonomic nervous system.

Uses: Many products are used to decrease secretions before surgery, to reverse neuromuscular blockade, and to decrease motility of GI, biliary, urinary tracts. Other products are used for parkinsonian symptoms, including dystonia associated with neuroleptic drugs.

Adverse effects: The most common side effects are dryness of the mouth and constipation, which can be prevented by frequent rinsing of the mouth and increasing water and bulk in the diet.

Contraindications: Hypersensitivity can occur, and allergies should be identified before administering these products. Persons with GI and GU obstruction should not use these products, since constipation and urinary retention may occur. They are also contraindicated in angle closure glaucoma and myasthenia gravis.

Precautions: Caution must be used when these products are given G to the elderly, since metabolism is slowed. Also, persons with tachycardia or prostatic hypertrophy should use these products with caution.

Pharmacokinetics: Onset, peak, and duration vary with route.

Interactions: Increase in anticholinergic effect occurs when used with narcotics, barbiturates, antihistamines, MAOIs, phenothiazines, amantadine.

NURSING CONSIDERATIONS
Assessment
- Assess I&O ratio; be alert for urinary retention, frequency, dysuria; drug should be discontinued if these occur
- Assess urinary hesitancy, retention; palpate bladder if retention occurs
- Assess constipation; increase fluids, bulk, exercise
- Assess for tolerance over long-term therapy; dosage may need to be changed
- Assess mental status: affect, mood, CNS depression, worsening of mental symptoms during early therapy

Nursing diagnoses

☑Impaired physical mobility (uses)

☑Pain (uses)

Implementation

- Give with food or milk to decrease GI symptoms
- Give parenteral dose with patient recumbent to prevent postural hypotension; give dose slowly, monitoring VS
- Give hard candy, gum, frequent rinsing of mouth for dryness

Evaluation

- Therapeutic response: absence of cramps, absence of EPS

Patient/family education

- Caution patient to avoid driving and other hazardous activity if drowsiness occurs
- Advise patient to avoid concurrent use of cough, cold preparations with alcohol, antihistamines unless directed by prescriber
- Caution patient to use with caution in hot weather, since medication may increase susceptibility to heat stroke

---

Generic Names

⚷ atropine

⚷ benztropine

biperiden

glycopyrrolate

scopolamine

trihexyphenidyl

CORTICOSTEROIDS

Action: Corticosteroids are divided into glucocorticoids and mineralocorticoids. Glucocorticoids decrease inflammation by the suppression of migration of polymorphonuclear leukocytes, fibroblasts, increased capillary permeability, and lysosomal stabilization. They also have varied metabolic effects and modify the body's immune responses to many different stimuli. Mineralocorticoids act by increasing resorption of sodium by increasing hydrogen and potassium excretion in the distal tubule.

Uses: Glucocorticoids are used to decrease inflammation and for immunosuppression. In addition, some products may be given for allergy, adrenal insufficiency, or cerebral edema. Mineralocorticoids are given for adrenal insufficiency or adrenogenital syndrome.

Adverse effects: The most common side effects include change in behavior, including insomnia and euphoria; GI irritation, including peptic ulcer; metabolic reactions; including hypokalemia, hyperglycemia, and carbohydrate intolerance; and sodium and fluid retention. Most adverse reactions are dose dependent.

Contraindications: Hypersensitivity may occur and should be identified before administering. Since these products mask infection, they should not be used in systemic fungal infections or amebiasis. Mothers taking pharmacologic doses of corticosteroids should not nurse.

Precautions: Caution must be used when these products are prescribed for diabetic patients, since hyperglycemia may occur. Also, patients with glaucoma, seizure disorders, peptic ulcer, impaired renal function, CHF, hypertension, ulcerative colitis, or myasthenia gravis should be monitored closely if corticosteroids are given. Use with caution in children and the elderly and during pregnancy.

Pharmacokinetics: For oral preparations the onset of action occurs between 1-2 hr, and duration can be up to 2 days, with a half-life of 2-4 days. Pharmacokinetics vary widely among products. These products cross the placenta and appear in breast milk.

Interactions: Decreased corticosteroid effect may occur with barbiturates, rifampin, phenytoin; corticosteroid dosage may need to be increased. There is a possibility of GI bleeding when used with salicylates, indomethacin. Steroids may reduce salicylate levels. When using with digitalis glycosides, potassium-depleting diuretics, and amphotericin, serum potassium levels should be monitored.

NURSING CONSIDERATIONS
Assessment
- Monitor potassium, blood sugar, urine glucose while on long-term therapy; hypokalemia and hyperglycemia are common
- Monitor weight daily; notify prescriber if weekly gain of >5 lb, since these products alter fluid and electrolyte balance
- Assess for potassium depletion, including paresthesias, fatigue, nausea, vomiting, depression, polyuria, dysrhythmias, weakness
- Assess for mental status, including affect, mood, behavioral changes, aggression; if severe personality changes occur, including depression, drug may need to be tapered and then discontinued
- Monitor I&O ratio; be alert for decreasing urinary output and increasing edema
- Monitor plasma cortisol levels during long-term therapy (normal level is 138-635 nmol/L when drawn at 8 AM)
- Assess for infection, including increased temp, WBC, even after withdrawal of medication; drug masks symptoms of infection
- Assess for adrenal insufficiency: nausea, anorexia, fatigue, dizziness, dyspnea, weakness, joint pain

Nursing diagnoses

☑ Risk for infection (adverse reactions)
☑ Body image disturbance (adverse reactions)
☑ Risk for violence: self-directed (suicide) (adverse reactions)

Implementation

• Give with food or milk to decrease GI symptoms

Evaluation

• Therapeutic response: decreased inflammation

Patient/family education

• Advise patient that ID as steroid user should be carried
• Advise patient not to discontinue this medication abruptly or adrenal crisis can result
• Teach patient all aspects of drug use, including cushingoid symptoms
• Instruct patient that single daily or alternate-day doses should be taken in the morning before 9 AM (for replacement therapy)
• Instruct patient to take with meals or a snack

Generic Names

Glucocorticoids:
beclomethasone
betamethasone
⚷ cortisone
flunisolide
hydrocortisone
methylprednisolone

prednisolone
⚷ prednisone
rimexolone
triamcinolone

Mineralocorticoid:
fludrocortisone

DIURETICS

Action: Diuretics are divided into subgroups: thiazides and thiazide-like diuretics, loop diuretics, carbonic anhydrase inhibitors, osmotic diuretics, and potassium-sparing diuretics. Each one of these subgroups differs in its mechanism of action. Thiazides and thiazide-like diuretics increase excretion of water and sodium by inhibiting resorption in the early distal tubule. Loop diuretics inhibit resorption of sodium and chloride in the thick ascending limb of the loop of Henle. Carbonic anhydrase inhibitors increase sodium excretion by decreasing sodium-hydrogen ion exchange throughout the renal tubule. Carbonic anhydrase inhibitors also decrease secretion of aqueous humor in the eye and thus decrease intraocular pressure. Osmotic diuretics increase the osmotic pressure of glomerular filtrate, thus decreasing net absorption of sodium. The potassium-sparing diuretics interfere with sodium resorption at the distal tubule, thus decreasing potassium excretion.

Uses: Blood pressure is reduced in hypertension; edema is reduced in CHF; intraocular pressure is decreased in glaucoma.

Adverse effects: Hypokalemia, hyperuricemia, and hyperglycemia occur most frequently with thiazide diuretics. Aplastic anemia, blood dyscrasias, volume depletion, and dehydration may occur when thiazide-like diuretics, loop diuretics, or carbonic anhydrase inhibitors are given. Side effects and adverse reactions vary widely for the miscellaneous products.

Contraindications: Persons with electrolyte imbalances (sodium, chloride, potassium), dehydration, or anuria should not be given these products until the problem is corrected.

Precautions: Caution must be used when diuretics are given to the elderly, since electrolyte disturbances and dehydration can occur rapidly. Hepatic and renal disorders may cause poor metabolism and excretion of the drug.

Pharmacokinetics: Onset, peak, and duration vary widely among the different subgroups of these drugs.

Interactions: Cholestyramine and colestipol decrease the absorption of thiazide diuretics. Concurrent use of thiazides with diazoxide may increase hyperuricemia, hyperglycemia, and antihypertensive effects of thiazides. Ototoxicity may occur when loop diuretics are used with aminoglycosides. Thiazide and loop diuretics may increase therapeutic and toxic effects of lithium.

NURSING CONSIDERATIONS
Assessment

- Monitor weight, I&O daily to determine fluid loss; check skin turgor for dehydration
- Monitor electrolytes: potassium, sodium, chloride: include BUN, blood sugar, CBC, serum creatinine, blood pH, ABGs, uric acid, calcium; electrolyte imbalances may occur quickly
- Monitor B/P with patient lying, standing; postural hypotension may occur, since fluid loss occurs from intravascular spaces first
- Assess for signs of metabolic alkalosis, including drowsiness and restlessness
- Assess for signs of hypokalemia with some products, including postural hypotension, malaise, fatigue, tachycardia, leg cramps, weakness

Nursing diagnoses
- ✓ Fluid volume excess (uses)
- ✓ Decreased cardiac output (adverse reactions)

Implementation
- Give in AM to avoid interference with sleep if using drug as a diuretic
- Give potassium replacement if potassium is less than 3 mg/dl

Evaluation
- Therapeutic reponse: improvement in edema of feet, legs, sacral area daily if medication is being used in CHF; improvement in B/P if medication is being used as a diuretic; improvement in intraocular pressure if medication is being used to decrease aqueous humor in the eye

Patient/family education
- Teach patient to take drug early in the day (diuretic) to prevent nocturia

---

Generic Names

Thiazides:
○━ hydrochlorothiazide

Thiazide-like:
chlorthalidone
indapamide
metolazone

Loop:
bumetanide
○━ furosemide
torsemide

Carbonic anhydrase inhibitors:
acetazolamide

Potassium-sparing:
amiloride
spironolactone
triamterene

Osmotic:
mannitol

HISTAMINE H$_2$ ANTAGONISTS

Action: Histamine H$_2$ antagonists act by inhibiting histamine at H$_2$ receptor site in parietal cells, which inhibits gastric acid secretion.

Uses: Histamine H$_2$ antagonists are used for short-term treatment of duodenal and gastric ulcers and maintenance therapy for duodenal ulcer; and for gastroesophageal reflux disease.

Adverse effects: The most serious adverse reactions are agranulocytosis, thrombocytopenia, neutropenia, aplastic anemia, exfoliative dermatitis. The most common side effects are confusion (not with rantidine), headache and diarrhea.

Contraindications: Persons with hypersensitivity should not use these products.

P Precautions: Caution should be used in pregnancy, lactation, children <16 yr, organic brain syndrome, hepatic disease, renal disease.

Pharmacokinetics: Onset, peak, and duration vary widely among products. Most products are metabolized in the liver and excreted in urine.

Interactions: Antacids interfere with absorption of histamine H$_2$ antagonists. Check individual monographs for other interactions.

NURSING CONSIDERATIONS
Assessment
- Monitor gastric pH (>5 should be maintained)
- Monitor I&O ratio, BUN, creatinine

Nursing diagnoses
☑Pain (uses)
☑Risk for injury (bleeding)
☑Knowledge deficit (teaching)

Implementation
- Give with meals for prolonged drug effect
- Give antacids 1 hr before or 1 hr after cimetidine
- Give **IV** slowly; bradycardia may occur; give over 30 min
- Store diluted sol at room temp for up to 48 hr

Evaluation
- Therapeutic response: decreased pain in abdomen

Patient/family education
- Advise patient that gynecomastia, impotence may occur, but is reversible
- Caution patient to avoid driving and other hazardous activities until patient is stabilized on this medication
- Caution patient to avoid black pepper, caffeine, alcohol, harsh spices, extremes in temp of food
- Caution patient to avoid OTC preparations: aspirin, cough, cold preparations
- Inform patient that drug must be continued for prescribed time to be effective
- Advise patient to report bruising, fatigue, malaise; blood dyscrasias may occur

Generic Names

cimetidine   ranitidine
famotidine

IMMUNOSUPPRESSANTS

Action: Immunosuppressants produce immunosuppression by inhibiting T lymphocytes.

Uses: Most products are used for organ transplants to prevent rejection.

Adverse effects: The most serious adverse reactions are albuminuria, hematuria, proteinuria, renal failure, and hepatotoxicity. The most common side effects are oral *Candida* infection, gum hyperplasia, tremors, and headache. The most serious adverse reactions for azathioprine are hematologic (leukopenia and thrombocytopenia) and GI (nausea and vomiting). There is a risk of secondary infection.

Contraindications: Products are contraindicated in hypersensitivity.

Precautions: Caution should be used in severe renal disease, severe hepatic disease, and pregnancy.

Pharmacokinetics: Onset, peak, and duration vary widely among products. Most products are metabolized in the liver and excreted in urine.

Interactions: Please check individual monographs, since interactions vary widely among products.

NURSING CONSIDERATIONS
Assessment
- Monitor renal studies: BUN, creatinine at least monthly during treatment, 3 mo after treatment
- Monitor liver function studies: alkaline phosphatase, AST, ALT, bilirubin
- Monitor drug blood levels during treatment
- Assess for hepatotoxicity: dark urine, jaundice, itching, light-colored stools; drug should be discontinued

Nursing diagnoses
☑ Risk for infection (adverse reactions)
☑ Risk for injury (uses)
☑ Knowledge deficit (teaching)

Implementation
- Give for several days before transplant surgery
- Give with meals for GI upset or place drug in chocolate milk
- Give with oral antifungal for *Candida* infections

Evaluation
- Therapeutic response: absence of rejection

Patient/family education
- Advise patient to report fever, chills, sore throat, fatigue, since serious infections may occur
- Caution patient to use contraceptive measures during treatment and for 12 wk after ending therapy

---

Generic Names

☛ azathioprine
basiliximab
cyclosporine

muromonab-CD3
sirolimus
tacrolimus

LAXATIVES

Action: Laxatives are divided into bulk products, lubricants, osmotics, saline laxative stimulants, and stool softeners. Bulks work by absorbing water and expanding to increase moisture content and bulk in the stool. Lubricants increase water retention in the stool, causing reabsorption of water in the bowel. Stimulants act by increasing peristalsis by direct effect on the intestine. Saline draws water into the intestinal lumen. Osmotics increase distention and promote peristalsis. Stool softeners reduce surface tension of liq in the bowel.

Uses: Laxatives are used as a preparation for bowel, rectal examination, constipation, or as stool softeners.

Adverse effects: The most common side effects are nausea, abdominal cramps, and diarrhea.

Contraindications: Persons with GI obstruction, perforation, gastric retention, toxic colitis, megacolon, abdominal pain, nausea, vomiting, and fecal impaction should not use these products.

Precautions: Caution should be used in rectal bleeding, large hemorrhoids, and anal excoriation.

Pharmacokinetics: Onset, peak, and duration vary among products.

Interactions: Please check individual monographs, since interactions vary widely among products.

NURSING CONSIDERATIONS
Assessment
- Monitor blood, urine electrolytes if drug is used often by patient
- Monitor I&O ratio: to identify fluid loss
- Determine cause of constipation; identify whether fluids, bulk, or exercise is missing from lifestyle
- Assess for cramping, rectal bleeding, nausea, vomiting; if these symptoms occur, drug should be discontinued

Nursing diagnoses
☑ Constipation (uses)
☑ Diarrhea (adverse reactions)
☑ Knowledge deficit (teaching)

Implementation
- Give alone only with water for better absorption; do not take within 1 hr of antacids, milk, or cimetidine

Evaluation
- Therapeutic response: decrease in constipation

Patient/family education
- Teach patient to swallow tab whole; do not chew
- Caution patient not to use laxatives for long-term therapy; bowel tone will be lost; that normal bowel movements do not always occur daily
- Caution patient not to use in presence of abdominal pain, nausea, vomiting
- Advise patient to notify prescriber of abdominal pain, nausea, vomiting
- Advise patient to notify prescriber if constipation is unrelieved or if symptoms of electrolyte imbalance occur: muscle cramps, pain, weakness, dizziness

---

Generic Names

Bulk laxative:
psyllium

Osmotic agents:
glycerin
lactulose

Saline:
magnesium salts
sodium phosphate/biphosphate

Stimulants:
bisacodyl
cascara
phenolphthalein
senna

Stool softeners:
docusate

NEUROMUSCULAR BLOCKING AGENTS

Action: Neuromuscular blocking agents are divided into depolarizing and nondepolarizing blockers. They act by inhibiting transmission of nerve impulses by binding with cholinergic receptor sites.

Uses: Neuromuscular blocking agents are used to facilitate endotracheal intubation and skeletal muscle relaxation during mechanical ventilation, surgery, or general anesthesia.

Adverse effects: The most serious adverse reactions are prolonged apnea, bronchospasm, cyanosis, respiratory depression, and malignant hyperthermia. The most common side effects are bradycardia and decreased motility.

Contraindications: Persons that are hypersensitive should not be given this product.

Precautions: Caution should be used in pregnancy, thyroid disease, collagen disease, cardiac disease, lactation, children <2 yr, electrolyte imbalances, dehydration, neuromuscular disease (myasthenia gravis), and respiratory disease.

Pharmacokinetics: Onset, peak, and duration vary widely among products. Most products are metabolized in the liver and excreted in urine.

Interactions: Aminoglycosides potentiate neuromuscular blockade. See individual monographs.

NURSING CONSIDERATIONS
Assessment
- Monitor for electrolyte imbalances (potassium, magnesium); may lead to increased action of this drug
- Monitor VS (B/P, pulse, respirations, airway) q15 min until fully recovered; rate, depth, pattern of respirations, strength of hand grip
- Monitor I&O ratio; check for urinary retention, frequency, hesitancy
- Assess for recovery: decreased paralysis of face, diaphragm, leg, arm, rest of body
- Assess for allergic reactions: rash, fever, respiratory distress, pruritus; drug should be discontinued

Nursing diagnoses
- ☑ Ineffective breathing pattern (uses)
- ☑ Risk for injury (adverse reactions)
- ☑ Knowledge deficit (teaching)

Implementation

- Administer using nerve stimulator by anesthesiologist to determine neuromuscular blockade
- Administer anticholinesterase to reverse neuromuscular blockade
- Administer **IV** undiluted over 1-2 min (only by qualified person, usually an anesthesiologist)
- Store in light-resistant, cool area
- Reassure if communication is difficult during recovery from neuromuscular blockade

Evaluation

- Therapeutic response: paralysis of jaw, eyelid, head, neck, rest of body

---

Generic Names

atracurium
cisatracurium
doxacurium
gallamine
metocurine
mivacurium

pancuronium
pipecuronium
succinylcholine
⚷ tubocurarine
vecuronium

NONSTEROIDAL ANTIINFLAMMATORIES

Action: Nonsteroidal antiinflammatories decrease prostaglandin synthesis by inhibiting an enzyme needed for biosynthesis.

Uses: Nonsteroidal antiinflammatories are used to treat mild to moderate pain, osteoarthritis, rheumatoid arthritis, and dysmenorrhea.

Adverse effects: The most serious adverse reactions are nephrotoxicity (dysuria, hematuria, oliguria, azotemia), blood dyscrasias, and cholestatic hepatitis. The most common side effects are nausea, abdominal pain, anorexia, dizziness, and drowsiness.

Contraindications: Persons with hypersensitivity, asthma, severe renal disease, and severe hepatic disease should not use these products.

P Precautions: Caution should be used in pregnancy, lactation, children, bleeding disorders, GI disorders, cardiac disorders, hypersensitivity to other antiinflammatory agents, and the elderly.

G

Pharmacokinetics: Onset, peak, and duration vary widely among products. Most products are metabolized in the liver and excreted in urine.

Interactions: Please check individual monographs, since interactions vary widely among products.

NURSING CONSIDERATIONS
Assessment
- Monitor renal, liver, blood studies: BUN, creatinine, AST, ALT, Hgb, before treatment, periodically thereafter
- Monitor audiometric, ophth examination before, during, and after treatment.
- Check for eye, ear problems: blurred vision, tinnitus, may indicate toxicity

Nursing diagnoses
☑ Chronic pain (uses)
☑ Impaired physical mobility (uses)
☑ Knowledge deficit (teaching)
☑ Noncompliance (teaching)

Implementation
- Give with food to decrease GI symptoms; however, best to take on empty stomach to facilitate absorption
- Store at room temp

Evaluation
- Therapeutic response: decreased pain, stiffness in joints, decreased swelling in joints, ability to move more easily

Patient/family education
- Advise patient to report blurred vision, ringing, roaring in ears; may indicate toxicity
- Caution patient to avoid driving, other hazardous activities if **G** dizziness, drowsiness occurs, especially elderly
- Advise patient to report change in urine pattern, increased weight, edema, increased pain in joints, fever, blood in urine; indicate nephrotoxicity
- Inform patient that therapeutic effects may take up to 1 mo

---

Generic Names
celecoxib
diclofenac
etodolac
fenoprofen
flurbiprofen
⚷ ibuprofen
indomethacin
ketoprofen

ketorolac
meclofenamate
nabumetone
naproxen
piroxicam
rofecoxib
sulindac
tolmetin

OPIOID ANALGESICS

Action: These agents depress pain impulse transmission at the spinal cord level by interacting with opioid receptors. Products are divided into opiates and nonopiates.

Uses: Most products are used to control moderate to severe pain and are used before and after surgery.

Adverse effects: GI symptoms, including nausea, vomiting, anorexia, constipation, and cramps are the most common side effects. Other common side effects include lightheadedness, dizziness, sedation. Serious adverse reactions such as respiratory depression, respiratory arrest, circulatory depression, and increased intracranial pressure may result, but are less common and usually dose dependent.

Contraindications: Hypersensitive reactions occur frequently. Check for sensitivity before administering. These drugs should not be used if narcotic addiction is suspected, and they are also contraindicated in acute bronchial asthma and upper airway obstruction.

Precautions: Caution must be used when these products are given to persons with an addictive personality, since the possibility of addiction is so great. Also, persons with increased intracranial pressure may experience an even greater increase in intracranial pressure. Persons with severe heart disease, hepatic or renal disease, respiratory conditions, and seizure disorders should be monitored closely for worsening condition.

Pharmacokinetics: Onset of action is immediate by **IV** route and rapid by IM and PO routes. Peak occurs from 1-2 hr, depending on route, with a duration of 2-8 hr. These agents cross the placenta and appear in breast milk.

Interactions: Barbiturates, other narcotics, hypnotics, antipsychotics, or alcohol can increase CNS depression when taken with narcotics.

NURSING CONSIDERATIONS
Assessment

- Monitor I&O ratio; be alert for urinary retention, frequency, dysuria; drug should be discontinued if these occur
- Assess for respiratory dysfunction, including respiratory depression, rate, rhythm, character; notify prescriber if respirations are <12/min
- Assess for CNS changes: dizziness, drowsiness, hallucinations, euphoria, LOC, pupil reaction
- Assess for allergic reactions: rash, urticaria
- Assess for need for pain medication, use pain scoring

Nursing diagnoses
✓ Pain (uses)
✓ Impaired gas exchange (adverse reactions)

Implementation
- Give with antiemetic if nausea or vomiting occurs
- Give when pain is beginning to return; determine dosage interval by patient response
- Provide assistance with ambulation; patient should not be ambulating during drug peak

Evaluation
- Therapeutic response: decrease in pain

Patient/family education
- Advise patient to report any symptoms of CNS changes, allergic reactions, or shortness of breath
- Caution patient that physical dependency may result when used for extended periods
- Teach patient that withdrawal symptoms may occur, including nausea, vomiting, cramps, fever, faintness, anorexia
- Advise patient to avoid alcohol and other CNS depressants

Generic Names

alfentanil
buprenorphine
butorphanol
☠ codeine
fentanyl
fentanyl transdermal
hydromorphone
levorphanol tartrate

☠ meperidine
methadone HCl
☠ morphine
oxycodone
oxymorphone
pentazocine
propoxyphene
remifentanil
sufentanil

SALICYLATES

Action: Salicylates have analgesic, antipyretic, and antiinflammatory effects. The antiinflammatory and analgesic activities may be mediated through the inhibition of prostaglandin synthesis. Antipyretic action results from inhibition of the hypothalamic heat-regulating center.

Uses: The primary uses of salicylates are relief of mild to moderate pain and fever and in inflammatory conditions such as arthritis, thromboembolic disorders, and rheumatic fever.

Adverse effects: The most common side effects are GI symptoms and rash. Serious blood dyscrasias and hepatotoxicity may result when used for long periods at high doses. Tinnitus or impaired hearing may indicate that blood salicylate levels are reaching or exceeding the upper limit of the therapeutic range.

Contraindications: Hypersensitivity to salicylates is common. Check for sensitivity before administering. Persons with bleeding disorders, GI bleeding, and vitamin K deficiency should not use these products, since salicylates increase prothrombin time. Children should not use these products, since salicylates have been associated with Reye's syndrome.

Precautions: Caution is needed when salicylates are given to patients with anemia, hepatic or renal disease, or Hodgkin's disease. Caution should also be exercised in pregnancy and lactation.

Pharmacokinetics: Onset of action occurs in 15-30 min, with a peak of 1-2 hr and a duration up to 6 hr. These drugs are metabolized by the liver and excreted by the kidneys.

Interactions: Increased effects of anticoagulants, insulin, methotrexate, heparin, valproic acid, and oral sulfonylureas may occur when used with salicylates. Aspirin may decrease serum concentrations of nonsteroidal antiinflammatory agents.

NURSING CONSIDERATIONS
Assessment

- Monitor hepatic and renal studies: AST, ALT, bilirubin, creatinine, LDH, alkaline phosphatase, BUN if patient is on long-term therapy, since these products are metabolized and excreted by the liver and kidney
- Monitor blood studies: CBC, Hct, Hgb, and prothrombin time if patient is on long-term therapy, since these products increase the possibility of bleeding and blood dyscrasias
- Assess for hepatotoxicity: dark urine, clay-colored stools, jaundice skin and sclera, itching, abdominal pain, fever, diarrhea, which may occur with long-term use
- Assess for ototoxicity: tinnitus, ringing, roaring in ears; audiometric testing is needed before and after long-term therapy

Nursing diagnoses

- ✓ Pain (uses)
- ✓ Impaired physical mobility (uses)
- ✓ Activity intolerance (uses)
- ✓ Sensory-perceptual alteration: auditory (adverse reactions)
- ✓ Thermoregulation (uses)

Implementation
- Give with food or milk to decrease gastric irritation; give 30 min ac or 1 hr pc with a full glass of water

Evaluation
- Therapeutic response: decreased pain, fever

Patient/family education
- Advise patient that blood sugar levels should be monitored closely, if patient is diabetic
- Caution patient not to exceed recommended dosage; acute poisoning may result
- Inform patient that therapeutic response takes 2 wk in arthritis
- Caution patient to avoid use of alcohol, since GI bleeding may result
- Advise patient to notify prescriber if ringing in the ears or persistent GI pain occurs
- Advise patient to take with full glass of water to reduce risk of lodging in esophagus

---

Generic Names

⟳ aspirin
choline salicylate

magnesium salicylate
salsalate

THROMBOLYTICS

Action: Thrombolytics activate conversion of plasminogen to plasmin (fibrinolysin): plasmin is able to break down clots (fibrin).

Uses: Thrombolytics are used to treat deep vein thrombosis, pulmonary embolism, arterial thrombosis, arterial embolism, arteriovenous cannula occlusion, lysis of coronary artery thrombi after MI, acute evolving transmural MI.

Adverse effects: Serious adverse reactions include GI, GU, intracranial, and retroperitoneal bleeding, and anaphylaxis. The most common side effects are decreased Hct, urticaria, headache, and nausea.

Contraindications: Persons with hypersensitivity, active bleeding, intraspinal surgery, neoplasms of the CNS, ulcerative colitis/enteritis, severe hypertension, renal disease, hepatic disease, hypocoagulation, COPD, subacute bacterial endocarditis, rheumatic valvular disease, cerebral embolism/thrombosis/hemorrhage, intraarterial diagnostic procedure or surgery (10 days), and recent major surgery should not use these products.

Precautions: Caution should be used in arterial emboli from left side of heart and pregnancy.

Pharmacokinetics: Onset, peak, and duration vary widely among products. Most products are metabolized in the liver and excreted in urine.

Interactions: Please check individual monographs, since interactions vary widely among products.

NURSING CONSIDERATIONS
Assessment
- Monitor VS, B/P, pulse, respirations, neurologic signs, temp at least q4h, temp is an indicator of internal bleeding, cardiac rhythm following intracoronary administration; systolic pressure increase of >25 mm Hg should be reported to prescriber
- Assess for neurologic changes that may indicate intracranial bleeding
- Assess retroperitoneal bleeding: back pain, leg weakness, diminished pulses
- Assess for allergy: fever, rash, itching, chill; mild reaction may be treated with antihistamines
- Assess for bleeding during 1st hr of treatment: hematuria, hematemesis, bleeding from mucous membranes, epistaxis, ecchymosis
- Monitor blood studies (Hct, platelets, PTT, PT, TT, APTT) before starting therapy; PT or APTT must be less than 2 times control before starting therapy TT or PT q3-4h during treatment

Nursing diagnoses
☑ Risk for injury (uses)

Implementation
- Administer as soon as thrombi identified; not useful for thrombi over 1 wk old
- Administer cryoprecipitate or fresh, frozen plasma if bleeding occurs
- Administer loading dose at beginning of therapy; may require increased loading doses
- Give heparin after fibrinogen level is over 100 mg/dl; heparin inf to increase PTT to 1.5-2 times baseline for 3-7 days
- About 10% of patients have high streptococcal antibody titers requiring increased loading doses
- Give **IV** therapy using 0.8-μm filter
- Store reconstituted sol in refrigerator; discard after 24 hr
- Provide bed rest during entire course of treatment
- Avoid venous or arterial puncture, injection, rec temp
- Provide treatment of fever with acetaminophen or aspirin

- Apply pressure for 30 sec to minor bleeding sites; inform prescriber if this does not attain hemostasis; apply pressure dressing

Evaluation
- Therapeutic response: resolution of thrombosis, embolism

Generic Names

alteplase

anistreplase

○━ streptokinase

urokinase

THYROID HORMONES

Action: Increase metabolic rates, resulting in increased cardiac output, O_2 consumption, body temp, blood volume, growth, development at cellular level, respiratory rate, enzyme system activity

Uses: Products are used for thyroid replacement.

Adverse effects: The most common side effects include insomnia, tremors, tachycardia, palpitations, angina, dysrhythmias, weight loss, and changes in appetite. Serious adverse reactions include thyroid storm.

Contraindications: Persons with adrenal insufficiency, myocardial infarction, or thyrotoxicosis should not use these products.

G Precautions: The elderly and patients with angina pectoris, hypertension, ischemia, cardiac disease, or diabetes mellitus or insipidus should be watched closely when using these products. Caution should be used in pregnancy and lactation.

Pharmacokinetics: Pharmacokinetics vary widely among products; check specific monographs.

Interactions
- Impaired absorption of thyroid products may occur when administered with cholestyramine (separate by 4-5 hr)
- Increased effects of anticoagulants, sympathomimetics, tricyclic antidepressants, catecholamines may occur
- Decreased effects of digitalis, glycosides, insulin, hypoglycemics may occur
- Decreased effects of thyroid products may occur with estrogens

NURSING CONSIDERATIONS
Assessment
- Monitor B/P, pulse before each dose
- Monitor I&O ratio

- Monitor weight qd in same clothing, using same scale, at same time of day
- **P** Monitor height, growth rate if given to a child
- Monitor T_3, T_4, which are decreased; radioimmunoassay of TSH, which is increased; ratio uptake, which is decreased if patient is on too low a dosage of medication
- Assess for increased nervousness, excitability, irritability; may indicate too high doses of medication usually after 1-3 wk of treatment
- Assess for cardiac status: angina, palpitation, chest pain, change in VS

Nursing diagnoses
✓ Knowledge deficit (teaching)
✓ Noncompliance (teaching)
✓ Body image disturbance (adverse reactions)

Implementation
- Give at same time each day to maintain drug level
- Give only for hormone imbalances; not to be used for obesity, male infertility, menstrual conditions, lethargy
- Remove medication 4 wk before RAIU test

Evaluation
- Therapeutic response: absence of depression; increased weight loss, diuresis, pulse, appetite; absence of constipation, peripheral edema, cold intolerance, pale, cool, dry skin, brittle nails, alopecia, coarse hair, menorrhagia, night blindness, paresthesias, syncope, stupor, coma, rosy cheeks

Patient/family education
- **P** Advise patient that hair loss will occur in child and is temporary
- Advise patient to report excitability, irritability, anxiety; indicates overdose
- Caution patient not to switch brands unless directed by prescriber
- **P** Caution patient that hypothyroid child will show almost immediate behavior/personality change
- Advise patient that treatment drug is not to be taken to reduce weight
- Advise patient to avoid OTC preparations with iodine; read labels; to avoid iodine-containing food, iodinized salt, soybeans, tofu, turnips, some seafood, some bread

---

Generic Names
⟲ levothyroxine (T_4)   liotrix
liothyronine (T_3)   thyroid USP

VASODILATORS

Action: Vasodilators act in various ways. Please check individual monograph for specific action.

Uses: Vasodilators are used to treat intermittent claudication, arteriosclerosis obliterans, vasospasm and muscular ischemia, ischemic cerebral vascular disease, hypertension, and angina.

Adverse effects: The most common side effects are headache, nausea, hypotension or hypertension, and ECG changes.

Contraindications: Some drugs are contraindicated in acute MI, paroxysmal tachycardia, and thyrotoxicosis.

Precautions: Caution should be used in uncompensated heart disease or peptic ulcer disease.

Pharmacokinetics: Onset, peak, and duration vary widely among products. Most products are metabolized in the liver and excreted in urine.

Interactions: Please check individual monographs, since interactions vary widely among products.

NURSING CONSIDERATIONS
Assessment
• Assess bleeding time in individuals with bleeding disorders
• Assess cardiac status: B/P, pulse, rate, rhythm, character; watch for increasing pulse

Nursing diagnoses
☑Decreased cardiac output (uses)
☑Altered tissue perfusion: cardiovascular/pulmonary (uses)
☑Knowledge deficit (teaching)

Implementation
• Give with meals to reduce GI symptoms
• Store in tight container at room temp

Evaluation
• Therapeutic response: ability to walk without pain, increased temp in extremities, increased pulse volume

Patient/family education
• Inform patient that medication is not cure, may need to be taken continuously
• Advise patient that it is necessary to quit smoking to prevent excessive vasoconstriction
• Advise patient that improvement may be sudden, but usually occurs gradually over several wk

- Instruct patient to report headache, weakness, increased pulse, since drug may need to be decreased or discontinued
- Instruct patient to avoid hazardous activities until stabilized on medication; dizziness may occur

---

Generic Names

amyl nitrite

dipyridamole

hydralazine

minoxidil

papaverine

tolazoline

VITAMINS

Action: Action varies widely among products and classes; check specific monographs.

Uses: Vitamins are used to correct and prevent vitamin deficiencies.

Adverse effects: There is an absence of side effects or adverse reactions with the water-soluble vitamins (C, B). However, fat-soluble vitamins (A, D, E, K) may accumulate in the body and cause adverse reactions (refer to specific monographs).

Contraindications: Hypersensitive reactions may occur, and allergies should be identified before these products are given.

Pharmacokinetics: Onset, peak, and duration vary widely among products; check individual monograph for specific information.

NURSING CONSIDERATIONS
Nursing diagnoses

☑ Altered nutrition, less than body requirements (uses)

Implementation
- Give PO with food for better absorption
- Store in tight, light-resistant container

Evaluation
- Therapeutic response: absence of vitamin deficiency

Patient/family education
- Advise patient not to take more than prescribed amount

Generic Names

Fat-soluble:
phytonadione
vitamin A
vitamin D
vitamin E

Water-soluble:
ascorbic acid (C)

pyridoxine (B_6)
riboflavin (B_2)
thiamine (B_1)

Miscellaneous:
multivitamins

Appendix A

Selected New Drugs

abacavir (℞)
(aba-ka′veer)
Ziagen
Func. class.: Antiviral
Chem. class.: Nucleoside analog
Pregnancy category C

Action: A synthetic, nucleoside analog with inhibitory action against HIV. Inhibits replication of HIV by incorporating into cellular DNA by viral reverse transcriptase, thereby terminating the cellular DNA chain

➡ **Therapeutic Outcome:** Decreased symptoms of HIV

Uses: In combination with other antiretroviral agents for HIV-1 infection

Dosage and routes
Adult: PO 300 mg bid with other antiretrovirals

🄿 *Adolescents and children ≥3 mo:* PO 8 mg/kg bid, max 300 mg bid with other antiretrovirals

Available forms: Tabs 300 mg; oral sol 20 mg/ml

Adverse effects
CNS: Fever, headache, malaise, insomnia, paresthesia
GI: Nausea, vomiting, diarrhea, anorexia, cramps, abdominal pain
HEMA: Granulocytopenia, anemia
INTEG: Rash, **fatal hypersensitivity reactions,** urticaria

META: **Lactic acidosis**
RESP: Dyspnea

Contraindications: Hypersensitivity

Precautions: Granulocyte count <1000/mm³ or Hgb <9.5 g/dl, pregnancy **C**, lacta-🄿 tion, children, severe renal disease, severe hepatic function

Pharmacokinetics	
Absorption	Well absorbed (PO)
Distribution	50% plasma protein binding
Metabolism	To inactive metabolite
Excretion	Kidneys, feces
Half-life	1½-2 hr

Pharmacodynamics
Unknown

Interactions
Individual drugs
Alcohol: ↑ abacavir levels

NURSING CONSIDERATIONS
Assessment
• Assess for lactic acidosis and severe hepatomegaly with steatosis
⬥• Assess for fatal hypersensitivity reactions: fever, rash, nausea, vomiting, diarrhea, abdominal discomfort; treatment should be discontinued and not restarted
⬥• Assess for pancreatitis: abdominal pain, nausea, vomiting, elevated liver enzymes; drug should be discontinued because condition can be fatal
• Monitor CBC, differential, platelet count qmo; withhold

drug if WBC is <4000 or plate-let count is <75,000; notify prescriber of results
• Monitor renal function studies; BUN, serum uric acid, urine CrCl before, during, therapy; these may be elevated throughout treatment
• Monitor temp q4h, may indicate beginning infection
• Monitor liver function tests before, during therapy (bilirubin, AST, ALT, amylase, alkaline phosphatase prn or qmo)

Nursing diagnoses
☑ Infection, risk for (uses)
☑ Injury, risk for physical injury (adverse reactions)
☑ Knowledge deficit (teaching)

Implementation
PO route
• Give on empty stomach, q12h around the clock
• Give in combination with other antiretrovirals with food

Patient/family education
• Advise patient to report signs of infection: increased temp, sore throat, flu symptoms; to avoid crowds and those with known infections
• Instruct patient to report signs of anemia: fatigue, headache, faintness, shortness of breath, irritability
• Advise patient to report bleeding; avoid use of razors or commercial mouthwash
• Inform patient that drug is not a cure, but will control symptoms
• Inform patient that major toxicities may necessitate discontinuing drug
• Instruct patient to use contraception during treatment
• Caution patient to avoid OTC products or other medications without approval of prescriber

• Caution patient not to have any sexual contact without use of a condom, needles should not be shared, blood from infected individual should not come in contact with another's mucus membranes
• Give Medication Guide and Warning Card; discuss points on guide

Evaluation
Positive therapeutic outcome
• Decreased infection; symptoms of HIV

---

alitretinoin (Rx)
(al-ee-tret'i-noyn)
Panretin
Func. class.: Retinoid, 2nd generation
Pregnancy category   D

Action: Controls cellular differentiation and proliferation of neoplastic and healthy cells

➡ **Therapeutic Outcome:** Decreased size and number of lesions

Uses: Kaposi's sarcoma cutaneous lesions

Dosage and routes
Adult: TOP apply enough gel to cover lesions with a generous coating, allow to dry for 3-5 mins before covering with clothing, do not apply near mucosal areas, apply as long as benefit occurs

Available forms: Top gel 0.1%

Adverse effects
INTEG: Rash, stinging, pain, warmth, redness, erythema, blistering, crusting, peeling, dermatitis

Contraindications: Hypersen-

☑ Herb/drug   Ⓢ Do Not Crush   ◆ Alert   ↻ Key Drug   Ⓖ Geriatric   Ⓟ Pediatric

sitivity to retinoids, pregnancy **D**
Precautions: Lactation, eczema, sunburn, elderly, cutaneous T-cell lymphoma

Pharmacokinetics

Absorption	Small amounts
Distribution	Unknown
Metabolism	Unknown
Excretion	Kidneys
Half-life	Unknown

Pharmacodynamics

Unknown

Interactions
Individual drugs
DEET: Do not use around DEET (an insect repellant)

NURSING CONSIDERATIONS
Assessment
• Assess part of body involved, including time involved, what helps or aggravates condition, cysts, dryness, itching
Nursing diagnoses
✓ Skin integrity, impaired (uses)
✓ Body image disturbances (uses)
✓ Knowledge deficit (teaching)
Implementation
• Apply bid initially to lesions, can be increased to tid-qid according to tolerance, discontinue for a few days if severe reactions occur
• Store at room temp
• Wash hands after application
Patient/family education
• Instruct patient to avoid application on normal skin, and to avoid getting cream in eyes, nose, other mucous membranes
• Advise patient to avoid sunlight, sunlamps or to use protective clothing or sunscreen to prevent burns

• Advise patient that treatment may cause warmth, stinging; dryness; peeling will occur
• Caution patient that drug does not cure condition; only relieves symptoms; that therapeutic results may be seen in 2-3 wk but may not be optimal until after 6 wk
Evaluation
Positive therapeutic outcome
• Decrease in size and number of lesions

aminolevulinic acid (℞)
(a-meen'oh-lev-uu-lin-ik)
Levulan KerasticK
Func. class.: Photochemotherapy
Pregnancy category   **C**

Action: ALA is the 1st step resulting in heme synthesis. A protoporphyrin IX precursor that is a photosensitizer
➤**Therapeutic Outcome:** Decreased signs/symptoms of non-hyperkeratotic actinic keratoses

Uses: Face/scalp non-hyperkeratotic actinic keratoses
Dosage and routes
Adult: TOP 1 application of solution and 1 dose of illumination/treatment site × 8wk

Available forms: Top solution 20% (354 mg)
Adverse effects
INTEG: Crusting, ulceration, pain, itching, bleeding, pustules, hypopigmentation, hyperpigmentation
Contraindications: Hypersensitivity to porphyrins

Precautions: Pregnancy **C**, lactation, inherited or acquired coagulation defects

Pharmacokinetics
Absorption	Unknown
Distribution	Unknown
Metabolism	Unknown
Excretion	Unknown
Half-life	Unknown

Pharmacodynamics
Unknown

Interactions
Drug classifications
Phenothiazines: may ↑ photosensitivity
Sulfonylureas: may ↑ photosensitivity
Tetracyclines: may ↑ photosensitivity
Thiazides: may ↑ photosensitivity

NURSING CONSIDERATIONS
Assessment
• Assess part of body involved, including time involved, what helps or aggravates condition

Nursing diagnoses
☑ Skin integrity, impaired (uses)
☑ Body image disturbances (uses)
☑ Knowledge deficit (teaching)

Implementation
• Prepare ALA top sol by holding applicator cap pointing up, crush the bottom ampule containing sol vehicle by applying pressure to position A on cardboard sleeve; crush top ampule containing ALA powder by applying pressure to position B on sleeve; hold applicator between thumb and forefinger, point away from the face, shake gently for about 3 min to dissolve powder; sol is applied to lesions after cleaning and drying

Patient/family education
• Advise patient to avoid sunlight, sunlamps or to use protective clothing or sunscreen to prevent burns
• Advise patient that treatment may cause burning, crusting
• After application, patient is told to return the next day for treatment

Evaluation
Positive therapeutic outcome
• Decrease in size and number of lesions

---

amprenavir (℞)
(am-pren′-a-ver)
Agenerase
Func. class.: Antiviral
Chem. class.: Protease inhibitor

Pregnancy category   C

Action: Inhibits human immunodeficiency virus (HIV) protease

⇒**Therapeutic Outcome:** Prevents maturation of the infectious virus

Uses: HIV in combination with other antiretroviral agents

Dosage and routes
Adult: PO (cap) 1200 mg bid
P *Child 13-16 yr:* PO (cap) 1200 mg bid
P *Child 4-12 yr or wt <50 kg:* PO (cap) 20 mg/kg qd or 15 mg/kg tid, max 2400 mg; PO (oral sol) 22.5 mg/kg bid or 17 mg/kg tid qd, max 2800 mg

Available forms: Cap 50, 150 mg; oral sol 15 mg/ml

Adverse effects
CNS: Paresthesia
ENDO: New onset diabetes,

hyperglycemia, exacerbation of preexisting diabetes mellitus
GI: Diarrhea, abdominal pain, nausea
HEMA: Acute hemolytic anemia
INTEG: Rash, **Stevens-Johnson syndrome**

Contraindications: Hypersensitivity

Precautions: Liver disease, pregnancy **C**, lactation, children, hemophilia, sulfonamide sensitivity, elderly

Pharmacokinetics	
Absorption	Unknown
Distribution	Unknown
Metabolism	Unknown
Excretion	Unknown
Half-life	Unknown

Pharmacodynamics
Unknown

Interactions
Individual drugs
Amiodarone: Serious/life threatening reactions
Carbamazepine: ↓ amprenavir levels
Cimetidine: ↑ amprenavir levels
Clarithromycin: ↑ amprenavir levels
Erythromycin: ↑ amprenavir levels
Indinavir: ↑ amprenavir levels
Itraconazole: ↑ amprenavir levels
Lidocaine: Serious/life threatening reactions
Loratadine: Do not use together
Midazolam: Do not use together
Phenobarbital: ↓ amprenavir levels
Quinidine: Serious/life threatening reactions

Rifamycin: ↓ amprenavir levels
Ritonavir: ↑ amprenavir levels
Drug classifications
Antacids: Decreased amprenavir levels
Ergots: Do not use together
Tricyclics: Serious life threatening reactions
Lab test interferences
Interference: CPK, glucose (low)
⊘*Herb/drug*
St. John's Wort: ↓ amprenavir

NURSING CONSIDERATIONS
Assessment
• Assess signs of infection, anemia
• Monitor liver studies: ALT, AST
• Monitor C&S before drug therapy; drug may be taken as soon as culture is taken; repeat C&S after treatment; determine the presence of other sexually transmitted diseases
• Assess bowel pattern before, during treatment; if severe abdominal pain with bleeding occurs, drug should be discontinued; monitor hydration
• Assess skin eruptions, rash, urticaria, itching
• Assess allergies before treatment, reaction of each medication; place allergies on chart

Nursing diagnoses
☑ Infection, risk for (uses)
☑ Knowledge deficit (teaching)

Implementation
• Caps and oral sol are not interchangeable on a mg/mg basis

Patient/family education
• Advise patient to take as prescribed with or without

food; if dose is missed, take as soon as remembered up to 1 hr before next dose; do not double dose

• Advise patient that drug must be taken in equal intervals around the clock to maintain blood levels for duration of therapy

• Instruct patient that caps and sol are not interchangeable

Evaluation
Positive therapeutic outcome
• Prevention of spread of infection

---

bexarotene (R)
(bex-air'-oo-teen)
Targretin
Func. class.: Retinoid, 2nd generation

Pregnancy category   X

Action: Selectively binds and activates retinoid X receptors (RXRs) that are partially responsible for cellular proliferation and differentiation. Inhibits some tumor cells

➡ **Therapeutic Outcome:** Decreased size and number of lesions

Uses: Cutaneous T-cell lymphoma

Investigational uses: Breast cancer

Dosage and routes
Adult: PO 300 mg/day/mm², may increase to 400 mg/day with proper monitoring

Available forms: Cap 75 mg

Adverse effects
CNS: Headache, fatigue, lethargy
GI: Nausea, abdominal pain, diarrhea, **acute pancreatitis**

HEMA: **Leukopenia, neutropenia, anemia**
INTEG: Rash, asthenia, dry skin
SYST: Infection, hypothyroidism

Contraindications: Hypersensitivity to retinoids, pregnancy **X**

Precautions: Lactation, sunburn, hepatic, renal disease

Pharmacokinetics	
Absorption	Unknown
Distribution	Unknown
Metabolism	Unknown
Excretion	Kidneys
Half-life	Unknown

Pharmacodynamics
Unknown

Interactions
Individual drugs
Vit A: limit intake to ≤15,000 IU/day
Drug classifications
Azole antiinfectives: ↑ bexarotene levels
Barbiturates: ↓ bexarotene levels
Rifampins: ↓ bexarotene levels
Drug/food
Grapefruit juice: ↑ bexarotene levels

NURSING CONSIDERATIONS
Assessment
• Assess part of body involved, including time involved, what helps or aggravates condition, cysts, dryness, itching
• Assess cholesterol, HDL, triglycerides; these may be elevated
• Monitor CBC for leukopenia, neutropenia, anemia

Nursing diagnoses
☑ Skin integrity, impaired (uses)
☑ Body image disturbances (uses)
☑ Knowledge deficit (teaching)

☑ Herb/drug   🚫 Do Not Crush   ◆ Alert   ⟜ Key Drug   Ⓖ Geriatric   Ⓟ Pediatric

Implementation
• Administer with food

Patient/family education
• Advise patient to avoid sunlight, sunlamps or to use protective clothing or sunscreen to prevent burns

Evaluation
Positive therapeutic outcome
• Decrease in size and number of lesions

---

cilostazol
(sil-oo-stay'zole)
Pletal
Func. class.: Platelet aggregation inhibitor
Chem. class.: Quinolinone derivative

Pregnancy category   C

Action: Inhibits cellular phosphodiesterase. Reversibly inhibits thrombin, ADP, collagen

➔ Therapeutic Outcome: Increased walking distance

Uses: Intermittent claudication

Dosage and routes
Adult: PO 100 mg bid taken ≥30 mins ac or 2 hrs pc breakfast and dinner or 50 mg bid, if using drugs that inhibit CYP3A4; 12 wks of treatment may be needed

Available forms: Tab 50, 100 mg

Adverse effects
CNS: Dizziness, vertigo, anxiety, insomnia, neuralgia
CV: Palpitations, tachycardia, **atrial fibrillation/flutter, cerebral infarct, cerebral ischemia, CHF, heart arrest, MI, nodal dysrhythmia**
GI: Nausea, vomiting, diarrhea, GI disorder, colitis, cholelithiasis, ulcer, esophagitis, gastritis
HEMA: **Bleeding (epistaxis, hematuria, conjunctival hemorrhage, GI bleeding), agranulocytosis, neutropenia, thrombocytopenia**
INTEG: Rash
MISC: Back pain, headache, infection, myalgia, peripheral edema, chills, fever, malaise, diabetes mellitus
RESP: Cough, pharyngitis, rhinitis

Contraindications: Hypersensitivity, CHF, active liver disease, blood dyscrasias

Precautions: Past liver disease, **G** renal disease, elderly, pregnancy **P** C, lactation, children, increased bleeding risk

Pharmacokinetics	
Absorption	Unknown
Distribution	95%-98% protein binding
Metabolism	Hepatic extensively by cytochrome P450 enzymes
Excretion	Urine (74%), feces (20%)
Half-life	11-13 hrs

Pharmacodynamics
Unknown

Interactions
Individual drugs
Aspirin: may ↑ bleeding tendencies
Diltiazem: ↑ cilostazol levels
Erythromycin: ↑ cilostazol levels
Fluconazole: ↑ cilostazol levels
Fluoxetine: ↑ cilostazol levels
Fluvoxamine: ↑ cilostazol levels
Itraconazole: ↑ cilostazol levels
Ketoconazole: ↑ cilostazol levels
Miconazole: ↑ cilostazol levels

Nefazodone: ↑ cilostazol levels
Omeprazole: ↑ cilostazol levels
Sertraline: ↑ cilostazol levels
Drug classifications
Anticoagulants: May ↑ bleeding tendencies
Macrolides: ↑ cilostazol levels
Food/drug
• Do not use with grapefruit juice

NURSING CONSIDERATIONS
Assessment
• Assess for underlying CV disease since cardiovascular risk is great
• Assess for CV lesions with repeated oral administration
• Monitor liver function studies: AST, ALT, bilirubin, creatinine
• Monitor blood studies: CBC, Hct, Hgb, pro-time if patient is on long-term therapy; thrombocytopenia, neutropenia may occur

Nursing diagnoses
☑ Injury, risk for (uses)
☑ Knowledge deficit (teaching)

Implementation
• Give bid ≥30 mins ac or 2 hrs pc

Patient/family education
• Advise patient that blood work will be necessary during treatment
• Advise patient to report any unusual bleeding to prescriber
• Caution patient to report side effects such as diarrhea, skin rashes, subcutaneous bleeding
• Teach patient that effects may take 2-4 wks, treatment of up to 12 wks may be required for necessary effect
• Teach patient about poten-

tial CV risks in patients with cardiac disease
• Advise patient to take ≥30 mins ac or 2 hrs pc
• Advise patient that reading patient package insert is necessary

Evaluation
Positive therapeutic outcome
• Increased walking distance

---

coagulation factor VIIa, recombinant (℞)
NovoSeven
Func. class.: Antihemophilic

Pregnancy category   C

Action: Promotes hemostasis by activating the intrinsic pathway of coagulation

Uses: Bleeding in hemophilia A or B, with inhibitors to Factor VIII or IX

Dosage and routes
Adult: **IV** BOL 90 μg/kg q2h until hemostasis occurs, or until therapy is deemed to be inadequate; post hemostatic doses q3-6h may be required

Available forms: Lyophilized powder 1.2 mg/vial (1200 μg/vial) recombinant human coagulation factor VIIa (rFVIIa); 4.8 mg/vial (4800 μg/vial) recombinant human coagulation factor VIIa (rFVIIa)

Adverse effects
CNS: Fever, headache
INTEG: Pain, redness at inj site, pruritus, purpura, rash
SYST: **Hemorrhage NOS, hemarthrosis, fibrinogen plasma decreased,** hypertension, bradycardia, **DIC, coagulation disorder, thrombosis**

☑ Herb/drug ⑤ Do Not Crush ◆ Alert ⟨ᴛᴛ Key Drug ⑥ Geriatric ⑫ Pediatric

Contraindications: Hypersensitivity to this product or mouse, hamster, or bovine products

Precautions: Pregnancy **C**, lactation, children

Pharmacokinetics	
Half-life	2-3 hr

Pharmacodynamics	
Unknown	

Interactions
Individual drugs
Activated prothrombin complex concentrate: Do not use together
Prothrombin complex concentrate: Do not use together

NURSING CONSIDERATIONS
Assessment
• Assess VS, B/P, pulse, respirations, neurologic signs, temperature at least q4h, temperature 104° F (40° C) or indicators of internal bleeding, cardiac rhythm
• Monitor pro time, aPTT, plasma FVII clotting
• Monitor for thrombosis, dose should be reduced or stopped

Implementation
IV route
• Bring to room temp; for 1.2 mg vial/2.2 ml sterile water for inj; 4.8 mg vial/8.5 ml sterile water for injection; remove caps from stop, cleanse stopper with alcohol, allow to dry, draw back plunger of sterile syringe and allow air into syringe, insert needle of syringe into sterile water for inj, inject the air and withdraw amount required, insert syringe needle with diluent into drug vial, aim

to side so liquid runs down vial wall, gently swirl until dissolved, use within 3 hrs, give by bol over 3-5 mins
• Do not admix, keep refrigerated until ready to use, avoid sunlight

Evaluation
Positive therapeutic outcome
• Therapeutic response: hemostasis

---

denileukin diftitox (℞)
(den-ih-loo'kin dif'tih-tox)
Ontak
Func. class.: Antineoplastic misc agent
Pregnancy category C

Action: A recombinant DNA-derived cytotoxic protein. Inhibits cellular protein synthesis

Therapeutic Outcome: Prevention of rapidly growing malignant cells

Uses: Cutaneous T-cell lymphoma that express CD25 component of the IL-2 receptor

Dosage and routes
Adult: **IV** 9-18 µg/kg/day given for 5 days q21 days, give over ≥15 mins

Available forms: Sol for inj, frozen 150 µg/ml

Adverse effects
CNS: Dizziness, paresthesia, nervousness, confusion, insomnia
CV: Hypotension, vasodilation, tachycardia, thrombosis, hypertension, dysrhythmia
GI: Nausea, anorexia, vomiting, diarrhea, constipation, dyspepsia, dysphagia

---

GU: **Hematuria,** albuminuria, pyuria, creatinine increase
HEMA: **Thrombocytopenia, leukopenia,** anemia
INTEG: *Rash, pruritus, sweating*
META: Hypoalbuminemia, edema, hypocalcemia, weight decrease, dehydration, hypokalemia
MISC: Fever, chills, asthenia, infection, pain, headache, chest pain, flu-like symptoms
MS: Myalgia, arthralgia
RESP: Dyspnea, cough, pharyngitis, rhinitis

Contraindications: Hypersensitivity to denileukin, diphtheria toxin, interleukin-2

Precautions: Radiation therapy, pregnancy **C,** elderly, lactation, children

Pharmacokinetics

Absorption	Complete bioavailability (**IV**)
Distribution	Widely distributed; concentrates in liver/kidneys
Metabolism	Proteolytic degradation
Excretion	Unknown
Half-life	Unknown

Pharmacodynamics

Unknown

Interactions
Individual drugs
Radiation: ↑ toxicity, bone marrow suppression
Drug classifications
Antineoplastics: ↑ toxicity, bone marrow suppression
Bone marrow-suppressing drugs: ↑ bone marrow suppression
Live vaccines: ↑ adverse reactions, ↓ antibody reaction

NURSING CONSIDERATIONS
Assessment
• Assess symptoms indicating severe allergic reaction: rash, pruritus, urticaria, purpuric skin lesions, itching, flushing; drug should be discontinued
• Assess for vascular leak syndrome after 2 wk of treatment: hypotension, edema, hypoalbuminemia; monitor weight, B/P, serum albumin, edema
• Obtain CD25 expression on skin biopsy samples
• Monitor CBC, differential, platelet count weekly; withhold drug if WBC count is <4000/mm³ or platelet count is <100,000/mm³
• Monitor renal function studies: BUN, creatinine, urine CrCl before and during therapy; I&O ratio; report fall in urine output to <30 ml/hr
• Monitor temp q4h (may indicate beginning of infection)
• Monitor liver function tests before and during therapy (bilirubin, AST, ALT, LDH) as needed or monthly; note jaundice skin or sclera, dark urine, clay-colored stools, itchy skin, abdominal pain, fever, diarrhea; hepatoxicity can be serious and fatal
• Assess for bleeding: hematuria, stool guaiac, bruising or petechiae, mucosa or orifices q8h; check for inflammation of mucosa, breaks in skin

Nursing diagnoses
☑ Injury, risk for (adverse reactions)
☑ Body image disturbance (adverse reactions)
☑ Infection, risk for (adverse reactions)
☑ Knowledge deficit (teaching)

☒ Herb/drug ◌ Do Not Crush ⬥ Alert ⊶ Key Drug 🄶 Geriatric 🄿 Pediatric

Implementation

- Give fluids **IV** or PO before chemotherapy to hydrate patient
- Give antiemetic 30-60 min before giving drug to prevent vomiting, and prn; antibiotics for prophylaxis of infection
- Provide liquid diet: carbonated beverages; gelatin may be added if patient is not nauseated or vomiting
- Prepare and hold sol in plastic syringes or soft plastic **IV** bags only
- Draw calculated dose from vial, inject into empty **IV** infusion bag, for each 1 ml of drug removed from vial, no more than 9 ml of sterile saline without preservative should be added to **IV** bag; infuse over ≥15 mins; do not give by bolus; do not admix with other drugs; do not use a filter
- Use within 6 hr, discard unused portions
- Watch for extravasation; give 3-5 ml of mixture of 4 ml sodium thiosulfate 10% plus 5 ml sterile water SC as prescribed

Patient/family education

- Teach patient to avoid use of products containing aspirin or NSAIDs, razors, commercial mouthwash, since bleeding may occur; to report symptoms of bleeding (hematuria, tarry stools)
- Instruct patient to report signs of anemia (fatigue, headache, irritability, faintness, shortness of breath)
- Caution patient not to have any vaccinations without the advice of prescriber; serious reactions can occur
- Advise patient contraception is needed during treatment and for several months after the completion of therapy; drug has teratogenic properties

Evaluation

Positive therapeutic outcome

- Prevention of rapid division of malignant cells

---

dexmedetomidine (℞)
(deks-med-ee-tome′a-dine)
Precedex
Func. class.: Sedative, alpha₂ adrenoceptor agonist
Pregnancy category   C

Action: Produces $alpha_2$ activity as seen at low and moderate doses; also, $alpha_1$ at high doses

Uses: Sedation in mechanically ventilated, intubated patients in ICU

Dosage and routes

Adult: **IV** Loading dose of 1 μg/kg over 10 mins, then 0.2-0.7 μg/kg/hr, do not use for over 24 hrs

Available forms: Inj 100 μg/ml

Adverse effects

CV: Bradycardia, hypotension, hypertension, **atrial fibrillation, infarction**
GI: Nausea, thirst
GU: Oliguria
HEMA: Leukocytosis, anemia
RESP: **Pulmonary edema, pleural effusion, hypoxia**

Contraindications: Hypersensitivity

Precautions: Elderly, renal disease, respiratory depression, severe respiratory disorders, cardiac dysrhythmias, pregnancy **C**, lactation, children

---

Pharmacokinetics

Half-life   8 min

Interactions
Drug classifications
Anesthetics: ↑ CNS depression
Antipsychotics: ↑ CNS depression
Opiates: ↑ CNS depression
Sedative/hypnotics: ↑ CNS depression
Skeletal muscle relaxants: ↑ CNS depression

NURSING CONSIDERATIONS
Assessment
• Assess injection site: phlebitis, burning, stinging
• Monitor ECG for changes: atrial fibrillation
• Assess CNS changes: movement, jerking, tremors, dizziness, LOC, pupil reaction
• Assess respiratory dysfunction: respiratory depression, character, rate, rhythm; notify prescriber if respirations are <10/min

Implementation
IV route
• Give after diluting with D_5W 0.9% NaCl, withdraw 2 ml of drug and add to 48 ml of 0.9% NaCl to a total of 50 ml, shake to mix well
• Give only with resuscitative equipment available
• Give only by qualified persons trained in management of ICU sedation

Solution compatibilities: LR, D_5W, 0.9% NaCl, 20% mannitol

Additive compatibilities:
Atracurium, atropine, etomidate, fentanyl, glycopyrrolate, midazolam, mivacurium, morphine, pancuronium, phenyl-

ephrine, succinyl choline, thiopental, vecuronium
• Provide safety measures: side rails, nightlight, call bell within easy reach

Evaluation
• Therapeutic response: induction of sedation

---

dofetilide
(doff-ee-till'-lide)
Tikosyn
Func. class.: Antidysrhythmic (Class III)
Pregnancy category   C

Action: Blocks cardiac ion channel carrying the rapid component of delayed potassium current, no effect on sodium channels

➡ **Therapeutic Outcome:**
Absence of atrial fibrillation

Uses: Atrial fibrillation, flutter

Dosage and routes
Adult: PO initial dose for CrCl > 60 mg/ml 500 μg bid; CrCl 40-60 mg/min 250 μg bid; CrCl 20-39 mg/min 125 μg bid; CrCl <20 mg/min do not use 2-3 hr after initial dose Measure QTc, if >15% compared with baseline, then give ½ initial dose except 125 μg bid, give same dose

Available forms: Caps 125, 250, 500 μg

Adverse effects
CNS: Syncope, dizziness, headache
CV: Hypotension, postural hypotension, bradycardia, chest pain, angina, PVCs, substernal pressure, precipitation of angina
GI: Nausea, vomiting, severe diarrhea, anorexia

Contraindications: Hypersensitivity, digitalis toxicity, aortic stenosis, pulmonary **P** hypertension, children

Precautions: Renal disease, pregnancy **C**, lactation

Pharmacokinetics	
Absorption	>90%
Distribution	Unknown
Metabolism	Not metabolized
Excretion	Kidneys 80%
Half-life	Unknown

Pharmacodynamics
Unknown

Interactions
Individual drugs
Cimetidine: Do not use together
Ketoconazole: Do not use together
Prochlorperazine: Do not use together
Trimethoprim/ sulfamethoxazole: Do not use together
Verapamil: Do not use together

NURSING CONSIDERATIONS
Assessment
• Monitor ECG continuously to determine drug effectiveness; measure PR, QRS, QT intervals; check for PVCs, other dysrhythmias; monitor B/P continuously
• Prior to administration, QTc must be determined using an average of 5-10 beats, if the QTc >440 msec or 500 msec in ventricular conduction abnormalities, do not use; do not use if heart rate <60 bpm
• Prior to dosing, identify CrCl, using CrCl to determine dosing

Nursing diagnoses
✓ Cardiac output, decreased (uses)
✓ Gas exchange, impaired (adverse reactions)
✓ Knowledge deficit (teaching)

Implementation
PO route
• Give for 3 days with patient hospitalized

Patient/family education
• Notify prescriber if fast heartbeats with fainting or dizziness occur
• Notify all prescribers of all medications and supplements taken

Evaluation
Positive therapeutic outcome
• Decreased atrial fibrillation

doxercalciferol (R̶)
(dox-er-kal′-cif-er-ol)
Hectorol
Func. class.: Parathyroid agent (calcium regulator)
Chem. class.: Vitamin D hormone
Pregnancy category   C

➡ **Therapeutic Outcome:** Calcium at normal level

Uses: To lower high parathyroid hormone levels in patients undergoing chronic kidney dialysis

Dosage and routes
Adult: PO 10 μg 3×/wk at dialysis

Available forms: Caps 2.5 μg

Adverse effects
CNS: Drowsiness, headache, lethargy
GI: Nausea, diarrhea, vomiting, anorexia, dry mouth, constipation, cramps, metallic taste

GU: Polyuria, hypercalciuria, hyperphosphatemia, hematuria
MS: Myalgia, arthralgia, decreased bone development
RESP: SOB

Contraindications: Hypersensitivity, hyperphosphatemia, hypercalcemia, vitamin D toxicity

Precautions: Pregnancy **C**, renal calculi, lactation, CV disease

Pharmacokinetics	
Absorption	Unknown
Distribution	Unknown
Metabolism	Unknown
Excretion	Unknown
Half-life	Unknown

Pharmacodynamics
Unknown

Interactions
Individual drugs
Cholestyramine: ↓ doxercalciferol levels, do not use together
Magnesium antacids: Do not use together
Mineral oil: ↓ doxercalciferol levels, do not use together

NURSING CONSIDERATIONS
Assessment
• Assess GI symptoms, polyuria, flushing, head swelling, tingling, headache; may indicate hypercalcemia
• Identify nutritional status; check diet for sources of vitamin D (milk, some seafood), calcium (dairy products, dark green vegetables), phosphates
• Monitor BUN, creatinine, uric acid, chloride electrolytes, urine pH, urinary calcium, magnesium, phosphate, urinalysis (calcium should be kept at 9-10 mg/dl; vitamin D 50-

135 IU/dl), alkaline phosphatase baseline and q3-6 mo
◆• Assess for increased drug level, since toxic reactions occur rapidly; have calcium chloride on hand if calcium level drops too low; check for tetany

Nursing diagnoses
☑ Injury, risk for (adverse reactions)
☑ Pain, chronic (uses)
☑ Knowledge deficit (teaching)

Implementation
• Give with meals for GI symptoms
🚫• Do not crush or chew caps

Patient/family education
• Teach patient the symptoms of hypercalcemia and about foods rich in calcium
• Advise patient to avoid products with sodium: cured meats, dairy products, cold cuts, olives, beets, pickles, soups, meat tenderizers in chronic renal failure
• Advise patient to avoid products with potassium: oranges, bananas, dried fruit, peas, dark green leafy vegetables, milk, melons, beans in chronic renal failure
• Advise patient to avoid OTC products containing calcium, potassium, or sodium in chronic renal failure
• Instruct patient to avoid all preparations containing Vit D
• Instruct patient to monitor weight weekly

Evaluation
Positive therapeutic outcome
• Calcium levels 9-10 mg/dl

---

entacapone (℞)
(en-ta'-ka-pone)
Comtan
Func. class.: Antiparkinsonian agent
Chem. class.: COMT
Pregnancy category   C

Action: Inhibits COMT (catecho-O-methyltransferase) and alters the plasma pharmacokinetics of levodopa. Given with levodopa/carbidopa

➡ **Therapeutic Outcome:** Decreased symptoms of Parkinson's disease (involuntary movements)

Uses: Parkinsonism in those experiencing end of dose, decreased effect

Dosage and routes
Adult: PO 200 mg given with carbidopa/levodopa, max 1600 mg/day

Available forms: Tabs 200 mg film coated

Adverse effects
CNS: Involuntary choreiform movements, dyskinesia, hypokinesia, hyperkinesia, hand tremors, fatigue, headache, anxiety, twitching, numbness, weakness, confusion, agitation, nightmares, psychosis, hallucinations, hypomania, severe depression, dizziness
CV: Orthostatic hypotension
GI: Nausea, vomiting, anorexia, abdominal distress, dry mouth, flatulence, dyspepsia, gastritis, GI disorder, *diarrhea, constipation*
INTEG: Rash, sweating, alopecia
MISC: Dark urine, back pain, taste perversion, dyspnea, purpura, fatigue, asthenia, infection-bacterial

Contraindications: Hypersensitivity

Precautions: Renal disease, hepatic disease, pregnancy **C,** affective disorders, psychosis, lactation, children

Pharmacokinetics	
Absorption	Well absorbed
Distribution	Protein binding 98%
Metabolism	Liver extensively
Excretion	Kidneys, feces; breast milk
Half-life	of levodopa is extended

Pharmacodynamics
Unknown

Interactions
Individual drugs
Ampicillin: ↓ excretion
Apomorphine: ↑ CV reactions, avoid use
Bitolterol: ↑ CV reactions, avoid use
Chloramphenicol: ↓ excretion
Cholestyramine: ↓ excretion
Dobutamine: ↑ CV reactions, avoid use
Dopamine: ↑ CV reactions, avoid use
Epinephrine: ↑ CV reactions, avoid use
Erythromycin: ↓ excretion
Isoetharine: ↑ CV reactions, avoid use
Methyldopa: ↑ CV reactions, avoid use
Norepinephrine: ↑ CV reactions, avoid use
Probenecid: May decrease excretion
Rifampin: ↓ excretion
Drug classifications
MAOIs: Prevents catecholamine metabolism, do not use together

---

🍁 Canada Only   Adverse effects: *italic* = common; **bold** = life-threatening

NURSING CONSIDERATIONS
Assessment

• Monitor B/P, respiration during initial treatment; hypotension should be reported

• Assess mental status: affect, mood, behavioral changes, depression; complete suicide assessment

• Monitor liver function enzymes: AST, ALT, alkaline phosphatase; also check LDH, bilirubin, CBC

• Assess for involuntary movements in parkinsonism: akinesia, tremors, staggering gait, muscle rigidity, drooling; these symptoms should improve with therapy when given with levodopa/carbidopa

Nursing diagnoses
☑ Mobility, impaired (uses)
☑ Injury, risk for (uses)
☑ Knowledge deficit (teaching)
☑ Noncompliance (teaching)

Implementation

• Adjust dosage to patient response

• Give with meals to decrease GI upset; limit protein taken with drug

• Give only after MAOIs have been discontinued for 2 wk

Patient/family education

• Advise patient that hallucinations, mental changes, nausea, dyskinesia can occur

• Caution patient to change positions slowly to prevent orthostatic hypotension; not to drive or operate machinery until stabilized on medication and mental performance is not affected

• Instruct patient to use drug exactly as prescribed

• Inform patient that urine, sweat may darken

• Inform patient to notify prescriber if pregnancy is suspected; or if lactating, drug is excreted in breast milk

Evaluation
Positive therapeutic outcome

• Decreased akathisia, other involuntary movements when used with levodopa/carbidopa

• Increased mood when used with levodopa/carbidopa

---

epirubicin (℞)
(ep-i-roo′-bi-sin)
Ellence
Func. class.: Antineoplastic, antibiotic
Chem. class.: Anthracycline
Pregnancy category   D

Action: Inhibits DNA synthesis primarily; replication is decreased by binding to DNA, which causes strand splitting; maximum cytotoxic effects at S and G_2 phases; a vesicant

Therapeutic Outcome: Prevention of rapidly growing malignant cells

Uses: Breast cancer as an adjuvant therapy, with axillary node involvement, following resection

Dosage and routes
Adult: **IV** infusion: 100-120 mg/m^2 initially given with other antineoplastics; given in repeated cycles; 3-4 wk cycles

Available forms: Inj 2 mg/ml

Adverse effects
CV: Increased B/P, **sinus tachycardia, PVCs,** chest pain, **bradycardia, extrasystole**
GI: Nausea, vomiting, diarrhea, anorexia, mucositis
GU: Hot flashes, amenorrhea, hyperuricemia

HEMA: **Thrombocytopenia, leukopenia, anemia, neutropenia, secondary AML**
INTEG: Rash, necrosis at inj site, alopecia
MISC: Infection, febrile neutropenia, lethargy, fever, conjunctivitis

Contraindications: Hypersensitivity to this drug, anthracyclines, anthracenediones, pregnancy **D**, lactation, systemic infections, severe hepatic disease, baseline neutrophil count <1500 cell/mm^3, severe myocardial insufficiency, recent MI

Precautions: Renal, hepatic, cardiac disease, gout, bone marrow suppression (severe), elderly, children

Pharmacokinetics

Absorption	Complete bioavailability
Distribution	Widely distributed, crosses placenta
Metabolism	Liver, extensively
Excretion	Bile (60%)
Half-life	3 min; 2.5 hr; 33 hrs

Pharmacodynamics

Unknown

Interactions
Individual drugs
Cimetidine: ↑ epirubicin level, stop cimetidine before giving epirubicin
Radiation: ↑ toxicity, bone marrow suppression
Drug classifications
Antineoplastics: ↑ toxicity, bone marrow suppression
Live virus vaccines: ↑ adverse reactions, ↓ antibody response

NURSING CONSIDERATIONS
Assessment
• Monitor LVEF, MUCA scan or ECHO, ECG; watch for ST-T wave changes, low QRS and T; possible dysrhythmias (sinus tachycardia, heart block, PVCs) may occur; assess tachypnea, ECG changes, dyspnea, edema, fatigue
• Assess symptoms indicating severe allergic reaction: rash, pruritus, urticaria, purpuric skin lesions, itching, flushing; drug should be discontinued
• Monitor CBC, differential, platelet count weekly; withhold drug if WBC count is <4000/mm^3 or platelet count is <100,000/mm^3; notify prescriber of results if WBC <20,000/mm^3, platelets <150,000/mm^3
• Assess for increased uric acid levels, swelling, joint pain, primarily extremities; patient should be well hydrated to prevent urate deposits
• Monitor renal function studies: BUN, creatinine, serum uric acid, urine CrCl before and during therapy; I&O ratio; report fall in urine output to <30 ml/hr; dosage adjustment is needed if serum creatinine >5 mg/dl
• Monitor temp q4h (may indicate beginning of infection)
• Monitor liver function tests before and during therapy (bilirubin, AST, ALT, LDH) as needed or monthly; note jaundice of skin or sclera, dark urine, clay-colored stools, itchy skin, abdominal pain, fever, diarrhea
• Assess for bleeding: hematuria, stool guaiac, bruising or petechiae, mucosa or orifices q8h; inflammation of mucosa, breaks in skin
• Identify effects of alopecia on body image; discuss feeling about body changes

---

♣ Canada Only   Adverse effects: *italic* = common; **bold** = life-threatening

Nursing diagnoses

☑ Injury, risk for (adverse reactions)

☑ Body image disturbance (adverse reactions)

☑ Infection, risk for (adverse reactions)

☑ Knowledge deficit (teaching)

Implementation

• Avoid contact with skin; very irritating; wash completely to remove; give fluids **IV** or PO before chemotherapy to hydrate patient

• Give antiemetic 30-60 min before giving drug to prevent vomiting and prn

• Administer prophylactic antibiotic with a fluoroquinolone or trimethoprim/sulfamethoxazole if dose of epirubicin is 120 mg/m²

• Provide liq diet: carbonated beverages; gelatin may be added if patient is not nauseated or vomiting

• Drug should be prepared by experienced personnel using proper precautions

• Give into tubing of free flowing **IV** infusion 0.9% NaCl or D_5 give over 3-5 min

• Use hydrocortisone, dexamethasone, or sodium bicarbonate (1 mEq/1 ml) for extravasation: apply ice compress

Patient/family education

• Advise patient to avoid use of products containing aspirin or NSAIDs, razors, commercial mouthwash, since bleeding may occur; to report symptoms of bleeding (hematuria, tarry stools)

• Instruct patient to report signs of anemia (fatigue, headache, irritability, faintness, shortness of breath)

• Inform patient that hair may be lost during treatment; a wig or hair piece may make patient feel better; new hair may be different in color, texture

• Caution patient not to have any vaccinations without the advice of the prescriber; serious reactions can occur

• Advise patient to use contraception during treatment

Evaluation

Positive therapeutic outcome

• Prevention of rapid division of malignant cells

---

exemestane (℞)

(x-ee-mes'-tane)

Aromasin

Func. class.: Antineoplastic

Chem. class.: Aromatase inhibitor

Pregnancy category **D**

Action: Lowers serum estradiol concentrations; many breast cancers have strong estrogen receptors

Therapeutic Outcome: Prevention of rapidly growing malignant cells

Uses: Advanced breast carcinoma that has not responded to other therapy in estrogen-receptor-positive patients (postmenopausal)

Dosage and routes

Adult: PO 25 mg qd, pc

Available forms: Tabs 25 mg

Adverse effects

CNS: Hot flashes, headache, fatigue, depression, insomnia, anxiety

CV: Hypertension

GI: Nausea, vomiting, in-

---

creased appetite, diarrhea, constipation, abdominal pain
RESP: Cough, dyspnea

Contraindications: Hypersensitivity, premenopausal women, pregnancy **D**

P Precautions: Lactation, **G** children, elderly, liver disease, renal disease

Pharmacokinetics	
Absorption	Rapidly absorbed
Distribution	Unknown
Metabolism	Liver
Excretion	Feces, urine
Half-life	24 hr

Pharmacodynamics
Unknown

NURSING CONSIDERATIONS
Assessment
• Assess B/P, hypertension may occur

Nursing diagnoses
✓ Injury, risk for (adverse reactions)
✓ Knowledge deficit (teaching)

Implementation
• Give with food or fluids for GI upset
• Store in light-resistant container at room temp

Patient/family education
• Instruct patient to report any complaints, side effects to health care prescriber; if dose is missed, do not double next dose
• Advise patient that hot flashes can occur, and are reversible after discontinuing treatment
• Inform patient about who should be told about therapy

Evaluation
Positive therapeutic outcome
• Decreased spread of malignant cells in breast cancer

ganirelix (℞)
(gan-i-rell′-ex)
Antagon
Func. class.: Gonadotropin-releasing hormone antagonist
Chem. class.: Synthetic decapeptide
Pregnancy category   X

Action: Inhibitor of pituitary gonadotropin secretion; initially increases LH and FSH, induces a rapid suppression of gonadotropin secretion

Therapeutic Outcome: Pregnancy

Uses: For inhibition of premature LH surges in women undergoing controlled ovarian hyperstimulation

Dosage and routes
Adult: SC 250 µg qd during early to mid follicular phase, continue until day of hCG administration

Available forms: Inj 250 µg/0.5 ml

Adverse effects
CNS: Headache
ENDO: Ovarian hyperstimulation syndrome, abdominal pain (Gyn)
GI: Nausea
INTEG: Pain on inj
SYST: **Fetal death**

Contraindications: Hypersensitivity, pregnancy **X**, latex allergy, lactation

---

Pharmacokinetics

Absorption	Unknown
Distribution	Unknown
Metabolism	To metabolites
Excretion	Unknown
Half-life	13-16 hr

Pharmacodynamics

Onset	Unknown
Peak	Unknown
Duration	Treatment length

Interactions: None

NURSING CONSIDERATIONS
Assessment
• Assess for suspected pregnancy, drug should not be used
• Assess for latex allergy, drug should not be used

Nursing diagnoses
☑ Sexual dysfunction (uses)
☑ Knowledge deficit (teaching)

Implementation
• Administer by SC using abdomen, around navel or upper thigh, swab inj area with disinfectant, clean a 2 in circle and allow to dry, pinch up area between thumb and finger, insert needle at 45-90° to surface, if positioned correctly, no blood will be drawn back into syringe, if blood is drawn into syringe, reposition needle without removing it
• Protect from light

Patient/family education
• Teach patient to report abdominal pain, vaginal bleeding

Evaluation
Positive therapeutic outcome
• Pregnancy

---

gatifloxacin (℞)
(gat-i-floks'-a-sin)
Tequin
Func. class.: Urinary anti-infectives
Chem. class.: Fluoroquinolone antibacterial
Pregnancy category   C

Action: Interferes with conversion of intermediate DNA fragments into high-molecular-weight DNA in bacteria; DNA gyrase inhibitor

➤**Therapeutic Outcome:** Bactericidal action against the following: gram-positive organisms methicillin-resistant strains of S. *aureus,* S. *pneumoniae;* gram-negative organisms *Escherichia coli, Haemophilus influenzae, H. parainfluenzae, Klebsiella pneumoniae, Moraxella catarrhalis, Neisseria gonorrhoeae, Proteus mirabilis;* and other microorganisms: *Chlamydia pneumoniae, Legionella pneumophilia, Mycoplasma pneumoniae*

Uses: Adult urinary tract infections (including complicated); lower respiratory, skin, bone, joint infections, acute bacterial exacerbation of chronic bronchitis, acute sinusitis, community-acquired pneumonia, gonorrhea

Dosage and routes
Renal dose
CrCl ≥40 ml/min 400 mg qd; CrCl <40 ml/min 200 mg qd after 400 mg initially; hemodialysis 200 mg qd after 400 mg initially

---

Uncomplicated urinary tract infections
Adult: PO/**IV** 400 mg single dose

Complicated/severe urinary tract infections
Adult: PO/**IV** 400 mg × 7-10 days

Chronic bronchitis
Adult: PO/**IV** 400 mg × 7-10 days

Acute sinusitis
Adult: PO/**IV** 400 mg × 10 days

Community acquired pneumonia
Adult: PO/**IV** 400 mg × 7-14 days

Gonorrhea
Adult: PO/**IV** 400 mg single dose

Available forms: Tabs 200, 400; inj 20 ml (200 mg), 40 ml (400 mg)

Adverse effects
CNS: Headache, dizziness, insomnia, paresthesia, tremor, vasodilation
GI: Nausea, constipation, increased ALT, AST, diarrhea, **pseudomembranous colitis**
INTEG: Rash, pruritus, urticaria, photosensitivity, flushing, fever, chills
RESP: Dyspnea, pharyngitis

Contraindications: Hypersensitivity to quinolones

Precautions: Pregnancy **C**, lactation, children, renal disease

Pharmacokinetics	
Absorption	Well absorbed (PO); complete (**IV**)
Distribution	Protein binding 20%
Metabolism	Liver
Excretion	Kidneys unchanged (70%)
Half-life	1 hr

Pharmacodynamics		
	PO	IV
Onset	Rapid	Immediate
Peak	1 hr	Infusion's end

Interactions
Individual drugs
Probenecid: ↑ blood levels of gatifloxacin
Sucralfate: ↓ absorption of gatifloxacin
Drug classifications
Antacids: ↓ absorption of gatifloxacin

NURSING CONSIDERATIONS
Assessment
• Assess patient for previous sensitivity reaction
• Assess patient for signs and symptoms of infection including characteristics of wounds, sputum, urine, stool, WBC >10,000, fever; obtain baseline information before and during treatment
• Obtain C&S before beginning drug therapy to identify if correct treatment has been initiated
• Assess for allergic reactions: rash, urticaria, pruritus, chills, fever, joint pain; may occur a few days after therapy begins; epinephrine and resuscitation equipment should be available for anaphylactic reaction
• Identify urine output; if decreasing, notify prescriber (may indicate nephrotoxicity); also check for increased BUN, creatinine
• Monitor blood studies: AST, ALT, CBC, Hct, bilirubin, LDH, alkaline phosphatase, Coombs' test monthly if patient is on long-term therapy
• Monitor electrolytes: potassium, sodium, chloride monthly if patient is on long-term therapy

- Assess bowel pattern qd; if severe diarrhea occurs, drug should be discontinued
- Monitor for bleeding: ecchymosis, bleeding gums, hematuria, stool guaiac daily if on long-term therapy
- Assess for overgrowth of infection: perineal itching, fever, malaise, redness, pain, swelling, drainage, rash, diarrhea, change in cough, sputum

Nursing diagnoses

☑ Infection, risk for (uses)
☑ Diarrhea (side effects)
☑ Injury, risk for (side effects)
☑ Knowledge deficit (teaching)
☑ Noncompliance (teaching)

Implementation

IV IV route

- Check for irritation, extravasation, phlebitis daily
- Do not use flexible containers in series connections, air embolism may occur
- Do not use if particulate matter is present
- Do not admix with other drugs
- Dilute with compatible sol to 2 mg/ml before administration

Solution compatibilities:
D_5, 0.9% NaCl, D_5/0.9% NaCl
LR/D_5, water for inj

Patient/family education

- Teach patient to report sore throat, bruising, bleeding, joint pain; may indicate blood dyscrasias (rare)
- Advise patient to contact prescriber if vaginal itching, loose, foul-smelling stools, furry tongue occur; may indicate superinfection; report itching, rash, pruritus, urticaria
- Instruct patient to take all medication prescribed for the length of time ordered; drug must be taken around the clock

to maintain blood levels: do not give medication to others
- Advise patient to notify prescriber of diarrhea with blood or pus

Evaluation

Positive therapeutic outcome

- Absence of signs/symptoms of infection (WBC <10,000, temp WNL, absence of red draining wounds)
- Reported improvement in symptoms of infection

**interferon alfa-n 1
lymphoblastoid** (℞)
(in-ter-feer'on)
Wellferon
Func. class.: Recombinant type I interferon
Pregnancy category   UK

Action: Induces biologic responses and has antiviral, antiproliferative and immunomodulatory effects; mixture of alpha interferons isolated from human cells after induction with parainfluenza virus

Uses: Chronic hepatitis C infections

Dosage and routes
Adult: SC/IM 3 Mu × 3×/ wk × 48 wks

Available forms: Solution 3 Mu/ml

Adverse effects
CNS: Headache, fever, insomnia, dizziness
GI: Abdominal pain, nausea, diarrhea, anorexia, vomiting
HEMA: Granulocytopenia, thrombocytopenia, leukopenia, ecchymosis
INTEG: Alopecia, pruritus, rash, erythema, dry skin
MS: Back pain

☑ Herb/drug ◎ Do Not Crush ◆ Alert ⚭ Key Drug ◪ Geriatric ℙ Pediatric

PSYCH: Nervousness, depression, anxiety, lability, abnormal thinking
RESP: Pharyngitis, upper respiratory infection, cough, dyspnea, bronchitis

Contraindications: Hypersensitivity to alpha interferons, history of anaphylaxis to bovine or ovine immunoglobulins, egg protein, polymyxin B, neomycin sulfate

Precautions: Thyroid disorders, myelosuppression, hepatic, cardiac disease, lactation, **P** children <18 yr, depression/suicidal tendencies

Pharmacokinetics	
Peak	24-36 hr

Interactions
Individual drugs
Theophylline: Use cautiously
Drug classifications
Myelosuppressive agents: Use together cautiously

NURSING CONSIDERATIONS
Assessment
• Monitor ALT, HCV viral load, patients that show no reduction in ALT, HCV are unlikely to show benefit to treatment after 16 wks
• Monitor platelet counts, heme concentration, ANC, serum creatinine concentration, albumin, bilirubin, TSH, T4
• Monitor for myelosuppression, hold dose if neutrophil count is $<500 \times 10^6$/L or if platelets are $<50 \times 10^9$/L
• Assess for hypersensitivity: discontinue immediately if hypersensitivity occurs
Implementation
• Give the same brand of

product during the course of treatment
Patient/family education
• Provide patient or family member with written, detailed information about drug
• Teach patient instructions for home use if appropriate
Evaluation
Positive therapeutic outcome
• Decrease chronic hepatitis C signs/symptoms

levalbuterol (℞)
(lev-al-bute′er-ole)
Xopenex
Func. class.: Bronchodilator
Chem. class.: Adrenergic β_2-agonist
Pregnancy category   C

Action: Causes bronchodilation by action on β_2 (pulmonary) receptors by increasing levels of cyclic adenosine monophosphate (cAMP), which relaxes smooth muscle; produces bronchodilatation; CNS, cardiac stimulation, increased diuresis, and increased gastric acid secretion; longer acting than isoproterenol

➤**Therapeutic Outcome:** Increased ability to breathe because of bronchodilatation

Uses: Treatment or prevention of bronchospasm (reversible obstructive airway disease)
Dosage and routes
P *Adult and child ≥12 yr:* INH 0.63 mg tid, q6-8h by nebulization
Available forms: Sol, inh 0.63 mg/3 ml, 1.25 mg/3 ml

Adverse effects

CNS: Tremors, anxiety, insomnia, headache, dizziness, stimulation, *restlessness,* hallucinations, flushing, irritability

CV: Palpitations, tachycardia, hypertension, angina, hypotension, dysrhythmias

EENT: Dry nose, irritation of nose and throat

GI: Heartburn, nausea, vomiting

MS: Muscle cramps

Contraindications: Hypersensitivity to sympathomimetics, tachydysrhythmias, severe cardiac disease

Precautions: Lactation, pregnancy **C**, cardiac disorders, hyperthyroidism, diabetes mellitus, hypertension, prostatic hypertrophy, narrow angle glaucoma, seizures

Pharmacokinetics

Absorption	Unknown
Distribution	Unknown
Metabolism	Liver extensively, tissues
Excretion	Unknown, breast milk
Half-life	Unknown

Pharmacodynamics

	INH
Onset	5-15 min
Peak	1-1½ hr
Duration	6-8 hr

Interactions
Drug classifications

β-Adrenergic blockers: Block therapeutic effect

Bronchodilators, aerosol: ↑ action of bronchodilator

MAOIs: ↑ chance of hypertensive crisis

Sympathomimetics: ↑ adrenergic side effects

NURSING CONSIDERATIONS
Assessment

• Assess respiratory function: vital capacity, forced expiratory volume, ABGs, lung sounds, heart rate, rhythm (baseline and during therapy)

• Determine that patient has not received theophylline therapy before giving dose, to prevent additive effect; client's ability to self-medicate

• Monitor for evidence of allergic reactions; paradoxic bronchospasm; withhold dose; notify prescriber

Nursing diagnoses

☑Airway clearance, ineffective (uses)

☑Impaired gas exchange (uses)

☑Knowledge deficit (teaching)

Implementation

• Give by nebulization q6-8h

Patient/family education

• Tell patient not to use OTC medications before consulting prescriber; extra stimulation may occur; instruct patient to use this medication before other medications and allow at least 5 min between each to prevent overstimulation; to limit caffeine products such as chocolate, coffee, tea, and cola

◆• Teach patient that if paradoxic bronchospasm occurs to stop drug immediately and notify prescriber

Evaluation
Positive therapeutic outcome

• Absence of dyspnea and wheezing after 1 hr

• Improved airway exchange

• Improved ABGs

Treatment of overdose: Administer a β₁-adrenergic blocker

☑ Herb/drug 🚫 Do Not Crush ◆ Alert ⚷ Key Drug 🅖 Geriatric 🅟 Pediatric

levetiracetam (℞)

(lev-ee-tye'ra-see-tam)

Keppra

Func. class.: Anticonvulsant

Pregnancy category C

Action: Inhibits nerve impulses by limiting influx of sodium ions across cell membrane in motor cortex

▶**Therapeutic Outcome:** Absence of seizures

Uses: Partial onset seizures

Dosage and routes
Adult: PO 500 mg bid

Available forms: Tabs 250, 500, 750 mg

Adverse effects
CNS: Dizziness, somnolence, asthenia
HEMA: ↓ Hct, Hgb, infection

Contraindications: Hypersensitivity

Precautions: Hepatic disease, renal disease, cardiac disease, pregnancy C, lactation, 🅿 children

Pharmacokinetics	
Absorption	Rapidly absorbed
Distribution	Widely distributed, not protein bound
Metabolism	Small amount liver
Excretion	Kidneys (66%) unchanged
🅖 Half-life	6-8 hr or more in elderly

Pharmacodynamics	
Unknown	

Interactions
None known

NURSING CONSIDERATIONS
Assessment
• Monitor liver function tests AST, ALT, and urine function tests, BUN, urine protein periodically during treatments
• Assess seizure activity including type, location, duration, and character; provide seizure precaution

Nursing diagnoses
☑ Injury, risk for (side effects)
☑ Knowledge deficit (teaching)

Implementation
• Give with food for GI symptoms

Patient/family education
• Teach patient to carry Medic Alert ID stating patient's name, drugs taken, condition, prescriber's name, phone number
• Caution patient to avoid driving, other activities that require alertness until stabilized on medication
• Teach patient not to discontinue medication quickly after long-term use
• Teach patient to use a nonhormonal type of contraception to prevent harm to the fetus
• Teach patient to take exactly as prescribed, do not double or omit doses

Evaluation
Positive therapeutic outcome
• Decreased seizure activity

levobupivacaine (℞)

(lee-voh-bu-piv'ah-kane)

Chirocaine

Func. class.: Local anesthetic

Chem. class.: Amide

Pregnancy category B

Action: Competes with calcium for sites in nerve membrane that control sodium transport across cell membrane; decreases rise of depolarization phase of action potential

➔ **Therapeutic Outcome:** Anesthesia, decreased pain

Uses: Local, regional anesthesia, surgical anesthesia, pain management, continuous epidural analgesia

Dosage and routes
Varies with route of anesthesia

Available forms: Inj 2.5, 5, 7.5 mg/ml

Adverse effects
CNS: Anxiety, restlessness, **convulsions, loss of consciousness,** drowsiness, disorientation, tremors, shivering
CV: **Myocardial depression, cardiac arrest, dysrhythmias,** bradycardia, hypotension, hypertension, **fetal bradycardia**
EENT: Blurred vision, tinnitus, pupil constriction
GI: Nausea, vomiting
INTEG: Rash, urticaria, allergic reactions, edema, burning, skin discoloration at injection site, tissue necrosis
RESP: **Status asthmaticus, respiratory arrest, anaphylaxis**

Contraindications: Hypersensitivity, child <12 yr, ☐ elderly, severe liver disease

Precautions: Severe drug allergies, pregnancy **B**

Pharmacokinetics

Absorption	Unknown
Distribution	Unknown
Metabolism	Liver
Excretion	Urine (metabolites)
Half-life	Unknown

Pharmacodynamics

Onset	2-8 min
Peak	Unknown
Duration	3-6 hr

Interactions
Drug classifications
Anesthetics, halothane: ↑ dysrhythmias
Antidepressants, tricyclics: ↑ hypertension
MAOIs: ↑ hypertension
Phenothiazines: ↑ hypertension

NURSING CONSIDERATIONS
Assessment
• Monitor B/P, pulse, respiration during treatment
• Monitor fetal heart tones during labor
• Monitor allergic reactions: rash, urticaria, itching
• Monitor cardiac status: ECG for dysrhythmias, pulse, B/P during anesthesia

Nursing diagnoses
✓ Pain, (uses)
✓ Knowledge deficit (teaching)

Implementation
• Administer only with crash cart, resuscitative equipment nearby
• Administer only drugs without preservatives for epidural or caudal anesthesia
• Discard unused portions

Evaluation
Positive therapeutic outcome
• Anesthesia necessary for procedure

Treatment of overdose: Airway, O_2, vasopressor, **IV** fluids, anticonvulsants for seizures

---

☑ Herb/drug ⊘ Do Not Crush ◆ Alert ☛ Key Drug ☐ Geriatric ☐ Pediatric

lymphocyte immune globulin, (anti-thymocyte) (℞)
Atgam
Func. class.: Immune globulins-immuno-suppressant
Pregnancy category C

Action: Produces immunosuppression by inhibiting the function of T-lymphocytes

→**Therapeutic Outcome:** Absence of transplant rejection; hematologic remission (aplastic anemia)

Uses: Organ transplants to prevent rejection, aplastic anemia

Dosage and routes
Adult: IV 10-30 mg/kg/day
P *Child:* IV 5-25 mg/kg/day

Available forms: Inj 50 mg/ml

Adverse effects
Renal transplant
CNS: Fever, chills, headache, dizziness, weakness, faintness, seizures
CV: Chest pain, hypertension, tachycardia
GI: Diarrhea, nausea, vomiting, epigastric pain
INTEG: Rash, pruritus, urticaria, wheal
SYST: Anaphylaxis

Aplastic anemia
CNS: Fever, chills, headache, seizures, lightheadedness, encephalitis, postviral encephalopathy
CV: Bradycardia, myocarditis, irregularity
GI: Nausea, LFT abnormality

Contraindications: Hypersensitivity

Precautions: Severe renal disease, severe hepatic disease, pregnancy **C,** lactation, **P** children

Pharmacokinetics

Absorption	Unknown
Distribution	Unknown
Metabolism	Unknown
Excretion	Unknown
Half-life	5.7 days

Pharmacodynamics

Onset	Rapid
Peak	Unknown
Duration	Unknown

Interactions
None known

NURSING CONSIDERATIONS
Assessment
• Assess for infection, if infection occurs evaluation will be needed to continue treatment
• Monitor renal studies: BUN, creatinine at least monthly during treatment, 3 mo after treatment
• Monitor liver function studies: alk phosphatase, AST, ALT, bilirubin
Nursing diagnoses
✓ Mobility, impaired (uses)
✓ Infection, risk for (uses)
✓ Knowledge deficit (teaching)
Implementation
IV IV route
• Do not infuse <4 hrs
Delaying the onset of allograft rejection
• For 14 doses qod over 28 days. Start 1st dose within 24 hrs of transplant
Treatment of rejection
• For 14 days, alternate day therapy up to 21 days
Aplastic anemia
• For 8-14 days, or alternate day treatment up to 21 days

• Keep emergency equipment nearby for severe allergic reactions
• Skin testing must be completed prior to treatment; use intradermal inj of 0.1 ml of a 1:1000 dilution (5 µg horse IgG) in 0.9% NaCl, if a wheal or rash >10 mm or both, use caution during inf
• Dilute in saline sol before inf; invert **IV** bag, so undiluted drug does not contact the air inside, concentration should not be >1 mg/ml

Patient/family education
• Advise patient to report fever, rash, chills, sore throat, fatigue, since serious infections may occur
• Caution patient to use contraceptive measures during treatment and for 12 wk after ending therapy; drug is teratogenic
• Caution patient to avoid crowds and persons with known infections to reduce risk of infection

Evaluation
Positive therapeutic outcome
• Absence of graft rejection
• Hematologic recovery (aplastic anemia)

---

modafinil (R)
(mod-aa-fen'ill)
Provigil
Func. class.: Cerebral stimulant
Pregnancy category   C

Action: Promotes wakefullness, exact mechanism is unknown

➡**Therapeutic Outcome:** Increased alertness, decreased fatigue, ability to stay awake (narcolepsy)

Uses: Narcolepsy

Dosage and routes
Adult: PO 200 mg qd in the AM, may increase to 400 mg qd if needed

Hepatic dose
Reduce dose by 50%

Available forms: Tabs 100, 200 mg

Adverse effects
CNS: Hyperactivity, insomnia, restlessness, dizziness, headache, chills, stimulation
CV: Palpitations, tachycardia, hypertension, dysrhythmias
EENT: Abnormal vision, amblyopia
GI: Anorexia, dry mouth, diarrhea, nausea, vomiting, mouth ulcer, gingivitis, thirst
GU: Urinary retention, abnormal ejaculation
INTEG: Herpes simplex, dry skin
META: Hyperglycemia, albuminuria
RESP: Rhinitis, pharyngitis, lung disorder, dyspnea, asthma, epistaxis

Contraindications: Hypersensitivity, hyperthyroidism, hypertension, glaucoma, severe arteriosclerosis, drug abuse, cardiovascular disease, anxiety

Precautions: Gilles de la Tourette's disorder, elderly, pregnancy **C**, lactation, children <16 yr

---

Pharmacokinetics

Absorption	Rapid
Distribution	Well distributed; protein binding 60%; crosses placenta
Metabolism	Liver extensively
Excretion	10%
Half-life	15 hrs with multiple dosing

Pharmacodynamics

Onset	Unknown
Peak	2-4 hr
Duration	Unknown

Interactions
Individual drugs
Clomipramine: ↑ levels of clomipramine
Cyclosporine: ↓ level of cyclosporine
Methylphenidate: ↓ modafinil absorption
Phenytoin: ↑ phenytoin toxicity
Warfarin: ↑ warfarin level
Drug classifications
Antidepressants, tricyclics: ↑ levels, reduce dose
Contraceptives, oral: ↓ oral contraceptive effect
MAOIs: Use caution when giving together

NURSING CONSIDERATIONS
Assessment
• Assess for improvement in narcolepsy

Nursing diagnoses
☑ Sleep pattern disturbance (uses)
☑ Knowledge deficit (teaching)

Implementation
• Titrate to patient's response; lowest dosage should be used to control symptoms

• Give gum, hard candy, frequent sips of water for dry mouth at beginning of treatment; these symptoms tend to lessen with time

Patient/family education
• Advise patient to decrease caffeine consumption (coffee, tea, cola, chocolate), which may increase irritability and stimulation; to avoid OTC preparations unless approved by prescriber; to avoid alcohol ingestion; these may cause serious drug interactions
• Inform patient to notify prescriber if rash or other symptoms of allergy occur
• Advise patient to notify prescriber if pregnancy is suspected, or if breast-feeding; another form of contraception is needed if using hormonal contraception while on this drug and for a month afterward
• Caution patient to avoid hazardous activities until patient is stabilized on medication
• Instruct patient/family to notify prescriber if significant side effects occur: tremors, insomnia, palpitations, restlessness, drug changes may be needed

Evaluation
Positive therapeutic outcome
• Absence of sleeping during day in narcolepsy

---

moxifloxacin (R)
(mox-i-floks'a-sin)
Avelox
Func. class.: Antiinfective
Chem. class.: Fluoroquin-
olone
Pregnancy category C

Action: Interferes with conversion of intermediate DNA
fragments into high-molecular-
weight DNA in bacteria; DNA
gyrase inhibitor

Therapeutic Outcome: Bactericidal action against the
following: *Staphylococcus aureus, Streptococcus pneumoniae,
Haemophilus influenza, H.
parainfluenzae, Moraxella
catarrhalis, Klebsiella pneumoniae, Mycoplasma pneumoniae,
Chlamydia pneumoniae*

Uses: Acute bacterial sinusitis,
acute bacterial exacerbation
of chronic bronchitis,
community-acquired pneumoniae (mild to moderate)

Dosage and routes
Adult: 400 mg qd × 5-10 days
depending on condition

Available forms: Tabs
400 mg

Adverse effects
CNS: Headache, dizziness,
fatigue, insomnia, depression,
restlessness
CV: Prolonged QT interval
GI: Nausea, constipation,
increased ALT, AST, flatulence, insomnia, heartburn,
vomiting, diarrhea, oral candidiasis, dysphagia
INTEG: Rash, pruritus, urticaria, photosensitivity, flushing,
fever, chills
MS: Blurred vision, tinnitus

Contraindications: Hypersensitivity to quinolones

Precautions: Pregnancy **C**,
lactation, children, renal disease, uncorrected hypokalemia,
prolonged QT interval, patients receiving class IA, III
antidysrhythmics

Pharmacokinetics

Absorption	Well absorbed (75%) (PO)
Distribution	Widely distributed
Metabolism	Liver
Excretion	Kidneys
Half-life	Increased in renal disease

Pharmacodynamics

	PO
Onset	Rapid
Peak	1 hr

Interactions
Individual drugs
Caffeine: ↓ effect of moxi-
floxacin
Cyclosporine: ↑ nephrotoxi-
city
Nitrofurantoin: ↓ effective-
ness
Probenecid: ↑ blood levels
Sucralfate: ↓ absorption of
moxifloxacin
Theophylline: ↑ toxicity
Warfarin: ↑ warfarin effect
Zinc sulfate: ↓ absorption of
moxifloxacin
Drug classifications
Antacids: ↓ absorption of
moxifloxacin
Anticoagulants, oral: ↑ effect
of anticoagulants
Antidysrhythmics IA, III:
Prolonged QT interval
Antineoplastics: ↓ moxiflox-
acin
Iron salts: ↓ absorption of
moxifloxacin
Lab test interferences
↑ AST, ↑ ALT, ↑ BUN, ↑
creatinine, ↑ alkaline phospha-
tase

NURSING CONSIDERATIONS
Assessment
- Assess patient for previous sensitivity reaction
- Assess patient for signs and symptoms of infection including characteristics of wounds, sputum, urine, stool, WBC >10,000, fever; obtain baseline information before and during treatment
- Obtain C&S before beginning drug therapy to identify if correct treatment has been initiated
- Assess for allergic reactions: rash, urticaria, pruritus, chills, fever, joint pain; may occur a few days after therapy begins; epinephrine and resuscitation equipment should be available for anaphylactic reaction
- Identify urine output; if decreasing, notify prescriber (may indicate nephrotoxicity); also check for increased BUN, creatinine
- Monitor blood studies: AST, ALT, CBC, Hct, bilirubin, LDH, alkaline phosphatase, Coombs' test monthly if patient is on long-term therapy
- Monitor electrolytes: potassium, sodium chloride monthly if patient is on long-term therapy
- Assess bowel pattern qd; if severe diarrhea occurs, drug should be discontinued
- Monitor for bleeding: ecchymosis, bleeding gums, hematuria, stool guaiac daily if on long-term therapy
- Assess for overgrowth of infection: perineal itching, fever, malaise, redness, pain, swelling, drainage, rash, diarrhea, change in cough, sputum

Nursing diagnoses
- ☑ Infection, risk for (uses)
- ☑ Diarrhea (side effects)
- ☑ Injury, risk for (side effects)
- ☑ Knowledge deficit (teaching)
- ☑ Noncompliance (teaching)

Implementation
PO route
- Give once a day for 5-10 days depending on condition

Patient/family education
- Teach patient to report sore throat, bruising, bleeding, joint pain; may indicate blood dyscrasias (rare)
- Advise patient to contact prescriber if vaginal itching, loose, foul-smelling stools, furry tongue occur; may indicate superinfection; report itching, rash, pruritus, urticaria
- Instruct patient to take all medication prescribed for the length of time ordered; do not give medication to others
- Advise patient to notify prescriber of diarrhea with blood or pus

Evaluation
Positive therapeutic outcome
- Absence of signs/symptoms of infection (WBC <10,000, temp WNL)
- Reported improvement in symptoms of infection

---

nitric oxide (℞)
INOmax
Func. class.: Respiratory inhalant

Pregnancy category   C

Action: Increases partial pressure of arterial oxygen (PaO_2) by dilating pulmonary vessels, and redistributing pulmonary blood flow

---

➡ **Therapeutic Outcome:** Ability of neonate to breathe without assistance

Uses: Treatment of term and near term (>34 wks) neonates with hypoxic respiratory failure associated with pulmonary hypertension; used with other agents and ventilatory support

Dosage and routes
P *Neonate:* INH 20 ppm × up to 2 wks until O₂ desaturation has been resolved and is ready to be weaned from therapy

Available forms: Cylinders side D, size 88

Adverse effects
CV: Hypotension
GU: Hematuria
OTHER: **Hyperglycemia**, *sepsis, infection, cellulitis, stridor, withdrawal syndrome,* **methemoglobinemia, intracranial hemorrhage, cerebral infarction, seizures, pulmonary/GI hemorrhage**
RESP: Atelectasis

Contraindications: Dependence on right to left shunting of blood, hypersensitivity

Precautions: Bradycardia, rales, infections, pregnancy **C**

Pharmacokinetics	
Absorption	Unknown
Distribution	Lung
Metabolism	Unknown
Excretion	Unknown
Half-life	Unknown

Pharmacodynamics
Unknown

Interactions
Individual drugs
Nitroglycerin: ↑ effect possible
Nitroprusside: ↑ effect possible

NURSING CONSIDERATIONS
Assessment
• Assess respiratory rate, rhythm, character, chest expansion, color, transcutaneous saturation, ABGs; monitor ECG; for methemoglobinemia

Nursing diagnoses
☑ Gas exchange, impaired (uses)
☑ Knowledge deficit (teaching)

Implementation
P • Use only in neonates, not indicated for other populations
P • Neonate must be weaned off therapy; do not discontinue abruptly

Patient/family education
• Explain disease process and purpose of medication to parents; communicate
P neonate's progress

Evaluation
Positive therapeutic outcome
• Significant improvement of hypoxia, pulmonary hypertension

---

octreotide (℞)
(ok-tree'-o-tide)
Sandostatin, Sandostatin LAR Depot
Func. class.: Hormone, antidiarrheal
Chem. class.: Octapeptide
Pregnancy category   B

Action: Action similar to somatostatin

➡ **Therapeutic Outcome:** Decreased diarrheal. Decreased symptoms of acromegaly, carcinoid tumors, VIPomas

Uses: Sandostatin: Acromegaly, carcinoid tumors, vasoactive intestinal peptide tumors (VIPomas); LAR depot: Long-term maintenance of

---

acromegaly, carcinoid tumors, VIPomas

Investigational uses: GI fistula, variceal bleeding, diarrheal conditions, pancreatic fistula, irritable bowel syndrome, dumping syndrome

Dosage and routes
Initial dose
Adult: **IV**/SC 50 µg bid-tid CSI (continuous SC inf) has been used but is not approved

Acromegaly
Adult: SC 50 µg tid, adjust q2wk based on Somatomedin C

VIPomas
Adult: SC 0.2-0.3 mg qd in 2-4 doses for 2 wks, not to exceed 0.45 mg qd

Carcinoid tumors
Adult: SC 0.1-0.6 mg qd in 2-4 doses for 2 wks, titrated to patient response

GI fistula
Adult: SC 50-200 µg q8hr

Irritable bowel syndrome
Adult: SC 100 µg single dose to 125 µg bid

Dumping syndrome
Adult: SC 50-150 µg/day

Variceal bleeding
Adult: **IV** 25-50 µg/hr cont IV Inf for 18 hrs - 5 days

Available forms: Sandostatin: inj 0.05, 0.1, 0.2, 0.5, 1 mg/ml; LAR depot: inj 10 mg, 20, 30 mg/5 ml

Adverse effects
CNS: Headache, dizziness, fatigue, weakness, depression, anxiety, tremors, **seizures,** paranoia
CV: Sinus bradycardia, conduction abnormalities, **dysrhythmias,** chest pain, SOB, throm-bophlebitis, ischemia, **CHF,** hypertension, palpitations
ENDO: Hyperglycemia, ketosis, hypothyroidism, hypoglycemia, galactorrhea, diabetes insipidus
GI: Diarrhea, nausea, abdominal pain, vomiting, flatulence, distension, constipation, **hepatitis,** increased LFTs, **GI bleeding, pancreatitis**
GU: UTI, pollakiuria
HEMA: Hematoma of inj site, bruise
INTEG: Rash, urticaria, pain, inflammation at injection site
MS: Joint and muscle pain

Contraindications: Hypersensitivity

Precautions: Diabetes mellitus, hypothyroidism, pregnancy **B,** elderly, lactation, children, renal disease

Pharmacokinetics	
Absorption	Rapidly, completely
Distribution	Unknown
Metabolism	Little
Excretion	Urine, unchanged
Half-life	1.7 hr

Pharmacodynamics	
Onset	Unknown
Peak	½ hr
Duration	12 hr

Interactions
Individual drugs
Cyclosporine: Possible ↑ rejection
Food/drug
↓ absorption of dietary fat
↓ B_{12} levels

NURSING CONSIDERATIONS
Assessment
• Identify growth hormone antibodies, IGF-1, 1-4 hr intervals for 8-12 hrs post dose in acromegaly; 5-HIAA, plasma

---

serotonin, plasma substance P in carcinoid; VIP in VIPomas
• Fecal fat, serum carotene
• Monitor thyroid function tests: T_3, T_4, T_7, TSH to identify hypothyroidism
• Assess for allergic reaction: rash, itching, fever, nausea, wheezing
• Assess for cardiac status: bradycardia, conduction abnormalities, dysrhythmias; monitor ECG for QT prolongation, low voltage, axis shifts, early repolarization, R/S transition, early wave progression

Nursing diagnoses
✓ Body image disturbance (uses)
✓ Knowledge deficit (teaching)

Implementation
• Store in refrigerator unopened amps, vials; or room temp for 2 wks, protect from light do not use discolored or cloudy sol
SC route
• Rotate inj sites

Patient/family education
• Explain reason for medication and expected results
• Advise patient that routine follow-up is needed
• Instruct parents on procedure for medication preparation and inj use—request demonstration, return demonstration; provide written instructions

Evaluation
Positive therapeutic outcome
• Decreased symptoms of acromegaly, carcinoid, VIPoma
• Decreased diarrhea

---

orlistat (℞)
(or-li′-stat)
Xenical
Func. class.: Lipase inhibitor
Pregnancy category B

Action: Inhibits the absorption of dietary fat

➡ **Therapeutic Outcome:** Decrease in weight

Uses: Obesity management

Dosage and routes
Adult: PO 120 mg tid with each main meal containing fat

Available forms: Caps 120 mg

Adverse effects
CNS: Insomnia, dizziness, headache, depression, anxiety, fatigue
GI: Oily spotting, flatus with discharge, fecal urgency, fatty/oily stool, oily evacuation, fecal incontinence, nausea, vomiting, abdominal pain, infectious diarrhea, rectal pain, tooth disorder
GU: UTI, vaginitis, menstrual irregularity
INTEG: Dry skin, rash
MS: Back pain, arthritis, myalgia, tendinitis
RESP: Influenza, URI, LRI, EENT symptoms

Contraindications: Hypersensitivity, malabsorption syndrome, cholestasis

Precautions: Hypothyroidism, other organic causes of obesity, lactation, children, pregnancy **B**

☑ Herb/drug ◎ Do Not Crush ◆ Alert ⚷ Key Drug ⑥ Geriatric ⑫ Pediatric

Pharmacokinetics

Absorption	Minimal
Distribution	99% protein binding
Metabolism	Unknown
Excretion	Feces
Half-life	1-2 hr

Pharmacodynamics

Onset	Unknown
Peak	8 hr
Duration	Unknown

Interactions
Individual drugs
Cyclosporine: ↓ absorption
Pravastatin: ↑ lipid-lowering effect
Drug classifications
Fat soluble vitamins: ↓ absorption

NURSING CONSIDERATIONS
Assessment
• Monitor weight weekly, diabetic patients may need reduction in oral hypoglycemics
• Assess for misuse in certain populations (anorexia nervosa, bulimia)

Nursing diagnoses
☑ Knowledge deficit (teaching)
☑ Noncompliance (teaching)

Implementation
• Patient should be on a diet with 30% of calories from fat, omit dose of orlistat if a meal contains no fat

Patient/family education
• Warn patient that safety and effectiveness beyond 2 yrs have not been determined
• Instruct patient to read patient's information sheet
• Advise patient to avoid hazardous activities until stabilized on medication
• Instruct patient to take a multivitamin containing fat-soluble vitamins, take 2 hrs before or after orlistat
• Instruct patient/family to notify health care provider if significant side effects occur

Evaluation
Positive therapeutic outcome
• Decreased weight

---

oseltamivir (℞)
(oo-sell-tam′ii-ver)
Tamiflu
Func. class.: Antiviral
Chem. class.: Ethyl ester prodrug
Pregnancy category　**C**

Action: Inhibits influenza virus neuraminidase with possible alteration of virus particle aggregation and release

➡ Therapeutic Outcome: Decreased symptoms of influenza type A

Uses: Treatment of influenza type A

Dosage and routes
Adult: PO 75 mg × 5 days, begin treatment within 2 days of onset of symptoms

Available forms: Caps 75 mg

Adverse effects
CNS: Headache, fatigue, insomnia, vertigo
GI: Nausea, *vomiting,* diarrhea, abdominal pain
RESP: Cough

Contraindications: Hypersensitivity

Precautions: Hepatic disease, renal disease, lactation,
P children <18 yr, pregnancy **C**

Pharmacokinetics

Absorption	Rapidly absorbed
Distribution	Protein binding is low
Metabolism	Converted to oseltamivir carboxylate
Excretion	Eliminated by conversion
Half-life	1-3 hr

Pharmacodynamics

Unknown

NURSING CONSIDERATIONS
Assessment
• Assess for symptoms of influenza A: increased temperature, malaise, aches and pains

Nursing diagnoses
✓ Infection, risk for (uses)
✓ Knowledge deficit (teaching)

Implementation
• Give within 2 days of symptoms of influenza; continue for 5 days
• Give at least 4 hr before hs to prevent insomnia
• Administer after meals for better absorption, to decrease GI symptoms: caps may be opened and mixed with food for easy swallowing
• Store in tight, dry container

Patient/family education
• Teach patient about aspects of drug therapy: the need to report dyspnea, weight gain, dizziness, poor concentration, dysuria, behavioral changes
• Teach patient to avoid hazardous activities if dizziness occurs

Evaluation
Positive therapeutic outcome
• Absence of fever, malaise, cough, dyspnea in influenza A

---

perindopril (℞) ⚷
(per-in-doe-pril)
Aceon
Func. class.: Antihypertensive
Chem. class.: Angiotensin-converting enzyme inhibitor

Pregnancy category C (1st trimester), D (2nd/3rd trimesters)

Action: Selectively suppresses renin-angiotensin-aldosterone system; inhibits ACE; prevents conversion of angiotensin I to angiotensin II, resulting in dilatation of arterial and venous vessels

⇒**Therapeutic Outcome:** Decreased B/P in hypertension

Uses: Hypertension alone or in combination

Dosage and routes
Adult: PO 4 mg/day, may increase or decrease to desired response; range 4-8 mg/day may give in 2 divided doses or as a single dose

Patients on diuretics
Discontinue diuretic 2-3 days prior to perindopril, then resume diuretic if needed

Renal impairment
CrCl >30 ml/min 2 mg/day, max 8 mg/day

Available forms: Tabs 2, 4, 8 mg scored

Adverse effects
CNS: Insomnia, dizziness, paresthesias, headache, fatigue, anxiety
CV: Hypotension, chest pain, tachycardia, dysrhythmias
EENT: Tinnitus, visual changes, sore throat, double vision, dry burning eyes

---

🌿 Herb/drug 🚫 Do Not Crush ◆ Alert ⚷ Key Drug G Geriatric P Pediatric

GI: Nausea, vomiting, colitis, cramps, diarrhea, constipation, flatulence, dry mouth, loss of taste
GU: **Proteinuria, renal failure,** increased frequency of polyuria or oliguria
HEMA: **Agranulocytosis, neutropenia**
INTEG: Rash, purpura, alopecia, hyperhidrosis
META: Hyperkalemia
RESP: Dyspnea, cough, rales, angioedema

Contraindications: Pregnancy **D** (2nd/3rd trimesters), lactation

Precautions: Renal disease, hyperkalemia, pregnancy **C** (1st trimester)

Pharmacokinetics

Absorption	Well absorbed
Distribution	Unknown
Metabolism	Liver
Excretion	Kidneys
Half-life	Unknown

Pharmacodynamics

Unknown

Interactions
Individual drugs
Alcohol: ↑ hypotension (large amounts)
Allopurinol: ↑ hypersensitivity
Digoxin: ↑ serum levels
Hydralazine: ↑ toxicity
Indomethacin: ↓ antihypertensive effect
Lithium: ↑ serum levels
Prazosin: ↑ toxicity
Drug classifications
Adrenergic blockers: ↑ hypotension
Antacids: ↓ absorption
Antihypertensives: ↑ hypotension
Diuretics: ↑ hypotension
Diuretics, potassium-sparing: ↑ toxicity

Ganglionic blockers: ↑ hypotension
Potassium supplements: ↑ toxicity
Sympathomimetics: ↑ toxicity
Lab test interferences
Interference: Glucose/insulin tolerance tests

NURSING CONSIDERATIONS
Assessment
- Monitor blood studies: neutrophils, decreased platelets
- Monitor B/P, orthostatic hypotension, syncope; if changes occur dosage change may be required
- Monitor renal studies: protein, BUN, creatinine; increased levels may indicate nephrotic syndrome and renal failure
- Monitor renal symptoms: polyuria, oliguria, frequency, dysuria
- Establish baselines in renal, liver function tests before therapy begins
- Check potassium levels throughout treatment, although hyperkalemia rarely occurs
- Check for edema in feet, legs daily
- Assess for allergic reactions: rash, fever, pruritus, urticaria; drug should be discontinued if antihistamines fail to help

Nursing diagnoses
☑ Cardiac output, decreased (uses)
☑ Injury, potential for (adverse reactions)
☑ Knowledge deficit (teaching)
☑ Noncompliance (teaching)

Implementation
PO route
- Store in air-tight container at 86° F (30° C) or less
- Severe hypotension may

✦ Canada Only   Adverse effects: *italic* = common; **bold** = life-threatening

occur after 1st dose of this medication; decreased hypotension may be prevented by reducing or discontinuing diuretic therapy 3 days before beginning benazepril therapy

• Give by **IV** inf of 0.9% NaCl (as ordered) to expand fluid volume if severe hypotension occurs

Patient/family education

• Advise patient not to discontinue drug abruptly; advise patient to tell all persons associated with health care

• Teach patient not to use OTC products (cough, cold, allergy medications) unless directed by physician; serious side effects can occur; xanthines, such as coffee, tea, chocolate, cola can prevent action of drug

• Instruct patient on the importance of complying with dosage schedule, even if feeling better; to continue with medical regimen to decrease B/P: exercise, cessation of smoking, decreasing stress, diet modifications

• Emphasize the need to rise slowly to sitting or standing position to minimize orthostatic hypotension; not to exercise in hot weather, which can cause increased hypotension

• Advise patient to notify prescriber of mouth sores, sore throat, fever, swelling of hands or feet, irregular heartbeat, chest pain, coughing, shortness of breath

• Caution patient to report excessive perspiration, dehydration, vomiting, diarrhea; may lead to fall in B/P

• Caution patient that drug may cause dizziness, fainting, light-headedness; may occur during 1st few days of therapy; to avoid activities that may be hazardous

• Teach patient how to take B/P, and normal readings for age group

Evaluation

Positive therapeutic outcome

• Decreased B/P in hypertension

Treatment of overdose:

Lavage, **IV** atropine for bradycardia, **IV** theophylline for bronchospasm, digitalis, O_2; diuretic for cardiac failure, hemodialysis

---

pioglitazone (℞)
(pie-oh-glye′ta-zone)
Actos
Func. class.: Antidiabetic, oral
Chem. class.: Thiazolidinedione
Pregnancy category   C

Action: Improves insulin resistance by hepatic glucose metabolism, insulin receptor kinase activity, insulin receptor phosphorylation

➡ **Therapeutic Outcome:** Decreased symptoms of diabetes mellitus

Uses: Stable adult-onset diabetes mellitus (type II) NIDDM

Dosage and routes
Monotherapy
Adult: PO 15-30 mg qd, may increase to 45 mg/day

Combination therapy
Adult: PO 15-30 mg qd with a sulfonylurea, metformin or insulin. Decrease sulfonylurea dose if hypoglycemia occurs. Decrease insulin dose by 10-

---

25% if hypoglycemia occurs or if plasma glucose is <100 mg/dl max 45 mg/day

Hepatic dose
Do not use in active liver disease or if ALT >2.5 times ULN

Available forms: Tab 15, 30, 45 mg

Adverse effects
CNS: Headache
ENDO: Aggravated diabetes mellitus
MISC: Myalgia, sinusitis, URI, pharyngitis

Contraindications: Hypersensitivity to thiazolidinediones, diabetic ketoacidosis, lactation, ℙ children

Precautions: Pregnancy C, 🄶 elderly, thyroid disease, hepatic, renal disease

Pharmacokinetics	
Absorption	Unknown
Distribution	Unknown
Metabolism	Unknown
Excretion	Kidneys
Half-life	3-7 hr, total 16-24 hrs

Pharmacodynamics	
Onset	Unknown
Peak	6-12 wk
Duration	Unknown

Interactions
Drug classifications
Oral contraceptives: ↓ effect, use an alternate contraceptive method

NURSING CONSIDERATIONS
Assessment
• Assess for hypoglycemic reactions (sweating, weakness, dizziness, anxiety, tremors, hunger), hyperglycemic reactions soon after meals
• Assess CBC (baseline, q3mo) during treatment; check liver function tests periodically;

AST, LDH, FBS, glycosylated Hgb, fasting plasma insulin, plasma lipids, lipoproteins, B/P, body weight during treatment

Nursing diagnoses
☑ Nutrition, altered: more than body requirements (uses)
☑ Knowledge deficit (teaching)

Implementation
• Convert from other oral hypoglycemic agents; change may be made without gradual dosage change; monitor serum or urine glucose and ketones tid during conversion
• Give once a day; give with meals to decrease GI upset and provide best absorption
• Give tabs crushed and mixed with meal or fluids for patients with difficulty swallowing
• Store in tight container in cool environment

Patient/family education
• Teach patient to use capillary blood glucose test or Chemstrip tid
• Teach patient symptoms of hypo/hyperglycemia, what to do about each
• Advise patient that drug must be continued on daily basis; explain consequence of discontinuing drug abruptly
• Advise patient to avoid OTC medications or herbal preparations unless approved by the prescriber
• Advise patient that diabetes is life-long illness; that this drug is not a cure, only controls symptoms
• Advise patient that all food included in diet plan must be eaten to prevent hypoglycemia
• Advise patient to carry Medic Alert ID and glucagon emergency kit for emergencies
• Instruct patient to notify

prescriber if oral contraceptives are used
• Teach patient not to use if breast-feeding

Evaluation
Positive therapeutic outcome
• Decrease in polyuria, polydipsia, polyphagia; clear sensorium; absence of dizziness; stable gait; blood glucose at normal level

poractant alfa (Ŗ)
(poor-ak'tant al'fah)
Curosurf
Func. class.: Lung surfactant

Pregnancy category   UK

Action: Replenishes surfactant and restores surface activity to the lungs in premature infants

→Therapeutic Outcome: Ability of neonate to breathe without assistance

Uses: Treatment (rescue) of respiratory distress syndrome in premature infants

Investigational uses: Prophylaxis RDS, adult RDS due to viral pneumonia, HIV-infected infants with *Pneumocystis carinii* pneumonia, treatment of adult RDS in near drowning

Dosage and routes
Intratracheal instill: 2.5 ml/kg birth weight, up to 2 subsequent doses of 1.25 ml/kg birthweight can be administered at 12 hr intervals, max 5 ml kg

Available forms: Susp 120 mg (1.5 ml); 240 mg (3 ml)

Adverse effects
RESP: Pulmonary air leaks, pulmonary interstitial emphysema, apnea, pulmonary hemorrhage
SYST: Patent ductus arteriosus, intracranial hemorrhage, severe intracranial hemorrhage, necrotizing entercolitis, posttreatment sepsis, posttreatment infection, bradycardia, oxygen desaturation, pallor, vasoconstriction, hypotension, hypertension

Precautions: Bradycardia, rales, infections

Pharmacokinetics	
Absorption	Unknown
Distribution	Lung
Metabolism	Recycled
Excretion	Unknown
Half-life	Unknown

Pharmacodynamics	
Onset	Few min
Peak	Unknown
Duration	Becomes lung associated within hours of administration

Interactions: None

NURSING CONSIDERATIONS
Assessment
• Assess respiratory rate, rhythm, character, chest expansion, color, transcutaneous saturation, ABGs; monitor ECG
• Check endotracheal tube placement before dosing; monitor for apnea after endotracheal administration
• Check for reflux of drug into the endotracheal tube during administration; stop drug administration if this occurs, and if needed increase peak inspiratory pressure on the ventilator by 4-5 cm H_2O until tube is cleared
• Assess infant for repeat dosing using radiographic confir-

mation of respiratory distress syndrome; repeat doses should be given as noted above; ventilator settings for repeat doses FIO_2 are decreased by 0.2 or amount to prevent cyanosis; ventilator rate of 30/min; inspiratory time <1 sec; if infant's pretreatment rate was >30, leave unchanged during dosing; resume usual ventilator management after dosing

Nursing diagnoses
☑ Gas exchange, impaired (uses)
☑ Knowledge deficit (teaching)

Implementation
• Administer after suctioning; give by endotracheal administration only by persons trained 🅟 in neonatal intubation and ventilation

• Use a no. 5 Fr end-hole catheter inserted into the endotracheal tube with the tip at distal end of endotracheal tube; shorten the catheter before insertion; insert the drug into the main bronchi by positioning infant with either right or left side dependent

• Determine the dosing by 🅟 weight of infant; slowly withdraw the contents into the plastic syringe through a 20-G needle; do not filter or shake; attach the premeasured no. 5 Fr catheter to syringe; fill with drug and discard excess through the catheter so only dose to be given remains in syringe

• For **prevention dosing,** stabilize, weigh, and intubate 🅟 the infant; give drug within 15 min of birth if possible; position infant and inj first quarter dose through catheter over 2-3 sec; remove catheter and manually ventilate with O_2 to prevent cyanosis (60 bpm) and

sufficient positive pressure to promote adequate air exchange and chest wall excursion

• For **rescue dosing,** give 🅟 drug as soon as infant is placed on ventilator after birth; immediately before administering dose, change ventilator settings to 60/min, inspiratory time 🅟 0.5 sec, FIO_2 l; position infant and inj first quarter through catheter over 2-3 sec; remove catheter; return to mechanical ventilator

🅟 • Ventilate infant for >30 sec or until stable after prevention or rescue strategy; reposition for next dose; same procedure for subsequent dosing; do not suction for at least 1 hr after dosing unless airway obstruction is evident; resume ventilator therapy after dosing

• Reduce peak ventilator inspiratory pressure immediately if chest expansion improves substantially after dose

• Reduce in FIO_2 in small, 🅟 repeated steps when infant becomes pink and transcutaneous oxygen saturation is in excess of 95%; oxygen saturation should remain between 90% and 95%

🅟 • Suction all infants before administration to prevent mucus plugging; if endotracheal tube obstruction is suspected, remove the obstruction and replace tube immediately

• Store in refrigerator; protect from light; warm to room temp for ≥20 min or warm in hand 8 min before giving; do not use artificial warming methods; enter a vial only once; unopened, unused vials that have been warmed to room temp may be rerefrigerated within 8 hr of warming;

do not warm and return to refrigerator more than once

Patient/family education
• Explain disease process and purpose of medication to parents; communicate
P neonate's progress

Evaluation
Positive therapeutic outcome
• Significant improvement in respiratory status (oxygenation, arterial blood gases, WNL)

---

rabeprazole (℞)
(rab-ee-pray′zole)
Aciphex
Func. class.: Proton pump inhibitor
Chem. class.: Benzimidazole
Pregnancy category C

Action: Suppresses gastric secretion by inhibiting hydrogen/potassium ATPase enzyme system in the gastric parietal cell; characterized as a gastric acid pump inhibitor, since it blocks the final step of acid production

➤**Therapeutic Outcome:** Absence of duodenal ulcers; decreased gastroesophageal reflux

Uses: Gastroesophageal reflux disease (GERD), severe erosive esophagitis, poorly responsive systemic GERD, pathologic hypersecretory conditions (Zollinger-Ellison syndrome, systemic mastocytosis, multiple endocrine adenomas); possibly effective for treatment of duodenal ulcers

Dosage and routes
Healing of duodenal ulcers
Adult: PO 20 mg qd × ≤4 wk, to be taken after breakfast

Erosive esophagitis/ gastroesophageal reflux disease
Adult: PO 20 mg qd × 4-8 wk

Pathologic hypersecretory conditions
Adult: PO 60 mg/day; may increase to 120 mg in 2 divided doses

Available forms: Tab, delayed rel 20 mg

Adverse effects
CNS: Headache, dizziness, asthenia
CV: Chest pain, angina, tachycardia, bradycardia, palpitations, peripheral edema
EENT: Tinnitus, taste perversion
GI: Diarrhea, abdominal pain, vomiting, nausea, constipation, flatulence, acid regurgitation, abdominal swelling, anorexia, irritable colon, esophageal candidiasis, dry mouth
GU: UTI, frequency, increased creatinine, **proteinuria, hematuria,** testicular pain, glycosuria
HEMA: **Pancytopenia, thrombocytopenia, neutropenia, leukocytosis,** anemia
INTEG: Rash, dry skin, urticaria, pruritus, alopecia
META: Hypoglycemia, increased hepatic enzymes, weight gain
MISC: Back pain, fever, fatigue, malaise
RESP: Upper respiratory tract infections, cough, epistaxis

Contraindications: Hypersensitivity

Precautions: Pregnancy **C,**
P lactation, children

Pharmacokinetics

Absorption	Unknown
Distribution	Unknown
Metabolism	Liver, extensively
Excretion	Kidneys, feces
Half-life	Unknown

Pharmacodynamics

Unknown

Interactions
Individual drugs
Clarithromycin: ↑ levels of rapeprazole
Diazepam: ↑ serum levels of rapeprazole
Phenytoin: ↑ serum levels of rapeprazole
Sucralfate: ↓ rapeprazole levels
Drug classifications
Benzodiazepines: ↑ levels of rapeprazole

NURSING CONSIDERATIONS
Assessment
• Assess GI system: bowel sounds q8h, abdomen for pain and swelling, anorexia
• Monitor hepatic enzymes: AST, ALT, increased alkaline phosphatase during treatment

Nursing diagnoses
☑ Pain (uses)
☑ Knowledge deficit (teaching)

Implementation
• Give after breakfast qd; do not crush, break, chew delayed rel tab

Patient/family education
• Advise patient to report severe diarrhea; drug may have to be discontinued
• Caution patient to avoid driving and other hazardous activities until response to drug is known
• Caution patient to avoid alcohol, salicylates, NSAIDs; may cause GI irritation

Evaluation
Positive therapeutic outcome
• Absence of epigastric pain, swelling, fullness

---

rapacuronium (℞)
(rap-a-kure-oh′nee-um)
Raplon
Withdrawn from market
Questions should be directed to 800-241-8812

Action: Inhibits transmission of nerve impulses by competing for cholinergic receptor sites; no analgesic response

▶**Therapeutic Outcome:** Paralysis of all skeletal muscles

Uses: Facilitation of endotracheal intubation, skeletal muscle relaxation during mechanical ventilation, surgery, or general anesthesia

Dosage and routes
Tracheal intubation
Adult: **IV** 1.5 mg/kg for short procedures, max block 90 secs, lasting about 15 mins

Repeat dosing in adults
Adult: **IV** after intubating dose, may give up to 3 maintenance doses of 0.5 mg/kg
P *Child 1 mo-12 yrs:* **IV** 2 mg/kg under halothane anesthesia

Available forms: Inj 100, 200 mg

Adverse effects
CV: Bradycardia, tachycardia, increased, decreased B/P, extrasystoles
INTEG: Rash, flushing, pruri-

---

tus, urticaria, sweating, salivation
MS: Weakness
RESP: **Prolonged apnea, bronchospasm, cyanosis, respiratory depression**

Contraindications: Hypersensitivity

Precautions: Pregnancy **C,** renal disease, cardiac disease, lactation, electrolyte imbalances, dehydration, neuromuscular disease, respiratory disease, ICP, malignant hyperthermia

Pharmacokinetics

Absorption	Complete bioavailability
Distribution	Crosses placenta
Metabolism	Plasma, protein binding, 50-80%
Excretion	Kidneys
Half-life	Elimination: Up to 22 days

Pharmacodynamics

Unknown

Interactions
Individual drugs
Lithium: ↑ paralysis length and intensity
Magnesium: ↑ paralysis length and intensity
Procainamide: ↑ paralysis length and intensity
Quinidine: ↑ paralysis length and intensity
Succinylcholine: ↑ paralysis length and intensity
Drug classifications
Antibiotics: ↑ neuromuscular blockade
Anticonvulsants: ↓ neuromuscular blockage
General anesthesia: ↑ paralysis length and intensity
Local anesthetics: ↑ neuromuscular blockade

NURSING CONSIDERATIONS
Assessment
• Monitor vital signs (B/P, pulse, respirations, airway) until fully recovered; note rate, depth, pattern of respirations, strength of hand grip; patient should be intubated before use
• Monitor for electrolyte imbalances (potassium, magnesium) before drug is used; electrolyte imbalances may lead to increased action of this drug
• Monitor for recovery: decreased paralysis of face, diaphragm, leg, arm, rest of body; residual weakness and respiratory problems may occur during recovery period
• Assess for hypersensitive reactions: rash, fever, respiratory distress, pruritus; drug should be discontinued

Nursing diagnoses
☑ Breathing pattern, ineffective (uses)
☑ Communication, impaired verbal (adverse reactions)
☑ Fear (adverse reactions)
☑ Knowledge deficit (teaching)

Implementation
• Use peripheral nerve stimulator (anesthesiologist) to determine neuromuscular blockade; deep tendon reflexes should be monitored during extended periods
• Should be administered only by qualified person, usually an anesthesiologist; do not administer IM
• Store in light-resistant area
• Give anticholinesterase to reverse neuromuscular blockade

Additive compatibilities:
Alfentanil, atropine, droperidol, epinephrine, fentanyl, gentamicin, glycopyrrolate, heparin, ketamine, labetalol,

---

☑ Herb/drug   🚫 Do Not Crush   ◆ Alert   ⟳π Key Drug   G Geriatric   P Pediatric lidocaine, methohexital, metoclopramide, midazolam, morphine, potassium chloride, propranolol, ranitidine, remifentanil, sufentanil, verapamil

Solution compatibilities:
0.9% NaCl, D_5W, D_5 NaCl, sterile water for inj, LR, bacteriostatic water for inj

Patient/family education
• Provide reassurance if communication is difficult during recovery from neuromuscular blockade
• Provide explanation to patients regarding all procedures or treatments; patient will remain conscious if anesthesia is not given also

Evaluation
Positive therapeutic outcome
• Paralysis of jaw, eyelid, head, neck, rest of body as evaluated by peripheral nerve stimulator

Treatment of overdose:
Edrophonium or neostigmine, atropine; monitor VS; may require mechanical ventilation

---

rofecoxib (℞)
(roe-fi-coks'ib)
Vioxx
Func. class.: Nonsteroidal antiinflammatory
Pregnancy category   C

Action: May inhibit prostaglandin synthesis by decreasing enzyme needed for biosynthesis; analgesic, antiinflammatory, antipyretic properties

➔ Therapeutic Outcome: Decreased pain, inflammation

Uses: Acute, chronic osteoarthritis, pain, primary dysmenorrhea

Dosage and routes
Osteoarthritis
Adult: PO 12.5 mg/day as a single dose may increase to 25 mg if needed

Primary dysmenorrhea
Adult: PO 50 mg qd, use for <5 days

Available forms: Tabs 12.5, 25 mg; susp 12.5, 25 mg/5 ml

Adverse effects
CNS: Fatigue, anxiety, depression, nervousness, paresthesia
CV: **Tachycardia,** angina, **MI,** *palpitations,* **dysrhythmias,** *hypertension, fluid retention*
EENT: Tinnitus, hearing loss, blurred vision, glaucoma, cataract, conjunctivitis, eye pain
GI: Nausea, anorexia, vomiting, constipation, dry mouth, diverticulitis, gastritis, gastroenteritis, hemorrhoids, hiatal hernia, stomatitis, **GI bleeding**
GU: **Nephrotoxicity:** *dysuria,* **hematuria, oliguria, azotemia, cystitis, UTI**
HEMA: **Blood dyscrasias,** *epistaxis, bruising, anemia*
INTEG: Purpura, *rash, pruritus, sweating, erythema, petechiae, photosensitivity, alopecia*
RESP: Pharyngitis, shortness of breath, pneumonia, coughing

Contraindications: Hypersensitivity to aspirin, iodides, other NSAIDs, asthma

Precautions: Pregnancy **C,** lactation, children, bleeding disorders, GI disorders, cardiac disorders, hypersensitivity to other antiinflammatory agents

---

Pharmacokinetics	
Absorption	Well absorbed (PO)
Distribution	Crosses placenta, bound to plasma proteins
Metabolism	Liver
Excretion	Kidneys
Half-life	Unknown

Pharmacodynamics
Unknown

Interactions
Individual drugs
Aspirin: ↓ effectiveness, ↑ adverse reactions
Coumadin: ↑ anticoagulant effects
Lithium: ↑ toxicity
Drug classifications
ACE inhibitors: may ↓ effects of ACE inhibitors
Anticoagulants: ↑ risk of bleeding
Antineoplastics: ↑ risk of hematologic toxicity
Diuretics: ↓ effectiveness of diuretics
Glucocorticoids: ↑ adverse reactions
NSAIDs: ↑ adverse reactions

NURSING CONSIDERATIONS
Assessment
• Assess for pain of osteoarthritis; check ROM, inflammation of joints, characteristics of pain
• Assess for pain, discomfort of dysmenorrhea
• Monitor blood counts during therapy; watch for decreasing platelets; if low, therapy may need to be discontinued, restarted after hematologic recovery; and for blood dyscrasias (thrombocytopenia): bruising, fatigue, bleeding, poor healing

Nursing diagnoses
☑ Pain (uses)
☑ Mobility, impaired physical (uses)
☑ Injury, risk for (side effects)
☑ Knowledge deficit (teaching)
Implementation
PO route
• Administer with food or milk to decrease gastric symptoms
◌ •Do not crush, dissolve, or chew

Patient/family education
• Teach patient that drug must be continued for prescribed time to be effective; to avoid other NSAIDs
• Caution patient to report bleeding, bruising, fatigue, malaise, since blood dyscrasias do occur
• Teach patient to take with a full glass of water to enhance absorption

Evaluation
Positive therapeutic outcome
• Decreased pain and inflammation in arthritic conditions
• Decrease pain in dysmenorrhea

rosiglitazone (℞)
(roes-i-glye′ta-zone)
Avandia
Func. class.: Antidiabetic, oral
Chem. class.: Thiazolidinedione
Pregnancy category C

Action: Improves insulin resistance by hepatic glucose metabolism, insulin receptor kinase activity, insulin receptor phosphorylation

⇒**Therapeutic Outcome:** Decreased symptoms of diabetes mellitus

---

☑ Herb/drug ◌ Do Not Crush ◆ Alert ☞ Key Drug 🄶 Geriatric 🄿 Pediatric

Uses: Stable adult-onset diabetes mellitus (type II) NIDDM

Dosage and routes
Monotherapy
Adult: PO 4 mg qd or in 2 divided doses, may increase to 8 mg qd or in 2 divided doses after 12 wks

Combination therapy
Adult: PO this drug should be added to metformin at the adult dose

Available forms: Tab 2, 4, 8 mg

Adverse effects
CNS: Fatigue, headache
ENDO: Hyper/hypoglycemia
MISC: Accidental injury, URI, sinusitis, anemia, back pain, diarrhea, edema

Contraindications: Hypersensitivity to thiazolidinediones, **P** children, lactation, diabetic ketoacidosis

Precautions: Pregnancy **C**, **G** elderly, thyroid disease, hepatic, renal disease

Pharmacokinetics	
Absorption	Unknown
Distribution	Protein binding 99.8%
Metabolism	Unknown
Excretion	Urine, feces
Half-life	Elimination 3-4 hrs

Pharmacodynamics	
Onset	Unknown
Peak	6-12 wk
Duration	Unknown

Interactions
Drug classification
Oral contraceptives: May decrease effect of oral contraceptive, alternate method advised

NURSING CONSIDERATIONS
Assessment
• Assess for hypoglycemic reactions (sweating, weakness, dizziness, anxiety, tremors, hunger), hyperglycemic reactions soon after meals
• Assess CBC (baseline, q3mo) during treatment; check liver function tests periodically; AST, LDH, FBS, glycosylated Hgb, fasting plasma insulin, plasma lipids, lipoproteins, B/P, body weight during treatment

Nursing diagnoses
☑ Nutrition, altered: more than body requirements (uses)
☑ Knowledge deficit (teaching)

Implementation
• Convert from other oral hypoglycemic agents if needed; change may be made without gradual dosage change; monitor serum or urine glucose and ketones tid during conversion
• Give once or in 2 divided doses
• Give tabs crushed and mixed with meal or fluids for patients with difficulty swallowing
• Store in tight container in cool environment

Patient/family education
• Teach patient to use capillary blood glucose test or Chemstrip tid
• Teach patient symptoms of hypo/hyperglycemia, what to do about each
• Advise patient that drug must be continued on daily basis; explain consequence of discontinuing drug abruptly
• Advise patient to avoid OTC medications or herbal preparations unless approved by the prescriber
• Advise patient that diabetes is life-long illness; that this

drug is not a cure, only controls symptoms
• Advise patient that all food included in diet plan must be eaten to prevent hypoglycemia
• Advise patient to carry Medic Alert ID and glucagon emergency kit for emergencies
• Instruct patient to notify prescriber if oral contraceptives are used
• Teach patient not to use if breast-feeding

Evaluation
Positive therapeutic outcome
• Decrease in polyuria, polydipsia, polyphagia; clear sensorium; absence of dizziness; stable gait; blood glucose at normal level

---

sirolimus (℞)
(seer-roe'-li-mus)
Rapamune
Func. class.: Immunosuppressant
Chem. class.: Macrolide
Pregnancy category   C

Action: Produces immunosuppression by inhibiting T lymphocytes activation and proliferation

Therapeutic Outcome: Prevention of rejection in organ transplant

Uses: Organ transplants—to prevent rejection, recommended use is with cyclosporine and corticosteroids

Investigational uses: Psoriasis

Dosage and routes
Adult: PO 2 mg qd with a 6 mg loading dose, may use 5 mg qd with a 15 mg loading dose

P *Child >13 yr weighing <40 kg (88 lbs):* PO/mg/m²/day, 3 mg/m²/loading dose

Hepatic dose
Reduce by 33% in maintenance dose

Available forms: Oral sol 1 mg/ml

Adverse effects
CNS: Tremors, headache, insomnia, paresthesia
CV: Hypertension, **atria fibrillation, CHF,** hypotension, palpitations, **tachycardia**
EENT: Blurred vision, photophobia
GI: Nausea, vomiting, diarrhea, *oral Candida, gum hyperplasia,* **hepatotoxicity,** constipation
GU: Urinary tract infections, **albuminuria, hematuria, proteinuria, renal failure**
HEMA: Anemia, **thrombocytopenia purpura, leukopenia**
INTEG: Rash, *acne*
META: Creatinine, edema, hypercholesterolemia, hyperlipemia, hypophosphatemia, weight gain, hyperglycemia, hyperkalemia, hyperuricemia, hypokalemia, hypomagnesemia
RESP: **Pleural effusion, atelectasis,** *dyspnea*
SYST: **Lymphoma**

Contraindications: Hypersensitivity to this drug or to components of the drug

Precautions: Severe renal disease, severe hepatic disease, pregnancy C, diabetes mellitus, hyperkalemia, hyperuricemia, lymphomas, lactation, **P** child <13 yrs, hypertension

---

Pharmacokinetics	
Absorption	Rapidly absorbed
Distribution	92% protein binding
Metabolism	Liver
Excretion	Unknown
Half-life	Unknown

Pharmacodynamics	
	PO
Onset	Unknown
Peak	1 hr single dose, 2 hr multiple dosing
Duration	Unknown

Interactions
Individual drugs
Bromocriptine: ↑ blood level
Carbamazepine: ↓ blood levels
Cimetidine: ↑ blood levels
Cyclosporine: ↑ blood levels
Danazol: ↑ blood levels
Erythromycin: ↑ blood levels
Metoclopramide: ↑ blood level
Phenobarbital: ↓ blood levels
Phenytoin: ↓ blood levels
Rifamycin: ↓ blood levels
Drug classifications
Antifungals: ↑ sirolimus levels
Calcium channel blockers: ↑ sirolimus levels
HIV-protease inhibitors: ↑ blood levels
Vaccines: ↓ effect of vaccines
Food/drug
Food: Alters bioavailability, use consistently with or without food
Grapefruit juice: Do not use with grapefruit juice

NURSING CONSIDERATIONS
Assessment
• Monitor blood studies: Hgb, WBC, platelets during treatment monthly; if leukocytes are <3000/mm³, or platelets <100,000/mm³, drug should be discontinued or reduced; decreased hemoglobulin level may indicate bone marrow suppression
• Monitor blood levels in those that may have altered metabolism, trough level ≥15 ng/ml are associated with increased adverse reactions
• Monitor lipid profile: cholesterol, triglycerides, a lipid-lowering agent may be needed
• Assess for infection and development of lymphoma
• Monitor liver function studies: alk phosphatase, AST, ALT, amylase, bilirubin, and for hepatotoxicity: dark urine, jaundice, itching, light-colored stools; drug should be discontinued

Nursing diagnoses
☑ Infection, risk for (uses)
☑ Knowledge deficit (teaching)

Implementation
• Administer prophylaxis for *Pneumocystis carinii* pneumonia for 1 yr after transplantation; prophylaxis for cytomegalovirus (CMV) is recommended for 90 days after transplantation in those at increased risk for CMV
• Use amber oral dose syringe and withdraw amount needed of oral sol from the bottle, empty correct dose into plastic/glass container holding 60 ml of water/orange juice, stir vigorously and have patient drink at once, refill container with additional 120 ml water/orange juice stir vigorously and drink at once, if using a pouch squeeze entire contents into container and follow above directions
• Give all medications PO if possible; avoid IM inj because bleeding may occur
• Give for 3 days before transplant surgery; patients should

be placed in protective isolation

• Store protected from light, refrigerate, stable for 24 months

Patient/family education

• Instruct patient to report fever, rash, severe diarrhea, chills, sore throat, fatigue because serious infections may occur; clay-colored stools, cramping may indicate hepatotoxicity

• Caution patient to avoid crowds or persons with known infections to reduce risk of infection

• To use contraception before, during, and 12 wk after drug has been discontinued

Evaluation

Positive therapeutic outcome

• Absence of graft rejection

---

temozolomide (℞)
(tem-oo-zole'oo-mide)
Temodar
Func. class.: Antineoplastic misc agent
Chem. class.: Imidazo-tetrazine derivative
Pregnancy category   **D**

Action: A pro-drug that undergoes conversion to MTIC. MTIC action prevents DNA transcription

Therapeutic Outcome: Prevention of rapidly growing malignant cells

Uses: Anaplastic astrocytoma with relapse

Dosage and routes
Adult: PO adjust dose based on nadir neutrophil and platelet counts 150 mg/m²/day × 5 days during 28-day cycle

Available forms: Caps 5, 20, 100, 250 mg

Adverse effects

CNS: **Seizures,** *hemiparesis, dizziness, poor coordination, amnesia, insomnia, paresthesia, somnolence, paresis, ataxia, anxiety, dysphagia, depression, confusion*

GI: *Nausea, anorexia, vomiting*

GU: *Urinary incontinence, UTI, frequency*

HEMA: **Thrombocytopenia, leukopenia,** anemia

INTEG: *Rash, pruritus*

MISC: *Headache, fatigue, asthenia, fever, edema, back pain, wt increase, diplopia*

RESP: *URI, pharyngitis, sinusitis, coughing*

Contraindications: Hypersensitivity to this drug or dacarbazine, pregnancy **D**, lactation

Precautions: Radiation therapy, renal, hepatic disease

Pharmacokinetics

Absorption	Rapid, complete
Distribution	Crosses blood-brain barrier
Metabolism	To MTIC and metabolite
Excretion	Urine, feces
Half-life	1.8 hr

Pharmacodynamics

Onset	Unknown
Peak	1 hr
Duration	Unknown

Interactions
Individual drugs
Radiation: ↑ toxicity, bone marrow suppression
Drug classifications
Antineoplastics: ↑ toxicity, bone marrow suppression
Bone marrow-suppressing drugs: ↑ bone marrow suppression

Live vaccines: ↑ adverse reactions, ↓ antibody reaction
Food/drug
↓ absorption

NURSING CONSIDERATIONS
Assessment
• Assess symptoms indicating severe allergic reaction: rash, pruritus, urticaria, purpuric skin lesions, itching, flushing; drug should be discontinued
• Obtain CBC on day 22 (21 days after 1st dose), CBC weekly until recovery if ANC is $<1.5 \times 10^9$/L and platelets $<100 \times 10^9$/L, do not administer to patients that do not tolerate 100 mg/m², myelosuppression usually occurs late in the treatment cycle
• Monitor renal function studies: BUN, creatinine, urine CrCl before and during therapy; I&O ratio; report fall in urine output to <30 ml/hr
• Monitor temp q4h (may indicate beginning of infection)
• Monitor liver function tests before and during therapy (bilirubin, AST, ALT, LDH) as needed or monthly; note jaundice of skin or sclera, dark urine, clay-colored stools, itchy skin, abdominal pain, fever, diarrhea; hepatotoxicity can be serious and fatal
• Assess for bleeding: hematuria, stool guaiac, bruising or petechiae, mucosa or orifices q8h; check for inflammation of mucosa, breaks in skin

Nursing diagnoses
☑ Injury, risk for (adverse reactions)
☑ Body image disturbance (adverse reactions)
☑ Infection, risk for (adverse reactions)
☑ Knowledge deficit (teaching)

Implementation
• Give fluids **IV** or PO before chemotherapy to hydrate patient
• Give antiemetic 30-60 min before giving drug to prevent vomiting, and prn; antibiotics for prophylaxis of infection
• Provide liquid diet: carbonated beverages; gelatin may be added if patient is not nauseated or vomiting
• Capsules should not be opened, if accidentally damaged, do not allow contact with skin, or inhale
• Give on empty stomach to prevent nausea/vomiting

Patient/family education
• Teach patient to avoid use of products containing aspirin or NSAIDs, razors, commercial mouthwash, since bleeding may occur; to report symptoms of bleeding (hematuria, tarry stools)
• Instruct patient to report signs of anemia (fatigue, headache, irritability, faintness, shortness of breath)
• Caution patient not to have any vaccinations without the advice of prescriber; serious reactions can occur
• Advise patient contraception is needed during treatment and for several months after the completion of therapy; drug has teratogenic properties

Evaluation
Positive therapeutic outcome
• Prevention of rapid division of malignant cells

♣ Canada Only   Adverse effects: *italic* = common; **bold** = life-threatening

zaleplon (℞)
(zale′plon)
Sonata
Func. class.: Sedative-hypnotic
Chem. class.: Pyrazolopyrimidine
Pregnancy category C

Action: Binds selectively to omega-1 receptor of the $GABA_A$ receptor complex; results are sedation, hypnosis, skeletal muscle relaxation, anticonvulsant activity, anxiolytic action

⇒**Therapeutic Outcome:** Ability to sleep

Uses: Insomnia

Dosage and routes
Adult: PO 10 mg hs; may increase dose to 20 mg hs if needed; 5 mg may be used in low weight persons

G *Elderly:* PO 15 mg hs; may increase if needed

Available forms: Caps 5, 10 mg

Adverse effects
CNS: Drowsiness, amnesia, depersonalization, hallucinations, hypesthesia, paresthesia, somnolence, tremor, vertigo, dizziness, anxiety
EENT: Vision changes, ear/eye pain, hyperacusis, parosmia
GI: Nausea, anorexia, colitis, dyspepsia, dry mouth, constipation
MISC: Abdominal pain, asthenia, fever, headache, myalgia, dysmenorrhea

Contraindications: Hypersensitivity

Precautions: Hepatic disease,
G renal disease, elderly, psychosis,

P child <15 yr, pregnancy **C**, lactation

Pharmacokinetics	
Absorption	Rapidly absorbed
Distribution	Extravascular tissues crosses blood-brain barrier; crosses placenta
Metabolism	Extensively, liver to inactive metabolites
Excretion	Kidneys
Half-life	1 hr

Pharmacodynamics	
Onset	Rapid
Peak	1 hr
Duration	Unknown

Interactions
Individual drugs
Cimetidine: ↑ action of zaleplon
Rifampin: ↓ zaleplon levels
Food/drug
Prolonged absorption
High fat/heavy meal: Sleep onset reduced

NURSING CONSIDERATIONS
Assessment
• Assess for previous drug dependence or tolerance; if drug dependent or tolerant, amount of medication should be restricted
• Monitor patient's mental status: mood, sensorium, affect, sleeping patterns, drowsiness, dizziness, suicidal tendencies

Nursing diagnoses
☑ Sleep pattern disturbance (uses)
☑ Knowledge deficit (teaching)
☑ Noncompliance (teaching)

Implementation
• Give ½-1 hr before hs for sleeplessness; give on empty stomach
• Advise patient that drug may cause memory problems, de-

pendence (if used for longer periods of time), changes in behavior/thinking

Patient/family education
• Inform patient that drug is for short term use only
• Teach patient to take immediately before going to bed
• Advise patient not to ingest a high fat/heavy meal before taking
• Advise patient to avoid OTC preparations unless approved by a physician, to avoid alcohol ingestion or other psychotropic medications unless prescribed by a health care provider, that 1-2 wk of therapy may be required before therapeutic effects occur
• Caution patient to avoid driving, activities requiring alertness—drowsiness may occur; until medication response is known, tell patient that drowsiness may worsen at beginning of treatment
• Instruct patient not to discontinue medication abruptly after long-term use

Evaluation
Positive therapeutic outcome
• Decreased sleeplessness

zanamivir (R)
(zan-a-mee'veer)
Relenza
Func. class.: Antiviral
Pregnancy category **B**

Action: Inhibits the enzyme needed for influenza virus replication

➤ **Therapeutic Outcome:** Decreased symptoms of influenza type A for those that have been symptomatic for no more than 2 days

Uses: Treatment of influenza type A

Dosage and routes
P **Adult and child >12 yr:** inh 2 inhalations (two 5 mg blisters) q12h × 5 days, on the 1st day 2 doses should be taken at least 2 hrs between doses

Available forms: Blisters of powder for inhalation: 5 mg

Adverse effects
CNS: Headache, dizziness, fatigue
EENT: Ear, nose, throat infections
GI: Nausea, vomiting, diarrhea
RESP: Nasal symptoms, cough, sinusitis, bronchitis

Contraindications: Hypersensitivity

G **Precautions:** Elderly, lactation,
P children <12 yr, respiratory disease, pregnancy **B**

Pharmacokinetics	
Absorption	4-17% absorbed
Distribution	<10% protein binding
Metabolism	Not metabolized
Excretion	Kidneys unchanged
Half-life	2½-5 hr

Pharmacodynamics
Unknown

Interactions
None known

NURSING CONSIDERATIONS
Assessment
• Assess for symptoms of influenza A: increased temperature, malaise, aches and pains
• Assess for skin eruptions, photosensitivity after administration of drug
• Monitor respiratory status: rate, character, wheezing, tightness in chest

- Assess for allergies before initiation of treatment, reaction of each medication

Nursing diagnoses

✓ Infection, risk for (uses)

✓ Knowledge deficit (teaching)

Implementation

- Give before exposure to influenza; continue for 5 days after contact
- Store in tight, dry container

Patient/family education

- Give patient "Patient's instruction for use" and review all points before using delivery system
- Teach patient to avoid hazardous activities if dizziness occurs

- Teach patient to take drug exactly as prescribed; to use for the entire 5 days
- Inform patient that this drug does not reduce transmission risk of influenza to others
- Advise patients with asthma or COPD to carry a fast-acting inhaled bronchodilator since bronchospasm may occur; to use scheduled inhaled bronchodilators before using this drug

Evaluation

Positive therapeutic outcome

- Absence of fever, malaise, cough, dyspnea in influenza A

Appendix B

Recent FDA Drug Approvals

GENERIC NAME	TRADE NAME	USE
alosetron	Lotronex	Irritable bowel syndrome
cevimeline	Evoxac	Dry mouth in Sjögren's syndrome
linezolid	Zyvox	Antibiotic-resistant infections
oxcarbazepine	Trileptal	Partial seizures
pemirolast	Alamast	Allergic conjunctivitis
pneumococcal 7-valent conjugate vaccine	Prevnar	Immunization against *Streptococcus pneumoniae*
progestogen emergency contraceptive	Plan B	Prevention of pregnancy

Appendix C

Ophthalmic, Otic, Nasal, and Topical Products

OPHTHALMIC PRODUCTS

α-ADRENERGIC BLOCKER
dapiprazole (℞)
(da-pip′ra-zole)
Rev-Eyes

ANESTHETICS
proparacaine (℞)
(proe-par′a-kane)
AK-Taine, Alcaine,
Diocaine ✤, Ocu-Caine,
Ophthaine, Ophthestic,
Specto-Caine
tetracaine
(tet′ra-kane)
Minims Tetracaine,
Pontocaine Eye, Pontocaine
Hcl

ANTIHISTAMINES
emedastine
(ee-med′-a-steen)
Emadine
levocabastine (℞)
(lee-voh-cab′ah-steen)
Livostin
olopatadine (℞)
(oh-loh-pat′ah-deen)
Patanol

ANTIINFECTIVES
bacitracin (℞)
(bass-i-tray′sin)
AK-Tracin, Bacitracin
Ophthalmic
brimonidine
(bri-moe′ni-deen)
Alphagan

chloramphenicol (℞)
(klor-am-fen′i-kole)
AK-Chlor, Chloramphenicol,
Chloramphenicol
Ophthalmic, Chloromycetin
Ophthalmic, Chloroptic,
Chloroptic S.O.P., Fenicol ✤,
Isopto Fenical ✤,
Pentamycin ✤
ciprofloxacin (℞)
(sip-ro-floks′a-sin)
Ciloxan
erythromycin (℞)
(er-ith-roe-mye′sin)
AK-Mycin, erythromycin,
Ilotycin
gentamicin (℞)
(jen-ta-mye′sin)
Garamycin Ophthalmic,
Genoptic Ophthalmic,
Genoptic S.O.P., Gentacidin,
Gent-AK, gentamicin,
Gentamicin Ophthalmic
Liquifilm, Gentak
idoxuridine-IDU (℞)
(eye-dox-yoor′i-deen)
Herplex, Stoxil
natamycin (℞)
(nat-a-mye′sin)
Natacyn
norfloxacin (℞)
(nor-floks′a-sin)
Chibroxin
ofloxacin (℞)
(oh-floks′a-sin)
Ocuflox

�*Z* Herb/drug ⓢ Do Not Crush ◆ Alert ⟳ Key Drug Ⓖ Geriatric Ⓟ Pediatric

polymyxin B (℞)
(pol-ee-mix'in)
Aerosporin, polymyxin B sulfate
silver nitrate 1% (℞)
sulfacetamide sodium (℞)
(sul-fa-seet'a-mide)
AK-Sulf, Bleph-10 Liquifilm, Bleph-10 S.O.P., Isopto Cetamide, Ophthacet, Sodium Sulamyd, sodium sulfacetamide 10%, sodium sulfacetamide 15%, sodium sulfacetamide 30%, SOSS-10, Sulfair 15
tetracycline (℞)
(tet-ra-sye'kleen)
Achromycin Ophthalmic
tobramycin (℞)
(toe-bra-mye'sin)
Tobrex
trifluridine (℞)
(trye-floor'i-deen)
Viroptic
vidarabine (℞)
(vye-dare'a-been)
Vira-A

β-ADRENERGIC BLOCKERS
betaxolol (℞)
(beh-tax'oh-lole)
Betoptic, Betoptic S
carteolol (℞)
(kar-tee'oh-lole)
Ocupress
levobunolol (℞)
(lee-voe-byoo'no-lole)
Betagen
metipranolol (℞)
(met-ee-pran'oh-lole)
Optipranolol
timolol (℞)
(tym'-moe-lole)
Apo-Timop ❖, Betimol, Timoptic

CHOLINERGICS
(Direct-acting)
carbachol (℞)
(kar'ba-kole)
Iosopto Carbachol, Miostat
pilocarpine (℞)
(pye-loe-kar'peen)
Adsorbocarpine, Akarpine, Isopto Carpine, Ocu-Carpine, Ocusert-Pilo, Pilagan, Pilocar, pilocarpine, Pilopine HS, Piloptic-1, Piloptic-2, Pilostat, Pilopto-Carpine

(cholinesterase inhibitors)
demecarium (℞)
(dem-e-kare'ee-um)
Humorsol
ecothiophate (℞)
(ek-oh-thye'eh-fate)
Ecostigmine Iodide, Phospholine Iodide
isoflurophate
(eye-soe-floor'oh-fate)
Floropryl
physostigmine (℞)
(fi-zoe-stig'meen)
Eserine Salicylate, Isopto Eserin

CYCLOPLEGIC MYDRIATICS
atropine (℞)
(a'troe-peen)
Atropine-1, Atropine Care Ophthalmic, Atropine Sulfate Ophthalmic, Atropine Sulfate S.O.P., Atropisol, Isopto Atropine
cyclopentolate (℞)
(sye-kloe-pen'toe-late)
AK-Pentolate, Cyclogly, I-Pentolate

❖ Canada Only   Adverse effects: *italic* = common; **bold** = life-threatening

homatropine (Ŗ)
(home-a'troe-peen)
AK-Homatropine,
l-Homatrine, Isopto
Homatropine, Minims
Homatropine ✽, Spectro-
Homatropine
physostigmine (Ŗ)
(fi-zoe-stig'meen)
Fisostin, Isopto Eserine
Solution/Eserine Sulfate
Ointment
scopolamine (Ŗ)
(skoe-pol'a-meen)
Isopto-Hyoscine
tropicamide (Ŗ)
(troe-pik'a-mide)
Mydriacyl, Tropicacyl,
l-Piramide

GLUCOCORTICOIDS
dexamethasone
(dex-a-meth'a-sone)
AK-Dex, Decadron
Phosphate, Dexamethasone
Ophthalmic Suspension,
Maxidex
fluorometholone (Ŗ)
(flure-oh-meth'oh-lone)
Flarex, Fluor-Op, FML, FML
Forte, FML Liquifilm
medrysone (Ŗ)
(me'dri-sone)
HMS
prednisolone (Ŗ)
(pred-niss'oh-lone)
Econopred, Econopred Plus,
AK-Pred, Inflamase Forte,
Inflamase Mild Ophthalmic,
Metreton Ophthalmic, Pred-
Forte, Pred-Mild
rimexolone (Ŗ)
(ri-mex'a-lone)
Vexol

NONSTEROIDAL
ANTIINFLAMMATORIES
diclofenac (Ŗ)
(dye-kloe'fen-ak)
Voltaran
flurbiprofen (Ŗ)
(flure-bi'-pro-fen)
Ocufen
ketorolac (Ŗ)
(kee-toe'role-ak)
Acular
suprofen
(soo-proe'fen)
Profenal

SYMPATHOMIMETICS
apraclonidine
(a-pra-klon'i-deen)
Iopidine
brimonidine (Ŗ)
(brem-on'-ii-dine)
Alphagan
dipivefrin
(dye-pi'vef-rin)
Propine
**epinephrine bitartrate/
epinephrine HCl/
epinephryl borate** (Ŗ)
(ep-i-nef'rin)
Epitrate, Mytrate/Epifrin,
Glaucon/Epinal, Eppy ✽

OPHTHALMIC
DECONGESTANTS/
VASOCONSTRICTORS
naphazoline (OTC, Ŗ)
(naf-az'oh-leen)
AK-Con Ophthalmic, Albalon
Liquifilm Ophthalmic,
Allerest Eye Drops, Clear
Eyes, Comfort Eye Drops,
Degest 2, Nafazair,
naphazoline HCl, Naphcon,
Naphcon Forte, Opcon,
Vasoclear, Vasocon Regular,
Estivin II

☒ Herb/drug ⬆ Do Not Crush ◆ Alert ⬤╍ Key Drug ᴳ Geriatric ᴾ Pediatric

oxymetazoline (℞, OTC)
(ox-i-met-ah-zoh′leen)
OcuClear, Visine LR
phenylephrine (OTC)
(fen-ill-ef′rin)
AK-Dilate Ophthalmic, AK-Nefrin Ophthalmic, Isopto Frin, Neo-Synephrine 2.5%, Neo-Synephrine 10% Plain, Neo-Synephrine Viscous, phenylephrine HCl, 2.5% Mydfrin Ophthalmic, Phenoptic Relief, Prefrin
tetrahydrozoline (OTC)
(tet-ra-hye-dro′zoe-leen)
Collyrium Fresh Eye Drops, Eyesine, Murine Plus Eye Drops, Optigene 3 Eye Drops, Soothe Eye Drops, tetrahydrozoline HCl, Tyzine HCl, Tyzine Pediatric, Visine Eye Drops

MISCELLANEOUS OPHTHALMICS
brinzolamide (℞)
(brin-zole′aa-mide)
Azopt
dorzolamide (℞)
(dor-zol′a-mid)
Trusopt
ketotifen
(ke-toe-tie′fen)
Zaditor
latanoprost (℞)
(la-tan′oh-proest)
Xalatan
lodoxamide
(loe-dox′ah-mide)
Alomide
Pregnancy category: demecarium, isofluro-phate **X;** apraclonidine, cyclopentolate, ecothipate, glucocorticoids,✷levobuna-

lol, metipranolol, pilo-carpine, proparacaine, suprofen, tetracaine **C;** dapiprazole, dipivefrin **B**

β-*Adrenergic blockers*
Action: Reduces production of aqueous humor by unknown mechanism

Uses: Ocular hypertension, chronic open-angle glaucoma

Anesthetics
Action: Decreases ion permeability by stabilizing neuronal membrane

Uses: Cataract extraction, tonometry, gonioscopy, removal of foreign objects, corneal suture removal, glaucoma surgery (ophth); pruritus, sunburn, toothache, sore throat, cold sores, oral pain, rectal pain and irritation, control of gagging (top)

Antiinfectives
Action: Inhibits folic acid synthesis by preventing PABA use, which is necessary for bacterial growth

Uses: Conjunctivitis, superficial eye infections, corneal ulcers, prophylaxis against infection after removal of foreign matter from the eye

Antiinflammatories
Action: Decreases inflammation, resulting in decreased pain, photophobia, hyperemia, cellular infiltration

Uses: Inflammation of eye, eyelids, conjunctiva, cornea; uveitis, iridocyclitis, allergic conditions, burns, foreign bodies, postoperatively in cataract

---

✷ Canada Only   Adverse effects: *italic* = common; **bold** = life-threatening

Carbonic anhydrase inhibitor

Action: Converted to epinephrine, which decreases aqueous production and increases outflow

Uses: Open-angle glaucoma, ocular hypertension

Direct-acting miotic

Action: Acts directly on cholinergic receptor sites; induces miosis, spasm of accommodation, fall in intraocular pressure, caused by stimulation of ciliary, pupillary sphincter muscles, which leads to pulling away of iris from filtration angle, resulting in increased outflow of aqueous humor

Uses: Primary glaucoma, early stages of wide-angle glaucoma (less useful in advanced stages), chronic open-angle glaucoma, acute narrow-angle glaucoma before emergency surgery; also neutralizes mydriatics used during eye exam; may be used alternately with mydriatics to break adhesions between iris and lens

———

Adverse effects

CNS: Headache

CV: Hypertension, tachycardia, dysrhythmias

EENT: Burning, stinging

GI: Bitter taste

Contraindications: Hypersensitivity

Precautions: Pregnancy, lactation, children, aphakia, hypersensitivity to carbonic anhydrase inhibitors, sulfonamides, thiazide diuretics, ocular inhibitors, hepatic and renal insufficiency

NURSING CONSIDERATIONS

Assessment

• Monitor ophth exams and intraocular pressure readings

• Monitor blood counts; liver, renal function tests and serum electrolytes during long-term treatment

Nursing diagnoses

☑ Sensory-perceptual alteration: visual (uses)

☑ Knowledge deficit (teaching)

Implementation

• Storage at room temp away from light

Patient/family education

• Teach how to instill drops

• Advise patient that drug may cause burning, itching, blurring, dryness of eye area

Evaluation

Positive therapeutic outcome

• Absence of increased intraocular pressure

NASAL AGENTS

NASAL DECONGESTANTS
azelastine (℞)
(ay-zell'ah-steen)
Astelin
desoxyephedrine (OTC)
(des-oxy-e-fed'rin)
Vicks Inhaler
ephedrine (OTC)
(e-fed'rin)
Kondon's Nasal Jelly,
Pretz-D, Vicks Vatronol
epinephrine (OTC)
(ep-i-neff'rin)
Adrenalin
naphazoline (OTC)
(naff-a-zoe'leen)
Privine

———

☑ Herb/drug 🚫 Do Not Crush ⬥ Alert ⊶ Key Drug G Geriatric P Pediatric

oxymetazoline (OTC)
(ox-i-met-az'oh-leen)
Afrin, Afrin Children's Nose Drops, Allerest 12-Hour Nasal, Chlorphed-LA, Coricidin Nasal Mist, Dristan Long Lasting, Duramist Plus, Duration, Genasal, NTZ Long-Acting Nasal, Nafrine ✦, Neo-Synephrine 12 Hour, Nostrilla, oxymetazoline HCl, Sinarest 12-Hour, Sinex Long-Acting, Twice-A-Day Nasal, 4-Way Long Acting Nasal
phenylephrine (OTC)
(fen-ill-eff'rin)
Alconefrin 12, Children's Nostril, Neo-Synephrine, Sinex
propylhexadrine (OTC)
(proe-pil-hex'a-dreen)
Benzedrex Inhaler
tetrahydrozoline (OTC)
(tet-ra-hye-dro'zoe-leen)
Tyzine
xylometazoline (OTC)
(zye-loh-meh-tazz'oh-leen)
Otrivin, Otrivin Pediatric Nasal Drops, xylometazoline HCl

NASAL STEROIDS
beclomethasone (Ŗ)
(be-kloe-meth'a-sone)
Beconase AQ Nasal, Beconase Inhalation, Vancenase AQ Nasal, Vancenase Nasal
dexamethasone (Ŗ)
(dex-a-meth'a-sone)
Decadron Phosphate Turbinaire
Pregnancy category **C**

Action: Produces vasoconstriction (rapid, long acting) of arterioles, thereby decreasing fluid exudation, mucosal engorgement by stimulation of α-adrenergic receptors in vascular smooth muscle

⇒ **Therapeutic Outcome:** Absence of nasal congestion

Uses: Nasal congestion

Dosage and routes
Desoxyephedrine
▣ *Adult and child >6 yr:* 1-2 **INH** in each nostril q2h or less
Ephedrine
Adult: Fill dropper to the level marked, then use in each nostril q4h or less
Epinephrine
▣ *Adult and child >6 yr:* Apply with swab, drops, spray prn
Naphazoline
▣ *Adult and child >6 yr:* 1-2 drops/spray q6h or less
Oxymetazoline
▣ *Adult and child >6 yr:* **INSTILL** 2-3 gtt or sprays to each nostril bid
▣ *Child 2-6 yr:* **INSTILL** 2-3 gtt or sprays 0.025 sol bid, not to exceed 3 days
Phenylephrine
▣ *Adult and child >12 yr:* 2-3 drops/spray (0.25-0.5) in each nostril: q3-4h or less; or 2-3 drops/spray (1%) in each nostril q4h or less
▣ *Child 6-12 yr:* 2-3 drops/spray (0.25%) in each nostril q3-4h
▣ *Infant >6 mo:* 1-2 drops (0.16%) in each nostril q3h
Propylhexadrine
▣ *Adult and child >6 yr:* 1-2 **INH** in each nostril q2h or less
Tetrahydrozoline
▣ *Adult and child >6 yr:* 2-4 drops (0.1%) q3-4h prn or 3-4 sprays in each nostril q4h prn

---

✦ Canada Only   Adverse effects: *italic* = common; **bold** = life-threatening

P *Child 2-6 yr:* 2-3 drops
(0.05%) in each nostril q4-
6h prn

Xylometazoline
P *Adult and child >12 yr:* 2-3
drops/spray (0.1%) in each
nostril q8-10h

P *Child 2-12yr:* 2-3 drops
(0.05%) in each nostril q8-10h

Available forms: Nasal sol
0.025%, 0.05%

Adverse effects
CNS: Anxiety, restlessness,
tremors, weakness, insomnia,
dizziness, fever, headache
EENT: Irritation, burning,
sneezing, stinging, dryness,
rebound congestion
GI: Nausea, vomiting, anorexia
INTEG: Contact dermatitis

Contraindications: Hypersensitivity to sympathomimetic
amines

P **Precautions:** Children <6 yr,
G elderly, diabetes, cardiovascular
disease, hypertension, hyperthyroidism, increased intracranial pressure, prostatic hypertrophy, pregnancy **C,** glaucoma

NURSING CONSIDERATIONS
Assessment
• Assess for redness, swelling,
pain in nasal passages before
and during treatment
• Assess for syst absorption;
hypertension, tachycardia;
notify prescriber; syst absorption occurs at high doses or
after prolonged use

Nursing diagnoses
✓Airway clearance, ineffective
(uses)
✓Knowledge deficit (teaching)
✓Noncompliance (teaching)

Implementation
• Have patient tilt head back,
squeeze bulb to create a vac-
uum, and draw correct amount
of sol into dropper; insert 2 gtt
of sol into nostril; repeat in
other nostril
• Store in light-resistant
container; do not expose to
high temp or let sol come into
contact with aluminum
• Give for <4 consecutive days
• Provide environmental humidification to decrease nasal
congestion, dryness

Patient/family education
• Advise patient that stinging
may occur for several
applications; drying of mucosa
may be decreased by environmental humidification
• Caution patient to notify
prescriber if irregular pulse,
insomnia, dizziness, or tremors
occur
• Teach patient proper administration to avoid syst absorption
• Advise patient to rinse dropper with very hot water to
prevent contamination

Evaluation
Positive therapeutic outcome
• Decreased nasal congestion

**TOPICAL
GLUCOCORTICOIDS**

alclometasone (℞)
(al-kloe-met′a-sone)
Adovate
amcinonide (℞)
(am-sin′oh-nide)
Cyclocort

---

betamethasone (℞)
(bay-ta-meth′a-sone)
Alphatrex, Beben ✤,
Betacort ✤, Betaderm,
Betatrex, Beta-Val,
Bethovate ✤, Betmethacort,
Celestoderm ✤, Dermabet,
Diprolene, Diprosone,
Ectosonel ✤, Maxivate,
Metaderm ✤,
Novobetamet, Psorion,
Uticort, Valisone, Valnac
clobetasol (℞)
(kloe-bay′ta-sol)
Dermovate ✤, Temovate
clocortolone (℞)
(kloe-kore′toe-lone)
Cloderm
desonide (℞)
(dess′oh-nide)
Des Owen, Tridesilon
desoximetasone (℞)
(dess-ox-i-met′a-sone)
Topicort
dexamethasone (℞)
(dex-a-meth′a-sone)
Aeroseb-Dex, Decaderm,
Decaspray
diflorasone (℞)
(dye-flor′a-sone)
Florone, Maxiflor, Psorcon
fluocinolone (℞)
(floo-oh-sin′oh-lone)
Fluocin, Licon, Lidemol ✤,
Lidex, Lyderm ✤, Topsyn ✤,
Vasoderm
flurandrenolide (℞)
(flure-an-dren′oh-lide)
Cordran, Cordran SP,
Cordran Tape, Drenison
1/4 ✤, Drenison Tape ✤
fluticasone (℞)
(floo-tik′a-sone)
Cutivate

halcinonide (℞)
(hal-sin′oh-nide)
Halog, Halog-E
halobetasol (℞)
(hal-oh-bay′ta-sol)
Ultravate
hydrocortisone (℞)
(hye-droe-kor′ti-sone)
Actiocort, Aeroseb-HC, Ala-
Cort, Allercort, Alphaderm,
Anusol HC, Bactine, Barriere-
HC ✤, Calde-CORT Anti-Itch,
Carmol HC, Cetacort,
Cortacet ✤, Cortaid,
Cortate ✤, Cort-Dome,
Cortef ✤, Corticaine,
Corticreme ✤, Cortifair,
Cortizone, Cortoderm ✤,
Cortril, Delcort, Dermacort,
DemiCort, Dermtex HC, Emo-
Cort, Epifoam, FoilleCort,
Gly-Cort, Gynecort, Hi-Cor,
Hycort, Hyderm ✤, Hydro-
Tex, Hytone, Lacti-Care-HC,
Lanacort, Lemoderm, Locoid,
My Cort, Novoehydrocort ✤,
Nutracort Pharm,
Pharmacort, Pentacort,
Rederm, Rhulicort S-T Cort,
Synacort, Sarna HC ✤, Texa-
Cort, Unicort ✤, Westcort
methylprednisolone (℞)
(meth-ill-pred-niss′oh-lone)
Depo-Medrol
mometasone (℞)
(moe-met′a-sone)
Elocon
prednicarbate (℞)
(pred-ni-kar′bate)
Dermatop
triamcinolone (℞)
(trye-am-sin′oh-lone)
Aristocort, Flutex, Kenac,
Kenalog, Kenonel,
Triaderm ✤, Trianide ✤,
Triderm, Trymex
Pregnancy category   **C**

✤ Canada Only   Adverse effects: *italic* = common; **bold** = life-threatening

Action: Antipruritic, antiinflammatory

→**Therapeutic Outcome:** Decreased itching, inflammation

Uses: Psoriasis, eczema, contact dermatitis, pruritus; usually reserved for severe dermatoses that have not responded
to less potent formulation

Dosage and routes
P *Adult and child:* Apply to
affected area

Adverse effects
*INTEG: Acne, atrophy, epider-
mal thinning, purpura, striae*

Contraindications: Hypersensitivity, viral infections,
fungal infections

Precautions: Pregnancy **C**

NURSING CONSIDERATIONS
Assessment
• Temp; if fever develops, drug
should be discontinued
• For systemic absorption,
increased temp, inflammation,
irritation

Nursing diagnoses
✓ Pain, chronic (uses)
✓ Knowledge deficit (teaching)
✓ Skin integrity, impaired (uses)

Implementation
• Apply only to affected areas;
do not get in eyes
• Apply and leave site uncov-
ered or lightly covered; occlusive dressing is not recommended—systemic absorption
may occur
• Use only on dermatoses; do
not use on weeping, denuded,
or infected area
• Cleanse area before application of drug
• Continue treatment for a few
days after area has cleared
• Store at room temp

Patient/family education
• Teach patient to avoid sunlight on affected area, burns
may occur
• Teach patient to limit treatment to 14 days

Evaluation
Positive therapeutic outcome
• Absence of severe itching,
patches on skin, flaking

TOPICAL ANTIFUNGALS

amphotericin B
(OTC)
(am-foe-ter′i-sin)
Fungizone
butenafine (℞)
(byoo-tin′a-feen)
Mentex
ciclopirox **(OTC)**
(sye-kloe-peer′ox)
Loprox
clioquinol **(OTC)**
(klye-oh-kwin′ole)
Vioforim
clotrimazole **(OTC)**
(kloe-trye′ma-zole)
Canestew ✦, Clotrimaderm
✦, Lotrimin, Lotrimin AF,
Mycelex, Mycelex OTC,
Myclo ✦, Neozol ✦
econazole **(OTC)**
(ee-kon′a-zole)
Spectazole
haloprogin **(OTC)**
(hal-oh-proe′jin)
Halotex
ketoconazole **(OTC)**
(kee-toe-kon′a-zole)
Nizoral
miconazole **(OTC)**
(mye-kon′a-zole)
Micatin, Monistat-Derm
naftifine **(OTC)**
(naff′ti-feen)
Naftin

☑ Herb/drug   ⓢ Do Not Crush   ◆ Alert   ⚷ Key Drug   ⓖ Geriatric   P Pediatric

nystatin (OTC)
(nye-stat'in)
Mycostatin, Nodostine ✚,
Nilstat, Nyoderm ✚, Nystex
oxiconazole (OTC)
(ox-i-kon'a-zole)
Oxistat
selenium (OTC)
(see-leen'ee-um)
Exsel, Head and Shoulders
Intensive Treatment,
Selenium Sulfide, Selsun,
Selsun Blue
terbinafine (OTC)
(ter-bin'a-feen)
Lamisil
tolnaftate (OTC)
(tole-naf'tate)
Absorbine Antifungal,
Absorbine Jock Itch,
Absorbine Jr. Antifungal,
Aftate For Athlete's Foot,
Aftate for Jock Itch, Desenex
Spray, Genaspor, NP-27,
Quinsana Plus, Tinactin,
Ting, tolnaftate, Zeasorb-AF
undecylenic acid (OTC)
(un-deh-sih-len'ik)
Caldesene, Cruex, Decylenes,
Desenex, Desenex Maximum
Strength, Protectol
Pregnancy category   **B**

Action: Interferes with fungal
cell membrane permeability

➔**Therapeutic Outcome:** Absence of itching and white
patches of the skin

Uses: Tinea cruris, tinea pedis,
diaper rash, minor skin
irritations; amphotericin B is
used for *Candida* infections

Dosage and routes
Massage into affected area,
surrounding area qd or bid,
continue for 7-14 days, not to
exceed 4 wk

Adverse effects
INTEG: Burning, stinging,
dryness, itching, local irritation

Contraindications: Hypersensitivity

Precautions: Pregnancy **B**,
lactation, children

Interactions: None

NURSING CONSIDERATIONS
Assessment
• Assess skin for fungal
infections; peeling, dryness,
itching before and throughout
treatment
• Assess for continuing
infection; increased size, number of lesions

Nursing diagnoses
✓ Skin integrity, impaired (uses)
✓ Infection, risk for (uses)
✓ Knowledge deficit (teaching)

Implementation
Top route
• Apply to affected area, surrounding area; do not cover
with occlusive dressings
• Store below 30° C (86° F)

Teach patient/family
• Instruct to apply with glove
to prevent further infection;
not to cover with occlusive
dressings
• Teach patient that long-term
therapy may be needed to clear
infection (2 wk-6 mo depending on organism); compliance
is needed even after feeling
better
• Teach patient proper
hygiene; hand-washing technique, nail care, use of concomitant top agents if prescribed
• Caution patient to avoid use
of OTC creams, ointments,
lotions unless directed by
prescriber
• Instruct patient to use med-

✚ Canada Only   Adverse effects: *italic* = common; **bold** = life-threatening ical asepsis (hand washing) before, after each application; to change socks and shoes once a day during treatment of tinea pedis

• Advise patient to report to health care prescriber if infection persists or recurs; if blisters, burning, oozing, swelling occur

• Caution patient to avoid alcohol because nausea, vomiting, hypertension may occur

• Caution patient to use sunscreen or avoid direct sunlight to prevent photosensitivity

• Advise patient to notify health-care prescriber of sore throat, fever, skin rash, which may indicate overgrowth of organisms

Evaluation
Positive therapeutic outcome
• Decrease in size, number of lesions

TOPICAL ANTIINFECTIVES

bacitracin (OTC)
(bass-i-tray′sin)
Baciguent, Bacitin ✦, Bacitracin
chloramphenicol (Ŗ)
(klor-am-fen′i-kole)
Chloromycetin
erythromycin (OTC)
(er-ith-roe-mye′sin)
A/T/S, Akne-Mycin, C-Solve 2, Erycette, Eryderm, Erygel, Erymax, Erythromycin, E-Solve 2, ETS-2%, Staticin, Theramycin Z, T-Statd
gentamicin (Ŗ)
(jen-ta-mye′sin)
G-Myticin, Garamycin, gentamicin
mafenide (Ŗ)
(ma′fe-nide)
Sulfamylon

mupirocin (Ŗ)
(myoo-peer′oh-sin)
Bactroban, Pseudomonic Acid A
neomycin (OTC)
(nee-oh-mye′sin)
Myciguent, Neomycin Sulfate
nitrofurazone (Ŗ)
(nye-troe-fyoor′a-zone)
Furacin, Nitrofurazone
silver sulfadiazine (Ŗ)
(sul-fa-dye′a-zeen)
Flamazine ✦, Silvadene, SSD, SSD AF, Thermazene
sodium sulfacetamide lotion 10% (Ŗ)
(sul-fa-see′ta-mide)
Klaron
tetracycline (Ŗ)
(tet-ra-sye′kleen)
Achromycin, Topicycline
Pregnancy category **C**

Action: Interferes with bacterial protein synthesis

▶**Therapeutic Outcome:** Resolution of infection

Uses: Skin infections, minor burns, wounds, skin grafts, primary pyodermas, otitis externa

Adverse effects
INTEG: Rash, urticaria, scaling, redness

Contraindications: Hypersensitivity, large areas, burns, ulcerations

Precautions: Pregnancy **C**, lactation, impaired renal function, external ear or perforated eardrum

---

☑ Herb/drug 🚫 Do Not Crush ♦ Alert ⛫ Key Drug **G** Geriatric **P** Pediatric

NURSING CONSIDERATIONS
Assessment
• Assess for allergic reaction: burning, stinging, swelling, redness
• Assess for signs of nephrotoxicity or ototoxicity

Nursing diagnoses
☑ Infection, risk of (uses)
☑ Skin integrity (uses)
☑ Knowledge deficit (teaching)

Implementation
• Apply enough medication to cover lesions completely
• Apply after cleansing with soap, water before each application; dry well
• Apply to less than 20% of body surface area when patient has impaired renal function
• Store at room temp in dry place

Evaluation
Positive therapeutic outcome
• Decrease in size, number of lesions

TOPICAL ANTIVIRALS

acyclovir (℞)
(ay-sye′kloe-ver)
Zovirax
penciclovir (℞)
(pen-sye′kloe-ver)
Denavir
Pregnancy category   C

Action: Interferes with viral DNA replication

➡**Therapeutic Outcome:** Resolution of infection

Uses: Simple mucocutaneous herpes simplex, in immunocompromised clients with initial herpes genitalis

Adverse effects
INTEG: Rash, urticaria, stinging, burning, pruritus, vulvitis

Contraindications: Hypersensitivity

Precautions: Pregnancy **C**, lactation

NURSING CONSIDERATIONS
Assessment
• Assess for allergic reaction: burning, stinging, swelling, redness, rash, vulvitis, pruritus
• Assess for signs of nephrotoxicity or ototoxicity

Nursing diagnoses
☑ Infection, risk of (uses)
☑ Skin integrity (uses)
☑ Knowledge deficit (teaching)

Implementation
• Using finger cot or rubber glove to prevent further infection
• Apply enough medication to cover lesions completely
• Apply after cleansing with soap, water before each application; dry well
• Storage at room temp in dry place

Patient/family education
• Teach patient not to use in eyes or when there is no evidence of infection
• Advise patient to apply with glove to prevent further infection
• Advise patient to avoid use of OTC creams, ointments, lotions unless directed by prescriber
• Advise patient to use medical asepsis (hand washing) before, after each application and avoid contact with eyes
• Advise patient to adhere strictly to prescribed regimen to maximize successful treatment outcome
• Advise patient to begin taking drug when symptoms arise

Evaluation
Positive therapeutic outcome
• Decrease in size, number of lesions

TOPICAL ANESTHETICS

benzocaine (OTC)
(ben′zoe-kane)
Anbesol Maximum Strength, Baby Anbesol, Children's Chloraseptic, Medamint, Orabase Baby, Oracin, Ora-Jel, Oratect, Spec-T Anesthetic, T-Caine, Tyrobenz
dibucaine (OTC)
(dye′byoo-kane)
dibucaine, Nupercainal
lidocaine (OTC, ℞)
(lye′doe-kane)
Aloe Extra, Anestacon, Burn Relief, Derma Flex, lidocaine HCl topical, lidocaine viscous, Solarcaine, Xylocaine, Xylocaine Viscous, Zilactin-L
pramoxine (OTC)
(pra-mox′een)
Fleet Relief, Prax, ProctoFoam, Tronolane, Tronothane
tetracaine (OTC)
(tet′ra-cane)
Pontocaine
Pregnancy category   **C**

Action: Inhibits conduction of nerve impulses from sensory nerves

▷Therapeutic Outcome: Decreasing inflammation, itching, pain

Uses: Oral irritation, sore throat, toothache, cold sore, canker sore, sunburn, minor cuts, insect bites, pain, itching

Dosage and routes
P *Adult and child:* **TOP** apply qid as needed; **RECT** insert tid and after each BM

Adverse effects
INTEG: Rash, irritation, sensitization

Contraindications: Hypersen-
P sitivity, infants <1 yr, application to large areas

P Precautions: Child <6 yr, sepsis, pregnancy **C,** denuded skin

NURSING CONSIDERATIONS
Assessment
• Assess pain: location, duration, characteristics before and after administration
• Assess for infection: redness, drainage, inflammation; this drug should not be used until infection is treated

Implementation
• Store in tight, light-resistant container; do not freeze, puncture, or incinerate aerosol container

Patient/family education
• Teach patient to avoid contact with eyes
• Teach patient not to use for prolonged periods: use for <1 wk; if condition remains, prescriber should be contacted

Evaluation
Positive therapeutic outcome
• Decreased redness, swelling, pain

VAGINAL ANTIFUNGALS

butoconazole (OTC)
(byoo-toh-kone'ah-zole)
Femstat
clotrimazole (OTC)
(kloe-trye'ma-zole)
Canesten ✤, Gyne-Lotrimin,
Mycelex G, Mycelex Twin
Pak, Myclo ✤
miconazole (OTC)
(mye-kon'a-zole)
Monistat, Monistat 3,
Monistat 7, Monistat Dual
Pak
nystatin (OTC)
(nye-stat'in)
mycostatin, Nadostine ✤,
Nilstat, Nyoderm ✤, O-V
Statin
terconazole (OTC)
(ter-kone'ah-zole)
Terazol
tioconazole (OTC)
(tye-oh-kone'ah-zole)
Gyne-Trosyd ✤, Vagistat
Pregnancy category: Ny-
statin **A;** clotrimazole
B; butoconazole,
terconazole, tioconazole **C**

Action: Interferes with fungal
DNA replication; binds sterols
in fungal cell membranes,
which increases permeability,
leaking of nutrients

→**Therapeutic Outcome:**
Fungistatic/fungicidal against
susceptible organisms: *Candida* only

Uses: Vaginal, vulval, vulvovaginal candidiasis (moniliasis)

Dosage and routes
Butoconazole
Adult: VAG 5 g (1 applicator)
hs × 3-6 days

Clotrimazole
Adult: 100 mg (1 vag tab, 100
mg) hs × 1 wk, or 200 mg (2
vag tab, 100 mg) hs × 3 nights,
or 500 mg (1 vag tab, 500
mg); or 5 g (1 applicator) hs ×
1-2 wks

Miconazole
Adult: 200 mg supp hs × 3
days or 100 mg supp × 1 wk

Nystatin
Adult: 100,000 U qd × 2 wk

Terconazole
Adult: VAG 5 g (1 applicator)
hs × 7 days

Tioconazole
Adult: 1 applicator hs × 1 wk

Adverse effects
GU: Vulvovaginal burning,
itching, pelvic cramps
INTEG: Rash, urticaria, sting-
ing, burning
MISC: Headache, body pain

Contraindications: Hypersensitivity

P Precautions: Children <2 yr,
pregnancy, lactation

Interactions: None

NURSING CONSIDERATIONS
Assessment
• Assess for allergic reaction:
burning, stinging, itching,
discharge, soreness
Nursing diagnoses
☑ Skin integrity, impaired (uses)
☑ Infection, risk for (uses)
☑ Knowledge deficit (teaching)
Implementation
Topical route
• Administer one full applica-
tor every night high into the
vagina
• Store at room temp in dry
place

Teach patient/family
• Instruct patient in asepsis (hand washing) before, after each application
• Teach patient to apply with applicator only; to avoid use of any other vaginal product unless directed by prescriber; sanitary napkin may prevent soiling of undergarments
• Instruct patient to abstain from sexual intercourse until treatment is completed; reinfection and irritation may occur
• Advise patient to notify prescriber if symptoms persist

Evaluation
Positive therapeutic outcome
• Decrease in itching or white discharge (vaginal)

OTIC STEROIDS

hydrocortisone
(hye-droe-kor'ti-sone)
Cortamed ✦, Otall (℞)
Pregnancy category   C

Action: Antiinflammatory, antipruritic

⊃**Therapeutic Outcome:** Decreased otic inflammation

Uses: Ear canal inflammation

Adverse effects
EENT: Itching, irritation in ear
INTEG: Rash, urticaria

Contraindications: Hypersensitivity, perforated eardrum

Precautions: Pregnancy C

NURSING CONSIDERATIONS
Assessment
• Assess for redness, swelling, fever, pain in ear, which indicates infection

Nursing diagnoses
☑ Pain (uses)
☑ Knowledge deficit (teaching)

Implementation
• Administer after removing impacted cerumen by irrigation
• Administer after cleaning stopper with alcohol
• Administer after restraining child if necessary
• Instill after warming sol to body temp

Patient/family education
• Teach patient the correct method of instillation using aseptic technique, including not touching dropper to ear
• Advise patient that dizziness may occur after instillation

Evaluation
Positive therapeutic outcome
• Decreased ear pain, inflammation

OTIC ANTIINFECTIVES

chloramphenicol (℞)
(klor-am-fen'i-kole)
Chloromycetin Otic,
Sopamycetin ✦
neomycin (℞)
(nee-oh-mye'sin)
Drotic, Otocort
Pregnancy category   C

Action: Inhibits protein synthesis in susceptible microorganisms

⊃**Therapeutic Outcome:** Decreased redness, swelling, fever, and/or pain in ear

Uses: Ear infection (external), short-term use

Adverse effects
EENT: Itching, irritation in ear
INTEG: Rash, urticaria

☑ Herb/drug   ⊗ Do Not Crush   ◆ Alert   ☞ Key Drug   ⏚ Geriatric   ⏚ Pediatric

Contraindications: Hypersensitivity, perforated eardrum

Precautions: Pregnancy **C**

NURSING CONSIDERATIONS
Assessment
• Assess for redness, swelling, fever, pain in ear, which indicates superinfection

Nursing diagnoses
☑ Pain (uses)
☑ Infection, risk for (uses)
☑ Knowledge deficit (teaching)

Implementation
• Administer after removing impacted cerumen by irrigation
• Administer after cleaning stopper with alcohol
• Administer after restraining child if necessary
• Instill after warming sol to body temp

Patient/family education
• Teach patient the correct method of instillation using aseptic technique, including not touching dropper to ear
• Advise patient that dizziness may occur after instillation

Evaluation
Positive therapeutic outcome
• Decreased ear pain

Appendix D

Combination Products

A-200 Shampoo:
0.33% pyrethrins
4% piperonyl butoxide
Uses: Scabicide, pediculicide
Acid-X:
acetaminophen 500 mg
calcium carbonate 250 mg
Uses: Analgesic, antacid
Actifed:
pseudoephedrine 60 mg
triprolidine 2.5 mg
Uses: Decongestant
Actifed, Allergy, Nighttime:
pseudoephedrine 30 mg
diphenhydramine 25 mg
Uses: Decongestant, antihistamine
Actifed Plus:
pseudoephedrine 30 mg
triprolidine 1.25 mg
acetaminophen 500 mg
Uses: Decongestant, antihistamine
Actifed Sinus Daytime:
pseudoephedrine 30 mg
acetaminophen 500 mg
Uses: Decongestant
Actifed Sinus Nighttime:
pseudoephedrine 30 mg
diphenhydramine 25 mg
acetaminophen 500 mg
Uses: Decongestant, antihistamine
Adderall 10 mg:
dextroamphetamine sulfate 5 mg
dextroamphetamine saccharate 2.5 mg
amphetamine sulfate 2.5 mg
amphetamine aspartate 2.5 mg
Uses: CNS stimulant
Adderall 20 mg:
dextroamphetamine sulfate 5 mg
dextroamphetamine saccharate 5 mg
amphetamine sulfate 5 mg
amphetamine aspartate 5 mg
Uses: CNS stimulant
Advil Cold & Sinus Caplets:
pseudoephedrine 30 mg
ibuprofen 200 mg
Uses: Decongestant
**AK-Cide Ophthalmic Suspension/
Ointment:**
10% sulfacetamide sodium

0.5% prednisolone acetate
Uses: Ophth antiinfective, antiinflammatory
Aldactazide 25/25:
spironolactone 25 mg
hydrochlorothiazide 25 mg
Uses: Diuretic
Aldactazide 50/50:
spironolactone 50 mg
hydrochlorothiazide 50 mg
Uses: Diuretic
Aldoclor-150:
methyldopa 250 mg
chlorothiazide 150 mg
Uses: Antihypertensive
Aldoclor-250:
methyldopa 250 mg
chlorothiazide 250 mg
Uses: Antihypertensive
Aldoril-15:
methyldopa 250 mg
hydrochlorothiazide 15 mg
Uses: Antihypertensive
Aldoril-25:
methyldopa 250 mg
hydrochlorothiazide 25 mg
Uses: Antihypertensive
Alka-Seltzer Effervescent, Original:
sodium bicarbonate 1916 mg
citric acid 1000 mg
aspirin 325 mg
Uses: Antacid, adsorbent, antiflatulent
Alka-Seltzer Plus Allergy Liqui-Gels:
pseudoephedrine 30 mg
chlorpheniramine 2 mg
acetaminophen 325 mg
Uses: Decongestant, antihistamine
**Alka-Seltzer Plus Night-Time Cold
Liqui-Gels:**
doxylamine 6.25 mg
dextromethorphan 10 mg
pseudoephedrine 30 mg
acetaminophen 250 mg
Uses: Antitussive, decongestant
**Alka-Seltzer Plus Cold & Cough
Liqui-Gels:**
dextromethorphan 10 mg
pseudoephedrine 30 mg
chlorpheniramine 2 mg

acetaminophen 250 mg
Uses: Antitussive, decongestant
Alka-Seltzer Plus Cold & Cough:
phenylpropanolamine 20 mg
chlorpheniramine 2 mg
dextromethorphan 10 mg
aspirin 325 mg
Uses: Antitussive, decongestant
Alka-Seltzer Plus Cold Liqui-Gels:
pseudoephedrine 30 mg
chlorpheniramine 2 mg
acetaminophen 250 mg
Uses: Decongestant, antihistamine
Alka-Seltzer Plus Cold Medicine:
chlorpheniramine 2 mg
phenylpropanolamine 20 mg
aspirin 325 mg
Uses: Antihistamine, analgesic
Alka-Seltzer Plus Flu & Body Aches
 Non-Drowsy Liqui-Gels:
pseudoephedrine 30 mg
dextromethorphan 10 mg
acetaminophen 250 mg
Uses: Decongestant, antitussive, analgesic
Alka-Seltzer Plus Night-Time Cold:
phenylpropanolamine 20 mg
doxylamine 6.25 mg
dextromethorphan 15 mg
aspirin 500 mg
Uses: Antitussive, analgesic
Alka-Seltzer Plus Sinus:
phenylpropanolamine 20 mg
aspirin 325 mg
Uses: Analgesic
Allerest Headache Strength Advanced
 Formula:
pseudoephedrine 30 mg
chlorpheniramine 2 mg
acetaminophen 325 mg
Uses: Decongestant, antihistamine
Allerest Maximum Strength
 Caplets:
pseudoephedrine 30 mg
chlorpheniramine 2 mg
Uses: Decongestant, antihistamine
Allerest Maximum Strength
 12 Hour Caplets:
phenylpropanolamine 75 mg
chlorpheniramine 12 mg
Uses: Antihistamine
Allerest No-Drowsiness:
pseudoephedrine 30 mg
acetaminophen 325 mg
Uses: Decongestant, analgesic
Allerest Sinus Pain Formula:
pseudoephedrine 30 mg
chlorpheniramine 2 mg

acetaminophen 500 mg
Uses: Decongestant, antihistamine,
 analgesic
All-Nite Cold Formula Liquid:
Per 5 ml:
pseudoephedrine 10 mg
doxylamine 1.25 mg
dextromethorphan 5 mg
acetaminophen 167 mg
Uses: Decongestant, antihistamine,
 analgesic
Alor 5/500:
hydrocodone 5 mg
aspirin 500 mg
Uses: Analgesic
Amaphen:
acetaminophen 325 mg
butalbital 50 mg
caffeine 40 mg
Uses: Analgesic, barbiturates
Ambenyl Cough Syrup:
Per 5 ml:
bromodiphenhydramine 12.5 mg
codeine 10 mg
5% alcohol
Uses: Antihistamine, opioid analgesic
Anacin:
aspirin 400 mg
caffeine 32 mg
Uses: Analgesic
Anacin Maximum Strength:
aspirin 500 mg
caffeine 32 mg
Uses: Analgesic
Anacin PM (Aspirin Free):
diphenhydramine 25 mg
acetaminophen 500 mg
Uses: Analgesic
Anaplex HD Syrup:
Per 5 ml:
hydrocodone 1.7 mg
phenylephrine 5 mg
chlorpheniramine 2 mg
Uses: Analgesic, adrenergic, antihistamine
Anaplex Liquid:
Per 5 ml:
chlorpheniramine 2 mg
pseudoephedrine 30 mg
Uses: Antihistamine, decongestant
Anatuss:
guaifenesin 100 mg
dextromethorphan 15 mg
phenylpropanolamine 25 mg
acetaminophen 325 mg
Uses: Antitussive, expectorant, analgesic
Anatuss DM:
guaifenesin 400 mg

pseudoephedrine 60 mg
dextromethorphan 20 mg
Uses: Expectorant, adrenergic, antitussive
Anatuss DM Syrup:
Per 5 ml:
guaifenesin 100 mg
pseudoephedrine 30 mg
dextromethorphan 10 mg
Uses: Expectorant, adrenergic, antitussive
Anatuss LA:
pseudoephedrine 120 mg
guaifenesin 400 mg
Uses: Adrenergic, expectorant
Anatuss Syrup:
Per 5 ml:
guaifenesin 100 mg
dextromethorphan 15 mg
phenylpropanolamine 25 mg
Uses: Expectorant, antitussive
Anexsia 5/500:
hydrocodone 5 mg
acetaminophen 500 mg
Uses: Analgesic
Anexsia 7.5/650:
hydrocodone 7.5 mg
acetaminophen 650 mg
Uses: Analgesic
Anexsia 10/660:
hydrocodone 10 mg
acetaminophen 660 mg
Uses: Analgesic
Antihist-D:
clemastine 1.34 mg
phenylpropanolamine 75 mg
Uses: Antihistamine
Antrocol Elixir:
Per 5 ml:
atropine 0.195 mg
phenobarbital 16 mg
alcohol 20%
Uses: Anticholinergic, barbiturate
Apresazide 25/25:
hydralazine 25 mg
hydrochlorothiazide 25 mg
Uses: Antihypertensive
Aprodine w/Codeine Syrup:
Per 5 ml:
pseudoephedrine 30 mg
triprolidine 1.25 mg
codeine 10 mg
Uses: Adrenergic, analgesic
Aprodine Syrup:
Per 5 ml:
pseudoephedrine 30 mg
triprolidine 1.25 mg
Uses: Adrenergic, analgesic

A.R.M.:
phenylpropanolamine 25 mg
chlorpheniramine 4 mg
Uses: Antihistamine
Arthritis Pain Formula:
aspirin 500 mg
aluminum hydroxide 27 mg
magnesium hydroxide 100 mg
Uses: Analgesic, antacid
Arthrotec:
diclofenac 50 or 75 mg
misoprostol 200 μg
Uses: NSAID, gastric protectant
Asbron G Elixir:
theophylline 150 mg
guaifenesin 100 mg
alcohol 15%
Uses: Bronchodilator, expectorant
Asbron G Inlay:
theophylline 150 mg
guaifenesin 100 mg
sucrose
Uses: Bronchodilator, expectorant
Ascriptin A/D:
aspirin 325 mg
aluminum hydroxide 75 mg
magnesium hydroxide 75 mg
calcium carbonate 75 mg
Uses: Analgesic
Aspirin-Free Bayer Select Allergy Sinus:
pseudoephedrine 30 mg
chlorpheniramine 2 mg
acetaminophen 500 mg
Uses: Adrenergic, antihistamine, analgesic
**Aspirin-Free Bayer Select Head &
    Chest Cold:**
pseudoephedrine 30 mg
guaifenesin 100 mg
dextromethorphan 10 mg
acetaminophen 325 mg
Uses: Adrenergic, antitussive, expectorant, analgesic
Aspirin Free Excedrin:
acetaminophen 500 mg
caffeine 65 mg
Uses: Analgesic
Aspirin Free Excedrin Dual:
acetaminophen 500 mg
calcium carbonate 111 mg
magnesium carbonate 64 mg
magnesium oxide 30 mg
Uses: Analgesic, antacid
Augmentin 250:
amoxicillin 250 mg
clavulanic acid 125 mg
Uses: Antiinfective

Augmentin 500:
amoxicillin 500 mg
clavulanic acid 125 mg
Uses: Antiinfective
Augmentin 875:
amoxicillin 875 mg
clavulanic acid 125 mg
Uses: Antiinfective
Augmentin 125 Chewable:
amoxicillin 125 mg
clavulanic acid 31.25 mg
Uses: Antiinfective
Augmentin 250 Chewable:
amoxicillin 250 mg
clavulanic acid 62.5 mg
Uses: Antiinfective
Augmentin 125 mg/5 ml Suspension:
Per 5 ml:
amoxicillin 125 mg
clavulanic acid 31.25 mg
Uses: Antiinfective
Augmentin 250 mg/5 ml Suspension:
Per 5 ml:
amoxicillin 250 mg
clavulanic acid 62.5 mg
Uses: Antiinfective
Auralgan Otic Solution:
5.4% antipyrine
1.4% benzocaine
Uses: Otic analgesic
B&O Supprettes No. 15A Supps:
belladonna extract 15 mg
opium 30 mg
Uses: Anticholinergic, narcotic analgesic
B&O Supprettes No. 16A Supps:
belladonna extract 16.2 mg
opium 60 mg
Uses: Anticholinergic, narcotic analgesic
Bactrim:
trimethoprim 80 mg
sulfamethoxazole 400 mg
Uses: Antiinfective
Bactrim DS:
trimethoprim 160 mg
sulfamethoxazole 800 mg
Uses: Antiinfective
Bactrim I.V.:
trimethoprim 80 mg
sulfamethoxazole 400 mg
Uses: Antiinfective
Bancap HC:
acetaminophen 500 mg
hydrocodone 5 mg
Uses: Analgesic
Bayer Plus, Extra Strength:
aspirin 500 mg
calcium carbonate
magnesium carbonate

magnesium oxide
Uses: Analgesic, antacid
Bayer Select Chest Cold:
dextromethorphan 15 mg
acetaminophen 500 mg
Uses: Antitussive, analgesic
Bayer Select Flu Relief:
acetaminophen 500 mg
pseudoephedrine 30 mg
dextromethorphan 15 mg
chlorpheniramine 2 mg
Uses: Analgesic, adrenergic, antitussive,
antihistamine
Bayer Select Head & Chest Cold, Aspirin Free Caplets:
pseudoephedrine 30 mg
dextromethorphan 10 mg
guaifenesin 100 mg
acetaminophen 325 mg
Uses: Adrenergic, antitussive, expectorant, analgesic
Bayer Select Head Cold:
pseudoephedrine 30 mg
acetaminophen 500 mg
Uses: Adrenergic, analgesic
Bayer Select Maximum Strength Headache:
acetaminophen 500 mg
caffeine 65 mg
Uses: Nonnarcotic analgesic
Bayer Select Maximum Strength Menstrual:
acetaminophen 500 mg
pamabrom 25 mg
Uses: Nonnarcotic analgesic
Bayer Select Maximum Strength Night-Time Pain Relief:
acetaminophen 500 mg
diphenhydramine 25 mg
Uses: Analgesic, antihistamine
Bayer Select Maximum Strength Sinus Pain Relief:
acetaminophen 500 mg
pseudoephedrine 30 mg
Uses: Analgesic, adrenergic
Bayer Select Night Time Cold:
acetaminophen 500 mg
pseudoephedrine 30 mg
dextromethorphan 15 mg
triprolidine 1.25 mg
Uses: Analgesic, adrenergic, antitussive,
antihistamine
Bellatal:
phenobarbital 16.2 mg
hyoscyamine sulfate 0.1037 mg
atropine sulfate 0.0194 mg
scopolamine hydrobromide 0.0065 mg
Uses: Barbiturate, anticholinergic

Bellergal-S:
ergotamine 0.6 mg
belladonna alkaloids 0.2 mg
phenobarbital 40 mg
Uses: α-Adrenergic blocker, anticholinergic, barbiturate

Bel-Phen-Ergot-SR:
phenobarbital 40 mg
ergotamine tartrate 0.6 mg
belladonna alkaloids 0.2 mg
Uses: α-Adrenergic blocker, anticholinergic, barbiturate

Benadryl Allergy Decongestant Liquid:
Per 5 ml:
diphenhydramine 12.5 mg
pseudoephedrine 30 mg
Uses: Antihistamine, adrenergic

Benadryl Allergy/Sinus Headache Caplets:
diphenhydramine 12.5 mg
pseudoephedrine 30 mg
acetaminophen 500 mg
Uses: Antihistamine, adrenergic, analgesic

Benadryl Decongestant Allergy:
pseudoephedrine 60 mg
diphenhydramine 25 mg
Uses: Adrenergic, antihistamine

Benylin Expectorant Liquid:
Per 5 ml:
dextromethorphan 5 mg
guaifenesin 100 mg
5% alcohol
Uses: Expectorant, antitussive

Benylin Multi-Symptom Liquid:
Per 5 ml:
dextromethorphan 5 mg
pseudoephedrine 15 mg
guaifenesin 100 mg
Uses: Antitussive, adrenergic, expectorant

Betoptic-Pilo:
0.25% betaxolol
1.75% pilocarpine
Uses: Ophthalmic

Biohist-LA Tablets:
pseudoephedrine 120 mg
carbinoxamine 8 mg
Uses: Adrenergic

Blephamide Ophthalmic Suspension/ Ointment:
0.2% prednisolone
10% sodium sulfacetamide
Uses: Ophthalmic antiinfective, antiinflammatory

Bromatapp Tablets:
phenylpropanolamine 75 mg
brompheniramine 12 mg
Uses: Decongestant, antihistamine

Bromfed Capsules:
pseudoephedrine 120 mg
brompheniramine 12 mg
Uses: Antihistamine, adrenergic

Bromfed-PD Capsules:
pseudoephedrine 60 mg
brompheniramine 6 mg
Uses: Adrenergic, antihistamine

Bromfed Tablets:
pseudoephedrine 60 mg
brompheniramine 4 mg
Uses: Antihistamine, adrenergic

Bromfenex:
brompheniramine 12 mg
pseudoephedrine 120 mg
Uses: Antihistamine, adrenergic

Bromfenex PD:
brompheniramine 6 mg
pseudoephedrine 60 mg
Uses: Antihistamine, adrenergic

Bromo-Seltzer:
sodium bicarb 2781 mg
acetaminophen 325 mg
citric acid 2224 mg
Uses: Antacid, analgesic

Bromophen T.D.:
phenylephrine 15 mg
phenylpropanolamine 15 mg
brompheniramine 12 mg
Uses: Antihistamine, decongestant

Brondelate Elixir:
theophylline 192 mg
guaifenesin 150 mg
Uses: Bronchodilator, expectorant

Brontex:
codeine 10 mg
guaifenesin 300 mg
Uses: Analgesic, expectorant

Bufferin:
aspirin 325 mg
calcium carbonate 158 mg
magnesium oxide 63 mg
magnesium carbonate 34 mg
Uses: Analgesic, antacid

Bufferin AF Nite-Time:
acetaminophen 500 mg
diphenhydramine 38 mg
Uses: Analgesic, antihistamine

Butibel:
belladonna extract 15 mg
butabarbital 15 mg
Uses: Anticholinergic, barbiturate

Cafatine PB:
ergotamine 1 mg
caffeine 100 mg
belladonna alkaloids 0.125 mg

pentobarbital 30 mg
Uses: Migraine agent
Cafergot:
ergotamine 1 mg
caffeine 100 mg
Uses: Adrenergic blocker
Cafergot Suppositories:
ergotamine 2 mg
caffeine 100 mg
Uses: Adrenergic blocker
Caladryl:
8% calamine, camphor
2.2% alcohol
1% pramoxine
Uses: Top antihistamine
Caladryl Clear:
1% pramoxine
0.1% zinc acetate
2% alcohol
camphor
Uses: Top antihistamine
Calcet:
calcium 152.8 mg
vitamin D 100 IU
Uses: Supplement
Calcidrine Syrup:
Per 5 ml:
codeine 8.4 mg
calcium iodide 152 mg
Uses: Analgesic
Caltrate 600+D:
vitamin D 200 IU
calcium 600 mg
Uses: Supplement
Cama Arthritis Pain Reliever:
aspirin 500 mg
magnesium oxide 150 mg
aluminum hydroxide 125 mg
Uses: Nonnarcotic analgesic, antacid
Capozide 25/15:
captopril 25 mg
hydrochlorothiazide 15 mg
Uses: Antihypertensive
Capozide 25/25:
captopril 25 mg
hydrochorothiazide 25 mg
Uses: Antihypertensive
Capozide 50/15:
captopril 50 mg
hydrochlorothiazide 15 mg
Uses: Antihypertensive
Capozide 50/25:
captopril 50 mg
hydrochlorothiazide 25 mg
Uses: Antihypertensive
Cardec DM Syrup:
Per 5 ml:
pseudoephedrine 60 mg

carbinoxamine 4 mg
dextromethorphan 15 mg
Uses: Adrenergic, antitussive
Cetacaine Topical:
14% benzocaine
2% tetracaine
0.5% benzalkonium chloride
0.005% cetyl dimethyl ethyl ammonium
  bromide
Uses: Local analgesic
Ceta Plus:
hydrocodone 5 mg
acetaminophen 500 mg
Uses: Analgesic
Cetapred Ophthalmic Ointment:
0.25% prednisolone
10% sodium sulfacetamide
Uses: Ophthalmic antiinfective, antiinflammatory
Cheracol Syrup:
Per 5 ml:
codeine 10 mg
guaifenesin 100 mg
Uses: Analgesic, expectorant
Cheracol Plus Liquid:
Per 5 ml:
phenylpropanolamine 8.3 mg
chlorpheniramine 1.3 mg
dextromethorphan 6.7 mg
8% alcohol
Uses: Antihistamine, antitussive
Children's Cepacol Liquid:
Per 5 ml:
acetaminophen 160 mg
pseudoephedrine 15 mg
Uses: Analgesic, adrenergic
**Chlor-Trimeton Allergy-Sinus
  Caplets:**
phenylpropanolamine 12.5 mg
chlorpheniramine 2 mg
acetaminophen 500 mg
Uses: Antihistamine, analgesic
Chlor-Trimeton 4 Hour Relief:
pseudoephedrine 60 mg
chlorpheniramine 4 mg
Uses: Antihistamine, adrenergic
Chlor-Trimeton 12 Hour Relief:
pseudoephedrine 120 mg
chlorpheniramine 8 mg
Uses: Antihistamine, adrenergic
Chromagen:
ferrous fumarate 66 mg
vitamin B_{12} 10 μg
vitamin C 250 mg
intrinsic factor 100 mg
Uses: Supplement
Claritin-D:
loratidine 5 mg

pseudoephedrine 120 mg
Uses: Antihistamine, adrenergic
Claritin-D 24-Hour:
loratidine 10 mg
pseudoephedrine 240 mg
Uses: Antihistamine, adrenergic
Clindex:
chlordiazepoxide 5 mg
clidinium 2.5 mg
Uses: Antianxiety, anticholinergic
Clomycin Ointment:
bacitracin 500 U
neomycin sulfate 3.5 g
polymyxin B sulfate 500 U
lidocaine 40 mg
Uses: Antiinfective, local anesthetic
Co-Apap:
pseudoephedrine 30 mg
chlorpheniramine 2 mg
dextromethorphan 15 mg
acetaminophen 325 mg
Uses: Adrenergic, antihistamine, antitussive, analgesic
Co-Gesic:
acetaminophen 500 mg
hydrocodone 5 mg
Uses: Analgesic
Codamine Syrup:
Per 5 ml:
hydrocodone 5 mg
phenylpropanolamine 25 mg
Uses: Analgesic
Codehist DH Elixir:
Per 5 ml:
pseudoephedrine 30 mg
chlorpheniramine 2 mg
codeine 10 mg
Uses: Adrenergic, antihistamine, analgesic
Codiclear DH Syrup:
Per 5 ml:
hydrocodone 5 mg
guaifenesin 100 mg
Uses: Analgesic, expectorant
Codimal:
pseudoephedrine 30 mg
chlorpheniramine 2 mg
acetaminophen 500 mg
Uses: Adrenergic, antihistamine, analgesic
Codimal DH Syrup:
Per 5 ml:
hydrocodone 1.66 mg
phenylephrine 5 mg
pyrilamine 8.33 mg
Uses: Analgesic, adrenergic
Codimal DM Syrup:
Per 5 ml:
phenylephrine 5 mg
pyrilamine 8.33 mg

dextromethorphan 10 mg
Uses: Adrenergic, antitussive
Codimal LA:
chlorpheniramine 8 mg
pseudoephedrine 120 mg
Uses: Antihistamine, adrenergic
Codimal PH Syrup:
Per 5 ml:
codeine 10 mg
phenylephrine 5 mg
pyrilamine 8.33 mg
Uses: Analgesic, adrenergic
Col-Probenecid:
probenecid 500 mg
colchicine 0.5 mg
Uses: Antigout agent
ColBenemid:
probenecid 500 mg
colchicine 0.5 mg
Uses: Antigout agent
Coldrine:
pseudoephedrine 30 mg
acetaminophen 500 mg
Uses: Decongestant, nonnarcotic analgesic
Coly-Mycin S Otic Suspension:
1% hydrocortisone
neomycin base 3.3 mg/ml
colistin 3 mg/ml
0.05% thonzonium bromide
Uses: Otic antiinfective
Combipres 0.1:
chlorthalidone 15 mg
clonidine 0.1 mg
Uses: Antihypertensive
Combipres 0.2:
chlorthalidone 15 mg
clonidine 0.2 mg
Uses: Antihypertensive
Combipres 0.3:
chlorthalidone 15 mg
clonidine 0.3 mg
Uses: Antihypertensive
Combivent:
ipratropium bromide 18 μg
albuterol 103 μg/actuation
Uses: Bronchodilator
Combivir:
lamivudine 150 mg
zidovudine 300 mg
Uses: Antiviral
Comhist Tablets:
phenylephrine 10 mg
chlorpheniramine 2 mg
phenyltoloxamine 25 mg
Uses: Adrenergic, antihistamine
Comhist LA:
phenylephrine 20 mg
chlorpheniramine 4 mg

phenyltoloxamine 50 mg
Uses: Adrenergic, antihistamine
Comtrex Liquid:
Per 5 ml:
chlorpheniramine 0.67 mg
acetaminophen 108.3 mg
dextromethorphan 3.3 mg
pseudoephedrine 10 mg
Uses: Antihistamine, analgesic, antitussive, decongestant
Comtrex Allergy-Sinus:
chlorpheniramine 2 mg
acetaminophen 500 mg
pseudoephedrine 30 mg
Uses: Antihistamine, analgesic, decongestant
Comtrex Liqui-Gels:
acetaminophen 325 mg
phenylpropanolamine 12.5 mg
chlorpheniramine 2 mg
dextromethorphan 10 mg
Uses: Analgesic, decongestant, antihistamine, antitussive
Comtrex Maximum Strength Caplets:
acetaminophen 500 mg
pseudoephedrine 30 mg
chlorpheniramine 2 mg
dextromethorphan 15 mg
Uses: Analgesic, decongestant, antihistamine, antitussive
Comtrex Maximum Strength Liqui-Gels:
acetaminophen 500 mg
phenylpropanolamine 12.5 mg
chlorpheniramine 2 mg
dextromethorphan 15 mg
Uses: Analgesic, decongestant, antihistamine, antitussive
Comtrex Maximum Strength Multi-Symptom Cold, Flu Relief:
pseudoephedrine 30 mg
dextromethorphan 15 mg
chlorpheniramine 2 mg
acetaminophen 500 mg
Uses: Analgesic, decongestant, antihistamine, antitussive
Comtrex Maximum Strength Multi-Symptom Cold & Flu Relief Liqui-Gels:
acetaminophen 500 mg
phenylpropanolamine 12.5 mg
chlorpheniramine 2 mg
dextromethorphan 15 mg
Uses: Analgesic, decongestant, antihistamine, antitussive

Comtrex Maximum Strength Non-Drowsy Caplets:
acetaminophen 500 mg
pseudoephedrine 30 mg
dextromethorphan 15 mg
Uses: Analgesic, decongestant, antitussive
Congess SR:
guaifenesin 250 mg
pseudoephedrine 120 mg
Uses: Expectorant, decongestant
Congestac:
guaifenesin 400 mg
pseudoephedrine 60 mg
Uses: Expectorant, decongestant
Contac Cough & Chest Cold Liquid:
Per 5 ml:
pseudoephedrine 15 mg
dextromethorphan 5 mg
guaifenesin 50 mg
acetaminophen 125 mg
Uses: Decongestant, antitussive, expectorant, analgesic
Contac Cough & Sore Throat Liquid:
Per 5 ml:
dextromethorphan 5 mg
acetaminophen 125 mg
Uses: Antitussive, analgesic
Contac Day Allergy/Sinus:
pseudoephedrine 60 mg
acetaminophen 650 mg
Uses: Decongestant, analgesic
Contac Day Cold and Flu:
pseudoephedrine 60 mg
dextromethorphan 30 mg
acetaminophen 650 mg
Uses: Decongestant, antitussive, analgesic
Contac 12 Hour Capsules:
phenylpropanolamine 75 mg
chlorpheniramine 8 mg
Uses: Antihistamine
Contac Maximum Strength 12 Hour:
phenylpropanolamine 75 mg
chlorpheniramine 12 mg
Uses: Antihistamine
Contac Night Allergy Sinus:
pseudoephedrine 60 mg
diphenhydramine 50 mg
acetaminophen 650 mg
Uses: Decongestant, antihistamine, analgesic
Contac Night Cold and Flu Caplets:
pseudoephedrine 60 mg
diphenhydramine 50 mg

acetaminophen 650 mg
Uses: Decongestant, antihistamine, antitussive, analgesic
Contac Severe Cold & Flu Nighttime Liquid:
Per 5 ml:
pseudoephedrine 10 mg
chlorpheniramine 0.67 mg
dextromethorphan 5 mg
acetaminophen 167 mg
18.5% alcohol
Uses: Decongestant, antihistamine, antitussive, analgesic
Contuss Liquid:
Per 5 ml:
phenylpropanolamine 20 mg
phenylephrine 5 mg
guaifenesin 100 mg
Uses: Adrenergic, expectorant
Coricidin:
chlorpheniramine 2 mg
acetaminophen 325 mg
Uses: Antihistamine, analgesic
Coricidin 'D':
phenylpropanolamine 12.5 mg
chlorpheniramine 2 mg
acetaminophen 325 mg
Uses: Antihistamine, analgesic
Coricidin Maximum Strength Sinus Headache Caplets:
phenylpropanolamine 12.5 mg
chlorpheniramine 2 mg
acetaminophen 500 mg
Uses: Antihistamine, analgesic
Cortisporin Ophthalmic/Otic Suspension:
0.35% neomycin polymyxin B 10,000 U/ml
1% hydrocortisone
Uses: Ophthalmic antiinfective, antiinflammatory
Cortisporin Ophthalmic Ointment:
0.35% neomycin base
bacitracin 400 U
polymyxin B 10,000 U
hydrocortisone 1%
Uses: Ophthalmic antiinfective
Cortisporin Topical Cream:
0.5% neomycin sulfate
polymyxin B 10,000 U
0.5% hydrocortisone
Uses: Topical antiinfective
Cortisporin Topical Ointment:
0.5% neomycin sulfate
bacitracin 400 U
polymyxin B 5,000 U
1% hydrocortisone
Uses: Topical antiinfective

Corzide 40/5:
nadolol 40 mg
bendroflumethiazide 5 mg
Uses: Antihypertensive
Cough-X:
dextromethorphan 5 mg
benzocaine 2 mg
Uses: Antitussive, local anesthetic
Creon:
lipase 8,000 U
amylase 30,000 U
protease 13,000 U
pancreatin 300 mg
Uses: Digestive enzyme
Cyclomydril Ophthalmic Solution:
0.2% cyclopentolate
1% phenylephrine
Uses: Mydriatic
Dallergy Caplets:
chlorpheniramine 8 mg
phenylephrine 20 mg
methscopolamine 2.5 mg
Uses: Antihistamine, adrenergic
Dallergy Syrup:
Per 5 ml:
chlorpheniramine 2 mg
phenylephrine 10 mg
methscopolamine 0.625 mg
Uses: Antihistamine, adrenergic
Dallergy Tablets:
chlorpheniramine 4 mg
phenylephrine 10 mg
methscopolamine 1.25 mg
Uses: Antihistamine, adrenergic
Dallergy-D Syrup:
Per 5 ml:
phenylephrine 5 mg
chlorpheniramine 2 mg
Uses: Antihistamine, adrenergic
Damason-P:
hydrocodone 5 mg
aspirin 500 mg
Uses: Analgesic
Darvocet-N 100:
propoxyphene-N 100 mg
acetaminophen 650 mg
Uses: Analgesic
Darvon Compound-65:
propoxyphene 65 mg
aspirin 389 mg
caffeine 32.4 mg
Uses: Analgesic
Deconamine:
pseudoephedrine 60 mg
chlorpheniramine 4 mg
Uses: Antihistamine, decongestant
Deconamine CX:
hydrocodone 5 mg

pseudoephedrine 30 mg
guaifenesin 300 mg
Uses: Analgesic, decongestant, expectorant

Deconamine SR:
pseudoephedrine 120 mg
chlorpheniramine 8 mg
Uses: Antihistamine, decongestant

Deconamine Syrup:
Per 5 ml:
pseudoephedrine 30 mg
chlorpheniramine 2 mg
Uses: Antihistamine, decongestant

Defen-LA:
pseudoephedrine 60 mg
guaifenesin 600 mg
Uses: Decongestant, expectorant

Demazin:
phenylpropanolamine 25 mg
chlorpheniramine 4 mg
Uses: Antihistamine

Demi-Regroton:
chlorthalidone 25 mg
reserpine 0.125 mg
Uses: Antihypertensive

Demulen 1/50:
ethinyl estradiol 50 µg
ethynodiol diacetate 1 mg
Uses: Oral contraceptive

**Dexacidin Ophthalmic Ointment/
   Suspension:**
Per ml:
0.1% dexamethasone
0.35% neomycin
polymyxin B 10,000 U/g
Uses: Ophth, antiinfective/antiinflammatory

Dexasporin Ophthalmic Ointment:
Per gram:
0.1% dexamethasone
0.35% neomycin
polymyxin B 10,000 U
Uses: Ophth, antiinfective/antiinflammatory

DHC Plus:
dihydrocodeine 16 mg
acetaminophen 356.4 mg
caffeine 30 mg
Uses: Analgesic

Dialose Plus:
docusate sodium 100 mg
yellow phenolphthalein 65 mg
Uses: Laxative

Dieutrim T.D.:
benzocaine 9 mg
phenylpropanolamine 75 mg
carboxymethylcellulose 75 mg
Uses: Top anesthetic

Di-Gel Advanced Formula:
magnesium hydroxide 128 mg
calcium carbonate 280 mg
simethicone 20 mg
Uses: Antacid, adsorbent, antiflatulent

Di-Gel Liquid:
Per 5 ml:
aluminum hydroxide 200 mg
magnesium hydroxide 200 mg
simethicone 20 mg
Uses: Antacid, adsorbent, antiflatulent

Dihistine DH Liquid:
Per 5 ml:
pseudoephedrine 30 mg
chlorpheniramine 2 mg
codeine 10 mg
Uses: Decongestant, antihistamine,
   analgesic

Dilaudid Cough Syrup:
Per 5 ml:
guaifenesin 100 mg
hydromorphone 1 mg
5% alcohol
Uses: Expectorant, analgesic

Dilor-G Liquid:
dyphylline 300 mg
guaifenesin 300 mg
Uses: Bronchodilator, expectorant

Dilor-G Tablets:
dyphylline 200 mg
guaifenesin 200 mg
Uses: Bronchodilator, expectorant

Dimetane Decongestant:
brompheniramine 4 mg
phenylephrine 10 mg
Uses: Antihistamine, adrenergic

Dimetane-DC Cough Syrup:
Per 5 ml:
brompheniramine 2 mg
phenylpropanolamine 12.5 mg
codeine 10 mg
Uses: Antihistamine, analgesic

Dimetane-DX Cough Syrup:
Per 5 ml:
brompheniramine 2 mg
pseudoephedrine 30 mg
dextromethorphan 10 mg
Uses: Antihistamine, decongestant, antitussive

Dimetapp:
brompheniramine 4 mg
phenylpropanolamine 25 mg
Uses: Antihistamine

Dimetapp Cold & Allergy Chewable:
phenylpropanolamine 6.25 mg
brompheniramine 1 mg
Uses: Antihistamine

Dimetapp Cold & Flu:
phenylpropanolamine 12.5 mg
brompheniramine 2 mg
acetaminophen 500 mg
Uses: Antihistamine, analgesic

Dimetapp DM Elixir:
Per 5 ml:
phenylpropanolamine 12.5 mg
brompheniramine 2 mg
dextromethorphan 10 mg
Uses: Antihistamine, antitussive

Dimetapp Elixir:
Per 5 ml:
phenylpropanolamine 12.5 mg
brompheniramine 2 mg
Uses: Antihistamine

Dimetapp Extentabs:
phenylpropanolamine 75 mg
brompheniramine 12 mg
Uses: Antihistamine

Dimetapp Sinus:
pseudoephedrine 30 mg
ibuprofen 200 mg
Uses: Decongestant, analgesic

Diutensin-R:
methylclothiazide 2.5 mg
reserpine 0.1 mg
Uses: Antihypertensive

Doan's PM Extra Strength:
magnesium salicylate 500 mg
diphenhydramine 25 mg
Uses: Analgesic, antihistamine

Dolacet:
hydrocodone 5 mg
acetaminophen 500 mg
Uses: Analgesic

Donnatal:
phenobarbital 16.2 mg
hyoscyamine 0.1037 mg
atropine 0.0194 mg
scopolamine 0.0065 mg
Uses: Anticholinergic, barbiturate

Donnatal Elixir:
Per 5 ml:
phenobarbital 16.2 mg
hyoscyamine 0.1037 mg
atropine 0.0194 mg
scopolamine 0.0065 mg
23% alcohol
Uses: Anticholinergic, barbiturate

Donnatal Extentabs:
phenobarbital 48.6 mg
hyoscyamine 0.3111 mg
atropine 0.0582 mg
scopolamine 0.0195 mg
Uses: Anticholinergic, barbiturate

Donnazyme:
pancreatin 500 mg
lipase 1000 U
protease 12,500 U
amylase 12,500 U
Uses: Pancreatic enzymes

Dorcol Children's Cold Formula Liquid:
Per 5 ml:
pseudoephedrine 15 mg
chlorpheniramine 1 mg
Uses: Decongestant, antihistamine

Doxidan:
docusate calcium 60 mg
phenolphthalein 65 mg
Uses: Stool softener

Dristan Cold:
pseudoephedrine 30 mg
acetaminophen 500 mg
Uses: Decongestant, analgesic

Dristan Cold Maximum Strength Caplets:
pseudoephedrine 30 mg
brompheniramine 2 mg
acetaminophen 500 mg
Uses: Decongestant, antihistamine, analgesic

Dristan Cold Multi-Symptom Formula:
acetaminophen 325 mg
phenylephrine 5 mg
chlorpheniramine 2 mg
Uses: Analgesic, adrenergic, antihistamine

Dristan Sinus:
pseudoephedrine 30 mg
ibuprofen 200 mg
Uses: Decongestant, analgesic

Drixoral Allergy Sinus:
pseudoephedrine 60 mg
dexbrompheniramine 3 mg
acetaminophen 500 mg
Uses: Decongestant, antihistamine, analgesic

Drixoral Cold & Allergy:
pseudoephedrine 120 mg
dexbrompheniramine 6 mg
Uses: Decongestant, antihistamine

Drixoral Cold & Flu:
pseudoephedrine 60 mg
dexbrompheniramine 3 mg
acetaminophen 500 mg
Uses: Decongestant, antihistamine, analgesic

Drixoral Cough & Congestion Liquid Caps:
pseudoephedrine 60 mg
dextromethorphan 30 mg
Uses: Decongestant, antitussive

Drixoral Cough & Sore Throat Liquid Caps:
dextromethorphan 15 mg
acetaminophen 325 mg
Uses: Antitussive, analgesic
Drixoral Plus:
pseudoephedrine 60 mg
dexbrompheniramine 3 mg
acetaminophen 500 mg
Uses: Decongestant, antihistamine, analgesic
DT:
Per 5 ml dose:
diphtheria toxoid 2LfU
tetanus toxoid 5LfU
Uses: Vaccine
DTP:
Per 0.5 ml dose:
diphtheria toxoid 6.5LfU
tetanus toxoid 5LfU
pertussis 4LfU
Uses: Vaccine
Dura-Vent:
phenylpropanolamine 75 mg
guaifenesin 600 mg
Uses: Expectorant
Dura-Vent/A:
phenylpropanolamine 75 mg
chlorpheniramine 10 mg
Uses: Antihistamine
Dura-Vent/DA:
phenylephrine 20 mg
chlorpheniramine 8 mg
methscopolamine 2.5 mg
Uses: Adrenergic, antihistamine
Dyazide:
hydrochlorothiazide 25 mg
triamterene 37.5 mg
Uses: Diuretic
Dylline-GG Liquid:
dyphylline 300 mg
quaifenesin 300 mg
Uses: Bronchodilator, expectorant
Dynafed Asthma Relief:
ephedrine 25 mg
guaifenesin 200 mg
Uses: Adrenergic, expectorant
Dynafed Plus Maximum Strength:
pseudoephedrine 30 mg
acetaminophen 500 mg
Uses: Decongestant, analgesic
Dyphylline-GG Elixir:
Per 5 ml:
dyphylline 100 mg
guaifenesin 100 mg
Uses: Bronchodilator, expectorant
E-Pilo-1 Ophthalmic Solution:
1% epinephrine bitartrate

1% pilocarpine
Uses: Miotic
E-Pilo-2 Ophthalmic Solution:
1% epinephrine bitartrate
2% pilocarpine
Uses: Miotic
E-Pilo-4 Ophthalmic Solution:
1% epinephrine bitartrate
4% pilocarpine
Uses: Miotic
Elase-Chloromycetin Ointment:
Per gram:
fibrinolysin 1 U
desoxyribonuclease 666.6 U
chloramphenicol 10 mg
Uses: Enzyme, antiinfective
Elase Ointment:
Per gram:
fibrinolysin 1 U
desoxyribonuclease 666.6 U
Uses: Enzyme
Elixophyllin GG Liquid:
Per 5 ml:
theophylline 100 mg
guaifenesin 100 mg
Uses: Expectorant, bronchodilator
EMLA Cream:
lidocaine 2.5 mg
prilocaine 2.5 mg
Uses: Local anesthetic
Empirin w/Codeine #3:
aspirin 325 mg
codeine phosphate 30 mg
Uses: Analgesic
Empirin w/Codeine #4:
aspirin 325 mg
codeine phosphate 60 mg
Uses: Analgesic
Enduronyl:
methyclothiazide 5 mg
deserpidine 0.25 mg
Uses: Diuretic
Entex:
phenylephrine 5 mg
phenylpropanolamine 45 mg
guaifenesin 200 mg
Uses: Adrenergic, expectorant
Entex LA:
phenylpropanolamine 75 mg
guaifenesin 400 mg
Uses: Adrenergic, expectorant
Entex PSE:
pseudoephedrine 120 mg
guaifenesin 600 mg
Uses: Adrenergic, expectorant
Epifoam Aerosol Foam:
1% hydrocortisone

1% pramoxine
Uses: Topical corticosteroid
Esgic-Plus:
butalbital 50 mg
acetaminophen 500 mg
caffeine 40 mg
Uses: Barbiturate, analgesic
Esimil:
guanethidine 10 mg
hydrochlorothiazide 25 mg
Uses: Antihypertensive
Estratest:
esterified estrogens 1.25 mg
methyltestosterone 2.5 mg
Uses: Androgen, estrogen
Etrafon:
perphenazine 2 mg
amitriptyline 25 mg
Uses: Antipsychotic, antidepressant
Etrafon Forte:
perphenazine 4 mg
amitriptyline 25 mg
Uses: Antipsychotic, antidepressant
Excedrin Migraine:
aspirin 250 mg
acetaminophen 250 mg
caffeine 65 mg
Uses: Migraine agent
Excedrin P.M.:
acetaminophen 500 mg
diphenhydramine citrate 38 mg
Uses: Analgesic, antihistamine
Excedrin P.M. Liquid:
Per 30 ml:
acetaminophen 1000 mg
diphenhydramine 50 mg
Uses: Analgesic, antihistamine
Excedrin P.M. Liquigels:
acetaminophen 500 mg
diphenhydramine 25 mg
Uses: Analgesic, antihistamine
Excedrin Sinus Extra Strength:
pseudoephedrine 30 mg
acetaminophen 500 mg
Uses: Decongestant, analgesic
Fansidar:
sulfidoxine 500 mg
pyrimethamine 25 mg
Uses: Antimalarial
Fedahist:
pseudoephedrine 60 mg
chlorpheniramine 4 mg
Uses: Decongestant, antihistamine
Fedahist Expectorant Syrup:
Per 5 ml:
guaifenesin 200 mg
pseudoephedrine 20 mg
Uses: Expectorant, decongestant

Fedahist Gyrocaps:
pseudoephedrine 65 mg
chlorpheniramine 10 mg
Uses: Decongestant, antihistamine
Fedahist Timecaps:
pseudoephedrine 120 mg
chlorpheniramine 8 mg
Uses: Decongestant, antihistamine
Feen-A-Mint Pills:
docusate sodium 100 mg
phenolphthalein 65 mg
Uses: Laxative
Fem-1:
acetaminophen 500 mg
pamabrom 25 mg
Uses: Nonnarcotic analgesic
Ferro-Sequels:
docusate sodium 100 mg
ferrous fumarate 150 mg
Uses: Laxative, hematinic
Fioricet:
acetaminophen 325 mg
caffeine 40 mg
butalbital 50 mg
Uses: Analgesic, barbiturate
Fioricet w/Codeine:
acetaminophen 325 mg
caffeine 40 mg
butalbital 50 mg
codeine 30 mg
Uses: Analgesic, barbiturate
Fiorinal:
aspirin 325 mg
caffeine 40 mg
butalbital 50 mg
Uses: Analgesic, barbiturate
Fiorinal with Codeine:
aspirin 325 mg
caffeine 40 mg
butalbital 50 mg
codeine 30 mg
Uses: Analgesic, barbiturate
FML-S Ophthalmic Suspension:
0.1% flurometholone
10% sulfacetamide
Uses: Ophth, antiinfective/antiinflam-
matory
Gas-Ban:
calcium carbonate 500 mg
simethicone 40 mg
Uses: Antiflatulent, antacid
Gas-Ban DS Liquid:
Per 5 ml:
aluminum hydroxide 400 mg
magnesium hydroxide 400 mg
simethicone 40 mg
Uses: Antiflatulent, antacid

Gaviscon:
magnesium trisilicate 20 mg
aluminum hydroxide 80 mg
Uses: Antacid, adsorbent, antiflatulent
Gaviscon Liquid:
Per 5 ml:
aluminum hydroxide 31.7 mg
magnesium carbonate 119.3 mg
Uses: Antacid, adsorbent, antiflatulent
Gelprin:
acetaminophen 125 mg
aspirin 240 mg
caffeine 32 mg
Uses: Analgesic
Gelusil:
aluminum hydroxide 200 mg
magnesium hydroxide 200 mg
simethicone 25 mg
Uses: Antacid, adsorbent, antiflatulent
Genatuss DM Syrup:
Per 5 ml:
guaifenesin 100 mg
dextromethorphan 10 mg
Uses: Expectorant, antitussive
Granulex Aerosol:
Per 0.82 ml:
trypsin 0.1 mg
balsam peru 72.5 mg
castor oil 650 mg
Uses: Top enzyme
Guaifenex PPA 75:
guaifenesin 600 mg
phenylpropanolamine 75 mg
Uses: Expectorant, decongestant
Guaifenex PSE 60:
pseudoephedrine 60 mg
guaifenesin 600 mg
Uses: Decongestant, expectorant
Guaifenex PSE 120:
pseudoephedrine 120 mg
guaifenesin 600 mg
Uses: Decongestant, expectorant
Haley's M-O Liquid:
Per 15 ml:
magnesium hydroxide 900 mg
mineral oil 3.75 ml
Uses: Laxative
Halotussin-DM Sugar Free Liquid:
Per 5 ml:
guaifenesin 100 mg
dextromethorphan 10 mg
Uses: Expectorant, antitussive
Helidac:
In a compliance package:
bismuth subsalicylate 262.4 mg tabs
metronidazole 250 mg tabs
tetracycline 500 mg caps
Uses: Antiinfective

Humibid DM Sprinkle Caps:
dextromethorphan 15 mg
guaifenesin 300 mg
Uses: Expectorant, antitussive
Humibid DM Tablets:
dextromethorphan 30 mg
guaifenesin 600 mg
Uses: Expectorant, antitussive
Hycodan:
hydrocodone 5 mg
homatropine 1.5 mg
Uses: Analgesic, mydriatic
Hycodan Syrup:
Per 5 ml:
hydrocodone 5 mg
homatropine 1.5 mg
Uses: Analgesic, mydriatic
Hycomine Compound:
chlorpheniramine 2 mg
acetaminophen 250 mg
phenylephrine 10 mg
hydrocodone 5 mg
caffeine 30 mg
Uses: Antihistamine, analgesic, adrenergic
Hycomine Syrup:
Per 5 ml:
hydrocodone 5 mg
phenylpropanolamine 25 mg
Uses: Analgesic, decongestant
Hycotuss Expectorant:
Per 5 ml:
guaifenesin 100 mg
hydrocodone 5 mg
10% alcohol
Uses: Expectorant
Hydro-Serp:
hydrochlorothiazide 50 mg
reserpine 0.125 mg
Uses: Antihypertensive
Hydrocet:
hydrocodone 5 mg
acetaminophen 500 mg
Uses: Narcotic, opioid analgesic
Hydrogesic:
hydrocodone 5 mg
acetaminophen 500 mg
Uses: Narcotic, opioid analgesic
Hydropres-50:
hydrochlorothiazide 50 mg
reserpine 0.125 mg
Uses: Antihypertensive
Hydroserpin #1:
hydrochlorothiazide 25 mg
reserpine 0.125 mg
Uses: Antihypertensive
Hyzaar:
losartan potassium 50 mg

hydrochlorothiazide 12.5 mg
potassium 4.24 mg
Uses: Antihypertensive
Iberet Filmtab:
ferrous sulfate 105 mg
ascorbic acid 150 mg
B-complex vitamins
Uses: Supplement
Iberet Liquid:
Per 5 ml:
ferrous sulfate 78.75 mg
ascorbic acid 112.5 mg
B-complex vitamins
Uses: Supplement
Imodium Advanced:
loperamide 2 mg
simethicone 125 mg
Uses: Antidiarrheal, antiflatulent
Inderide 40/25:
propranolol 40 mg
hydrochlorothiazide 25 mg
Uses: Antihypertensive
Innovar:
Per ml:
droperidol 2.5 mg
fentanyl 0.05 mg
Uses: Narcotic analgesic, general
    anesthetic
Iofed:
brompheniramine 12 mg
pseudoephedrine 120 mg
Uses: Antihistamine, adrenergic
Iofed PD:
brompheniramine 6 mg
pseudoephedrine 60 mg
Uses: Antihistamine, adrenergic
Iophen-C Liquid:
Per 5 ml:
iodinated glycerol 30 mg
codeine 10 mg
Uses: Expectorant, analgesic
Iophen-DM Liquid:
Per 5 ml:
iodinated glycerol 30 mg
dextromethorphan 10 mg
Uses: Expectorant, antitussive
Kondremul with Phenolphthalein:
Per 15 ml:
phenolphthalein 150 mg
55% mineral oil
Irish moss
Uses: Laxative
Lactinex:
Mixed culture of:
Lactobacillus acidophilus and
Lactobacillus bulgaricus
Uses: Supplement

Levsin PB Drops:
Per ml:
hyoscyamine 0.125 mg
phenobarbital 15 mg
5% alcohol
Uses: Anticholinergic, barbiturate
Levsin with Phenobarbital:
hyoscyamine 0.125 mg
phenobarbital 15 mg
Uses: Anticholinergic, barbiturate
Lexxel:
enalapril 5 mg
felodipine 5 mg
Uses: Antihypertensive
Librax:
chlordiazepoxide 5 mg
clidinium 2.5 mg
Uses: Antianxiety, anticholinergic
Lida-Mantel-HC-Cream:
0.5% hydrocortisone
3% lidocaine
Uses: Antiinflammatory, analgesic
Limbitrol DS 10-25:
chlordiazepoxide 10 mg
amitriptyline 25 mg
Uses: Antidepressant, antianxiety
Lobac:
salicylamide 200 mg
phenyltoloxamine 20 mg
acetaminophen 300 mg
Uses: Skeletal muscle relaxant, analgesic
Loestrin Fe 1.5/30:
norethindrone acetate 1.5 mg
ethinyl estradiol 30 µg
Uses: Oral contraceptive
Lomotil:
diphenoxylate 2.5 mg
atropine 0.025 mg
Uses: Antidiarrheal, anticholinergic
Lomotil Liquid:
Per 5 ml:
diphenoxylate 2.5 mg
atropine 0.025 mg
Uses: Antidiarrheal, anticholinergic
Lo Ovral:
ethinyl estradiol 30 µg
norgestrel 0.3 mg
Uses: Oral contraceptive
Lopressor HCT 50/25:
metoprolol 50 mg
hydrochlorothiazide 25 mg
Uses: Antihypertensive
Lopressor HCT 100/25:
metoprolol 100 mg
hydrochlorothiazide 25 mg
Uses: Antihypertensive
Lopressor HCT 100/50:
metoprolol 100 mg

hydrochlorothiazide 50 mg
Uses: Antihypertensive
Lorcet 10/650:
acetaminophen 650 mg
hydrocodone 10 mg
Uses: Analgesic
Lortab 2.5/500:
hydrocodone 2.5 mg
acetaminophen 500 mg
Uses: Analgesic
Lortab 5/500:
hydrocodone 5 mg
acetaminophen 500 mg
Uses: Analgesic
Lortab 7.5/500:
hydrocodone 7.5 mg
acetaminophen 500 mg
Uses: Analgesic
Lortab 10/500:
hydrocodone 10 mg
acetaminophen 500 mg
Uses: Analgesic
Lortab ASA:
aspirin 500 mg
hydrocodone 5 mg
Uses: Analgesic
Lortab Elixir:
Per 5 ml:
hydrocodone 2.5 mg
acetaminophen 167 mg
Uses: Analgesic
Lotensin HCT 5/6.25:
benazepril 5 mg
hydrochlorothiazide 6.25 mg
Uses: Antihypertensive
Lotensin HCT 10/12.5:
benazepril 10 mg
hydrochlorothiazide 12.5 mg
Uses: Antihypertensive
Lotensin HCT 20/12.5:
benazepril 20 mg
hydrochlorothiazide 12.5 mg
Uses: Antihypertensive
Lotensin HCT 20/25:
benazepril 20 mg
hydrochlorothiazide 25 mg
Uses: Antihypertensive
Lotrel 2.5/10:
amlopidine 2.5 mg
benazepril 10 mg
Uses: Antihypertensive
Lotrel 5/10:
amlodipine 5 mg
benazepril 10 mg
Uses: Antihypertensive
Lotrel 5/20:
amlodipine 5 mg

benazepril 20 mg
Uses: Antihypertensive
Lotrisone Topical:
0.05% betamethasone
1% clotrimazole
Uses: Local antiinfective, antiinflammatory
Lufyllin-EPG Elixir:
Per 5 ml:
dyphylline 150 mg
ephedrine 24 mg
guaifenesin 300 mg
phenobarbital 24 mg
Uses: Bronchodilator, expectorant
Lufyllin-EPG Tablets:
dyphylline 100 mg
ephedrine 16 mg
guaifenesin 200 mg
phenobarbital 16 mg
Uses: Bronchodilator, adrenergic, expectorant, barbiturate
Lufyllin-GG:
dyphylline 200 mg
guaifenesin 200 mg
Uses: Bronchodilator, expectorant
Lufyllin-GG Elixir:
dyphylline 100 mg
guaifenesin 100 mg
alcohol 17%
Uses: Bronchodilator, expectorant
M-M-R-II:
measles
mumps
rubella
Uses: Vaccine, toxoid
M-R Vax II:
measles
rubella
Uses: Vaccine, toxoid
Maalox:
aluminum hydroxide 200 mg
magnesium hydroxide 200 mg
Uses: Antacid, adsorbent, antiflatulent
Maalox Plus:
aluminum hydroxide 200 mg
magnesium hydroxide 200 mg
simethicone 25 mg
Uses: Antacid, adsorbent, antiflatulent
**Maalox Plus Extra Strength Suspen-
sion:**
Per 5 ml:
aluminum hydroxide 500 mg
magnesium hydroxide 450 mg
simethicone 40 mg
Uses: Antacid, adsorbent, antiflatulent
Maalox Suspension:
Per 5 ml:
aluminum hydroxide 225 mg

magnesium hydroxide 200 mg
Uses: Antacid, adsorbent, antiflatulent
Mapap Cold Formula:
acetaminophen 325 mg
chlorpheniramine 2 mg
pseudoephedrine 30 mg
dextromethorphan 15 mg
Uses: Bronchodilator, expectorant
Marax:
ephedrine 25 mg
theophylline 130 mg
hydroxyzine 10 mg
Uses: Bronchodilator, sedative/hypnotic
Maxitrol Ophthalmic Suspension/ Ointment:
Per ml:
0.35% neomycin
0.1% dexamethasone
polymyxin B 10,000 U
Uses: Ophthalmic antiinfective, antiin- flammatory
Maxzide:
hydrochlorothiazide 50 mg
triamterene 75 mg
Uses: Antihypertensive, diuretic
Maxzide-25 MG:
hydrochlorothiazide 25 mg
triamterene 37.5 mg
Uses: Diuretic
Medi-Flu Liquid:
Per 5 ml:
pseudoephedrine 10 mg
chlorpheniramine 0.67 mg
dextromethorphan 5 mg
acetaminophen 167 mg
18.5% alcohol
Uses: Decongestant, antihistamine, anti- tussive, analgesic
Mepergan Fortis:
meperidine 50 mg
promethazine 25 mg
Uses: Analgesic, antihistamine
Mepergan Injection:
meperidine 25 mg
promethazine 25 mg
Uses: Analgesic
Metimyd Ophthalmic Suspension/ Ointment:
0.5% prednisolone
10% sodium sulfacetamide
Uses: Ophthalmic antiinfective, antiin- flammatory
Midol Maximum Strength Multi- Symptom Menstrual Gelcaps:
acetaminophen 500 mg
pyrilamine 15 mg
caffeine 60 mg
Uses: Analgesic

Midol PM:
acetaminophen 500 mg
diphenhydramine 25 mg
Uses: Analgesic, antihistamine
Midol PMS Maximum Strength Caplets:
acetaminophen 500 mg
pyrilamine 15 mg
pamabrom 25 mg
Uses: Analgesic
Midol, Teen:
acetaminophen 400 mg
pamabrom 25 mg
Uses: Analgesic
Midrin:
isometheptene 65 mg
acetaminophen 325 mg
dichloralphenazone 100 mg
Uses: Analgesic
Minizide 1:
prazosin 1 mg
polythiazide 0.5 mg
Uses: Antihypertensive
Minizide 2:
prazosin 2 mg
polythiazide 0.5 mg
Uses: Antihypertensive
Minizide 5:
prazosin 5 mg
polythiazide 0.5 mg
Uses: Antihypertensive
Modane Plus:
docusate sodium 100 mg
phenolphthalein 65 mg
Uses: Laxative
Moduretic:
hydrochlorothiazide 50 mg
amiloride 5 mg
Uses: Diuretic
Motrin IB Sinus:
pseudoephedrine 30 mg
ibuprofen 200 mg
Uses: Adrenergic, analgesic
Murocoll-2 Ophthalmic Drops:
0.3% scopolamine
10% phenylephrine
Uses: Ophth anticholinergic, mydriatic
Mycolog II Topical:
Per gram:
0.1% triamcinolone acetonide
nystatin 100,000 U
Uses: Local antiinfective, antiinflamma- tory
Mylanta:
aluminum hydroxide 200 mg
magnesium hydroxide 200 mg
simethicone 20 mg
Uses: Antacid, adsorbent, antiflatulent

Mylanta Double Strength Liquid:
Per 5 ml:
aluminum hydroxide 400 mg
magnesium hydroxide 400 mg
simethicone 40 mg
Uses: Antacid, adsorbent, antiflatulent
Mylanta Gelcaps:
calcium carbonate 311 mg
magnesium carbonate 232 mg
Uses: Antacid, adsorbent, antiflatulent
Naldecon Tablets:
phenylpropanolamine 40 mg
phenylephrine 10 mg
phenyltoloxamine 15 mg
chlorpheniramine 5 mg
Uses: Antihistamine, decongestant
Naldecon CX Adult Liquid:
Per 5 ml:
guaifenesin 200 mg
phenylpropanolamine 12.5 mg
codeine 10 mg
Uses: Antihistamine
Naldecon DX Adult Liquid:
Per 5 ml:
dextromethorphan 10 mg
guaifenesin 200 mg
phenylpropanolamine 12.5 mg
Uses: Expectorant, decongestant
Naldecon DX Children's Syrup:
Per 5 ml:
dextromethorphan 5 mg
guaifenesin 100 mg
phenylpropanolamine 6.25 mg
Uses: Antihistamine, decongestant
Naldecon DX Pediatric Drops:
Per ml:
phenylpropanolamine 6.25 mg
dextromethorphan 5 mg
guaifenesin 50 mg
Uses: Antihistamine, decongestant
Naldecon EX Children's Syrup:
Per 5 ml:
guaifenesin 100 mg
phenylpropanolamine 6.25 mg
Uses: Antihistamine, decongestant
Naldecon EX Pediatric Drops:
Per ml:
phenylpropanolamine 6.25 mg
guaifenesin 50 mg
Uses: Antihistamine, decongestant
Naldecon Pediatric Drops:
Per ml:
phenylpropanolamine 5 mg
phenylephrine 1.25 mg
chlorpheniramine 0.5 mg
phenyltoloxamine 2 mg
Uses: Antihistamine, decongestant

Naldecon Pediatric Syrup:
Per 5 ml:
phenylpropanolamine 5 mg
phenylephrine 1.25 mg
chlorpheniramine 0.5 mg
phenyltoloxamine 2 mg
Uses: Antihistamine, decongestant
Naldecon Senior DX Liquid:
Per 5 ml:
dextromethorphan 10 mg
guaifenesin 200 mg
Uses: Expectorant, antitussive
Naldecon Syrup:
Per 5 ml:
chlorpheniramine 2.5 mg
phenylephrine 5 mg
phenylpropanolamine 20 mg
phenyltoloxamine 7.5 mg
Uses: Antihistamine, decongestant
Naphcon-A Ophthalmic Solution:
0.25% naphazoline
0.3% pheniramine
Uses: Ophth vasoconstrictor
Nasatab LA:
guaifenesin 500 mg
pseudoephedrine 120 mg
Uses: Expectorant, decongestant
**NeoDecadron Ophthalmic
Ointment:**
0.35% neomycin
0.05% dexamethasone
Uses: Ophth antiinfective, antiinflamma-
tory
**NeoDecadron Ophthalmic
Solution:**
0.35% neomycin
0.1% dexamethasone
Uses: Ophth antiinfective, antiinflamma-
tory
NeoDecadron Topical:
neomycin 0.5%
dexamethasone 0.1%
Uses: Top antiinfective, antiinflammatory
Neosporin Cream:
Per gram:
polymyxin B 10,000 U
neomycin 3.5 mg
Uses: Top antiinfective
Neosporin G.U. Irrigant:
Per ml:
neomycin 40 mg
polymyxin B 200,000 U
Uses: Antiinfective
Neosporin Ointment:
Per gram:
polymyxin B 5000 U
bacitracin zinc 400 U

neomycin 3.5 mg
Uses: Top antiinfective
Neosporin Ophthalmic Solution:
Per ml:
neomycin 1.75 mg
polymyxin B 10,000 U
gramicidin 0.025 mg
Uses: Ophthalmic antiinfective
Neosporin Ophthalmic Ointment:
Per gram:
neomycin 3.5 mg
polymyxin B 10,000 U
bacitracin zinc 400 U
Uses: Ophthalmic antiinfective
Neosporin Plus Cream:
polymyxin B 10,000 U
neomycin 3.5 mg
lidocaine 40 mg
Uses: Top antiinfective
Niferex-150 Forte:
ferrous sulfate 150 mg
vitamin B_{12} 25 μg
folic acid 1 mg
Uses: Supplement
Norgesic:
orphenadrine 25 mg
aspirin 385 mg
caffeine 30 mg
Uses: Skeletal muscle relaxant, analgesic
Norgesic Forte:
orphenadrine 50 mg
aspirin 770 mg
caffeine 60 mg
Uses: Skeletal muscle relaxant, analgesic
Novacet Lotion:
sodium sulfacetamine 10%
sulfur 5%
Uses: Acne agent
Novafed A:
pseudoephedrine 120 mg
chlorpheniramine 8 mg
Uses: Adrenergic, antihistamine
NuLytely:
PEG 3350/420 g
sodium bicarbonate 5.72 g
sodium chloride 11.2 g
potassium chloride 1.48 g
Uses: Laxative
NyQuil Hot Therapy:
Per packet:
acetaminophen 1000 mg
pseudoephedrine 60 mg
dextromethorphan 30 mg
doxylamine 12.5 mg
Uses: Analgesic, adrenergic, antitussive
**NyQuil Nightime Cold/Flu Medicine
  Liquid:**
Per 5 ml:

pseudoephedrine 10 mg
doxylamine 1.25 mg
dextromethorphan 5 mg
acetaminophen 167 mg
25% alcohol
Uses: Adrenergic, antitussive, analgesic
Octicair Otic Suspension:
hydrocortisone 1%
neomycin 5 mg/ml
polymyxin B 10,000 U/ml
Uses: Otic antiinflammatory, antiinfective
Opcon-A Ophthalmic Solution:
0.027% naphazoline
0.315% pheniramine
Uses: Ophth vasoconstrictor
Ornade:
phenylpropanolamine 75 mg
chlorpheniramine 12 mg
Uses: Antihistamine, decongestant
Ornex:
pseudoephedrine 30 mg
acetaminophen 500 mg
Uses: Adrenergic, analgesic
Ornex No Drowsiness Caplets:
acetaminophen 325 mg
pseudoephedrine 30 mg
Uses: Adrenergic, analgesic
Ortho-cept:
ethinyl estradiol 30 μg
desogestrel 0.15 mg
Uses: Oral contraceptive
Ortho-Novum 7/7/7:
Phase I:
0.5 mg norethindrone
35 μg ethinyl estradiol
Phase II:
0.75 mg norethindrone
35 μg ethinyl estradiol
Phase III:
1 mg norethinidrone
35 μg estradiol
Uses: Oral contraceptive
Otocort Otic Suspension:
hydrocortisone 1%
neomycin 5 mg/ml
polymyxin B 10,000 U
Uses: Otic antiinflammatory, antiinfective
Pain-X Topical:
0.05% capsaicin
5% menthol
4% camphor
Uses: Top analgesic
Pamprin Maximum Pain Relief:
acetaminophen 250 mg
pamabrom 25 mg
magnesium salicylate 250 mg
Uses: Analgesic

Pamprin Multi-Symptom:
acetaminophen 500 mg
pamabrom 25 mg
pyrilamine 15 mg
Uses: Analgesic
Panacet 5/500:
hydrocodone 5 mg
acetaminophen 500 mg
Uses: Analgesic
Panasal 5/500:
hydrocodone 5 mg
aspirin 500 mg
Uses: Analgesic
Pancrease Capsules:
amylase 20,000 U
protease 25,000 U
lipase 4500 U (microspheres)
Uses: Digestive enzyme
Pedia Care Cold-Allergy Chewable:
pseudoephedrine 15 mg
chlorpheniramine 1 mg
Uses: Adrenergic, antihistamine
Pedia Care Cough-Cold Liquid:
Per 5 ml:
pseudoephedrine 15 mg
chlorpheniramine 1 mg
dextromethorphan 5 mg
Uses: Adrenergic, antihistamine, antitussive
Pedia Care NightRest Cough-Cold Liquid:
Per 5 ml:
pseudoephedrine 15 mg
chlorpheniramine 1 mg
dextromethorphan 7.5 mg
Uses: Adrenergic, antihistamine, antitussive
Pediacof Syrup:
Per 5 ml:
codeine 5 mg
phenylephrine 2.5 mg
chlorpheniramine 0.75 mg
potassium iodide 75 mg
5% alcohol
Uses: Opioid, narcotic analgesic, antihistamine
Pediacon DX Children's Syrup:
Per 5 ml:
phenylpropanolamine 6.25 mg
guaifenesin 100 mg
dextromethorphan 5 mg
Uses: Expectorant, antitussive
Pediacon DX Pediatric Drops:
Per ml:
phenylpropanolamine 6.25 mg
guaifenesin 50 mg
dextromethorphan 5 mg
Uses: Expectorant, antitussive

Pediacon EX Drops:
phenylpropanolamine 6.25 mg
guaifenesin 50 mg
Uses: Antitussive, decongestant
Pediazole Suspension:
Per 5 ml:
erythromycin 200 mg
sulfisoxazole 600 mg
Uses: Antiinfective
Percocet:
oxycodone 5 mg
acetaminophen 325 mg
Uses: Analgesic
Percodan:
oxycodone 4.88 mg
aspirin 325 mg
Uses: Analgesic
Percogesic:
phenyltoloxamine 30 mg
acetaminophen 325 mg
Uses: Analgesic
Perdiem Granules:
Per teaspoon:
senna 0.74 g
psyllium 3.25 g
sodium 1.8 mg
potassium 35.5 mg
Uses: Laxative
Peri-Colace Capsules:
docusate sodium 100 mg
casanthranol 30 mg
Uses: Laxative
Peri-Colace Syrup:
Per 15 ml:
docusate sodium 60 mg
casanthranol 30 mg
Uses: Laxative
Phenerbel-S:
ergotamine tartrate 0.6 mg
belladonna alkaloids 0.2 mg
phenobarbital 40 mg
Uses: α-Adrenergic blocker, anticholinergic
Phenergan VC Syrup:
Per 5 ml:
phenylephrine 5 mg
promethazine 6.25 mg
Uses: Adrenergic, antihistamine
Phenergan VC w/Codeine Syrup:
Per 5 ml:
phenylephrine 5 mg
promethazine 6.25 mg
codeine 10 mg
Uses: Adrenergic, antihistamine, opioid analgesic
Phenergan w/Codeine Syrup:
Per 5 ml:
promethazine 6.25 mg

codeine 10 mg
Uses: Antihistamine, analgesic
Phenylfenesin LA:
phenylpropanolamine 75 mg
guaifenesin 400 mg
Uses: Decongestant, expectorant
Pherazine DM Syrup:
Per 5 ml:
dextromethorphan 15 mg
promethazine 6.25 mg
7% alcohol
Uses: Antitussive, antihistamine
Phillips' Laxative Gelcaps:
docusate sodium 83 mg
phenolphthalein 90 mg
Uses: Laxative
PMB-400:
conjugated estrogens 0.45 mg
meprobamate 400 mg
Uses: Oral contraceptive
Polaramine Expectorant Liquid:
Per 5 ml:
guaifenesin 100 mg
dexchlorpheniramine 2 mg
pseudoephedrine 20 mg
7.5% alcohol
Uses: Expectorant
Polycillin-PRB Oral Suspension:
Per single dose:
ampicillin 3.5 g
probenecid 1 g
Uses: Antiinfective
Polycitra Syrup:
Per 5 ml:
potassium citrate 550 mg
sodium citrate 500 mg
citric acid 334 mg
Uses: Laxative
Poly-Histine Elixir:
Per 5 ml:
pheniramine 4 mg
pyrilamine 4 mg
phenyltoloxamine 4 mg
4% alcohol
Uses: Antihistamine
Poly-Histine DM Syrup:
Per 5 ml:
brompheniramine 2 mg
phenylpropanolamine 12.5 mg
dextromethorphan 10 mg
Uses: Antihistamine, antitussive
Poly-Histine CS Syrup:
Per 5 ml:
phenylpropanolamine 12.5 mg
brompheniramine 2 mg
codeine 10 mg
Uses: Antihistamine, analgesic

Poly-Pred Ophthalmic Suspension:
Per ml:
0.5% prednisolone acetate
0.35% neomycin
polymyxin B 10,000 U
Uses: Ophth antiinflammatory, antiinfective
Polysporin Ointment:
Per gram:
polymyxin B 10,000 U
bacitracin zinc 500 U
Uses: Top antiinfective
Polysporin Ophthalmic Ointment:
Per gram:
polymyxin B 10,000 U
bacitracin zinc 500 U
Uses: Ophthalmic antiinfective
Polytrim Ophthalmic:
Per ml:
trimethoprim 1 mg
polymyxin B 10,000 U
Uses: Ophthalmic antiinfective
Premphase:
In a compliance package:
conjugated estrogens 0.625 mg
medroxyprogesterone 5 mg
Uses: Oral contraceptive
Prempro:
In a compliance package:
conjugated estrogens 0.625 mg
medroxyprogesterone 2.5 mg
Uses: Oral contraceptive
Premsyn PMS:
acetaminophen 500 mg
pamabrom 25 mg
pyrilamine 15 mg
Uses: Analgesic
Prevpac:
In a compliance package:
amoxicillin 500 mg caps
clarithromycin 500 mg tabs
lansoprazole 30 mg caps
Uses: Antiinfective
Primatene:
theophylline 130 mg
ephedrine 24 mg
phenobarbital 7.5 mg
Uses: Bronchodilator, barbiturate
Primatene Dual Action:
theophylline 60 mg
ephedrine 12.5 mg
guaifenesin 100 mg
Uses: Bronchodilator, expectorant, adrenergic
Primaxin 250 mg
I.V. for Injection:
imipenem 250 mg

cilastatin sodium 250 mg
Uses: Antiinfective
Primaxin 500 mg
I.V. for Injection:
imipenem 500 mg
cilastatin sodium 500 mg
Uses: Antiinfective
Prinzide 10-12.5:
lisinopril 10 mg
hydrochlorothiazide 12.5 mg
Uses: Antihypertensive
Prinzide 20-12.5:
lisinopril 20 mg
hydrochlorothiazide 12.5 mg
Uses: Antihypertensive
Prinzide 20-25:
lisinopril 20 mg
hydrochlorothiazide 25 mg
Uses: Antihypertensive
Probampacin Oral Suspension:
Per single dose:
ampicillin 3.5 g
probenecid 1 g
Uses: Antiinfective
Proben-C:
colchicine 0.5 mg
probenecid 500 mg
Uses: Antigout agent
Proctofoam-HC Aerosol Foam:
1% hydrocortisone
1% pramoxine
Uses: Topical corticosteroid
Propacet 100:
propoxyphene-N 100 mg
acetaminophen 650 mg
Uses: Analgesic
Pseudo-Chlor:
pseudoephedrine 120 mg
chlorpheniramine 8 mg
Uses: Antihistamine
Pseudo-Gest Plus:
pseudoephedrine 60 mg
chlorpheniramine 4 mg
Uses: Antihistamine
P-V-Tussin:
phenindamine 25 mg
guaifenesin 200 mg
hydrocodone 5 mg
Uses: Antihistamine, analgesic
Quadrinal:
ephedrine 24 mg
theophylline 65 mg
potassium iodide 320 mg
phenobarbital 24 mg
Uses: Adrenergic, bronchodilator, barbiturate
Quelidrine Cough Syrup:
Per 5 ml:

dextromethorphan 10 mg
phenylephrine 5 mg
ephedrine 5 mg
chlorpheniramine 2 mg
ammonium chloride 40 mg
ipecac 0.005 ml
Uses: Expectorant, adrenergic, antihistamine
Quibron-300:
theophylline 300 mg
guaifenesin 180 mg
Uses: Bronchodilator, expectorant
Quibron:
theophylline, 150 mg
guaifenesin 90 mg
Uses: Bronchodilator, expectorant
R&C Shampoo:
0.3% pyrethrins
3% piperonyl butoxide
Uses: Scabicide, pediculicide
Rauzide:
bendroflumethiazide 4 mg
powdered rauwolfia serpentina 50 mg
Uses: Diuretic, antihypertensive
Regroton:
chlorthalidone 50 mg
reserpine 0.25 mg
Uses: Diuretic, antihypertensive
Regulace:
docusate sodium 100 mg
casanthranol 30 mg
Uses: Laxative
Renese-R:
polythiazide 2 mg
reserpine 0.25 mg
Uses: Diuretic, antihypertensive
Respahist:
pseudoephedrine 60 mg
brompheniramine 6 mg
Uses: Adrenergic, antihistamine
Respaire-60:
guaifenesin 200 mg
pseudoephedrine 60 mg
Uses: Expectorant, adrenergic
RID Shampoo:
0.3% pyrethrins
3% piperonyl butoxide
Uses: Scabicide, pediculicide
Rifamate:
isoniazid 150 mg
rifampin 300 mg
Uses: Antitubercular, antileprotic
Rifater:
rifampin 120 mg
isoniazid 50 mg
pyrazinamide 300 mg
Uses: Antitubercular

Riopan Plus Suspension:
Per 5 ml:
magaldrate 540 mg
simethicone 40 mg
Uses: Antacid, adsorbent, antiflatulent
Robaxisal:
methocarbamol 400 mg
aspirin 325 mg
Uses: Skeletal muscle relaxant, analgesic
Robitussin A-C Syrup:
Per 5 ml:
codeine 10 mg
guaifenesin 100 mg
3.5% alcohol
Uses: Analgesic, expectorant
Robitussin-CF Liquid:
Per 5 ml:
guaifenesin 100 mg
dextromethorphan 10 mg
phenylpropanolamine 12.5 mg
4.75% alcohol
Uses: Antitussive, expectorant
Robitussin Cold & Cough Liqui-Gels:
pseudoephedrine 30 mg
guaifenesin 200 mg
dextromethorphan 10 mg
Uses: Antitussive, expectorant
Robitussin-DAC Syrup:
Per 5 ml:
codeine 10 mg
guaifenesin 100 mg
pseudoephedrine 30 mg
1.4% alcohol
Uses: Analgesic, expectorant, adrenergic
Robitussin-DM Liquid:
Per 5 ml:
guaifenesin 100 mg
dextromethorphan 10 mg
Uses: Expectorant, antitussive
Robitussin Maximum Strength Cough and Cold Liquid:
dextromethorphan 15 mg
pseudoephedrine 30 mg
Uses: Antitussive, adrenergic
Robitussin Night Relief Liquid:
dextromethorphan 5 mg
pyrilamine 8.3 mg
pseudoephedrine 10 mg
acetaminophen 108.3 mg
Uses: Antitussive, adrenergic
Robitussin Pediatric Cough & Cold Liquid:
Per 5 ml:
pseudoephedrine 15 mg
dextromethorphan 7.5 mg
Uses: Antitussive, adrenergic
Robitussin-PE Syrup:
guaifenesin 100 mg

pseudoephedrine 30 mg
1.4% alcohol
Uses: Expectorant, adrenergic
Robitussin Severe Congestion Liqui-Gels:
guaifenesin 200 mg
pseudoephedrine 30 mg
Uses: Expectorant, adrenergic
Rolaids Calcium Rich:
magnesium hydroxide 80 mg
calcium carbonate 412 mg
Uses: Antacid, adsorbent, antiflatulent
Rondec:
pseudoephedrine 60 mg
carbinoxamine 4 mg
Uses: Adrenergic
Rondec DM Drops:
Per ml:
pseudoephedrine 25 mg
carbinoxamine 2 mg
dextromethorphan 4 mg
Uses: Adrenergic, antitussive
Rondec DM Syrup:
Per 5 ml:
pseudoephedrine 60 mg
carbinoxamine 4 mg
dextromethorphan 15 mg
Uses: Adrenergic, antitussive
Rondec Oral Drops:
Per 5 ml:
pseudoephedrine 25 mg
carbinoxamine 2 mg
Uses: Adrenergic
Roxicet:
Per 5 ml:
acetaminophen 325 mg
oxycodone 5 mg
Uses: Opioid analgesic
Roxicet 5/500:
oxycodone 5 mg
acetaminophen 500 mg
Uses: Opioid analgesic
Ru-Tuss:
phenylephrine 25 mg
phenylpropanolamine 50 mg
chlorpheniramine 8 mg
hyoscyamine 0.19 mg
atropine 0.04 mg
scopolamine 0.01 mg
Uses: Antihistamine, anticholinergic
Ru-Tuss DE:
pseudoephedrine 120 mg
guaifenesin 600 mg
Uses: Adrenergic, expectorant
Ru-Tuss Expectorant Liquid:
Per 5 ml:
guaifenesin 100 mg
pseudoephedrine 30 mg

dextromethorphan 10 mg
10% alcohol
Uses: Adrenergic, expectorant, antitussive
Ru-Tuss w/Hydrocodone Liquid:
Per 5 ml:
hydrocodone 1.7 mg
phenylephrine 5 mg
pyrilamine 3.3 mg
pheniramine 3.3 mg
phenylpropanolamine 3.3 mg
5% alcohol
Uses: Analgesic, adrenergic, decongestant
Ryna-C Liquid:
Per 5 ml:
pseudoephedrine 30 mg
chlorpheniramine 2 mg
codeine 10 mg
Uses: Adrenergic, antihistamine, analgesic
Ryna Liquid:
Per 5 ml:
pseudoephedrine 30 mg
chlorpheniramine 2 mg
Uses: Adrenergic, antihistamine
Rynatan:
phenylephrine 25 mg
chlorpheniramine 8 mg
pyrilamine 25 mg
Uses: Adrenergic, antihistamine
Rynatan Pediatric Suspension:
Per 5 ml:
phenylephrine 5 mg
chlorpheniramine 2 mg
pyrilamine 12.5 mg
Uses: Adrenergic, antihistamine
Rynatuss:
ephedrine 10 mg
carbetapentane 60 mg
chlorpheniramine 5 mg
phenylephrine 10 mg
Uses: Adrenergic, antihistamine
Salutensin:
hydroflumethiazide 50 mg
reserpine 0.125 mg
Uses: Antihypertensive
Salutensin Demi:
hydroflumethiazide 25 mg
reserpine 0.125 mg
Uses: Antihypertensive
Scot-Tussin DM Liquid:
Per 5 ml:
chlorpheniramine 2 mg
dextromethorphan 15 mg
Uses: Antihistamine, antitussive
Scot-Tussin Original 5-Action
Liquid:
phenylephrine 4.2 mg
pheniramine 13.3 mg
sodium citrate 83.3 mg

sodium salicylate 83.3 mg
caffeine citrate 25 mg
Uses: Adrenergic, analgesic
Scot-Tussin Senior Clear Liquid:
Per 5 ml:
guaifenesin 200 mg
dextromethorphan 15 mg
Uses: Antitussive, expectorant
Sedapap-10:
acetaminophen 650 mg
butalbital 50 mg
Uses: Analgesic, barbiturate
Semprex-D:
acrivastine 8 mg
pseudoephedrine 60 mg
Uses: Adrenergic, bronchodilator
Senokot-S:
docusate 50 mg
senna concentrate 187 mg
Uses: Laxative
Septra:
sulfamethoxazole 400 mg
trimethroprim 80 mg
Uses: Antiinfective
Septra DS:
sulfamethoxazole 800 mg
trimethroprim 160 mg
Uses: Antiinfective
Septra I.V. for Injection:
Per 5 ml:
trimethoprim 80 mg
sulfamethoxazole 400 mg
Uses: Antiinfective
Septra Suspension:
Per 5 ml:
trimethoprim 40 mg
sulfamethoxazole 200 mg
Uses: Antiinfective
Ser-Ap-Es:
hydrochlorothiazide 15 mg
reserpine 0.1 mg
hydralazine 25 mg
Uses: Diuretic, antihypertensive
Silafed Syrup:
Per 5 ml:
pseudoephedrine 30 mg
triprolidine 1.25 mg
Uses: Adrenergic, antihistamine
Silaminic Cold Syrup:
Per 5 ml:
phenylpropanolamine 12.5 mg
chlorpheniramine 2 mg
Uses: Antihistamine
Silaminic Expectorant Liquid:
Per 5 ml:
phenylpropanolamine 12.5 mg
guaifenesin 100 mg
Uses: Expectorant

Sinarest Extra Strength:
pseudoephedrine 30 mg
chlorpheniramine 2 mg
acetaminophen 500 mg
Uses: Adrenergic, antihistamine, analgesic
Sinarest No Drowsiness:
pseudoephedrine 30 mg
acetaminophen 500 mg
Uses: Adrenergic, analgesic
Sinarest Sinus:
pseudoephedrine 30 mg
chlorpheniramine 2 mg
acetaminophen 325 mg
Uses: Adrenergic, antihistamine, analgesic
Sine-Aid IB:
pseudoephedrine 30 mg
ibuprofen 200 mg
Uses: Adrenergic, analgesic
Sine-Aid Maximum Strength:
pseudoephedrine 30 mg
acetaminophen 500 mg
Uses: Adrenergic, analgesic
Sinemet 10/100:
carbidopa 10 mg
levodopa 100 mg
Uses: Antiparkinsonian
Sinemet 25/100:
carbidopa 25 mg
levodopa 100 mg
Uses: Antiparkinsonian
Sinemet 25/250:
carbidopa 25 mg
levodopa 250 mg
Uses: Antiparkinsonian
Sinemet CR 25-100:
carbidopa 25 mg
levodopa 100 mg
Uses: Antiparkinsonian
Sinemet CR 50-200:
carbidopa 50 mg
levodopa 200 mg
Uses: Antiparkinsonian
Sine-Off Maximum Strength No Drowsiness Formula Caplets:
pseudoephedrine 30 mg
acetaminophen 500 mg
Uses: Adrenergic, analgesic
Sine-Off Sinus Medicine:
pseudoephedrine 30 mg
chlorpheniramine 2 mg
acetaminophen 500 mg
Uses: Adrenergic, antihistamine, analgesic
Sinutab Maximum Strength Sinus Allergy:
acetaminophen 500 mg
pseudoephedrine 30 mg
chlorpheniramine 2 mg
Uses: Analgesic, adrenergic, antihistamine

Sinutab Maximum Strength Without Drowsiness:
acetaminophen 500 mg
pseudoephedrine 30 mg
Uses: Analgesic, adrenergic
Sinutab Non-Drying:
pseudoepedrine 30 mg
guaifenesin 200 mg
Uses: Adrenergic, expectorant
Slo-Phyllin GG Syrup:
theophylline 150 mg
guaifenesin 90 mg
Uses: Bronchodilator, expectorant
Synophylate-GG Syrup:
theophylline 150 mg
guaifenesin 100 mg
alcohol 15%
Uses: Bronchodilator, expectorant
Soma Compound:
carisoprodol 200 mg
aspirin 325 mg
Uses: Skeletal muscle relaxant, analgesic
Spec-T Lozenge:
dextromethorphan 10 mg
benzocaine 10 mg
Uses: Antitussive, topical anesthetic
St. Joseph Cold Tablets for Children:
phenylpropanolamine 3.125 mg
acetaminophen 80 mg
Uses: Decongestant, analgesic
Sudafed Cold & Cough Liquicaps:
pseudoephedrine 30 mg
dextromethorphan 10 mg
guaifenesin 100 mg
acetaminophen 250 mg
Uses: Adrenergic, antitussive, expectorant, analgesic
Sudafed Plus:
pseudoephedrine 60 mg
chlorpheniramine 4 mg
Uses: Adrenergic, antihistamine
Sudafed Severe Cold:
pseudoephedrine 30 mg
dextromethorphan 15 mg
Uses: Adrenergic, antitussive
Sudafed Sinus Maximum Strength:
pseudoephedrine 30 mg
acetaminophen 500 mg
Uses: Adrenergic, analgesic
Sudal 60/500:
pseudoephedrine 60 mg
guaifenesin 500 mg
Uses: Adrenergic, expectorant
Sudal 120/600:
pseudoephedrine 120 mg
guaifenesin 600 mg
Uses: Adrenergic, expectorant

Sultrin Triple Sulfa Vaginal Cream:
3.42% sulfathiazole
2.86% sulfacetamine
3.7% sulfabenzamide
Uses: Antiinfective

Sultrin Triple Sulfa Vaginal Tablets:
sulfathiazole 172.5 mg
sulfacetamide 143.75
sulfabenzamide 184 mg
Uses: Antiinfective

Synalgos-DC:
aspirin 356.4 mg
caffeine 30 mg
dihydrocodeine 16 mg
Uses: Analgesic

Synercid:
quinupristin 150 mg
dalfopristin 350 mg
Uses: Antiinfective

Talacen:
acetaminophen 650 mg
pentazocine 25 mg
Uses: Analgesic

Talwin Compound:
aspirin 325 mg
pentazocine 12.5 mg
Uses: Analgesic

Talwin NX:
pentazocine 50 mg
naloxone 0.5 mg
Uses: Analgesic, opioid antagonist

Tarka 182:
trandolapril 2 mg (immed rel)
verapamil 180 mg (sus rel)
Uses: Antihypertensive, calcium channel blocker

Tarka 241:
trandolapril 1 mg (immed rel)
verapamil 240 mg (sus rel)
Uses: Antihypertensive, calcium channel blocker

Tarka 242:
trandolapril 2 mg (immed rel)
verapamil 240 mg (sus rel)
Uses: Antihypertensive, calcium channel blocker

Tarka 244:
trandolapril 4 mg (immed rel)
verapamil 240 mg (sus rel)
Uses: Antihypertensive, calcium channel blocker

Tavist-D:
clemastine 1.34 mg
phenylpropanolamine 75 mg
Uses: Antihistamine, decongestant

Tavist Sinus:
acetaminophen 500 mg
pseudoephedrine 30 mg
Uses: Analgesic, adrenergic

Teczem:
enalapril 5 mg (extended release)
diltiazem 180 mg (extended release)
Uses: Antihypertensive, calcium channel blocker

Tedrigen:
ephedrine 22.5 mg
theophylline 120 mg
phenobarbital 7.5 mg
Uses: Adrenergic, bronchodilator, barbiturate

Tegrin-LT Shampoo:
0.33% pyrethrins
3.15% piperonyl butoxide
Uses: Scabicide, pediculicide

Tenoretic 50:
atenolol 50 mg
chlorthalidone 25 mg
Uses: Antihypertensive

Tenoretic 100:
atenolol 100 mg
chlorthalidone 25 mg
Uses: Antihypertensive

Terra-Cortril Ophthalmic Suspension:
1.5% hydrocortisone acetate
0.5% oxytetracycline
Uses: Ophth antiinflammatory, antiinfective

Terramycin with Polymycin B Sulfate Ophthalmic Ointment:
Per gram:
polymyxin B 10,000 units
oxytetracycline 5 mg
Uses: Ophth antiinfective

T-Gesic:
hydrocodone 5 mg
acetaminophen 500 mg
Uses: Analgesic

Theodrine:
ephedrine 22.5 mg
theophylline 120 mg
Uses: Adrenergic, bronchodilator

Theolate Liquid:
theophylline 150 mg
guaifenesin 90 mg
Uses: Bronchodilator, expectorant

Theophylline Kl Elixir:
theophylline 80 mg
potassium iodide 130 mg
Uses: Bronchodilator, expectorant

Thera-Flu, Flu & Cold Medicine Powder:
Per packet:
pseudoephedrine 60 mg
chlorpheniramine 4 mg

acetaminophen 650 mg
Uses: Adrenergic, antihistamine, analgesic
Thera-Flu, Flu, Cold & Cough Powder:
Per packet:
pseudoephedrine 60 mg
chlorpheniramine 4 mg
dextromethorphan 20 mg
acetaminophen 650 mg
Uses: Adrenergic, antihistamine, antitussive, analgesic
Thera-Flu NightTime Powder:
Per packet:
pseudoephedrine 60 mg
chlorpheniramine 4 mg
dextromethorphan 30 mg
acetaminophen 1000 mg
Uses: Adrenergic, antihistamine, antitussive, analgesic
Thera-Flu Non-Drowsy Flu, Cold & Cough Maximum Strength Powder
Per packet:
pseudoephedrine 60 mg
dextromethorphan 30 mg
acetaminophen 1000 mg
Uses: Adrenergic, antitussive, analgesic
Thera-Flu Non-Drowsy Formula Maximum Strength Caplets:
pseudoephedrine 30 mg
dextromethorphan 15 mg
acetaminophen 500 mg
Uses: Adrenergic, antitussive, analgesic
Timentin for Injection:
Per 3.1-g vial:
ticarcillin 3 g
clavulanic acid 0.1 g
Uses: Antiinfective
Timolide 10/25:
timolol 10 mg
hydrochlorothiazide 25 mg
Uses: Antihypertensive
Titralac Plus:
calcium carbonate 420 mg
simethicone 21 mg
Uses: Antacid, adsorbent, antiflatulent
Tobra Dex Ophthalmic Suspension/ Ointment:
tobramycin 0.3%
dexamethasone 0.1%
Uses: Ophth antiinfective, antiinflammatory
Triacin-C Cough Syrup:
Per 5 ml:
codeine 10 mg
pseudoephedrine 30 mg
triprolidine 1.25 mg
Uses: Analgesic, adrenergic, antihistamine

Tri-Hydroserpine:
hydralazine 25 mg
hydrochlorothiazide 15 mg
reserpine 0.1 mg
Uses: Antihypertensive
Tri-Levlen:
Phase I:
levonorgestrel 0.05 mg
ethinyl estradiol 30 µg
Phase II:
levonorgestrel 0.075 mg
ethinyl estradiol 40 µg;
Phase III:
levonorgestrel 0.125 mg
ethinyl estradiol 30 µg
Uses: Oral contraceptive
Triaminic Allergy:
phenylpropanolamine 25 mg
chlorpheniramine 4 mg
Uses: Antihistamine
Triaminic AM Cough & Decongestant Formula Liquid:
Per 5 ml:
pseudoephedrine 15 mg
dextromethorphan 7.5 mg
Uses: Adrenergic, antitussive
Triaminic Cold:
phenylpropanolamine 12.5 mg
chlorpheniramine 2 mg
Uses: Decongestant, antihistamine
Triaminic-DM Syrup:
Per 5 ml:
dextromethorphan 5 mg
phenylpropanolamine 6.25 mg
Uses: Antitussive, decongestant
Triaminic Expectorant Liquid:
Per 5 ml:
guaifenesin 50 mg
phenylpropanolamine 6.25 mg
Uses: Expectorant, decongestant
Triaminic Expectorant DH Liquid:
Per 5 ml:
guaifenesin 100 mg
hydrocodone 1.67 mg
phenylpropanolamine 12.5 mg
pheniramine 6.25 mg
pyrilamine 6.25 mg
5% alcohol
Uses: Analgesic, expectorant, decongestant
Triaminic Expectorant w/Codeine Liquid:
Per 5 ml:
phenylpropanolamine 12.5 mg
codeine 10 mg
guaifenesin 100 mg
Uses: Expectorant, decongestant, analgesic

Triaminic Nite Light Liquid:
Per 5 ml:
pseudoephedrine 15 mg
chlorpheniramine 1 mg
dextromethorphan 7.5 mg
Uses: Adrenergic, antihistamine, antitussive

Triaminic Oral Infant Drops:
Per ml:
phenylpropanolamine 20 mg
pyrilamine 10 mg
pheniramine 10 mg
Uses: Decongestant, antihistamine

Triaminic Sore Throat Formula Liquid:
Per 5 ml:
pseudoephedrine 15 mg
dextromethorphan 7.5 mg
acetaminophen 160 mg
Uses: Adrenergic, antitussive

Triaminic Syrup:
Per 5 ml:
phenylpropanolamine 6.25 mg
chlorpheniramine 1 mg
Uses: Decongestant, antihistamine

Triaminicin Cold, Allergy, Sinus:
phenylpropanolamine 25 mg
chlorpheniramine 4 mg
acetaminophen 650 mg
Uses: Decongestant, antihistamine analgesic

Triaminicol Multi-Symptom Cough, Cold:
phenylpropanolamine 12.5 mg
chlorpheniramine 2 mg
dextromethorphan 10 mg
Uses: Decongestant, antihistamine, antitussive

Triaminicol Multi-Symptom Relief Liquid:
Per 5 ml:
phenylpropanolamine 12.5 mg
chlorpheniramine 2 mg
dextromethorphan 10 mg
Uses: Decongestant, antihistamine, antitussive

Triavil 2-10:
perphenazine 2 mg
amitriptyline 10 mg
Uses: Antidepressant, antipsychotic

Triavil 4-10:
perphenazine 4 mg
amitriptyline 10 mg
Uses: Antidepressant, antipsychotic

Triavil 2-25:
perphenazine 2 mg
amitriptyline 25 mg
Uses: Antidepressant, antipsychotic

Triminol Cough Syrup:
Per 5 ml:
dextromethorphan 10 mg
chlorpheniramine 2 mg
phenylpropanolamine 12.5 mg
Uses: Antitussive, antihistamine, decongestant

Trinalin Repetabs:
azatadine maleate 1 mg
pseudoephedrine 120 mg
Uses: Antihistamine

Triphasil:
Phase I:
levonorgestrel 0.05 mg
ethinyl estradiol 30 μg
Phase II:
levonorgestrel 0.075 mg
ethinyl estradiol 40 μg
Phase III:
levonorgestrel 0.125 mg
ethinyl estradiol 30 μg
Uses: Oral contraceptive

Triple Antibiotic Ophthalmic Ointment:
Per gram:
polymyxin B 10,000 U
neomycin 3.5 mg
bacitracin 400 U
Uses: Antiinfective

Tuinal 100 mg:
amobarbital 50 mg
secobarbital 50 mg
Uses: Sedative-hypnotic

Tuinal 200 mg:
amobarbital 100 mg
secobarbital 100 mg
Uses: Sedative-hypnotic

Tusibron-DM Syrup:
Per 5 ml:
guaifenesin 100 mg
dextromethorphan 15 mg
Uses: Expectorant, antitussive

Tussionex Pennkinetic Suspension:
Per 5 ml:
chlorpheniramine 8 mg
hydrocodone 10 mg
Uses: Antihistamine, analgesic

Tussi-Organidin NR Liquid:
Per 5 ml:
codeine 10 mg
guaifenesin 100 mg
Uses: Analgesic, expectorant

Tussi-Organidin DM NR Liquid:
Per 5 ml:
guaifenesin 100 mg
dextromethorphan 10 mg
Uses: Expectorant, antitussive

Tylenol Allergy Sinus, Maximum Strength Gelcaps:
acetaminophen 500 mg
chlorpheniramine 2 mg
pseudoephedrine 30 mg
Uses: Antihistamine, adrenergic, analgesic
Tylenol Children's Cold:
acetaminophen 80 mg
chlorpheniramine 0.5 mg
pseudoephedrine 7.5 mg
Uses: Antihistamine, adrenergic, analgesic
Tylenol Children's Cold Liquid:
Per 5 ml:
acetaminophen 160 mg
chlorpheniramine 1 mg
pseudoephedrine 15 mg
Uses: Antihistamine, adrenergic, analgesic
Tylenol Children's Cold Multi-Symptom Plus Cough Liquid:
Per 5 ml:
acetaminophen 160 mg
dextromethorphan 5 mg
chlorpheniramine 1 mg
pseudoephedrine 15 mg
Uses: Antihistamine, adrenergic, analgesic
Tylenol Children's Cold Plus Cough Chewable:
acetaminophen 80 mg
pseudoephedrine 7.5 mg
dextromethorphan 2.5 mg
chlorpheniramine 0.5 mg
Uses: Antihistamine, adrenergic, analgesic
Tylenol Cold Multi-Symptom:
acetaminophen 325 mg
chlorpheniramine 2 mg
pseudoephedrine 30 mg
dextromethorphan 15 mg
Uses: Antihistamine, adrenergic, analgesic
Tylenol Cold No Drowsiness:
acetaminophen 325 mg
pseudoephedrine 30 mg
dextromethorphan 15 mg
Uses: Analgesic, adrenergic, antitussive
Tylenol Flu Maximum Strength Gelcaps:
dextromethorphan 15 mg
pseudoephedrine 30 mg
acetaminophen 500 mg
Uses: Analgesic, adrenergic, antitussive
Tylenol Flu NightTime Maximum Strength Gelcaps:
pseudoephedrine 30 mg
chlorpheniramine 2 mg
acetaminophen 500 mg
Uses: Adrenergic, antihistamine, analgesic
Tylenol Flu NightTime Maximum Strength Powder:
pseudoephedrine 60 mg

diphenhydramine 50 mg
acetaminophen 1000 mg
Uses: Adrenergic, antihistamine, analgesic
Tylenol Headache Plus, Extra Strength:
acetaminophen 500 mg
calcium carbonate 250 mg
Uses: Analgesic, antacid
Tylenol Multi-Symptom Cough Liquid:
Per 5 ml:
dextromethorphan 10 mg
acetaminophen 216.7 mg
5% alcohol
Uses: Antitussive, analgesic
Tylenol Multi-Symptom Cough w/Decongestant Liquid:
Per 5 ml:
dextromethorphan 10 mg
acetaminophen 200 mg
pseudoephedrine 20 mg
Uses: Antitussive, analgesic, adrenergic
Tylenol Multi-Symptom Hot Medication:
Per packet:
acetaminophen 650 mg
chlorpheniramine 4 mg
pseudoephedrine 60 mg
dextromethorphan 30 mg
Uses: Analgesic, antihistamine, adrenergic, antitussive
Tylenol PM, Extra Strength:
acetaminophen 500 mg
diphenhydramine 25 mg
Uses: Analgesic, antihistamine
Tylenol Severe Allergy:
diphenhydramine 12.5 mg
acetaminophen 500 mg
Uses: Analgesic, antihistamine
Tylenol Sinus Maximum Strength:
pseudoephedrine 30 mg
acetaminophen 500 mg
Uses: Adrenergic, analgesic
Tylenol with Codeine Elixir:
Per 5 ml:
acetaminophen 120 mg
codeine 12 mg
Uses: Analgesic
Tylenol with Codeine No. 2:
acetaminophen 300 mg
codeine 15 mg
Uses: Analgesic
Tylenol with Codeine No. 3:
acetaminophen 300 mg
codeine 30 mg
Uses: Analgesic
Tylenol with Codeine No. 4:
acetaminophen 300 mg

codeine 60 mg
Uses: Analgesic
Tylox:
oxycodone 5 mg
acetaminophen 500 mg
Uses: Analgesic
Tyrodone Liquid:
Per 5 ml:
hydrocodone 5 mg
pseudoephedrine 60 mg
5% alcohol
Uses: Analgesic, adrenergic
Unasyn for Injection 1.5 g:
ampicillin 1 g
sulbactam 0.5 g
Uses: Antiinfective
Unasyn for Injection 3 g:
ampicillin 2 g
sulbactam 1 g
Uses: Antiinfective
Uniretic:
moexipril 7.5 mg
hydrochlorothiazide 12.5 mg
or moexipril 15 mg
hydrochlorothiazide 25 mg
Uses: Antihypertensive, diuretic
Unituss HC Syrup:
hydrocodone 2.5 mg
phenylephrine 5 mg
chlorpheniramine 2 mg
Uses: Analgesic, adrenergic, antihistamine
Urised:
methenamine 40.8 mg
phenylsalicylate 18.1 mg
atropine 0.03 mg
hyoscyamine 0.03 mg
benzoic acid 4.5 mg
methylene blue 5.4 mg
Uses: Antiinfective
Ursinus Inlay:
pseudoephedrine 30 mg
aspirin 325 mg
Uses: Adrenergic, analgesic
Vanquish:
aspirin 227 mg
acetaminophen 194 mg
caffeine 33 mg
Uses: Nonnarcotic analgesic
Vaseretic 10-25:
enalapril 10 mg
hydrochlorothiazide 25 mg
Uses: Antihypertensive, diuretic
Vasocidin Ophthalmic Ointment:
sulfacetamide 10%
prednisolone 0.5%
Uses: Ophthalmic antiinfective, antiinflammatory

Vasocidin Ophthalmic Solution:
sulfacetamide 10%
prednisolone 0.25%
Uses: Ophthalmic antiinfective, antiinflammatory
Vasocon-A Ophthalmic Solution:
naphazoline 0.05%
antazoline 0.5%
Uses: Ophthalmic vasoconstrictor
**Vicks 44D Cough & Head Congestion
Liquid:**
Per 5 ml:
dextromethorphan 10 mg
pseudoephedrine 20 mg
Uses: Antitussive, adrenergic
Vicks 44E Liquid:
Per 5 ml:
dextromethorphan 6.7 mg
guaifenesin 66.7 mg
Uses: Antitussive, expectorant
**Vicks 44M Cold, Flu, & Cough
LiquiCaps:**
dextromethorphan 10 mg
pseudoephedrine 30 mg
chlorpheniramine 2 mg
acetaminophen 250 mg
Uses: Antitussive, adrenergic, antihistamine, analgesic
**Vicks 44 Non-Drowsy Cold & Cough
LiquiCaps:**
dextromethorphan 30 mg
pseudoephedrine 60 mg
Uses: Antitussive, adrenergic
**Vicks Children's NyQuil Nighttime
Cough/Cold Liquid:**
Per 5 ml:
pseudoephedrine 10 mg
chlorpheniramine 0.67 mg
dextromethorphan 5 mg
Uses: Adrenergic, antihistamine, antitussive
Vicks Cough Silencers:
dextromethorphan 2.5 mg
benzocaine 1 mg
Uses: Antitussive, top anesthetic
**Vicks DayQuil Allergy Relief
4 Hour:**
phenylpropanolamine 25 mg
brompheniramine 4 mg
Uses: Decongestant, antihistamine
**Vicks DayQuil Allergy Relief
12 Hour ER:**
phenylpropanolamine 75 mg
brompheniramine 12 mg
Uses: Decongestant, antihistamine
Vicks DayQuil Liquid:
Per 5 ml:

dextromethorphan 3.3 mg
pseudoephedrine 10 mg
acetaminophen 108.3 mg
guaifenesin 33.3 mg
Uses: Antitussive, adrenergic, analgesic,
expectorant
**Vicks DayQuil Sinus Pressure & Pain
Relief:**
pseudoephedrine 30 mg
acetaminophen 500 mg
Uses: Adrenergic, analgesic
Vicks NyQuil Liquicaps:
pseudoephedrine 30 mg
doxylamine 6.25 mg
dextromethorphan 10 mg
acetaminophen 250 mg
Uses: Adrenergic, antihistamine, antitussive, analgesic
**Vicks NyQuil Multi-Symptom Cold Flu
Relief Liquid:**
pseudoephedrine 10 mg
doxylamine 2.1 mg
dextromethorphan 5 mg
acetaminophen 167 mg
Uses: Adrenergic, antihistamine, antitussive, analgesic
**Vicks Pediatric Formula 44e
Liquid:**
Per 5 ml:
dextromethorphan 3.3 mg
guaifenesin 33.3 mg
Uses: Expectorant, antitussive
**Vicks Pediatric Formula 44 m Multi-
Symptom Cough & Cold Liquid:**
pseudoephedrine 10 mg
chlorpheniramine 0.67 mg
dextromethorphan 5 mg
Uses: Adrenergic, antihistamine, antitussive
Vicodin:
acetaminophen 500 mg
hydrocodone 5 mg
Uses: Analgesic
Vicodin ES:
acetaminophen 750 mg
hydrocodone 7.5 mg
Uses: Analgesic

Vicodin HP:
hydrocodone 10 mg
acetaminophen 660 mg
Uses: Analgesic
VicodinTuss:
Per 5 ml:
hydrocodone 5 mg
guaifenesin 100 mg
Uses: Analgesic, expectorant
Vicoprofen:
hydrocodone 7.5 mg
ibuprofen 200 mg
Uses: Analgesic
Wigraine Suppositories:
ergotamine 2 mg
caffeine 100 mg
Uses: α-adrenergic blocker
Zestoretic 10/12.5:
lisinopril 10 mg
hydrochlorothiazide 12.5 mg
Uses: Antihypertensive
Zestoretic 20/12.5:
lisinopril 20 mg
hydrochlorothiazide 12.5 mg
Uses: Antihypertensive
Zestoretic 20/25:
lisinopril 20 mg
hydrochlorothiazide 25 mg
Uses: Antihypertensive
Ziac 2.5:
bisoprolol 2.5 mg
hydrochlorothiazide 6.25 mg
Uses: Antihypertensive
Ziac 5:
bisoprolol 5 mg
hydrochlorothiazide 6.25 mg
Uses: Antihypertensive
Ziac 10:
bisoprolol 10 mg
hydrochlorothiazide 6.25 mg
Uses: Antihypertensive
Zydone:
hydrocodone 5 mg
acetaminophen 500 mg
Uses: Analgesic

Appendix E

Rarely Used Drugs

abciximab (℞)
Func. class.: Platelet aggregation inhibitor

Dosage and routes
Adult: **IV** 250 µg (0.25 mg)/kg bolus 10-60 min prior to PTCA, followed by 10 µg/min CONT INF for 12 hr

Uses: Used with heparin and aspirin to prevent acute cardiac ischemia following percutaneous transluminal angioplasty (PTCA) in patients at high risk for reclosure of affected arteries

Contraindications: Hypersensitivity to this drug or murine protein; GI, GU bleeding; CVA within 2 yr, bleeding disorders, intracranial neoplasm, intracranial arteriovenous malformations, intracranial aneurysm, platelet count <100,000 cells/mm³, recent surgery, aneurysm, uncontrolled severe hypertension, vasculitis

aminocaproic acid (℞)
Func. class.: Hemostatic

Dosage and routes
Adult: PO/**IV** 5-g loading dose, then 1-1.25 g q1h if needed, not to exceed 30 g/day

Uses: Hemorrhage from hyperfibrinolysis; adjunctive therapy in hemophilia, amegakaryocytic thrombocytopenia, hereditary angioneurotic edema

Investigational uses: Prevention of recurrent subarachnoid hemorrhage

Contraindications: Hypersensitivity, abnormal bleeding, postpartum bleeding, DIC, upper urinary tract bleeding, new burns

amyl nitrite (℞)
Func. class.: Coronary vasodilator (antianginal, antidote for cyanide)

Dosage and routes
Angina
Adult: INH 0.18-0.3 ml as needed, 1-6 inhalations from 1 cap; may repeat in 3-5 min

Cyanide poisoning
Adult: INH 0.3-ml ampule 15 sec until preparation of sodium nitrite infusion is ready

Uses: Acute angina pectoris

Contraindications: Hypersensitivity to nitrites, severe anemia, increased intracranial pressure, hypertension, pregnancy **X**

aurothioglucose/gold sodium thiomalate (℞)
Func. class.: Antiinflammatory (gold)

Dosage and routes
Adult: IM 10 mg; then 25 mg weekly × 2-3 wk; then 50 mg/wk until total of 1 g is administered; then 25-50 mg q3-4 wk if there is improvement without toxicity (aurothioglucose); total of 800 mg-1 g

Adult: IM 10 mg, then 25 mg after 1 wk, then 50 mg weekly for total of 14-20 doses; then 50 mg q2 wk × 4; then 50 mg q3 wk × 4; then 50 mg monthly for maintenance (gold sodium thiomalate)

P *Child 6-12 yr:* IM 1 mg/kg/wk × 20 wk, or ¼ of adult dosage (aurothioglucose)

P *Child <6 yr:* IM 1 mg/kg/wk × 20 wk, then q3-4 wk if improvement without toxicity (gold sodium thiomalate), not to exceed 2.5 mg

Uses: Rheumatoid arthritis resistant to other treatment, psoriatic arthritis

Contraindications: Hypersensitivity to gold, SLE, uncontrolled diabetes mellitus, marked hypertension, recent radiation therapy, CHF, lactation, renal disease, liver disease

benzquinamide (℞)
Func. class.: Antiemetic

Dosage and routes
Adult: IM 50 mg or 0.5-1 mg/kg; may be repeated in 1 hr, then q3-4h prn; **IV** 25 mg or 0.2-0.4 mg/kg as a one-time dose

Uses: To inhibit nausea, vomiting associated with anesthetic

Contraindications: Hypersensitivity, hypertension

P beractant (℞)
Func. class.: Natural lung surfactant

Dosage and routes
Intratracheal instill: 4 doses can be administered in the 1st
P 48 hr of life; give doses no more frequently than q6h; each dose is 100 mg of phospholipids/kg birth weight (4 ml/kg)

Uses: Prevention and treatment (rescue) of respiratory distress syndrome in premature
P infants

cabergoline (℞)
Func. class.: Dopamine receptor/agonist

Dosage and routes:
Hyperprolactinemic indications
Adult: PO 0.25 mg 2×/wk, may increase by 0.25 mg 2×/wk at 4 wk intervals, max 1 mg 2×/wk; maintenance therapy may be needed for 6 mo

Uses: Reduced prolactin/secretion in postpartum lactation

Investigational uses: Parkinson's disease, normalization of androgen levels and improved menstrual cycles in polycystic ovarian syndrome

Contraindications: Hypersensitivity to uncontrolled hypertension

---

chlorpropamide (℞)
Func. class.: Antidiabetic, oral

Dosage and routes
Adult: PO 100-250 mg qd initially, then 100-500 mg maintenance according to response; not to exceed 750 mg/day

Uses: Stable adult-onset diabetes mellitus (type II; NIDDM)

Contraindications: Hypersensitivity to sulfonylureas, ☐ juvenile or brittle diabetes, pregnancy **C,** renal failure

clioquinol (OTC)
Func. class.: Local antiinfective

Dosage and routes
Top apply to affected area bid or tid × 7 days only

Uses: Cutaneous infections: athlete's foot, eczema, and other fungal infections

Contraindications: Hypersensitivity to iodine, chloroxine

clobetasol (℞)
Func. class.: Topical corticosteroid

Dosage and routes
☐ *Adult and child:* Top apply to affected area bid

Uses: Psoriasis, eczema, contact dermatitis, pruritus; usually reserved for severe dermatoses that have not responded to less potent formulation

Contraindications: Hypersensitivity to corticosteroids, fungal infections

clocortolone (℞)
Func. class.: Topical corticosteroid

Dosage and routes
☐ *Adult and child:* Top apply to affected area tid or qid

Uses: Psoriasis, eczema, contact dermatitis, pruritus

Contraindications: Hypersensitivity to corticosteroids, fungal infections

clotrimazole (℞) (OTC)
Func. class.: Local antiinfective

Dosage and routes
☐ *Adult and child:* Top rub into affected area bid × 1-4 wk; loz dissolve in mouth 5 times/ day × 2 wk; intravag 1 applicator/1 tab × 1-2 wk hs; oral troches 10 mg 5 times/ day × 14 days

Uses: Tinea pedis, tinea cruris, tinea corporis, tinea versicolor, *C. albicans* infection of the vagina, vulva, throat, mouth

Contraindications: Hypersensitivity

colfosceril (R)
Func. class.: Synthetic lung surfactant

Dosage and routes
Prophylactic treatment
Endotracheally: 5 ml/kg as soon as possible after birth and repeat doses 12 and 24 hr later
P to infants remaining on mechanical ventilation

Rescue treatment
Endotracheally: Administer in two half doses of 5 ml/kg doses; give initial dose after treatment of RDS, then second dose in 12 hr

Uses: Treatment of respiratory distress syndrome (RDS) in
P premature infants

cosyntropin (R)
Func. class.: Pituitary hormone

Dosage and routes
P *Adult and child >2 yr:* IM/**IV** 0.25-1 mg between blood sampling
P *Child <2 yr:* IM/**IV** 0.125 mg

Uses: Testing adrenocortical function

Contraindications: Hypersensitivity

deferoxamine (R)
Func. class.: Heavy metal antagonist

Dosage and routes
Acute iron toxicity
P *Adult and child:* IM/**IV** 1 g; then 500 mg q4h × 2 doses; then 500 mg q4-12h × 2 doses, not to exceed 15 mg/kg/hr or 6 g/24 hr

Chronic iron toxicity
P *Adult and child:* IM 500 mg-1 g/day plus **IV** inf 2 g given by separate line with each blood transfusion, not to exceed 15 mg/kg/hr or 6 g/24 hr; SC 1-2 g over 8-24 hr by SC infusion pump

Uses: Acute, chronic iron intoxication, hemochromatosis, hemosiderosis

Contraindications: Hypersensitivity, anuria, severe renal disease

dienestrol (R)
Func. class.: Estrogen

Dosage and routes
Adult: Vag cream 1-2 applications qd × 2 wk, then ½ dose × 2 wk, then 1 application

Uses: Atrophic vaginitis, kraurosis vulvae

Contraindications: Breast cancer, thromboembolic disorders, reproductive cancer, genital bleeding (abnormal, undiagnosed), pregnancy **X**

dimercaprol (R)
Func. class.: Heavy metal antagonist

Dosage and routes
Severe gold/arsenic poisoning
Adult: IM 3 mg/kg q4h × 2 days; then qid × 1 day; then bid × 10 days

Mild gold/arsenic poisoning
Adult: IM 2.5 mg/kg qid × 2 days; then bid × 1 day; then qd × 10 days

Acute lead poisoning
Adult: IM 4 mg/kg; then q4h

with edetate calcium disodium 12.5 mg/kg IM; not to exceed 5 mg/kg/dose

Mercury poisoning
Adult: IM 5 mg/kg; then 2.5 mg/kg/day or bid × 10 days

Uses: Arsenic, gold, mercury, lead poisoning; adjunct in severe lead poisoning with encephalopathy

Contraindications: Hypersensitivity, anuria, hepatic insufficiency, poisoning with other metals, severe renal disease, **P** child <3 yr, pregnancy **D**

---

disulfiram (℞)
Func. class.: Alcohol deterrent

Dosage and routes
Adult: PO 250-500 mg qd × 1-2 wk, then 125-500 mg qd until fully socially recovered

Uses: Chronic alcoholism (as adjunct)

Contraindications: Hypersensitivity, alcohol intoxication, psychoses, CV disease, pregnancy **X**

---

edetate calcium disodium (℞)
Func. class.: Heavy metal antagonist; antidote

Dosage and routes
Acute lead encephalopathy
P *Adult and child:* 1.5 g/m²/ day × 3-5 days, with dimercaprol; may be given again after 4 days off drug

Lead poisoning
Adult: IV 1 g/250-500 ml D₅W or 0.9% NaCl over 1-2 hr or q12h × 3-5 days; may repeat

after 2 days; not to exceed 50 mg/kg/day; may be given as a continuous inf over 8-24 hr

Adult: IM 35 mg/kg bid
P *Child:* IM 35 mg/kg/day in divided doses q8-12h, not to exceed 50 mg/kg/day; may give for 3-5 days, off 4 days before next course

Uses: Lead poisoning, acute lead encephalopathy

Contraindications: Hypersensitivity, anuria, poisoning of other metals, severe renal disease, **P** child <3 yr

---

felbamate (℞)
Func. class.: Anticonvulsant

Dosage and routes
Adjunctive therapy
Adult: PO add 1.2 g/day in 3-4 divided doses; reduce other anticonvulsants (valproic acid, phenytoin, carbamazepine, and derivatives) by 20% to control plasma concentrations; may increase felbamate in 1.2 g/day increments qwk, up to 3.6 g/day

Monotherapy
Adult: PO 1.2 g/day in 3-4 divided doses; titrate with close supervision; increase dose in 600-mg increments q2wk to 3.6 g/day if needed

Lennox-Gastaut syndrome
P *Child (2-14 yr):* PO add 15 mg/kg/day in 3-4 divided doses; reduce other anticonvulsants (valproic acid, phenytoin, carbamazepine, and derivatives) by 20% to control plasma concentrations; may increase felbamate 15 mg/kg/day qwk up to 45 mg/day

---

♣ Canada Only   Adverse effects: *italic* = common; **bold** = life-threatening

Uses: Partial seizures, with or without generalization in adults; partial and generalized seizures in children with Lennox-Gastaut syndrome

Contraindications: Hypersensitivity to this drug, other carbamates

---

floxuridine (℞)
Func. class.: Antineoplastic, antimetabolite

Dosage and routes
Adult: Intraarterial by continuous inf 0.1-0.6 mg/kg/day × 1-6 wk; hepatic artery inj 0.4-0.6 mg/kg/day × 1-6 wk

Uses: GI adenocarcinoma metastatic to liver; cancer of breast, head, neck, liver, brain, gallbladder, bile duct

Contraindications: Hypersensitivity, myelosuppression, pregnancy **D**, poor nutritional status, serious infections

---

fludarabine (℞)
Func. class.: Antineoplastic, antimetabolite

Dosage and routes
Adult: IV 25 mg/m² over 30 min qd × 5 days, may repeat q28 days; reconstitute with 2 ml of sterile water for inj; dissolution should occur in <15 sec

Uses: Chronic lymphocytic leukemia; non-Hodgkin's lymphoma

Contraindications: Hypersensitivity, pregnancy **D**

---

flunisolide (℞)
Func. class.: Steroid, intranasal

Dosage and routes:
Adult: Instill 2 sprays in each nostril bid, then increase to tid if needed, not to exceed 8 sprays/day in each nostril

P *Child 6-14 yr:* Instill 1 spray in each nostril tid or 2 sprays bid, not to exceed 4 sprays/day in each nostril

P *Adult and child >6 yr:* Spray 2 puffs bid, not to exceed 4 puffs bid

Uses: Rhinitis (seasonal or perennial), nasal polyps; chronic steroid-dependent asthma (inh)

Contraindications: Hypersensitivity, child <12 yr; fungal, bacterial infection of nose

---

hydroxychloroquine (℞)
Func. class.: Antimalarial, antiarthritic

Dosage and routes
Malaria
P *Adult and child:* PO 5 mg/kg/wk on same day of week, not to exceed 400 mg; treatment should begin 2 wk before entering endemic area; continue 8 wk after leaving; if treatment begins after exposure, 800 mg for adult, 10 mg/kg for children in 2 divided doses 6 hr apart

Lupus erythematosus
Adult: PO 400 mg qd-bid; length depends on patient response; maintenance 200-400 mg qd

Rheumatoid arthritis
Adult: PO 400-600 mg qd,

☑ Herb/drug 🚫 Do Not Crush ◆ Alert ⛐ Key Drug G Geriatric P Pediatric then 200-300 mg qd after good response

Uses: Malaria caused by *Plasmodium vivax, P. malariae, P. ovale, P. falciparum* (some strains); SLE, rheumatoid arthritis

Contraindications: Hypersensitivity, retinal field changes, P porphyria, children (long-term)

hydroxyprogesterone (R)
Func. class.: Progestin, hormone

Dosage and routes
Menstrual disorders
Adult: IM 125-375 mg q4wk; discontinue after 4 cycles
Uterine cancer
Adult: IM 1 g 5-7 times/wk

Uses: Uterine carcinoma, menstrual disorders (abnormal uterine bleeding, amenorrhea)

Contraindications: Breast cancer, hypersensitivity, thromboembolic disorders, reproductive cancer, genital bleeding (abnormal, undiagnosed), pregnancy

isotretinoin (R)
Func. class.: Dermatologic antiacne agent

Dosage and routes
Adult: PO 0.5-2 mg/kg/day in 2 divided doses × 15-20 wk; if relapse occurs, repeat after 8 wk off drug

Uses: Severe recalcitrant cystic acne

Contraindications: Hypersensitivity, inflamed skin, pregnancy **X**

ketamine (R)
Func. class.: General anesthetic

Dosage and routes
P *Adult and child:* **IV** 1-4.5 mg/kg over 1 min
P *Adult and child:* IM 6.5-13 mg/kg
Maintenance: ½ to full induction dose may be repeated

Uses: Short anesthesia for diagnostic/surgical procedures; as an adjunct with other anesthetics

Contraindications: Hypersensitivity, CVA, increased intracranial pressure, severe hypertension, cardiac decompen-
P sation, child <2 yr

methohexital (R)
Func. class.: General anesthetic

Dosage and routes
Induction
P *Adult and child:* **IV** 50-120 mg given 1 ml/5 sec
Maintenance
P *Adult and child:* **IV** 20-40 mg q4-7 min of a 0.1% sol

Uses: General anesthesia for electroshock therapy, reduction of fractures, adjunct with other anesthetics, balanced anesthesia

Contraindications: Hypersensitivity, status asthmaticus, hepatic/intermittent porphyrias

---

mitotane (R)
Func. class.: Antineoplastic

Dosage and routes
Adult: PO 9-10 g/day in divided doses tid or qid; may have to decrease dosage if severe reactions occur
Uses: Adrenocortical carcinoma
Investigational uses: Pituitary disorders with cushingoid symptoms
Contraindications: Hypersensitivity

papaverine (R)
Func. class.: Peripheral vasodilator

Dosage and routes
Adult: PO 100-300 mg 3-5 times day; sus rel cap 150-300 mg q8-12h; IM/**IV** 30-120 mg q3h prn; Intracavernosal (IC) 30 mg/0.5-1 mg phentolamine or 60 mg alone
Uses: Arterial spasm resulting in cerebral and peripheral ischemia, myocardial ischemia associated with vascular spasm or dysrhythmias, angina pectoris, peripheral pulmonary embolism, visceral spasm as in ureteral, biliary, GI colic, peripheral vascular disease
Contraindications: Hypersensitivity, complete AV heart block

phenoxybenzamine (R)
Func. class.: Antihypertensive

Dosage and routes
Adult: PO 10 mg qd; increase by 10 mg qod; usual range 20-40 mg bid-tid
P *Child:* PO 0.2 mg/kg or 6 mg/m^2/day, max 10 mg, may increase at 4-day intervals; maintenance dosage 0.4-1.2 mg/kg/day or 12-36 mg/m^2/day given in divided doses tid or qid
Uses: Pheochromocytoma
Contraindications: Hypersensitivity, CHF, angina, cerebral vascular insufficiency, coronary arteriosclerosis

pralidoxime (R)
Func. class.: Cholinesterase reactivator

Dosage and routes
Anticholinesterase overdose
Adult: **IV** 1-2 g, then 250 mg q5 min until desired response
Organophosphate poisoning
Adult: **IV** inf 1-2 g/100 ml 0.9% NaCl over 15-30 min; may repeat in 1 hr; PO 1-3 g q5h
P *Child:* **IV** inf 20-40 mg/kg/dose diluted in 100 ml 0.9% NaCl over 15-30 min
Uses: Cholinergic crisis in myasthenia gravis, organophosphate poisoning antidote, early relief of paralysis of respiratory muscles; used as an adjunct to systemic atropine administration

---

☑ Herb/drug 🚫 Do Not Crush ◆ Alert ⚷ Key Drug **G** Geriatric **P** Pediatric

Contraindications: Hypersensitivity, carbamate insecticide poisoning

---

prazepam (℞)
Func. class.: Sedative/hypnotic; antianxiety agent

Dosage and routes
Adult: PO 10 mg tid; 20-60 mg in divided doses or 20 mg at hs

G *Elderly:* PO 10-15 mg/day in divided doses

Uses: Anxiety

Contraindications: Hypersensitivity to benzodiazepines, narrow-angle glaucoma, psy-**P** chosis, pregnancy **D**, child <18 yr

---

teniposide (℞)
Func. class.: Antineoplastic

Dosage and routes
P *Child* IV inf: Combo teniposide 165 mg/m² and cytarabine 300 mg/m² 2 ×/wk × 8-9 doses or combo teniposide 250 mg/m² and vincristine 1.5 mg/m² qwk × 4-8 wk and prednisone 40 mg/m² PO × 28 days

Uses: Childhood acute lymphoblastic leukemia (ALL), refractory childhood acute lymphocytic leukemia

Contraindications: Hypersensitivity, bone marrow depression, severe hepatic disease, severe renal disease, bacterial infection, pregnancy **D**

---

thiopental (℞)
Func. class.: General anesthetic

Dosage and routes
Induction
Adult: **IV** 210-280 mg or 3-5 ml/kg
General anesthetic
Adult: **IV** 50-75 mg given at 20-40 sec intervals
Narcoanalysis
Adult: **IV** 100 mg/min, not to exceed 50 ml/min
Sedation or narcosis
Adult: Rec 12-20 mg/lb
Increased intracranial pressure
Adult: 1.5-3.5 mg/kg

Uses: Short general anesthesia, narcoanalysis, induction anesthesia before other anesthetics

Investigational uses: Increased intracranial pressure

Contraindications: Hypersensitivity, status asthmaticus, hepatic/intermittent porphyrias

---

tolazamide (℞)
Func. class.: Antidiabetic, oral

Dosage and routes
Adult: PO 100 mg/day for FBS <200 mg/dl or 250 mg/day for FBS >200 mg/dl; dose should be titrated to patient response (1 g or less/day)

Uses: Type II (NIDDM) diabetes mellitus

Contraindications: Hypersensitivity to sulfonylureas, juvenile or brittle diabetes

---

tolbutamide ⚷ (℞)
Func. class.: Antidiabetic

Dosage and routes
Adult: PO 1-2 g/day in divided doses, titrated to patient response; **IV** 1 g (Fajan's test)

Uses: Type II (NIDDM) diabetes mellitus

Contraindications: Hypersensitivity to sulfonylureas, juvenile or brittle diabetes

vasopressin ⚷ (℞)
Func. class.: Pituitary hormone

Dosage and routes
Diabetes insipidus
Adult: IM/SC 5-10 units bid-qid prn; IM/SC 2.5-5 units q2-3 days (Pitressin Tannate) for chronic therapy
P *Child:* IM/SC 2.5-10 units bid-qid prn; IM/SC 1.25-2.5 units q2-3 days (Pitressin Tannate) for chronic therapy

Abdominal distention
Adult: IM 5 units, then q3-4h, increasing to 10 units if needed (aqueous)

Uses: Diabetes insipidus (nonnephrogenic/nonpsychogenic), abdominal distention postoperatively, bleeding esophageal varices

Contraindications: Hypersensitivity, chronic nephritis

xylometazoline (OTC)
Func. class.: Nasal decongestant

Dosage and routes
P *Adult and child >12 yr:* Instill 2-3 gtt or 2 sprays q8-10h (0.1%)
P *Child <12 yr:* Instill 2-3 gtt or 1% spray q8-10h (0.05%)

Uses: Nasal congestion; adjunct in otitis media

Contraindications: Hypersensitivity to sympathomimetic amines

---

Appendix F Less frequently used antihistamines

GENERIC NAME	TRADE NAME(S)	USES	DOSAGES AND ROUTES	AVAILABLE FORMS	INTERACTIONS	CONTRAINDICATIONS
acrivastine/ pseudoephedrine (R)	Semprex-D	• Rhinitis • Allergy symptoms • Chronic idiopathic urticaria	• Adult, child >12 yr: PO 8 mg q4-6h	• Caps 8 mg/60 mg	• Increased CNS depression: alcohol, narcotics, sedatives, hypnotics • Hypertensive crisis: MAOIs ☑ May increase CNS depression: kava ☑ May increase anticho-linergic effect: henbane leaf	• Hypersensitivity to this drug or triprolidine • Severe hypertension • Cardiac disease
azatadine (R)	Optimine	• Allergy symptoms • Rhinitis • Chronic urticaria	• Adult: PO 1-2 mg bid, not to exceed 4 mg/ day • Elderly: PO 1 mg qd-bid	• Tabs 1 mg	• Increased CNS depression: barbitu-rates, narcotics, hyp-notics, tricyclic antide-pressants, alcohol • Decreased effect of: oral anticoagulants • Increased effect of azatadine: MAOIs ☑ Increased CNS depression: kava ☑ Increased anticholiner-gic effect: henbane leaf	• Hypersensitivity to H₁-receptor antagonists • Acute asthma attack • Lower respiratory tract disease • Child <12 yr
buclizine (R)	Bucladin-S, Softabs	• Motion sickness • Dizziness • Nausea • Vomiting • Antihistamine	• Adult: PO 25-50 mg prn ½ hr before travel; may be repeated q4-6h prn	• Tabs 50 mg	☑ Increased anticholin-ergic effect: henbane leaf ☑ Increased CNS depression: kava	• Hypersensitivity to cyclizines • Shock

Continued

KEY: ✦ = Canada only; ☑ = herb-drug interaction

1445

Appendix F Less frequently used antihistamines—cont'd

GENERIC NAME	TRADE NAME(S)	USES	DOSAGES AND ROUTES	AVAILABLE FORMS	INTERACTIONS	CONTRAINDICATIONS
cyclizine (OTC, ℞)	Marezine	• Motion sickness • Prevention of post-operative vomiting • Antihistamine	*Vomiting* • Adult: IM 25-50 mg ½ hr before termination of surgery, then q4-6h prn (lactate) • Child: IM 3 mg/kg divided in 3 equal doses *Motion sickness* • Adult: PO 50 mg then q4-6h prn, not to exceed 200 mg/day (HCl) • Child: PO 25 mg q4-6h prn	• Tabs (HCl) 50 mg • Inj (lactate) 50 mg/ml	• May increase CNS effect: alcohol, tranquilizers, narcotics ☑ Increased CNS depression: kava	• Hypersensitivity to cyclizines • Shock
dexchlorpheniramine (℞)	Dexchlor, dexchlorpheniramine maleate, Poladex, Polaramine	• Allergy symptoms • Rhinitis • Pruritus • Contact dermatitis	• Adult: PO 1-2 mg tid-qid; repeat action 4-6 mg bid-tid • Child 6-11 yr: PO 1 mg q4-6h, or time rel 4 mg hs • Child 2-5 yr: PO 0.5 mg q4-6h; do not use repeat action form	• Tabs 2 mg • Repeat action tabs 4, 6 mg • Syr 2 mg/5 ml	• Increased CNS depression: barbiturates, narcotics, hypnotics, tricyclic antidepressants, alcohol • Decreased effect: oral anticoagulants, heparin • Increased effect of dexchlorpheniramine: MAOIs ☑ Increased anticholinergic effect: henbane leaf	• Hypersensitivity to H₁-receptor antagonists • Acute asthma attack • Lower respiratory tract disease

trimeprazine (B)	Panectyl ✦, Temaril	• Pruritus	• Adult: PO 2.5 mg qid; time-rel 5 mg bid • Elderly: PO 2.5 mg bid • Child 3-12 yr: PO 2.5 mg tid or hs • Child 6 mo-1 yr: PO 1.25 mg tid or hs	• Tabs 2.5 mg • Time-rel spanules 5 mg • Syr 2.5 mg/ 5 ml	• Increased CNS depression: barbiturates, narcotics, hypnotics, tricyclic antidepressants, alcohol • Decreased effect of oral anticoagulants, heparin • Increased effect of trimeprazine: MAOIs ☑ Increased anticholinergic effect: henbane leaf	• Hypersensitivity to H₁-receptor antagonists • Acute asthma attack • Lower respiratory tract disease
tripelennamine (B)	PBZ, PBZ-SR, Pelamine, tripelennamine HCl	• Rhinitis • Allergy symptoms	• Adults: PO 25-50 mg q4-6h, not to exceed 600 mg/day; time-rel 100 mg bid-tid, not to exceed 600 mg/day • Child >5 yr: PO time-rel 50 mg q8-12h, not to exceed 300 mg/day • Child <5 yr: PO 5 mg/kg/day in 4-6 divided doses, not to exceed 300 mg/day	• Tabs 25, 50 mg • Time-rel tabs 100 mg • Elix 37.5 mg/5 ml	• Increased CNS depression: barbiturates, narcotics, hypnotics, tricyclic antidepressants, alcohol • Increased effect of tripelennamine: MAOIs ☑ Increased anticholinergic effect: henbane leaf	• Hypersensitivity to H₁-receptor antagonists • Acute asthma attack • Lower respiratory tract disease

KEY: ✦ = Canada only; ☑ = herb-drug interaction

Appendix G

Herbal Products

agrimony

Uses: Mild diarrhea, gastroenteritis, intestinal mucous secretion, inflammation of the mouth and throat, cuts and scrapes, amenorrhea

alfalfa

Uses: Poor appetite, hay fever and asthma, high cholesterol, nutrient source

aloe

Uses of aloe vera gel:
External: Minor burns, skin irritations, minor wounds, frostbite, radiation-caused injuries

Internal: To heal intestinal inflammation and ulcers, as a digestive aid to stimulate bile secretion

angelica

Uses: Heartburn, indigestion, gas, colic, poor blood flow to the extremities, bronchitis, poor appetite, psoriasis, vitiligo, as an antiseptic

arnica

Uses: Topical application for muscle and joint inflammation and swelling; in homeopathic preparations as a remedy for shock, injury, pain

astragalus

Uses: Immune stimulant, viral infections, HIV/AIDS, cancer, vascular disorders, improve circulation, lower blood pressure, possible efficacy in myasthenia gravis

bilberry

Uses: Diabetic retinopathy, macular degeneration, glaucoma, cataract, capillary fragility, varicose veins, hemorrhoids, mild diarrhea

black cohosh

Uses:
Menopause: Hot flashes, nervous conditions associated with menopause
Dysmenorrhea: Menstrual cramps, pain, inflammation

Adapted from: Dubusk, Ruth, and Treadwell, Phillip. *Serious Drug/Herb Interactions.* Skidmore-Roth Publishing, Inc. 1999.

black haw (cramp bark)

Uses: Dysmenorrhea, menstrual cramps and pain, menopausal metrorrhagia, hysteria, asthma, lower blood pressure, heart palpitations

blessed thistle

Uses: Loss of appetite, indigestion, intestinal gas

blue cohosh

Uses: Menopausal symptoms, uterine and ovarian pain, improve flow of menstrual blood, anti-inflammatory, antirheumatic, popular remedy in black ethnic medicine

borage

Uses: Antiinflammatory for premenstrual syndrome, rheumatoid arthritis, Raynaud's disease, other inflammatory conditions, atopic dermatitis, infant cradle cap, cystic fibrosis, high blood pressure, diabetes

burdock root

Uses: Skin diseases, inflammation, rashes, cold and fever, cancer, gout, arthritis

calendula

Uses:
External: Minor skin ailments
Internal: Inflammation

throughout the gastrointestinal tract, toxic liver and gallbladder, menstrual bleeding and pain, yeast infections

capsicum (cayenne)

Uses: Muscle spasms, pain of inflammation, neuromas, psoriasis, dry mouth, as an antioxidant food, as a food seasoning

cascara

Uses: Chronic constipation, hepatitis, gallstones

cat's claw

Uses: Cancer, herpes, HIV/AIDS, rheumatoid arthritis, gastritis, gout, wounds, gastric ulcers

chamomile

Uses:
External: As an antiseptic and soothing agent for inflamed skin and minor wounds
Internal: As an antispasmodic, gas-relieving, and antiinflammatory agent for the treatment of digestive problems; light sleep aid and sedative for adults and children; possible anticancer agent

chaparral

Uses: Not recommended—potentially toxic to the liver and kidneys

chicory

Uses: Coffee substitute, source of fructo-oligosaccharides, mild laxative for children, gout, rheumatism, loss of appetite, digestive distress

comfrey

Uses: Bruises, sprains, broken bones, acne, boils

cranberry

Uses: Urinary tract infections (UTIs); susceptibility to kidney stones

dong quai

Uses: To restore vitality to tired women; for a variety of gynecologic, menstrual, and menopausal symptoms; cirrhosis of the liver

echinacea

Uses: Low immune status, hard-to-heal superficial wounds, sun protection

elder (elderberry)

Uses: Susceptibility to colds, flu, yeast infections; nasal and chest congestion; earache associated with chronic congestion; hay fever

eleuthero (See siberian ginseng)

ephedra *(ma huang)*

Uses: Seasonal and chronic asthma, nasal congestion, cough

evening primrose

Uses: Premenstrual syndrome, arthritis and inflammatory disorders in general, dry skin, eczema, asthma, diabetes, migraines, chronic fatigue syndrome, heart disease and stroke, circulatory disorders, Raynaud's disease, NSAID use, multiple sclerosis

fenugreek

Uses: Loss of appetite, inflamed areas of the skin, water retention, cancer, constipation, diarrhea, high cholesterol, high blood sugar, calcium oxalate stones

feverfew

Uses: Migraines, cluster headaches, fever, psoriasis, inflammation

flaxseed

Uses: Constipation, as a source of omega-3 fatty acids

fo-ti

Uses: Tiredness, constipation, elevated cholesterol

garcinia cambogia

Uses: Appetite control, weight loss, high cholesterol

garlic

Uses: Vascular disease, elevated LDL, elevated triglycerides, low HDL, high blood pressure, poor circulation, risk of cancer, inflammatory disorders, childhood ear infection, yeast infection

ginger

Uses: Nausea, motion sickness, indigestion, inflammation

ginkgo

Uses: Poor circulation; age-related decline in cognition, memory; diabetes; vascular disease; cancer; inflammatory disorders; impotence; degenerative nerve conditions

ginseng

Uses: Physical and mental exhaustion, stress, viral infections, diabetes, sluggishness, fatigue, weak immunity, convalescence

goldenseal

Uses: High blood pressure, poor appetite, infections, menstrual problems, minor sciatic pain, muscle spasms, eye washes

gotu kola

Uses: Chronic wounds, psoriasis

grape seed

Uses: Antioxidant, chronic disease prevention, inflammation

green tea

Uses: Cancer prevention, heart disease prevention, hypercholesterolemia, diarrhea

guggul

Uses: High LDL cholesterol, elevated triglycerides, weight loss

gymnema sylvestre

Uses: High blood sugar levels

hawthorn

Uses: Poor circulation, chest pain, irregular heartbeat, high blood fats, high blood pressure

hops

Uses: Mild sedative, diuretic, weak antibiotic, insomnia, hyperactivity, pain, fever, jaundice, improve appetite

horse chestnut

Uses: Fever, fluid retention, frostbite, hemorrhoids, inflammation, lower extremity swelling, phlebitis, varicose veins, wounds

horsetail

Uses: Diuretic, genitourinary astringent, anti-hemorrhagic, Bell's Palsy, healing broken bones

kava

Uses: Anxiety, restlessness, sleep disturbances, stress

khat

Uses: Obesity, gastric ulcers, stimulant

kombucha

Uses: Numerous claims for a wide variety of ills; none has been substantiated to date

konjac

Uses: Blood sugar control, constipation, high blood fats, high blood pressure, excessive appetite

kudzu

Uses: Alcohol cravings, menopausal symptoms

lapacho (pau d'arco)

Uses: Cancer, inflammation, infection

lemon balm (melissa)

Uses: Abdominal gas and cramping, cold sores

licorice

Uses: Allergies, arthritis, asthma, constipation, esophagitis, gastritis, hepatitis, inflammatory conditions, peptic ulcers, poor adrenal function, poor appetite

maitake

Uses: Immunostimulant activity, diabetes, hypertension, high cholesterol, obesity

maté

Uses: Diuretic, depurative

melatonin

Uses: Jet lag, insomnia, cancer protection, oral contraceptive

milk thistle

Uses: Protection for alcoholic cirrhosis and hepatitis, antiinflammatory

monascus

Uses: Maintaining acceptable cholesterol levels

morinda

Uses: Headache, digestive, heart and liver conditions, arthritis

nettle

Uses: Diuretic, hay fever

octacosanol

Uses: Herpes, inflammation of the skin, physical endurance

passionflower

Uses: Antifungal, hypertension, sedative, group A hemolytic streptococcus

peppermint

Uses: GI disorders

pygeum

Uses: Benign prostate hypertrophy, antiinflammatory

raspberry leaves

Uses: Facilitation of childbirth, dysmenorrhea, uterine tonic, fever, vomiting

red clover

Uses: Antispasmodic, expectorant, sedative, psoriasis, eczema, amenorrhea

rose hips

Uses: Source of vit C, cold, fever, mild infection

st. john's wort

Uses: Depression, antiviral

sarsaparilla

Uses: Anti-inflammatory, antiseptic, syphilis, skin diseases, rheumatism, necrosis, mercury poisoning

sassafras

Uses: Banned in the United States

saw palmetto

Uses: Benign prostatic hypertrophy

schisandra

Uses: GI disorders, liver protection, tonic

scull cap

Uses: Antibacterial, sedative

senna

Uses: Laxative

siberian ginseng (eleuthero)

Uses: Improve appetite, memory loss, hypertension, insomnia, rheumatism, improving circulation, heart ailments, diabetes, headache

tea tree oil

Uses: Topical use for infections; inhaled for respiratory disorders

uva ursi

Uses: Diuretic, urinary tract infections, contact dermatitis, arthritis

valerian

Uses: Sedative

vitex

Uses: Premenstrual and menstrual disorders, spasms, estrogen gestagen imbalance

yarrow

Uses: To decrease bleeding, Gi disorders, hypertension, thrombi, to improve circulation

yohimbine

Uses: Male organic impotence

Appendix H

FDA Pregnancy Categories

A No risk demonstrated to the fetus in any trimester

B No adverse effects in animals, no human studies available

C Only given after risks to the fetus are considered; animal studies have shown adverse reactions, no human studies available

D Definite fetal risks, may be given in spite of risks if needed in life-threatening conditions

X Absolute fetal abnormalities; not to be used anytime during pregnancy

Controlled Substance Chart

DRUGS	UNITED STATES	CANADA
Heroin, LSD, peyote, marijuana, mescaline	Schedule I	Schedule H
Opium (morphine), meperidine, amphetamines, cocaine, short-acting barbiturates (secobarbital)	Schedule II	Schedule G
Glutethimide, paregoric, phendimetrazine	Schedule III	Schedule F
Chloral hydrate, chlordiazepoxide, diazepam, mazindol, meprobamate, phenobarbital (Canada-G)	Schedule IV	Schedule F
Antidiarrheals with opium (Canada-G), antitussives	Schedule V	Schedule F

Appendix J

Commonly Used Abbreviations

abd abdomen
ABG arterial blood gas
ac before meals
ACE angiotensin-converting enzyme
ACT activated clotting time
ADA American Diabetes Association
ADH antidiuretic hormone
ALT alanine aminotransferase
ANA antinuclear antibody
AP anteroposterior
APTT activated partial thromboplastin time
ASA acetylsalicylic acid, aspirin
ASHD arteriosclerotic heart disease
AST aspartate aminotransferase (SGOT)
AV atrioventricular
bid twice a day
BM bowel movement
BMR basal metabolic rate
B/P blood pressure
BPH benign prostatic hypertrophy
BPM beats per minute
BS blood sugar
BUN blood urea nitrogen
C Celsius (centigrade)
Ca cancer
CAD coronary artery disease
cap capsule
Cath catheterization or catheterize

CBC complete blood cell count
CC chief complaint
cc cubic centimeter
CHF congestive heart failure
cm centimeter
CNS central nervous system
CO$_2$ carbon dioxide
CONT continuous
COPD chronic obstructive pulmonary disease
CPAP continuous positive airway pressue
CPK creatinine phosphokinase
CPR cardiopulmonary resuscitation
CrCl creatinine clearance
C&S culture and sensitivity
C sect cesarean section
CSF cerebrospinal fluid
CV cardiovascular
CVA cerebrovascular accident
CVP central venous pressure
D&C dilatation and curettage
DIR INF direct infusion
dr dram
D$_5$W 5% glucose in distilled water
ECG electrocardiogram (EKG)
EDTA ethylenediamine tetraacetic acid
EEG electroencephalogram

EENT	ear, eye, nose, and throat
EPS	extrapyramidal symptom
ESR	erythrocyte sedimentation rate
EXT REL	extended release
EXTRA STREN	extra strength
SUSP	suspension
FBS	fasting blood sugar
FHT	fetal heart tones
FSH	follicle-stimulating hormone
g	gram
GABA	γ-aminobutyric acid
GI	gastrointestinal
gr	grain
GTT	glucose tolerance test
gtt	drops
GU	genitourinary
H$_2$	histamine$_2$
HCG	human chorionic gonadotropin
Hct	hematocrit
HDCV	human diploid cell rabies vaccine
Hgb	hemoglobin
H & H	hematocrit and hemoglobin
5-HIAA	5-hydroxindoleacetic acid
HIV	human immunodeficiency virus (AIDS)
H$_2$O	water
HOB	head of bed
HR	heart rate
hr	hour
hs	at bedtime
IgG	immunoglobulin G
IM	intramuscular
INF	infusion
INH	inhalation
inj	injection
I&O	intake and output
IPPB	intermittent positive-pressure breathing

ITP	idiopathic thrombocytopenic purpura
IUD	intrauterine device
IV	intravenous
IVP	intravenous pyelogram
K	potassium
kg	kilogram
L	liter
lb	pound
LDH	lactic dehydrogenase
LE	lupus erythematosus
LH	luteinizing hormone
LLQ	left lower quadrant
LMP	last menstrual period
LOC	level of consciousness
LR	lactated Ringer's solution
LUQ	left upper quadrant
M	meter
m	minim
m^2	square meter
MAOI	monoamine oxidase inhibitor
mEq	milliequivalent
mg	milligram
μg	microgram
MI	myocardial infarction
min	minute
ml	milliliter
mm	millimeter
mo	month
Na	sodium
neg	negative
NPO	nothing by mouth (Lat. *nulla per os*)
NS	normal saline
O$_2$	oxygen
OBS	organic brain syndrome
OD	right eye
OR	operating room
os	left eye
OTC	over-the-counter
OU	each eye
oz	ounce
p̄	after
P56	plasma-lyte 56

PaCO₂ arterial carbon dioxide tension (pressure)
PaO₂ arterial oxygen tension (pressure)
PAT paroxysmal atrial tachycardia
PBI protein-bound iodine
PCWP pulmonary capillary wedge pressure
PEEP positive end-expiratory pressure
PERRLA pupils equal, round, react to light and accommodation
pH hydrogen ion concentration
PO by mouth
postop postoperative
PP postprandial
preop preoperative
prn as required
PT prothrombin time
PTT partial thromboplastin time
PVC premature ventricular contraction
q every
qAM every morning
qd every day
qh every hour
q2h every 2 hours
q3h every 3 hours
q4h every 4 hours
q6h every 6 hours
q12h every 12 hours
qid four times daily
qod every other day
qPM every night
qs sufficient quantity
qt quart
R right
RAIU radioactive iodine uptake
RBC red blood count or cell
RLQ right lower quadrant
ROM range of motion
RUQ right upper quadrant

SC subcutaneous
SIMV synchronous intermittent mandatory ventilation
SL sublingual
SLE systemic lupus erythematosus
SOB shortness of breath
sol solution
ss one half
suppos suppository
sus rel sustained release
Syr syrup
T&A tonsillectomy and adenoidectomy
tab tablet
tbsp tablespoon
temp temperature
tid three times daily
tinc tincture
TPN total parenteral nutrition
top topical
TRANS transdermal
TSH thyroid-stimulating hormone
tsp teaspoon
TT thrombin time
U unit
UA urinalysis
UTI urinary tract infection
UV ultraviolet
vag vaginal
VMA vanillylmandelic acid
vol volume
VS vital sign
WBC white blood cell count
wk week
wt weight
yr year
> greater than
< less than
= equal
° degree
% percent
γ gamma
β beta

Appendix K

IV Drug/Solution Compatibility Chart

	D_5	D_{10}	D_5 ½S	D_5 S	NS	R	LR	OTHER
Acetazolamide	C	C	C	C	C	C	C	
Acyclovir	C							
Alpha₁-proteinase inhibitor								Sterile water for inj
Alprostadil	C	C			C			
Alteplase								Sterile water for inj
Amdinocillin	C	C	C	C	C	C	C	D_5 in R
Amikacin	C				C			
Aminocaproic acid			C	C	C	C		D in distilled water
Ammonium Cl					C			May add KCl to solution
Amphotericin B	C							
Ampicillin	C				C			
Amrinone lactate					C			0.45% saline
Antithrombin III	C				C			Sterile water for inj
Ascorbic acid	C				C	C	C	Sodium lactate
Azlocillin	C		C		C			
Atenolol	C				C			0.45% saline
Aztreonam	C	C			C	C	C	Normosol-R
Bretylium tosylate	C				C			
Cefamandole	C				C			
Cefazolin	C				C			
Cefotetan	C				C			
Cefoxitin	C	C			C	C	C	Aminosol
Ceftrazidime	C		C	C	C	C	C	M/G Sodium lactate
Ceftriaxone	C				C			
Cefuroxime	C		C	C		C		M/G Sodium lactate
Cephalothin	C				C	C	C	M/G Sodium lactate

This chart is not inclusive and is based on manufacturers' recommendations.

Key

C = Compatible
C_5 = Dextrose 5%
D_{10} = Dextrose 10%
D_5½S = Dextrose 5% in saline 0.45%

D_5S = Dextrose 5% in saline 0.9%
NS = Sodium chloride 0.9% (normal saline)
R = Ringer's solution
LR = Lactated Ringer's solution

	D_5	D_{10}	D_5 ½S	D_5 S	NS	R	LR	OTHER
Cephapirin	C				C			
Ciprofloxacin	C				C			
Cyclosporine	C				C			Use only glass containers
Dobutamine					C			Sodium lactate
Dopamine	C		C	C	C		C	M/G Sodium lactate
Doxycycline	C				C			Invert sugar 10%
Edetate Na	C	C						Isotonic saline
Ganciclovir	C				C	C	C	
Gentamicin	C				C			Normosol-R
Heparin Na	C	C			C	C		
Ifosfamide	C				C		C	Sterile water for inj
Isoproterenol	C			C	C	C		Invert sugar 5% & 10%
Kanamycin	C				C			
Metaraminol	C			C	C	C	C	Normosol-R
Methicillin	C			C				
Metoclopramide	C			C		C	C	
Mezlocillin	C	C	C	C	C	C	C	Fructose 5%
Moxalactam	C	C	C	C	C	C	C	M/G Sodium lactate
Netilmicin	C	C		C	C	C	C	Normosol-R
Norepinephrine	C	C		C			C	
Nitroglycerin	C	C			C			
Piperacillin	C			C	C		C	
Ritodrine	C							
Ticarcillin	C				C		C	
Tobramycin	C				C			
Vidarabine	C	C			C			

Appendix L

Nomogram for Calculation of Body Surface Area

Place a straight edge from the patient's height in the left column to his or her weight in the right column. The point of intersection on the body surface area column indicates the body surface area (BSA). Reproduced from Behrman RE, and Vaughn VC (editors): Nelson's textbook of pediatrics, ed 12, Philadelphia, 1983. WB Saunders.

Disorders Index

Index

Entries can be identified as follows: generic name, Trade Name, DRUG CATEGORY, *Combination Product.*

Entries can be identified as follows: generic name, Trade Name, DRUG CATEGORY, *Combination Product.*

Entries can be identified as follows: generic name, Trade Name, DRUG CATEGORY, *Combination Product*.

Entries can be identified as follows: generic name, Trade Name, DRUG CATEGORY, *Combination Product.*

Entries can be identified as follows: generic name, Trade Name, DRUG CATEGORY, *Combination Product.*

Entries can be identified as follows: generic name, Trade Name, DRUG CATEGORY, *Combination Product.*

Entries can be identified as follows: generic name, Trade Name, DRUG CATEGORY, *Combination Product*.

Entries can be identified as follows: generic name, Trade Name, DRUG CATEGORY, *Combination Product.*

Entries can be identified as follows: generic name, Trade Name, DRUG CATEGORY, *Combination Product.*

Entries can be identified as follows: generic name, Trade Name, DRUG CATEGORY, *Combination Product*.

Entries can be identified as follows: generic name, Trade Name, DRUG CATEGORY, *Combination Product.*

Entries can be identified as follows: generic name, Trade Name, DRUG CATEGORY, *Combination Product*.

Entries can be identified as follows: generic name, Trade Name, DRUG CATEGORY, *Combination Product.*

Entries can be identified as follows: generic name, Trade Name, DRUG CATEGORY, *Combination Product.*

Entries can be identified as follows: generic name, Trade Name, DRUG CATEGORY, *Combination Product.*

Entries can be identified as follows: generic name, Trade Name, DRUG CATEGORY, *Combination Product.*

Entries can be identified as follows: generic name, Trade Name, DRUG CATEGORY, *Combination Product.*

Entries can be identified as follows: generic name, Trade Name, DRUG CATEGORY,
Combination Product.

Entries can be identified as follows: generic name, Trade Name, DRUG CATEGORY, *Combination Product*.

2002 Update to Mosby's Drug Guide for Nurses
Fourth Edition

Following are monographs for 21 drugs that have received FDA approval since the publication of *Mosby's Drug Guide for Nurses,* 4th edition. These monographs follow the same format as those in the book. They are arranged in alphabetical order by generic name, and trade names are given for all medications in common use. Each monograph contains the same subsections as those listed and described on pages v through viii of the preface to this book.

Drug Monographs in This Insert

GENERIC	TRADE
argatroban	Acova
arsenic trioxide	Trisenox
balsalazide	Colazal
bivalirudin	Angiomax
cetrorelix	Cetrotide
choriogonadotropin	Ovidrel
colesevelam	Welchol
gemtuzumab	Mylotarg
insulin aspart/insulin glargine	NovoLog/Lantus
iron sucrose	Venofer
linezolid	Zyvox
meloxicam	Mobic
mifepristone	Mifeprex
pantoprazole	Protonix
rivastigmine	Exelon
tenecteplase	TNKase
tinzaparin	Innohep
triptorelin	Trelstar Depot
verteporfin	Visadyne
ziprasidone	Geodon
zonisamide	Zonegran

Key recent FDA drug approvals

GENERIC NAME	TRADE NAME	USE
ammonium lactate	Lac-Hydrin	Ichthyosis vulgaris and xerosis in children
botulinum toxins	Botox Myobloc	Cervical dystonia Cervical dystonia
caspofungin	Cancidas	Invasive aspergillosis
esomeprazole	Nexium	Erosive esophagitis, GERD
formoterol fumarate	Foradil	Long-term, twice-daily administration in the maintenance treatment of asthma and prevention of bronchospasm
imatinib	Gleevec	Chronic myeloid leukemia (CML)
levonorgestrel-releasing intrauterine system	Mirena	Intrauterine contraception for 5 yr
nateglinide	Starlix	Type 2 diabetes
pantoprazole sodium	Protonix	Short-term treatment of GERD
peginterferon alfa-2b	PEG-Intron	Chronic hepatitis C

argatroban (℞)
(are-ga-troe'ban)
Acova
Func. class.: Anticoagulant
Chem. class.: Thrombin inhibitor
Pregnancy Category   B

Action: Direct inhibitor of thrombin that is derived from L-arginine; it reversibly binds to the thrombin active site

▷**Therapeutic Outcome:** Absence or decrease of thrombosis

Uses: Thrombosis, prophylaxis or treatment

Dosage and routes
Adult: IV 2 µg/kg/min (1 mg/ml) give at 6 ml/hr for 50 kg of weight, at 8 ml/hr for 70 kg of weight, at 11 ml/hr for 90 kg of weight, at 13 ml/hr for 110 kg of weight, at 16 ml/hr for 130 kg of weight

Available forms: Inj 100 mg/ml

Adverse effects
CV: Atrial fibrillation, ventricular tachycardia
SYST: Sepsis
CNS: Fever
GI: Nausea, vomiting, abdominal pain, diarrhea, **GI bleeding**
GU: Hematuria, abnormal kidney function, UTI
HEMA: Hemorrhage, thrombocytopenia
RESP: Pneumonia, dyspnea

Contraindications: Hypersensitivity, overt major bleeding

Precautions: Intracranial bleeding, renal function impairment, lactation, children, hepatic disease, pregnancy **B**

Pharmacokinetics
Absorption	Unknown
Distribution	Unknown
Metabolism	Liver
Excretion	Feces
Half-life	39-51 min

Pharmacodynamics
Unknown

Interactions
Drug classifications
Anticoagulants: ↑ risk of bleeding
Thrombolytics: ↑ action of argatroban

NURSING CONSIDERATIONS
Assessment
• Obtain baseline in aPTT before treatment; do not start treatment if aPTT ratio ≥ 2.5, then aPTT 4 hr after initiation of treatment and at least qd thereafter; if aPTT above target, stop inf for 2 hr, then restart at 50%, take aPTT in 4 hr; if below target, increase inf rate by 20%, take aPTT in 4 hr, do not exceed inf rate of 0.21 mg/kg/hr without checking for coagulation abnormalities
• Monitor aPTT, which should be 1.5-3 × control
◆Assess for bleeding gums, petechiae, ecchymosis, black tarry stools, hematuria/epistaxis, B/P, vaginal bleeding and possible hemorrhage
• Fever, skin rash, urticaria

Nursing diagnoses
☑Decreased cardiac output (uses)
☑Diarrhea (adverse reactions)
☑Knowledge deficit (teaching)

Implementation
• Avoid all IM injections that may cause bleeding

☑ Herb/drug 🚫 Do Not Crush ◆ Alert   Key Drug **G** Geriatric **P** Pediatric

IV INF
• Dilute in 0.9% NaCl, D$_5$, LR to a final conc 1 mg/ml. Dilute each 2.5 ml vial 100-fold by mixing with 250 ml of diluents, mix by repeated inversion of the diluent bag for 1 min; may be slightly hazy
• Dosage adjustment may be made after review of aPTT, not to exceed 10 µg/kg/min

Patient/family education
• Advise to use soft-bristle toothbrush to avoid bleeding gums, avoid contact sports, use electric razor, avoid IM injection
• Instruct to report any signs of bleeding: gums, under skin, urine, stools

Evaluation
Positive therapeutic outcome
• Absence or decrease of thrombosis

arsenic trioxide (R)
Trisenox
Func. class.: Antineoplastic-miscellaneous
Pregnancy category   D

Action: Not understood, causes morphological changes and DNA fragmentation

▶**Therapeutic Outcome:** Decrease in malignant cells

Uses: Acute promyelocytic leukemia

Dosage and routes
Induction
Adult: IV 0.15 mg/kg/day until bone marrow remission, max 60 doses
Consolidation treatment
Wait 3-6 wk after completion of induction

Adult: IV 0.15 mg/kg/day × 25 doses over a period of up to 5 wk

Available forms: Inj 1 mg/ml

Adverse effects
META: Increased ALT/AST, hyperkalemia, hypokalemia, hypomagnesemia, hyperglycemia
GU: Vaginal hemorrhage, **renal failure,** incontinence
HEMA: Leukocytosis, anemia, thrombocytopenia, neutropenia, DIC
CV: Hypotension, hypertension, ECG prolonged QT interval, other ECG changes, chest pain, *tachycardia*
GI: Abdominal pain, constipation, diarrhea, dyspepsia, fecal incontinence, **GI hemorrhage,** dry mouth, *nausea, vomiting, anorexia*
CNS: Anxiety, confusion, insomnia, headache, paresthesia, depression, dizziness, tremor, **seizures,** agitation, **coma,** weakness
RESP: Pleural effusion, dyspnea, cough, epistaxis, hypoxia, sinusitis, wheezing, rales, tachypnea
MISC: Weight gain or decrease, fatigue, severe edema, rigors, herpes simplex/zoster

Contraindications: Hypersensitivity, pregnancy **D**

G **Precautions:** Elderly, lacta-
P tion, children

Pharmacokinetics	
Absorption	Unknown
Distribution	Stored in liver, kidney, heart, lung, hair, nails
Metabolism	Liver
Excretion	Kidneys
Half-life	Unknown

Pharmacodynamics
Unknown

Interactions
None known

NURSING CONSIDERATIONS
Assessment
◆ Monitor for APL differentiation syndrome: fever, dyspnea, pulmonary infiltrates, pleural or pericardial effusions, weight gain; this condition can be fatal; give high-dose steroids
• Assess for ECG changes: QT interval prolongation, complete AV block; obtain baseline ECG prior to drug therapy
• Monitor electrolytes: potassium, calcium, magnesium, creatine

Nursing diagnoses
☑ Risk for infection (adverse reactions)
☑ Altered nutrition: less than body requirements (adverse reactions)
☑ Knowledge deficit (teaching)

Implementation
IV
• Dilute with 100-250 ml D₅ or 0.9% NaCl immediately after withdrawing from ampule, give over 1-2 hr; may give over 4 hr if reactions occur

Patient/family education
• Teach to report planned or suspected pregnancy
• Inform that fertility impairment has not been studied

Evaluation
Positive therapeutic outcome
• Decrease in malignant cells

Treatment of overdose:
• Dimercaprol 3 mg/kg IM q4hr, then 250 mg penicillamine PO, max 4 ×/day (≤1 g/day)

---

balsalazide (℞)
(ball-sal'a-zide)
Colazal
Func. class.: Antiinflammatory
Chem. class.: Salicylate derivative

Pregnancy category   B

Action: Delivered intact to the colon, bioconverted to 4-aminobenzoyl-β-alanine

▶**Therapeutic Outcome:** Decreased inflammation in colon

Uses: Active, mild to moderate ulcerative colitis

Dosage and routes
Adult: PO 750 mg tid × 8 wk, may take up to 12 wk

Available forms: Tabs 750 mg

Adverse effects
EENT: Dry mouth, dry eyes, rhinitis, sinusitis, watery eyes, blurred vision
SYST: Anaphylaxis
GI: Nausea, vomiting, abdominal pain, diarrhea, rectal bleeding, flatulence, dyspepsia, dry mouth, constipation
CNS: Headache, insomnia, fatigue, fever, dizziness
MS: Arthralgia, back pain, myalgia

Contraindications: Hypersensitivity to salicylates

Precautions: Pregnancy **B**, P child <14 yr, lactation, pyloric stenosis

Pharmacokinetics

Absorption	Low, variable
Distribution	Plasma protein binding 99%
Metabolism	Unknown
Excretion	Kidneys, as metabolites
Half-life	Unknown

☑ Herb/drug   🚫 Do Not Crush   ◆ Alert   Key Drug   **G** Geriatric   **P** Pediatric

Pharmacodynamics

Unknown

Interactions
None known

Lab test interferences
False positive: Urinary glucose test

NURSING CONSIDERATIONS
Assessment
• Monitor kidney function studies: BUN, creatinine, urinalysis (long-term therapy)
• Assess for allergic reaction: rash, dermatitis, urticaria, pruritus, dyspnea, bronchospasm

Nursing diagnoses
☑ Injury, risk for (uses)
☑ Knowledge deficit (teaching)

Implementation
• Give with food in evenly divided doses
• Use with resuscitative equipment available; severe allergic reactions may occur
• Give total daily dose evenly spaced to minimize GI intolerance
• Store in tight, light-resistant container at room temp

Evaluation
Positive therapeutic outcome
• Absence of fever, mucus in stools, resolution of symptoms of ulcerative colitis

bivalirudin (℞)
(bye-val-i-rue'din)
Angiomax
Func. class.: Anticoagulant
Chem. class.: Thrombin inhibitor
Pregnancy category B

Action: Direct inhibitor of thrombin that is highly specific

➡**Therapeutic Outcome:** Anticoagulation in PTCA

Uses: Unstable angina in patients undergoing percutaneous transluminal coronary angioplasty (PTCA)

Dosage and routes
Adult: **IV** BOL 1 mg/kg, then **IV** INF 2.5 mg/kg/hr for 4 hr; another **IV** INF may be used at 0.2 mg/kg/hr for ≤20 hr; this drug is intended to be used with aspirin (325 mg qd) adjusted to body weight

Available forms: Inj, lyophilized 250 mg

Adverse effects
CV: Hypo/hypertension, bradycardia
CNS: Headache, insomnia, anxiety, nervousness, fever
GI: Nausea, vomiting, abdominal pain, dyspepsia
HEMA: Hemorrhage
MS: Back pain
MISC: Pain at inj site, pelvic pain, urinary retention

Contraindications: Hypersensitivity, active bleeding

Precautions: Renal function
🅿 impairment, lactation, children, hepatic disease, pregnancy **B**

Pharmacokinetics	
Absorption	Unknown
Distribution	Unknown
Metabolism	Unknown
Excretion	Kidneys
Half-life	25 min

Pharmacodynamics
Unknown

cetrorelix (℞)
(set-roe-ree'lix)
Cetrotide
Func. class.:
Gonadotropin-releasing
hormone antagonist
Chem. class.: Synthetic
decapeptide
Pregnancy category   X

Action: Inhibitor of pituitary gonadotropin secretion; initially increases LH and FSH, induces a rapid suppression of gonadotropin secretion

▶**Therapeutic Outcome:** Pregnancy

Uses: For inhibition of premature LH surges in women undergoing controlled ovarian hyperstimulation

Dosage and routes
Single-dose regimen
Adult: SC 3 mg when serum estradiol level is at appropriate stimulation response, usually on stimulation day 7; if hCG has not been given within 4 days after inj of 3 mg cetrorelix, give 0.25 mg qd until day of hCG administration
Multiple-dose regimen
Adult: SC 0.25 mg is given on stimulation day 5 (either morning or evening) or 6 (morning) and continued qd until day hCG is given

Available forms: Inj 0.25, 3 mg

Adverse effects
CNS: Headache
ENDO: Ovarian hyperstimulation syndrome, abdominal pain (gyn)
GI: Nausea

Interactions
Drug classifications
Anticoagulants: ↑ risk of bleeding
Thrombolytics: ↑ risk of bleeding

NURSING CONSIDERATIONS
Assessment
◆Assess for fall in B/P or Hct that may indicate hemorrhage
• Assess for fever, skin rash, urticaria
Nursing diagnoses
☑ Decreased cardiac output (uses)
☑ Knowledge deficit (teaching)
Implementation
• To each 250 mg vial add 5 ml of sterile water for inj, swirl until dissolved, further dilute reconstituted vial with 50 ml of D₅W or 0.9% NaCl (5 mg/ml); the dose is adjusted to body weight
• Give reduced dose in renal impairment

Patient/family education
• Explain reason for drug and expected results

Evaluation
Positive therapeutic outcome
• Anticoagulation in PTCA

INTEG: Pain on injection; local site reactions
SYST: Fetal death

Contraindications: Hypersensitivity, pregnancy **X**, latex allergy, lactation

Pharmacokinetics

Absorption	Unknown
Distribution	Protein binding 86%
Metabolism	Liver to metabolites
Excretion	Feces/urine
Half-life	Depends on dosage

Pharmacodynamics

Unknown

Interactions
None known

NURSING CONSIDERATIONS
Assessment
• Assess for suspected pregnancy; drug should not be used
• Assess for latex allergy; drug should not be used
• Monitor ALT, AST, GGT, alk phosphatase

Nursing diagnoses
☑ Knowledge deficit (teaching)

Implementation
• Give SC using abdomen, around navel or upper thigh, swab inj area with disinfectant, clean a 2 in circle and allow to dry, pinch up area between thumb and finger, insert needle at 45-90° to surface; if blood is drawn into the syringe, reposition needle without removing it
• Do not administer if patient is pregnant
• Protect from light

Patient/family education
• Instruct to report abdominal pain, vaginal bleeding
• Teach self-administration technique if needed

Evaluation
Positive therapeutic outcome
• Pregnancy

---

choriogonadotropin
(℞)
(chore-i-oh-gon′a-doe-troe-pin)
Ovidrel
Func. class.: Ovulation stimulant
Pregnancy category X

Action: hCG is an analog of LH and binds to LH/hCG receptor

➡ **Therapeutic Outcome:** Fertility

Uses: Final follicular maturation ovulation induction

Dosage and routes
Infertile women undergoing OI
Adult: SC 250 µg single dose following last dose of FS agent
Infertile women undergoing ART
Adult: SC 250 µg/day following last dose of FS agent

Available forms: Powder for inj, lyophilized 285 µg r-hCG

Adverse effects
CV: Vasomotor flushing, phlebitis, **deep-vein thrombosis**
CNS: Headache, depression, restlessness, anxiety, nervousness, fatigue, insomnia, dizziness, flushing, lability
GI: Nausea, vomiting, abdominal pain, bloating, diarrhea
INTEG: Rash
GU: Polyuria, urinary frequency, birth defects, spontaneous abortions, multiple ovulation, breast pain, oliguria, abnormal uterine bleeding

---

Contraindications: Hypersensitivity, pregnancy **X**, hepatic disease, undiagnosed uterine bleeding, uncontrolled thyroid or adrenal dysfunction, intracranial lesion, ovarian cysts

Precautions: Hypertension, depression, convulsions, diabetes mellitus

Pharmacokinetics

Absorption	Unknown
Distribution	Unknown
Metabolism	Unknown
Excretion	Unknown
Half-life	29 hrs

Pharmacodynamics

Unknown

Interactions
None known

Lab test interferences:
↑ FSH/LH, ↑ ALT

NURSING CONSIDERATIONS
Nursing diagnoses
☑ Knowledge deficit (teaching)

Implementation
• After reconstituting with 1 ml sterile water for inj, discard unused portion, store vial at room temp, protect from light

Patient/family education
• Advise that multiple births are common
• Advise to notify prescriber immediately if low abdominal pain occurs; may indicate ovarian cyst, cyst rupture
• Teach the method for taking, recording basal body temp to determine whether ovulation has occurred
• Teach if ovulation can be determined (there is a slight decrease in temp, then a sharp increase for ovulation), to attempt coitus 3 days before and qod until after ovulation

• Teach if pregnancy is suspected, to notify prescriber immediately

Evaluation
Positive therapeutic outcome
• Fertility

---

colesevelam (Ŗ)
(coal-see-vel'am)
Welchol
Func. class.: Antilipemic
Chem. class.: Bile acid sequestrant
Pregnancy category   C

Action: Absorbs, combines with bile acids to form insoluble complex that is excreted through feces; loss of bile acids lowers cholesterol levels

➡**Therapeutic Outcome:** Decreasing LDL cholesterol

Uses: Elevated LDL cholesterol, alone or in combination with HMG-CoA reductase inhibitor

Dosage and routes
Adult: PO Monotherapy: 3 625 mg tabs bid with meals or 6 tabs qd with a meal; may increase to 7 tabs if needed

Combination therapy
3 tabs bid with meals or 6 tabs qd with a meal given with an HMG-CoA reductase inhibitor

Available forms: Tabs 625 mg

Adverse effects
CNS: Headache, dizziness, drowsiness, vertigo, tinnitus
MS: Muscle, joint pain
GI: Constipation, abdominal pain, nausea, fecal impaction, hemorrhoids, flatulence, vomiting, steatorrhea, peptic ulcer

---

INTEG: Rash, irritation of perianal area, tongue, skin
HEMA: Decreased vit A, D, K, red cell folate content; *hyperchloremic acidosis, bleeding,* decreased protime

Contraindications: Hypersensitivity, biliary obstruction

Precautions: Pregnancy **C**, **P** lactation, children

Pharmacokinetics

Absorption	Unknown
Distribution	Unknown
Metabolism	Unknown
Excretion	Feces
Half-life	Unknown

Pharmacodynamics

Unknown

Interactions
Individual drugs
Cephalexin: ↓ absorption of this drug
Chenodiol: ↓ absorption of this drug
Clindamycin: ↓ absorption of this drug
Digitalis: ↓ absorption of this drug
Folic acid: ↓ absorption of this drug
Iron: ↓ absorption of this drug
Penicillin G: ↓ absorption of this drug
Phenobarbital: ↓ absorption of this drug
Phenylbutazone: ↓ absorption of this drug
Thyroid: ↓ absorption of this drug
Trimethoprim: ↓ absorption of this drug
Warfarin: ↓ absorption of this drug
Drug classifications
Fat-soluble vitamins: ↓ absorption of this drug

Tetracyclines: ↓ absorption of this drug
Thiazides: ↓ absorption of this drug
Lab test interferences
↑ Liver function studies, ↑ Cl, ↑ PO_4

NURSING CONSIDERATIONS
Assessment
• Assess cardiac glycoside level, if both drugs are being administered
• Assess for signs of vit A, D, K deficiency
• Monitor fasting LDL, HDL, total cholesterol, triglyceride levels, electrolytes if on extended therapy
• Monitor bowel pattern daily; increase bulk, H_2O in diet for constipation

Nursing diagnoses
☑ Constipation (adverse reactions)
☑ Knowledge deficit (teaching)
☑ Noncompliance (teaching)

Implementation
• Give drug ac, hs; give all other medications 1 hr before colesevelam or 4 hr after colesevelam to avoid poor absorption
• Give supplemental doses of vit A, D, K, if levels are low

Patient/family education
◆Teach the symptoms of hypoprothrombinemia: bleeding mucous membranes, dark tarry stools, hematuria, petechiae; report immediately
• Teach the importance of compliance; toxicity may result if doses missed
• Teach that risk factors should

---

be decreased: high-fat diet, smoking, alcohol consumption, absence of exercise
• Advise not to discontinue suddenly

Evaluation
Positive therapeutic outcome
• Decreased cholesterol level (hyperlipidemia); diarrhea, pruritus (excess bile acids)

gemtuzumab (℞)
(gem-tue-zue′mab)
Mylotarg
Func. class.: Misc. antineoplastic
Chem. class.: Monoclonal antibody
Pregnancy category **D**

Action: Composed of recombinant humanized IgG$_4$ kappa antibody, binds to CD33 antigen that is released in myeloid cells

➲Therapeutic Outcome: Decreasing signs/symptoms of leukemia

Uses: Acute myeloid leukemia (AML)

Dosage and routes
Adult: **IV** 9 m/m^2 as a 2 hr inf; before giving inf, give diphenhydramine 50 mg PO, acetaminophen 650-1000 mg PO 1 hr prior to inf; then use acetaminophen 650-1000 mg q1-4h prn

Available forms: Powder for inj, lyophilized 5 mg

Adverse effects
CNS: Dizziness, insomnia, depression
CV: Hypertension, **hemorrhage,** tachycardia, hypotension

INTEG: Rash, herpes simplex, local reaction, petechiae
GI: Anorexia, diarrhea, constipation, nausea, stomatitis, vomiting
GU: Hematuria, **vaginal hemorrhage**
MISC: Fever, myalgias, headache, chills
RESP: Cough, pneumonia, epistaxis, rhinitis
META: Hypokalemia, hypomagnesemia

Contraindications: Hypersensitivity, pregnancy **D,** severe myelosuppression

P **Precautions:** Lactation, children, severe renal or hepatic disease

Pharmacokinetics	
Absorption	Unknown
Distribution	Unknown
Metabolism	Unknown
Excretion	Unknown
Half-life	45, 100 hr respectively

Pharmacodynamics
Unknown

Interactions
None known

NURSING CONSIDERATIONS
Assessment
• Assess for symptoms of infection; chills, fever, headache, may be masked by drug fever
• Assess CNS reaction: LOC, mental status, dizziness, confusion
• Assess cardiac status: Lung sounds; ECG before and during treatment, especially in those with cardiac disease
• Assess bone marrow depression: bruising, bleeding, blood in stools, urine, sputum, emesis

insulin aspart 13

Nursing diagnoses
- ☑ Risk for infection (adverse reactions)
- ☑ Altered nutrition: less than body requirements (adverse reactions)
- ☑ Altered oral mucous membrane (adverse reactions)

Implementation
- Do not give **IV** push or bolus
- Protect from light, use biologic safety hood, allow to come to room temp
- Reconstitute each vial with 5 ml sterile water for inj using sterile syringes, swirl each vial, check for discoloration or particulate matter, give over 2 hr, use a separate line with 1.2 micron terminal filter
- Store reconstituted sol for ≤8 hr in refrigerator

Patient/family education
- Advise to take acetaminophen for fever
- Instruct to avoid hazardous tasks, since confusion, dizziness may occur; avoid prolonged sunlight, use sunscreen
- Instruct to report signs of infection: sore throat, fever, diarrhea, vomiting

Evaluation
Positive therapeutic outcome
- Decrease in size, number of lesions

insulin aspart (℞)
NovoLog
insulin glargine
Lantus
Func. class.: Pancreatic hormone
Pregnancy category   C

Action: Decreases blood sugar; by transport of insulin into cells and the conversion of glucose to glycogen, indirectly increases blood pyruvate and lactate, decreases phosphate and potassium; insulin may be beef, pork, human (processed by recombinant DNA technologies)

➡ **Therapeutic Outcome:** Resolution of signs/symptoms of diabetes

Uses: Adult-onset diabetes, juvenile diabetes, ketoacidosis types 1 and 2, type 2 (non–insulin-dependent) diabetes mellitus, type 1 (insulin-dependent) diabetes mellitus

Dosage and routes
Lantus
Adult: SC 10 IU qd, range 2-100 IU/day

P *Child ≥6 yr:* Same as adults

Available forms: Lantus (inj 100 IU); NovoLog (inj 100 U/ml human insulin aspart (rDNA)

Adverse effects
EENT: Blurred vision, dry mouth
INTEG: Flushing, rash, urticaria, warmth, *lipodystrophy,* lipohypertrophy, swelling, redness
META: *Hypoglycemia,* rebound

hyperglycemia (Somogyi effect 12-72 hr or longer)
SYST: Anaphylaxis

Contraindications: Hypersensitivity to protamine

Precautions: Pregnancy **C**

Pharmacokinetics

Absorption	Unknown
Distribution	Unknown
Metabolism	Liver, muscles, kidneys
Excretion	Kidneys
Half-life	Lantus 1½

Pharmacodynamics

	NOVOLOG	LANTUS
Onset	0.25 hr	1.1 hr
Peak	1-3 hr	no peak
Duration	3-5 hr	24 hr

Interactions
Individual drugs
Alcohol: ↑ hypoglycemia
Diltiazem: ↑ insulin need
Dobutamine: ↑ insulin need
Fenfluramine: ↓ insulin need
Guanethidine: ↓ insulin need
Phenylbutazone: ↓ insulin need
Rifampin: ↑ insulin need
Sulfinpyrazone: ↓ insulin need
Tetracycline: ↓ insulin need
Drug classifications
Anabolic steroids: ↓ insulin need
β-Adrenergic blockers: Signs/symptoms of hypoglycemia may be masked
Estrogens: ↑ insulin need
Glucocorticoid steroids: ↑ insulin need
MAOIs: ↓ insulin need
Oral anticoagulants: ↓ insulin need
Oral hypoglycemics: ↑ hypoglycemia
Thiazide diuretics: ↑ insulin need

Thyroid hormones: ↑ insulin need
☑ *Herb/drug*
Broom: ↓ hypoglycemic effect
Buchu: ↓ hypoglycemic effect
Chromium: ↓ or ↑ hypoglycemic effect
Dandelion: ↓ hypoglycemic effect
Fenugreek: ↓ or ↑ hypoglycemic effect
Ginseng: ↓ or ↑ hypoglycemic effect
Juniper: ↓ hypoglycemic effect
Karela: ↑ glucose tolerance
Smoking
↑ insulin need
Lab test interferences
↑ VMA
↓ Potassium, ↓ magnesium, ↓ inorganic phosphate
Interference: Liver function studies, thyroid function studies

NURSING CONSIDERATIONS
Assessment
• Monitor fasting blood glucose, 2 hr PP (80-150 mg/dl, normal fasting level; 70-130 mg/dl, normal 2-hr level); also glycosylated Hgb may be drawn to identify treatment effectiveness
• Monitor urine ketones during illness; insulin requirements may increase during stress, illness, surgery
• Assess for hypoglycemic reaction that can occur during peak time (sweating, weakness, dizziness, chills, confusion, headache, nausea, rapid weak pulse, fatigue, tachycardia, memory lapses, slurred speech, staggering gait, anxiety, tremors, hunger)
• Assess for hyperglycemia: acetone breath, polyuria, fatigue, polydipsia, flushed, dry skin, lethargy

---

Nursing diagnoses
- ☑ Injury, risk for (adverse reactions)
- ☑ Knowledge deficit (teaching)
- ☑ Noncompliance (teaching)

Implementation
SC route
- Give after warming to room temp by rotating in palms to prevent injecting cold insulin; use only insulin syringes with markings or syringe matching U/ml; rotate inj sites within one area: abdomen, upper back, thighs, upper arm, buttocks; keep record of sites
- Give increased dosages if tolerance occurs; give human insulin to those allergic to beef or pork
- Store at room temp for <1 mo; keep away from heat and sunlight; refrigerate all other supply; do not use if discolored; do not freeze

Patient/family education
- Advise that blurred vision occurs; not to change corrective lens until vision is stabilized 1-2 mo
- Advise to keep insulin, equipment available at all times
- Teach that drug does not cure diabetes but controls symptoms
- Teach to carry Medic Alert ID as diabetic
- Teach to recognize hypoglycemia reaction: headache, tremors, fatigue, weakness
- Teach the dosage, route, mixing instructions, if any diet restrictions, disease process
- Advise to carry candy or lump sugar to treat hypoglycemia
- Advise the symptoms of ketoacidosis: nausea, thirst, polyuria, dry mouth, decreased B/P, dry, flushed skin, acetone breath, drowsiness, Kussmaul respirations
- Inform that a plan is necessary for diet, exercise; all food on diet should be eaten; exercise routine should not vary
- Teach about blood glucose testing; make sure patient is able to determine glucose level
- Advise to avoid OTC drugs unless directed by prescriber

Evaluation
Positive therapeutic outcome
- Decrease in polyuria, polydipsia, polyphagia, clear sensorium, absence of dizziness, stable gait

Treatment of overdose:
Glucose 25 g **IV**, via dextrose 50% sol, 50 ml or glucagon 1 mg

iron sucrose (℞)
Venofer
Func. class.: Hematinic
Chem. class.: Ferric hydroxide complex with dextran

Pregnancy category B

Action: Iron is carried by transferrin to the bone marrow, where it is incorporated into hemoglobin

▶**Therapeutic Outcome:** Improved signs/symptoms of iron deficiency anemia; iron levels improved

Uses: Iron deficiency anemia

Investigational uses: Dystrophic epidermolysis bullosa (DEB)

Dosage and routes
Adult: IV 5 ml (100 mg of elemental iron) given during dialysis, most will need 1000

mg of elemental iron over 10 dialysis sessions

Available forms: Inj 20 mg/ml

Adverse effects
CNS: Headache, dizziness
GI: Nausea, vomiting, abdominal pain
INTEG: Rash, pruritus, urticaria, fever, sweating, chills
CV: Chest pain, hypo/hypertension, hypervolemia
RESP: Dyspnea, pneumonia, cough
OTHER: Anaphylaxis

Contraindications: Hypersensitivity, all anemias excluding iron deficiency anemia, iron overload

G **Precautions:** Lactation, (**IV**),
P pregnancy **B**, elderly, children

Pharmacokinetics	
Absorption	Unknown
Distribution	Unknown
Metabolism	Unknown
Excretion	Urine
Half-life	6 hr

Pharmacodynamics
Unknown

Interactions
Individual drugs
Oral iron: ↑ toxicity, do not use together

NURSING CONSIDERATIONS
Assessment
• Monitor blood studies: Hct, Hgb, reticulocytes, transferrin, plasma iron concentrations, ferritin, total iron-binding, bilirubin before treatment, at least monthly
• Assess for allergy: anaphylaxis, rash, pruritus, fever, chills, wheezing; notify prescriber immediately, keep emergency equipment available

• Assess cardiac status: hypotension, hypertension, hypervolemia
• Assess for toxicity: nausea, vomiting, diarrhea, fever, abdominal pain (early symptoms), cyanotic-looking lips and nailbeds, seizures, CV collapse (late symptoms)

Nursing diagnoses
☑ Nutrition, less than body requirements (uses)
☑ Knowledge deficit (teaching)

Implementation
◆ Give only with epinephrine available in case of anaphylactic reaction during dose
IV
• Give directly in dialysis line by slow inj or inf; give by slow inj at 1 ml/min (5 min/vial); inf dilute each vial exclusively in a maximum of 100 ml of 0.9% NaCl, give at rate of 100 mg of iron/15 min, discard unused portions
• Store at room temp in cool environment, do not freeze

Patient/family education
• Teach that iron poisoning may occur if increased beyond recommended level; not to take oral iron preparation

Evaluation
Positive therapeutic outcome
• Increased serum iron levels, Hct, Hgb

Treatment of overdose:
Discontinue drug, treat allergic reaction, give diphenhydramine or epinephrine as needed, give iron-chelating drug in acute poisoning

linezolid (℞)
(line-zoe'lide)
Zyvox
Func. class.: Broad-spectrum antiinfective
Chem. class.: Oxalodinone
Pregnancy category C

Action: Binds to bacterial 235 ribosomal RNA of the 50S subunit preventing formation of the bacterial translation process

Therapeutic Outcome: Negative blood cultures, absence of signs/symptoms of infection

Uses: Vancomycin-resistant *Enterococcus faecium* infections, nosocomial pneumonia, uncomplicated or complicated skin and skin structure infections, community-acquired pneumonia

Dosage and routes
Vancomycin-resistant Enterococcus faecium infections
Adult: **IV** 600 mg q12h × 14-28 days PO
Nosocomial pneumonia/ complicated skin infections/ community-acquired pneumonia/concurrent bacterial infection
Adult: **IV**/PO 600 mg q12h × 10-14 days
Uncomplicated skin infections
Adult: **IV**/PO 400 mg q10-14 days

Available forms: Tab 400, 600 mg; powder for reconstitution 100 mg/5 ml; inj 2 mg/ml

Adverse effects
CNS: Headache, dizziness, confusion
GI: Nausea, diarrhea, increased ALT, AST, *vomiting,* taste change, tongue color change
MISC: Vaginal moniliasis, fungal infection, oral moniliasis

Contraindications: Hypersensitivity

Precautions: Pregnancy **C**, lactation, children, thrombocytopenia

Pharmacokinetics

Absorption	Rapidly, excessively
Distribution	Protein binding 31%
Metabolism	Oxidation of the morpholine ring
Excretion	Unknown
Half-life	Unknown

Pharmacodynamics

Unknown

Interactions
Drug classifications
MAOIs: ↓ effects of MAOIs
Adrenergics: ↑effects of adrenergics

NURSING CONSIDERATIONS
Assessment
• Assess CNS symptoms: headache, dizziness
• Monitor liver function studies: AST, ALT
• Monitor allergic reactions: fever, flushing, rash, urticaria, pruritus

Nursing diagnoses
☑ Infection, potential for (uses)
☑ Knowledge deficit (teaching)

Implementation
PO
• Store reconstituted oral suspension at room temperature, use within 3 wk
IV
• Give over 30-120 min; do not use IV infusion bag in series connections, do not use with additives in sol, do not

use with another drug, administer separately

Solution compatibilities: D_5, 0.9% NaCl, LR

Patient/family education
- Advise if dizziness occurs, to ambulate, perform activities with assistance
- Advise to complete full course of drug therapy
- Advise to contact prescriber if adverse reaction occurs

Evaluation
Positive therapeutic outcome
- Decreased symptoms of infection, blood cultures negative

---

meloxicam (℞)
(mel-ox'i-kam)
Mobic
Func. class.: Nonsteroidal antiinflammatory/ nonopioid analgesic
Chem. class.: Oxicam
Pregnancy category   C

Action: Inhibits prostaglandin synthesis by decreasing an enzyme needed for biosynthesis; analgesic, antiinflammatory, antipyretic effects

Therapeutic Outcome: Decreased pain, swelling of joints; improved mobility

Uses: Osteoarthritis

Dosage and routes
Adult: PO 7.5 mg qd, may increase to 15 mg qd

Available forms: Tabs 7.5 mg

Adverse effects
CV: Hypertension, angina, *cardiac failure, MI,* hypotension, palpitations, *dysrhythmias,* tachycardia
CNS: Dizziness, drowsiness, tremors, headache, nervousness, malaise, fatigue, insomnia, depression, *seizures*
EENT: Tinnitus, hearing loss
GI: Pancreatitis, nausea, colitis, GERD, vomiting, diarrhea, constipation, flatulence, cramps, dry mouth, peptic ulcer, *GI bleeding, perforation*
GU: Nephrotoxicity: dysuria, hematuria, oliguria, azotemia
HEMA: Blood dyscrasias, anemia, prolonged bleeding
INTEG: Rash, urticaria, photosensitivity
SYST: Angioedema, anaphylaxis

Contraindications: Hypersensitivity, asthma, severe renal disease, severe hepatic disease, peptic ulcer disease, L&D, lactation, CV bleeding

Precautions: Pregnancy **C,** children, bleeding disorders, GI disorders, cardiac disorders, hypersensitivity to other antiinflammatory agents, elderly, CrCl <25 ml/min

Pharmacokinetics

Absorption	Unknown
Distribution	Unknown
Metabolism	Liver <50%
Excretion	Breast milk, kidneys
Half-life	6 hr

Pharmacodynamics

	PO	IM
Onset	Unknown	Unknown
Peak	4-5 hr	50 min
Duration	Unknown	Unknown

Interactions
Individual drugs
Cholestyramine: ↓ action of meloxicam
Cyclosporine: ↑ nephrotoxicity
Phenytoin: ↑ action of meloxicam

Drug classifications
Aminoglycosides: ↑ action of aminoglycosides
Anticoagulants: ↑ action of anticoagulants
β-Adrenergic blockers: ↓ action of beta blockers
Diuretics: ↑ action of diuretics
Hydantoins: ↑ action of hydantoins
Salicylates: ↑ action of meloxicam
Sulfonamides: ↑ action of meloxicam

NURSING CONSIDERATIONS
Assessment
• Monitor renal, liver, blood studies: BUN, creatinine, AST, ALT, Hgb before treatment, periodically thereafter
• Assess for bleeding times; check for bruising, bleeding; test for occult blood in urine
⚠Assess for anaphylaxis and angioedema; emergency equipment should be nearby
⚠Assess for hepatic dysfunction: jaundice, yellow sclera and skin, clay-colored stools
• Assess for audiometric, ophthalmic exam before, during, after treatment
• Assess for GI condition, hypertension, cardiac conditions

Nursing diagnoses
☑ Impaired mobility (uses)
☑ Pain (uses)
☑ Knowledge deficit (teaching)

Implementation
• May take without regard to meals, to take with food for GI upset
• Store at room temp

Patient/family education
• Advise to report blurred vision or ringing, roaring in ears (may indicate toxicity)
• Advise to avoid driving, other hazardous activities if dizziness or drowsiness occurs
• Teach to report change in urine pattern, weight increase, edema, pain increase in joints, fever, blood in urine (indicates nephrotoxicity); to report rash, black stools, or continuing headache
• Teach to avoid alcohol, ASA

Evaluation
Positive therapeutic outcome
• Decreased pain, stiffness, swelling in joints, able to move more easily

mifepristone (℞)
(mif-ee-press'tone)
Mifeprex
Func. class.: Abortifacient
Pregnancy category C

Action: Stimulates uterine contractions, causing complete abortion

Therapeutic Outcome: Termination of pregnancy

Uses: Abortion through 49 days gestation

Investigational uses: Postcoital contraception/contragestation, intrauterine fetal death, endometriosis, Cushing's syndrome, unresectable meningioma

Dosage and routes
Available forms: Tabs 200 mg

Adverse effects
CNS: Dizziness, insomnia, anxiety, syncope, fainting, headache
GI: Nausea, vomiting, diarrhea, dyspepsia
GU: Uterine cramping, uterine hemorrhage, vaginitis, pelvic pain

MISC: Fatigue, back pain, fever, viral infections, chills, sinusitis

Contraindications: Hypersensitivity, severe hepatic disease, severe renal disease, PID, respiratory disease, cardiac disease

Precautions: Asthma, anemia, jaundice, diabetes mellitus, convulsive disorders, past uterine surgery, pregnancy **C**

Pharmacokinetics

Absorption	Rapidly
Distribution	98% protein binding, albumin, glycoprotein
Metabolism	Unknown
Excretion	Feces, urine
Half-life	Unknown

Pharmacodynamics

Onset	Unknown
Peak	90 min
Duration	Unknown

Interactions
Individual drugs
Erythromycin: ↓ metabolism of erythromycin
Itraconazole: ↓ metabolism of itraconazole
Ketoconazole: ↓ metabolism of ketoconazole

NURSING CONSIDERATIONS
Assessment
• Monitor B/P, pulse; watch for change that may indicate hemorrhage
• Monitor respiratory rate, rhythm, depth; notify prescriber of abnormalities
• Assess for length, duration of contraction; notify prescriber of contractions lasting over 1 min or absence of contractions
• Assess for incomplete abortion, pregnancy must be terminated by another method; drug is teratogenic

Nursing diagnoses
☑ Pain (adverse reactions)
☑ Knowledge deficit (teaching)

Implementation
• Provide emotional support before and after abortion

Patient/family education
• Advise to report increased blood loss, abdominal cramps, increased temperature, foul-smelling lochia
• Teach some methods of comfort control and pain control
• Advise must continue with follow-up
• Advise that cramping and vaginal bleeding will occur

Evaluation
Positive therapeutic outcome
• Expulsion of fetus

---

pantoprazole (℞)
(pan-toe-pray′zole)
Protonix
Func. class.: Proton pump inhibitor
Chem. class.: Benzimidazole

Pregnancy category C

Action: Suppresses gastric secretion by inhibiting hydrogen/potassium ATPase enzyme system in gastric parietal cell; characterized as gastric acid pump inhibitor, since it blocks final step of acid production

Therapeutic Outcome: Absence of epigastric fullness, pain, swelling

Uses: Gastroesophageal reflux disease (GERD), severe erosive esophagitis

---

Dosage and routes
Adult: PO 40 mg qd × 8 wk, may repeat course

Available forms: Tabs, delayed rel 40 mg

Adverse effects
CNS: Headache, insomnia
GI: Diarrhea, abdominal pain, flatulence
INTEG: Rash
META: Hyperglycemia

Contraindications: Hypersensitivity

Precautions: Pregnancy **C**,
🅿 lactation, children

Pharmacokinetics	
Absorption	Unknown
Distribution	Protein binding 97%
Metabolism	Unknown
🅖 Excretion	Urine-metabolites, feces, ↓ rate in elderly
Half-life	1½ hr

Pharmacodynamics	
Onset	Unknown
Peak	2.4 hr
Duration	>24 hr

Interactions
Individual drugs
Clarithromycin: ↑ levels of pantoprazole
Diazepam: ↑ level of pantoprazole
Flurazepam: ↑ level of pantoprazole
Phenytoin: ↑ level of pantoprazole
Sucralfate: ↓ absorption of pantoprazole
Triazolam: ↑ level of pantoprazole
Warfarin: ↑ risk of bleeding

NURSING CONSIDERATIONS
Assessment
• Assess GI system: bowel sounds q8h, abdomen for pain, swelling, anorexia
• Monitor hepatic enzymes: AST, ALT, alk phosphatase during treatment

Nursing diagnoses
☑ Knowledge deficit (teaching)

Implementation
• May take with or without food
🚫• Do not crush del rel tabs

Patient/family education
• Advise to report severe diarrhea; drug may have to be discontinued
• Advise that diabetic patient should know hypoglycemia may occur
• Advise to avoid hazardous activities; dizziness may occur
• Advise to avoid alcohol, salicylates, ibuprofen; may cause GI irritation

Evaluation
Positive therapeutic outcome
• Absence of epigastric pain, swelling, fullness

rivastigmine (℞)
(riv-as-tig′mine)
Exelon
Func. class.: Cholinesterase inhibitor
Pregnancy category   B

Action: May enhance cholinergic functioning by increasing acetylcholine

➡**Therapeutic Outcome:** Decreased signs and symptoms of Alzheimer's dementia

Uses: Alzheimer's dementia

Dosage and routes
Adult: PO 1.5 mg bid for 2 wk or more, may increase to 3 mg bid after 2 wk or more;

---

may increase to 4.5 mg bid and thereafter 6 mg

Available forms: Caps 1.5, 3, 4.5, 6 mg; solution 2 mg/ml

Adverse effects

CNS: Tremors, confusion, insomnia, psychosis, hallucination, depression, dizziness, headache, anxiety, somnolence, fatigue, syncope

GI: Nausea, vomiting, anorexia, abdominal distress, flatulence, diarrhea, constipation

MISC: Urinary tract infection, asthenia, increased sweating, hypertension, influenza-like syncope, weight change

Contraindications: Hypersensitivity, narrow-angle glaucoma, undiagnosed skin lesions

Precautions: Renal disease, hepatic disease, respiratory disease, seizure disorder, peptic ulcer, pregnancy **B**, asthma, **P** lactation, children

Pharmacokinetics	
Absorption	Rapidly, completely
Distribution	Not known
Metabolism	To decarbamylated metabolite
G Excretion	Kidney-metabolites, clearance lowered in elderly, hepatic disease, ↑ nicotine use
Half-life	1½ hr

Pharmacodynamics
Unknown

Interactions
Drug classifications
Cholinomimetics: ↑ synergistic effect
Food/drug
↓ rivastigmine absorption

NURSING CONSIDERATIONS
Assessment
• Monitor liver function enzymes: AST, ALT, alk phosphatase, LDH, bilirubin, CBC
• Assess for severe GI effects: nausea, vomiting, anorexia, weight loss
• Monitor B/P, respiration during initial treatment; hypo-/hypertension should be reported
• Assess mental status: affect, mood, behavioral changes, depression; complete suicide assessment

Nursing diagnoses
☑ Knowledge deficit (teaching)
☑ Cognitive impairment (uses)

Implementation
• Give with meals; take with morning and evening meal
• Provide assistance with ambulation during beginning therapy

Patient/family education
• Teach the procedure for giving oral solution; use instruction sheet provided
• Teach to notify prescriber of severe GI effects

Evaluation
Positive therapeutic outcome
• Increased coherence, decreased symptoms of Alzheimer's disease

---

☑ Herb/drug   ⊘ Do Not Crush   ◆ Alert   Key Drug   **G** Geriatric   **P** Pediatric

tenecteplase (℞)
(ten-ek'ta-place)
TNKase
Func. class.: Thrombolytic enzyme
Chem. class.: β-hemolytic streptococcus filtrate (purified)
Pregnancy category **C**

Action: Activates conversion of plasminogen to plasmin (fibrinolysin): plasmin breaks down clots (fibrin), fibrinogen, factors V, VII; occlusion of venous access lines

▶**Therapeutic Outcome:** Resolution of myocardial infarction

Uses: Acute myocardial infarction

Dosage and routes
Adult <60 kg: IV BOL 30 mg, give over 6 sec

Adult ≥60-<70 kg: IV BOL 35 mg, give over 7 sec

Adult ≥70-<80 kg: IV BOL 40 mg, give over 8 sec

Adult ≥80-<90 kg: IV BOL 45 mg, give over 9 sec

Adult ≥90 kg: IV BOL 50 mg, give over 10 sec

Available forms: Powder for inj, lyophilized 50 mg

Adverse effects
CV: Dysrhythmias, hypotension, pulmonary edema, *pulmonary embolism, cardiogenic shock, cardiac arrest, heart failure, myocardial reinfarction, myocardial rupture, tamponade, pericarditis, pericardial effusion, thrombosis*
HEMA: Decreased Hct, *bleeding*
INTEG: Rash, urticaria, phlebitis at* **IV** *inf site, itching, flushing
SYST: GI, GU, intracranial, retroperitoneal bleeding, surface bleeding, anaphylaxis

Contraindications: Hypersensitivity, active bleeding, intraspinal surgery, CNS neoplasms, ulcerative colitis, enteritis, severe hypertension, severe renal disease, hepatic disease, hypocoagulation, COPD, subacute bacterial endocarditis, rheumatic valvular disease, cerebral embolism/thrombosis/hemorrhage, intraarterial diagnostic procedure or surgery (10 days), recent major surgery

Precautions: Arterial emboli from left side of heart, pregnancy **C**, lactation, children

Pharmacokinetics	
Absorption	Unknown
Distribution	Unknown
Metabolism	Liver
Excretion	Unknown
Half-life	20-24 min

Pharmacodynamics	
Onset	Immediate
Peak	Unknown
Duration	Unknown

Interactions
Individual drugs
Aspirin: ↑ bleeding potential
Indomethacin: ↑ bleeding potential
Phenylbutazone: ↑ bleeding potential
Drug classifications
Anticoagulants: ↑ bleeding potential
Antithrombolytics: ↑ bleeding potential
Lab test interferences
↑ PT, ↑ aPTT, ↑ TT
↓ Plasminogen, ↓ fibrinogen

NURSING CONSIDERATIONS
Assessment

• Assess for allergy: fever, rash, itching, chills; mild reaction may be treated with antihistamines

◆Assess for bleeding during 1st hr of treatment; hematuria, hematemesis, bleeding from mucous membranes, epistaxis, ecchymosis; may require transfusion (rare), continue to assess for bleeding for 24 hr

• Monitor blood studies (Hct, platelets, PTT, PT, TT, aPTT) before starting therapy; PT or aPTT must be less than 2× control before starting therapy; PTT or PT q3-4h during treatment

• Assess for hypersensitive reactions: fever, rash, dyspnea; drug should be discontinued; for streptokinase reactions previously

• Monitor VS, B/P, pulse, respirations, neuro signs, temp at least q4h; temp >104° F (40° C) indicates internal bleeding; cardiac rhythm following intracoronary administration; systolic pressure increase >25 mm Hg should be reported to prescriber

◆Assess for neurologic changes that may indicate intracranial bleeding

◆Assess for retroperitoneal bleeding: back pain, leg weakness, diminished pulses

• Assess for respiratory depression

Nursing diagnoses

☑ Knowledge deficit (teaching)
☑ Decreased cardiac output (uses)

Implementation
IV

• Give as soon as thrombi identified; not useful for thrombi over 1 wk old

• Administer cryoprecipitate or fresh frozen plasma if bleeding occurs

• Administer loading dose at beginning of therapy; may require increased loading doses

• Give heparin after fibrinogen level >100 mg/dl; heparin infusion to increase PTT to 1.5-2 × baseline for 3-7 days; **IV** heparin with loading dose is recommended after discontinuing streptokinase to prevent redevelopment of thrombi

• Aseptically withdraw 10 ml of sterile H_2O for inj from diluent vial, use red cannula syringe-filling device, inject all contents of syringe into drug vial, direct into powder, swirl, withdraw correct dose, discard any unused solution; stand the shield with dose vertically on flat surface and passively recap the red cannula, remove entire shield assembly by twisting counter-clockwise, give by **IV** BOL

• About 10% of patients have high streptococcal antibody titers requiring increased loading doses

• **IV** therapy: use upper extremity vessel that is accessible to manual compression

Y-site compatibilities:

Dobutamine, dopamine, heparin, lidocaine, nitroglycerin

• Provide bed rest during entire course of treatment

• Avoid venous or arterial puncture, inj, rectal temp; any invasive treatment

• Treat fever with acetaminophen or aspirin

• Apply pressure for 30 sec to minor bleeding sites; inform prescriber if this does not attain hemostasis; apply pressure dressing

Evaluation
Positive therapeutic outcome
• Resolution of myocardial infarction

---

tinzaparin (R)
(tin-zay-par′in)
Innohep
Func. class.: Anticoagulant
Chem. class.: Unfractionated porcine heparin
Pregnancy category   C

Action: Prevents conversion of fibrinogen to fibrin and prothrombin to thrombin by enhancing inhibitory effects of antithrombin III; produces higher ratio of antifactor Xa to antifactor IIa

Therapeutic Outcome: Resolution of deep vein thrombosis

Uses: Treatment of deep-vein thrombosis, pulmonary emboli when given with warfarin

Dosage and routes
Adult: SC 175 anti-Xa IU/kg qd ≥6 days and until adequate anticoagulation with warfarin (INR ≥2 for 2 consecutive days)

Available forms: Inj 40,000 IU/2 ml

Adverse effects
CNS: Fever, confusion
GI: Nausea
GU: Edema, peripheral edema
HEMA: Hypochromic anemia, thrombocytopenia, bleeding
INTEG: Ecchymosis

Contraindications: Hypersensitivity to this drug, heparin, or pork; hemophilia, leukemia with bleeding, peptic ulcer disease, thrombocytopenic purpura, heparin-induced thrombocytopenia

Precautions: Alcoholism, elderly, pregnancy **C**, hepatic disease (severe), renal disease (severe), blood dyscrasias, severe hypertension, subacute bacterial endocarditis, acute nephritis, lactation, children

Pharmacokinetics	
Absorption	Unknown
Distribution	Unknown
Metabolism	Unknown
Excretion	Unknown
Half-life	4.5 hr

Pharmacodynamics	
Onset	Unknown
Peak	3-5 hrs (max antithrombin activity)
Duration	Unknown

Interactions
Drug classifications
Oral anticoagulants: ↑ tinzaparin action
Salicylates: ↑ tinzaparin action
Herb/drug
Bromelain: ↑ risk of bleeding
Cinchona bark: ↑ risk of bleeding

NURSING CONSIDERATIONS
Assessment
• Monitor blood studies (Hct, platelets, occult blood in stools), anti-Xa; thrombocytopenia may occur
• Assess for bleeding gums, petechiae, ecchymosis, black tarry stools, hematuria

---

Nursing diagnoses

✓ Cardiac output, decreased (uses)

✓ Knowledge deficit (teaching)

Implementation

• Give only after screening patient for bleeding disorders

• Give SC only; do not give IM

• Give to recumbent patient; give SC; rotate inj sites (left/right anterolateral, left-right posterolateral abdominal wall)

• Insert whole length of needle into skin fold held with thumb and forefinger

◆ Use only this drug when ordered; not interchangeable with heparin

• Give at same time each day to maintain steady blood levels

• Do not massage area or aspirate when giving SC injection

• Avoid all IM injections that may cause bleeding

• Store at 77° F (25° C); do not freeze

Patient/family education

• Advise to use soft-bristle toothbrush to avoid bleeding gums, to use electric razor

• Instruct to report any signs of bleeding: gums, under skin, urine, stools

Evaluation

Positive therapeutic outcome

• Resolution of deep vein thrombosis

Treatment of overdose: Protamine SO₄ 1% sol; dose should equal dose of enoxaparin

---

triptorelin (℞)

(trip-toe′rel-in)

Trelstar Depot

Func. class.: Gonadotropin-releasing hormone antagonist

Chem. class.: Synthetic decapeptide analog of LHRH

Pregnancy category   X

Action: Inhibitor of pituitary gonadotropin secretion; initially increases LH and FSH, with increases in testosterone, reduction in sex steroid levels

▶ **Therapeutic Outcome:** Decreased signs/symptoms of advanced prostate cancer

Uses: Advanced prostate cancer

Dosage and routes

Adult: IM 3.75 mg qmo

Available forms: Microgranules, depot inj 3.75 mg

Adverse effects

CNS: Headache, insomnia, dizziness, lability, fatigue

CV: Hypertension

ENDO: Gynecomastia, breast tenderness, hot flashes

GI: Nausea, vomiting, diarrhea

GU: Impotence, urinary retention, UTI

INTEG: Rash, pain on injection, pruritus, hypersensitivity

MS: Osteoneuralgia

Contraindications: Hypersensitivity to this product or other LHRH agonists or LHRH, pregnancy **X**, lactation

Pharmacokinetics	
Absorption	Unknown
Distribution	Unknown
Metabolism	CYP/450
Excretion	Liver, kidneys
Half-life	3 hrs

Pharmacodynamics
Unknown

Lab test interferences
↑ Alk phosphatase, ↑ estradiol, ↑ FSH, ↑ LH, ↑ testosterone levels
↓ Testosterone levels, ↓ progesterone

NURSING CONSIDERATIONS
Assessment
• Assess for severe hypersensitivity: discontinue drug and give antihistamines, have emergency equipment nearby
• Monitor I&O ratios; palpate bladder for distention in urinary obstruction
• Monitor for relief of bone pain (back pain)
• Assess levels of testosterone and PSA

Nursing diagnoses
✓ Diarrhea (adverse reactions)
✓ Knowledge deficit (teaching)

Implementation
• Give IM using implant, inserted by qualified person
• Use syringe with 20-G needle, withdraw 2 ml sterile water for inj, inject into vial, shake well, withdraw vial contents, inject immediately

Patient/family education
• Teach that postmenopausal symptoms may occur but will decrease after treatment is dicontinued

Evaluation
Positive therapeutic outcome
• More normal levels of prostate-specific antigen, acid phosphatase, alk phosphatase; testosterone level of <25 ng/dl

verteporfin (℞)
(ver-tee-poor'fin)
Visudyne
Func. class.: Ophthalmic phototherapy
Pregnancy category C

Action: A light-activated drug for photodynamic therapy, using a 2-step process with this drug and nonthermal red light

⇨**Therapeutic Outcome:** Improved vision

Uses: Age-related macular degeneration

Dosage and routes
Adults: Initiate 689 nm wavelength laser light for 83 sec, 15 min after start of the 10 min infusion of verteporfin

Available forms: Lyophilized cake 15 mg

Adverse effects
CNS: Hypesthesia, vertigo, *insomnia*
CV: **Hypertension**, **atrial fibrillation**, *peripheral vascular disorder, varicose veins*
EENT: Cataracts, diplopia, dry eyes, ocular itching, severe vision loss
GI: Constipation, **GI cancers**, *nausea*
MS: Arthralgia, arthrosis, myesthenia
RESP: Pharyngitis, pneumonia
MISC: Asthenia, back pain, elevated LFTs, photosensitivity

Contraindications: Porphyria, hypersensitivity

Precautions: Elderly, pregnancy C, lactation, children

Pharmacokinetics	
Absorption	Unknown
Distribution	Unknown
Metabolism	Unknown
Excretion	Feces
Half-life	5-6 hrs

Pharmacodynamics
Unknown

Interactions
Drug classifications
Anticoagulants: ↓ action of verteporfin
Antiplatelets: ↓ action of verteporfin
Phenothiazines: ↑ photosensitivity
Sulfonamides: ↑ photosensitivity
Sulfonylureas: ↑ photosensitivity
Tetracyclines: ↑ photosensitivity
Thiazides: ↑ photosensitivity

NURSING CONSIDERATIONS
Assessment
• Assess for ocular sensitivity: sensitivity to sun, bright lights, car headlights; patients should wear dark sunglasses with an average light transmittance of <4%
• Assess for extravasation at inj site: take care to protect from light
Nursing diagnoses
☑ Knowledge deficit (teaching)
Implementation
• Give after reconstitution of each vial with 7 ml sterile water for inj for 2 mg/ml; protect from light and use within 4 hr; solution is dark green
• Wipe spills with damp cloth, avoid skin/eye contact, dispose of material in polyethylene bag according to policy
• Store between 68°-77° F

Patient/family education
• Advise to report eye sensitivity
• Advise to wear sunglasses with average white light transmittance of <4% for 5 days after treatment; also to use protective clothing
Evaluation
Positive therapeutic outcome
• Improved vision

---

ziprasidone (℞)
(zi-praz'ih-dohn)
Geodon
Func. class.: Antipsychotic/neuroleptic
Chem. class.: Benzisoxazole derivative
Pregnancy category C

Action: Unknown; may be mediated through both dopamine type 2 (D_2) and serotonin type 2 (5-HT_2) antagonism

➡ **Therapeutic Outcome:** Decreased signs/symptoms of psychosis

Uses: Schizophrenia

Dosage and routes
Adult: PO 20 mg bid with food, adjust dosage every 2 days upward to max of 80 mg bid

Available forms: Tabs 20, 40, 60, 80 mg

Adverse effects
CNS: EPS, pseudoparkinsonism, akathisia, dystonia, tardive dyskinesia; drowsiness, insomnia, agitation, anxiety, headache, seizures, neuroleptic malignant syndrome
CV: Orthostatic hypotension, tachycardia, prolonged QT/QTc, sudden death

---

EENT: Blurred vision
GI: Nausea, vomiting, *anorexia, constipation,* jaundice, weight gain
RESP: Rhinitis

Contraindications: Hypersensitivity, lactation, seizure disorders

🅟 **Precautions:** Children, renal disease, pregnancy **C**, hepatic
🅖 disease, elderly, breast cancer

Pharmacokinetics

Absorption	Unknown
Distribution	Protein binding 90%
Metabolism	Liver-extensively to metabolite
Excretion	Unknown
Half-life	Unknown

Pharmacodynamics

Unknown

Interactions
Individual drugs
Alcohol: ↑ sedation
Carbamazepine: ↑ excretion of ziprasidone
Lithium: ↑ EPS
Drug classifications
Antipsychotics: ↑ EPS
CNS depressants: ↑ sedation
🖉*Herb/drug*
Kava: ↑ CNS depression

NURSING CONSIDERATIONS
Assessment
• Assess mental status before initial administration
• Check swallowing of PO medication; check for hoarding or giving of medication to other patients
• Monitor I&O ratio; palpate bladder if urinary output is low
• Monitor bilirubin, CBC, liver function studies qmo
• Monitor urinalysis before, during prolonged therapy
• Assess affect, orientation, LOC, reflexes, gait, coordination, sleep pattern disturbances
• Monitor B/P standing and lying; also pulse, respirations; take these q4h during initial treatment; establish baseline before starting treatment; report drops of 30 mm Hg; watch for ECG changes
• Assess dizziness, faintness, palpitations, tachycardia on rising
• Assess EPS, including akathisia (inability to sit still, no pattern to movements), tardive dyskinesia (bizarre movements of the jaw, mouth, tongue, extremities), pseudoparkinsonism (rigidity, tremors, pill rolling, shuffling gait)
◆ Assess for neuroleptic malignant syndrome: hyperthermia, increased CPK, altered mental status, muscle rigidity
• Assess skin turgor qd
• Assess constipation, urinary retention qd; if these occur, increase bulk and water in diet

Nursing diagnoses
☑ Thought processes, altered (uses)
☑ Coping, ineffective individual (uses)
☑ Knowledge deficit (teaching)
☑ Noncompliance (teaching)

Implementation
🅖• Give reduced dose in elderly
• Give antiparkinsonian agent on order from prescriber, to be used for EPS
• Provide decreased stimulus by dimming lights, avoiding loud noises
• Provide supervised ambulation until patient is stabilized on medication; do not involve in strenuous exercise program because fainting is possible; patient should not stand still for a long time

• Provide increased fluids to prevent constipation
• Provide sips of water, candy, gum for dry mouth
• Store in tight, light-resistant container

Patient/family education
• Advise that orthostatic hypotension may occur and to rise from sitting or lying position gradually
• Advise to avoid hot tubs, hot showers, tub baths; hypotension may occur
• Inform to avoid abrupt withdrawal of this drug; EPS may result; drug should be withdrawn slowly
• Inform to avoid OTC preparations (cough, hay fever, cold) unless approved by prescriber, since serious drug interactions may occur; avoid use with alcohol, CNS depressants; increased drowsiness may occur
• Teach to avoid hazardous activities if drowsy or dizzy
• Teach compliance with drug regimen
• Teach to report impaired vision, tremors, muscle twitching
• Teach that in hot weather, heat stroke may occur; take extra precautions to stay cool

Evaluation
Positive therapeutic outcome
• Decrease in emotional excitement, hallucinations, delusions, paranoia; reorganization of patterns of thought, speech

Treatment of overdose: Lavage if orally ingested; provide airway; *do not induce vomiting*

---

zonisamide (℞)
(zone-is′a-mide)
Zonegran
Func. class.: Anticonvulsant
Chem. class.: Sulfonamides
Pregnancy category   C

Action: May act through at sodium and calcium channels, but exact action is unknown

⮕Therapeutic Outcome: Decreased seizures

Uses: Epilepsy, adjunctive therapy of partial seizures

Dosage and routes
P *Adults and child >16 yr:* 100 mg qd, may increase after 2 wk to 200 mg/day, may increase q2 wk, maximum dose >600 mg/day

Available forms: Caps 100 mg

Adverse effects
CNS: Dizziness, insomnia, paresthesias, depression, fatigue, headache, confusion
EENT: Diplopia, verbal difficulty, speech abnormalities, taste perversion
GI: Nausea, constipation, anorexia, weight loss, diarrhea, dyspepsia
INTEG: Rash

Contraindications: Hypersensitivity to this drug or sulfonamides, psychiatric condition, hepatic failure

Precautions: Allergies, hepatic
G disease, renal disease, elderly,
P pregnancy **C**, lactation, child <16 yr

Pharmacokinetics

Absorption	Unknown
Distribution	Unknown
Metabolism	Liver
Excretion	Kidneys
Half-life	63 hr

Pharmacodynamics

Onset	Unknown
Peak	2-6 hr
Duration	Unknown

Interactions
Drugs inducing CYP 450 enzyme: ↑ half-life of zonisamide

NURSING CONSIDERATIONS
Assessment
• Assess for seizures: duration, type, intensity, precipitating factors
• Monitor blood studies: CBC, platelets q2wk until stabilized, then qmo × 12, then q3mo; discontinue drug if neutrophils <1600/mm^3; renal function: albumin conc
• Assess mental status: mood, sensorium, affect, memory (long, short)

Nursing diagnoses
☑ Injury, risk for (uses, adverse reactions)
☑ Knowledge deficit (teaching)
☑ Noncompliance (teaching)

Patient/family education
• Advise not to discontinue drug abruptly; seizures may occur
• Advise to avoid hazardous activities until stabilized on drug
• Advise to carry Medic Alert ID stating drug use

Evaluation
Positive therapeutic outcome
• Decrease in severity of seizures

♣ Canada Only   Adverse effects: *italic* = common; **bold** = life-threatening